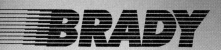

SIXTH EDITION

Prehospital Emergency Care

JOSEPH J. MISTOVICH, M. ED., NREMT-P
Chairperson and Associate Professor
Department of Health Professions
Youngstown State University
Youngstown, Ohio

BRENT Q. HAFEN, PH.D.
Professor, Department of Health Sciences
Brigham Young University
Provo, Utah

KEITH J. KARREN, PH.D.
Professor, Department of Health Sciences
Brigham Young University
Provo, Utah

MEDICAL EDITOR
Howard A. Werman, M.D.

BRADY
Prentice Hall Health
Upper Saddle River, New Jersey 07458

Library of Congress Cataloging-in-Publication Data

Mistovich, Joseph J.
  Prehospital emergency care / Joseph J. Mistovich,
Brent Q. Hafen, Keith J. Karren; medical editor,
Howard A. Werman.—6th ed.
    p.   cm.
  Includes index.
  ISBN 0-89303-763-X case. — ISBN 0-8359-6064-1
  (paper)
  1. Emergency medicine.   2. Emergency medical
technicians.   I. Hafen, Brent Q.   II. Karren, Keith J.
III. Werman, Howard A.   IV. Hafen, Brent Q. Prehospital
emergency care.   V. Title.
  [DNLM: 1. Emergency Medical Services.   2. Crisis
  Intervention.   3. Emergency Medicine.
    WX 215 M678p 2000]
RC86.7.H346   2000
616.02'5—dc21
DNLM/DLC
for Library of Congress   99-23560
                                                    CIP

Publisher: Julie Alexander
Acquisitions editor: Laura Edwards
Director of production and manufacturing: Bruce Johnson
Managing production editor: Patrick Walsh
Senior production manager: Ilene Sanford
Production liaison: Julie Boddorf
Production editor: Lisa Garboski, bookworks
Managing development editor: Lois Berlowitz
Project editor: Sandy Breuer
Proofreader: Wayne Beatty
Managing photography editor: Michal Heron
Assistant photography editor: Mary Jo Robertiello
Photographers: Michael Gallitelli, Michal Heron, Richard
  Logan, Carl Leet
Creative director: Marianne Frasco
Interior designer: Jill Yutkowitz
Cover designer: Bill Smith Studio
Cover photographer: Mark C. Ide
Marketing manager: Tiffany Price
Marketing coordinator: Cindy Frederick
Composition: The Clarinda Company
Printing and binding: Von Hoffman Press

Printed in the United States of America

10 9 8 7 6 5 4 3

ISBN 0-8359-5331-9
ISBN 0-8359-5705-5 (paper)

Prentice-Hall International (UK) Limited, London
Prentice-Hall of Australia Pty. Limited, Sydney
Prentice-Hall Canada Inc., Toronto
Prentice-Hall Hispanoamericana, S.A., Mexico
Prentice-Hall of India Private Limited, New Delhi
Prentice-Hall of Japan, Inc., Tokyo
Prentice-Hall Pte. Ltd., Singapore
Editora Prentice-Hall do Brasil Ltda., Rio de Janeiro

NOTICE ON CARE PROCEDURES

It is the intent of the authors and publisher that this textbook be used as part of a formal EMT-Basic education program taught by qualified instructors and supervised by a licensed physician. The procedures described in this textbook are based upon consultation with EMT and medical authorities. The authors and publisher have taken care to make certain that these procedures reflect currently accepted clinical practice; however, they cannot be considered absolute recommendations.

The material in this textbook contains the most current information available at the time of publication. However, federal, state, and local guidelines concerning clinical practices, including, without limitation, those governing infection control and universal precautions, change rapidly. The reader should note, therefore, that the new regulations may require changes in some procedures.

It is the responsibility of the reader to familiarize himself or herself with the policies and procedures set by federal, state, and local agencies as well as the institution or agency where the reader is employed. The authors and the publisher of this textbook and the supplements written to accompany it disclaim any liability, loss, or risk resulting directly or indirectly from the suggested procedures and theory, from any undetected errors, or from the reader's misunderstanding of the text. It is the reader's responsibility to stay informed of any new changes or recommendations made by any federal, state, or local agency as well as by his or her employing institution or agency.

NOTICE ON GENDER USAGE

The English language has historically given preference to the male gender. Among many words, the pronouns "he" and "his" are commonly used to describe both genders. Society evolves faster than language, and the male pronouns still predominate in our speech. The authors have made great effort to treat the two genders equally, recognizing that a significant percentage of EMTs are female. However, in some instances, male pronouns may be used to describe both males and females solely for the purpose of brevity. This is not intended to offend any readers of the female gender.

NOTICE RE "CASE STUDIES"

The names used and situations depicted in the case studies throughout this text are fictitious.

NOTICE ON MEDICATIONS

The authors and the publisher of this book have taken care to make certain that the equipment, doses of drugs, and schedules of treatment are correct and compatible with the standards generally accepted at the time of publication. Nevertheless, as new information becomes available, changes in treatment and in the use of equipment and drugs become necessary. The reader is advised to carefully consult the instruction and information material included in the page insert of each drug or therapeutic agent, piece of equipment, or device before administration. This advice is especially important when using new or infrequently used drugs. Prehospital care providers are warned that use of any drugs or techniques must be authorized by their medical director, in accord with local laws and regulations. The publisher disclaims any liability, loss, injury, or damage incurred as a consequence, directly or indirectly, of the use and application of any of the contents of this book.

To my best friend and wife, Andrea, for her unconditional love, continuous support, and inspiration to pursue my dreams. To my daughters, Katie, Kristyn, Chelsea, Morgan, and Kara, who are my never-ending sources of love, laughter, and adventure and remind me why life is so precious. To my father, Paul, and the memory of my mother, Marge, who provided me with encouragement and taught me the value of perseverance. I love you all.

JJM

Brief Contents

Detailed Contents

Assessment Summaries/ Emergency Care Protocols/Algorithms

DRUG PROFILES

Features of This Textbook

The following are special features of the Sixth Edition of *Prehospital Emergency Care*.

DOT Curriculum Objectives At the beginning of each chapter, the relevant cognitive, affective, and psychomotor objectives from the U.S. Department of Transportation 1994 EMT-Basic National Standard Curriculum are listed. The objective numbers are those that appear in the DOT curriculum. Following each objective, the numbers of the text pages where the objective is addressed are provided to allow the instructor or student the opportunity to proceed directly to that particular subject matter if desired.

Material that relates to the cognitive and affective objectives is found in the chapter. The psychomotor objectives refer to practical skills that will be presented and reinforced by the instructor in the classroom setting. Every objective in the DOT curriculum is listed in the textbook; every cognitive and affective objective from the DOT curriculum is covered in the text.

Case Studies Each chapter includes a two-part case study that provides a realistic scenario that reinforces the assessment and emergency care of a patient. Each case study is based on the information being presented in that particular chapter. The case study at the beginning of the chapter includes the "Dispatch"—a typical radio dispatch for a call. "On Arrival" sets the scene the EMT-B walks into, including details that would be discovered during scene size-up. It stimulates the student to use the senses—to think about what he or she would see, hear, and smell when entering that scene. It also describes scene characteristics that require the student to think about possible hazards and other considerations and precautions that must be taken prior to entering.

At the conclusion of the chapter, the student returns to a "Case Study Follow-Up" where the complete assessment and emergency care information are given. This section walks the student through the call, step by step, and provides an excellent method to review and reinforce assessment and emergency care techniques learned in the chapter in a realistic context.

Assessment Chapter In Chapter 9, "Patient Assessment," the patient assessment sequence is presented in six separate parts—each part a mini-chapter that covers one main step in the patient assessment. A small diagram appears at the beginning of each part in the chapter to remind students of the total patient assessment sequence with the step they are now studying highlighted in a different color. This helps the student, at each step, to remember what has come before and to anticipate what is coming next. In this way, the patient assessment is presented with continuity from beginning to end as well as with in-depth attention to each separate part of the assessment. To help the student address life threats, "Critical Findings" and appropriate "Interventions" are highlighted.

Assessment Summaries Assessment summaries reinforce assessment steps and processes as well as key assessment findings for specific medical and trauma emergencies. A student can go to the assessment summary and identify abnormal findings that may become evident during assessment of a patient with that particular complaint.

Emergency Care Protocols Emergency care protocols are provided in a concise step-by-step format similar to the formats encountered in protocols used by EMT-Basics. They provide brief summaries of emergency care for specific medical and trauma emergencies.

Algorithms The algorithms are graphic pathways that integrate assessment and care for a medical or trauma emergency. They are summaries that afford the student a visual flow of assessment and emergency medical care procedures. The algorithms are color coded to identify assessment steps, key decision points, and interventions.

Medications   There are six medications that EMT-Basics are permitted to administer or assist in administering, with approval from medical direction: oxygen, metered dose inhaler, nitroglycerin, oral glucose, epinephrine auto-injector, and activated charcoal. Because administering medications is a serious responsibility, each of these medications is given specially highlighted coverage in the text, including a complete drug profile for each of the five medications other than oxygen.

Enrichment   An Enrichment section is included in many chapters to present information that is valuable to the EMT-B but that goes substantially beyond the DOT 1994 EMT-Basic curriculum. This information is very useful for those students who will pursue further education and training in emergency medical services. Also, the material will be useful to those students who have a desire to learn additional information and expand their knowledge base.

Special Chapters   Several chapters are entirely devoted to special topics or material that either expands on or goes significantly beyond the DOT 1994 EMT-Basic curriculum. Some of these cover new topics. Others cover topics that have been included in prior editions of *Prehospital Emergency Care,* completely revised and updated. They include Chapter 10, "Assessment of the Geriatric Patient," Chapter 18, "Altered Speech, Sensory, or Motor Function: Stroke Emergency", Chapter 19, "Seizures and Syncope," Chapter 22, "Drug and Alcohol Emergencies," Chapter 23, "Acute Abdominal Pain," Chapter 28, "Mechanisms of Injury: Kinetics of Trauma," Chapter 35, "Eye, Face, and Neck Injuries," Chapter 36, "Chest, Abdomen, and Genitalia Injuries," and Chapter 37, "Agricultural and Industrial Emergencies."

Terms and Concepts   The important terms and concepts introduced in each chapter are set in bold type and defined in context within the chapters. All of the terms and concepts introduced within the chapter are then grouped and defined in a Terms and Concepts mini-glossary at the end of the chapter. The terms and concepts from the entire textbook are included in the Glossary of Terms at the end of the book, for general reference and review as students encounter the terms throughout the text or during their work as an EMT-Basic.

Photo Scans   Groupings of photographs throughout the chapters illustrate key information and step-by-step procedures.

Review Questions   A set of Review Questions, to help the student think back through key points and concepts, concludes each chapter. Answers to the questions appear in the Instructor's Resource Manual.

Basic Life Support Review   Appendix 1 reviews basic life support information that is a prerequisite to the EMT-Basic course, including CPR and foreign body airway obstruction techniques.

National Registry Skill Sheets   The practical skill sheets used at the EMT-Basic level by the National Registry of Emergency Medical Technicians are included in Appendix 2 as a tool to aid the students in practicing their practical skills. In addition, the skill sheets allow the instructor the opportunity to utilize a formal evaluation instrument when evaluating the students' performance. The skill sheets also contain the instructions provided to the candidate prior to practical testing. This should allay the students' fears and uncertainties about what criteria will be tested on the practical examination.

Website Links   Website links are correlated with specific chapter topics so that students can go to the Internet for additional information on particular items. This will allow students to seek the most current and up-to-date information available and also to enhance their foundation of knowledge. Look for the Web icon throughout the text.

Companion Website   for *Prehospital Emergency Care, Sixth Edition* contains chapter-by-chapter review quizzes, message boards, chat rooms, and additional student and instructor resources. (www.prenhall.com/mistovich)

Student CD-Rom   This brand new addition to the program contains case studies, patient assessment video footage, quizzes, games, links to EMS-related websites, and more.

THE REST OF EDUCATIONAL PACKAGE

Several ancillary components have been developed as aids to instruction, including a **Student Workbook** and an **Instructor's Resource Manual.** A **Test Manager** and a set of **slides** and **videos** are also available.

CONTINUING IMPROVEMENTS

Any student, practicing EMT-B, or EMS instructor who has suggestions for improving this textbook or EMT-Basic training and education should write to the authors at the following address:

Brady Marketing Department
c/o Tiffany Price
Prentice Hall
One Lake Street
Upper Saddle River, NJ 07458

If you have access to a computer with a modem, you can reach the authors through Internet at the following:

Joseph Mistovich
jjmistov@cc.ysu.edu

Brent Hafen
brent_hafen@byu.edu

Keith Karren
keith_karren@byu.edu

Acknowledgments

We wish to thank the following groups of people for their assistance on developing the Sixth Edition of *Prehospital Emergency Care*.

Medical Editor Our special thanks to Dr. Howard A. Werman, Associate Professor, Department of Emergency Medicine, The Ohio State University College of Medicine and Public Health, Columbus, Ohio. Dr. Werman reviewed material every step of the way in the development of this text. His reviews were carefully prepared, and we appreciate the advice and insight he offered.

Contributing Writers The Sixth Edition has built heavily on the foundation of the Fifth Edition. We would like to express special appreciation to Kathryn J. Frandsen, Novell, Inc., Provo, UT, for her writing assistance and to the following people who contributed chapters and ideas to the Fifth Edition.

Randall W. Benner, M.Ed., NREMT-P
Allied Health Department
Youngstown State University
Youngstown, OH

Chip Boehm, R.N., EMT-P
Training Coordinator
Maine Emergency Medical Services
August, ME

John B. Booth, Jr., EMT-B
Director, Human Resources
Gold Cross Ambulance
Youngstown, OH

Kenneth Bouvier, NREMT-I
Hazardous Materials Specialist
New Orleans, LA

Rick Buell
Department of Health
Office of EMS/Trauma System
Olympia, WA

John R. Clark, EMT-P
Pennstar Flight Program
University of Pennsylvania Medical Center
Philadelphia, PA

Alice (Twink) Dalton
Faculty-Prehospital Education
Creighton University
Omaha, NE

Bob Elling, MPA, REMT-P
Director, Institute of Prehospital Emergency
    Medicine
Troy, NY

Paul L. Hillers
Rescue Concepts
Newton, IA

Kathryn Lewis, R.N., Ph.D.
Department Chair
EMT/Fire Science
Phoenix College
Phoenix, AZ

Scott Martin, B.S., REMT-P
Akron General Paramedic Program
Akron, OH

Dane Williams
Captain
Sycamore Fire/Rescue/EMS
Cincinnati, OH

Thanks also to Dan Bloom, Wayne Watson, and Baxter Larmon.

Reviewers The following reviewers of Sixth Edition material provided invaluable feedback and suggestions:

Linda Abrahamson, EMT-P, RN
EMS Education Coordinator
Silver Cross Hospital
Joliet, IL

DeAnn Barnson, BSN, EMT-B
President, EMEDCO
Coordinator, University of Utah EMT Program
Utah

Kathryn R. Allen
Hill Country EMS Training
Johnson City, TX

William F. Drees, BS, LP
Assistant Professor
The University of Texas Health Science Center
    At San Antonio
San Antonio, TX

James A. Christopher
EMS Coordinator, St. Francis Hospital &
    Health Centers
Indiana

J. R. Behan, MICT I/C
Morton County Emergency Services
Elkhart, KS 67950

Steven B. English
EMS/Critical Care Education
Owensboro Mercy Health Systems
Kentucky

J. Bret McGill, BS, NREMT-P
Director, Emergency Medicine Program
Northwest Shoals Community College
Alabama

C. Scott Dembrowski, MBA, NREMT-P
EMS Program Director
Columbus State Community College
Columbus, OH

Marlene L. Beckman, RN, EMT-P
Southeastern Community College
West Burlington, IA

Sam R. Cary
Grand Prairie Fire Department
Grand Prairie, TX

Robert D. Cook, EMT-P I/C
St Johns Educational Programs
Springfield, MO

Mark S. Decker, BA, NREMT-P
Tidewater EMS Council, Inc
Norfolk, VA

David R. Chase
Gateway Technical College
Kenosha, WI

Avery Borntrager
Montgomery, AL

David M. Ediger
Ulysses, KS

M. Elliott Nelson
Learn Life Support
Grand Haven, MI

John Senft, Deputy Chief
Department of Fire/Rescue Services
City of York, PA

Mark Goodlett
Indiana Fire Instructors Association
Indiana

Photo Acknowledgments
All photographs not credited adjacent to the photograph were photographed on assignment for Brady/ Prentice Hall Health.

Organizations We wish to thank the following organizations for their valuable assistance in creating the photo program for this edition.

American Medical Response, Hemet Valley
Ambulance Service, Hemet, CA: Laurie Hunter,
Director of Government Affairs; Jacke Hansen,
Manager of Operations; Art Durbin, EMT-P,
RN, BS, Clinical Manager

Reichhold Chemicals, Inc., Newark, NJ: Ron
Kurtz, Jack Connolly, EMS Technician

TACTRON Incident Control Products,
Sherwood, Oregon

Youngstown State University, Youngstown, OH:
Carl Leet, Media Services

Technical Advisors Our thanks to the following people for providing extraordinary assistance and valuable technical support during the photo shoots:

Art Durbin, EMT-P, RN, BS, Clinical Manager
Hemet Valley Ambulance Service
American Medical Response, Hemet, CA

Jack Connolly, EMS Technician
Reichhold Chemicals, Inc., Newark, NJ

Daniel Pohan, Savox Lifeline Communications, Ridgefield, NJ

Brian Rathbone, Hazmat/Rescue Training Consultant
The Mechanical Advantage
Hackettstown, NJ

CHAPTER 1

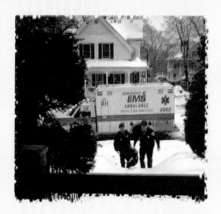

Introduction to Emergency Medical Care

INTRODUCTION

One of the most critical health problems in the United States today is the sudden loss of life and disability caused by catastrophic accidents and illnesses. Every year thousands of people in this country die or suffer permanent harm because of the lack of adequate and available emergency medical services. As an Emergency Medical Technician-Basic (EMT-Basic), you can make a positive difference.

This course is designed to help you gain the knowledge, skills, and attitudes necessary to be a competent, productive, and valuable member of the Emergency Medical Services (EMS) team. As you begin, your instructor will provide the necessary paperwork, describe the expectations for the course and the job, inform you of required or available immunizations, and outline your state and local provisions for certification as an EMT-Basic.

Objectives

Numbered objectives are from the United States Department of Transportation 1994 EMT-Basic National Standard Curriculum. Asterisked objectives, if any, pertain to material that is supplemental to the DOT curriculum.

Cognitive

1-1.1 Define Emergency Medical Services (EMS) systems. (pp. 3–5)

1-1.2 Differentiate the roles and responsibilities of the EMT-Basic from other prehospital care providers. (pp. 4–7)

1-1.3 Describe the roles and responsibilities related to personal safety. (pp. 5–6)

1-1.4 Discuss the roles and responsibilities of the EMT-Basic toward the safety of the crew, the patient, and bystanders. (pp. 5–6)

1-1.5 Define quality improvement and discuss the EMT-Basic's role in the process. (p. 9)

1-1.6 Define medical direction and discuss the EMT-Basic's role in the process. (p. 8)

1-1.7 State the specific statutes and regulations in your state regarding the EMS system. (pp. 3, 5, 8)

Affective

1-1.8 Assess areas of personal attitude and conduct of the EMT-Basic. (p. 9)

1-1.9 Characterize the various methods used to access the EMS system in your community. (pp. 3–4)

Case Study

The Dispatch

EMS Unit 121—respond to 10915 Pine Lake Road in Perry Township—you have an elderly male at that location—victim of a fall—Perry Township Fire Department has been notified and is en route—time out 1032 hours.

En Route

While you confirm the address with dispatch, your partner pulls out the county map. "I know that location," he says. "Yes, here. We need to head north on Lincoln." You pull your unit out of the garage. Your partner operates the emergency lights and sirens. Within 8 minutes, you turn onto Pine Lake Road and spot a police car and a fire truck.

On Arrival

You position your ambulance in the driveway of the residence to afford an easy exit. As you leave the unit, the police officer—a First Responder who radioed for EMS help—tells you that a 65-year-old male fell about 30 feet down a very steep embankment behind his house. He's been at the bottom for about 30 minutes. The patient, Edgar Robinson, is conscious and is able to tell you that his right arm and leg are injured. The rescue squad from the fire department is preparing to rappel down the embankment to extricate the patient.

How would you proceed?

During this chapter, you will read about the roles and responsibilities of an EMT-B. Later, we will return to the case study and put in context some of the information you learned.

THE EMERGENCY MEDICAL SERVICES SYSTEM

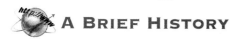 **A BRIEF HISTORY**

Emergency medical care has developed from the days when the local funeral home was the ambulance provider and patient care did not begin until arrival at the hospital. By contrast, the modern, sophisticated **EMS system** (Emergency Medical Services system) permits patient care to begin at the scene of the injury or illness, and EMS is part of a continuum of patient care that extends from the time of injury or illness until rehabilitation or discharge. Today when a person becomes ill or suffers an injury, he has easy access to EMS by telephone, gets a prompt response, and can depend on getting high-quality prehospital emergency care from trained professionals.

What happens to an injured person before he reaches a hospital is of critical importance. Wars helped to teach us this lesson. During the Korean and Vietnam conflicts, for example, it became obvious that injured soldiers benefited from emergency care in the field prior to transport. In time this realization helped the civilian EMS system evolve from a load-and-go operation to a system that provides professional care at the scene and en route to the hospital.

The modern EMS system has evolved from its beginnings in the 1960s. During that decade the National Academy of Sciences Research Council advocated professional training for prehospital emergency personnel. More significantly, the federal government and the American Heart Association made two important changes.

- The National Highway Safety Act charged the Department of Transportation with developing an Emergency Medical Services (EMS) system and upgrading prehospital emergency care. The emergency medical technician programs now available have gradually evolved from this charge.
- The American Heart Association began to teach cardiopulmonary resuscitation (CPR) and basic life support to the public. Completion of a CPR course is now a prerequisite to the EMT-Basic course.

Advances continue to be made in emergency medical services, in equipment design, and in the education of EMTs. Many lives have been saved and unnecessary disabilities avoided because the EMS system extends the services of the hospital into the community.

CURRENT STANDARDS

FEDERAL RECOMMENDATIONS

Each state has control of its own EMS system, independent of the federal government. However, the National Highway Traffic Safety Administration (NHTSA) provides a set of recommended standards called the "Technical Assistance Program Assessment Standards." A brief description of these standards follows. They will be discussed in much more detail throughout this text and in your EMT-Basic course.

- ***Regulation and Policy.*** Each state must have laws, regulations, policies, and procedures that govern its EMS system. A state-level EMS agency is also required to provide leadership to local jurisdictions.
- ***Resource Management.*** Each state must have central control of EMS resources so that each locality and all patients have equal access to acceptable emergency care.
- ***Human Resources and Training.*** All personnel who staff ambulances and transport patients must be trained to at least the EMT-Basic level.
- ***Transportation.*** Patients must be provided with safe, reliable transportation by ground or air ambulance.
- ***Facilities.*** Each seriously ill or injured patient must be delivered in a timely manner to an appropriate medical facility.
- ***Communications.*** A system of communications must be in place to provide public access to the system and communication among dispatcher, EMS personnel, and hospital.
- ***Public Information and Education***. EMS personnel should participate in programs designed to educate the public in the prevention of injuries and how to properly and appropriately access the EMS system.
- ***Medical Direction.*** Each EMS system must have a physician as a medical director to oversee patient care and delegate appropriate medical practices to EMT-Basics and other EMS personnel.
- ***Trauma Systems.*** Each state must develop a system of specialized care for trauma patients, including one or more trauma centers and rehabilitation programs, plus systems for assigning and transporting patients to those facilities.
- ***Evaluation.*** Each state must have a quality improvement system for the continuing evaluation and upgrading of the system.

ACCESS TO THE SYSTEM

There are two general systems by which the public can access the emergency medical system: 9-1-1 and non-9-1-1.

Often called the universal number, 9-1-1 is the telephone number used in many areas of the nation to access emergency services, including police, fire, rescue, EMS, and others. While exact procedures may vary, the basic process is always the same. Calls are received by a public service answering point (PSAP), who records information about the emergency, decides which service must respond, and alerts that service (Figure 1-1).

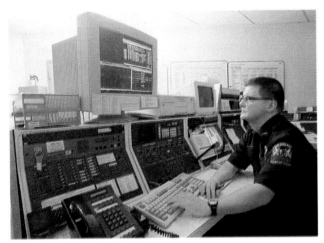

Figure 1-1 Communications play a vital role in the Emergency Medical Services (EMS) system.

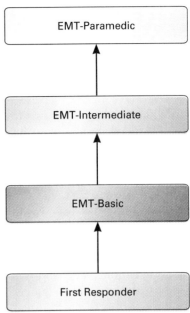

Figure 1-2 Various levels of training are found within the EMS system.

There are two main benefits to a universal number:

- The public service answering point is generally staffed by trained communications personnel. They may be able to offer medical help while the patient waits for emergency personnel to arrive. This capability is referred to as Emergency Medical Dispatching (EMD).
- The universal number minimizes the risk of delays. Callers do not have to look up a number—it is easy enough to be remembered by even the youngest callers. The chance of dialing a wrong number is slim, and there is no chance that the caller will reach the wrong service (fire instead of police, for example) or that the call-taker/dispatcher will misdirect the call.

In areas not served by 9-1-1, callers either phone a dispatch center by dialing a seven-digit number or directly call the emergency service they need. Probably the most serious drawback of the non-9-1-1 system is the delay in reaching the appropriate services.

LEVELS OF TRAINING

There are four nationally accepted levels of prehospital emergency medical training: First Responder, EMT-Basic, EMT-Intermediate, and EMT-Paramedic (Figure 1-2).

First Responder The **First Responder** is typically the first person on the scene with emergency care training. He may be a police officer, for example, or a firefighter, industrial health officer, truck driver, schoolteacher, or a volunteer associated with the community emergency care system. The U.S. Department of Transportation publishes a curriculum and guidelines for First Responder training, just as it does for EMTs.

First Responders can provide information valuable in patient care, including how the emergency came about, what was observed during patient assessment by the First Responder, and what emergency care they have provided before the ambulance arrived.

EMT-Basic The **EMT-Basic** (EMT-B) level of certification is held by those who successfully complete a course based on the U.S. Department of Transportation curriculum and who have been certified as EMT-Basics by the state emergency medical services division.

The basic course prepares an EMT-Basic to function in three areas:

- Controlling life-threatening situations, including maintaining an open airway, providing artificial ventilation, controlling severe bleeding, and treating shock.
- Stabilizing non-life-threatening situations, including dressing and bandaging wounds, splinting injured extremities, delivering and caring for infants, and dealing with the psychological stress of the patient, family members, neighbors, and colleagues.
- Using nonmedical skills, such as driving, maintaining supplies and equipment in proper order, using good communication skills, keeping good records, knowing proper extrication techniques, and coping with related legal issues.

EMT-Intermediate The **EMT-Intermediate** (EMT-I) is an EMT-Basic who completes additional training prescribed by the U.S. Department of Transportation EMT-Intermediate curriculum. This training includes emphasis on roles and responsibilities, EMS systems, medical/legal considerations, medical terminology, EMS communications, patient assessment, and initial assessment and management of shock. Additional skills include intravenous therapy, defibrillation, medication administration, endotracheal intubation, and ECG interpretation. In some states, advanced training qualifies EMT-Intermediates as cardiac technicians or cardiac rescue technicians.

EMT-Paramedic The title **EMT-Paramedic** (EMT-P) is assigned to those who are trained in all aspects of prehospital emergency care, including or equal to the U.S. Department of Transportation paramedic curriculum, and who have received the appropriate certification. Paramedics have a broad foundation of knowledge in emergency care. They also can perform advanced interventions including starting intravenous lines, administering medications, inserting endotracheal tubes (which EMT-Basics may also be trained to do in some areas), decompressing the chest cavity, reading electrocardiograms, using manual defibrillators to restore heart rhythm, cardiac pacing, cricothyroidotomy, and advanced cardiac life support.

The Health Care System

First Responders and EMTs are an integral part of a community's health care system—a network of medical care that begins in the field and extends to hospitals and other treatment centers. In essence, EMT-Basics provide **prehospital care**—emergency medical treatment given to patients before they are transported to a hospital or other facility. (In some areas the term out-of-hospital care is preferred, reflecting a trend toward providing care on the scene with or without subsequent transport to a hospital. Your instructor can provide information on how or if this term may apply to your EMS system.)

The EMT-Basic may be required to decide on the facility to which the patient must be transported. The most familiar destination is the hospital emergency department, which is staffed by physicians, nurses, and others trained in emergency trauma and emergency medical treatment. Here patients are stabilized and prepared for further care elsewhere in the hospital. Special facilities to which some patients may need to be transported include:

- A trauma center for specialized treatment of injuries that generally exceeds hospital emergency department capabilities
- A burn center for specialized treatment of serious burns, often including long-term care and rehabilitation
- An obstetrical center for high-risk obstetric patients
- A pediatric center for specialized treatment of infants and children
- A poison center for specialized treatment of poisoning victims

You will often be called to emergencies where you are the only trained emergency personnel involved. At other times, two or more emergency services will be

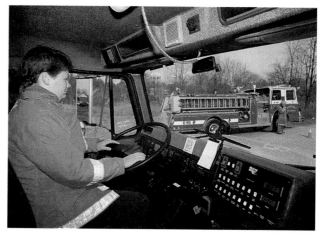

Figure 1-3   The EMT-Basic works closely with other public safety personnel.

needed at the scene (Figure 1-3). Specialized rescue teams and fire personnel, as well as law enforcement, all may be involved. As a member of the team that stabilizes and transports a patient, you will be in a unique position to serve as the liaison between the community's medical services and those public safety workers.

THE EMT-BASIC

ROLES AND RESPONSIBILITIES

While specific responsibilities may vary from one area to another, your general responsibilities as an EMT-Basic include personal safety and the safety of others, patient assessment and emergency medical care, safe lifting and moving, patient transport and transfer, record keeping and data collection, and patient advocacy. (All of these will be covered in greater detail in later chapters.)

The Americans with Disabilities Act (ADA) of 1990 protects individuals who have a documented disability from being denied initial or continued employment based on their disability. The employer must make necessary and reasonable adjustments so that the disabled are not precluded from employment. Check with your state EMS office and ADA representative to seek further information.

Personal Safety and the Safety of Others

Your first and most important priority is to protect your own safety (Figure 1-4). Remember this rule: You cannot help the patient, other rescuers, or yourself if you are injured. You also do not want to endanger other rescuers by forcing them to rescue you—instead of the patient. Once scene safety is assured, the patient's needs become your priority.

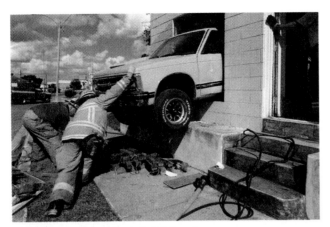

Figure 1-4   The EMT-Basic must assure personal safety at all times. (Tracy Mack/In the Dark Photography)

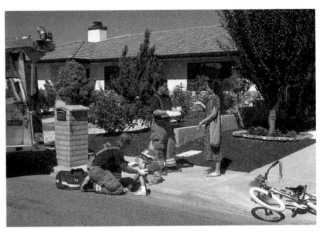

Figure 1-5   The EMT-Basic is responsible for providing competent patient care.

Drive safely at all times, using proper precautions to avoid traffic accidents. Use a seat belt whenever you drive or ride, unless you need to remove it to care for the patient. Remove yourself from potentially hazardous sites, such as high-traffic areas, gasoline leaks, fires, chemical spills, radiation leaks, and so on. Never enter a volatile crowd situation, such as a riot, crime scene, or hostage situation, until it has been controlled by law enforcement. Take extra precautions when you suspect that a victim, relative, or bystander has committed a violent crime.

At the scene, follow directions from police, fire, utility, and other expert personnel. Create a safe area in which the patient can be treated (away from the threat of fire or explosion, for example). Remove debris that poses a threat to patients or bystanders. Redirect traffic for the safety of patients and bystanders.

Wear reflective emblems or clothing at night, and provide adequate lighting at an accident scene. Minimize personal injury from jagged metal or broken glass at an accident scene by wearing a firefighter's helmet or hard hat, turnout gear, eye protection, and leather gloves. In addition, wear protective clothing, such as latex gloves, eye protection, mask, and gown, to avoid infectious diseases.

PATIENT ASSESSMENT AND EMERGENCY CARE

Once you have ensured scene safety, you must gain access to patients, recognize and evaluate problems, and provide emergency care (Figure 1-5)—often in situations that involve more than one patient. First, always perform an initial assessment to help you identify and care for immediately life-threatening problems, such as airway blockage, respiratory or cardiac arrest, or severe bleeding. Then complete a focused history and physical exam, after which you can stabilize and treat other emergency injuries or conditions

you discover or suspect. Work as quickly as possible while avoiding undue haste, carelessness, and mishandling of the patient.

SAFE LIFTING AND MOVING

Prevent further injury of patients by always using the easiest and safest recommended moves and equipment. Prevent injuring yourself by always using proper body mechanics and by making sure you have sufficient help to lift and move patients and equipment.

TRANSPORT AND TRANSFER OF CARE

Before leaving the scene, determine which facility (local emergency department, children's hospital, burn center, or other) will be most appropriate. Consider the patient's condition, the extent of injuries, the relative locations, and hospital staffing when making transport decisions. Consult medical direction if necessary, and follow your local transport protocols.

Use the communications equipment in your ambulance correctly to notify the receiving facility of the number of patients, the destination(s), and the nature and extent of injuries. Alert the hospital emergency department about high-priority patients and what will be needed immediately upon arrival, such as a trauma team or a cardiac arrest team. Report changes in the patient's condition, and consult medical direction during transport as appropriate (Figures 1-6 and 1-7).

Drive in a way that will minimize further injury and maximize patient comfort. Obey appropriate laws and regulations, and use lights and sirens properly. Once you reach the destination, help remove the wheeled stretcher and maneuver it into the emergency department (Figure 1-8).

Report both verbally and in writing to the appropriate receiving facility personnel what injuries were identified and what care has been given the patient.

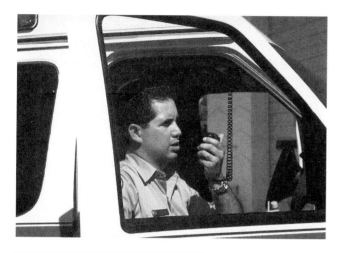

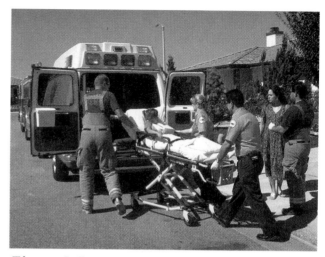

Figure 1-7   Assessment and emergency care are continued en route to the medical facility.

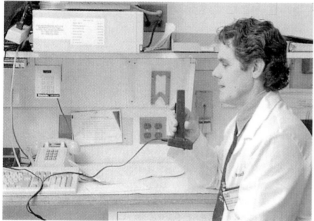

Figure 1-6   The EMT-Basic can get on-line medical direction by telephone, cellular phone, or radio.

Provide other assistance as needed and do not leave before the patient has been properly transferred to the care of hospital personnel.

RECORD KEEPING AND DATA COLLECTION

Throughout your shift, maintain an up-to-date log of calls. Before leaving the hospital, complete the written prehospital care report. This report will become part of the hospital's permanent record on the patient and part of your EMS system's records.

PATIENT ADVOCACY

As an emergency care provider, you are also responsible for protecting the patient's rights. At the scene, collect and safeguard a patient's valuables, transport them with the patient, and obtain a receipt when you give them to emergency department personnel. In the field protect the patient's privacy, shield the patient as much as possible from curious bystanders, and answer questions truthfully. Conceal from curious onlookers the body of a patient who has died until appropriate authorities arrive.

Make sure that the patient's friends or loved ones at the scene know how to get to the hospital. In some systems a relative may be transported in the operator's section of the ambulance. At the hospital, act as the patient's advocate by making certain you have provided necessary information, especially about circumstances hospital personnel have not witnessed. Honor any patient requests that you reasonably can, such as notifying a relative or ensuring that the patient's home is secure.

PROFESSIONAL ATTRIBUTES

A number of professional attributes are important to maximize your effectiveness as an EMT-Basic. They include appearance, knowledge, skills, and the ability to meet physical demands, as well as your general interests and temperament.

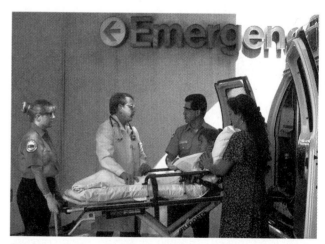

Figure 1-8   The EMT-Basic is responsible for properly transferring the care of the patient to the appropriate medical personnel.

APPEARANCE

Excellent personal grooming and a neat, clean appearance help instill confidence in patients treated by EMT-Basics—and help protect them from contamination that could be caused by dirty hands, dirty fingernails, or soiled clothing. Respond to the scene in complete uniform, or appropriate dress, to portray the positive image you want to communicate. Remember, you are on a medical team. Your appearance can send the message that you are competent and can be trusted to make the right decisions.

KNOWLEDGE AND SKILLS

To practice as an EMT-Basic, you need to successfully complete the basic training program for EMTs as outlined by the U.S. Department of Transportation. In addition to the required course work, you also need to know:

- How to use and maintain common emergency equipment, such as suction machines, oxygen-delivery systems, airway adjuncts, automated external defibrillators, spinal immobilization equipment, splints, obstetrical kits, various types of patient moving devices, and light rescue tools
- How and when to assist with the administration of medications approved by medical direction
- How to clean, disinfect, and sterilize nondisposable equipment
- Safety and security measures for yourself, your partner and other rescuers, as well as for the patient and bystanders
- The territory and terrain within the service area to allow expedient response to the scene and to the appropriate receiving facility
- State and local traffic laws and ordinances concerning emergency transportation of the sick and injured. By law ambulances are given certain privileges, but they are not immune to all laws

Use opportunities for continuing education to expand your knowledge and learn about advances in patient care, new equipment, or better ways of using existing equipment. Take refresher courses to renew your knowledge and skills. Finally, make an effort to maintain up-to-date knowledge of local, state, and federal legislation, regulations, standards, guidelines, and issues that affect the emergency medical systems in your area.

PHYSICAL DEMANDS

To be an EMT-Basic, you must be in good physical health. Your eyesight must be good (correction by lenses is permitted) and you must have good color vision in order to properly assess a patient as well as for driving safely.

TEMPERAMENT AND ABILITIES

In times of crisis, patients will look toward someone to reestablish order in a suddenly chaotic world. Chances are that someone will be you. It can bring out the best in you as well as cause you a great deal of stress. To be as effective as you can be as an EMT-Basic, you should have the following characteristics.

- *A pleasant personality.* As an EMT-Basic you will often be required to perform skills and procedures while speaking in a reassuring and calming voice to a patient who may be agitated, in shock, or in a great deal of pain.
- *Leadership ability.* You must be able to assess a situation quickly, step forward to take control when appropriate, set action priorities, give clear and simple directions, be confident and persuasive enough to be obeyed, and carry through with what needs to be done.
- *Good judgment.* You must be able to make appropriate decisions quickly, often in unsafe or stressful situations involving human beings in crisis.
- *Good moral character.* While there are many legal constraints on the profession, you also have ethical obligations. You are in a position of public trust that can never be wholly described by statute or case law alone.
- *Stability and adaptability.* Being an EMT-Basic can be quite stressful. Exhaustion, frustration, anger, and grief are part of the package. You must be able to learn how to delay expressing your feelings until the emergency is over. Just as important, you must also be able to understand that intense emotional reactions are normal and that seeking support from coworkers, counselors, friends, and family are important aspects of keeping yourself mentally and physically fit.

MEDICAL DIRECTION

As an EMT-Basic, you are the designated agent of the physician medical director of your EMS system. The care you render to patients is considered an extension of the medical director's authority. (Learn your own state laws, statutes, and regulations in regard to medical direction.)

The **medical director** is a physician who is legally responsible for the clinical and patient care aspects of an EMS system. Every ambulance service and rescue squad must have physician medical direction in place to provide guidance to all emergency care and rescue personnel, both on-line (by telephone or radio) and off-line (in the form of protocols and standing orders—see Figure 1-9). The physician responsible for medical direction is also responsible for reviewing quality improvement for the EMS system.

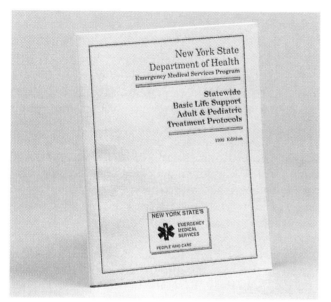

Figure 1-9 Off-line medical direction may take the form of standards protocols and standing orders.

QUALITY IMPROVEMENT

Quality improvement is a system of internal and external reviews and audits of all aspects of an emergency medical system. To ensure that the public receives the highest quality of prehospital care, the goals of quality improvement are to identify those aspects of the system that can be improved and to implement plans and programs that will remedy any shortcomings.

As an EMT-Basic, your role in quality improvement (Figure 1-10) is to:

• Carefully and thoroughly document each call. Information gathered from prehospital care reports that you prepare are studied by quality improvement committees to spot such things as excessive response times, which might be remedied by redeploying ambulances, or to identify seldom-used skills for refresher training.
• Perform reviews and audits as requested.
• Gather feedback from patients, other EMS personnel, and hospital staff.
• Conduct preventive maintenance on vehicles and equipment.
• Participate in refresher courses and continuing education to reinforce, update, and expand your knowledge and skills.
• Maintain skills in all aspects of patient care and equipment operation.

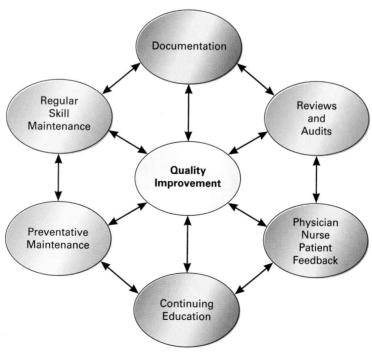

Figure 1-10 The EMT-Basic takes an active role in quality improvement.

CASE STUDY FOLLOW-UP

SCENE SIZE-UP

You have been dispatched to a 65-year-old male, Edgar Robinson, who fell down a steep embankment behind his house. Although the rescue squad officer informs you that you will be in no personal danger, you and your partner are cautious as you carry your equipment closer to the embankment. As your partner takes the patient's wife, Mrs. Robinson, aside, the rescue squad officer tells you that his crew all have First Responder training and will immobilize Mr. Robinson on a long spine board before bringing him up.

INITIAL ASSESSMENT

One First Responder reports her observations of the patient to you as the others place the patient where you indicate. She tells you that the patient's chief complaint is of pain to his right wrist and right thigh and that the patient has warm and dry skin, his airway is patent with respirations of 24 per minute, radial pulse is 90 beats per minute and strong.

As you begin your own initial assessment, you note that your general impression of Mr. Robinson is of an alert, robust older man. Mr. Robinson explains to you that while disposing of yard wastes, he got too close to the edge of the embankment and slipped.

FOCUSED HISTORY AND PHYSICAL EXAM

You perform a rapid trauma assessment while your partner takes vital signs, which indicate no change from those reported by the First Responder. Your physical exam reveals abrasions to the arms, with pain and a slight deformity to the right wrist. There are also superficial abrasions to the right leg, with deformity,

swelling and pain to the right thigh. You discover that the patient cannot feel or move the toes of his right foot. However, pulses are present in the foot.

You initiate oxygen therapy via nonrebreather mask.

The history you take, by asking questions of the patient, confirms sharp pain to the right wrist and thigh, which started immediately after he landed at the bottom of the embankment. Mr. Robinson also reports that he did not lose consciousness. He denies any other complaints, but informs you that he is allergic to sulfa drugs and takes medication for high blood pressure.

After checking the immobilization of the patient, you enlist the First Responders to help you apply a traction splint to the right leg. Then you splint the injured wrist. During these procedures, you speak quietly and reassuringly to the patient.

DETAILED PHYSICAL EXAM AND ONGOING ASSESSMENT

You move Mr. Robinson on the spine board to a wheeled stretcher, then transfer him to the ambulance. En route, you quickly perform a detailed head-to-toe physical exam to be sure that you have not overlooked any injuries. You notify the hospital that you are en route and give details of the patient's condition, then conduct an ongoing assessment every 5 minutes to monitor his condition until you arrive at the hospital.

Upon arrival, you transfer care of the patient without incident to the emergency department staff and give your verbal report. You carefully complete your written prehospital care report and prepare the unit for the next call.

CHAPTER REVIEW

TERMS AND CONCEPTS

You may wish to review the following terms and concepts included in this chapter.

EMS system—Emergency Medical Services system.
EMT-Basic—emergency medical technician trained to the basic level. Also EMT-B.
EMT-Intermediate—emergency medical technician trained to the intermediate level. Also EMT-I.

EMT-Paramedic—emergency medical technician trained to the paramedic level. Also EMT-P.
First Responder—a person typically trained to the first responder level who is likely to be the first person on the scene with emergency care training.
medical director—physician who is legally responsible for the clinical and patient care aspects of an EMS system.

prehospital care—emergency medical treatment given to patients before they are transported to a hospital or other facility. Also out-of-hospital care.

quality improvement—a system of internal and external reviews and audits of an EMS system to ensure a high quality of care.

REVIEW QUESTIONS

1. Describe the purpose of the modern EMS system.
2. Name two ways the public accesses the EMS system. Explain advantages or disadvantages of each.
3. List the four levels of emergency medical technician training.
4. List the general responsibilities of an EMT-Basic.
5. Describe the EMS physician medical director's primary responsibility.
6. List the goals of quality improvement.
7. Describe the EMT-B's role in quality improvement.

CHAPTER 2

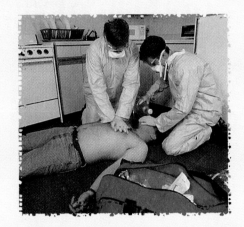

The Well-Being of the EMT-Basic

INTRODUCTION

As you proceed through your course and this text, you will study specific ways to safeguard your well-being—in the face of danger and under other high-stress circumstances. This chapter presents an overview. In it you will learn to recognize and deal with the stress that normally accompanies emergency work, to practice all appropriate body substance isolation precautions, and to wear the appropriate personal protective equipment at the scene of accidents and illness.

OBJECTIVES

Numbered objectives are from the United States Department of Transportation 1994 EMT-Basic National Standard Curriculum. Asterisked objectives, if any, pertain to material that is supplemental to the DOT curriculum.

COGNITIVE

1-2.1 List possible emotional reactions that the EMT-Basic may experience when faced with trauma, illness, death, and dying. (pp. 15–16)

1-2.2 Discuss the possible reactions that a family member may exhibit when confronted with death and dying. (p. 14)

1-2.3 State the steps in the EMT-Basic's approach to the family confronted with death and dying. (pp. 14–15)

1-2.4 State the possible reactions that the family of the EMT-Basic may exhibit due to their outside involvement in EMS. (p. 17)

1-2.5 Recognize the signs and symptoms of critical incident stress. (pp. 16, 17–18)

1-2.6 State possible steps that the EMT-Basic may take to help reduce/alleviate stress. (pp. 16–18)

1-2.7 Explain the need to determine scene safety. (p. 18)

1-2.8 Discuss the importance of body substance isolation (BSI). (p. 20)

1-2.9 Describe the steps the EMT-Basic should take for personal protection from airborne and bloodborne pathogens. (pp. 19–23)

1-2.10 List the personal protective equipment necessary for each of the following situations:
 – Hazardous materials (p. 23)
 – Rescue operations (pp. 23–24)
 – Violent scenes (pp. 24–25)
 – Crime scenes (pp. 24–25)
 – Exposure to bloodborne pathogens (pp. 19–23)
 – Exposure to airborne pathogens (pp. 19–23)

AFFECTIVE

1-2.11 Explain the rationale for serving as an advocate for the use of appropriate protective equipment. (p. 18)

PSYCHOMOTOR

1-2.12 Given a scenario with potential infectious exposure, the EMT-Basic will use appropriate personal protective equipment. At the completion of the scenario, the EMT-Basic will properly remove and discard the protective garments.

1-2.13 Given the above scenario, the EMT-Basic will complete disinfection/cleaning and all reporting documentation.

CASE STUDY

THE DISPATCH

EMS Units 111 and 112—both units respond to 327 Manchester Avenue—possible domestic dispute with reported gunfire—called in by the police department—time out 1441 hours.

ON ARRIVAL

You immediately identify three city police cruisers outside the house. Patrol officers are kneeling behind their units with guns drawn and pointed at the house.

One of the police officers is gesturing emphatically for you and your partner to keep back. Your partner stops the ambulance a good distance away. As you survey the scene with binoculars, you identify a downed police officer at the front door of the residence. He is not moving and seems to be bleeding profusely. You both hear gunfire.

How would you proceed?

During this chapter, you will learn about methods of safeguarding yourself from stress, body substances, and other hazards. Later, we will return to the case and apply the principles learned.

EMOTIONAL ASPECTS OF EMERGENCY CARE

In the course of providing emergency care, you will encounter family members, as well as patients, who are in distress—acute physical or mental suffering caused by pain, anxiety, strain, or sorrow. When such emotional pressures become too great for them to handle, emotional crisis occurs. The emergency care you provide can move those patients and family members toward reestablishing emotional equilibrium.

DEATH AND DYING

Death and dying are inherent parts of emergency medical care. You must care for the dying patient's emotional needs, as well as their injuries or illnesses. If the patient has suffered a sudden death, you may also need to help the family or bystanders deal with the situation.

Research into how people cope with death has identified five general stages that dying patients—and those close to them—will experience. However, each person is unique. Individuals will progress through the stages at their own rates and in their own ways. Note that while these stages usually apply to the dying patient, they also can apply to patients experiencing nonfatal emergencies. For example, a patient who loses both legs in an industrial accident will grieve the loss of the limbs.

FIVE EMOTIONAL STAGES

Characteristically, you will not witness all five stages during emergency treatment. For example, the critically injured patient who is aware that death is imminent typically displays denial, bargaining, or depression. The terminally ill patient may be more prepared and display acceptance. The key for you is to accept all these emotions as real and necessary, and respond accordingly.

- *Denial ("Not me.")*. At first, the patient may refuse to accept the possibility that death is near. This refusal, or denial, is a defense mechanism that creates a buffer between the shock of approaching death and the need to deal with the illness or injury.
- *Anger ("Why me?")*. As the patient moves through denial, anger generally follows—and you may be the target. Do not become defensive. That kind of anger is an aspect of the grieving process both dying patients and their families go through. Be empathetic, and use your best listening and communication skills.
- *Bargaining ("Okay, but first let me . . .")*. Following anger, the patient will likely try to "bargain,"

or make agreements that at least in the patient's mind will postpone death for a short time.
- *Depression ("Okay, but I haven't . . .")*. As reality settles in, the patient may become silent, distant, sad, and despairing—usually about those he will leave behind and things left undone.
- *Acceptance ("Okay, I am not afraid.")*. Finally, patients may appear to accept death, though not happy about it. At this stage, the family usually requires more support than the patient does.

DEALING WITH THE DYING PATIENT, FAMILY, AND BYSTANDERS

Although emergency care of the patient's illness or injury is your priority, you have an obligation to help patients and others through the grieving process. Keep in mind that patients, families, and bystanders may be progressing through the stages at different rates. Whatever stage they are in, their needs include dignity, respect, sharing, communication, privacy, and control. To help reduce their emotional burden:

- *Do everything possible to maintain the patient's dignity.* Avoid negative statements about the patient's condition. An unresponsive patient may hear what you say and feel the fear in your words. Even if the patient is unresponsive, talk to him as if he is fully alert and explain the care you are providing.
- *Show the greatest possible respect for the patient,* especially when death is imminent. Families will be extra sensitive to how the dying relative is treated. Even attitudes and unspoken messages are perceived. Allow family members to stay with the patient during resuscitation efforts, explain what you are doing, and assure them that you are making every possible effort to help the patient. It is important for the family to know with certainty that you never simply "gave up."
- *Communicate.* Help the patient become oriented to surroundings. Explain several times, if necessary, what has happened and where it has happened. Explain who you are and what you and others are planning to do. Assure the patient that you are doing everything possible and that you will see that the patient gets to a hospital as quickly as possible for further care. Without interrupting care for the patient, communicate the same message to the family. Explain any procedures you need to carry out. Give straightforward answers to questions. Report what you know to be true, but do not guess or make assumptions.
- *Allow family members to express themselves.* They should be able to scream, cry, or vent grief in a way that is not hazardous to you or others. This can help them progress through the stages of the grieving process. If they direct anger at you, remember

not to take the attack personally. Be tolerant and avoid getting defensive. Do not retaliate, get angry, or become hostile.

- *Listen empathetically.* Many dying people want messages delivered to survivors. Take notes and assure the patient that you will do whatever you can to honor his requests. Then, follow through on your promise. If possible, you or a member of your team should stay with the family to listen to their concerns and answer their questions.
- *Do not give false assurances,* but let the patient know that everything that can be done to help will be done. Allow for some hope. Be honest but tactful. If the patient asks if he is dying, do not confirm it. Patients who do the most poorly are often the ones who feel hopeless. Instead, say something like "We are doing everything we can for you. We need you to help us by not giving up." If the patient insists that death is imminent, say something like "That might be possible, but we can still try the best we can, can't we?"
- *Use a gentle tone of voice* with the patient and family. Explain the scope of the injury or problem, the procedures you are doing, and related information as kindly as you can in terms the family can understand.
- *Use a reassuring touch,* if appropriate. If family members want to touch or hold the body after death (and if local protocol allows), arrange for it. Do what you can to improve the appearance of the body. Clean vomitus, blood, or secretions from the face and hands. Elevate the head for a few minutes to allow fluids to drain. If the body is mutilated, warn the family first, and explain that you have covered the badly injured parts. If a possible crime is involved, do not clean the patient or remove any blood. Also, do not cover the patient with a sheet.
- *Do what you can to comfort the family.* Offer help to family members who are at the scene. Even if death is imminent, arrange for them briefly to see and talk to the patient. This should not interrupt your emergency care or delay transport. Encourage the family to talk to an unresponsive patient. Explain that the patient may still hear and understand. If the patient is deceased and the family asks you to pray with them, do so. Stay with the family until the medical examiner or coroner arrives. Finally, if a family member asks to accompany the patient in the ambulance, make the arrangements if at all possible.

HIGH STRESS SITUATIONS

Patients, families, and bystanders are not the only ones who experience extreme stress in an emergency situation. The EMT-B does too. Accepting and understanding that fact is the first step in learning how to handle it in healthy ways.

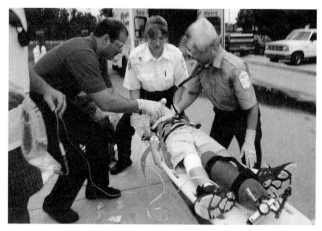

Figure 2-1 Responsibility for a life can be highly stressful. (Craig Jackson/In the Dark Photography)

Stress is any change in the body's internal balance. It occurs when external demands become greater than personal resources. Top sources of stress for the EMT-B include long hours, boredom between calls, working too much and too hard, getting little recognition, having to respond instantly, making life-and-death decisions, fearing serious errors, dealing with dying people and grieving survivors, and being responsible for someone's life (Figure 2-1).

Many emergency calls may be considered "routine" with a minimal level of stress. However, the nature of some calls may produce extreme levels of stress. Some of these situations include:

- Multiple-casualty incidents involving multiple patients at a single scene
- Abuse and neglect of infants, children, adults, and the elderly
- Emergencies involving infants and children
- Injury or death of a coworker
- Responding and providing emergency care to a relative or bystander
- Severe traumatic injuries such as amputations

 ## STRESS MANAGEMENT

Many EMT-Bs expose themselves to overwhelming stress in the desire to help meet the needs of patients. They feel completely responsible for everything that happens on a run, even things clearly out of their control. Some become so involved that their self-image becomes based on job performance.

Chronic stress brought about by work-related problems in an emotionally charged environment can lead to **burnout**—a state of exhaustion and irritability that can markedly decrease one's effectiveness in delivering emergency medical care. Beware. Even some of the very best EMS providers have had to leave the system because of it.

RECOGNIZE WARNING SIGNS

One of the best ways to prevent burnout is to recognize the warning signs of stress (Figure 2-2). The earlier they are recognized, the easier they are to remedy:

- Irritability with coworkers, family, and friends
- Inability to concentrate
- Difficulty sleeping and nightmares
- Anxiety
- Indecisiveness
- Guilt
- Loss of appetite
- Loss of sexual desire or interest
- Isolation
- Loss of interest in work

General categories of signs and symptoms also have been identified with stress. In addition to the warning signs listed above, they include:

- *Thinking*—confusion, inability to make judgments or decisions, loss of motivation, chronic forgetfulness, loss of objectivity
- *Psychological*—depression, excessive anger, negativism, hostility, defensiveness, mood swings, feelings of worthlessness
- *Physical*—persistent exhaustion, headaches, gastrointestinal distress, dizziness, pounding heart
- *Behavioral*—overeating, increased alcohol or drug use, grinding teeth, hyperactivity, lack of energy
- *Social*—increased interpersonal conflicts, decreased ability to relate to patients as individuals

MAKE LIFESTYLE CHANGES

The following lifestyle changes can help you deal with stress:

- *Take a look at your diet.* Certain foods tend to increase the body's stress response. So cut down on the amount of sugar, caffeine, and alcohol you consume. Increase the amount of protein and carbohydrates you eat, while decreasing fat intake. While at work, eat frequently but in small amounts.
- *Exercise more often.* Exercise has all sorts of benefits. One of the greatest is that it provides a physical release for the pent-up emotions that accompany many crises.
- *Learn to relax.* Practice relaxation techniques, such as taking a deep breath, holding it, and blowing out forcefully. Meditation and visual imagery techniques are also helpful ways to relax. You may also wish to try temporary diversions, such as watching a funny movie, reading a good book, or going to a concert with a friend. Cut loose a little bit.
- *Avoid self-medication.* Reaching for a bottle—whether it is filled with alcohol or pills—does not help you cope with stress. In fact, it will increase it. Your problems are still there when you come out of the stupor, and they probably will be worse because you did not act on them immediately.

KEEP BALANCE IN YOUR LIFE

One way to keep a balance of work, recreation, family, health, and other interests is to assess your priorities. Take a few minutes to list all your activities on

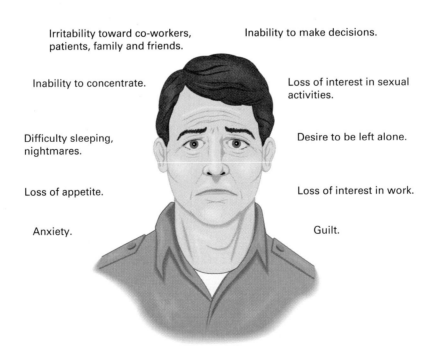

Figure 2-2   The warning signs of stress.

paper. Write "1" beside your first priority, "2" beside your second, and so on. Then address those activities—all of them—in order of the priority you have assigned them.

You can also share your worries with someone else. Talking to someone you trust and respect can help relieve stress. It can also help you to discover alternatives that might have otherwise escaped you. A good confidante can listen empathetically and ask questions that will help you explore your ideas honestly.

Still another way to help keep balance in your life is to accept the fact that you will occasionally make mistakes. Honestly admit to yourself that no person is right all of the time, and understand that a mistake does not reduce your value. You do not have to be perfect to do a good job.

RECOGNIZE THE RESPONSE OF YOUR FAMILY AND FRIENDS

The support of your family and friends is essential in helping you manage stress. However, you may find that they, too, suffer from a certain amount of stress as a result of your job. You may find:

- *Lack of understanding.* Families typically have little if any knowledge about prehospital emergency care.
- *Fear of separation or of being ignored.* Long hours and demanding physical labor can take their toll and increase your family's distress over your absences. Typically you may hear: "Your job is more important to you than your family!"
- *Worry about on-call situations.* Stress at home may increase because your family may overemphasize or exaggerate the danger you may face when you respond to emergency calls.
- *Inability to plan.* Family and friends may not understand why you cannot leave your call area or have to leave an event early. Typically you may hear: "You're not the only one on call. Let someone else go this time."
- *Frustrated desire to share.* You often find it too difficult to talk about what has happened during your shift. Your family and friends understand why, in a general way, but nevertheless feel frustrated in their desire to help and support you.

Help family and friends understand the nature of your work and what you do for patients. Talk to them. Describe how you feel about what you do. Answer their questions. Explaining the safety precautions you and coworkers take every day can ease their anxieties. Encouraging them to join you in staying fit (daily exercise and planning healthy meals, for example) also can help alleviate their concerns when you cannot be with them. Always include time with them on your list of priorities.

MAKE CHANGES IN YOUR WORK ENVIRONMENT

The following changes in your work environment can help you manage job-related stress:

- *Develop a "buddy" system with a coworker.* Keep an eye on each other, and suggest when breaks are advisable. Try to take a brief break whenever you find your effectiveness diminishing.
- *Encourage and support your coworkers.* Make positive remarks, and resist the temptation to criticize or dwell on the negative.
- *Periodically take a break* to get some exercise—do some aerobics at the station, take a brisk walk or similar activity.
- *Request work shifts that allow you more time to relax* with your family and friends.
- *Request a rotation of duty assignment* to a less busy area.

SEEK PROFESSIONAL HELP

You can also seek advice from mental-health professionals, who can help you realize that your reactions are normal, mobilize your best coping strategies, and arm you with more effective ways to deal with stress in the future.

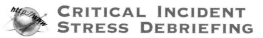

CRITICAL INCIDENT STRESS DEBRIEFING

A **critical incident** is any situation that causes you to experience emotions that are unusually strong and that may interfere with your ability to function, either during the critical incident or later. Common critical incidents include:

- The serious injury or death of an emergency team member in the line of duty
- Suicide of an emergency team member
- Injury or death of a friend or family member
- Death of a patient under especially tragic or emotional circumstances or after prolonged or intense rescue procedures
- Sudden death of an infant or child
- Injuries to children caused by child abuse
- Injuries or death to civilians that are caused by EMS personnel (such as an ambulance colliding with an automobile)
- An event that threatens your life
- An event that attracts unusual media attention
- An event that has distressing sights, sounds, or smells
- A multiple-casualty incident, such as a plane crash

Rescuers who suffer critical incident stress develop many of the signs and symptoms of burnout. They also may suffer from repeated mental images of the incident, fear of continuing in EMS work, and the inability to function at the scene of subsequent emergencies. One of the best ways of dealing with these signs and symptoms is called **critical incident stress debriefing (CISD).** CISD is not professional counseling but a means to release stress.

The CISD process is ideally held within 24 to 72 hours of a critical incident. During CISD, a team of peer counselors and mental health professionals help rescuers work through seven phases:

- *Introduction.* Rescuers are assured that everything said at a CISD meeting will be kept confidential. What they say will in no way affect their job status.
- *Facts.* Participants review details of the event.
- *Feelings.* Participants explore how they feel about what happened.
- *Symptoms.* Rescuers are urged to explore any physical, mental, or emotional symptoms they may be experiencing.
- *Teaching.* Skilled professionals help participants sort through their feelings and symptoms. The professionals emphasize that these are normal reactions.
- *Re-entry.* CISD leaders and mental health professionals evaluate information and offer suggestions on overcoming the stress, including a plan of action for returning to the job. Rescuers may set goals and plan activities to help to diffuse the stress further.
- *Follow-up.* Several weeks or months later, participants can resolve lingering issues.

CISD should include anyone involved in the incident—law enforcement personnel, firefighters, EMS personnel, dispatch operators, and hospital emergency department personnel (Figure 2-3). In some cases, the debriefing may involve rescue worker family members, who are inevitably affected by the stress of the incident. In cases of multiple casualties, such as earthquakes or tornadoes, a number of CISD meetings involving hundreds of people may need to be conducted.

Defusing is a version of CISD held within 1 to 4 hours following a critical incident. It is attended only by those most directly involved in the critical incident and lasts only 30 to 45 minutes. Less structured than a CISD meeting, defusing gives the smaller group of rescuers an opportunity to vent their emotions and get information they may need before the larger group meets.

CISD is successful because it helps rescuers vent their feelings quickly and because the nonthreatening environment encourages rescuers to feel free to air their concerns and reactions. The most effective CISD teams are those that include preplanning and education in addition to post-incident support.

Ask your instructor about the CISD programs available through your EMS system. Comprehensive critical incident stress management should include:

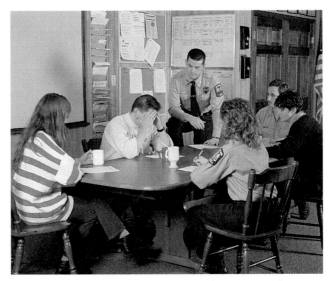

Figure 2-3 The critical incident stress debriefing (CISD) helps emergency personnel deal with particularly stressful incidents.

- Pre-incident stress education
- On-scene peer support
- One-on-one support
- Disaster support services
- Defusing
- CISD
- Follow-up services
- Spouse and family support
- Community outreach programs
- Other health and welfare programs, such as wellness programs

SCENE SAFETY

Keeping yourself safe at the scene of an illness or injury involves taking appropriate measures to protect yourself from infectious disease, following proper rescue procedures, and knowing how to handle violence, especially at a crime scene. It is also important to be an advocate for these protective measures—to help keep fellow rescuers, as well as yourself, safe and well.

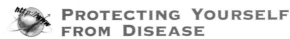

PROTECTING YOURSELF FROM DISEASE

How Diseases Spread

Diseases are caused by **pathogens,** or microorganisms such as bacteria and viruses. These pathogens can spread in a number of ways including by way of blood (bloodborne pathogens) or air (airborne pathogens). An infectious disease is one that spreads from person to person (Table 2-1). It can spread directly through blood-to-blood contact, contact with open wounds and exposed tissue, and contact with the mucous

TABLE 2-1

Infectious Diseases and Protective Measures

DISEASE	TRANSMITTED BY	PROTECTIVE CLOTHING	PROTECTIVE PROCEDURES	NOTES
AIDS	Blood and other body fluids by way of: –Sexual contact. –Infected needles. –Blood/blood products. –Mother/child.	–Disposable mask. –Disposable gloves. –Protective eyewear. –Waterproof apron, gown, or shoe covering if spraying or spattering body fluids. –Bandages on hands to cover cuts, lesions, scratches, hangnails, or other open sores and wounds.	–Wash hands thoroughly. –Use extreme care in suctioning. –Avoid unprotected artificial ventilation. –Use only disposable needles; do not cut, bend, or recap; seal in a clearly labeled, rigid, puncture-proof bag.	–Wash vehicle surfaces with CDC- or OSHA-approved germicidal. Rinse with diluted bleach. –Soak and disinfect all nondisposable equipment. –Immediately clean and disinfect any spills of blood and other body fluids. –Double-bag all soiled refuse. Dispose of properly. –Soak linens/clothing in hydrogen peroxide. Launder for 25 minutes in hot soapy water and bleach.
Hepatitis B	–Blood and other body fluids.	–Disposable gloves. –Bandages on hands to cover cuts, lesions, scratches, hangnails, or other open sores and wounds.	–Get hepatitis B vaccination series. –Get injection of HBIG within 7 days of exposure, and 1 month later if not previously immunized or inadequate antibody response. –Use only disposable needles; do not cut, bend, or recap; seal in a clearly labeled, rigid, puncture-proof bag. –Avoid unprotected artificial ventilation.	–Clean vehicle and nondisposable equipment with a diluted bleach solution. –Double-bag and seal all soiled refuse. Dispose of properly. –Double-bag all soiled clothing and linens. –Launder soiled clothing and linens in hot soapy water and bleach.
Tuberculosis	–Droplet spread (usually continual). –Direct contact with oral or nasal secretions.	–HEPA respirator.	–Wash hands thoroughly. –Avoid unprotected artificial ventilation. –Use HEPA respirator.	–Scrub vehicle surfaces and equipment contaminated by secretions. –Launder clothing and linens contaminated by secretions in hot soapy water and bleach. –Incinerate all disposable equipment used on patient.
Influenza	–Droplet spread.	–Disposable mask.	–Wash hands thoroughly. –Use care in suctioning mouth/nose. –Get annual immunization.	–Scrub surfaces of vehicle contacted by patient. –Disinfect all nondisposable equipment used for patient. –Launder contaminated clothing and linens in hot soapy water.
Common Childhood Diseases	–Droplet spread. –Oral and nasal secretions. –Indirect contact (rubella). –Direct contact with skin lesions (chickenpox).	–Disposable mask. –Disposable gloves (chickenpox).	–Get vaccination if not already immune (measles, mumps, rubella). –Use caution in suctioning mouth/nose. –Avoid touching skin lesions (chickenpox).	–Scrub vehicle surfaces and nondisposable equipment contaminated with secretions or lesions. –Boil nondisposable equipment or follow your system's recommendations. –Launder contaminated clothing and linens in hot soapy water. –Boil clothing and linens contaminated by patients with chickenpox or scarlet fever.

membranes of the eyes and mouth. It can also spread indirectly by way of a contaminated object such as a needle. Airborne pathogens are spread by infected droplets breathed into the respiratory tract.

BODY SUBSTANCE ISOLATION

For many years, U.S. Department of Labor Occupational Safety and Health Administration (OSHA) guidelines required emergency care workers to take universal precautions, or precautions against diseases transmitted by way of blood. However, in the late 1980s the Centers for Disease Control (CDC) of the U.S. Department of Health and Human Services published guidelines that set a new standard against infection. That standard assumes that all blood and body fluids are infectious and requires emergency workers to practice a strict form of infection control called **body substance isolation (BSI).** The following guidelines are required BSI precautions.

Handwashing *Handwashing is the single most important way you can prevent the spread of infection* (Figure 2-4). According to the U.S. Public Health Service, most contaminants can be removed from the skin with 10 to 15 seconds of vigorous lathering and scrubbing with plain soap. Note: *You should wash your hands even if you were wearing gloves.*

For maximum protection, begin by removing all jewelry from your hands and arms. Then proceed to vigorously lather and rub together all surfaces of your hands. Pay attention to creases, crevices, and the areas between your fingers. Use a brush to scrub under and around your fingernails. (It is recommended that you keep your nails short and unpolished.) If your

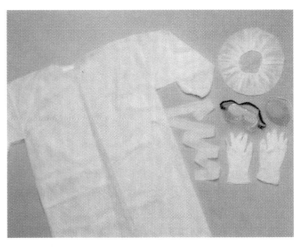

Figure 2-5 An infection control kit.

hands are visibly soiled, spend more time washing them. Wash your wrists and forearms if they were exposed or possibly contaminated. Rinse thoroughly under a stream of running water. Dry well, using a disposable towel if you can.

If you do not have access to soap and running water in the field, you can temporarily use a foam or liquid washing agent that requires no water. Then be sure to wash your hands again as soon as you can.

Personal Protective Equipment Always use **personal protective equipment** as a barrier against infection. It will help to prevent your skin and mucous membranes from coming in contact with a patient's blood and other body fluids. Personal protective equipment includes eye protection, protective gloves, gowns, and masks (Figure 2-5).

- *Eye protection.* Use eye shields to protect against blood and other body fluids splashing into your eyes. Several types are available (Figure 2-6): clear plastic shields that cover the eyes or cover the whole face, protective eyewear (safety glasses) with side shields, and if you wear prescription eyeglasses, there are removable side shields you can attach to your glasses. Form-fitting goggles also are available but are not required.

- *Protective gloves.* Wear high quality vinyl, latex, or other synthetic gloves whenever you care for a patient (Figure 2-7). If a glove accidentally tears while in use, remove it as soon as you can do so safely. Then wash your hands and replace the glove with a new one. Never reuse gloves. Put on a new pair of gloves between contact with different patients to avoid exposing one patient to another's infection. In addition, wear a good pair of utility gloves when cleaning vehicles and equipment.

- *Gowns.* Wear a gown in any situation where there may be significant contact with blood or other body fluids, such as during childbirth or major

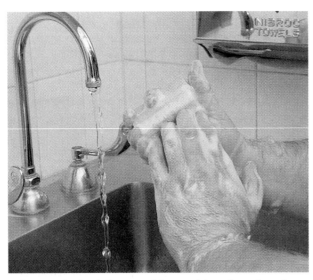

Figure 2-4 Thoroughly washing hands after patient contact is the first line of protection against infectious disease.

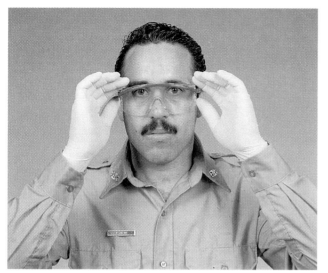

Figure 2-6   Protective eyewear. Removable side shields are also available for prescription glasses.

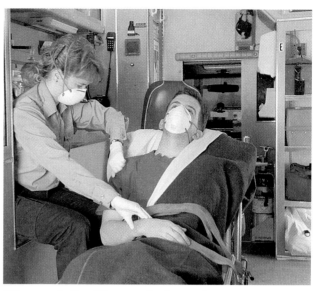

Figure 2-8   Use surgical masks to protect against blood splatters or airborne disease.

trauma. Whenever possible, use disposable gowns. If at all possible, also change your uniform after caring for a patient in a large-splash situation.

* *Masks.* Wear a disposable surgical-type face mask to prevent blood or other body fluids from being splashed into your nose or mouth. You may also put a surgical mask on the patient if an airborne disease is suspected (Figure 2-8). If you are treat-

ing a patient suspected of having tuberculosis, you need additional protection. Wear a high-efficiency particulate air (HEPA) respirator (Figure 2-9).

Additional Guidelines   The following guidelines should be observed as part of routine patient care:

* Whenever possible, use disposable equipment. Disinfect or sterilize nondisposable equipment according to local guidelines and protocols.
* Never reuse disposable equipment. Discard it after use with one patient. If you suspect that a patient may have an infectious disease, place used disposable equipment in a plastic bag clearly labeled as biohazardous or infectious waste. Then seal the bag.

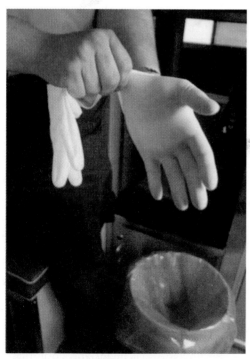

Figure 2-7   Wear protective gloves whenever you might be exposed to blood or other body fluids.

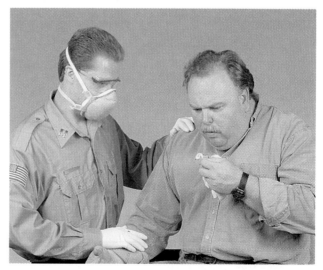

Figure 2-9   Wear a special high-efficiency particulate air (HEPA) respirator when you suspect tuberculosis.

Equipment used with HIV-infected or hepatitis B patients should be double-bagged.

- If your uniform gets soiled with body fluids, remove, bag, and label it. It should be washed in hot soapy water for at least 25 minutes. Take a hot shower yourself, and rinse thoroughly.
- After transferring care of a patient, gather all disposable equipment soiled by blood and other body fluids. Bag and seal it. Then label it as infectious waste (Figure 2-10).
- Document in your logbook or on your flowsheet any contact with blood or other body fluids and any cleaning you have done as a result.
- Sponge, wipe, or wash noncritical items that do not ordinarily touch the patient or only touch intact skin (such as blood pressure cuffs). Rinse with clear water and allow to dry thoroughly.
- Patient-care equipment that enters the body or that touches mucous membranes must be cleaned before each use with high-level disinfection or sterilization. Thoroughly clean to remove all blood, tissue, and other residue. Then follow local guidelines and local protocol for disinfection or sterilization.
- Dispose of all needles or sharp instruments in a rigid, puncture-proof container ("sharps container") immediately after you use them. Do not recap needles (Figure 2-11).
- Clean up blood and body fluids as soon as possible by routine cleaning with a hospital-grade disinfectant or a solution of household bleach and water.
- Walls, window coverings, and other non-horizontal surfaces in the ambulance do not need routine cleaning, but should be cleaned if visibly soiled.

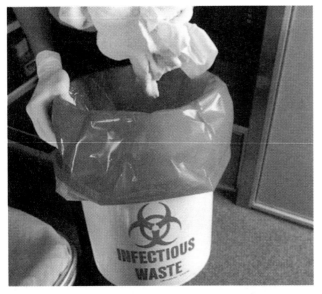

Figure 2-10 *Put linens in biohazard bag if infectious or contaminated with blood or other body fluids.*

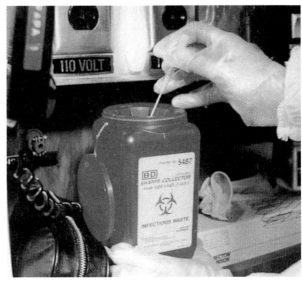

Figure 2-11 *Place all sharp instruments in a rigid, well mounted, puncture-resistant container.*

- Wash your hands thoroughly after cleaning the ambulance or disposing of equipment.

Cleaning, disinfecting, and sterilizing are all related terms. **Cleaning** is simply the process of washing a soiled object with soap and water. **Disinfecting** includes cleaning, but also involves using a disinfectant such as alcohol to kill many of the microorganisms that may be present on the surface of the object. **Sterilization** is the process by which an object is subject to a chemical or physical substance (typically, superheated steam in an autoclave) that kill all microorganisms on the surface of an object. Generally, disinfection is used for items that will come in contact with the intact skin of a patient, such as backboards, cervical collars, splints, and so on. However, if the object will come in contact with the body in any other way, it should be sterilized (laryngoscope blades, for example).

Advance Safety Precautions Before you begin active duty, have a physician make sure you are adequately protected against common diseases. Have a **purified protein derivative (PPD) test** for tuberculosis every year. In addition, the following immunizations are recommended for active-duty EMT-Bs:

- Tetanus prophylaxis (every ten years)
- Hepatitis B vaccine
- Influenza vaccine (annually)
- Polio immunization (if needed)
- Rubella (German measles) vaccine
- Measles vaccine (if needed)
- Mumps vaccine (if needed)

Because some immunizations have been found to offer only partial protection, have your physician verify your immune status against rubella, measles, and mumps. Remember, while immunizations offer protection against many diseases, BSI precautions must always be practiced, even by immunized EMTs.

Reporting Exposure State laws vary regarding the reporting of exposure to blood and other body fluids, especially if a patient is known to be HIV positive or have hepatitis B or is known to be in a high-risk category for infection. In general, promptly report any suspected exposure to your supervisor, including date and time of the exposure, type of body fluid involved, the amount of fluid, and details of the exposure. Follow local protocol.

PROTECTING YOURSELF FROM ACCIDENTAL INJURY

As an EMT-B you need to protect yourself during rescue operations involving hazardous materials, potentially life-threatening rescues, and violence. It is imperative that you not fall victim to the same hazards that affect your patients.

HAZARDOUS MATERIALS

Whenever you are called to a scene involving possible hazardous materials, use binoculars to try to identify the materials as hazardous before approaching. Look for signs or placards and compare them to those listed in Hazardous Materials: The Emergency Response Guidebook, published by the U.S. Department of Transportation (Figures 2-12 and 2-13). A copy of the handbook should be in every emergency vehicle.

In general, rescuers should wear protective clothing at a hazardous materials emergency, including self-contained breathing apparatus and "hazmat" suits (Figures 2-14 and 2-15). Whenever possible, a specialized hazardous materials team should be called to control the scene before you enter. EMT-Bs should provide basic emergency care only after the scene is safe and patient contamination is limited. See Chapter 42, "Hazardous Materials Emergencies," for detailed discussion.

RESCUE SITUATIONS

The following rescue situations involve potential threat to the life of both patients and rescuers:

- Downed power lines or other potential for electrocution
- Fire or threat of fire (including gasoline or chemical spills)
- Explosion or threat of explosion
- Hazardous materials
- Possible structural collapse
- Low oxygen levels in confined spaces
- Trenches that are not properly secured

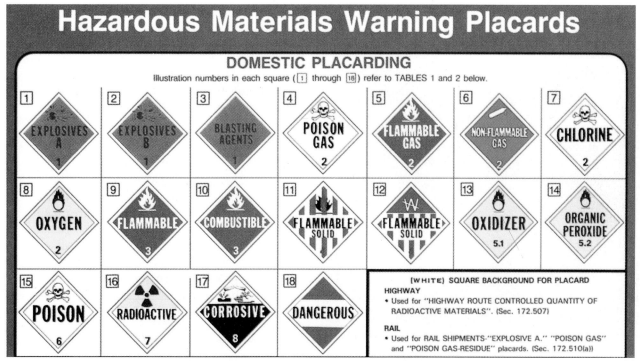

Figure 2-12 *Examples of hazardous materials warning placards.*

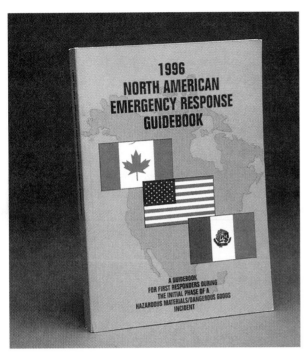

Figure 2-13 The Emergency Response Guidebook should be carried on all EMS vehicles. It helps to identify hazardous materials and provides guidelines for emergency care.

Generally, you should call for assistance from specialized teams from the power company or fire department, for example, before attempting rescue or patient treatment in a situation involving a life-threatening danger. If complex or extensive rescue is involved, also call for specialized rescue teams. Once a

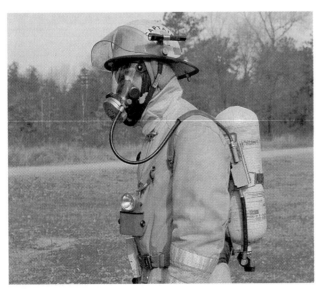

Figure 2-14 Self-contained breathing apparatus (SCBA).

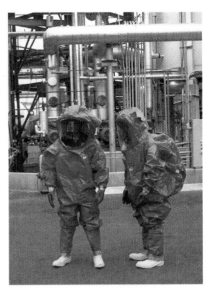

Figure 2-15 Typical hazardous materials protective suits.

scene is controlled, follow local protocol in wearing protective clothing, such as the kind of turnout gear firefighters wear, puncture-proof gloves, helmet, and protective eyewear (Figure 2-16).

Plenty of rescues take place outdoors in the dark and in bad weather. Therefore, an essential for every rescuer is reflective clothing or reflective tape on your clothing. Follow local protocol for other essential protective equipment for a rescuer. Depending on the situation, you might consider rubber or waterproof boots and slip-resistant waterproof gloves in wet weather. In cold weather, wear gloves, a warm hat, and long underwear, as well as several layers of clothing on your torso. In accidents involving grain, cement, or similar materials, wear a dust respirator. If there is any risk of falling debris, wear an impact-resistant protective helmet with reflective tape and a strap under the chin.

VIOLENCE AND CRIME

You may face violence without warning—from a patient, bystander, family member, or perpetrator of a crime during any patient rescue or treatment situation. Generally, if you suspect potential violence, you should call law enforcement before you enter the scene, especially if the perpetrator of a crime is or may still be present. Do not enter the scene to render patient care until it has been adequately controlled by law enforcement and until those with weapons (such as guns or knives) have been removed from the scene. Typical emergencies in which you should call law enforcement include domestic disputes, street or gang fights, bar fights, potential suicide, scenes with angry

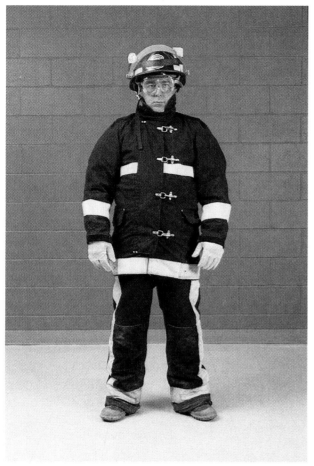

Figure 2-16 Full protective gear, including eye protection, helmet, turnout gear, and gloves.

family members or angry bystanders, and any type of crime scene.

Regardless of where you work, you may want to consider using body armor, sometimes called a "bullet-proof vest." Many metropolitan area EMS agencies issue body armor or provide some other means for personnel to be protected.

If you need to treat patients at a crime scene, take specific precautions to preserve the chain of evidence needed for investigation and prosecution. A general rule is to avoid disturbing the scene unless absolutely necessary for medical care. More specific details on crime scene behavior are listed in Chapter 3, "Medical, Legal, and Ethical Issues."

ENRICHMENT

The enrichment section contains information that is valuable as background for the EMT-B but that goes substantially beyond the U.S. Department of Transportation (DOT) EMT-Basic curriculum.

 ## DISEASES OF CONCERN

HEPATITIS B

Hepatitis B is one of the five viruses that directly affect the liver. A serious disease that can last for months, hepatitis B can be contracted through blood and body fluids. A major source of the virus is the chronic carrier, who usually has no signs or symptoms and is often unaware of being ill. These people can transmit the disease at any time.

Signs and symptoms of the hepatitis B virus include:

- Fatigue
- Nausea and loss of appetite
- Abdominal pain
- Headache
- Fever
- Yellowish color of the skin and whites of the eyes (jaundice)

Remember—hepatitis B infection may not cause symptoms. You can be unaware of infection and still pass it on to others. Protective procedure recommendations include the following:

- Wear disposable protective gloves whenever you care for patients to prevent contact with blood and other body fluids. Make sure you have bandaged all cuts, lesions, scratches, hangnails, and any other open wound on your hands.
- After removing gloves, wash your hands, wrists, and forearms thoroughly with hot soapy water and rinse well.
- Get vaccinated against hepatitis B before beginning EMS field work. These vaccines are offered by employers when employees have the potential to come in contact with blood and body fluids.
- Double-bag and seal all soiled refuse. Dispose of it according to local protocol.
- Clean, disinfect, or sterilize all nondisposable equipment. Launder your soiled clothing in hot soapy water and bleach.

If you suspect you have been exposed to hepatitis B, report the incident to your supervisor. Immediately contact a physician or your local public health agency for care. Care may include an injection of HBIG (hepatitis B immunoglobulin) immediately and again within a month. You may also receive a vaccination, if you have not already had one.

TUBERCULOSIS

Tuberculosis almost vanished once, but it has made a dramatic comeback. In fact, researchers are worried because new drug-resistant strains are developing. The pathogen that causes tuberculosis is found in the lungs and other tissues of the infected patient. You can be infected by droplets from the cough of a patient and from the patient's infected sputum.

The main signs and symptoms of tuberculosis include:

- Fever
- Cough
- Night sweats
- Weight loss

OSHA has adopted protective procedure standards for rescuers in areas of tuberculosis outbreaks. The standards include the use of special respirators. Recommendations include the following:

- Wear disposable protective gloves to avoid contact with infected sputum or mucus.
- Wear a HEPA (respirator) mask to avoid breathing infected droplets.
- Avoid mouth-to-mouth ventilation. Perform artificial ventilation with OSHA-approved equipment.
- After you remove your gloves, wash hands thoroughly with hot soapy water and rinse well.
- Scrub all nondisposable equipment that was contaminated by the patient's body fluids. See that all linens and clothing are laundered in hot soapy water and bleach.

ACQUIRED IMMUNE DEFICIENCY SYNDROME (AIDS)

Fortunately, AIDS is not spread through casual contact. It cannot be transmitted by coughing, sneezing, sharing eating utensils, linens, skin contact, or such indirect exposures. It is far more difficult to contract HIV (human immunodeficiency virus, the virus that causes AIDS) through occupational exposure than it is to contract the virus that causes hepatitis B. *HIV transmission requires intimate contact with the body fluids of infected persons.* The identified modes of transmission include the following:

- Sexual contact involving the exchange of semen, saliva, blood, urine, or feces

- Infected needles
- Infected blood or blood products
- Mother-child transmission, which occurs when an infected mother passes the virus to her child, sometimes as early as the twelfth week of gestation

Simply stated, AIDS is a syndrome of medical problems caused by HIV, a virus that destroys the body's ability to fight infections such as hepatitis B. Many patients infected with HIV do not exhibit signs or symptoms and do not know they are infected. AIDS victims become infected with what are called opportunistic infections (infections that take advantage of the "opportunity" provided by the body's lack of ability to fight them). These infections are caused by viruses, bacteria, parasites, and fungi. They are serious illnesses that either do not occur or occur only in milder forms among people with healthy immune systems.

AIDS can involve many organs and systems of the body. This results in a countless array of signs and symptoms. The most common include:

- Persistent, low-grade fever
- Night sweats
- Swollen lymph glands
- Loss of appetite
- Nausea
- Persistent diarrhea
- Headache
- Sore throat
- Fatigue
- Weight loss
- Shortness of breath
- Muscle and joint aches
- Rash
- Various opportunistic infections

Remember—not everyone who is infected by HIV has yet developed, or even will develop, AIDS. However, people who carry HIV are still capable of spreading the infection to others, even if they have no signs or symptoms. Follow BSI precautions at all times. They can significantly reduce your risk of becoming infected with HIV.

CASE STUDY FOLLOW-UP

SCENE SIZE-UP

You have been dispatched to the scene of a domestic dispute. You learn from the police that the husband is an unemployed alcoholic who is going through a "detox" program. He is holding his wife and two daughters hostage and threatens to harm them if the police don't back off. An officer is already down, and a special tactics team is working to bring the situation under control.

Two hours later you still are not permitted to approach the house. The husband has released the two children and they are transported by another

EMS unit to the hospital for evaluation. You can hear the husband and wife arguing again, when suddenly there is a single gunshot and silence. The husband appears at the front door, shooting randomly. The special tactics team returns fire. The man falls to the ground.

After the police secure the scene, you and your partner approach with full body substance isolation precautions.

PATIENT ASSESSMENT

Initial assessment shows that the downed police officer is dead, having received multiple gunshot wounds to the head and neck. The gunman is also dead, with multiple gunshot wounds to the head and chest. The wife inside the house is dead, having been beaten and shot once through the head. You and your partner slowly walk back to the ambulance and notify dispatch that there will be no additional transports.

There is nothing more you can do. The incident commander releases you and your partner from the scene.

CRITICAL INCIDENT FOLLOW-UP

During the drive back to the station, you notice that your partner is very quiet and tense. When he speaks, it is in anger. At the station, you try to get him to discuss the call. He responds angrily and tells you he is going to quit EMS. You both summon your supervisor, who initiates the procedure for a critical incident stress debriefing (CISD) session.

Less than 48 hours later, the police, special tactics team, and EMS personnel involved with the call are brought together. The CISD team leads the discussion. Sometime during the meeting, you and your partner express your feelings about the incident. Afterward additional counseling is set up for your partner, who returns to regular duty quickly.

CHAPTER REVIEW

TERMS AND CONCEPTS

You may wish to review the following terms and concepts included in this chapter.

body substance isolation (BSI)—a method of preventing infection by disease organisms based on the premise that all blood and body fluids are infectious.
burnout—a condition resulting from chronic job stress, characterized by a state of irritability and fatigue that can markedly decrease effectiveness.
cleaning—the process of washing a soiled object with soap and water.
critical incident—any situation that causes unusually strong emotions that interfere with the ability to function.
critical incident stress debriefing (CISD)—a session usually held within 24 to 72 hours of a critical incident, where a team of peer counselors and mental health professionals help rescuers work through the emotions that normally follow a critical incident.
defusing—a session held prior to a critical incident stress debriefing (CISD) for rescuers most directly involved to provide an opportunity to vent emotions and get information before the CISD.
disinfecting—in addition to cleaning, this process involves using a disinfectant such as alcohol or bleach to kill many of the microorganisms that may be present on the surface of an object.
pathogens—microorganisms such as bacteria and viruses that cause disease. Bloodborne pathogens can spread disease by way of the blood. Airborne pathogens can spread disease by way of spraying droplets through the air.
personal protective equipment—equipment an emergency rescuer uses or wears to protect against injury and spreading infectious disease.
purified protein derivative (PPD) test—a test for tuberculosis.
sterilization—the process by which an object is subject to certain chemical or physical substances (typically, superheated steam in an autoclave) that kill all microorganisms on the surface of an object.

REVIEW QUESTIONS

1. List the five stages through which a dying patient may pass.
2. Describe several things you can do—other than provide emergency medical care—to help dying patients.
3. List five of the signs and symptoms of chronic stress and burnout.
4. List four ways you can help deal with the stress in your life.

5. Identify some of the negative feelings families of EMT-Bs may have in response to the job. Describe some of the ways you can help.
6. Describe the safety precautions an EMT-B can take to prevent the spread of infectious disease.
7. List the personal protective equipment necessary for hazardous materials situations, rescue operations, and scenes of violence or crime.

CHAPTER 3

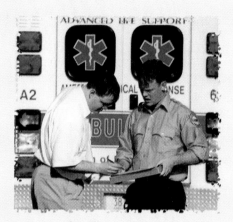

Medical, Legal, and Ethical Issues

INTRODUCTION

Medical, legal, and ethical issues are a vital element of the EMT-Basic's life, both on and off duty. You may already have some questions, such as: Should you stop to treat an accident victim when you are off duty? Should patient information be released to an attorney over the phone? May a child be treated without parents being present? You may begin to wonder if you can provide emergency care at all without being sued! The answers to questions like these require that you consider your scope of practice, advance directives, the issues surrounding patient consent, your duty to act, and other factors.

Objectives

Numbered objectives are from the United States Department of Transportation 1994 EMT-Basic National Standard Curriculum. Asterisked objectives, if any, pertain to material that is supplemental to the DOT curriculum.

Cognitive

1-3.1 Define the EMT-Basic scope of practice. (pp. 31–32)

1-3.2 Discuss the importance of Do Not Resuscitate (DNR) (advance directives) and local or state provisions regarding EMS application. (p. 32)

1-3.3 Define consent and discuss the methods of obtaining consent. (pp. 32–34)

1-3.4 Differentiate between expressed and implied consent. (pp. 33–34)

1-3.5 Explain the role of consent of minors in providing care. (p. 34)

1-3.6 Discuss the implications for the EMT-Basic in patient refusal of transport. (p. 34)

1-3.7 Discuss the issues of abandonment, negligence, and battery and their implications to the EMT-Basic. (pp. 32, 35)

1-3.8 State the conditions necessary for the EMT-Basic to have a duty to act. (pp. 31, 35)

1-3.9 Explain the importance, necessity, and legality of patient confidentiality. (pp. 35–36)

1-3.10 Discuss the considerations of the EMT-Basic in issues of organ retrieval. (p. 36)

1-3.11 Differentiate the actions that an EMT-Basic should take to assist in the preservation of a crime scene. (p. 37)

1-3.12 State the conditions that require an EMT-Basic to notify local law enforcement officials. (p. 37)

Affective

1-3.13 Explain the role of EMS and the EMT-Basic regarding patients with DNR orders. (p. 32)

1-3.14 Explain the rationale for the needs, benefits, and usage of advance directives. (p. 32)

1-3.15 Explain the rationale for the concept of varying degrees of DNR. (p. 32)

Case Study

The Dispatch

EMS Unit 105—proceed to 733 East Third Street—you have an elderly male at that location with abdominal pain—time out 1430 hours.

On Arrival

An elderly woman, who tells you she is Mrs. Schuman, meets you and your partner on the front porch of the home. She is wearing only a nightgown, and the temperature is only 13° F. She says, "It's my husband. Something is wrong. I just can't handle him anymore."

You quickly usher Mrs. Schuman inside while you scan the scene for hazards. As soon as you enter you notice that the house is in shambles. The rooms are so cluttered that you and your partner can barely pass through. Mrs. Schuman leads you to the bedroom, where you find the patient lying on the bed. Mr. Schuman's eyes are open, and he's moaning softly. His bed sheets and undergarments are stained with dried urine. The odor is very strong, and the temperature inside the room is very cold.

How would you proceed with this case?

During this chapter, you will learn about special legal and ethical considerations that have an impact on the medical care you administer to your patients. Later, we will return to the case and put in context some of the information you learned.

THE SCOPE OF PRACTICE

Prehospital emergency care has changed significantly since its early days. One improvement has been in the quality of training emergency medical personnel receive today. The public and the health care profession have come to expect a competent EMT-Basic who understands and accepts the legal and ethical responsibilities to the patient, to the medical director, and to the public.

 LEGAL DUTIES

In general, state law identifies the EMT-B's **scope of practice,** or the actions and care that are legally allowed. For example, providing oxygen under the appropriate circumstances is within the EMT-B's scope of practice. However, suturing a laceration is not and is therefore illegal—even if the EMT-B may actually know how to perform the skill.

Among the sources used to define the EMT-B's scope of practice is the U.S. Department of Transportation's "Emergency Medical Technician-Basic: National Standard Curriculum," which reflects minimum standards applied throughout the United States. Another source is your EMS system's medical director, who—within your state's scope of practice—establishes the day-to-day guidelines under which you will function through local protocols, standing orders, and telephone/radio communications.

DUTY TO ACT

The concept known as **duty to act** refers to your obligation to provide care. Legally, while you are on duty you are obligated to care for a patient who requires and consents to it, rendering the necessary emergency care to the best of your ability and training. If you are off duty, however, in most states you have no more legal obligation to act than any other citizen. Legally while off duty you could:

• Stop and help the accident victim at the scene
• Pass the scene and telephone for help at your earliest convenience
• Pass the scene and make no attempt to call for help

Note that some states do require EMTs to stop and render aid even when off duty. If you do stop and help, you assume certain legal responsibilities. For example, once you have begun to provide care, you cannot leave until someone with equal or more expertise takes over care. You are also legally responsible for any of the patient's personal property that you pick up.

GOOD SAMARITAN LAWS

Many states have "Good Samaritan" laws. The first of these laws was enacted in 1959 in California specifically to protect from liability "persons licensed (such as a physician or surgeon) who in good faith render emergency care at the scene of the emergency . . . for civil damages as a result of any acts or omissions." Most states have followed with laws of their own, some of which specifically cover prehospital emergency care providers.

Generally, a Good Samaritan law protects a person from liability for acts performed in good faith unless those acts constitute gross negligence. Therefore, the person suing must prove that the care provided was markedly below the **standard of care,** or that which would be expected to have been provided to the same patient under the same circumstances by another EMT who had received the same training. (This is called the "reasonable person" test.)

Most states have specific laws authorizing EMT-Bs to perform prehospital emergency medical procedures without a medical license. Most states also provide some form of immunity to nurses, physicians, supervisors, and other personnel who give directions to EMT-Bs by phone or radio. The laws governing private and public providers vary. Be sure to learn your local laws.

As you see, a Good Samaritan law does not prevent you from being sued, although it may provide you some protection against losing the lawsuit if you have performed according to the standard of care for an EMT-B. So while on duty or assisting off duty, your best defense to lawsuits is prevention. Always render care to the best of your ability, always working within your scope of practice. If you keep your patient's best interests in mind when rendering care, you will seldom, if ever, go wrong.

MEDICAL DIRECTION

Your legal right to function as an EMT-B is contingent upon medical direction. When providing emergency care you should:

• Follow standing orders and protocols, as approved by medical direction
• Establish telephone and radio communications with medical direction when appropriate
• Communicate clearly and completely with medical direction, and follow orders medical direction gives in response
• Any time there is a question about the scope or direction of care, consult medical direction

Most areas also have protocols for cooperation between EMS personnel and other public safety services.

ETHICAL RESPONSIBILITIES

A code of ethics is a list of rules of ideal conduct. The "Code of Ethics for EMTs" was issued by the National Association of Emergency Medical Technicians in 1978. Basically, if you place the welfare of the patient above all else when providing medical care, you will rarely commit an unethical act.

Your ethical responsibilities include these:

- Serve the needs of the patient with respect for human dignity, without regard to nationality, race, gender, creed, or status.
- Maintain skill mastery. Demonstrate respect for the competence of other medical professionals.
- Keep abreast of changes in EMS that affect patient care. Assume responsibility in defining and upholding professional standards.
- Critically review performances, seeking ways to improve response time, patient outcome, and communication. Assume responsibility for individual professional actions and judgment.
- Report with honesty. Hold in confidence all information obtained in the course of professional work unless required by law to divulge such information.
- Work harmoniously with other EMTs, nurses, physicians, and other members of the health care team.

ISSUES OF PATIENT CONSENT AND REFUSAL

 ### ADVANCE DIRECTIVES

You may be called to treat terminally ill patients. In some cases the patient may request—and a physician may order—that no resuscitation measures take place if the heart and lungs stop functioning. Legally, the patient has a right to refuse resuscitative efforts. An **advance directive** (instructions written in advance) against resuscitation, signed by the patient, is legally recognized in many states. This documents the wish of the chronically or terminally ill patient not to be resuscitated and legally allows the health care provider to withhold resuscitation.

Three types of advance directives are a Do Not Resuscitate (DNR) order, a living will, and a health care proxy. A DNR is a legal document or order that most often governs resuscitation issues only, whereas a living will is more often used to cover more general health care issues, including the use of long-term life support equipment such as ventilators and feeding tubes. A health care proxy is a person who is legally designated to make health care decisions for the signer of the document if he is unable to do so for himself. Decisions by health care proxies usually pertain only to in-hospital or long-term care facility situations.

When you are presented with a DNR, you must determine to the best of your ability that it is valid. Check to see that the physician's instructions are clear, concise, and unambiguous and typed or written in a clear hand on professional letterhead. Phrases like "no heroics" or "no extraordinary treatment" are not clear enough to meet legal requirements. In many jurisdictions, a standard legal form is used for Do Not Resuscitate (DNR) orders.

Different degrees of DNR (different kinds of resuscitation treatments refused) may exist based on various levels of chronic illness or terminal status. Some patients may request that only selected emergency care or comfort procedures be performed (Figure 3-1). Typically, oxygen administration is considered a standard comfort measure and should be provided for both the do-not-resuscitate and the modified-support patient. Be sure to learn your local protocol.

Advance directives may be filled with problems for prehospital providers. First, by its very nature, a living will is generally more useful in an institutional setting, such as a nursing home or hospital, where health care providers are aware of it and know the doctor who signed it. In addition, many advance directives require more than one physician to verify the patient's condition—a requirement that may be difficult to fulfill in the field, even if the advance directive is located. Finally, the time taken to scrutinize an advance directive can take precious moments away from providing resuscitative care.

Even if there is a signed and witnessed living will and a physician's written DNR order, most legal experts agree that you should consult medical direction before following or disregarding the order. (In some states, laws require that patients wear some sort of DNR insignia on their bodies, where EMS personnel will be sure to find it.) In the absence of the DNR and a physician's written instructions, or when in doubt, you are obligated to begin full resuscitation immediately.

TYPES OF CONSENT

Under the law, the patient has the right to accept or refuse emergency medical care. Therefore, it is necessary to obtain consent, or permission, before providing such care. Before emergency care is rendered, the patient must be informed of the care to be provided and the associated risks and consequences. Consent so obtained is termed *informed consent*. If you were to touch a patient's body or clothing without first obtaining the proper consent, you can be charged with assault and battery (placing a person in fear of immediate bodily harm and touching unlawfully). Assault and battery also applies to anyone who provides emergency care when the patient does not consent to the specific treatment.

PREHOSPITAL DO NOT RESUSCITATE ORDERS

<u>ATTENDING PHYSICIAN</u>

In completing this prehospital DNR form, please check part A if no intervention by prehospital personnel is indicated. Please check Part A and options from Part B if specific interventions by prehospital personnel are indicated. To give a valid prehospital DNR order, this form must be completed by the patient's attending physician and must be provided to prehospital personnel.

A) _____ **Do Not Resuscitate (DNR):**
    No Cardiopulmonary Resuscitation or Advanced Cardiac Life Support be performed by prehospital personnel

B) _____ **Modified Support:**
    Prehospital personnel administer the following checked options:
    _____Oxygen administration
    _____Full airway support: intubation, airways, bag/valve/mask
    _____Venipuncture: IV crystalloids and/or blood draw
    _____External cardiac pacing
    _____Cardiopulmonary resuscitation
    _____Cardiac defibrillator
    _____Pneumatic anti-shock garment
    _____Ventilator
    _____ACLS meds
    _____Other interventions/medications (physician specify)
    _____

Prehospital personnel are informed that (print patient name)_____
should receive no resuscitation (DNR) or should receive Modified Support as indicated. This directive is medically appropriate and is further documented by a physician's order and a progress note on the patient's permanent medical record. Informed consent from the capacitated patient or the incapacitated patient's legitimate surrogate is documented on the patient's permanent medical record. The DNR order is in full force and effect as of the date indicated below.

_____   _____

Attending Physician's Signature

_____   _____

Print Attending Physician's Name   Print Patient's Name and Location
                                                (Home Address or Health Care Facility)

_____

Attending Physician's Telephone

_____   _____

Date   Expiration Date (6 Mos from Signature)

Figure 3-1   Example of an EMS "Do Not Resuscitate" form.

There are three types of consent: **expressed consent, implied consent,** and **minor consent** (consent for a minor or mentally incompetent adult).

• *Expressed consent* must be obtained from every conscious, mentally competent adult before treatment is started. The patient must be of legal age, able to make a rational decision, and informed of the procedure you will be performing and all related risks. Basically, the patient must receive in terms that the patient understands all of the information that would affect a reasonable person's de-cision to accept or refuse treatment. Oral consent, a nod, or an affirming gesture constitutes valid expressed consent.

• *Implied consent* occurs when you assume that a patient who is unresponsive or unable to make a rational decision (e.g., a patient who is disoriented because of a head injury) would consent to life-saving emergency care. Implied consent also applies to the patient who initially refuses your care, but then becomes unresponsive or irrational because of illness or injury. In a true emergency where the patient is at significant risk of death, disability, or deterioration of condition, the law assumes that the unresponsive patient would give consent.

- ***Consent to treat a minor or a mentally incompetent adult*** must be obtained from a parent or legal guardian. Depending on state law, a minor usually is any person under age 18 or 21. However, you do not need consent of a parent or guardian to treat an emancipated minor—usually one who is married, pregnant, a parent, a member of the armed forces, or financially independent and living away from home. Note that if a life-threatening condition exists and the parent or legal guardian is unavailable for consent, you should render treatment under the principle of implied consent.

REFUSING TREATMENT

COMPETENCY

A competent adult is one who is lucid and capable of making an informed decision. People who display an altered mental status or who are mentally ill or under the influence of drugs or alcohol may be considered not competent. A competent adult has the right to refuse treatment—verbally, or by pulling away, shaking his head, gesturing you away, or pushing you away— or to withdraw from treatment after it has started.

Under the law, to refuse treatment or transport a patient must be informed of and fully understand the treatment and all risks and consequences of refusal. Once this has been accomplished, you must require that the patient sign an official "release from liability" form (Figure 3-2). The signed form—or a patient's witnessed refusal to the sign the form—must be part of the documentation of the case.

When in doubt, always err in favor of providing care to the patient.

PROTECTING YOURSELF

Complete and accurate documentation is a key factor in protecting yourself from liability for negligence or abandonment when a patient refuses treatment. Do the following before you leave the scene:

- ***Try again to persuade the patient to accept treatment or transport to a hospital.*** Tell the patient why treatment or transport is essential. Be especially clear in explaining the possible consequences of refusal. Document your attempts to convince the patient as well as the consequences of refusal, and have the patient read aloud from the report to verify understanding.
- ***Make sure that the patient is able to make a rational, informed decision.*** A patient who is emotionally, intellectually, or physically impaired by illness or injury may not be capable of absorbing all the information you give. Make sure that the patient is competent, not suicidal, and not under the influence of drugs, alcohol, or other mind-altering substances.
- ***Consult medical direction as required by local protocol.***
- ***If the patient still refuses, have him sign a refusal form.*** In some areas the form must be signed by witnesses (follow local protocol). If the patient refuses to sign the form, get signed statements of witnesses that the patient refused to sign.
- ***Before you leave the scene, encourage the patient to seek help if certain symptoms develop.*** If possible, be specific. Say things like "if you have a burning pain in your stomach" or "if you start seeing double." Avoid technical terms the patient might not understand. Document the fact that you encouraged the patient to seek help later.

> REFUSAL OF TREATMENT AND TRANSPORTATION
>
> I, THE UNDERSIGNED HAVE BEEN ADVISED THAT MEDICAL ASSISTANCE ON MY BEHALF IS NECESSARY AND THAT REFUSAL OF SAID ASSISTANCE AND TRANSPORTATION MAY RESULT IN DEATH, OR IMPERIL MY HEALTH. NEVERTHELESS, I REFUSE TO ACCEPT TREATMENT OR TRANSPORT AND ASSUME ALL RISKS AND CONSEQUENCES OF MY DECISION AND RELEASE GOLD CROSS AMBULANCE COMPANY AND ITS EMPLOYEES FROM ANY LIABILITY ARISING FROM MY REFUSAL.
>
> _____
> SIGNATURE OF PATIENT
>
> _____
> WITNESSED BY
>
> _____
> DATE SIGNED

Figure 3-2 Example of a patient refusal statement.

OTHER LEGAL ASPECTS OF EMERGENCY CARE

MORE ABOUT THE DUTY TO ACT

As noted earlier in this chapter, you are legally obligated to care for any patient who requires and requests your services while you are on duty. As an EMT-B, you are bound by either implied or formal obligation by virtue of the service that employs you.

In some cases the contractual or legal obligation may be implied. For example, a patient may call for an ambulance, and a dispatcher may confirm that an ambulance will be sent. As part of the ambulance team that responds, you then have a legal obligation to provide treatment to the patient.

In other cases, the obligation is formal. For example, an ambulance service may have a written contract with a municipality designating when ambulance service must be provided or may be refused.

In most states, while you are off duty or when you are driving the ambulance outside your company's service area, you may not have a legal duty to act. However, you may feel a certain moral or ethical obligation to provide emergency care to a patient. If you do, take extra precautions against legal risk. Carefully document all aspects of patient treatment, including a patient's possible refusal to accept treatment.

ABANDONMENT AND NEGLIGENCE

There are two different situations in which an EMT-B may be held legally liable for decisions made in the course of treatment: abandonment and negligence.

Abandonment means that you stopped providing care without ensuring that equivalent or better care would be provided. Under abandonment laws, once you start giving emergency care to a patient, you must continue until another health care professional with at least as much expertise as you takes over care.

You may be considered negligent by law if the care you provide deviates from the accepted standard of care and results in further injury to the patient. **Negligence** is defined as carelessness, inattention, disregard, inadvertence, or oversight that was accidental but avoidable. To establish negligence, the court must decide that all of the following are true:

- The EMT-B had a duty to act.
- The patient was injured, either physically or psychologically.
- The EMT-B violated the standard of care reasonably expected of an EMT-B with similar background and training.
- The EMT-B's action or lack of action in violating the standard of care caused or contributed to the patient's injury.

In determining negligence, the jury has to answer six critical questions:

- Did the EMT-B act or fail to act?
- Did the patient sustain physical, psychological, or financial injury?
- Did the action or inaction of the EMT-B cause or contribute to that injury by violating the standard of care reasonably expected of an EMT-B?
- Did the patient contribute to the injury?
- Did the EMT violate the duty to care for the patient?
- If the patient proves negligence, what damages should be awarded?

Your best defense against negligence is to display professional competence and a professional attitude, to provide a consistently high standard of care, and to correctly and completely document the care you provide.

 ## CONFIDENTIALITY

While many jurisdictions do not have specific laws about confidentiality, laws do exist that prevent the invasion of a person's privacy. Some of them apply to cases involving emergency care, specifically to information obtained while getting a patient history, performing a physical assessment, and treating the patient. In many states, the deliberate invasion of a patient's privacy by an EMT-B may lead to loss of certification or licensure and other legal actions.

Do not speak to the press, your family, friends, or other members of the public about details of the emergency care you provided to a patient. If you speak about the emergency, you must not relate specifics about what a patient said, who the patient was with, anything unusual about the patient's behavior or personal appearance. The same restrictions hold true of information you receive from another member of the EMS system. Confidentiality applies not only to cases of physical injury, but also to cases involving possible infectious diseases, illnesses, and emotional and psychological emergencies.

Releasing confidential information requires a written release form signed by the patient or a legal guardian. You should not release confidential written or spoken information about the patient to someone claiming to be a legal guardian until you have established legal guardianship. By law, you are allowed to release confidential patient information without a patient's or guardian's permission if:

- Another health care provider needs to know the information in order to continue medical care.
- You are requested by the police to provide the information as part of a potential criminal investigation. State laws, for example, require the reporting of incidents of rape, abuse, or certain other crimes.

- A third-party billing form requires the information.
- You are required by legal subpoena to provide the information in court.

 ## SPECIAL SITUATIONS

DONORS AND ORGAN HARVESTING

Organs can be donated only if there is a legal signed document giving permission to harvest the organs. A signed donor card is considered a legal document. The sticker affixed to the reverse side of a patient's driving license provides an intent to donate organs.

A potential organ donor should be treated no differently than any other patient requiring emergency care. The individual is a patient first, an organ donor last. In addition to providing appropriate care, you can assist the organ harvesting procedure as follows:

- Identify the patient as a potential donor based on the type of injuries or illness and treatment that was rendered. Patients who are about to die or who have died within hours are potential organ donors. In each case, however, hospital staff and the patient's family make the ultimate decision.
- Communicate with medical direction regarding the possibility of organ donation. You can initiate this process by alerting the receiving hospital's emergency department staff, who will in turn contact other necessary departments.
- Provide emergency care, such as CPR, that will help maintain vital organs in case harvesting is attempted. This is best accomplished by treating every patient equally well.

MEDICAL IDENTIFICATION INSIGNIA

A patient with a medical condition, such as an allergy, diabetes, or epilepsy, may be wearing or carrying a medical identification tag, such as a bracelet, necklace, or card (Figure 3-3). Look for them during assessment. Note that medical identification insignia may also list a phone number you can call for specific treatment and medication requirements.

RECOGNIZING DEATH IN THE FIELD

It is the ultimate responsibility of a physician to determine the cause of death. However, in some situations you may have to make a judgment as to whether to attempt resuscitation or not. As a general rule, if the patient is still warm and does not exhibit any obvious signs of death, begin resuscitation. An exception is hypothermia (low body temperature) where the patient's body is extremely cold and rigid. Hypothermic patients have survived long periods of cardiac arrest and cannot be considered dead until rewarmed

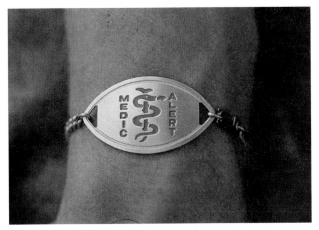

Figure 3-3   A medical identification tag.

When dealing with patients holding a do not resuscitate (DNR) order or those with terminal illness, it is necessary to determine the presumptive signs of death. These include:

- Absence of a pulse, breathing, and breath sounds
- Complete unresponsiveness to any stimuli
- No eye movement or pupil response
- Absence of a blood pressure
- No reflexes
- Dependent lividity (discoloration of the skin due to blood pooling effected by gravity)

There are some situations in which signs of death are obvious and resuscitative efforts are not necessary. The obvious signs of death include:

- Decapitation
- Rigor mortis (body becomes stiff within 2 to 12 hours)
- Decomposition of the body
- Dependent lividity

Cases involving violent, unusual, or suspicious causes of death usually require investigation by the medical examiner or coroner. The medical examiner or coroner is usually called for.

- Homicides
- Suicides
- Violent deaths
- Crash-related deaths (auto, motorcycle, all-terrain vehicle, snowmobile)
- Unusual scene characteristics (e.g., burns, electrocution)
- Sudden Infant Death Syndrome (SIDS)
- Dead on arrival (depending on your local protocol)

It is important to understand your local protocol related to death-in-the-field situations. It is better to err to benefit the patient and begin resuscitation if you have any doubt. Also, be sure you understand the situations in which the medical examiner or coroner must be called to investigate a field death.

CRIME SCENES

Whenever an EMS is called to a potential crime scene, dispatch should also notify the police. Recognizing a possible crime scene requires a high index of suspicion. As a general guideline, a potential crime scene is any scene that may require police support, including a potential or actual suicide, homicide, drug overdose, domestic dispute, rape, abuse, hit-and-run accident, riot, robbery, gunfire, or potentially dangerous weapons.

Your first concern upon approaching a crime scene should be for your own safety. *If you suspect that a crime is in progress or a criminal is still active at the scene, do not attempt to provide care to any patient.* Wait until the police declare that the scene is safe.

Once the scene is secure, your priority is emergency care of the patient. However, also try to avoid disturbing anything that may be considered evidence:

- Touch only what you need to touch.
- Move only what you need to move to protect the patient and to provide proper emergency care.
- Do not use the telephone unless the police give you permission to do so.
- In the absence of police permission, move the patient only if the patient is in danger or must be moved in order for you to provide care.
- Observe and document anything unusual.
- If possible, do not cut through holes in clothing possibly caused by bullets or stabbing.
- Do not cut through any knot in a rope or tie (a possible clue). Cut away from the knot. Do not cover the patient with a sheet.
- If the crime is rape, do not wash the patient or allow the patient to wash. Ask the patient not to change clothing, use the bathroom, or take anything by mouth, because doing so may destroy evidence. While you cannot force a person to avoid

these activities, explain your reasons. Most will cooperate.

As an EMT-B, you may have a legal duty to report situations in which injury may have resulted from commission of a crime. Learn your local protocols.

SPECIAL REPORTING SITUATIONS

You may be required to report certain conditions. Familiarize yourself with the requirements in your state. Commonly required reporting situations include:

- *Abuse.* Many states require people to report suspected child abuse. Some states have very broad requirements, while others require reporting only from physicians. Such statutes frequently grant immunity from liability for libel, slander, or defamation of character as long as the report is made in good faith. In some states, laws also exist regarding the reporting of other kinds of abuse, such as abuse of the elderly and spouse abuse.
- *Crime.* Many states require EMT-Bs to report an injury that may have resulted from a crime or to report injuries such as gunshot wounds, knife wounds, and poisonings. Your state may also require you to report any injury that you suspect was caused by sexual assault.
- *Drug-related injuries.* Some states require you to report drug-related injuries. However, the U.S. Supreme Court has ruled that drug addiction—not drug possession—is an illness, not a crime.

Other situations you may be required to report include suspected infectious disease exposure, use of patient restraints to treat or transport patients against their will, cases in which a patient appears to be mentally incompetent or intoxicated, attempted suicides, and dog bites. Learn the laws in your state regarding situations you are required to report.

CASE STUDY FOLLOW-UP

SCENE SIZE-UP

You and your partner are dispatched to the scene of an elderly male complaining of abdominal pain. As you scan for hazards, you notice that there is clutter everywhere in the house and that the inside temperature is not much warmer than the outside. Although the patient's wife is alert, she seems confused. She changes the subject often and keeps asking your partner if she is her daughter Ellen.

PATIENT ASSESSMENT

Your general impression of Mr. Schuman is that he is conscious but disoriented and experiencing abdominal pain. His wife is unsure of his age, so you estimate that he is in his mid 80s. He responds to questions with unintelligible mumbled words. His airway is open, breathing and circulation appear normal. He does not appear to be in acute distress.

Trying to obtain a complete history is impossible, since the patient cannot respond coherently. Instead you perform a rapid assessment, a quick head-to-toe physical exam. Upon palpation of the abdomen, Mr. Schuman tries to force your hand away. If he were competent, you might take this gesture as a refusal of care. However, because of his disorientation, you continue providing care. You measure and record baseline vital signs—breathing rate; pulse; pupils; skin color, temperature, and condition; and blood pressure. Meanwhile, your partner applies an oxygen mask to provide Mr. Schuman high-flow oxygen, which may help his mental condition as well as his apparent abdominal condition.

When you try to obtain a medical history from Mrs. Schuman, she does not understand. All she wants to do is show you her porcelain doll collection.

You prepare Mr. Schuman for transport and help his wife find a coat. During transport, you reassess the patient and find no change in his condition.

An Ethical Obligation

After transferring Mr. Schuman to hospital personnel, you contact the hospital's social service department, as you are required to do in case of elderly abuse or neglect. While you saw no signs of intentional abuse or neglect, you do believe that the Schumans are not capable of caring for themselves, and you understand that you are therefore ethically responsible to report the situation in order to assure their safety after discharge.

Two weeks later you see the social worker who tells you that Mr. Schuman was diagnosed with a gastric ulcer and organic brain syndrome. Additionally, Mrs. Schuman has been diagnosed with Alzheimer's disease. Both are now residents of a local extended-care nursing home, under 24-hour supervision. The social worker thanks you and your partner for bringing this case to his attention.

CHAPTER REVIEW

TERMS AND CONCEPTS

You may wish to review the following terms and concepts included in this chapter.

abandonment—the act of discontinuing emergency care without ensuring that another health care professional with equivalent or better training will take over.

advance directive—instructions, written in advance, such as a living will or Do Not Resuscitate (DNR) order.

duty to act—the obligation to care for a patient who requires it.

expressed consent—permission which must be obtained from every conscious, mentally competent adult before emergency treatment may be provided.

implied consent—the assumption that, in a true emergency where a patient who is unresponsive or unable to make a rational decision is at significant risk of death, disability, or deterioration of condition, that patient would agree to emergency treatment.

minor consent—permission obtained from a parent or legal guardian for emergency treatment of a minor or a mentally incompetent adult.

negligence—the act of deviating from an accepted standard of care through carelessness, inattention, disregard, inadvertence, or oversight, which results in further injury to the patient.

scope of practice—the actions and care that are legally allowed to be provided by an EMT-Basic.

standard of care—emergency care that would be expected to be given to a patient by any trained EMT-B under similar circumstances.

REVIEW QUESTIONS

1. Define a "Do Not Resuscitate (DNR)" order, and explain how an EMT-B should respond if presented with such an order.
2. Define the three types of consent that must be obtained before emergency care is provided.
3. Explain how to handle a refusal of treatment.
4. Describe what must happen for the EMT-B to be liable for abandonment or negligence.
5. Describe what it means for an EMT-B to have a duty to act.
6. List the conditions under which an EMT-B may release confidential patient information.
7. List some ways in which an EMT-B can preserve evidence at a crime scene.
8. List situations that an EMT-B may be required to report.

CHAPTER 4

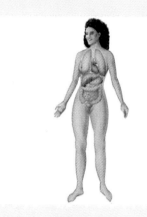

The Human Body

INTRODUCTION

Your ability to develop a foundation of knowledge of the human body and its systems is essential to high quality patient assessment and emergency care. That understanding will help you recognize when the body is working as it should and when there are life-threatening deviations to normal function. Your ability to use proper terminology to describe the human body will also allow you to communicate necessary patient information to other health care professionals concisely and accurately.

OBJECTIVES

COGNITIVE

1-4.1   Identify the following topographic terms: medial, lateral, proximal, distal, superior, inferior, anterior, posterior, midline, right and left, midclavicular, bilateral, and midaxillary. (pp. 41–42)

1-4.2   Describe the anatomy and function of the following major body systems: respiratory (pp. 51–54), circulatory (pp. 55–59), musculoskeletal (pp. 42, 44–51), nervous (pp. 59–61, 62), and endocrine (p. 61).

- Identify and define other common descriptive anatomical terms. (pp. 40–42, 43)
- Describe the anatomy and function of the skin. (pp. 61–62, 63)

CASE STUDY

THE DISPATCH

EMS Unit 108—respond to Centennial Park on Highland Avenue—you have a female patient at that location who suffered a burn. Time out 1306 hours.

ON ARRIVAL

After positioning the ambulance out of the flow of traffic, you scan the scene for hazards and exit. A woman runs up to you and says, "A woman over here was trying to refuel her son's model airplane when the gas tank blew up or something." You approach the patient and find that she is sitting on a patch of grass about 15 feet away from a smoldering model plane.

How would you proceed to assess and care for this patient?

During this chapter, you will read a brief overview of the human body. Later, we will return to the case study and put in context some of the information you learned.

ANATOMICAL TERMS

Basic knowledge of the human body includes the study of anatomy and physiology. The word **anatomy** refers to the structure of the body and the relationship of its parts to each other (how the body is made). The word **physiology** refers to the function of the living body and its parts (how the body works).

As you proceed through your course, you will encounter descriptive terms you may not have heard or used before. Study and learn them. It is essential that you use them correctly to describe position, direction, and location of a patient and his illness or injury. Using correct terms minimizes confusion and helps to communicate the exact extent of a patient's problem based on a careful physical assessment.

One important term that is essential for you to understand and use is the **normal anatomical position.** Unless otherwise indicated, all references to the human body assume the normal anatomical position: The patient is standing erect, facing forward, with arms down at the sides and palms forward. This basic position is used as the point of reference whenever terms of direction and location are used. Other terms of position include (Figures 4-1a to f):

- **Supine.** The patient is lying face up on his back.
- **Prone.** The patient is lying face down on his stomach.
- **Lateral recumbent (recovery) position.** The patient is lying on his left or right side.
- **Fowler's position.** The patient is lying on his back with his upper body elevated at a 45° to 60° angle.
- **Trendelenburg position.** The patient is lying on his back with the lower part of his body elevated approximately 12 inches. (Note: This is sometimes called "shock position," but its use for shock pa-

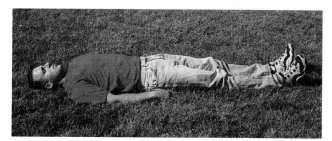

Figure 4-1a   Supine position.

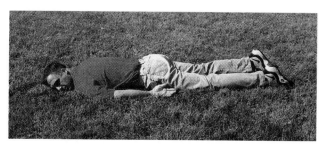

Figure 4-1b   Prone position.

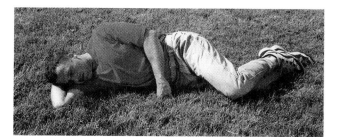

Figure 4-1c   Right lateral recumbent position.

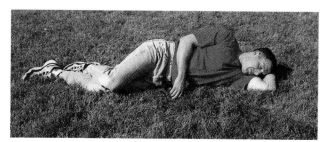

Figure 4-1d   Left lateral recumbent position.

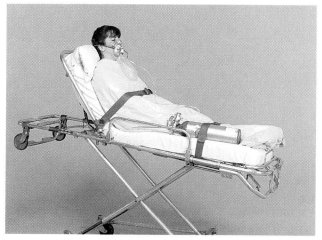

Figure 4-1e   Fowler's position.

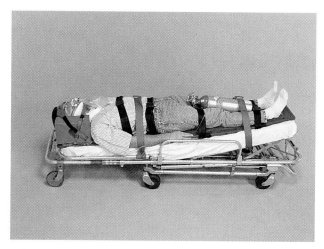

Figure 4-1f   Trendelenburg position.

tients is controversial. See Chapter 29, "Bleeding and Shock," for detailed discussion on caring for suspected shock patients.)

In assessing a patient's condition, it is important to know certain external and internal landmarks, or the anatomical regions of the body and related parts (Figures 4-2 through 4-8). Referring to these landmarks makes your description of the patient's condition more understandable, especially when you are seeking medical direction over the phone or radio.

Imaginary straight-line divisions of the body are called **anatomical planes.** These planes indicate the internal body structure and the relationship of different groups of organs to others. Anatomical planes are delineated by the following (Figure 4-2):

- **Midline.** Visualize the normal anatomical position (the patient is facing you). Now imagine a line drawn vertically through the middle of the patient's body, beginning at the top of the head and continuing down through the nose and the navel and to the ground between the legs. This line divides the body into **right plane** and **left plane.**

- **Midaxillary line.** Visualize a patient standing in profile. Now draw an imaginary line vertically from the middle of the patient's armpit down to the ankle. This is the midaxillary line, which divides the body into the **anterior plane** (the patient's front) and the **posterior plane** (the patient's back).

- **Transverse line.** Visualize the normal anatomical position. Draw an imaginary line horizontally through the patient's waist. This is the transverse line, which divides into the superior plane (above the waist) and the inferior plane (below the waist).

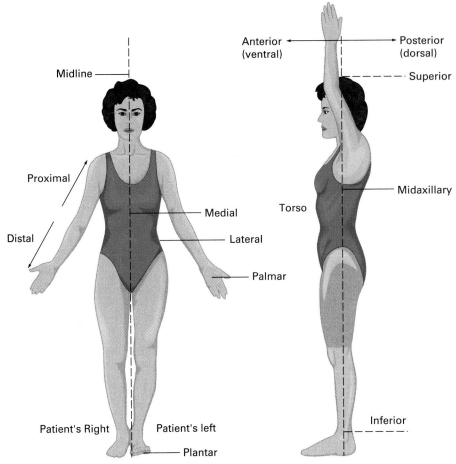

Figure 4-2   Terms of direction.

Other descriptive terms include (Figure 4-2):

- **Anterior** and **posterior.** *Anterior* is toward the front. *Posterior* is toward the back.
- **Superior** and **inferior.** *Superior* means toward the head or above the point of reference. *Inferior* means toward the feet or below the point of reference.
- **Dorsal** and **ventral.** *Dorsal* means toward the back or backbone (spine). *Ventral* means toward the front or belly (abdomen).
- **Medial** and **lateral.** *Medial* means toward the midline or center of the body. *Lateral* refers to the left or right of the midline, or away from the midline of the body. Note that **bilateral** refers to both left and right, meaning "on both sides."
- **Proximal** and **distal.** *Proximal* means near the point of reference. *Distal* is distant, or far from the point of reference.
- **Right** and **left.** These terms always refer to the *patient's* right and left.
- **Midclavicular** and **midaxillary.** *Midclavicular* refers to the center of each of the collarbones (clavicle). The **midclavicular line** (Figure 4-4) extends from the center of either collarbone down the anterior thorax. *Midaxillary* refers to the center of the armpit (axilla). The **midaxillary line** (Figure

4-6), as defined on page 41, extends from the middle of the armpit to the ankle.
- **Plantar** and **palmar.** *Plantar* refers to the sole of the foot. Palmar refers to the palm of the hand.

The abdomen may be referred to as if it were divided by horizontal and vertical lines drawn through the umbilicus (navel). The four parts, or **abdominal quadrants** (Figure 4-9), are the right upper quadrant (RUQ), right lower quadrant (RLQ), left upper quadrant (LUQ), and left lower quadrant (LLQ).

BODY SYSTEMS

 THE MUSCULOSKELETAL SYSTEM

The **musculoskeletal system** of the human body consists of a bony framework, or skeleton, held together by *ligaments* that connect bone to bone, layers of muscles, *tendons* that connect muscles to bones, and various other connective tissues. The system must be strong to provide support and protection, jointed to permit motion, and flexible to withstand stress.

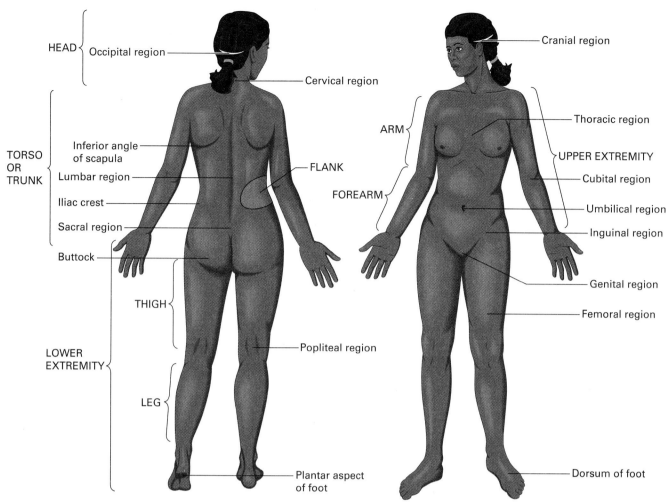

Figure 4-3   Regions of the body.

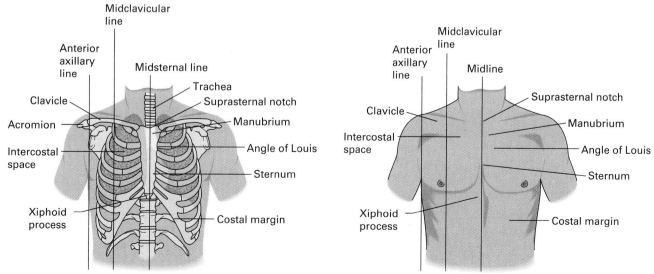

Figure 4-4   Terms describing the anterior chest.

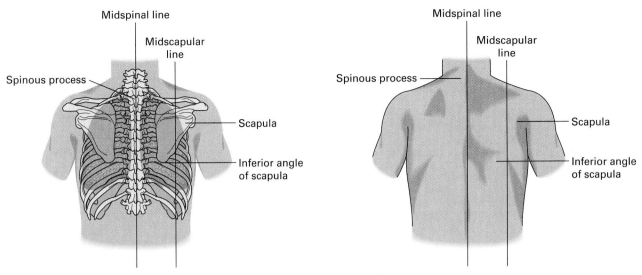

Figure 4-5   Anatomical terms describing the posterior chest.

THE SKELETAL SYSTEM

The skeletal system serves three functions. It:

- Gives the body its shape
- Protects the vital internal organs
- Allows for movement

The skeletal system has six basic components: the skull, spinal column, thorax, pelvis, and the upper and lower extremities (Figure 4-10). The bones of the adult skeleton are classified by size and shape (long, short, flat, or irregular).

The Skull   The **skull** rests at the top of the spinal column and houses and protects the brain. It has two parts: the cranium and the face.

The **cranium** forms the top, back, and sides of the skull plus the forehead. The interlocking bones of the cranium—the *occipital*, two *parietal*, two *temporal*, and the *frontal*—are typical flat bones. The outer layer of the cranium is thick and tough. The inner layer is thinner and more brittle. Though this arrangement

provides for maximum strength, lightness, and elasticity, the cranium may still be fractured. The brain is commonly lacerated by the bony projections and ridges on the inferior surface of the skull. Impact also can bruise the brain and cause it to bleed and swell. Because the cranium cannot expand, bleeding and swelling increase pressure within the brain and can cause unresponsiveness or death.

The area between the brow and chin—the **face**—has fourteen bones, thirteen of which are immovable and interlocking. The immovable bones form the bony settings of the eyes, nose, cheeks, and mouth. Among them are the **orbits** (the eye sockets), the **nasal bones** (the bed of the nose), the **maxillae** (fused bones of the upper jaw), and the **zygomatic bones** (cheek bones). The **mandible** (lower jaw) moves freely on hinge joints. Shaped like a horseshoe, it is the largest and strongest bone of the face.

The Spinal Column   The **spinal column** is the principal support system of the body. Ribs originate from it to form the thoracic (chest) cavity. The rest of the

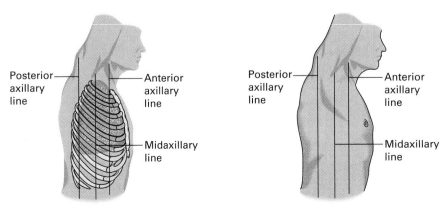

Figure 4-6   Terms describing the lateral chest.

TOPOGRAPHIC ANATOMY

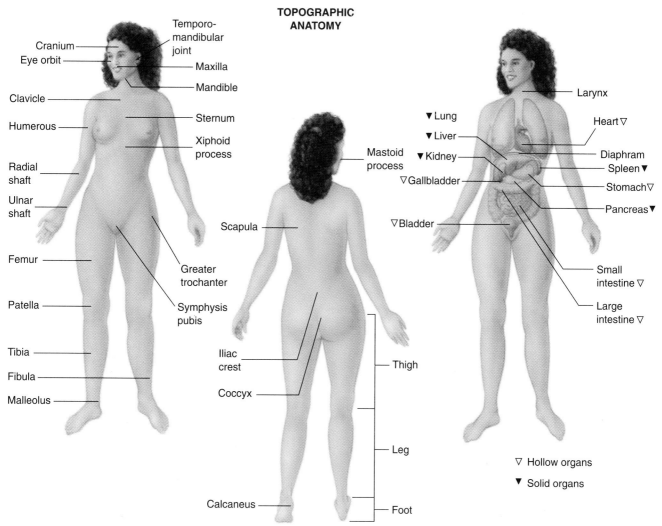

Figure 4-7 Topographic anatomy.

human skeleton is directly or indirectly attached to the spine as well.

The spinal column is made up of irregularly shaped blocks of bone called **vertebrae** and has a great deal of mobility. Lying one on top of the other to form a column, the vertebrae are bound firmly together by strong ligaments. If any vertebrae are crushed or displaced, the spinal cord (which is housed inside the spinal column) may be squeezed, stretched, torn, or severed.

Between each two vertebrae is a fluid-filled pad of tough elastic cartilage called the *intervertebral disc.* The intervertebral discs act as shock absorbers and allow for movement of the spine. The discs are extremely susceptible to injury from twisting, grinding, or improper lifting of heavy objects.

The spinal column is composed of thirty-three vertebrae divided into the following five parts: cervical, thoracic, lumbar, sacral, and the coccyx.

- **Cervical spine** (neck). The first seven vertebrae form the cervical spine, which is the most prone to injury.

- **Thoracic spine** (upper back). The twelve thoracic vertebrae that are directly inferior to the cervical spine form the upper back. The twelve pairs of thoracic ribs are attached to the spine posteriorly and help support the vertebrae.
- **Lumbar spine** (lower back). The next five vertebrae form the lower back, and are the least mobile of the vertebrae. Most lower-back injuries involve muscles, not vertebrae.
- **Sacral spine** (back wall of the pelvis). The next five vertebrae are fused together to form the rigid part of the posterior side of the pelvis.
- **Coccyx** (tailbone). The last four vertebrae are fused together and do not have the protrusions characteristic of the other vertebrae.

The Thorax The **thorax,** or chest, is composed of the ribs, the **sternum** (the breastbone), and the thoracic spine. The twenty-four ribs are semiflexible arches of bone, which are arranged in twelve pairs and are attached posteriorly by ligaments to the

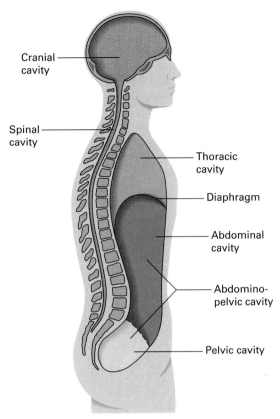

Cranial cavity

Spinal cavity

Thoracic cavity

Diaphragm

Abdominal cavity

Abdomino-pelvic cavity

Pelvic cavity

Figure 4-8 Main body cavities.

twelve thoracic vertebrae. The first seven pairs of ribs are attached to the sternum by cartilage and are called the *true ribs*. The next three pairs are attached to the ribs above them with cartilage. The front ends of the last two pairs—the floating ribs—are not attached to the sternum. These last five pairs of ribs are referred to as *false ribs*.

The sternum is a flat, narrow bone in the middle of the anterior chest. The **clavicle** (collarbone) is attached to the superior portion of the sternum called the **manubrium.** The ribs are attached to the middle of the sternum. The inferior portion of the sternum is the **xiphoid process.**

The Pelvis   The **pelvis** is a doughnut-shaped structure that consists of several bones, including the sacrum and the coccyx. At each side of the pelvis is an **iliac crest.** The iliac crests form the "wings" of the pelvis. The **pubis** is in the anterior and inferior portion of the pelvis, and the **ischium** is in the posterior and inferior portion. The pelvis forms the floor of the abdominal cavity. The pelvic cavity supports the intestines and houses the bladder, rectum, and internal reproductive organs.

The Lower Extremities   The limbs of the body, the arms and legs, are known as the **extremities.** The legs from the hip to the toes are called the *lower extremi-*

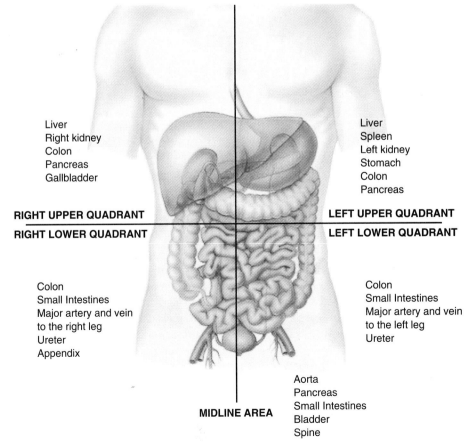

Liver
Right kidney
Colon
Pancreas
Gallbladder

Liver
Spleen
Left kidney
Stomach
Colon
Pancreas

RIGHT UPPER QUADRANT

LEFT UPPER QUADRANT

RIGHT LOWER QUADRANT

LEFT LOWER QUADRANT

Colon
Small Intestines
Major artery and vein
to the right leg
Ureter
Appendix

Colon
Small Intestines
Major artery and vein
to the left leg
Ureter

Aorta
Pancreas
Small Intestines
Bladder
Spine

MIDLINE AREA

Figure 4-9 The abdominal cavity.

THE SKELETON

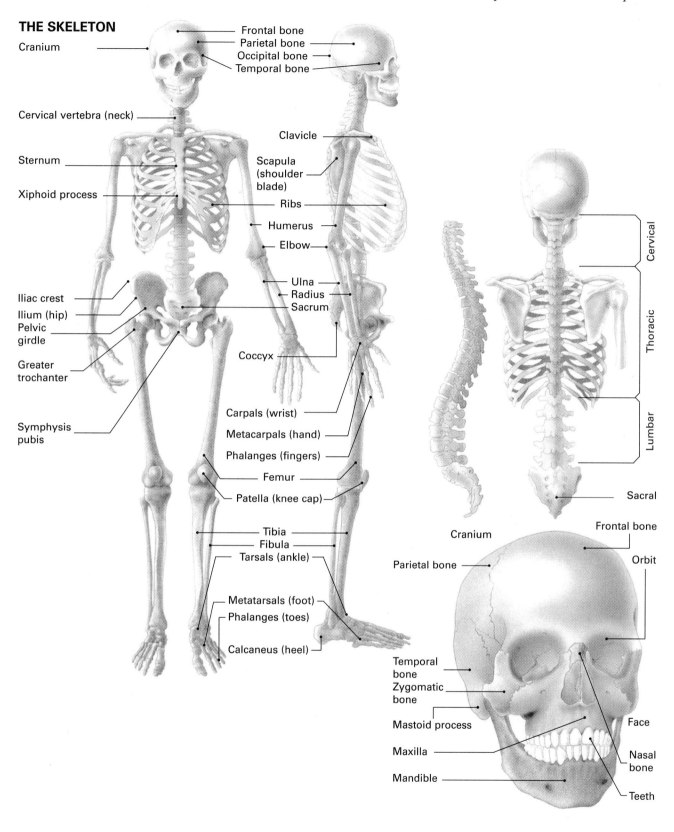

Cranium
Frontal bone
Parietal bone
Occipital bone
Temporal bone

Cervical vertebra (neck)

Clavicle

Sternum

Scapula (shoulder blade)

Xiphoid process

Ribs

Humerus

Elbow

Ulna
Radius
Sacrum

Iliac crest
Ilium (hip)
Pelvic girdle

Greater trochanter

Coccyx

Symphysis pubis

Carpals (wrist)

Metacarpals (hand)

Phalanges (fingers)

Femur

Patella (knee cap)

Tibia
Fibula
Tarsals (ankle)

Metatarsals (foot)
Phalanges (toes)

Calcaneus (heel)

Cervical

Thoracic

Lumbar

Sacral

Cranium

Parietal bone

Frontal bone

Orbit

Temporal bone
Zygomatic bone

Mastoid process

Maxilla

Mandible

Face

Nasal bone

Teeth

THE SKULL

Figure 4-10 *The skeletal system.*

ties. On the lateral aspect of each hip is the hip joint. The joint is made up of the pelvic socket, called the **acetabulum,** into which fits the rounded top, or head, of the **femur** (thigh bone).

The bottom of the femur is flat with two projections that help to form the hinged knee joint, which like the elbow allows angular movement only. The knee joint is protected and stabilized in front by the **patella** (kneecap), a small, triangular-shaped bone. Because the patella usually receives the force of falls or blows to the knee, it is often bruised and can be fractured.

The two bones of the lower leg are the **tibia** (shin) and the **fibula.** The tibia is the weight-bearing bone located at the anterior and medial side of the leg. Its broad upper surface receives the rounded end of the distal femur to form the knee joint. The much smaller distal end of the tibia forms the medial knob of the ankle. The fibula is attached to the tibia at the top and is located at the lateral side of the leg parallel to the tibia.

The bony prominences at the ends of the tibia and fibula form the ankle joint socket. The medial and lateral **malleolus** are the knobby surface landmarks of the ankle joint. A group of bones, including the **calcaneus** (heel bone), are called the **tarsals** and make up the posterior portion of the foot. Five **metatarsals** form the substance of the foot, and fourteen **phalanges** on each foot form the toes (two in the big toe and three in each other toe).

The Upper Extremities   The upper limbs, including the shoulders, arms, forearms, wrists, and hands, are called the *upper extremities.* Each clavicle (collar bone) and **scapula** (shoulder blade) form a shoulder girdle, the tip of which is called the **acromion.** The powerful muscles of the shoulder girdle help attach the arms to the trunk and extend from it to the arms, thorax, neck, and head.

The proximal portion of the arm is the **humerus,** the largest bone in the upper extremity. Its shaft is roughly cylindrical, its upper end is round, and its lower end is flat. The round head of the humerus fits into a shallow cup in the shoulder blade, forming a ball-and-socket joint that is the most freely movable joint in the body.

The hinged elbow joint is made up of the distal end of the humerus plus the proximal ends of the **radius** (the lateral bone of the forearm) and the **ulna** (the medial bone of the forearm). The radius is located on the thumbside and the ulna is found on the little-finger side of the forearm. The **olecranon** is a part of the ulna that forms the bony prominence of the elbow. While the ulna can be felt through the skin with your fingertips, the upper two-thirds of the radius cannot because it is sheathed in muscle tissue. Only the lower third of the radius, which enlarges to form most of the wrist joint, can be felt through the skin.

The wrist consists of eight bones called the **carpals.** The structural strength of the hand comes from the **metacarpals.** The bones that make up the fingers and thumbs are the **phalanges** (three per finger, two per thumb).

The Joints   The place where one bone connects to another is called a **joint.** Some joints are immovable (as in the skull), others are slightly movable (as in the spine), and the remaining joints such as the elbow and knee are movable (Figure 4-11). Movable joints allow changes of position and motion as follows:

- *Flexion*—bending toward the body
- *Extension*—straightening away from the body
- *Abduction*—movement away from the midline
- *Adduction*—movement toward the midline
- *Circumduction*—a combination of all four of the above motions
- *Pronation*—turning the forearm so the palm of the hand is turned toward the back

Immovable 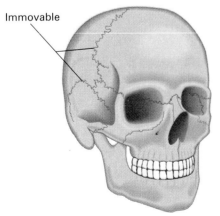 Slightly movable 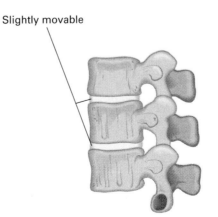 Freely movable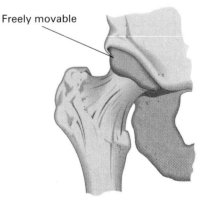

Figure 4-11   Three types of joints.

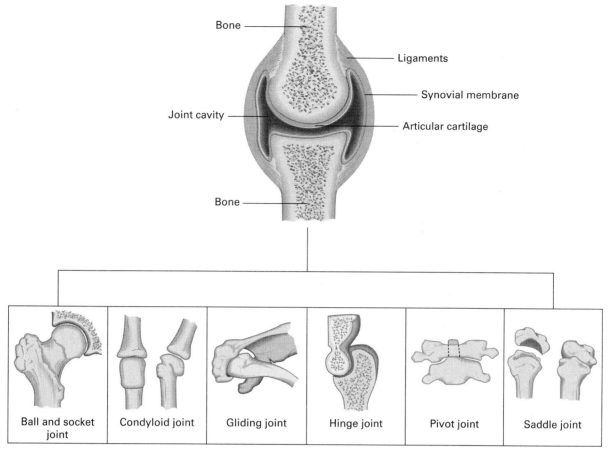

Figure 4-12 Types of freely movable joints.

- *Supination*—turning the forearm so the palm of the hand is turned toward the front

The structure of the joint determines the kind of movement that is possible. Types of joints include the following, the most common of which are the ball-and-socket joint and hinged joint (Figure 4-12).

- *Ball and socket joint.* This type of joint permits the widest range of motion—flexion, extension, abduction, adduction, and rotation. Examples: joints at the shoulder and hip.
- *Hinged joint.* Hinged joints (such as those in the elbow, knee, and finger) permit flexion and extension. Elbow joints have forward movement (the anterior bone surfaces approach each other), while knee joints have backward movement (the posterior bone surfaces approach each other).
- *Pivot joint.* This type of joint allows for a turning motion, and includes the joints between the head and neck at the first and second cervical vertebrae and those in the wrist.
- *Gliding joint.* The simplest movement between bones occurs in a gliding joint, where one bone slides across another to the point where surrounding structures restrict the motion. Gliding joints connect the small bones in the hands and the feet.

- *Saddle joint.* This joint is shaped to permit combinations of limited movements along perpendicular planes. For example, the ankle allows the foot to turn inward slightly as it moves up and down.
- *Condyloid joint.* This is a modified ball-and-socket joint that permits limited motion in two directions. In the wrist, for example, it allows the hand to move up and down and side to side, but not to rotate completely.

THE MUSCULAR SYSTEM

Movement of the body is due to work performed by the muscles (Figure 4-13). What enables muscle tissue to work is its ability to contract (to become shorter and thicker) when stimulated by a nerve impulse. The cells of a muscle are called *fibers,* because they are usually long and threadlike. Each muscle has countless bundles of closely packed, overlapping fibers bound together by connective tissue.

Muscles can be injured in many ways. Overexerting a muscle may tear fibers, and muscles subjected to trauma can be bruised, crushed, cut, torn, or otherwise injured, even if the skin is not broken. Muscles injured in any way tend to become swollen, tender, painful, or weak.

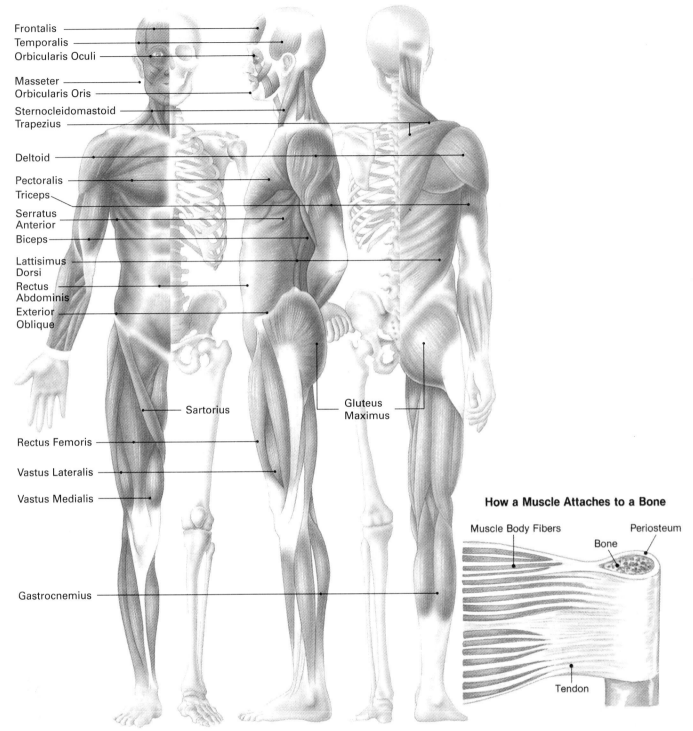

Figure 4-13 The muscular system.

There are three kinds of muscle: voluntary (skeletal), involuntary (smooth), and cardiac muscle (Figure 4-14).

Voluntary Muscle Under the control of the brain and nervous system, **voluntary muscle** can be contracted and relaxed by will of the individual. This type of muscle makes possible all deliberate movement, such as walking, chewing, swallowing, smiling, frowning, talking, or moving the eyeballs. It forms the major muscle mass of the body, helps to shape it, and forms its walls.

Voluntary muscle, often referred to as *skeletal muscle,* is generally attached at one or both ends to bone by tendons. A few are attached to skin, cartilage, organs (such as the eyeball), or other muscles (such as

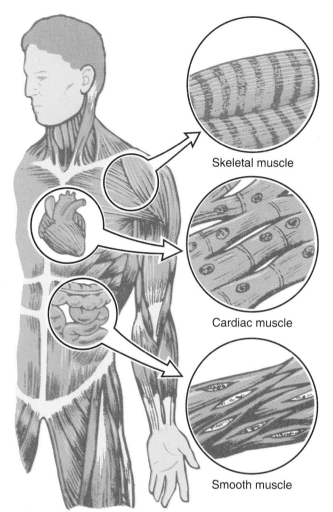

Figure 4-14 *Three types of muscle.*

- Skeletal muscle
- Cardiac muscle
- Smooth muscle

the tongue). In the trunk, voluntary muscles are broad, flat, and expanded to help form the walls of the cavities they enclose—the abdomen and the chest. In the extremities, the voluntary muscles are long and more rounded, somewhat resembling spindles.

Involuntary Muscle Also called *smooth muscle,* **involuntary muscle** is made up of large fibers that carry out the automatic muscular functions of the body. Through rhythmic wavelike movements, for example, involuntary muscles move blood through the veins, bile from the gallbladder, and food through the digestive tract. The individual has no direct control over this type of muscle, though it responds to stimuli such as stretching, heat, and cold.

Involuntary muscle is found in the walls of tubelike organs, ducts, the respiratory tract, and blood vessels and forms much of the walls of the intestines and urinary system.

Cardiac Muscle Found only in the walls of the heart, **cardiac muscle** is a special kind of involuntary muscle particularly suited for the work of the heart. It has *automaticity.* That is, it has the ability to generate

an impulse on its own, even when disconnected from the central nervous system.

Smooth like involuntary muscle but striated (stringlike) like voluntary muscle, cardiac muscle is made up of a cellular meshwork unlike either. It has its own blood supply furnished by the coronary artery system and cannot tolerate interruption of the blood supply for even very short periods.

THE RESPIRATORY SYSTEM

BASIC ANATOMY

The body can store food for weeks and water for days, but it can store enough oxygen to last only a few minutes. Simple inhalation normally provides the body with the oxygen it needs. However, if the oxygen supply is cut off, as in a drowning or choking patient, brain cells will ordinarily begin to die in about five minutes.

Oxygen from the air is transported to the blood through the **respiratory system** (Figure 4-15). The major components of the respiratory system include those described below.

The Nose and Mouth Air normally enters the body through the nose and mouth. There it is warmed, moistened, and filtered as it flows over the damp, sticky mucous membranes.

The Pharynx From the back of the nose or mouth, the air enters the **pharynx** (throat), the common passageway for food and air. Air from the mouth enters through the oral portion of the pharynx, or the **oropharynx.** Air from the nose enters the nasal portion of the pharynx, or the **nasopharynx.** At its lower end the pharynx divides into two structures—the **esophagus,** which leads to the stomach, and the **trachea** (windpipe), which leads to the lungs.

The Epiglottis The trachea is protected by a small leaf-shaped flap called the **epiglottis.** Usually, this flap automatically covers the entrance of the larynx during swallowing to keep food and liquid from entering the trachea and lungs. However, during an altered mental status or unresponsiveness reflexes may not work properly. If liquid, blood, vomit, or another substance is in the mouth of an unresponsive patient, it may be aspirated into the trachea and lungs and cause impaired exchange of oxygen and carbon dioxide.

The Trachea and Larynx The trachea carries air from the nose and mouth to the lungs. Immediately superior to the trachea is the **larynx,** which houses the vocal cords and is commonly called the "voice box." The "Adam's apple" or **thyroid cartilage** is the anterior cartilage that covers the larynx. The larynx can be easily felt through the skin with your fingertips

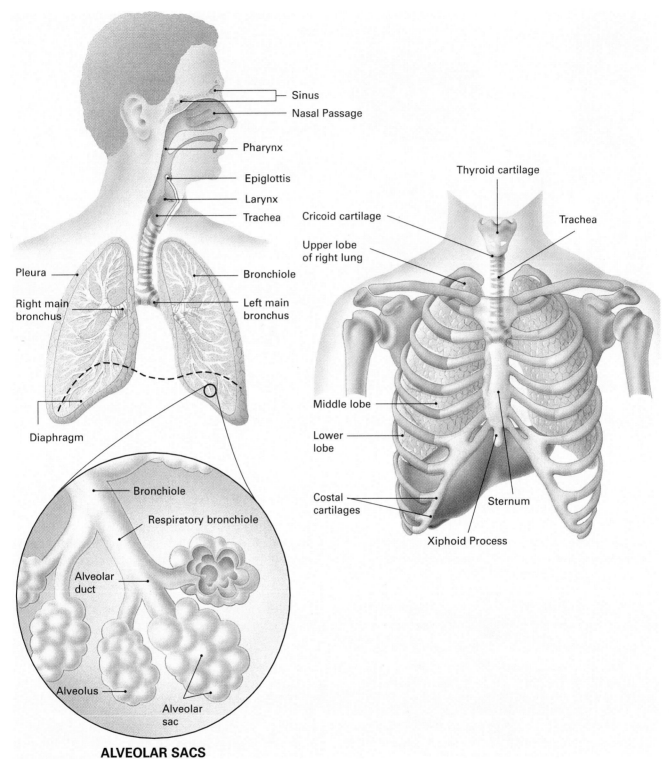

ALVEOLAR SACS

Figure 4-15 The respiratory system.

at the front of the neck. The most inferior part of the larynx is the **cricoid cartilage,** a firm, full ring of cartilage that forms the lower edge of the larynx.

The Bronchi The distal portion of the trachea branches into two main tubes, or **bronchi,** one branching off to each lung. Each bronchus divides and subdivides into smaller **bronchioles,** somewhat like the branches of a tree. At the ends are thousands of tiny air sacs called **alveoli,** each enclosed in a network of capillaries (tiny blood vessels). This is the site of gas exchange in the lungs.

The Lungs The principal organs of respiration are the **lungs,** two large, lobed organs that house thousands of tiny alveolar sacs responsible for the ex-

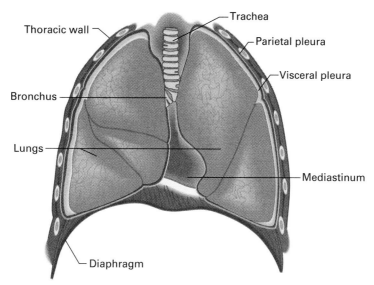

Figure 4-16   The pleural lining of the lung.

change of oxygen and carbon dioxide (as will be explained later). A thin layer of connective tissue called the *visceral pleura* covers the outer surface of the lungs. A layer of thicker, more elastic tissue called the *parietal pleura* covers the internal chest wall. Between the two layers is the *interpleural space*, a tiny space with negative pressure that allows the lungs to stay inflated with air. (See Figure 4-16.)

The Diaphragm   A powerful dome-shaped muscle essential to breathing, the **diaphragm** also separates the thoracic cavity from the abdominal cavity. During inhalation the diaphragm and the **intercostal muscles** (the muscles between the ribs) contract, increasing the size of the thoracic cavity. The diaphragm moves slightly downward, flaring the lower portion of the rib cage, which moves upward and outward. This de-

creases pressure in the chest and causes air to flow into the lungs. During exhalation the diaphragm and intercostal muscles relax, decreasing the size of the thoracic cavity. The diaphragm moves upward, the ribs move downward and inward, and air flows out of the lungs. (See Figure 4-17.)

ANATOMY IN INFANTS AND CHILDREN

When treating infants or children, remember the anatomical differences in the respiratory system:

- The mouth and nose are smaller than those of adults and are more easily obstructed by even small objects, blood, or swelling. Therefore, extra attention to keeping the airway open is required when treating an infant or child.

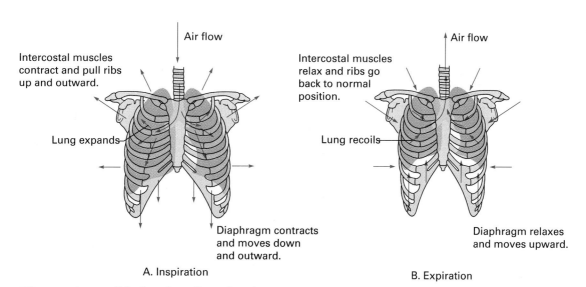

Figure 4-17   Mechanics of respiration.

- The tongue of an infant or child takes up proportionally more space in the pharynx and it can block the pharynx more easily, again with implications for care of the infant or child's airway.
- Infants and children have narrower tracheas that may be obstructed more easily by swelling. The trachea is also softer and more flexible than that of an adult. Therefore, hyperextension of the head (tipping the head back), or flexion (allowing the head to tip forward), can occlude the trachea. Because the head of an infant or young child is quite large relative to the body, it is necessary to place a folded towel or similar item about one inch thick under the shoulders to keep the trachea aligned and open ("sniffing" position).
- Like other cartilage in the body, the cricoid cartilage in an infant or child is less developed and much less rigid. Therefore, the maneuver of pressing on the cricoid cartilage to help in placing a tube into the trachea, often used on adults, is not appropriate for an infant or child, since it can depress the soft cartilage and result in obstruction.
- Because the chest wall is softer, infants and children rely more heavily on the diaphragm for breathing. Excessive movement of the diaphragm is a sign of respiratory distress in an infant or child.

PHYSIOLOGY OF RESPIRATION

In the lungs, oxygen and carbon dioxide are exchanged through the thin walls of the alveoli and the capillaries (Figures 4-18 and 4-19). In alveolar/capillary exchange, oxygen-rich air enters the alveoli during each inspiration and passes through the capillary walls into the bloodstream. Carbon dioxide and other waste gases move from the blood through the capillary walls into the alveoli and are exhaled. In capillary/cellular exchange throughout the body, carbon dioxide moves from the cells to the capillaries and oxygen moves from th capillaries to the cells.

Adequate breathing is characterized by an adequate respiratory rate and volume. Normal respiratory rates are: adults—12 to 20 breaths per minute; children—15 to 30 breaths per minute; and infants—25 to 50 breaths per minute. Also, the respirations are regular in rhythm and free of unusual sounds, such as wheezing. The chest should expand adequately and equally with each breath, the depth (tidal volume) of breaths should be adequate, and breathing should be virtually effortless (accomplished without the use of accessory muscles of the neck and abdomen).

Inadequate breathing may be characterized by:

- Rates that are either slower or faster than normal
- Irregular pattern of breathing
- Diminished or absent breath sounds
- Unequal or inadequate chest expansion
- Depth (tidal volume) that is inadequate or shallow
- Pale or bluish mucous membranes or skin that may also be cool and clammy
- Use of accessory muscles during breathing, especially among infants and children
- Retractions above the clavicles, between the ribs, and below the rib cage, especially in children
- Nasal flaring, especially in children
- "Seesaw" breathing in infants (the chest and abdomen move in opposite directions)
- *Agonal* respirations (occasional gasping breaths) that may be seen just before death

For the breathing to be considered adequate, both rate and tidal volume must be adequate. If *either* rate or tidal volume is inadequate, the breathing is considered inadequate, and immediate intervention is necessary.

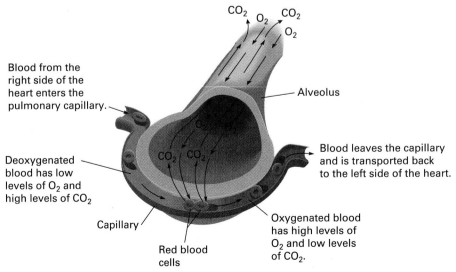

Figure 4-18 Alveolar/capillary gas exchange.

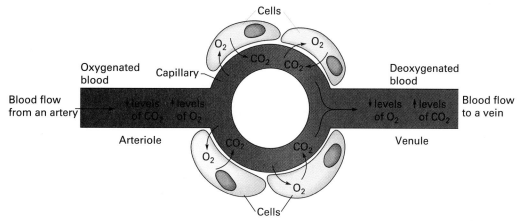

Figure 4-19   Capillary/cell gas exchange.

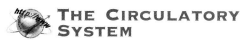

THE CIRCULATORY SYSTEM

The **circulatory system** is composed of the heart, blood vessels, and blood (Figure 4-20). It is a closed system that transports blood to all parts of the body. Blood brings oxygen, nutrients, and other essential chemical elements to tissue cells, and removes carbon dioxide and other waste products resulting from cell metabolism.

BASIC ANATOMY

The Heart   The **heart,** a highly efficient pump, is a chambered muscular organ that lies within the chest in the thoracic cavity between the two lungs. In size and shape, it resembles a closed fist. About two-thirds of its mass is located to the left of the midline of the body. Its lower point, the apex, lies just above the diaphragm.

The *pericardium* is a double-walled sac that encloses the heart, gives support, and prevents friction as the heart moves within this protective sac. The surfaces of the pericardial sac produce a small amount of fluid lubrication needed to facilitate the normal movements of the heart.

The heart has four chambers. The upper chambers, called the **atria,** receive blood from the veins. The right atrium receives oxygen-depleted blood from the veins of the body. The left atrium receives oxygen-rich blood from the pulmonary veins from the lungs.

The lower chambers are called **ventricles.** They pump blood out to the arteries. The right ventricle pumps oxygen-depleted blood to the pulmonary arteries which transport the blood to the lungs where it will be oxygenated. The left ventricle pumps oxygen-rich blood to the major artery from the heart, the aorta (see below), from which the blood is gradually delivered to all body cells.

A series of **valves** between the chambers of the heart keep the blood flowing in one direction and prevent the backflow of blood. The four valves are:

* *Tricuspid valve*—between the right atrium and the right ventricle
* *Pulmonary valve*—at the base of the pulmonary artery in the right ventricle
* *Mitral valve,* also known as the *bicuspid valve*—between the left atrium and the left ventricle
* *Aortic valve*—at the base of the aortic artery in the left ventricle

The heart is composed of specialized contractile and conductive muscle that responds to electrical impulses. A sophisticated cardiac conduction system causes the *myocardium,* or middle layer of muscle, to contract and eject blood from the heart. The electrical impulse originates at the *sinoatrial (SA) node* and travels to the *atrioventricular (AV) node,* which is located between the atria and the ventricles, and finally through the *bundle of His* to the *Purkinje fibers* to the ventricles. As the heart muscle contracts, blood is propelled through the pulmonary arteries and to the lungs and into the aorta. From the aorta, it is eventually circulated throughout the body.

The Arteries   An **artery** carries blood away from the heart. All arteries except the pulmonary arteries (see page 58) carry oxygen-rich blood. The major arteries include the following:

* **Aorta**—The major artery from the heart, the aorta, lies in front of the spine and passes through the thoracic and abdominal cavities. At about the level of the navel, the aorta divides into the iliac arteries, allowing blood to travel down each leg. The aorta and its branches supply all other arteries with blood.
* **Coronary arteries**—The coronary arteries are the vessels that supply the heart with blood.

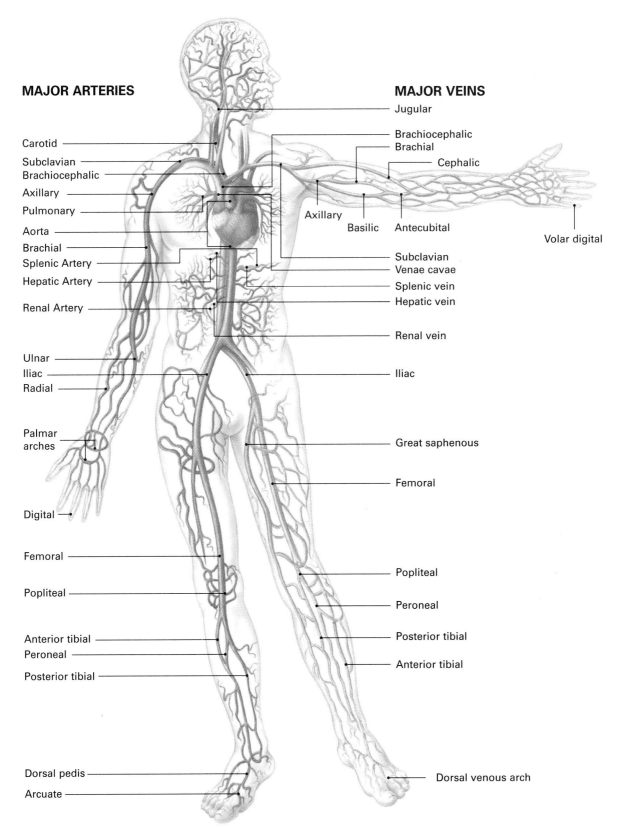

MAJOR ARTERIES

Carotid
Subclavian
Brachiocephalic
Axillary
Pulmonary
Aorta
Brachial
Splenic Artery
Hepatic Artery
Renal Artery
Ulnar
Iliac
Radial
Palmar arches
Digital
Femoral
Popliteal
Anterior tibial
Peroneal
Posterior tibial
Dorsal pedis
Arcuate

MAJOR VEINS

Jugular
Brachiocephalic
Brachial
Cephalic
Axillary
Basilic
Antecubital
Volar digital
Subclavian
Venae cavae
Splenic vein
Hepatic vein
Renal vein
Iliac
Great saphenous
Femoral
Popliteal
Peroneal
Posterior tibial
Anterior tibial
Dorsal venous arch

Figure 4-20a The circulatory system.

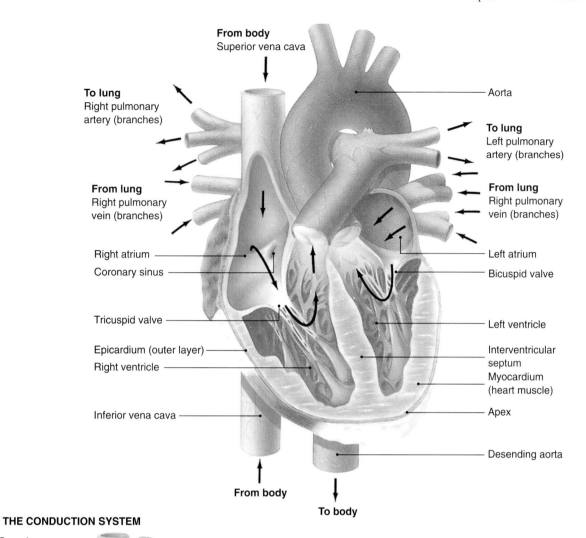

From body
Superior vena cava

To lung
Right pulmonary
artery (branches)

From lung
Right pulmonary
vein (branches)

Right atrium

Coronary sinus

Tricuspid valve

Epicardium (outer layer)

Right ventricle

Inferior vena cava

Aorta

To lung
Left pulmonary
artery (branches)

From lung
Right pulmonary
vein (branches)

Left atrium

Bicuspid valve

Left ventricle

Interventricular
septum

Myocardium
(heart muscle)

Apex

Desending aorta

From body

To body

THE CONDUCTION SYSTEM

Superior
vena cava

Sinoatrial node
(pacemaker)

Right atrium

Right ventricle

Purkinje fibers

Inferior vena cava

Aorta

Left atrium

Atrioventricle
node

Left
ventricle

Right and left branches of the bundle of His

THE CORONARY ARTERIES

Base (superior)

Right coronary
artery

Left coronary
artery

Apex (inferior)

Anterior descending branch

Figure 4-20b   The circulatory system (continued).

- **Carotid arteries**—The carotid arteries (one on each side of the neck) supply the brain and head with blood. Pulsations of the carotid arteries can be felt on either side of the neck.
- **Femoral arteries**—The femoral artery is the major artery of the thigh and supplies the groin and leg with blood. Pulsations of the femoral artery can be felt in the groin at the crease between abdomen and thigh.
- **Dorsalis pedis arteries**—Pulsations of the dorsalis pedis, an artery in the foot, can be felt on the top surface of the foot on the big toe side.
- **Posterior tibial arteries**—The posterior tibial artery travels from the calf to the foot. Pulsations of this artery can be felt posterior to the medial malleolus (ankle bone).
- **Brachial arteries**—The brachial artery is the major artery of the upper arm. Its pulsations can be felt on the medial aspect of the arm, midway between the shoulder and the elbow. The brachial artery is used when determining blood pressure.
- **Radial arteries**—The radial artery is the major artery of the arm distal to the elbow joint. Its pulsations can be felt proximal to the thumb on the wrist. It is the artery that is usually assessed when taking a patient's pulse.
- **Pulmonary arteries**—The pulmonary arteries, which originate at the right ventricle of the heart, carry oxygen-depleted blood to the lungs, where the blood is oxygenated and returned to the heart for circulation throughout the body. Note: The pulmonary arteries are the only arteries that carry deoxygenated, or oxygen-depleted, blood.

The Arterioles   The arteries are smaller the farther they are from the heart. Each eventually branches into an **arteriole,** the smallest kind of artery. The arterioles carry blood from the arteries into the capillaries.

The Capillaries   A tiny blood vessel that connects an arteriole to a venule, a **capillary** has walls that allow for the exchange of gases, nutrients, and waste at the cellular level. All fluid, oxygen, and carbon dioxide exchange takes place between the blood and tissue cells through the walls of the capillaries in all parts of the body.

The Venules   The smallest branches of the veins, the **venules,** are connected to the distal ends of capillaries. Blood that has been depleted of oxygen flows from the capillaries into the venules, from which it is transported into larger veins.

The Veins   A **vein** carries blood back to the heart. All veins except the pulmonary veins (see the next column) carry oxygen-depleted blood. The major veins include the venae cavae and the pulmonary veins.

The **venae cavae** carry oxygen-depleted blood back to the right atrium, where it begins circulation through the heart and lungs. The *superior vena cava* enters the top of the right atrium, carrying oxygen-depleted blood from the upper body. The *inferior vena cava* enters the bottom of the right atrium, carrying oxygen-depleted blood from the lower body.

The **pulmonary veins** carry oxygen-rich blood from the lungs to the left atrium. They are the only veins that carry oxygenated blood.

Composition of the Blood

Blood is composed of red blood cells, white blood cells, platelets, and plasma.

- **Red blood cells**—The red cells give the blood its color, carry oxygen to the body cells, and carry carbon dioxide away from the cells.
- **White blood cells**—The white cells are part of the body's immune system and help to defend against infection.
- **Platelets**—Platelets are essential to the formation of blood clots, necessary to stop bleeding.
- **Plasma**—This is the liquid part of the blood, which carries blood cells and transports nutrients to all tissues. The plasma also transports waste products to organs where they can be excreted from the body.

Physiology of Circulation

Two ways of determining the adequacy of circulation are by assessing the pulse and by assessing the blood pressure.

When the left ventricle contracts, sending a wave of blood through the arteries, the **pulse,** or wave of propelled blood, can be felt at various points called *pulse points.* Simply, the pulse can be felt at the point where an artery passes over a bone near the skin surface.

The central pulses are the carotid and femoral—located centrally, closer to the heart. The peripheral pulses are the radial, brachial, tibial, and dorsalis pedis—located on the periphery of the body, farther from the heart. These pulses can be felt at the locations described earlier.

Blood pressure is the force exerted by the blood on the interior walls of the arteries. The **systolic blood pressure** is the pressure exerted against the walls of the arteries when the left ventricle contracts. The **diastolic blood pressure** is the pressure exerted against the walls of the arteries when the left ventricle is at rest, or between contractions.

Perfusion is the delivery of oxygen and other nutrients to the cells of all organ systems, and the elimination of carbon dioxide and other waste products, which results from the constant adequate circulation of blood through the capillaries.

Shock, or **hypoperfusion,** is the insufficient supply of oxygen and other nutrients to some of the body's cells and the inadequate elimination of carbon dioxide and other wastes that result from inadequate circulation of blood. It is a state of profound depression of the vital processes of the body. (Detailed information will be found in Chapter 29, "Bleeding and Shock.")

 ## THE NERVOUS SYSTEM

The **nervous system** (Figure 4-21) controls the voluntary and involuntary activity of the human body. It enables the individual to be aware of and to react to the environment. It also coordinates the responses of the body to stimuli and keeps body systems working together. Nerves carry impulses from tissues and organs to the nerve centers, and from nerve centers to other tissues and organs.

The nervous system is divided into two main structural divisions: the central nervous system and the peripheral nervous system.

THE CENTRAL NERVOUS SYSTEM

The **central nervous system** consists of the brain, which is located within the cranium, and the spinal cord, which is located within the spinal column (Figure 4-22). The three layers of protective membranes enclosing both the brain and the spinal cord are the *meninges.* In addition, nature provides a cushion of fluid around and within the brain and spinal cord called *cerebrospinal fluid.* It is formed and circulated constantly, and part of it is perpetually reabsorbed into the venous blood of the brain.

The brain, which is the control center of the nervous system, is probably the most highly specialized organ in the body. It weighs about three pounds in the average adult, is richly supplied with blood vessels, and requires considerable oxygen to perform effectively. It has three main subdivisions: the cerebrum, cerebellum, and medulla oblongata. A smaller subdivision of the brain, the pons, acts as a bridge that connects the three.

• *The cerebrum*—The outermost portion of the brain, the cerebrum occupies nearly all the cranial cavity. It controls specific body functions, such as sensation, thought, and associative memory. It also initiates and manages motions that are under the conscious control of the individual.

• *The cerebellum*—Also called the "small brain," the cerebellum is located in the posterior and inferior aspect of the cranium. It coordinates muscle activity and maintains balance through impulses from the eyes and the ears. Though it cannot initiate a muscle contraction, it can hold muscles in a state of partial contraction.

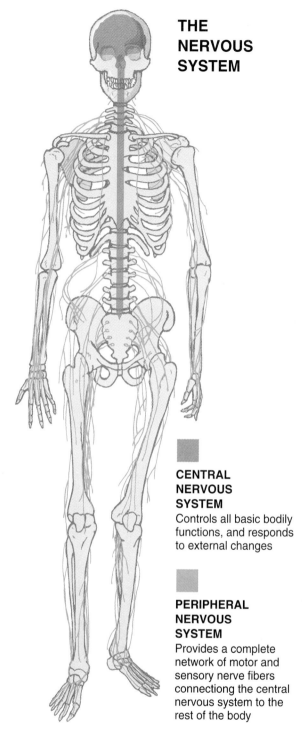

THE NERVOUS SYSTEM

CENTRAL NERVOUS SYSTEM
Controls all basic bodily functions, and responds to external changes

PERIPHERAL NERVOUS SYSTEM
Provides a complete network of motor and sensory nerve fibers connectiong the central nervous system to the rest of the body

Figure 4-21   The nervous system.

• *Medulla oblongata*—The medulla oblongata, a part of the brain stem, consists of three major control centers: the respiratory center, the cardiac center, and the vasomotor center. The *respiratory center* controls the rate and depth of respiration. The *cardiac center* is responsible for regulating the heart rate and force of contraction of the ventricles. The blood pressure is controlled by the *vasomotor cen-*

THE BRAIN

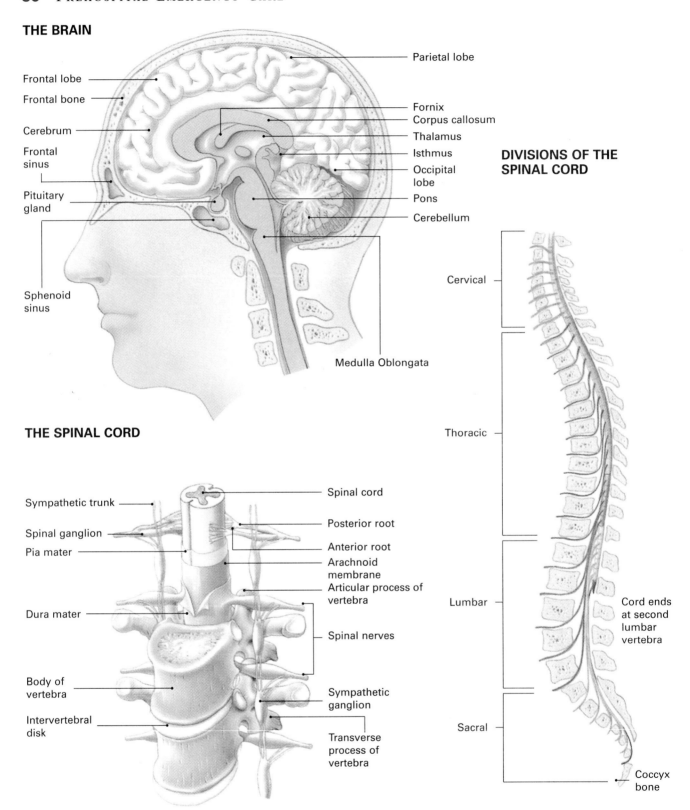

Parietal lobe

Frontal lobe

Frontal bone

Cerebrum

Frontal sinus

Pituitary gland

Sphenoid sinus

Fornix

Corpus callosum

Thalamus

Isthmus

Occipital lobe

Pons

Cerebellum

Medulla Oblongata

DIVISIONS OF THE SPINAL CORD

Cervical

Thoracic

Lumbar

Sacral

Cord ends at second lumbar vertebra

Coccyx bone

THE SPINAL CORD

Sympathetic trunk

Spinal ganglion

Pia mater

Dura mater

Body of vertebra

Intervertebral disk

Spinal cord

Posterior root

Anterior root

Arachnoid membrane

Articular process of vertebra

Spinal nerves

Sympathetic ganglion

Transverse process of vertebra

Figure 4-22 The central nervous system.

ter, which produces dilation (relaxation) and constriction of the blood vessels.

The spinal cord is about eighteen inches long and is an extension of the brain stem. The major function of the spinal cord is conduction of nerve impulses. Many nerves enter and leave the spinal cord at different levels. These nerves all connect with nerve centers located in the brain or spinal cord.

The Peripheral Nervous System

The **peripheral nervous system** is composed of the nerves located outside the spinal cord and brain. It also carries sensory information from the body to the spinal cord and brain. It carries motor information from the brain and spinal cord to the body.

Functional Divisions of the Nervous System

The functional divisions of the nervous system are:

- The *voluntary nervous system,* which influences the activity of voluntary (skeletal) muscles and movements
- The *autonomic nervous system,* which is automatic and influences the activities of involuntary muscles and glands. It is partly independent of the rest of the nervous system

The Autonomic Nervous System The autonomic nervous system is divided into the *sympathetic nervous system* and the *parasympathetic nervous system.* The two systems have opposite effects and act in a delicate balance. The sympathetic nervous system is activated when the body is challenged by stressors: trauma, blood loss, fright, and so on. Its actions are commonly known as the "fight or flight" response. The parasympathetic nervous system returns body processes to normal or depresses body function. Figure 4-23 illustrates the effects on various organs.

The Endocrine System

The **endocrine system** is made up of ductless glands, the body's regulators (Figure 4-24). Secretions from these glands are called *hormones,* chemical substances that have effects on the activity of certain organs. Hormones are carried by the bloodstream to all parts of the body, affecting physical strength, mental ability, build, stature, reproduction, hair growth, voice pitch, and behavior. How people think, act, and feel depends largely on these secretions.

The endocrine glands discharge secretions directly into the bloodstream. Good health depends on a well-balanced output of hormones. Endocrine imbalance yields profound changes in growth and serious changes in mental, emotional, physical, and sexual behavior.

The endocrine glands and their functions include the following:

- *Thyroid gland,* which is located in the neck, regulates metabolism, growth and development, and the activity of the nervous system.
- *Parathyroid glands,* behind the thyroid, produce a hormone necessary for the metabolism of calcium and phosphorus in the bones.
- *Adrenal glands,* which sit atop the kidneys, secrete adrenalin, postpone muscle fatigue, increase the storage of sugar, control kidney function, and regulate the metabolism of salt and water.
- *Gonads* (ovaries and testes) produce the hormones that govern reproduction and sex characteristics.
- *Islets of Langerhans,* which are in the pancreas, make insulin for sugar metabolism.
- *Pituitary gland,* which is at the base of the brain, is considered to be the "master gland." It regulates growth, the thyroid and parathyroid glands, the pancreas, the gonads, metabolism of fatty acids and some basic proteins, blood sugar reactions, and urinary excretion.

 ## The Skin

All the various tissues, organs, and systems that make up the human body are separated from the outside environment by the skin, which is the largest organ in the body (Figure 4-25). The skin has the following functions:

- Protects the body from the environment, bacteria, and other foreign organisms
- Regulates the temperature of the body
- Serves as a receptor for heat, cold, touch, pain, and pressure
- Aids in the regulation of water and electrolytes (sodium and chloride)

The skin has three basic layers: the epidermis, the dermis, and a subcutaneous layer. The **epidermis,** or outermost layer of skin, is actually composed of four layers of cells. The outer two layers are dying and dead cells that are sloughed off as new cells replace them. The skin's pigmentation—the *melanin*—is located in the deepest layers of the epidermis.

The **dermis,** or second layer of the skin, is much thicker than the epidermis. It contains the vast network of blood vessels that supply the skin as well as the hair follicles, sweat glands, oil glands, and sensory nerves. Composed of dense connective tissue, the dermis is what gives the skin its elasticity and strength.

Just below the dermis is a layer of fatty tissue called the **subcutaneous layer,** or *subcutaneous connective tissue.* It varies in thickness, depending on what part of the body it covers. Subcutaneous tissue

ORGAN EFFECT

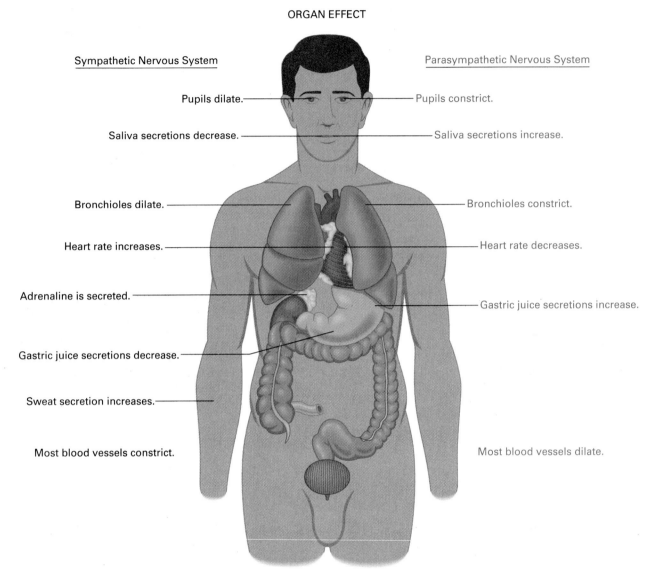

Sympathetic Nervous System

Pupils dilate.

Saliva secretions decrease.

Bronchioles dilate.

Heart rate increases.

Adrenaline is secreted.

Gastric juice secretions decrease.

Sweat secretion increases.

Most blood vessels constrict.

Parasympathetic Nervous System

Pupils constrict.

Saliva secretions increase.

Bronchioles constrict.

Heart rate decreases.

Gastric juice secretions increase.

Most blood vessels dilate.

Figure 4-23   The effects of the autonomic nervous system on organs.

of the eyelids, for example, is extremely thin, but that of the abdomen and buttocks is thick.

The four accessory structures of the skin are the nails, hair, sweat glands, and oil glands.

ENRICHMENT

The enrichment section contains information that is valuable as background for the EMT-B but that goes substantially beyond the U.S. Department of Transportation (DOT) EMT-Basic curriculum.

THE DIGESTIVE SYSTEM

BASIC ANATOMY

The digestive system is composed of the *alimentary tract* (the passage through which food travels) and the *accessory organs* (organs that help prepare food for

absorption and use by tissues of the body). The main functions of the digestive system are to ingest and carry food so that absorption can occur and waste can be eliminated.

The abdominal cavity contains all the major organs of the digestive system except for the mouth and the esophagus.

- *The stomach,* a large, hollow organ, is the main organ of the digestive system. While digestion actually begins in the mouth, where saliva begins to break down foods, the majority of digestion takes place in the stomach, which secretes *gastric juices* that begin converting ingested foods to a form that can be absorbed and used by the body.

- *The pancreas* is a flat, solid organ that lies just inferior and posterior to the stomach. It secretes *pancreatic juices* that aid in the digestion of fats, starches, and proteins. The islets of Langerhans, lo-

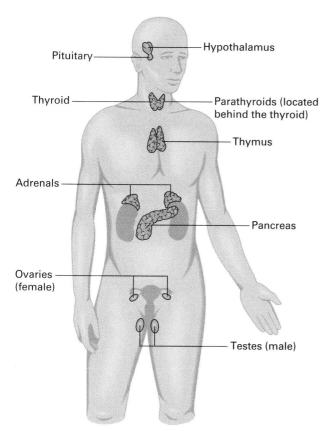

Figure 4-24   The endocrine system.

Pituitary
Hypothalamus
Thyroid
Parathyroids (located behind the thyroid)
Thymus
Adrenals
Pancreas
Ovaries (female)
Testes (male)

cated in the pancreas, produce the insulin that regulates the amount of sugar in the bloodstream.

• *The liver,* the largest solid organ in the abdomen, lies immediately beneath the diaphragm in the right upper quadrant of the abdominal cavity. The liver produces bile, which aids in the digestion of fat. It stores sugars until they are needed by the body. It also produces components necessary for immune function, blood clotting, and the production of plasma. Finally, the toxic substances produced by digestion are rendered harmless in the liver.

• *The spleen* is a solid organ located in the left upper quadrant of the abdominal cavity. It helps in the production of red blood cells and filtration of the blood. If the spleen is injured or removed, its function is assumed by the liver and bone marrow.

• *The gallbladder* is a hollow pouch. Part of the *bile duct* leading from the liver, the gallbladder acts as a reservoir for bile. When food enters the small intestine, contractions are stimulated that empty the gallbladder into the small intestine, where the bile aids in the digestion of fats.

• *The small intestine* is made up of the *duodenum, jejunum,* and *ileum.* It receives food from the stomach and secretions from the pancreas and liver. Digestion of food continues in the small intestine,

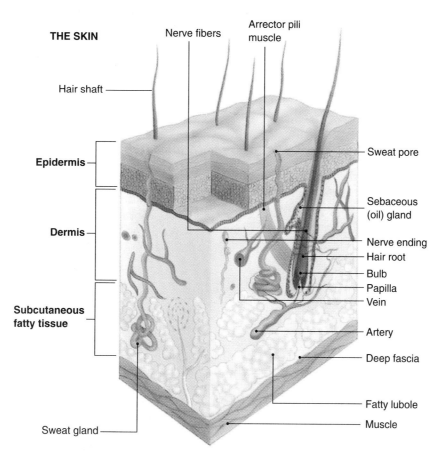

THE SKIN
Nerve fibers
Arrector pili muscle
Hair shaft
Epidermis
Dermis
Subcutaneous fatty tissue
Sweat gland
Sweat pore
Sebaceous (oil) gland
Nerve ending
Hair root
Bulb
Papilla
Vein
Artery
Deep fascia
Fatty lubole
Muscle

Figure 4-25   Anatomy of the skin.

ORGANS OF THE URINARY SYSTEM

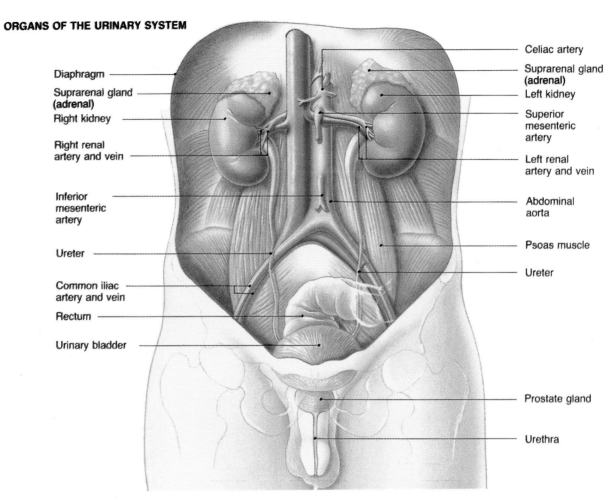

Figure 4-26 *The urinary system.*

where food is completely broken down into a form that can be used by the body. Nutrients are absorbed through the walls of the small intestine and circulated through the bloodstream to all parts of the body.

- *The large intestine* is also called the *colon*. The parts of food that cannot be absorbed by the body are passed as waste products from the small intestine to the large intestine. As these waste products move through the large intestine, their water is absorbed. What remains is the stool that is then passed through the rectum and the anus.

DIGESTIVE PROCESS

Digestion consists of two processes—one mechanical and the other chemical. The mechanical process includes chewing, swallowing, *peristalsis* (the rhythmic movement of matter through the digestive tract), and *defecation* (the elimination of digestive wastes). The chemical process of digestion occurs when *enzymes*, or digestive juices, break foods down into simple components that can be absorbed and used by the body. Carbohydrates are broken into glucose (simple

sugar), fats are changed into fatty acids, and proteins are converted to amino acids.

THE URINARY SYSTEM

The *urinary system* (Figure 4-26) filters and excretes wastes from the blood. It consists of two *kidneys*, which filter waste from the bloodstream and help control fluid balance; two *ureters*, which carry the wastes from the kidneys to the bladder; one *urinary bladder*, which stores the urine prior to excretion; and one *urethra*, which carries the urine from the bladder out of the body.

The urinary system helps the body maintain its delicate balance of water and various chemicals in the proportions needed for health and survival. During the process of urine formation, wastes are removed from the circulating blood for elimination, and useful products are returned to the blood.

THE REPRODUCTIVE SYSTEM

The *reproductive system* of women and men (Figure 4-27) consists of complementary organs that can function to accomplish reproduction. The male's

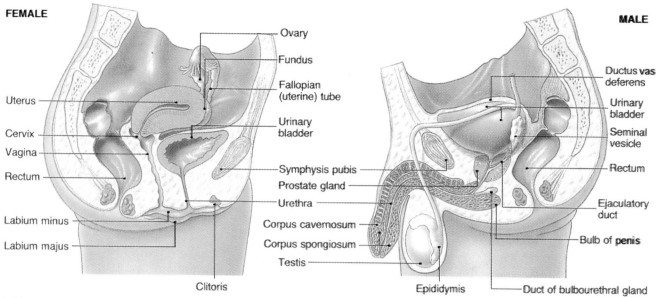

FEMALE

Uterus
Cervix
Vagina
Rectum
Labium minus
Labium majus
Clitoris

Ovary
Fundus
Fallopian (uterine) tube
Urinary bladder
Symphysis pubis
Prostate gland
Urethra
Corpus cavernosum
Corpus spongiosum
Testis

MALE

Ductus vas deferens
Urinary bladder
Seminal vesicle
Rectum
Ejaculatory duct
Bulb of penis
Duct of bulbourethral gland
Epididymis

Labium minus (singular), Labia minora (plural)
Labium majus (singular), Labia majora (plural)

Figure 4-27   The reproductive system.

sperm and the female's *ovum* contribute the genes that determine the hereditary characteristics of an offspring. Combination of a single sperm with a single ovum forms a fertilized ovum, which can grow into an *embryo*, then into a *fetus*, and finally into a newborn baby.

The reproductive system of the male includes two *testes*, a duct system, accessory glands (including the *prostate gland*), and the *penis*.

The female reproductive system consists of two *ovaries*, two *fallopian tubes*, the *uterus*, the *vagina*, and the external *genitals*.

CASE STUDY FOLLOW-UP

SCENE SIZE-UP

You have been dispatched to the scene of a 38-year-old woman who was burned when the fuel for a model airplane ignited. By the time you arrive, the fire has been extinguished and the fuel and airplane no longer pose a threat.

PATIENT ASSESSMENT

Your general impression is that the patient is experiencing extreme pain from burns to her right arm and the right side of her head. When you question the patient, she responds appropriately with her name—Sherry Washington—and is able to describe what happened. Her airway and breathing are adequate. You assess circulation and start oxygen therapy before proceeding with assessment and care.

Upon examining the injury sites, you find that the entire right arm from the elbow to the fingertips have been severely charred from the burning fuel. The burns to the head are minor but fairly extensive,

involving the right side of Ms. Washington's face and singing to the hair, and you notice some swelling of the mucous membranes in the mouth and singing of the nasal hair.

Pupils are equal and reactive to light. There are no other injuries noted to the head or neck. Breath sounds are equal bilaterally and the patient denies shortness of breath. You inspect the entire body for evidence of other burns. You find present pulses to all extremities, and the patient is able to move her extremities well.

While performing the physical exam, you also ask questions to gather the patient's history. The information you elicit is consistent with the burn injury. There is no other significant medical history.

Your partner readies the wheeled stretcher while you record the patient's vital signs. You find that blood pressure and heart rate are both slightly high while rate and depth of breathing are normal.

You gently place sterile burn sheets on the injury sites and try to help the patient relax as you and your partner prepare her for transport. You place her on the cot in a Fowler's position, which she finds is comfortable and helps her to breathe more easily.

En route to the hospital you reassess the patient's mental status, airway, respiration, and circulation, and ensure that the burn sheets are properly protecting the burned skin. Ms. Washington remains alert. You reassess vital signs and record your findings.

COMMUNICATION AND DOCUMENTATION

You notify the hospital en route, describing the types and locations of the burns. You tell the staff that there is a full thickness burn (through all layers of the skin) originating at the right elbow joint, which extends inferiorly and circumferentially to the distal fingers. The burn to the skull appears to be a superficial burn which involves the right cranium and face. The

facial burn involves the lateral aspect of the right mandible, maxilla, and zygomatic arch. The emergency department physician reminds you to stay alert to possible airway compromise from upper airway swelling secondary to the burns to the face.

When you arrive at the hospital, Ms. Washington is still alert and suffering severe pain but in no severe respiratory distress. You give a verbal report to the emergency department staff and help transfer the patient to a hospital bed. You and your partner then complete the prehospital care report, restock the ambulance, and prepare for another call.

Reflecting on this call, you are able to take pride in your ability to communicate clearly with the emergency department staff, and to document Ms. Washington's injuries in your prehospital care report, using correct anatomical terminology.

CHAPTER REVIEW

TERMS AND CONCEPTS

You may wish to review the following terms and concepts included in this chapter.

abdominal quadrants—the four parts of the abdomen as divided by imaginary horizontal and vertical lines through the umbilicus.
acetabulum (AS-i-TAB-u-lum)—the rounded cavity or socket on the external surface of the pelvis that receives the head of the femur.
acromion (ah-KRO-me-on)—the lateral triangular projection of the scapula that forms the point of the shoulder.
alveoli (al-VE-oh-le)—the air sacs of the lungs. Pl. of alveolus.
anatomical planes—imaginary straight-line divisions of the body.
anatomy—the study of the structure of the body and the relationship of its parts to each other.
anterior—toward the front. Opposite of *posterior.*
anterior plane—the front, or abdominal side of the body.
aorta (ay-OR-tah)—the major artery from the heart.
arteriole (ar-TE-re-ol)—the smallest branch of an artery, which at its distal end leads into a capillary.
artery—a blood vessel that carries blood away from the heart.

atria (AY-tre-uh)—the two upper chambers of the heart. Pl. of *atrium.*
bilateral—on both sides.
blood pressure—the force exerted by the blood on the interior walls of the blood vessels.
brachial (BRAY-ke-al) **artery**—the major artery of the upper arm.
bronchi (BRONG-ke)—the two main branches leading from the trachea to the lungs, providing the passageway for air movement. Pl. of *bronchus.*
bronchioles (BRONG-ke-olz)—small branches of the bronchi.
calcaneus (kal-KAY-ne-us)—the heel bone.
capillary (KAP-i-lair-e)—a tiny blood vessel that connects an arteriole to a venule.
cardiac muscle—a kind of involuntary muscle found only in the walls of the heart. Cardiac muscle has automaticity, the ability to generate an impulse on its own, separately from the central nervous system.
cardiovascular system—see *circulatory system.*
carotid (kah-ROT-id) **artery**—one of two major arteries of the neck, which supply the brain and head with blood.
carpals (KAR-pulz)—the eight bones that form the wrist.

central nervous system—the brain and the spinal cord. Abbr. CNS.

cervical (SER-vi-kal) **spine**—the first seven vertebrae, or the neck.

circulatory system—the body system that transports blood to all parts of the body. Includes the heart, blood vessels, and blood. Also called the *cardiovascular system*.

clavicle (KLAV-i-kul)—the collarbone, attached to the superior portion of the sternum.

coccyx (KOK-siks)—the last four vertebrae, or tailbone.

coronary (KOR-o-nair-e) **arteries**—blood vessels that supply the heart with blood.

cranium (KRAY-ne-um)—The bones that form the top, back, and sides of the skull plus the forehead.

cricoid (KRIK-oyd) **cartilage**—the lowermost cartilage of the larynx.

dermis—the second layer of the skin. See also *epidermis* and *subcutaneous layer*.

diaphragm (DI-ah-fram)—a powerful dome-shaped muscle essential to respiration that also separates the thoracic cavity from the abdominal cavity.

diastolic (di-as-TOL-ic) **blood pressure**—the pressure exerted against the walls of the arteries when the left ventricle is at rest. See also *systolic blood pressure*.

distal—distant, or far from the point of reference. Opposite of *proximal*.

dorsal—toward the back or spine. Opposite of *ventral*.

dorsalis pedis (dor-SAL-is PED-is) **artery**—an artery of the foot, which can be felt on the top surface of the foot.

endocrine (EN-do-krin) **system**—a system of ductless glands that produce hormones which regulate body functions.

epidermis (EP-i-DER-mis)—the outermost layer of the skin. See also *dermis* and *subcutaneous layer*.

epiglottis (EP-i-GLOT-is)—a small leaf-shaped flap of tissue, located immediately posterior to the root of the tongue, that covers the entrance of the larynx to keep food and liquid from entering the trachea and lungs.

esophagus (es-AH-fuh-gus)—a passageway at the lower end of the pharynx that leads to the stomach.

extremities—the limbs of the body. The lower extremities include the hips, thighs, legs, ankles, and feet. The upper extremities include the shoulder, arm, forearm, wrist, and hand.

face—the area of the skull between the brow and the chin.

femoral (FEM-or-al) **artery**—the major artery of the thigh that supplies the groin and leg with blood.

femur (FE-mer)—the thigh bone.

fibula (FIB-u-lah)—the lateral, smaller long bone of the lower leg.

Fowler's position—a position in which the patient is lying on the back with upper body elevated at a 45° to 60° angle.

heart—the muscular organ that contracts to force blood into circulation through the body.

humerus (HU-mer-us)—the largest bone in the upper extremity, located in the proximal portion of the upper arm.

hypoperfusion (HY-po-per-FU-zhun)—the insufficient delivery of oxygen and other nutrients to some of the body's cells and inadequate elimination of carbon dioxide and other wastes that results from inadequate circulation of blood. Also called *shock*.

iliac (IL-i-ak) **crest**—the upper margin of the bones of the pelvis.

inferior—beneath, lower, or toward the feet. Opposite to *superior*.

inferior plane—everything below the transverse line. Opposite to *superior plane*.

intercostal (in-ter-KOS-tal) **muscles**—the muscles between the ribs.

involuntary muscle—muscle that carries out the automatic muscular functions of the body. Also called *smooth muscle*.

ischium (IS-ke-um)—the posterior and inferior portion of the pelvis.

joint—a place where one bone meets another.

larynx (LAIR-inks)—structure that houses the vocal cords and is located inferior to the pharynx and superior to the trachea.

lateral (LAT-er-al)—refers to the left or right of the midline, or away from the midline, or to the side of the body. See also *medial*.

lateral recumbent—a position in which the patient is lying on the left or right side.

left—refers to the patient's left.

left plane—everything to the left of the midline.

lumbar (LUM-bar) **spine**—the five vertebrae that form the lower back, located between the sacral and the thoracic spine.

lungs—the principal organs of respiration.

malleolus (mal-E-o-lus)—the knobby surface landmark of the ankle. There is a medial malleolus and a lateral malleolus.

mandible (MAN-di-bl)—the lower jaw.

manubrium (ma-NU-bre-um)—the superior portion of the sternum where the clavicle is attached.

maxillae—the fused bones of the upper jaw.

medial—toward the midline or center of the body. See also *lateral*.

metacarpals (MET-uh-KAR-pulz)—the bones of the hand.

metatarsals (MET-uh-TAR-sulz)—the bones that form the arch of the foot.

midaxillary (mid-AX-uh-lar-e)—refers to the center of the armpit (axilla).

midaxillary line—an imaginary line that divides the body into anterior and posterior planes; the imaginary line from the middle of the armpit to the ankle.

midclavicular (mid-klav-IK-u-ler)—refers to the center of the collarbone (clavicle).

midclavicular line—the imaginary line from the center of either clavicle down the anterior thorax.

midline—an imaginary line drawn vertically through the middle of the patient's body, dividing it into right and left planes.

musculoskeletal (MUS-kyu-lo-SKEL-uh-tul) **system**—the system of bones and muscle plus connective tissue that provides support and protection to the body and permits motion.

nasal bones—the bones that form the bed of the nose.

nasopharynx (NA-zo-FAIR-inks)—nasal portion of the pharynx situated above the soft palate.

nervous system—the body system including the brain, spinal cord, and nerves, that controls the voluntary and involuntary activity of the human body.

normal anatomical position—a position in which the patient is standing erect, facing forward, with arms down at the sides and palms forward.

olecranon (o-LEK-ran-on)—the part of the ulna that forms the bony prominence of the elbow.

orbits—the eye sockets.

oropharynx (OR-o-FAIR-inks)—the central portion of the pharynx lying between the soft palate and the epiglottis with the mouth as the opening.

palmar—relates to the palm of the hand.

patella—the kneecap.

pelvis—the bones that form the floor of the abdominal cavity: the sacrum and coccyx of the spine, the iliac crests, the pubis, and the ischium.

perfusion—the delivery of oxygen and other nutrients to the cells of all organ systems, which results from the constant adequate circulation of blood through the capillaries.

peripheral nervous system—that portion of the nervous system located outside the brain and spinal cord. Abbr. PNS.

phalanges (fa-LAN-jez)—bones of the fingers, thumbs, and toes. Pl. of *phalanx*.

pharynx (FAIR-inks)—the throat, or passageway for air from the nasal cavity to the larynx and passageway for food from the mouth to the esophagus.

physiology (FIZ-e-OL-o-je)—the study of the function of the living body and its parts.

plantar—refers to the sole of the foot.

plasma—the liquid part of the blood.

platelets (PLATE-lets)—components of blood that are essential to the formation of blood clots.

posterior (pos-TE-re-or)—toward the back. Opposite of *anterior*.

posterior plane—the back or dorsal side of the body.

posterior tibial artery—a major artery that travels from the calf to the foot and that can be felt on the lateral surface of the ankle bone.

prone—lying on the stomach.

proximal (PROK-sim-al)—near the point of reference. Opposite of *distal*.

pubis (PYU-bis)—bone of the groin.

pulmonary artery—artery that leads from the right ventricle of the heart to the lungs.

pulmonary vein—vein that drains the lungs and returns the blood to the left atrium of the heart.

pulse—the wave of blood propelled through the arteries as a result of the contraction of the left ventricle.

radial artery—a major artery of the arm, distal to the elbow joint.

radius—the lateral bone of the forearm.

red blood cells—part of the blood that gives it its color, carries oxygen to body cells, and carries carbon dioxide away from body cells.

respiratory system—the organs involved in the exchange of gases between an organism and the atmosphere.

right—refers to the patient's right.

right plane—everything to the right of the midline.

sacral (SAY-krul) **spine**—five vertebrae which are fused together to form the rigid part of the posterior side of the pelvis. Also *sacrum*.

scapula (SKAP-u-la)—the shoulder blade.

shock—see *hypoperfusion*.

skull—the bony structure at the top of the spinal column that houses and protects the brain. The skull has two parts, the cranium and the face.

spinal column—the column of vertebrae that encloses the spinal cord.

sternum—the breastbone.

subcutaneous (SUB-kyu-TAY-ne-us) **layer**—a layer of fatty tissue just below the dermis. See also *dermis* and *epidermis*.

superior—above; toward the head. Opposite to *inferior*.

superior plane—everything above the transverse line. Opposite to *inferior plane*.

supine—lying on the back.

systolic (sis-TOL-ik) **blood pressure**—the pressure exerted against the walls of the arteries when the left ventricle contracts. See also *diastolic blood pressure*.

tarsals—the bones of the ankle, hind foot, and midfoot.

thoracic (tho-RAS-ik) **spine**—the upper back, or the twelve thoracic vertebrae directly inferior to the cervical spine.

thorax (THO-raks)—the chest, or that part of the body between the base of the neck and the diaphragm.

thyroid cartilage—the Adam's apple; the anterior cartilage that covers the larynx.

tibia—the medial, larger bone of the lower leg; the shinbone.

trachea (TRAY-ke-ah)—the windpipe.

transverse line—an imaginary line drawn horizontally through the waist to divide the body into the superior and inferior planes.

Trendelenburg (tren-DEL-en-burg) **position**—lying on the back with the lower part of the body elevated up to 12 inches.

ulna—the medial bone of the forearm.

valves—structures within the heart and circulatory system that keep blood flowing in one direction and prevent backflow.

vein—a blood vessel that carries blood back to the heart.

venae cavae—the principal veins that carry deoxygenated blood to the heart. Pl. of *vena cava*. The *superior vena cava* carries blood from the upper body; the *inferior vena cava* carries blood from the lower body.

ventral—toward the front, or toward the anterior portion of the body. Opposite of *dorsal*.

ventricles—the two lower chambers of the heart.

venule—the smallest branch of a vein.

vertebrae (VER-te-bray)—The 33 bony segments of the spinal column. Pl. of *vertebra*.

voluntary muscle—any muscle that can be consciously controlled by the individual. Also called *skeletal muscle*.

white blood cells—the part of the blood that helps the body's immune system defend against infection.

xiphoid (ZI-foyd) **process**—inferior portion of the sternum.

zygomatic (ZI-go-MAT-ic) **bones**—the cheek bones.

REVIEW QUESTIONS

1. Describe the following six positions: normal anatomical position, supine, prone, lateral recumbent, Fowler's, and Trendelenburg.
2. Define the following five descriptive terms: midline, midclavicular line, midaxillary line, plantar, and palmar. Also define the following five terms and name and define the opposite of each term: anterior, superior, dorsal, lateral, and distal.
3. Briefly describe the anatomy and physiology of the musculoskeletal system.
4. Briefly describe the anatomy and physiology of the respiratory system.
5. Briefly describe the anatomy and physiology of the circulatory system.
6. Identify the central and peripheral pulse points and their locations.
7. Define shock (hypoperfusion).
8. Briefly describe the anatomy and physiology of the nervous system.
9. Briefly describe the anatomy and physiology of the endocrine system.
10. Briefly describe the anatomy and physiology of the skin.

CHAPTER 5

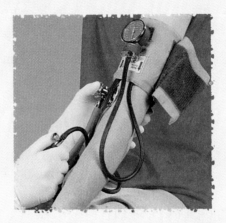

Baseline Vital Signs and History Taking

INTRODUCTION

As an EMT-B, you will perform a variety of skills necessary to manage a patient's injuries or illness. There is one skill, however, that you will perform on each and every one of your patients—one skill that is in fact the basis for all the emergency care you will provide. That skill is patient assessment.

Like putting together the pieces of a puzzle, the EMT-B uses each detail revealed by the assessment to help build a picture of the patient's condition and to make informed decisions on emergency care.

One set of details—accurate measurement and recording of vital signs over a period of time—may reveal a trend in the patient's condition that provides valuable information in the continuum of care. The patient history is just as important. It can guide your pace, shine light on underlying problems, and in the event that the patient loses consciousness, it can be the only source of patient information available to hospital personnel.

OBJECTIVES

Numbered objectives are from the United States Department of Transportation 1994 EMT-Basic National Standard Curriculum. Asterisked objectives, if any, pertain to material that is supplemental to the DOT curriculum.

COGNITIVE

1-5.1 Identify the components of vital signs. (p. 72)

1-5.2 Describe the methods to obtain a breathing rate. (p. 73)

1-5.3 Identify the attributes that should be obtained when assessing breathing. (p. 73)

1-5.4 Differentiate between shallow, labored, and noisy breathing. (p. 73)

1-5.5 Describe the methods to obtain a pulse rate. (pp. 73–74)

1-5.6 Identify the information obtained when assessing a patient's pulse. (pp. 74–75)

1-5.7 Differentiate between a strong, weak, regular, and irregular pulse. (p. 75)

1-5.8 Describe the methods to assess the skin color, temperature, and condition (capillary refill in infants and children). (pp. 75–77)

1-5.9 Identify the normal and abnormal skin colors. (p. 76)

1-5.10 Differentiate between pale, blue, red, and yellow skin color. (p. 76)

1-5.11 Identify the normal and abnormal skin temperature. (p. 76)

1-5.12 Differentiate between hot, cool, and cold skin temperature. (p. 76)

1-5.13 Identify normal and abnormal skin conditions. (p. 76)

1-5.14 Identify normal and abnormal capillary refill in infants and children. (p. 77)

1-5.15 Describe the methods to assess the pupils. (p. 77)

1-5.16 Identify normal and abnormal pupil size. (p. 77)

1-5.17 Differentiate between dilated (big) and constricted (small) pupil size. (p. 77)

1-5.18 Differentiate between reactive and nonreactive pupils and equal and unequal pupils. (p. 77)

1-5.19 Describe the methods to assess blood pressure. (pp. 77–79)

1-5.20 Define systolic pressure. (pp. 77–78)

1-5.21 Define diastolic pressure. (p. 78)

1-5.22 Explain the difference between auscultation and palpation for obtaining a blood pressure. (p. 78)

1-5.23 Identify the components of the SAMPLE history. (pp. 79–80)

1-5.24 Differentiate between a sign and a symptom. (p. 79)

1-5.25 State the importance of accurately reporting and recording the baseline vital signs. (p. 72)

1-5.26 Discuss the need to search for additional medical identification. (p. 80)

AFFECTIVE

1-5.27 Explain the value of performing the baseline vital signs. (pp. 70, 72)

1-5.28 Recognize and respond to the feelings patients experience during assessment. (p. 72)

1-5.29 Defend the need for obtaining and recording an accurate set of vital signs. (pp. 70, 72)

1-5.30 Explain the rationale for recording additional sets of vital signs. (p. 72)

1-5.31 Explain the importance of obtaining a SAMPLE history. (pp. 70, 79)

PSYCHOMOTOR

1-5.32 Demonstrate the skills involved in assessment of breathing.

1-5.33 Demonstrate the skills associated with obtaining a pulse.

1-5.34 Demonstrate the skills associated with assessing skin color, temperature, condition, and capillary refill in infants and children.

1-5.35 Demonstrate the skills associated with assessing the pupils.

1-5.36 Demonstrate the skills associated with obtaining blood pressure.

1-5.37 Demonstrate the skills that should be used to obtain information from the patient, family, or bystanders at the scene.

CASE STUDY

THE DISPATCH

EMS Unit 114—proceed to 1895 East State Street for an unknown medical emergency called in by a family member—time out 1748 hours.

ON ARRIVAL

Upon arrival a woman approaches you. She says she is the patient's daughter, Ms. Kennedy. She adds that she has been trying to reach her father, Mr. Li, by phone all day, but he had not answered. After driving to her father's house, she says, she broke in and found her father lying on the floor in the kitchen. The daughter adds that Mr. Li seems pretty weak and in pain.

How would you proceed to assess and care for this patient?

During this chapter, you will learn about taking vital signs and a patient history. Later, we will return to the case and put in context some of the information you learned.

When you arrive at the scene of an emergency call, you will need to find out all you can about the patient's condition: What's wrong with the patient right now? What led up to the problem? and so on. The process of finding out is called assessment. Most of your EMT-B course and most of the chapters of this text will be devoted to teaching you how to assess, as well as how to care for, a patient in the prehospital setting.

Much of the information you gain during assessment is readily obvious or available. An open bottle of bleach may provide the clue to a poisoning. The patient or a family member may tell you the chief complaint—for example, "I can't catch my breath," or "I hurt my leg when I fell." The fact that the patient is answering questions clearly may tell you that he is alert, has an open airway, is breathing, and has a pulse. As you conduct a physical exam, you may spot swelling, cuts, bruises, or other signs of injury.

Other indications of the patient's condition require a bit of "detective work"—some special skills for finding out more than what is readily obvious. These skills include measuring the patient's vital signs and asking questions to obtain the patient's history.

Always be aware of the feelings, such as anxiety or embarrassment, that a patient may experience during assessment. Continually reassure the patient and respect his dignity.

BASELINE VITAL SIGNS

 You can't get inside the patient's body to see what is going on, but you can measure the **vital signs.** These are the "signs of life"—outward signs that give clues to what is happening inside the body. The vital signs that you will measure are:

- *Breathing*
- *Pulse*
- *Skin*
- *Pupils*
- *Blood pressure*

Correctly reading and interpreting the vital signs significantly impacts the success of prehospital emergency care as well as providing critical information for the hospital staff. Taking two or more sets of vital signs and comparing them will reveal changes in the patient's condition and may indicate how effectively you are managing the patient's injury or illness, or if the patient is deteriorating. The first set of measurements you take are known as the **baseline vital signs,** to which subsequent measurements can be compared.

While you can monitor most of the vital signs with your senses (looking, listening, feeling), it is best that you use and routinely carry the following equipment:

- A **sphygmomanometer** (blood pressure cuff) in adult and pediatric sizes to measure blood pressure
- A stethoscope to take blood pressure and listen to lung sounds
- A wristwatch that counts seconds to measure pulse and respiratory rates
- A penlight to examine pupils
- A pair of heavy-duty bandage scissors for cutting away clothing
- A pen and pocket notebook for entering vital signs and other findings
- Your personal protective equipment for body substance isolation, such as protective gloves, eyewear, and face mask

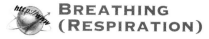 # BREATHING (RESPIRATION)

BREATHING (RESPIRATORY) RATE

The breathing (respiratory) rate is assessed by observing the patient's chest rise and fall (Figure 5-1). Normal ranges for the number of respirations per minute are (Table 5-1):

- Adults—12 to 20 per minute.
- Children—15 to 30 per minute.
- Infants—25 to 50 per minute.

Breathing, or respiratory, rate—the number of respirations per minute—is usually determined by counting the number of breaths in a 30-second period and multiplying by 2. (One breath = one inhalation + one exhalation.) If the patient knows you are counting, it can influence the rate. Instead, you can pretend you are checking the radial pulse and cross the patient's arm over the lower chest while actually counting respirations.

BREATHING (RESPIRATORY) QUALITY

Determining quality of breathing, or respiration, is as important as determining rate. It will tell you how much air is moving in and out of the lungs per minute and how well it is moving. The quality of breathing may be normal or abnormal. An abnormal quality of breathing may be shallow, labored, or noisy. You can assess the quality of breathing while you are counting the rate.

- *Normal breathing* involves average chest wall motion, which is at least one inch of expansion in an outward direction. The patient does not use the ac-

TABLE 5-1

Normal Breathing Rates

Patient	Normal Breathing Rate
Adult	12 to 20 per minute
Child	15 to 30 per minute
Infant	25 to 50 per minute

cessory muscles of the chest, neck, or abdomen while breathing. Rate is normal, and inhalations and exhalations are about the same length. Normal breathing is quiet; it does not produce abnormal sounds or noises.
- *Shallow breathing* is indicated by only slight chest or abdominal wall motion.
- *Labored breathing,* where the patient is working hard to breathe, is indicated by an abnormal sound of breathing that may include grunting or **stridor** (a harsh, high pitched sound), the use of accessory muscles to breathe, nasal flaring, and sometimes gasping. In infants and children there also may be retraction of the skin, muscles, and other tissues around the clavicle and between the ribs.
- *Noisy breathing,* or an abnormal sound of breathing (Table 5-2), may include snoring, wheezing, gurgling, crowing, or stridor. Auscultate the chest with a stethoscope to determine if breath sounds are present on both sides and to identify any noisy breathing sounds not audible to the ear alone.

Remember to record your observations.

BREATHING (RESPIRATORY) RHYTHM

The breathing, or respiratory, rhythm—the regularity or irregularity of respirations—can be easily affected by speech, activity, emotions, and other factors in the conscious and alert patient. However, an abnormal respiratory rhythm—that is, an irregular pattern of respiration—in the patient with an altered mental status is a serious concern. It may indicate a medical illness, a chemical imbalance, or a brain injury. It is important to assess for adequacy of breathing when faced with an irregular breathing pattern and to document and report your findings.

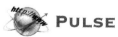 # PULSE

LOCATION OF PULSES

The pulse is the pressure wave generated by the contraction of the left ventricle. It directly reflects the rhythm, rate, and relative strength of the contraction of the heart, and it can be felt at any point where an artery crosses over a bone and is near the surface of skin. Central pulses (carotid and femoral) and periph-

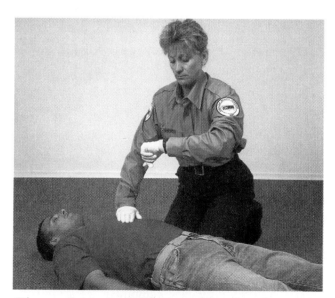

Figure 5-1 *Assess the breathing (respiratory) rate, quality, and rhythm.*

TABLE 5-2

Noisy Breathing

Sound	Potential Cause
Snoring	Tongue partially blocking the upper airway at the level of the pharynx
Wheezing	Constriction (narrowing) of the bronchioles in the lungs
Gurgling	Fluid in the upper airway
Crowing or stridor (Harsh, high-pitched sound)	Partial obstruction of the upper airway at the level of the larynx

eral pulses (radial, brachial, tibial, and dorsalis pedis) can be felt at the following locations:

- *Carotid artery,* on either side of the neck in the groove between the trachea and the muscle mass.
- *Femoral artery,* in the crease between the abdomen and the groin.
- *Radial artery,* proximal to the thumb on the wrist.
- *Brachial artery,* on the medial aspect of the arm, midway between the shoulder and the elbow.
- *Posterior tibial artery,* posterior to the lateral ankle bone.
- *Dorsalis pedis artery,* on the top of the foot.

A radial pulse should be assessed in all patients 1 year or older (Figure 5-2). In patients younger than 1 year, assess a brachial pulse (Figures 5-3a and b). When a peripheral pulse cannot be obtained, take the carotid pulse (Figure 5-4). In palpating the carotid pulse take care not to cut off circulation to the brain. Avoid excessive pressure in elderly patients and never assess the carotid pulse on both sides at once.

Always try to assess pulses in several areas, both central and peripheral locations, to determine how well the entire circulatory system is functioning. If the pulse is present, assess its rate and quality.

PULSE RATE

A pulse rate should be taken as soon as possible and frequently. The normal resting rate is 60 to 80 beats per minute for an adult, 60 to 105 for an adolescent, 60 to 120 for a school-age child, 80 to 150 for a preschooler, and 120 to 150 for an infant (Table 5-3).

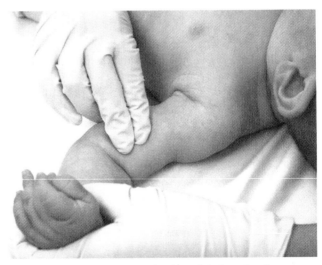

Figure 5-3a   Assess the brachial pulse in patients who are less than 1 year of age.

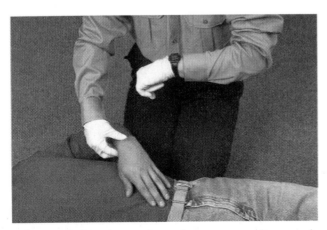

Figure 5-2   Assess the pulse rate, quality, and rhythm. The radial pulse is assessed in patients older than 1 year of age.

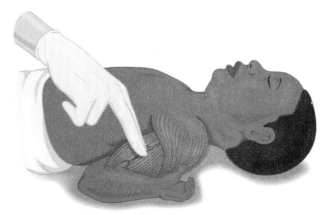

Figure 5-3b   Taking a brachial pulse.

The pulse can help you gauge what is happening to the patient. For example, a rapid pulse may indicate shock (hypoperfusion). Absence of a pulse indicates that the heart has stopped beating, the blood pressure is extremely low, or the artery has been blocked or injured. Absence of a pulse in a single extremity may indicate obstruction to the artery in that extremity and may be associated with bone or joint injuries. If so, the patient may complain of numbness, weakness, and tingling, and the skin may gradually turn mottled, blue, and cold.

PULSE QUALITY AND RHYTHM

The quality of the pulse can be characterized as strong or weak, the rhythm regular or irregular (Table 5-4).

- *Strong pulse* usually refers to a pulse that is both full and normally strong. A "bounding" pulse is one that is abnormally strong.
- *Weak pulse* is one that doesn't feel full or may be difficult to find and palpate. A weak pulse may also be quite rapid. The general term for a weak, rapid pulse is "thready."
- *Regular pulse* is usually a normal pulse that occurs at regular intervals with a smooth rhythm.
- *Irregular pulse* is one that occurs at irregular intervals, which may indicate a cardiac disease.

Remember to record the pulse quality.

SKIN

The appearance and condition of the skin (Table 5-5) is another important indicator of the body's perfusion status. In assessing the skin, you should check color, temperature, condition, and (in children under 6 years) capillary refill.

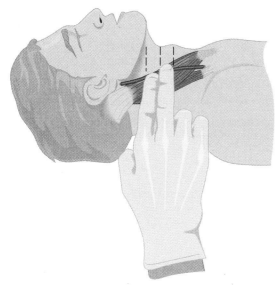

Figure 5-4   Locating and assessing the carotid pulse.

To take the pulse rate:

1. Position the patient. He should be sitting or lying down.
2. Using the tips of two or three fingers, palpate the artery (feel it gently). Avoid using your thumb, because it has a prominent pulse of its own.
3. Count the number of beats in a 30-second period. Then multiply by 2. An irregular pulse should be taken for a full minute.

TABLE 5-3

Normal and Abnormal Pulse Rates

Patient	Pulse Rate approx. per minute at rest	Description
Adult	60 to 80	Normal
	100+	Rapid
	Below 60	Slow
Adolescent	60 to 105	Normal
	Above 105	Rapid
	Below 60	Slow
Child (5-12 years)	60 to 120	Normal
	Above 120	Rapid
	Below 60	Slow
Child (1-5 years)	80 to 150	Normal
	Above 150	Rapid
	Below 80	Slow
Infant	120 to 150	Normal
	Above 150	Rapid
	Below 120	Slow

TABLE 5-4

Pulse Rate, Quality, Rhythm, and Related Problems

Pulse	Possible Problem
Rapid, regular, and full	Exertion, fright, fever, high blood pressure, or first stages of blood loss
Rapid, regular, and thready	Reliable sign of shock, often evident in later stage of blood loss
Slow	Head injury, barbiturate or narcotic use, some poisons, possible cardiac problems
No pulse	Cardiac arrest

TABLE 5-5

Skin Color, Temperature, and Condition

Color	Possible Problem
Pallor (white)	Vasoconstriction, blood loss, shock, heart attack, fright, anemia, fainting, emotional distress
Cyanosis (blue-gray)	Inadequate oxygenation or perfusion (shock), inadequate respiration; heart attack, poisoning
Flushing (red)	Heat exposure, carbon monoxide poisoning
Jaundice (yellow)	Liver disease
Temperature	**Possible Problem**
Hot	Fever, heat exposure
Cool	Inadequate circulation (shock), cold exposure
Cold	Extreme cold exposure
Condition	**Possible Problem**
Wet or moist	Shock, heat emergency, diabetic emergency
Abnormally dry	Spinal injury, dehydration

SKIN COLOR

Skin color indicates how well the blood is being oxygenated and circulated to the skin and, therefore, how well the lungs and heart, respiratory and circulatory system, are functioning. In all patients, check the color of the nail beds, **oral mucosa** (mucous membranes of the mouth), and **conjunctiva** (mucous membranes that line the eyelid). They all should be pink. In infants and children and dark-skinned people, check the palms of the hands and the soles of the feet. They should be pink, too.

Abnormal skin colors include:

- *Paleness,* or **pallor,** may be a sign of extreme vasoconstriction, blood loss, or both. It may indicate shock (hypoperfusion), heart attack, fright, anemia, fainting, or emotional distress.
- *Blue-gray color,* or **cyanosis,** indicates inadequate oxygenation or poor perfusion. It often appears first in the fingertips and around the mouth. It can indicate suffocation, inadequate respirations, lack of oxygen, heart attack, or poisoning. Cyanosis always indicates a serious problem but often is seen very late.
- *Red color,* or **flushing,** may be a sign of heat exposure or late carbon monoxide poisoning.
- *Yellow color,* or **jaundice,** may indicate liver disease.

SKIN TEMPERATURE

The most common measurement of temperature in the field is *relative skin temperature* (Figure 5-5). This can be assessed by placing the back of your hand against the patient's skin. Relative skin temperature is not a precise measurement but is a good indicator of abnormally low or high temperatures.

Normal skin feels warm to the touch. Abnormal skin temperatures include:

- *Hot,* which indicates a fever or exposure to heat
- *Cool,* which may be a sign of inadequate circulation, shock, or exposure to cold
- *Cold,* which indicates extreme exposure to cold

Changes in skin temperature over a period of time, or different temperatures in various parts of the body, can be significant. For example, circulatory problems can result in a cold foot, while an isolated "hot" area may indicate a localized infection.

SKIN CONDITION

Normally, skin is dry. Wet or moist skin may indicate shock (hypoperfusion), poisoning, a heat-related, cardiac, or diabetic emergency, or many other conditions. Skin that is abnormally dry may be a sign of spinal injury or severe dehydration.

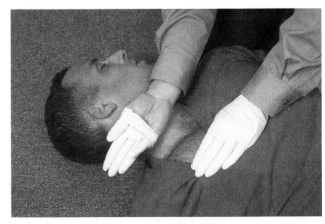

Figure 5-5 Assess relative skin temperature.

CAPILLARY REFILL

The time it takes for compressed capillaries to fill up again with blood is called **capillary refill** time. It is a reliable sign more in infants and children less than 6 years of age (Figure 5-6).

To measure capillary refill, press firmly on the skin or nail bed. When you remove your finger, the compressed area will be white. Count the time it takes to return to the original color. Normal capillary refill takes less than 2 seconds. When it takes longer, the circulation of blood through the capillaries may be inadequate, indicating that the patient is suffering from shock (hypoperfusion). Capillary refill alone does not provide enough information to determine shock. You need to look at the entire patient and other signs and symptoms. It is important also to look at the color of the mucous membranes inside the mouth, especially in an adult, as a reliable indicator of perfusion status.

PUPILS

To assess the pupils, briefly shine a light into the patient's eyes (Figure 5-7 and Table 5-6).

- **Size.** Pupils that are **dilated** (too large) may indicate cardiac arrest or the use of certain drugs including LSD, amphetamines, and cocaine. Pupils that are **constricted** (too small) may indicate a central nervous system disorder or the use of narcotics.
- **Equality.** Pupils of unequal size may indicate a stroke, head injury, or an artificial eye. A few people normally have unequal pupils; if it is a normal condition, however, the pupils remain reactive to light.
- **Reactivity.** Normally, pupils react to light by constricting. Nonreactive pupils may indicate cardiac

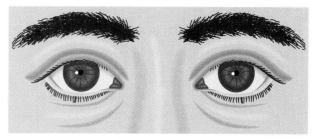

Constricted pupils

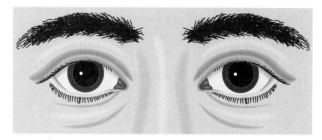

Dilated pupils

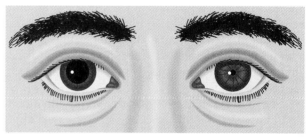

Unequal pupils

Figure 5-7   Assess pupils for size, equality, and reactivity.

arrest, brain injury, or the use of drugs. If one pupil reacts but the other does not, suspect stroke or head injury.

 BLOOD PRESSURE

Low blood pressure indicates that there is not enough pressure in the arteries to keep the organs supplied adequately with blood. This can lead to severe damage to the organs and death. Blood pressure can fall drastically due to blood loss, cardiac pump failure, or blood vessel dilation associated with conditions such as severe bleeding, heart attack, or spinal injury. Low blood pressures may be an indication of poor perfusion, also known as *hypoperfusion*, or *shock. High blood pressure* can result from a variety of factors. The abnormal pressure can rupture or damage arteries, including those in the brain and cause the heart to function poorly.

- **Systolic pressure** is the amount of pressure exerted against the walls of the arteries when the left ventricle of the heart contracts. It is assessed as the

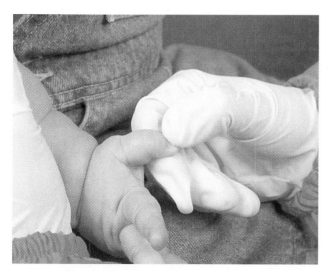

Figure 5-6   Assess capillary refill in infants and children less than 6 years of age.

TABLE 5-6

Pupil Size, Equality, and Reactivity

Factor	Possible Problem
Dilated	Cardiac arrest, drug use such as LSD, amphetamines, cocaine
Constricted	Central nervous system disorder, narcotics use
Unequal	Stroke, head injury, artificial eye (occasionally a normal finding), eye drops
Nonreactive	Cardiac arrest, brain injury, drug use

first distinct sound of blood flowing through the artery as the pressure in the sphygmomanometer (blood pressure cuff) is released.

- **Diastolic pressure** is the pressure exerted against the walls of the arteries while the left ventricle of the heart is at rest. It is assessed as the point during deflation of the sphygmomanometer when the beating or swooshing sounds are no longer heard.

The systolic and diastolic readings obtained when you measure blood pressure are expressed in millimeters of mercury (mmHg), the units that correspond to marks on the sphygmomanometer gauge. For example, a blood pressure with a systolic reading of 120 and a diastolic reading of 80 would be expressed as 120/80 mmHg.

The usual guide for normal systolic pressure in the adult male is 100 plus the patient's age, up to 150 mmHg. Normal diastolic pressure in the adult male is 60 to 90 mmHg. Normal systolic and diastolic pressures in the female are both 8 to 10 mmHg lower than in the male. A blood pressure of 120/80 in an adult is an average systolic and diastolic reading, not "the normal" blood pressure. The high end of a normal systolic blood pressure in an infant or child is 90 + (2 × the age in years). The lower end of a normal systolic blood pressure in the infant and child is 70 + (2 × the age in years) (Table 5-7). (Blood pressure is usually not measured in children less than 3 years of age; in these patients, pulse, skin, and mental status are better indicators of perfusion.) "Normal" blood pressures vary widely. Treat the patient, not the blood pressure.

With most diseases or injuries, the two pressures will either rise or fall together. However, there are ex-

ceptions: head injury, cardiac tamponade (a condition that occurs when the sac around the heart fills with blood), and tension pneumothorax (when one lung collapses and compresses the heart and the uninjured lung). Head injury may cause a rise in systolic pressure accompanied by a stable or falling diastolic pressure. Cardiac tamponade and tension pneumothorax cause a rise in diastolic pressure and a drop in systolic pressure.

There are two methods of measuring blood pressure with a sphygmomanometer: by **auscultation,** or listening for the systolic and diastolic sounds through a stethoscope (Figure 5-8), and by **palpation,** or feeling for the return of the pulse as the cuff is deflated (Figure 5-9).

To assess blood pressure by auscultation:

1. *Choose the proper size sphygmomanometer cuff.* It should completely encircle the patient's bare arm about one inch above the antecubital space (at the front of the elbow) without overlapping. The cuff should cover two-thirds of the upper arm. Its bladder should be centered over the brachial artery, and cover half the arm's circumference. Properly fitted, the cuff should fit snugly, but you should still be able to place one finger easily under its bottom edge.
2. *Inflate the cuff* to 30 mmHg above the point where you can no longer palpate the radial pulse.
3. *Apply the stethoscope* to the brachial pulse in the antecubital space. Hold the diaphragm of the stethoscope with your thumb or fingers.
4. *Deflate the cuff* at approximately 2 mmHg per second, watching the pressure indicator drop.
5. *As soon as you hear two or more consecutive beats*

TABLE 5-7

Normal Blood Pressure Ranges

Patient	Systolic	Diastolic
Adult male	Patient's age + 100 (up to 150 mmHg)	60 to 90 mmHg
Adult female	Patient's age + 90 (up to 140 mmHg)	50 to 80 mmHg
Infants and children	90 + (2 × age in years)—high end of normal	2/3 systolic
	70 + (2 × age in years)—low end of normal	

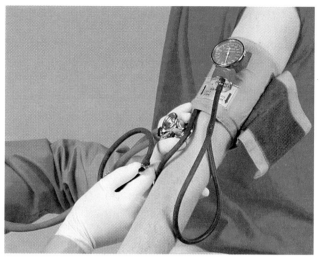

Figure 5-8 Taking blood pressure by auscultation.

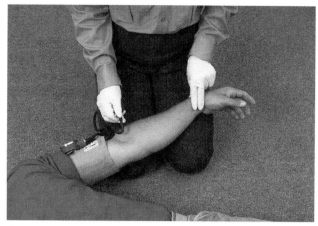

Figure 5-9 Taking blood pressure by palpation.

(clear but dull tapping sounds of increasing intensity), *record the pressure.* This is the systolic pressure.

6. *Continue releasing air from the bulb.* At the point where you hear the last sound, record the diastolic pressure. Continue to deflate slowly for at least 10 mmHg. With children and some adults, you may hear sounds all the way to zero. In those cases, record the pressure when the sound changes from a clear tapping to a soft, muffled tapping.

7. *After you have recorded the blood pressure, leave the cuff deflated but in place* so you can take more blood pressure readings during treatment and transport. Carefully record the blood pressure each time you take it. Changes can be significant.

To measure the blood pressure by palpation:

1. *Inflate the cuff rapidly* with the rubber bulb while palpating the radial pulse until you can no longer feel it. (Make a mental note of that reading.) Without stopping, continue to inflate the cuff to 30 mmHg above the level where the radial pulse could no longer be felt.

2. *Slowly deflate the cuff.* Make a note of the pressure at which the radial pulse returns. This is the systolic pressure as measured by palpation. In a noisy situation where you cannot hear well enough to measure the blood pressure by auscultation, this will be the only blood pressure measurement you can make. You will not be able to measure the diastolic pressure by palpation. Record the palpated blood pressure as, for example, 120/P.

Blood pressure should be measured in all patients older than 3 years of age. In infants or young children, however, the general appearance, physical assessment, and quality of pulse are more valuable than the blood pressure.

VITAL SIGN REASSESSMENT

If the patient is stable, vital signs should be taken and recorded at least every 15 minutes and as often as necessary to assure proper care. Take and record vital signs every 5 minutes if the patient is unstable. Reassess vital signs immediately following every medical intervention, regardless of how soon it follows your previous assessment of vital signs.

THE SAMPLE HISTORY

The **SAMPLE history** is a medical history of the patient that you gather by asking questions of the patient, family, and bystanders. *SAMPLE* is an acronym used to help you remember the information that must be included in a patient history. It spells out the first letters of the following categories:

• *Signs and symptoms.* **Signs** are any objective physical evidence of medical or trauma conditions that you can see, hear, feel, or smell. For example, you can hear stridor, you can see bleeding, and you can feel skin temperature. **Symptoms** are conditions that cannot be observed and must be described by the patient, such as pain in the abdomen or numbness in the legs. When you begin to question the patient, ask: What are you feeling? When and where did the first symptoms occur? What were you doing at the time? Another mnemonic used to evaluate the patient's symptoms is OPQRST (onset, provocation/palliation, quality, radiation, severity, and time). OPQRST questions will be discussed in detail in the section titled "Responsive Medical Patient" in Chapter 9.

- *Allergies.* Determine whether the patient has any allergies to medications, food, or environmental agents such as pollen, grass, ragweed, or molds. If you have not already done so during the physical exam, check for a medical alert tag, necklace, anklet, or bracelet, which can alert you to an allergy or other medical problem.
- *Medications.* Has the patient taken any medications recently? Is the patient taking any medications regularly? It is important to determine if the patient takes (1) prescription medications, (2) non-prescription or over-the-counter medications, (3) birth control pills, or (4) illicit drugs. If you suspect illegal drug use, you might say something like, "I'm an EMT, not a police officer. I need all the information you can give me so I can provide the proper care. Let's work on helping you right now." As with allergies, look for a medical alert tag if the patient is unresponsive.
- *Pertinent past history.* Find out about underlying medical problems like epilepsy, heart disease, diabetes, kidney disease, or emphysema. Ask if there have been past surgical procedures or trauma, and whether or not the patient is currently under a doctor's care. Again, look for a medical alert tag if the patient is unresponsive.
- *Last oral intake.* Find out when the patient last ingested a solid or liquid. Find out what it was, when it was consumed, and the quantity that was consumed. Ask: When did you last eat or drink anything?

- *Events leading to the injury or illness.* What occurred before the patient became ill or had the accident? Were there any unusual circumstances? What was the patient doing? Did the patient have any peculiar feelings or experiences?

As you conduct a SAMPLE history, try to get more detailed information about the conditions that are directly related to or that could adversely affect the present problem. If you are caring for a burn victim, for example, it would be important to learn if there are underlying cardiac or respiratory problems that might impair breathing. It would *not* be relevant to learn that the patient had a hernia surgery five years ago or had measles as a child.

To gather the most effective information, ask open-ended questions when you can—ones that cannot be answered merely yes or no but require a fuller response or description from the patient. Then wait for the patient's response. Whenever trauma is involved, try to identify the *mechanism of injury* (the manner by which the injury occurred) through observation or questioning. Pertinent negatives, things the patient denies, are also important to note. For example if you ask a patient with chest pain if he is short of breath and he says no, you would document "patient denies having shortness of breath." Finally, remember to write all pertinent findings from the SAMPLE history on the patient's record.

CASE STUDY FOLLOW-UP

SCENE SIZE-UP

You have been dispatched to the scene of an 86-year-old male who lives alone. His daughter, who found him, reports that the patient, Mr. Li, fell early this morning and was unable to get up. As you and your partner enter the home you note no safety hazards.

Upon entering the kitchen, you see Mr. Li supine on the floor, eyes closed, with a blanket covering him from shoulders to feet. The kitchen is very tidy and clean. The daughter, Ms. Kennedy, says she thinks he fell off a chair he had been standing on to reach the top of a cupboard.

PATIENT ASSESSMENT

You crouch next to Mr. Li as your partner provides manual stabilization of his head and neck and ask, "Are you okay?" He opens his eyes and responds, "I think so." You check for life-threatening problems with airway, breathing, or circulation and find none.

You determine that there is time to conduct a more thorough exam before you transport Mr. Li to the hospital.

You administer oxygen, conduct a head-to-toe physical exam (during which you discover that Mr. Li is wearing a bracelet identifying him as a diabetic), and apply a spinal cervical immobilization collar. Then you obtain a set of baseline vital signs. Your findings are: respirations 18 and normal; pulse 78 and regular; skin pink, warm, and dry; pupils normal, equal, and reactive; and blood pressure 168/82.

Finally, you gather a SAMPLE history. By questioning Mr. Li and his daughter, you learn that Mr. Li's main symptom is the pain in his left hip, which he says was brought on by the fall about an hour ago. In answer to your questions, he says the pain is especially severe when he tries to move his left leg, describes the pain as sharp, and says it does not radiate to any other location. Mr. Li also states that he is allergic to penicillin. Questioned about his medications, he says he takes insulin daily to help control blood sugar. When you ask about pertinent past history, the daughter confirms that Mr. Li has a history of diabetes and tells you that he had both hip joints replaced in 1989. You inquire about last oral intake—what Mr. Li last ate or drank—and Mr. Li says he has not eaten a meal since dinner last night. Ms. Kennedy adds that while they were waiting for the ambulance, she gave her father a glass of water. The patient describes the events that led to the injury by explaining that he slipped and fell from the chair at about 9 A.M.

You prepare your patient for transport by applying a splint to the left leg and hip, immobilizing him to a long spine board, securing him to your wheeled stretcher, and placing him in the ambulance.

En route to the hospital, you reassess Mr. Li's airway, breathing, and circulation and find no abnor-malities. You frequently check that he is comfortable, that he is properly secured to the splint, spine board, and stretcher, and that the oxygen mask is secure and oxygen flowing properly. You repeat the physical exam to the extent possible without interfering with immobilization. Mr. Li's condition seems stable. Because Mr. Li is considered stable, you repeat and record his vital signs every 15 minutes before reaching the hospital without finding any significant changes. You also repeat the SAMPLE history without discovering any significant additional details. Transport is uneventful, and you transfer Mr. Li to the emergency department personnel without a problem. After completing a prehospital care report, you and your partner prepare the ambulance for the next call.

CHAPTER REVIEW

TERMS AND CONCEPTS

You may wish to review the following terms and concepts included in this chapter.

auscultation—the process of listening for sounds within the body with a stethoscope.

baseline vital signs—the first set of vital signs measurements to which subsequent measurements can be compared. See *vital signs.*

capillary refill—the amount of time it takes for capillaries that have been compressed to refill with blood.

conjunctiva—mucous membranes that line the eyelid.

constricted—narrowed, made small.

cyanosis—a blue-gray color of the mucous membranes and/or skin, which indicates inadequate oxygenation or poor perfusion.

diastolic pressure—the pressure exerted against the walls of the arteries while the left ventricle of the heart is at rest. See also *systolic pressure.*

dilated—expanded, made large.

flushing—abnormally red skin color.

jaundice—a condition characterized by yellowness of skin, whites of eyes, mucous membranes, and body fluids.

oral mucosa—mucous membranes of the mouth.

pallor—pale or abnormally white skin color.

palpation—feeling, as for a pulse.

SAMPLE history—a type of patient history. *SAMPLE* is an acronym used to remember categories of information necessary to the patient history: signs and symptoms, allergies, medications, pertinent past history, last oral intake, and events leading to the injury or illness.

signs—any objective evidence of medical or trauma conditions that can be seen, heard, felt, or smelled in a patient. See also *symptoms.*

sphygmomanometer—instrument used to measure blood pressure. Also called a *blood pressure cuff.*

stridor—a harsh, high pitched sound resembling the blowing of the wind, associated with obstruction of upper air passages, usually heard on inspiration.

symptoms—conditions that must be described by the patient because they cannot be observed by another person. See also *signs.*

systolic pressure—the amount of pressure exerted against the walls of the arteries when the left ventricle of the heart contracts.

vital signs—the traditional signs of life; assessments related to breathing, pulse, skin, pupils, and blood pressure. See also *baseline vital signs.*

REVIEW QUESTIONS

1. Identify the components of vital signs, and state how often they should be taken.
2. Explain how to assess a patient's breathing rate and quality of breathing. Also state the normal ranges of respirations per minute for the adult, child, and infant.
3. Describe what you would observe when a patient is breathing normally and when a patient is breathing abnormally.
4. State the general circumstances under which you would choose to take a radial pulse, a brachial pulse, or a carotid pulse.
5. Explain how to take a pulse. Also identify normal resting pulse rates in an adult, adolescent, school-age child, preschool child, and infant.
6. Define the terms that you would use to describe pulse quality.
7. List the places on the body to check for skin color. Also identify normal and abnormal skin colors.
8. Explain how to assess a patient's pupils, and describe normal and abnormal findings.
9. Explain how to take a blood pressure by palpation and by auscultation. Also identify the normal ranges of systolic and diastolic blood pressure for an adult male and an adult female.
10. Name the categories of information you need to obtain through a SAMPLE history.

CHAPTER 6

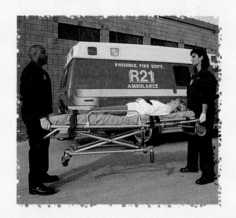

Preparing to Lift and Move Patients

INTRODUCTION

Many EMT-Basics are injured every year because they attempt to lift patients or equipment improperly. The knowledge and use of proper body mechanics are a necessary foundation for your health, longevity, and effectiveness as an EMT-B.

OBJECTIVES

Numbered objectives are from the United States Department of Transportation 1994 EMT-Basic National Standard Curriculum. Asterisked objectives, if any, pertain to material that is supplemental to the DOT curriculum.

COGNITIVE

1-6.1 Define body mechanics. (p. 84)
1-6.2 Discuss the guidelines and safety precautions that need to be followed when lifting a patient. (pp. 84–89)
1-6.4 Describe the guidelines and safety precautions for carrying patients and/or equipment. (pp. 87–90)
1-6.5 Discuss one-handed carrying techniques. (p. 89)

1-6.6 Describe correct and safe carrying procedures on stairs. (p. 89)
1-6.7 State the guidelines for reaching and their application. (pp. 89–90)
1-6.8 Describe correct reaching for log rolls. (p. 90)
1-6.9 State the guidelines for pushing and pulling. (p. 90)

AFFECTIVE

1-6.13 Explain the rationale for properly lifting and moving patients. (p. 84)

Additional objectives from DOT lesson 1-6 are addressed in Chapter 39, " Moving Patients."

CASE STUDY

THE DISPATCH

EMS Unit 101—proceed to Hunter complex on Main Street in Mountain Lakes—go to Apartment #21 for a nonemergency transport of a patient to the hospital—time out 0933 hours.

ON ARRIVAL

You are a probationary EMT-B accompanied by a training officer and an experienced EMT-B. As you work together to remove the wheeled stretcher from the ambulance, your training officer tells you that she is familiar with this patient, George Miller. He is a 26-year-old male who is in a full body cast (from the chest to the feet) and needs to be taken to the hospital for a routine evaluation.

She asks you: "How should we proceed?"

During this chapter, you will read about special considerations that can ensure your own well-being while moving patients and equipment safely. Later, we will return to the case study and apply the procedures learned.

BODY MECHANICS

As an EMT-Basic you are required to lift and carry patients and heavy equipment. If you perform these tasks improperly, bodily injury, strain, and life-long pain can be the result. With conscious planning, good health, and skill, you can perform these tasks with minimum risk to yourself. Apply the principles and techniques of proper lifting and moving every day. Practice often enough for them to become automatic. Make them a habit that increases your safety

and performance—even in the most stressful emergency situations.

FOUR BASIC PRINCIPLES

Body mechanics are defined as the safest and most efficient methods of using your body to gain a mechanical advantage. They are based on four simple principles.

- *Keep the weight of the object as close to the body as possible* (Figure 6-1). Back injury is much more likely

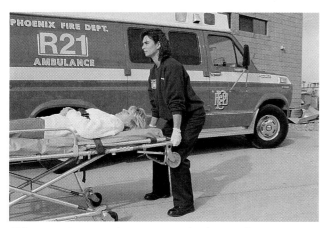

Figure 6-1   Using proper body mechanics, the weight is kept close to the body as it is lifted.

to occur while reaching a great distance to lift a light object than while reaching a short distance to lift a heavy object.

- *To move a heavy object use the leg, hip, and gluteal (buttocks) muscles plus contracted abdominal muscles.* The use of these muscles will help you generate a huge amount of power safely. Always avoid using back muscles to move a heavy object.
- *"Stack."* Visualize the shoulders stacked on top of the hips and the hips stacked on top of the feet (base). Then move them as a unit. If any of the three are not aligned with the others, you can create twisting forces that are potentially harmful to the lower back.
- *Reduce the height or distance through which the object must be moved.* Get closer to the object or reposition it before lifting (Figure 6-2). Lift in stages if necessary.

Lifting, carrying, moving, reaching, pushing, and pulling are all activities to which proper body mechanics should be applied. One important key to preventing injury is correct alignment of the spine. Maintaining a normal inward curve in the lower back significantly reduces the potential for spinal injury. Keeping wrists and knees in normal alignment can also help to prevent injury of the extremities. In addition, whenever possible, substitute equipment for manual force.

 POSTURE AND FITNESS

One much-overlooked aspect of proper body mechanics is posture. Because you will spend a great deal of time sitting or standing, poor posture can easily fatigue back and abdominal muscles, thereby making you vulnerable to back injury.

One extreme of poor posture is the swayback, or excessive **lordosis.** In this posture the stomach is too anterior and the buttocks are too posterior, causing excessive stress on the lumbar region of the back. Another extreme is the slouch, or excessive **kyphosis.** In this posture the shoulders are rolled forward, which results in fatigue of the lower back and increases pressure on every region of the spine (Figure 6-3).

Be aware of your posture. While standing, your ears, shoulders, and hips should be in vertical alignment, with knees slightly bent and pelvis slightly tucked forward (Figure 6-4). In the proper sitting position, your weight should be evenly distributed on both ischia (lower portion of the pelvic bones), with your ears, shoulders, and hips in vertical alignment, and your feet should be flat on the floor or crossed at your ankles. If possible, your lower back

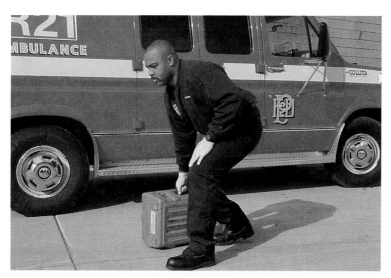

Figure 6-2   Reduce the height or distance through which the object must be moved. Get closer, reposition it, or move it in stages.

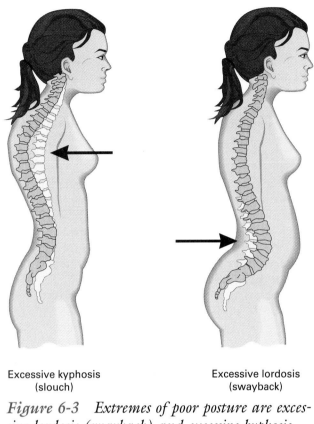

Excessive kyphosis
(slouch)

Excessive lordosis
(swayback)

Figure 6-3   Extremes of poor posture are excessive lordosis (swayback) and excessive kyphosis (slouch).

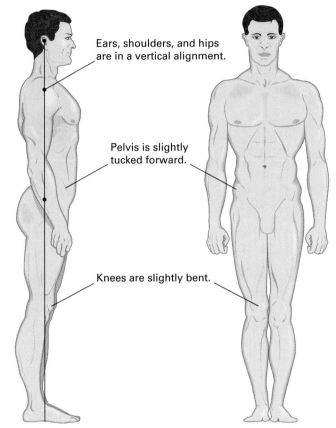

Ears, shoulders, and hips are in a vertical alignment.

Pelvis is slightly tucked forward.

Knees are slightly bent.

Figure 6-4   Proper standing posture.

should be in contact with the support of the chair (Figure 6-5).

Note that proper body mechanics cannot sufficiently protect you if you are not physically fit. A proactive, well-balanced physical fitness program should include flexibility training, cardiovascular conditioning, strength training, and nutrition. Such a program can help you prevent injury, enhance performance, and manage stress.

COMMUNICATION AND TEAMWORK

In an emergency, teamwork and effective communication among team members are essential. Patients come in all sizes, shapes, and strengths. Just as a football coach positions players according to their abilities, rescuers should capitalize on their abilities to ensure the best outcome in an emergency.

All team members should be trained in the proper techniques. Problems can occur when partners are greatly mismatched, and not only to the overloaded weaker partner. The stronger partner can also be injured if the weaker one fails to lift. Ideally, partners in lifting and moving a patient or object should have adequate and equal strength and height. Two adequately strong but weaker rescuers are as efficient and safe as the pairing of two stronger rescuers.

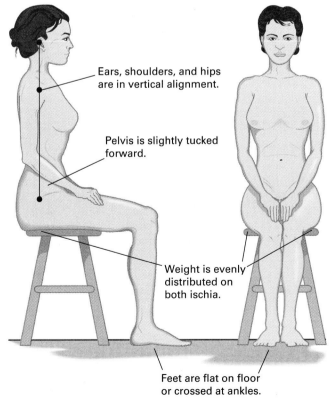

Ears, shoulders, and hips are in vertical alignment.

Pelvis is slightly tucked forward.

Weight is evenly distributed on both ischia.

Feet are flat on floor or crossed at ankles.

Figure 6-5   Proper sitting posture.

In order for team members to work together effectively, they need to communicate throughout all lifting and moving tasks. Use commands that are easy for team members to understand. Verbally coordinate each lift from beginning to end. Good teamwork will also allow you to:

- Size up the scene immediately and accurately
- Consider the weight of the patient and recognize the need for additional help
- Be aware of the physical abilities and limitations of each team member
- Select the most appropriate equipment for the job

Just as important as the communication between team members is the EMT-B's communication with the patient. If startled or frightened, the patient might shift body weight while you attempt the lift. Shifts in weight can cause disabling injury to rescuers as well as cause significant additional injury to the patient. So, whenever a patient is able to understand, explain the plan before any action is taken. This will improve patient confidence and can engage the patient in assisting in his own rescue.

GENERAL GUIDELINES FOR LIFTING AND MOVING

Know your own physical abilities and limitations. Do not overestimate yourself or other rescuers. Before lifting, know or find out the weight of the patient as well as the weight limitations of the equipment being used. Call for additional help whenever necessary. Even though your first impulse may be to jump in and help the patient, you must not proceed until you know you can do so safely.

Always try to use an even number of rescuers to maintain balance. Two-rescuer teams should carry heavy loads for one minute or less. More time can generate a high level of muscle fatigue, which can significantly increase the potential for injury. Whenever possible, transport patients and equipment on wheeled stretchers or other rolling devices.

When you must carry, keep the weight as close to your body as possible. Keep your back in a locked-in position. Do not hyperextend your back, or lean back from the waist. Refrain from twisting, and never lift and twist simultaneously. First lift, then turn as a unit.

THE POWER LIFT

The **power lift** is the technique that offers you the best defense against injury and protects the patient with a safe and stable move. It also is a useful technique for rescuers with weak knees or thighs. Remember, in performing this technique, keep your back locked and avoid bending at the waist. Follow these steps (Figure 6-6a to c):

1. Place your feet a comfortable distance apart. For the average-sized person, this is usually about shoulder width. Taller rescuers might prefer a little wider stance since this brings them closer to the object to be lifted.
2. Turn your feet slightly outward. Most people find that this helps them feel more comfortable and more stable.
3. Bend your knees to bring your center of gravity closer to the object to be lifted. As you bend your knees, you should feel as though you are sitting down, not falling forward.
4. Tighten the muscles of your back and abdomen to splint the vulnerable lower back. The back should remain as straight as comfortable (there is normally a slight inward curve), with your head facing forward in a neutral position.
5. Straddle the object. Keep your feet flat with your weight evenly distributed and just forward of the heels.
6. Place your hands a comfortable distance from each other to provide balance to the object as it is lifted. This is usually at least 10 inches apart.
7. Always use a **power grip** to get maximum force from the hands (Figure 6-7). That is, your palm and fingers should come in complete contact with the object and all fingers should be bent at the same angle.
8. As lifting begins, your back should remain locked in as the force is driven through the heels and arches of your feet. Your upper body should come up before the hips.
9. Reverse these steps to lower the wheeled stretcher or other object.

THE SQUAT LIFT

The squat lift is an alternative technique you can use if you have one weak leg, one weak ankle, or if both your knees and legs are strong and healthy (Figure 6-8). In performing this technique, *avoid bending at the waist.*

1. Place your weaker leg slightly forward. This foot should stay flat on the ground throughout the lift.
2. Squat down until you can grasp the cot, stretcher, or other patient moving device. Be sure to use the power grip.
3. Push yourself up with your stronger leg. Make sure your back is locked and your upper body goes up before your hips. Lead with your head.

While performing any lift, remember always to use your leg muscles—not your back—to lift, keep the weight as close to your body as possible, position yourself correctly, and communicate clearly and frequently with your partner.

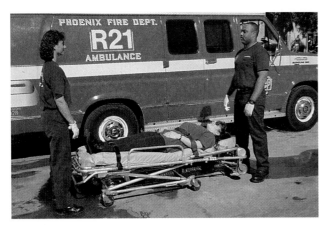

Figure 6-6a Get in position. Your feet should be about shoulder width apart, turned slightly outward, and flat on the ground.

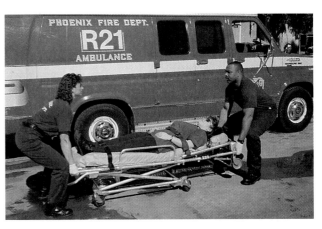

Figure 6-6b As lifting begins, your back should remain locked and your feet should remain flat. Tighten the muscles of your back and abdomen to splint the lower back.

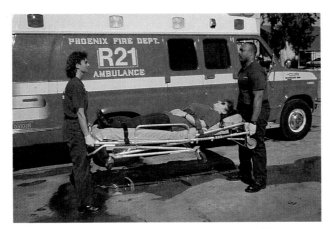

Figure 6-6c As you return to a standing position, make sure your back is locked in and your upper body comes up before your hips.

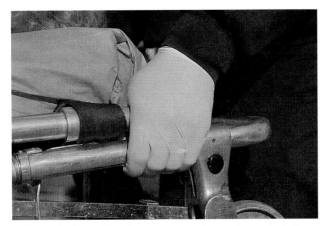

Figure 6-7 In the power grip, palms and fingers should come in complete contact with the object and fingers should be bent at the same angle.

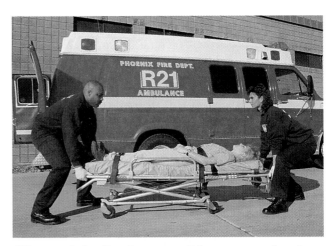

Figure 6-8 In the squat lift, your weaker leg stays slightly forward and you push up with your stronger leg.

ONE-HANDED CARRYING TECHNIQUE

There are times when you will want to lift and carry certain equipment with one hand. When you do, be sure to keep your back in a locked position. Maintain proper body mechanics and avoid leaning to the opposite side too much to compensate for the imbalance.

To use a one-handed carrying technique (Figure 6-9) to lift and move a patient carrying device, first stagger your feet with one knee up and one knee pointing toward the ground. Bend at the hips, not the waist, and do not let your trunk go any farther forward than 45°. On command from the rescuer at the patient's head, simultaneously drive upward through the arch and heel of the front foot and the ball of the back foot.

STAIR-CHAIR TECHNIQUE

Frequently patients will have to be moved up or down stairs. This challenge provides a huge potential for EMT-Bs to become injured. When possible, use a stair chair instead of a stretcher (Figure 6-10). With either a stretcher or a stair chair, use as many people to help as you need to support the patient. As the rescuers maneuver the stretcher or stair chair down stairs, a spotter should be placed to direct the move and navigate, frequently communicating information such as the number of stairs and the conditions ahead. Be sure to remember to keep your back in a locked position, flex at the hips and not at the waist, bend at the knees, and keep the weight and your arms as close to your body as possible. As long as you use proper body mechanics, stairs should be only a slight hindrance.

REACHING

Generally, a person can sustain a 100 percent effort for six seconds and a 50 percent effort for only one minute before becoming fatigued. After that minute, the potential for injury greatly increases. So, to mini-

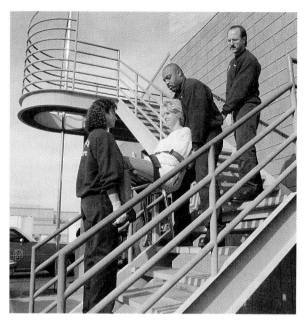

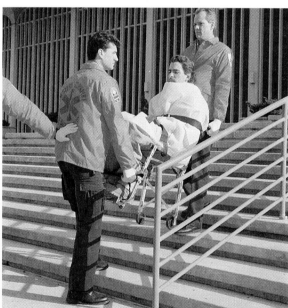

Figure 6-10   Whenever possible, use a stair chair instead of a stretcher when moving a patient up or down stairs.

mize effort, whenever possible reposition the object or get closer to the object to avoid or reduce reaching and lifting. Especially avoid situations in which prolonged strenuous effort (more than one minute) is required.

Many times EMT-Bs will find it necessary to reach for equipment or for a patient (as in a log roll). When it is necessary, reach no more than 15 to 20 inches in front of the body. If an object is more than 20 inches away, move closer to it before attempting to reach and lift. When reaching, keep the back in a locked position. Do not twist. Use your free arm to

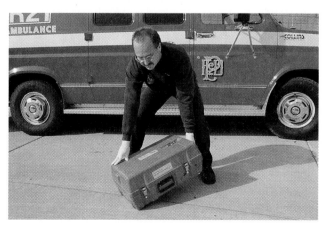

Figure 6-9   One-handed carrying technique.

support the weight of your upper body whenever possible. If you reach overhead, avoid hyperextending (that is, do not lean back from the waist).

When performing a log roll, lean from the hips, not the waist, and keep the back straight. Use the stronger shoulder muscles to assist whenever possible. (Log roll technique will be taught in Chapters 9, "Patient" Assessment, and 34, "Injuries to the Spine.")

PUSHING AND PULLING

Occasionally you will have to decide whether to push or pull an object. Whenever possible, push rather than pull. If the object must be pulled, keep the load between your shoulders and hips and close to your body. Keep your back straight and slightly bend your knees. This will help to keep the line of pull through the center of your body (Figure 6-11).

When pushing, push from the areas between your waist and shoulders. If the weight is below waist level, use the kneeling position to avoid bending. Keep your elbows bent, with your arms close to the

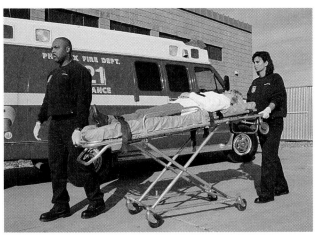

Figure 6-11   Proper pulling and pushing.

sides of your body. This will help to increase the force you can apply. Due to the inherent danger, even likelihood, of injury, avoid pushing or pulling an object that is overhead.

CASE STUDY FOLLOW-UP

SCENE SIZE-UP

As a probationary EMT-B, you have been dispatched—along with a training officer and experienced partners—to a 26-year-old patient in a full body cast for a nonemergency transport to the hospital. On your approach to the apartment complex, you scan the scene for hazards. Everything appears to be peaceful. There are children playing, adults going about their business, and a police officer walking his beat. The officer nods to you. You decide the scene is safe.

As you approach the patient's apartment building with a wheeled stretcher, you assess the potential obstacles to moving the patient. You look for curbs, sidewalks, steps, doors, and so on. Your assessment reveals that you will have to navigate the patient about 25 yards on a sidewalk, six steps outside the front door, and one flight of stairs.

When you enter the patient's apartment, you immediately see that the patient is alert and in a hospital bed in the middle of a large, nearly bare room.

PATIENT ASSESSMENT

Your general impression of the patient, George Miller, is that he is alert, has good color, and appears to be calm, cheerful, and cooperative. You see no IVs or other medical equipment or medications. Airway, breathing, and circulation appear normal. Mr. Miller

reports that there are no problems, and he tells you that he believes this will be his last visit to the hospital via ambulance. As your partners bring in and position the wheeled stretcher, you take and record vital signs and ask if he has any physical complaints.

LIFTING AND MOVING THE PATIENT

You and your partners decide to use the draw-sheet method of transferring the patient. This involves placing the stretcher between yourselves and the bed, then reaching across the stretcher to pull the loosened bottom sheet and patient toward the stretcher. You explain the procedure to Mr. Miller. As you begin the procedure—just as you lean over to reach across the stretcher—your training officer stops you.

"Your back," she says.

Reminded, you straighten up and complete the reach, supporting yourself by bracing your hips against the stretcher and your free hand on the edge of the bed. As you help slide Mr. Miller onto the wheeled stretcher, you contract your abdominal and gluteal muscles to splint your lower back.

After you check to make sure that Mr. Miller is comfortable, you push the stretcher out the door into the hallway. Two of you get in position, one at each end of the stretcher. The training officer moves to the top of the steps to "spot."

You open the space between your feet, tighten your muscles to lock your back, make sure your hands and fingers are properly positioned for a power grip, and bend from the hips. You use the power-lift technique to pick up the stretcher. You make sure you can keep the weight and arms as close to your body as possible. When you're both ready, you both say so.

The spotter tells you how many steps there are ahead and begins to count them out as you descend. You and the other carrier are keeping pace and checking in. The three of you sound like this:

One step. Okay. Okay.

Two step. Okay. Too fast, slow down.

Three step. Okay. Okay. (and so on)

The rest of the move is relatively simple. After a short rest, you proceed down the front steps. When you reach the sidewalk, you and your partners push the wheeled stretcher to the ambulance. You keep your elbows bent with arms as close to sides of the body as possible, aligning the force of the push through the center of your body.

You and your partner lift the stretcher into the ambulance. When you work the safety bar and latches, you remember to bend at the hips (not the waist) and move as a unit, avoiding twisting.

En route, you make certain that Mr. Miller is comfortable. You arrive at the hospital without any change in the patient's condition and use correct body mechanics to transfer him from the ambulance and to assist in moving him onto the hospital bed. You and your partners complete an EMS report and then proceed to ready the ambulance for the next call.

CHAPTER REVIEW

TERMS AND CONCEPTS

You may wish to review the following terms and concepts included in this chapter.

body mechanics—application of the study of muscles and body movement (kinesiology) to the use of the body and to the prevention and correction of problems related to posture and lifting. Principles of body mechanics focus on the most efficient methods of moving or using the body to gain a mechanical advantage when lifting objects.

kyphosis—abnormal curvature of the spine with convexity backward. Also called slouch.

lordosis—abnormal anterior convexity of the spine. Also called *swayback*.

power grip—recommended gripping technique. The palm and fingers come in complete contact with the object and all fingers are bent at the same angle.

power lift—recommended technique for lifting. Feet are apart, knees bent, back and abdominal muscles tightened, back as straight as possible, lifting force driven through heels and arches, upper body rising before hips.

REVIEW QUESTIONS

1. Explain why you should follow the principles of body mechanics.
2. List the four basic principles of body mechanics.
3. Explain how to perform the power grip, and when you should use it.
4. Explain how to perform the power lift, and when you should use it.
5. List some of the guidelines and safety precautions for carrying.
6. Explain the precautions you should take when performing a one-handed carrying technique.
7. Name the device that is recommended for carrying a patient up and down stairs, whenever possible, and explain the function of the spotter.
8. Name some precautions that can be taken when reaching to lift an object.
9. Explain the proper body mechanics for reaching while doing a log roll.
10. Explain the safety guidelines for pushing and pulling.

CHAPTER 7

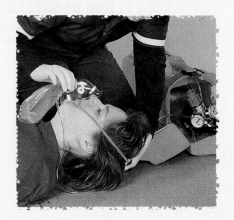

Airway Management, Ventilation, and Oxygen Therapy

INTRODUCTION

The most basic components of emergency medical care are to establish and maintain an airway, ensure effective ventilation, and provide oxygen to the patient. Without an open and clear airway, adequate breathing, or sufficient oxygenation all other emergency care is futile since the patient will rapidly deteriorate and die. Therefore, these components are part of the initial assessment that is conducted on every patient regardless of the injuries or illness. By understanding the mechanical and physiological processes of breathing and the various ways to assist patients with breathing, you will be able to quickly initiate and maintain an adequate airway and oxygenation in cases of emergency.

OBJECTIVES

Numbered objectives are from the United States Department of Transportation 1994 EMT-Basic National Standard Curriculum. Asterisked objectives, if any, pertain to material that is supplemental to the DOT curriculum.

COGNITIVE

2-1.1   Name and label the major structures of the respiratory system on a diagram. (pp. 94–96)

2-1.2   List the signs of adequate breathing. (p. 107)

2-1.3   List the signs of inadequate breathing. (pp. 107–108)

2-1.4   Describe the steps in performing the head-tilt, chin-lift. (p. 99)

2-1.5   Relate the mechanism of injury to opening the airway. (pp. 99–100)

2-1.6   Describe the steps in performing the jaw thrust. (p. 100)

2-1.7   State the importance of having a suction unit ready for immediate use when providing emergency care. (p. 100)

2-1.8   Describe the techniques of suctioning. (pp. 101–102)

2-1.9   Describe how to artificially ventilate a patient with a pocket mask. (pp. 110–111)

2-1.10   Describe the steps in performing the skill of artificially ventilating a patient with a bag-valve mask while using the jaw thrust. (pp. 113–114)

2-1.11   List the parts of a bag-valve-mask system. (p. 111)

2-1.12   Describe the steps in performing the skill of artificially ventilating a patient with a bag-valve mask for one and two rescuers. (pp. 111–112)

2-1.13   Describe the signs of adequate artificial ventilation using the bag-valve mask. (pp. 112–113)

2-1.14   Describe the signs of inadequate artificial ventilation using the bag-valve mask. (p. 113)

2-1.15   Describe the steps in artificially ventilating a patient with a flow restricted, oxygen-powered ventilation device. (p. 115)

2-1.16   List the steps in performing the actions taken when providing mouth-to-mouth and mouth-to-stoma artificial ventilation. (pp. 109–110, 123–124)

2-1.17   Describe how to measure and insert an oropharyngeal (oral) airway. (pp. 103–104)

2-1.18   Describe how to measure and insert a nasopharyngeal (nasal) airway. (pp. 105–106)

2-1.19   Define the components of an oxygen delivery system. (pp. 116–121)

2-1.20   Identify a nonrebreather face mask and state the oxygen flow requirements needed for its use. (pp. 119–120)

2-1.21   Describe the indications for using a nasal cannula versus a nonrebreather face mask. (p. 120)

2-1.22   Identify a nasal cannula and state the flow requirements needed for its use. (pp. 120–121)

AFFECTIVE

2-1.23   Explain the rationale for basic life support artificial ventilation and airway protective skills taking priority over most other basic life support skills. (p. 92)

2-1.24   Explain the rationale for providing adequate oxygenation through high inspired oxygen concentrations to patients who, in the past, may have received low concentrations. (p. 120)

PSYCHOMOTOR

2-1.25   Demonstrate the steps in performing the head-tilt, chin-lift.

2-1.26   Demonstrate the techniques in performing the jaw thrust.

2-1.27   Demonstrate the techniques of suctioning.

2-1.28   Demonstrate the steps in providing mouth-to-mouth artificial ventilation with body substance isolation (barrier shields).

2-1.29   Demonstrate how to use a pocket mask to artificially ventilate a patient.

2-1.30   Demonstrate the assembly of a bag-valve-mask unit.

2-1.31   Demonstrate the steps in performing the skill of artificially ventilating a patient with a bag-valve mask for one and two rescuers.

2-1.32   Demonstrate the steps in performing the skill of artificially ventilating a patient with a bag-valve mask while using the jaw thrust.

2-1.33   Demonstrate artificial ventilation of a patient with a flow restricted, oxygen-powered ventilation device.

2-1.34   Demonstrate how to artificially ventilate a patient with a stoma.

2-1.35   Demonstrate how to insert an oropharyngeal (oral) airway.

2-1.36   Demonstrate how to insert a nasopharyngeal (nasal) airway.

2-1.37   Demonstrate the correct operation of oxygen tanks and regulators.

2-1.38 Demonstrate the use of a nonrebreather face mask and state the oxygen flow requirements needed for its use.

2-1.39 Demonstrate the use of a nasal cannula and state the flow requirements needed for its use.

2-1.40 Demonstrate how to artificially ventilate the infant and child patient.

2-1.41 Demonstrate oxygen administration for the infant and child patient.

CASE STUDY

THE DISPATCH

EMS Unit 108—respond to the Twighlight Bar, 59 South Market Street. You have an unresponsive male patient—time out 1703 hours.

ON ARRIVAL

As your ambulance draws up to the bar, you and your partner recognize it as one you've been sent to several times in the past to handle injuries caused in fights. "They must have changed the name of the bar," you say to your partner. She contacts dispatch and inquires, "Is this patient's unresponsiveness a result of a fight or other violent act?"

Dispatch responds, "EMS Unit 108, be advised the bartender states the patient was drinking heavily this afternoon. He was found unresponsive in the bathroom by another patron."

You cautiously approach the scene and enter the bar. It is quite dark and a typical "bar smell" fills the air. You are directed to the men's bathroom at the end of a short hallway. You enter and find a man approximately 30 years of age lying prone on the bathroom floor. Vomitus surrounds the patient's face.

How would you proceed to assess and care for this patient?

During this chapter you will learn special considerations of assessment and management of the airway and breathing status and techniques of oxygen administration. Later we will return to the case and apply the procedures learned.

RESPIRATORY SYSTEM REVIEW

To ensure that you can establish and maintain an open airway and properly ventilate a patient, you should understand some basics of the anatomy and physiology of the respiratory system. What follows is a brief review of that system. You may also wish to review the material on the respiratory system in Chapter 4, "The Human Body."

ANATOMY OF THE RESPIRATORY SYSTEM

The respiratory system takes oxygen from air that is breathed in and supplies it to the blood. The blood then transports the oxygen to body cells through the circulatory system. If the oxygen supply is decreased by an obstructed airway, inadequate breathing, or ineffective oxygen exchange in the lungs, the body cells will die. Figure 7-1 illustrates the anatomy of the upper airway.

NOSE AND MOUTH

Air normally enters the body through the nostrils. It is warmed, moistened, and filtered as it flows over the damp, sticky **mucous membrane** lining the nose. Air also enters through the mouth; however, there is less filtration and warming by that route than through the nostrils. The tongue is a common cause of airway obstruction in the patient with an altered mental status.

PHARYNX

Air entering the body through the mouth and nostrils travels into the **pharynx** (throat). Air from the nasal passages enters through what is referred to as the **nasopharynx.** Air entering through the mouth travels through the **oropharynx.** Both the oropharynx and

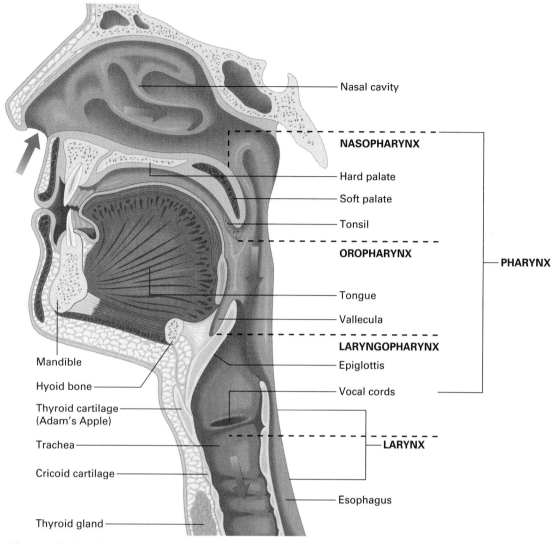

Figure 7-1 Anatomy of the upper airway.

nasopharynx enter into the pharynx at the back of the throat. The pharynx must be kept clear because obstructions in it can prevent air from traveling into the lower airways and interfere with oxygen and carbon dioxide exchange in the lungs.

Two passageways are found at the lower end of the pharynx—the **trachea** and the **esophagus.** The trachea is the passageway for air traveling into the lungs. Food and water are routed to the esophagus, which leads to the stomach.

EPIGLOTTIS

The trachea is protected by a small flap of tissue called the **epiglottis.** This acts as a valve that closes over the trachea while food and drink are being swallowed. At other times, the epiglottis is pulled away from the opening to the trachea, which permits breathing. This controlled diversion usually works automatically to keep food and drink out of the trachea and air from going into the esophagus.

At times, the epiglottis may fail to close, and food or liquids can enter the larynx and the upper portion of the trachea, causing a patient to choke. Also, if a patient is unresponsive, the protective reflexes may not work during swallowing, so that foreign objects, blood, secretions, and vomitus can enter the trachea and cause an airway obstruction or lung infection.

LARYNX AND TRACHEA

The trachea, commonly known as the windpipe, is the passageway for air entering the lungs. Just above the trachea and just below the epiglottis, is the **larynx,** or voice box, which contains the vocal cords. The anterior portion of the larynx, the **thyroid cartilage,** is more commonly known as the **Adam's apple;** it can be felt at the front of the throat. The **cricoid cartilage,** which forms the inferior portion of the larynx and is the only completely circular cartilagenous ring of the upper airway, is found at the lower portion of the larynx just below the thyroid cartilage. The larynx is a common site of airway obstruction in adults, infants, and children.

BRONCHI

The trachea descends into the chest cavity. There it branches into two main tubes, the left and right mainstem **bronchi.** Each bronchus goes into a lung, where it divides and subdivides into smaller **bronchioles,** somewhat like the branches of a tree.

LUNGS

The bronchioles terminate in thousands of tiny air sacs in the lungs. These are called the **alveoli.** Each air sac is wrapped in a web of thin-walled capillaries.

The lungs are made of an elastic tissue and are surrounded by two layers of connective tissue called the **pleura.** The **visceral pleura** is the innermost covering of the lung. The **parietal pleura** is a thicker, more elastic layer that adheres to the inner portion of the chest wall. Between the two layers is the **pleural space,** a small space that is at negative pressure. The pleural space contains a small amount of **serous fluid** that acts as a lubricant to reduce friction when the layers of the pleura rub against each other during breathing.

If a hole is made in either pleural layer, air may enter the pleural space increasing its size and pressure and collapsing the lung. This is frequently seen in blunt and penetrating injuries to the chest and can lead to severe respiratory distress and inadequate oxygenation of the cells.

DIAPHRAGM

The **diaphragm** is a muscle that separates the chest cavity from the abdominal cavity. It is the major muscle used in breathing. If contraction of the diaphragm is ineffective because of trauma or illness, the patient may show signs of significant respiratory distress due to inadequate breathing.

MECHANICS OF BREATHING

The passage of air into and out of the lungs is called **ventilation.** Ventilation is a mechanical process that creates pressure changes in the lungs to draw air in and force air out. **Inhalation** or **inspiration** is the process of breathing air in, and **exhalation** or **expiration** is the process of breathing air out.

INHALATION

During inhalation, the diaphragm and the **intercostal muscles,** or muscles between the ribs, contract. The diaphragm moves slightly downward and flares the lower portion of the rib cage outward. The intercostal muscles pull the ribs and sternum upward and outward. These actions increase the size of the chest cavity, creating negative pressure. This draws air by way of the nose, mouth, trachea, and bronchi into the lungs. Inhalation is an *active* process because it requires energy to contract the muscles.

EXHALATION

During exhalation, the diaphragm and intercostal muscles relax, moving the diaphragm upward and the ribs and sternum downward and inward back to their normal resting positions. The size of the chest cavity is reduced, the elastic lung tissue recoils to its normal position, and the pressure in the chest cavity becomes positive. This forces the air out of the lungs. Because this process involves relaxation of muscles and little energy is expended, it is considered to be *passive.*

In some respiratory diseases affecting the lower airway, such as asthma, the patient has a difficult time moving air out of the lungs. There is a loss of the elastic recoil of the chest wall and lungs. The patient has to contract muscles not only to draw air into the lungs but also to force air out of the lungs. Therefore, both inhalation and exhalation become active, requiring energy. Such patients have a tendency to become exhausted very quickly because of the amount of energy it takes to breathe. They are very prone to a rapid deterioration in their breathing status.

RESPIRATORY PHYSIOLOGY

Oxygenation is the process by which the blood and the cells become saturated with oxygen. This happens as a result of **respiration,** the process in which fresh oxygen replaces waste carbon dioxide, a gas exchange that takes place between the alveoli and the capillaries in the lungs, and also between the capillaries and the cells throughout the body.

A blocked airway or inadequate breathing will prevent oxygen from entering the lungs. This results in **hypoxia,** or inadequate oxygen being delivered to the cells. Hypoxia can also result from inadequate blood circulation, or **hypoperfusion.** The following are signs of hypoxia:

- An increased or decreased heart rate (decreased late in the adult but an early sign in the infant or child)
- Altered mental status ranging from confusion to complete unresponsiveness
- Agitation
- An elevation in blood pressure followed by a decrease
- **Cyanosis,** bluish skin and mucous membranes

Because cyanosis is often a late sign, it is much more important to recognize agitation or a decrease in the patient's mental status as an indicator of hypoxia. If signs of hypoxia are present, it is necessary to establish and maintain an open airway, provide positive pressure ventilation if the patient is breathing inadequately, and deliver high-flow oxygen.

ALVEOLAR/CAPILLARY EXCHANGE

Oxygen-rich air enters the alveoli during each inspiration. Surrounding the alveoli are capillaries that deliver blood to the alveoli. The blood moving into the capillaries is **deoxygenated,** that is with low oxygen concentration, but is high in carbon dioxide. The alveoli themselves contain an enriched supply of oxygen and very little carbon dioxide. Because both gases will move from areas of high concentration to areas of low concentration, the oxygen moves from the alveoli into the capillaries and the carbon dioxide moves from the capillaries into the alveoli. From this point, the blood in the capillaries is **oxygenated,** that is with high oxygen concentration and low in carbon dioxide. **Hemoglobin,** found on the surface of red blood cells, is responsible for picking up the oxygen in the blood and carrying it through the arterial system to the capillaries throughout the body. The carbon dioxide is exhaled from the alveoli and out of the lungs.

CAPILLARY/CELLULAR EXCHANGE

The blood entering the capillaries surrounding the body's cells has a high oxygen content and a very low carbon dioxide content. The cells have high levels of carbon dioxide and low levels of oxygen from normal metabolism. Again, because oxygen and carbon dioxide move from areas of high concentration to those of low concentration, the oxygen moves out of the capillaries and into the cells and the carbon dioxide moves out of the cells and into the capillaries. The blood, now low in oxygen and high in carbon dioxide, moves out of the capillaries and into the venous system where it is transported back to the lungs for gas exchange.

AIRWAY ANATOMY IN INFANTS AND CHILDREN

The causes of airway obstruction and inadequate breathing in infants and children are usually similar to those in adults. However, there are several anatomical features in infants and children that may cause them to deteriorate more rapidly than adults (Figure 7-2).

MOUTH AND NOSE

The noses and mouths of infants and children are smaller than those of adults. Thus, they are more easily obstructed by foreign bodies, swelling, blood, mucus, and secretions.

PHARYNX

Because the tongue of an infant or a child is relatively large in proportion to the size of the mouth, it takes up much more room. Therefore, an infant or a child is much more prone to airway obstruction by posterior displacement of the tongue at the level of the pharynx. Also, the epiglottis is more U-shaped and can protrude into the pharynx, contributing to obstruction.

TRACHEA AND LOWER AIRWAY

The trachea and lower airway passages of infants and children are narrower, softer, and more flexible than those of adults. Thus, airway obstructions occur more easily due to mucus, pus, blood, secretions, swelling (edema), and constriction. Very small reductions in the diameter of the lower airway result in significant

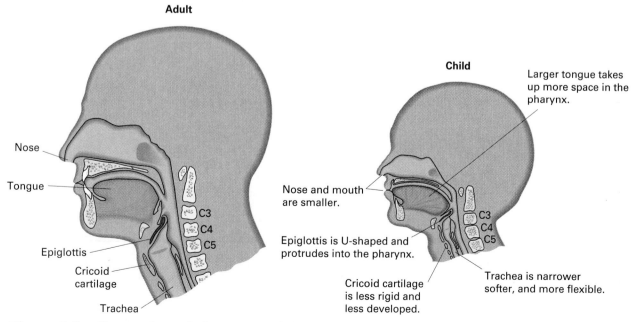

Figure 7-2 Comparison of airways of adult and infant or child.

airway obstruction and very high resistance to air flow, reducing effective breathing and oxygenation.

CRICOID CARTILAGE

The cricoid cartilage, like other cartilage in infants and children, is less developed and less rigid. Also, in infants and children less than 10 years of age, the cricoid cartilage is the narrowest portion of the upper airway.

CHEST WALL AND DIAPHRAGM

The chest wall in an infant or a child is much softer and more pliable than in an adult. This leads to a much greater compliance (elasticity; response to pressure) or movement during ventilation. Thus, infants and children rely much more on the diaphragm for breathing. When you perform artificial ventilation on an infant or child, the chest should expand and rise easily. If the chest is not rising, you should assume that the ventilation is inadequate. Also, because the chest expands so readily, it is much easier for the EMT-B to over-inflate the lungs and cause possible lung injury.

AIRWAY ASSESSMENT

An open airway is necessary for adequate breathing and oxygenation. Therefore, assessment of the airway is one of the first components in the initial assessment of the patient. An open airway is commonly referred to as a **patent airway.**

The mental status of a patient typically correlates well with the status of his airway. An alert, responsive patient who is talking to you in a normal voice has an open airway. It takes an open and clear airway, along with adequate breathing, to enable a patient to communicate easily.

A patient who has an altered mental status or is completely unresponsive commonly cannot protect his own airway and has the potential for airway occlusion, or obstruction. The tongue relaxes and falls back, blocking the pharynx. The epiglottis can also relax and obstruct the airway at the level of the larynx. Efforts by the patient to breathe will create a negative pressure; this may draw the tongue, epiglottis, or both into the airway to block airflow into the trachea and lungs.

When assessing the airway in the patient with an altered mental status, it is necessary to open it manually, inspect inside the mouth, and listen for any abnormal sounds. The following are sounds that may indicate airway obstruction:

- **Snoring** (sonorous sounds) occurs when the upper airway is partially obstructed by the base of the tongue or by relaxed tissues in the pharynx. The snoring and obstruction can be corrected by performing a head-tilt, chin-lift maneuver. This lifts the base of the tongue from the back of the pharynx (throat). In a patient with a suspected spinal injury, a jaw-thrust should be used. Both maneuvers are described below.
- **Crowing** is a sound like the cawing of a crow that occurs when the muscles around the larynx begin to spasm and narrow the opening into the trachea. Air rushing through the restricted passage causes the sound.
- **Gurgling,** a sound like gargling, usually indicates the presence of blood, vomitus, secretions, or other liquid in the airway. Immediately suction the substance from the airway.
- **Stridor** is a harsh, high-pitched sound heard during inspiration. It is characteristic of a significant upper airway obstruction from swelling in the larynx.

OPENING THE MOUTH

It may be necessary to open the mouth of a patient to adequately assess the airway. This is done by using the **crossed-finger technique** (Figure 7-3):

1. Kneel above and behind the patient.
2. Cross the thumb and forefinger of one hand.
3. Place the thumb on the patient's lower incisors and your forefinger on the upper incisors.
4. Use a scissors motion or finger-snapping motion to open the mouth.

Inspect inside the mouth for vomitus, blood, secretions, broken teeth or foreign bodies that can obstruct the airway. Suction any foreign substance from

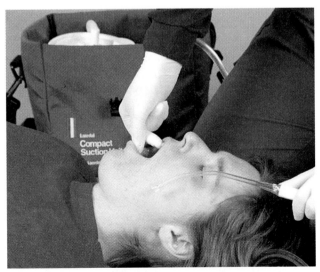

Figure 7-3 Open the mouth using a crossed-finger technique.

the mouth. If suction equipment is not immediately available, wipe the fluids away with your index and middle fingers wrapped in a cloth or gauze pad. If you can see foreign objects, such as food, broken teeth, or dentures, sweep the mouth with your index finger and remove them. Do this quickly. Be extremely cautious because the patient could bite down on your fingers, gag, or vomit.

OPENING THE AIRWAY

Before a patient who is breathing inadequately can receive positive pressure ventilation, or breathing assistance in which air is forced into his lungs, he must have an open airway. Open the airway manually by using either the head-tilt, chin-lift maneuver or the jaw-thrust maneuver. Generally, the head-tilt, chin-lift maneuver is used. *However, if you suspect that a patient may have suffered a spinal injury, then use the jaw-thrust maneuver in conjunction with in-line spinal stabilization.*

HEAD-TILT, CHIN-LIFT MANEUVER

The American Heart Association recommends the **head-tilt, chin-lift maneuver** for opening the airway in a non-trauma patient. The head-tilt, chin-lift is illustrated in Figure 7-4 and summarized below.

1. Place one hand on the patient's forehead, and apply firm, backward pressure with the palm of the hand to tilt the head back. Place the tips of the fingers of the other hand underneath the bony part of the lower jaw.
2. Bring the chin forward, supporting the jaw and tilting the head backward as far as possible. *Do not compress the soft tissues underneath the chin; they might obstruct the airway.*
3. Continue to press the other hand on the patient's forehead to keep the head tilted backward.
4. Lift the chin so that the teeth are brought nearly together. (If necessary, you can use your thumb to depress the lower lip; this will keep the patient's mouth slightly open. The thumb should not be used to lift the chin.)
5. If the patient has loose dentures, hold them in position, making obstruction by the lips less likely. A seal is easier to form when the dentures are in place. If the dentures cannot be managed, remove them.

HEAD-TILT, CHIN-LIFT IN INFANTS AND CHILDREN

The preferred method of opening the airway in infants and children without suspected spinal injury is the head-tilt, chin-lift maneuver.

ADULT

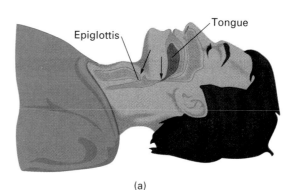

(a)

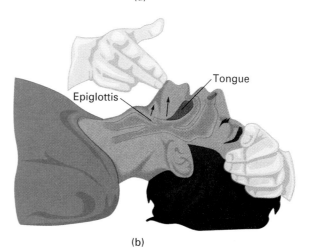

(b)

Figure 7-4 Head-tilt, chin-lift maneuver in the adult.

The hand positions and procedures for performing the head-tilt, chin-lift maneuver with infants and children are the same as with adults except for a variation in head positioning. With an infant, the head should be tilted back gently into a "sniffing" or neutral position (Figure 7-5). Because of the large size of the head, it may be necessary to place a pad behind the shoulders to keep the airway open. Because of the underdeveloped airway structures in the infant, care must be taken not to overextend the infant's head; this could lead to an obstruction of the trachea. With a child, the head is tilted only slightly back from the neutral position. Only the index finger of one hand lifts the chin and jaw.

JAW-THRUST MANEUVER

If a spinal injury is suspected, the patient's head and neck must be brought into and maintained in a neutral, in-line position. This means that the head is not turned to the side, tilted forward (flexed), or tilted backward (extended). The **jaw-thrust maneuver** is used to open the airway in such a patient because the head and neck are not tilted back during this maneu-

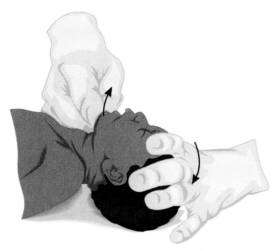

Figure 7-5 Head-tilt, chin-lift maneuver in the infant. Be sure to avoid overextension.

ver. The jaw (mandible) is displaced forward by the EMT-B's fingers; this causes the patient's tongue to be pulled forward, away from the back of the airway. If the head-tilt, chin-lift maneuver is unsuccessful in opening the airway of the non-spine-injured patient, perform the jaw-thrust maneuver. The procedure for the jaw thrust is illustrated in Figure 7-6. It involves the following steps:

1. Kneel at the top of the patient's head. Place your elbows on the surface on which the patient is lying, putting your hands at the side of the patient's head.
2. Grasp the angles of the patient's lower jaw on both sides. Move the jaw forward with both hands. This will move the tongue forward, away from the airway. If no spinal injury is suspected, the head could be tilted backward.

3. Retract the lower lip with your thumb if the lips close.

If the jaw thrust alone is not effective in establishing an open airway, reposition the jaw. If repositioning is not effective, insert an oral or nasal airway adjunct, as explained later in this chapter. The EMT-B holding the in-line stabilization can also establish and maintain the jaw thrust.

JAW-THRUST IN INFANTS AND CHILDREN

Follow the basic procedure described above when performing the jaw-thrust maneuver in infants and children. Place two or three fingers of each hand at the angle of the jaw to lift it up and forward while the other fingers guide the movement. Insert an airway adjunct if the jaw thrust does not clear the airway.

SUCTION EQUIPMENT AND TECHNIQUE

It is necessary to remove any blood, vomitus, secretions, and any other liquids, food particles, or objects from the mouth and airway since they can cause obstruction. Such substances are best removed through the use of suction devices. If a gurgling sound is heard when you are assessing the airway or during artificial ventilation, immediately apply suction to remove the liquid from the airway. Failure to do so will force the liquid substance farther down the airway and possibly into the lungs.

Some suction equipment is not very effective in removing very thick vomitus or solid objects, such as teeth, foreign bodies, or food, from the airway. In such situations, it may be necessary to use an alternative piece of suction equipment or to perform a finger sweep to remove the material.

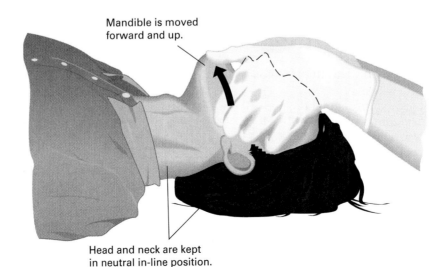

Mandible is moved forward and up.

Head and neck are kept in neutral in-line position.

Figure 7-6 The jaw-thrust maneuver is used to open the airway in patients with suspected spinal injury.

BODY SUBSTANCE ISOLATION DURING SUCTIONING

Because suctioning involves removal of body fluids and the potential for coughing and spatters, you must take appropriate body substance isolation precautions. Protective eyewear, a mask, and gloves should be used. If a patient is known to have tuberculosis or displays signs and symptoms consistent with tuberculosis, a HEPA (high-efficiency particulate air) respirator should be worn at all times in addition to eyewear and gloves.

SUCTION EQUIPMENT

Suction equipment includes the device that creates the suction as well as the catheters that are inserted in the airway. Various types of fixed and portable suction devices and catheters are available.

Mounted Suction Devices Fixed or installed units should be part of the required on-board ambulance equipment. They should be powerful enough to create a vacuum of more than 300 mmHg on the gauge when the tubing is clamped or kinked. The device should be adjustable to allow for a reduced vacuum when suctioning infants and children. Such fixed systems are powered by an electric vacuum pump or by the vacuum produced by the ambulance engine manifold.

Portable Suction Devices A portable unit must produce a vacuum adequate to suction substances from the pharynx. Portable suction units can be electric-, oxygen- or air-, or hand-powered (Figure 7-7). These suction units should be inspected before each shift or on a regular basis.

Electric suction devices must have fully charged batteries to function effectively. A low battery charge will reduce the effective vacuum and the length of time the unit can be used. Some units allow for constant charging so that the batteries are always fully charged when needed.

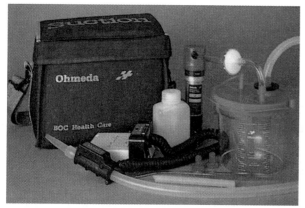

Figure 7-7 A portable suction unit.

Oxygen-powered devices function only as long as a source of oxygen is available. Once the oxygen source has run out, the vacuum is lost and suction becomes ineffective.

Hand-powered suction devices do not require any energy source other than an EMT-B to create the vacuum. Therefore, these devices lack some typical problems associated with electric- or oxygen-powered devices. Also, hand-powered units can more effectively suction heavier substances, such as thick vomitus.

Any type of portable suction device must have the following:

• Wide-bore, thick-walled, non-kinking tubing that fits standard rigid or soft suction catheters
• An unbreakable collection bottle or container and a supply of water for rinsing and clearing the tubes and catheters
• Enough vacuum pressure and flow to suction substances from the pharynx effectively

Suction Catheters Suction catheters must be disposable and capable of being connected to the suction unit's tubing. Two different types of suction catheters are available:

• **Hard or rigid catheter**—This type of catheter is a rigid plastic tube. It is commonly referred to as a **"tonsil tip"** or **"tonsil sucker."** It is used to suction the mouth and oropharynx of an unresponsive patient. It is more effective for particulate matter than a soft catheter. The catheter should be inserted only as far as you can see, typically not farther than the base of the tongue. If you are using it on an infant or child, be careful not to apply suction to the back of the airway, since doing so would likely cause soft tissue trauma.
• **Soft catheter**—The soft suction catheter consists of flexible tubing. It is also called a **"French"** **catheter.** It is used in suctioning the nose and nasopharynx and in other situations where the rigid catheter cannot be used. The length of catheter should be determined by measuring from the tip of the patient's nose to the tip of his ear if it is being inserted in the nasopharynx or from the corner of his mouth to the tip of his ear if it is being inserted in the mouth and oropharynx. The soft suction catheter should not be inserted beyond the base of the tongue.

TECHNIQUE OF SUCTIONING

There are many suctioning techniques. They vary depending on the device and type of catheter used. One technique is described below:

1. Position yourself at the patient's head (Figure 7-8a). If this is not possible, take a position in which you can observe the airway.
2. Turn on the suction unit.

SUCTIONING TECHNIQUE

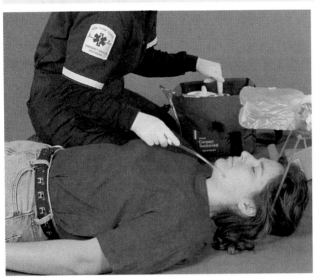

Figure 7-8a *Position yourself at the head of the patient and turn on the suction unit. Note: Apply suction only after the catheter is in place.*

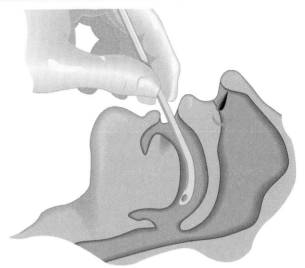

Figure 7-8b *Place the rigid tip so that the convex (bulging) side is against the roof of the mouth. Insert it to the beginning of the throat.*

3. Select the appropriate type of catheter. Use a rigid catheter when suctioning the mouth or oropharynx. If the nasal passages need to be suctioned, select a soft (French) catheter and use low to medium suction (80 to 120 mmHg). A bulb syringe may be used if a soft catheter is not available.

4. Measure the catheter and insert it into the oral cavity without suction, if possible. Place the rigid tip so that the convex (bulging) side is against the roof of the mouth. Insert it no farther down than the base of the tongue (Figure 7-8b).

5. Begin suction after the tip has been positioned, moving the catheter tip from side to side to clear material from the mouth. **Suction for no more than 15 seconds at a time in the adult; in infants and children, suction in shorter periods, approximately 5 seconds.**

6. If necessary, rinse the catheter with water to prevent obstruction of the tubing from dried or thick material. Do this by keeping a bottle of water available and applying suction to the water as necessary to clear the tubing.

SPECIAL CONSIDERATIONS WHEN SUCTIONING

The following are special considerations when suctioning the airway:

- If the patient has secretions or vomitus that cannot be removed quickly and easily by suctioning, the patient should be log rolled onto his side and the oropharynx cleared by finger sweeping the foreign material from the mouth.

- If the patient is producing frothy secretions as rapidly as suctioning can remove them, apply suction for 15 seconds, provide positive pressure ventilation with supplemental oxygen for 2 minutes, then apply suction for another 15 seconds. Repeat this sequence until the airway is cleared. Consult medical direction in such a situation.

- During suctioning, the residual air in the lungs between respirations is removed. This will cause a quick decrease in blood oxygen levels. Therefore, monitor the patient's pulse and heart rate while suctioning. If the heart rate drops during suctioning, especially in infants and children, immediately remove the catheter and begin positive pressure ventilation with supplemental oxygen.

    Stimulation of the back of the throat by the suction catheter may also cause a decrease in heart rate, especially in children and infants. In the adult patient, a rapid heart rate (tachycardia), slow heart rate (bradycardia), or an irregular heart rate may be seen during suctioning. These can occur from stimulation of the airway by the suction catheter or may be an indication that the oxygen level in the blood is getting dangerously low. Stop the suction procedure and resume positive pressure ventilation for at least 30 seconds if the patient is being artificially ventilated.

- Before suctioning mucus and small amounts of secretions in a patient who is being artificially ventilated, hyperventilate him at a rate greater than 24 ventilations per minute for 5 minutes to wash out the residual nitrogen and increase the functional oxygen reserve. After suctioning, hyperventilate him for another 5 minutes.

AIRWAY ADJUNCTS

Once the airway is opened by the head-tilt, chin-lift or jaw-thrust maneuver, and all foreign substances are removed by suctioning, it may be necessary to insert an airway adjunct to keep the airway open. There are two types of artificial airways: the oropharyngeal and nasopharyngeal. Both extend near to, but do not pass through, the larynx. These adjuncts are frequently used during artificial ventilation. When using these devices, keep the following points in mind:

• The adjunct must be clean and clear of obstructions.
• The proper size airway adjunct must be selected to avoid complications and ineffectiveness.
• The airway adjuncts do not protect the airway from aspiration of secretions, blood, vomitus, or other foreign substances into the lungs.
• The mental status of the patient will determine whether or not an adjunct can be used. The patient's mental status must be continually and carefully monitored. If the patient becomes more responsive or gags, remove the airway adjunct.
• A head-tilt, chin-lift or jaw-thrust maneuver must still be maintained, even when an airway adjunct is in place and properly positioned.

OROPHARYNGEAL (ORAL) AIRWAY

The **oropharyngeal airway,** also known as the **oral airway,** is a semicircular device of hard plastic or rubber that holds the tongue away from the back of the airway (Figure 7-9). The device also allows for suction of secretions. There are two common types of oropharyngeal airway: One is tubular and the other has a channeled side. Both are disposable and come in a variety of adult, child, and infant sizes.

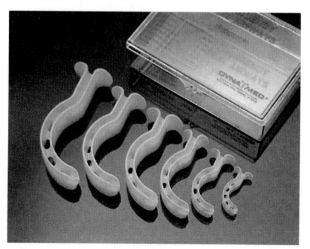

Figure 7-9 Oropharyngeal (oral) airways.

The patient must be completely unresponsive. *Do not use this device on a patient who is responsive or has a gag reflex.* If inserted in such a patient, it may cause vomiting or spasm of the vocal cords. This will further compromise the airway.

Use of an improperly sized airway adjunct can result in major complications. If the device is too long, it can push the epiglottis over the opening to the trachea causing a complete obstruction of the airway. Also, if the device is not inserted properly it may push the tongue back into the airway.

Even with the adjunct properly inserted, it is often necessary to maintain the position of patient's head with the head-tilt, chin-lift or jaw-thrust maneuver to ensure an open airway. Some patients improve significantly with placement of the adjunct.

Inserting the Oropharyngeal Airway The procedure for inserting an oropharyngeal airway is illustrated in Figures 7-10a to d. When inserting such a device, follow these steps:

1. Select the proper size airway. Measure the airway by holding it next to the patient's face. A properly sized airway should extend from the corner of the mouth (lips) to the bottom of the angle of the jaw or the tip of the earlobe.
2. Open the patient's mouth using the crossed-finger technique. In adults, insert the airway upside down, tip pointing to the roof of the mouth.
3. When the airway comes in contact with the soft palate at the back of the roof of the mouth, gently rotate it 180 degrees while continuing to advance it until the flat flange at the top of the airway rests on the patient's front teeth. The airway follows the natural curve of the tongue and the oropharynx (Figure 7-11). Following this procedure will reduce the chances of the tongue being pushed back and obstructing the airway. The airway can also be inserted sideways in the corner of the mouth and rotated 90 degrees while it is being advanced into position.

An alternative method of inserting the oropharyngeal airway involves the use of a tongue depressor (blade). The tongue depressor is inserted in the mouth until its tip is at the base of the tongue. The tongue is then pressed up and forward with the tongue depressor. The airway is inserted in its normal anatomic position until the flange is seated on the teeth (Figure 7-12). This is the preferred method of airway insertion in infants and children.

If a patient at any time gags during the insertion, remove the oropharyngeal airway. It may then be necessary to use a nasopharyngeal airway or no adjunct at all. If a patient tries to dislodge the device after it has been inserted, remove it by gently pulling it out and down. Because this airway adjunct commonly causes the patient to gag, be prepared for vomiting.

INSERTING AN OROPHARYNGEAL AIRWAY

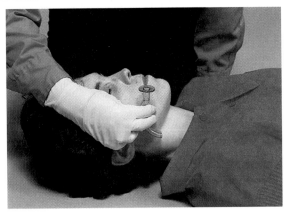

Figure 7-10a Measure to assure correct size.

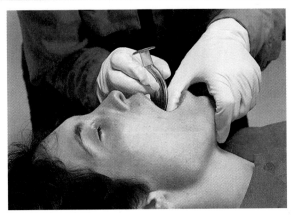

Figure 7-10b Insert with top pointing up toward roof of mouth.

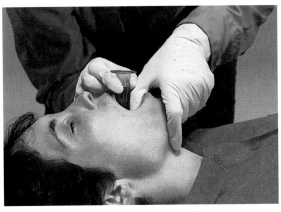

Figure 7-10c Advance while rotating 180°.

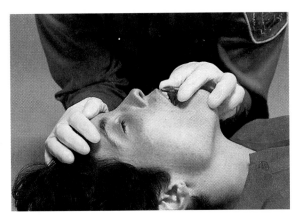

Figure 7-10d Continue until flange rests on the teeth.

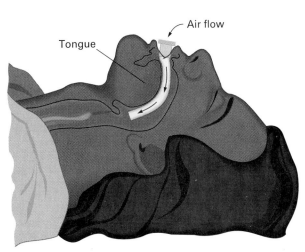

Figure 7-11 Oropharyngeal airway that is properly placed. The tongue is kept from falling back to occlude the patient's airway.

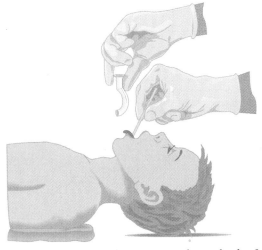

Figure 7-12 The preferred method of inserting the oropharyngeal airway in the infant or child is to use a tongue blade to hold the tongue forward and up as the airway is inserted.

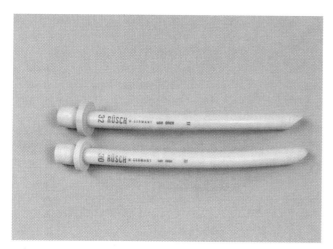

Figure 7-13   Nasopharyngeal (nasal) airways.

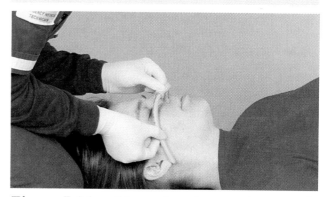

Figure 7-14a   Measuring the nasopharyngeal airway.

NASOPHARYNGEAL (NASAL) AIRWAY

The **nasopharyngeal airway,** or **nasal airway,** is a curved hollow tube of soft plastic or rubber with a flange or flare at the top end and a bevel at the distal end (Figure 7-13). This airway adjunct comes in a variety of sizes based on the diameter of the tube. Use of this airway is indicated if the patient is unable to tolerate an oropharyngeal airway or if the teeth are clenched shut and insertion of an oropharyngeal airway is impossible. The nasopharyngeal airway is less likely to stimulate vomiting because the soft tube moves and gives when the patient swallows. Therefore, it can be used on a patient who is not fully responsive and needs assistance in maintaining an open airway but who still has a gag reflex.

Be careful to select a nasopharyngeal airway of proper length. One that is too long can enter the esophagus during insertion, potentially causing massive **gastric distention** (inflation of the stomach), and inadequate ventilation.

Insertion and use of this device may still cause gagging, vomiting, and spasming of the vocal cords. Also, like the oropharyngeal airway, it does not completely protect the trachea and lungs from aspiration of blood, vomitus, secretions, or other foreign substances. Even though the tube is lubricated, insertion is painful and may cause injury to the nasal mucosa, causing the nose to bleed and allowing blood to enter the airway, resulting in possible obstruction or aspiration. It is still necessary to maintain a head-tilt, chin-lift or jaw-thrust maneuver once the airway is inserted.

Inserting the Nasopharyngeal Airway   The procedure for inserting the nasopharyngeal airway is illustrated in Figures 7-14a to c. When inserting such a device, follow these steps:

1. Measure the airway by placing it next to the patient's face. A properly sized airway should ex-

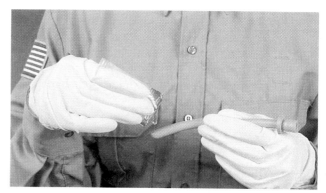

Figure 7-14b   Lubricate it with water-soluble lubricant.

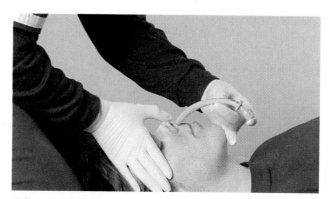

Figure 7-14c   Insert with the bevel toward the septum or base of the tonsil.

tend from the tip of the patient's nose to the tip of the earlobe. The diameter of the airway must be such that it can fit inside the patient's nostril without blanching the skin of the nose.

2. Lubricate the airway well with a sterile, water-soluble lubricant. This will ease the insertion and lessen the chance of trauma to the nasal mucous lining.

3. Insert the device in the larger or more open nostril. The bevel should be facing the septum (wall between the nostrils) or floor of the nostril. The device is inserted close to the midline, along the floor of the nostril, and straight back into the nasopharynx. If you meet resistance, rotate the device gently from side to side as you continue to insert it. If you still meet resistance, remove the airway and try the other nostril. When the device is properly inserted, the flange should lie against the flare of the nostril.

4. Check to be sure that air is flowing through the airway during inhalation and exhalation. If the patient is spontaneously breathing and no air movement is felt through the tube, remove it and attempt reinsertion in the other nostril.

ASSESSMENT OF BREATHING

After establishing a patent airway, it is necessary to assess the adequacy of the patient's breathing. Inadequate breathing leads to both poor gas exchange in the alveoli and ineffective delivery of oxygen to the cells. The rate, rhythm, quality, and depth of respirations should be assessed. This is done by looking, listening, feeling, and auscultating (listening with a stethoscope).

- *Look (inspect).* Inspection includes the following:
  1. *Inspect the chest.* Observe for adequate expansion by watching the chest wall rise and fall. Look for **retractions,** or pulling inward, of the intercostal muscles of the chest as well as excessive use of the neck muscles during inspiration. In the unresponsive patient, you should place your ear near the patient's mouth or nose while looking at the chest. You will simultaneously look, listen, and feel for air movement.

  2. *Observe the patient's general appearance.* Does he appear to be anxious, uncomfortable, or in distress? Is the patient lying down or sitting very erect? (Typically, a patient who has difficulty in breathing is sitting up, leaning forward.) Does it appear that the patient is straining to breathe?

  3. *Decide if the breathing pattern is regular or irregular.* Injuries to the brain commonly produce irregular breathing patterns that are ineffective.

  4. *Look at the nostrils* to see if they open wide during inhalation. Such flaring indicates difficulty in breathing.

- *Listen.* How does the patient speak to you? Does he speak only a few words at a time, then have to catch his breath? If the patient has an altered mental status or is unresponsive, place your ear next to the patient's nose and mouth and listen and feel for air escaping during exhalation. The sound or movement of air will indicate that the patient is breathing.

- *Feel.* With your ear next to the patient's nose and mouth, feel the volume of air escaping during exhalation. Feeling the air against your ear and cheek will provide you with a sense of the volume that the patient is breathing.

- *Auscultate.* Place your stethoscope at the second intercostal space, about two inches below the clavicle, at the midclavicular line. You can also auscultate at the fourth or fifth intercostal space on the anterior or midaxillary line, or at the fifth intercostal space next to the sternum on the anterior chest (Figure 7-15). Listen to one full inhalation and exhalation and determine if the breath sounds are present and equal **bilaterally** (on both sides). An adequate volume of air being inspired will produce full breath sounds that are equal on both

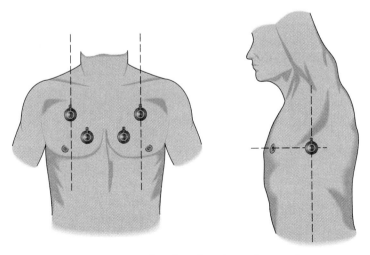

Figure 7-15 Auscultation landmarks on the anterior and lateral chest.

sides. Breath sounds that are diminished or absent indicate inadequate breathing.

The rate, rhythm, quality, and depth of the breathing must be checked during assessment. The rate is simply checked by counting the number of respirations in one minute (one inhalation + one exhalation = one respiration). The rhythm is checked by looking at the pattern of respirations (regular or irregular). The quality of breath sounds is assessed by auscultating the breath sounds, inspecting for adequate chest expansion, and the use of accessory muscles. The depth, or **tidal volume**, is determined by assessing the rise and fall of the chest, listening and feeling for air movement, and auscultating the breath sounds.

Either rate or depth by itself is not enough to determine that the breathing is adequate. You may, for example, determine that an adult patient is breathing at a rate of 16 respirations per minute, which falls within the normal limits. If you also note, however, that his chest shows only a slight rise and fall, that you hear and feel very little air being expelled, and that his breath sounds are diminished bilaterally, the patient's breathing is inadequate. On the other hand, you might find a patient who has very good tidal volume, but who is only breathing at six respirations per minute. This patient's breathing is also inadequate.

ADEQUATE BREATHING

The patient whose breathing is adequate will exhibit the following characteristics:

- *Rate*—The respiratory rate falls within normal limits: for an adult, 12 to 20 respirations a minute; for a child, 15 to 30 a minute; and for an infant, 25 to 50 a minute. In situations where the patient is frightened or nervous, the respiratory rate will be slightly elevated.
- *Rhythm*—The pattern is regular. Each breath is of about the same volume and comes at a regular interval. However, it is normal for a patient to sigh, which alters the pattern and makes it slightly irregular.
- *Quality*—The breath sounds are equal and full bilaterally, indicating good expansion of each lung. The chest rises and falls adequately and equally with each breath. No excessive accessory muscle use is seen with inhalation and exhalation. Note that it is normal for infants and children to use the abdominal muscles more than adults do in breathing; therefore, expect greater movement of the abdomen with these patients.
- *Depth (tidal volume)*—The volume of air felt and heard by placing your ear next to the patient's mouth and nose is adequate. The chest is rising and falling adequately and full breath sounds are heard on each side of the chest.

INADEQUATE BREATHING

Inadequate breathing leads to both inadequate oxygen exchange at the level of the alveoli and inadequate delivery of oxygen to the cells. It also causes inadequate elimination of carbon dioxide from the body. If the breathing remains inadequate, the cells become hypoxic and begin to die. The brain, heart, and liver are the organs most sensitive to hypoxia. The brain will begin to die in about 4 to 6 minutes without an oxygen supply.

It is very important for you to recognize the signs of inadequate breathing and to immediately begin positive pressure (artificial) ventilation when they are present. Some of the signs are subtle and require careful evaluation (Figure 7-16). If you are uncertain as to whether a patient requires breathing assistance, it is better to err on the side of safety and provide ventilation. Any time that ventilation is administered, oxygen must be connected and delivered with each ventilation.

SIGNS OF INADEQUATE BREATHING

Figure 7-16 summarizes the signs of inadequate breathing. Note how the rate, rhythm, quality, and depth differ from those of adequate breathing.

- *Rate*—The respiratory rate is either too fast or too slow—outside the normal rate ranges that were listed under Adequate Breathing. **Tachypnea** is an excessively rapid breathing rate and may indicate inadequate oxygenation and breathing, especially in an adult. **Bradypnea** is an abnormally slow breathing rate and an ominous sign of inadequate breathing and oxygenation in infants and children. Bradypnea may also be seen in adult patients, particularly those with drug or alcohol emergencies.
- *Rhythm*—An irregular breathing pattern may indicate a severe brain injury or medical illness. Most irregular breathing patterns also produce an inadequate depth and quality.
- *Quality*—Breath sounds that are decreased or absent indicate an inadequate volume of air moving in and out of the lungs with each breath. If the chest wall is not rising and falling adequately with each breath, or if the sides of the chest rise and fall unequally, the breathing is inadequate.
  - Inadequate breathing can lead to excessive use of the neck muscles and intercostal muscles during breathing. This can produce retractions, or depressions between the ribs, above the clavicles, around the muscles of the neck, and below the rib cage with inspiration. These retractions are seen more often in infants and children.
  - The abdomen may also move excessively in a patient breathing inadequately. Such a patient is using the abdomen to push up on the diaphragm in an effort to force air out of the lungs. Re-

Fast or slow respiratory rate.

Irregular rhythm.

Unequal or inadequate chest expansion.

Increased effort to breathe.

Retractions above clavicles, between ribs, below rib cage.

Shallow or inadequate depth of breathing.

Cool and clammy skin.

Cyanosis.

Occasional gasping breaths may be seen just before death.

Nasal flaring.

Use of accessory muscles to breathe.

Figure 7-16   Signs of inadequate breathing and severe respiratory distress.

member, however, that infants and children normally use their abdominal muscles in breathing.
- Infants may display a "seesaw" breathing motion in which the abdomen and chest move in opposite directions during breathing.
- The nostrils may flare during inspirations, an indication that a patient is working hard to breathe. Flaring is seen most often in children.
- *Depth*—The depth of breathing (tidal volume) is shallow and inadequate. Occasional gasping respirations with no regular pattern or depth, known as **agonal respirations,** are commonly seen as the patient goes into cardiac arrest or as a late sign of impending respiratory arrest.

It is important to note that not all of the signs of inadequate breathing will be present at the same time. *Any of these signs—a breathing rate that is too low or too high, a shallow depth, a poor quality, or an inadequate tidal volume—is by itself a reason to ventilate a patient without delay. Waiting for additional signs to appear would only risk further compromise in the patient's condition.*

TECHNIQUES OF ARTIFICIAL VENTILATION

The EMT-Basic can use several methods to artificially ventilate, or force air into, the patient who is breathing inadequately or not breathing at all. Because air is

being forced into the patient's lungs, the technique is referred to as **positive pressure ventilation (PPV).** The methods for providing positive pressure ventilation vary and require different levels of skill and different types of equipment. Each method has different advantages and disadvantages; the method you select should be based on the characteristics of the situation and the resources available.

BASIC CONSIDERATIONS

The methods that the EMT-B can use to artificially ventilate the patient are listed below in order of preference (Figure 7-17):

- Mouth-to-mask
- Bag-valve mask (BVM) operated by two people
- Flow-restricted, oxygen-powered ventilation device
- Bag-valve mask (BVM) operated by one person

There are three major considerations when using a device for artificial ventilation:

1. You must be able to maintain a good mask seal and not allow excessive air leakage from between the mask and the patient's face. An inadequate mask seal will lead to an insufficient volume of air being delivered.
2. The device must be able to deliver an adequate volume of air to sufficiently inflate the lungs.
3. There must be a connection to allow for simultaneous oxygen delivery while artificially ventilating.

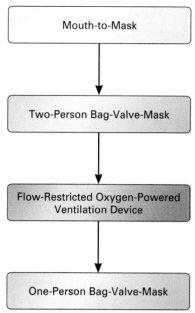

Figure 7-17 Order of preference for methods to ventilate a patient.

BODY SUBSTANCE ISOLATION

As with any technique being performed in which there is a risk of coming in contact with body fluids, it is necessary to take body substance isolation precautions when performing artificial ventilation. The risks of coming in contact with secretions, blood, or vomitus while ventilating are relatively high; therefore, the EMT-B must, at minimum, use gloves and eyewear. If large amounts of blood or secretions are present, use a face mask. If tuberculosis is suspected, use a HEPA respirator during the entire patient contact.

ADEQUATE VENTILATION

When performing artificial ventilation, regardless of the device being used, it is necessary to monitor the patient continuously to ensure that the ventilation is adequate. Inadequate ventilation may occur because of problems with the patient's upper or lower airway or because of improper use of a ventilation device. You must be completely familiar with any device you use to ventilate a patient. Keep in mind that ventilation must not be interrupted for greater than 30 seconds.

Indications that the patient is being adequately ventilated include the following:

• *The rate of ventilation is sufficient.* Infants and children must be ventilated at a minimum rate of once every 3 seconds (20 times per minute). The rate for adults is once every 5 seconds (12 times per minute).
• *The tidal volume must be consistent; it must also be sufficient to cause the chest to rise during each ventilation.*

• *The patient's heart rate returns to normal.* (Other underlying conditions may prevent return of a normal heart rate even when ventilations are being adequately performed.)
• *Color improves.*

INADEQUATE VENTILATION

Indications of inadequate ventilation include:

• *The chest does not rise and fall with artificial ventilation.* This is an indication that the volume being delivered is not adequate. This may be due to a failure to use the ventilation device properly or to an airway obstruction. A common cause of ineffective ventilation is a poor mask seal that allows a portion of the ventilation to escape. If the patient's chest does not fall, it may be a sign that the ventilation device or the upper or lower airway is obstructed, preventing adequate exhalation.
• *The ventilation rate is too fast or too slow.* Ventilating a patient too rapidly does not allow for adequate exhalation and can cause gastric distention. Too slow a rate of ventilation will not provide an adequate amount of oxygen.
• *The heart rate does not return to normal with artificial ventilation.* (Remember, however, to consider other sources of heart rate disturbance, e.g., blood loss, anxiety, heart problem.)

MOUTH-TO-MOUTH VENTILATION

The air we breathe contains 21 percent oxygen. Of this 21 percent, only 5 percent is used by the body; the remaining 16 percent is exhaled. Because the exhaled breath contains about 16 percent oxygen, a patient can be oxygenated with the rescuer's exhaled breath. This is the principle behind mouth-to-mouth ventilation taught in many first-aid and CPR courses.

The risk of contracting infectious diseases makes this technique too dangerous for regular use by EMT-Bs, who are expected to ventilate many patients as a part of their responsibilities.

MOUTH-TO-MOUTH AND MOUTH-TO-NOSE TECHNIQUE

The EMT-B forms a seal with his mouth around the patient's mouth or nose and uses his exhaled air to ventilate. The nose is pinched during mouth-to-mouth ventilation, and the mouth is closed during mouth-to-mouth nose ventilation. This technique provides adequate volumes of air for ventilating a patient. Its major limitations are its inability to deliver high concentrations of oxygen while ventilating and the risk posed to the EMT-B by contact with the patient's body fluids. To reduce risks, a barrier device must be used.

Use mouth-to-nose ventilation when the patient's mouth cannot be opened, severe soft tissue or bone injury has occurred to the mouth or around it, or you cannot achieve a tight mouth-to-mouth seal.

MOUTH-TO-MASK VENTILATION

The mouth-to-mask technique, like the mouth-to-mouth or mouth-to-nose technique, uses the exhaled breath of the EMT-B to ventilate the patient. But with this technique, a plastic **pocket mask** is used to form a seal around the patient's nose and mouth (Figure 7-18). The EMT-B then blows into a port at the top of the mask to deliver the ventilation.

Mouth-to-mask ventilation is the preferred method to use when performing artificial ventilation because of the following advantages:

- The mask eliminates direct contact with the patient's nose, mouth, and secretions.
- Use of a one-way valve at the ventilation port prevents exposure to the patient's exhaled air.
- The method can provide adequate tidal volumes and possibly greater tidal volumes than bag-valve-mask ventilation.
- Supplemental oxygen can be administered through the oxygen inlet that most pocket masks have in addition to the ventilation port.

The mask used to ventilate the patient must have the following characteristics:

- It should be of a transparent material to permit the detection of vomitus, secretions, blood, or other substances in the patient's mouth.
- It must be able to fit tightly on the patient's face and form a good seal.
- It must have an oxygen inlet to allow for high-flow oxygen delivery at 15 liters per minute (lpm).
- It should be available in one average adult size and additional sizes for infants and children.
- It must have or be connectable to a one-way valve at the ventilation port.

MOUTH-TO-MASK TECHNIQUE

Mouth-to-mask ventilation is illustrated in Figure 7-19. The procedure is described below:

1. Connect a one-way valve to the ventilation port of the mask and connect tubing that is attached to an oxygen supply to the oxygen inlet (Figure 7-19). Set the oxygen flow for 15 lpm.
2. Perform a head-tilt, chin-lift or jaw-thrust maneuver to open the airway. An oropharyngeal or nasopharyngeal airway can be inserted, if needed to maintain the airway.
3. Position yourself, if possible, at the top of the patient's head.
4. Place the mask on the patient's face. The narrower top portion of the mask should be seated on the bridge of the nose and the broader portion in the cleft of the chin. Place your thumbs on the top portion of the mask and the thumb side of the palms of both hands along the sides of the mask and the index fingers over the bottom of the mask to hold it down and form a good seal. With the middle, ring, and little fingers, grasp under the mandible just in front of the earlobes to pull upward to maintain the head tilt. If no oropharyngeal or nasopharyngeal airway is in place, be sure to keep the patient's mouth open.
5. Place your mouth around the one-way valve and blow into the ventilation port of the mask. **Each breath should be slow and steady and delivered over at least 1.5 to 2 seconds for an adult and 1 to 1.5 seconds for an infant or child.** When the chest rises adequately, stop the ventilation to allow for exhalation. If you cannot ventilate or if the chest does not rise adequately, reposition the patient's head and try again; improper head position is the most common cause of difficulty with ventilation. If the second try also fails,

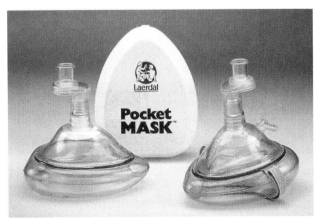

Figure 7-18   Pocket mask with one-way valve and oxygen connection. (Laerdal Medical Corporation)

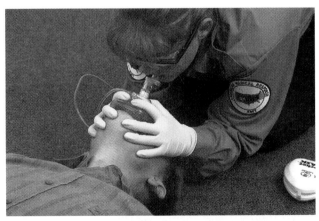

Figure 7-19   Mouth-to-mask ventilation. The mask should be connected to oxygen at a flow of 15 liters per minute (lpm).

assume the airway is blocked by a foreign object and follow the guidelines for removing a foreign-body airway obstruction found in Appendix 1.

6. **An adult should be ventilated once every 5 seconds and infants and children once every 3 seconds.**

BAG-VALVE-MASK VENTILATION

A **bag-valve-mask (BVM) device** (Figure 7-20) is a manual resuscitator used to provide positive pressure ventilation. The bag-valve mask consists of a self-inflating bag, a one-way nonrebreather valve, a face mask, an intake/oxygen reservoir valve, and an oxygen reservoir. Most adult-sized bag-valve-mask devices have a volume of approximately 1,600 milliliters. When used without an oxygen source, the device will only deliver 21 percent oxygen, the amount found in room air. By adding oxygen and a reservoir, you can deliver close to 100 percent oxygen to the patient, a major advantage of using the device.

The principal advantages of the bag-valve-mask device over mouth-to-mask ventilation are its convenience for the EMT-B and its ability to deliver enriched oxygen mixtures. However, the bag-valve mask rarely generates the tidal volumes that are possible with mouth-to-mask ventilation.

The bag-valve-mask device is harder to use than it looks and is fatiguing to the operator when performing a one-person technique. The EMT-B must simultaneously provide a tight mask seal, maintain an open airway by properly positioning the patient's head and chin, and squeeze the bag to deliver the ventilation. It takes frequent practice to maintain the skills needed to deliver adequate ventilation with the device. Because of the difficulty in working the bag-valve mask, use of the device by two persons is highly recommended but not always possible. A single-operator mask such as the pocket mask has few of these disadvantages, takes less skill and maintenance,

and is much easier to use by all practitioners, experienced or inexperienced.

A bag-valve mask should have these features:

• A self-refilling bag that is disposable or easy to clean and sterilize
• A nonjamming valve system that allows a minimum oxygen inlet flow of 15 lpm
• Either no pop-off valve or a pop-off valve that can be manually disabled. A pop-off valve that is not disabled may lead to inadequate ventilation.
• Standard 15/22 mm fittings to permit use with a variety of ventilation masks and other ventilation adjuncts
• An oxygen inlet and a reservoir that can be connected with an oxygen source to deliver high concentrations of oxygen during ventilation. An oxygen reservoir should be used when ventilating all patients.
• A true nonrebreather valve that vents the patient's exhalations and does not allow him to rebreathe any exhaled gas
• Adaptability to all environmental conditions and temperature extremes
• A variety of infant-, child-, and adult-sized masks. A properly sized mask will fit snugly over the bridge of the nose and into the cleft of the chin.
• Transparent masks to permit detection of vomitus, blood, or secretions during ventilation

Note that oropharyngeal or nasopharyngeal airway adjuncts can help in maintaining an open airway and should be used any time the bag-valve-mask device is used.

BAG-VALVE-MASK TECHNIQUE

A bag-valve-mask device can be used by one or two EMT-Bs. For reasons cited above, use of the device by two EMT-Bs is preferred. One EMT-B holds a

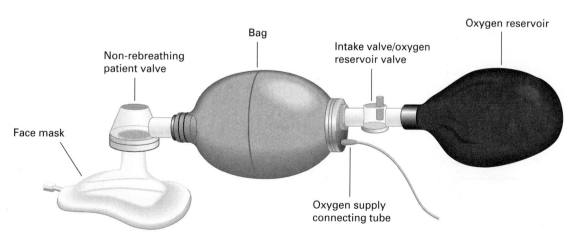

Figure 7-20 Bag-valve-mask unit with oxygen bag reservoir. Tubing-type reservoirs are also available.

tight mask seal with both hands while the second EMT-B uses both hands to squeeze the bag to deliver the full volume of oxygenated air inside it (Figure 7-21). This technique is considerably more effective than one-person use of the device and should always be employed unless the number of personnel or the circumstances of the run, such as an extremely cramped working area, do not allow it. Procedures to follow in use of the bag-valve mask are as follows:

1. If possible, position yourself at the top of the patient's head. If you do not suspect a spinal injury, open the airway using the head-tilt, chin-lift maneuver. Raise the patient's head slightly with a towel or pillow to achieve a better sniffing position. If a spinal injury is suspected, follow procedures described later under Bag-Valve-Mask Technique—Patient with Suspected Spinal Injury.

2. Select the correct size mask and bag-valve device. If the patient is unresponsive, an oropharyngeal or nasopharyngeal airway may be inserted to help maintain a patent airway.

3. Place the upper, narrower part of the mask over the bridge of the nose and lower it over the mouth and into the cleft of the chin. If the mask has a large round cuff surrounding the ventilation port, center the port over the mouth (Figure 7-22).

4. Position your thumbs over the top half of the mask and your index fingers over the bottom portion of the mask. Use your ring and little fingers to bring the patient's jaw up to the mask. The middle fingers, depending on the size of the EMT-B's hands, may be placed either under the mandible or over the mask. The thumbside edges of the palms are placed over both sides of the mask to hold it in place and form an airtight seal.

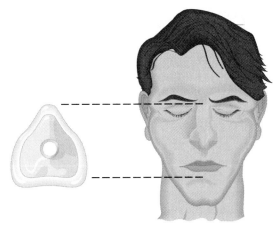

Figure 7-22   Always use the proper size mask. It should fit securely over the bridge of the nose and in the cleft of the chin.

5. Have another EMT-B connect the bag valve to the mask, if it is not already attached.

6. Begin ventilation as soon as possible. The other EMT-B or some qualified person should squeeze the bag with two hands while watching for adequate chest rise and fall. **Each ventilation should be delivered over a 1.5 to 2-second period for an adult, 1 to 1.5 seconds for an infant or child.** If you cannot ventilate or if the chest does not rise adequately, take the measures described under Bag-Valve Mask Problems, below.

7. **Ventilation should be delivered at a minimum of once every 5 seconds for adults and once every 3 seconds for infants and children.** The chest should be monitored continuously for adequate rise and fall.

8. If the bag-valve mask has not already been connected to the oxygen supply, the patient should receive positive pressure ventilation for one minute. At that point, the other EMT-B should make the connection, set the flow at 15 lpm, attach a reservoir if not already in place, and resume ventilation.

In those situations when you are operating the bag-valve mask alone, apply the mask to the patient's face with one hand. Your thumb should be placed over the part of the mask covering the bridge of the nose and your index finger over the part covering the cleft of the chin. Seal the mask firmly on the face by pushing down with the thumb and index finger while pulling up on the mandible with the other fingers to maintain a head-tilt, chin-lift. Squeeze the bag with the other hand while observing the chest rise to make certain the lungs are being inflated effectively (Figure 7-23). The bag may alternatively be compressed against your body or forearm to deliver a greater tidal volume to the patient.

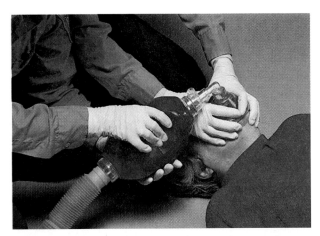

Figure 7-21   Two-person bag-valve-mask method.

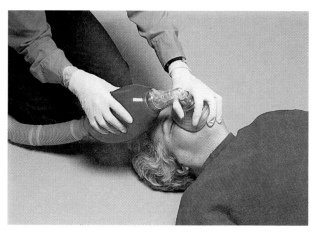

Figure 7-23   One-person bag-valve-mask method.

Bag-Valve-Mask Problems If the patient's chest does not rise and fall, reevaluate the bag-valve-mask device and the patient's airway, considering these possible problems and remedies:

1. Check the position of the head and chin. Reposition the airway and repeat your attempt at ventilation.
2. Check the mask seal to ensure that an excessive amount of air is not escaping from around the mask. Reposition your fingers and the mask to attain a tight seal.
3. Assess for an obstruction. If the airway is repositioned, the seal is adequate, and you are still unable to ventilate effectively, consider an airway obstruction. Inspect inside the mouth for evidence of an obstruction. If one is found, remove it with a finger sweep. If none is found, begin the foreign-body airway obstruction maneuver described in Appendix 1 until you are able to effectively ventilate.
4. Check the bag-valve-mask system to ensure that all the parts are properly connected and operational. Some systems with a bag-type oxygen reservoir will refill extremely slowly if the oxygen flow rate is inadequate. This causes a reduction in the tidal volume delivered to the patient and subsequently produces minimal chest rise and fall and leads to hypoxia.
5. If the chest still does not rise and fall, use an alternative method for positive pressure ventilation, e.g., a pocket mask or a flow-restricted, oxygen-powered ventilation device.
6. If you are having difficulty maintaining an open airway, insert an oropharyngeal or nasopharyngeal airway. Either device will help keep the tongue from falling back to block the airway.
7. If the patient's abdomen is rising with each ventilation or that it appears to be distended, it may be an indication of one of the following:

   - The head-tilt, chin-lift maneuver is not being performed properly and is allowing an excessive amount of air into the esophagus and stomach. Reposition the head and neck and resume ventilation.
   - The patient is being ventilated too rapidly or with too great a tidal volume. Such excessive ventilation increases the pressure in the esophagus and allows air to enter into the stomach. Squeeze the bag slowly to deliver the volume over a 2-second period and allow for adequate exhalation after each ventilation.

BAG-VALVE-MASK TECHNIQUE—PATIENT WITH SUSPECTED SPINAL INJURY

If you suspect a patient has a spinal injury, you must establish and maintain in-line spinal stabilization as a priority. The airway maneuvers and use of the bag-valve-mask technique must be performed with special care to avoid movement of the head or spine while maintaining in-line spinal stabilization until the patient is fully immobilized to a backboard. The procedures for using a bag-valve mask with a patient with suspected spinal injury are illustrated in Figures 7-24 a to c and are described below:

1. While following procedures for manual in-line stabilization of the head and neck (see Chapter 34, "Injuries to the Spine"), open the airway using a jaw-thrust maneuver.
2. Have another EMT-B or a trained assistant maintain the in-line stabilization of the head and neck while you select the correct size mask. If no other personnel are available, you can kneel at the patient's head and hold his head between your thighs and knees to prevent movement.
3. Position your thumbs over the top half of the mask and your index and middle fingers over the bottom half. Place the top of the mask over the bridge of the nose. Lower the mask over the mouth and until the bottom half of the mask fits snugly in the cleft of the chin.
4. Place your middle, ring, and little fingers under the mandible and bring the jaw up to the mask without tilting the head back or moving the neck.
5. Have another EMT-B connect the bag-valve device to the mask, if this has not already been done. Hold a mask seal with your thumbs at the bridge of the nose and the index fingers over the bottom half of the mask. The edges of the palms on the thumbside should hold the mask down on the face. The middle, ring, and little fingers are used to maintain the jaw thrust. EMT-Bs with smaller hands may be able to grasp the mandible only with the ring and little fingers.

IN-LINE STABILIZATION DURING BAG-VALVE VENTILATION

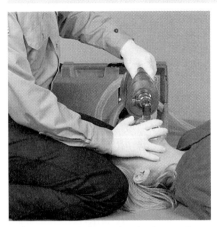

Figure 7-24a   Technique for one EMT-B to maintain in-line stabilization while performing one-person bag-valve-mask ventilation.

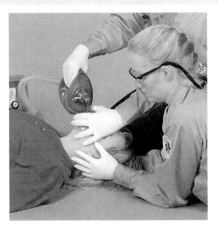

Figure 7-24b   Technique for two EMT-Bs to maintain in-line stabilization while performing bag-valve-mask ventilation.

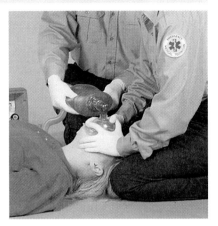

Figure 7-24c   Alternative technique for two EMT-Bs to maintain in-line stabilization while performing bag-valve-mask ventilation.

6. Begin ventilation as soon as possible. Have the other EMT-B or trained assistant squeeze the bag with two hands to deliver the volume over a 2-second period.

7. Ventilation should be repeated every 5 seconds for an adult and every 3 seconds for an infant or child. The rise and fall of the chest should be monitored continuously to ensure that ventilation is effective.

8. If the bag-valve mask has not already been connected to the oxygen supply, the patient should receive positive pressure ventilation for one minute without the oxygen supplement. At that point the other EMT-B should make the connection, set the flow at 15 lpm, attach a reservoir, and resume ventilation.

9. In-line manual stabilization must be maintained until the patient is completely immobilized to the backboard.

10. Once the patient is fully immobilized, follow the standard two-person bag-valve-mask technique, using the jaw-thrust maneuver to maintain a patent airway.

If only two EMT-Bs are at a scene, it may be necessary for one to hold the in-line stabilization with his thighs and knees, while performing all the additional steps of the one-person bag-valve-mask technique. This is the most ineffective method for providing bag-valve-mask ventilation and should be replaced with the two-person technique as soon as possible.

FLOW-RESTRICTED, OXYGEN-POWERED VENTILATION DEVICE (FROPVD)

Another method of providing positive pressure ventilation is through use of the **flow-restricted, oxygen-powered ventilation device** (**FROPVD**), also known as a demand-valve device (Figure 7-25). The device is powered by oxygen and, with a proper mask seal, will deliver 100 percent oxygen to the patient. In the

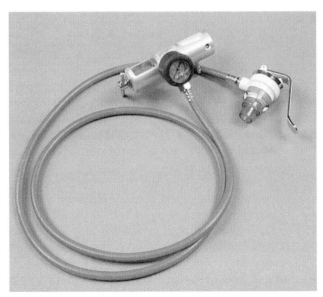

Figure 7-25   A flow-restricted, oxygen-powered ventilation device.

spontaneously breathing patient, the valve is opened automatically by the negative pressure created by the patient's inspiration. Oxygen flow ceases automatically when the inhalation ends.

This device is designed to be used only on adult patients. Because it delivers oxygen at high pressure and at a high flow rate, it cannot be used on infants or children.

The delivery rates and pressures also mean that gastric distention often occurs with use of the device. Additionally, improper use of the device can lead to rupture of a patient's lungs. Since the potential for complications is high, only those trained in its use should operate the device.

The flow-restricted, oxygen-powered ventilation device should have the following features:

- A peak flow rate of less than 40 lpm of 100 percent oxygen
- An inspiratory pressure relief valve that opens at approximately 60 centimeters of water pressure and vents any remaining volume to the atmosphere or ceases gas flow
- An audible alarm that sounds whenever the relief valve pressure is exceeded
- Adaptability to a variety of environmental conditions and extremes of temperature
- An activating trigger or on/off button positioned so that the EMT-B can keep both hands on the mask to hold a seal
- Standard 15/22 millimeter couplings for masks, endotracheal tubes, tracheostomy tubes, and other alternative airways
- A rugged design that is compact and easy to hold and operate

FROPVD Techniques

Follow the steps described below when using a flow-restricted, oxygen-powered ventilation device:

1. Check the unit to ensure that it is properly functioning. Also, check the oxygen source to ensure that there is an adequate supply to operate the unit effectively.
2. Open the airway using a head-tilt, chin-lift maneuver and insert an oropharyngeal or nasopharyngeal airway. Apply the adult mask to the patient's face in the same manner as for the bag-valve mask.
3. Connect the flow-restricted, oxygen-powered ventilation device to the mask if not already done.
4. Activate the valve by depressing the trigger or button on the valve. As soon as the chest begins to rise, deactivate the valve by releasing the trigger or button. The oxygen flow ceases and the

patient's exhaled gas is released through a one-way valve.
5. Repeat the ventilation a minimum of once every 5 seconds in the adult patient.

If you suspect that a patient has a spinal injury and two EMT-Bs are available, one can perform the in-line stabilization while the other holds a mask seal and triggers the device. If only one EMT-B is available, he can hold in-line stabilization of the head and neck with his thighs and knees while holding a mask seal and triggering the device.

FROPVD Problems If a patient's chest does not rise adequately during use of the flow-restricted, oxygen-powered ventilation device, reevaluate the position of the head and chin and the mask seal. If the chest does not rise after repositioning and the mask seal proves adequate, an airway obstruction is a possibility; follow the procedure for adult foreign-body airway obstruction in Appendix 1.

If the oxygen source that powers the device runs out or the user cannot effectively use the device, it is necessary to use an alternative means to ventilate the patient, e.g., pocket mask or bag-valve-mask device.

AUTOMATIC TRANSPORT VENTILATOR

Another device used for positive pressure ventilation is the **automatic transport ventilator** (**ATV**). Several different devices are currently available. They have been shown to be excellent at providing and maintaining a constant rate and tidal volume during ventilation, and maintaining adequate oxygenation of arterial blood. In addition, most ATVs use oxygen as their power source, thereby delivering 100 percent oxygen during ventilation.

The ATV can deliver oxygen at lower inspiratory flow rates and for longer inspiratory times. Therefore, the devices have a lesser likelihood of causing gastric distention compared with other methods of positive pressure ventilation, including mouth-to-mask, bag-valve mask, and flow-restricted, oxygen-powered ventilation devices. However, as with any other ventilation device, gastric distention can occur if the patient's head and neck are improperly positioned.

Among other advantages of the ATV are the following:

- The EMT-B is free to use both hands to hold the mask and maintain the airway position as the device delivers the ventilation automatically.
- The device can be set to provide a specific tidal volume, respiratory rate, and minute ventilation.
- Alarms indicate low pressure in the oxygen tank as well as accidental disconnection of the ventilator.

- One EMT-B can hold in-line stabilization with his thighs and knees and hold the mask seal with two hands while the ventilation is delivered.

  There are a few disadvantages associated with the ATV:

- Because the ATV is usually oxygen powered (although one type of ATV does use electric power), once the oxygen supply is depleted, the device cannot be used. A pocket mask or bag-valve-mask device should always be available when using an ATV in case of failure or oxygen depletion.
- The ATV cannot be used in children less than 5 years of age.
- When using the ATV device, it is not possible to feel an increase in airway resistance or a decrease in the compliance in the lungs.

ATV TECHNIQUES

It is necessary to consult with medical direction to determine the ventilator settings when using the ATV. Always follow the manufacturer's recommendations. The following are general guidelines for the operation of an ATV:

1. Check the ATV to ensure it is properly functioning.
2. Attach the ATV to a mask. Seal the mask on the face by using the same technique described earlier in the bag-valve mask section.
3. Select the appropriate tidal volume and rate to be delivered. On some models the tidal volume and rate are preset. Turn the unit on.
4. Observe the chest for adequate rise and fall. Adjust the tidal volume until adequate rise of the chest is achieved.
5. Continuously monitor both the device for proper functioning and the rise of the patient's chest for adequate ventilation. If a failure of the device is detected or suspected, immediately discontinue the use of the ATV and begin ventilation with a pocket mask or a bag-valve-mask device.

OXYGEN DELIVERY

Oxygen is a colorless, odorless gas normally present in the atmosphere in a concentration of approximately 21 percent. Pure or 100 percent oxygen is obtained commercially by fractional distillation, a process by which air is liquefied and the gases other than oxygen, primarily nitrogen, are boiled off. Liquid oxygen is then converted under high pressure to a gas and stored in steel or aluminum cylinders under a pressure of about 2,000 pounds per square inch (psi) (Figure 7-26).

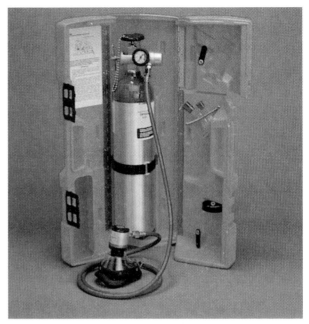

Figure 7-26   A basic portable resuscitator.

OXYGEN CYLINDERS

A number of different types of oxygen cylinders are available. They vary in size and in the volume of oxygen contained. Even though the volume of oxygen may vary, all of the cylinders when full are at the same pressure, about 2,000 psi. The cylinders are given letter designations according to their size. The following are sizes and related volumes of oxygen cylinders used in emergency medical care:

- D cylinder—350 liters
- E cylinder—625 liters
- M cylinder—3,000 liters
- G cylinder—5,300 liters
- H cylinder—6,900 liters

 ## SAFETY PRECAUTIONS

Because oxygen is a gas that acts as an accelerant for combustion and oxygen cylinders are under high pressure, they must be handled very carefully. Observe the following safety precautions:

- Never allow combustible materials such as oil or grease to touch the cylinder, regulator, fittings, valves, or hoses. Oil and oxygen under pressure will explode if they come into contact. This includes petroleum-based adhesive (adhesive tape) or lubricants such as petroleum jelly.
- Never smoke or allow others to smoke in any area where oxygen cylinders are in use or on standby. Because oxygen makes fires burn more rapidly, it greatly increases the risk of fire, not only from the tube but in towels, sheets, and clothing with which oxygen has come in contact.

- Store the cylinders below 125 degrees Fahrenheit.
- Never use an oxygen cylinder without a safe, properly fitting regulator valve. Never use a valve that has been modified from another gas.
- Keep all valves closed when the oxygen cylinder is not in use, even if the tank is empty.
- Keep oxygen cylinders secured to prevent their toppling over. In transit, they should be in a carrier rack or secured to the stretcher. An oxygen tank should never be left unsecured anywhere in the patient or driver compartment.
- When you are working with an oxygen cylinder, never place any part of your body over the cylinder valve. A full cylinder is at 2,000 to 2,200 psi. If the tank is punctured or if a valve breaks off, an oxygen cylinder can accelerate with enough force to penetrate concrete walls. A loosely fitting regulator can be blown off the cylinder with sufficient force to amputate a head or demolish any object in its path. Never stand an oxygen tank upright or in any position in which it may fall and possibly break off its valve. Lay the oxygen tank down next to the patient.

PRESSURE REGULATORS

Gas flow from an oxygen cylinder is controlled by a regulator that reduces the high pressure in the cylinder to a safe range, around 50 psi, and controls the flow of oxygen from 1 to 15 lpm. These regulators attach to the cylinder by a yoke, a series of pins configured to fit cylinders holding only one type of gas. The yoke prevents a regulator from being attached accidentally or purposefully to another type of gas. In addition, all gas cylinders are color-coded according to their contents. Oxygen cylinders in the United States are generally steel green or aluminum gray.

Two types of regulators may be attached to an oxygen cylinder: high-pressure regulators and therapy regulators. The **high-pressure regulator** can provide 50 psi to power a flow-restricted, oxygen-powered ventilation device. It has only one gauge, which registers the cylinder contents, and a threaded outlet. It cannot be used interchangeably with the therapy regulator because it has no mechanism for controlling and adjusting the flow rate. To use the high pressure regulator, attach the equipment supply line to the threaded outlet and open the cylinder valve fully; then turn it back one-half turn for safety.

The **therapy regulator** can administer oxygen up to 15 lpm. It typically has two gauges, one indicating the pressure in the tank and the other indicating the measured flow of oxygen being delivered to the patient. Some therapy regulators have only one gauge and a dial. The gauge shows the tank pressure. The dial, which has lpm markings, is used to select the flow of oxygen to be delivered to the patient. The various oxygen-delivery devices require different flow rates.

The pressure in the tank, about 2,000 psi when full, decreases proportionally as the volume of oxygen in the tank decreases. Therefore, a pressure reading of 1,000 psi would indicate that the tank is half full. The pressure in the tank will vary with changes in ambient temperature. An increase in ambient temperature would cause the pressure in the tank to increase, whereas, a decrease in ambient temperature would cause a decrease in tank pressure.

OXYGEN HUMIDIFIERS

Oxygen exits the tank in a dry gaseous form. The dryness can be irritating to a patient's respiratory tract if used over a long period of time. It is possible to add moisture to the oxygen by attaching an **oxygen humidifier** to the regulator. The humidifier, which consists of a container that is filled with sterile water, is connected directly to the regulator. The oxygen device tubing is attached directly to the humidifier. The oxygen leaving the regulator is forced through the water in the humidifier, picking up moisture before exiting and being delivered to the patient. Disposable humidifiers are available for one-time use.

For short periods of time, it is not harmful to deliver dry oxygen to the patient. Generally, a humidifier is not needed for prehospital administration of oxygen. If oxygen is to be delivered over a long period of time, as in a transport of an hour or more, a humidifier should be considered.

OXYGEN ADMINISTRATION PROCEDURES

To administer oxygen to a patient, it is necessary to prepare the oxygen tank and regulator. The oxygen system should be full and ready for patient use. However, in some situations, the tank must be changed and the regulator reattached. Follow the guidelines below when initiating oxygen administration (Figures 7-27a to h). Note that it is very important, before administering oxygen, to explain to the patient why the oxygen is needed, how it is to be administered, and how the oxygen delivery device will fit on the patient.

1. Check the cylinder to be sure it contains oxygen. Remove the protective seal on the tank valve.
2. Quickly open, then shut, the cylinder valve for 1 second to remove any dust or debris from the valve assembly.
3. Place the yoke of the regulator over the valve and align the pins. Be sure the regulator washer is present and in the proper place. Hand-tighten the T-screw on the regulator.
4. Slowly open the main cylinder valve about one-half turn to charge the regulator. Check the pressure gauge to be sure an adequate amount of oxygen is available.

INITIATING OXYGEN ADMINISTRATION

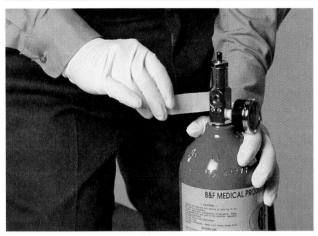

Figure 7-27a   Identify the cylinder as oxygen and remove the protective seal.

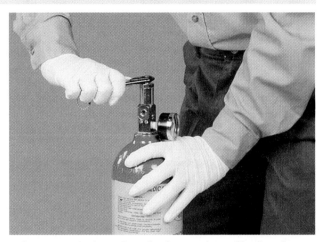

Figure 7-27b   Crack the main cylinder for one second to remove dust and debris.

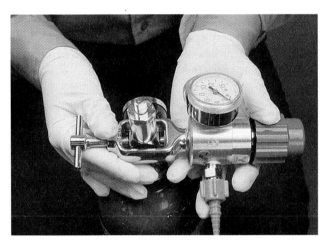

Figure 7-27c   Place the yoke of the regulator over the cylinder valve and align the pins.

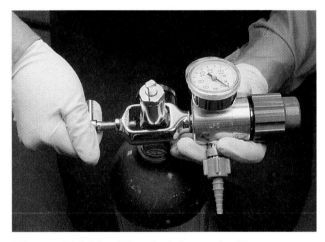

Figure 7-27d   Hand-tighten the T-screw on the regulator.

5. Attach the oxygen mask or nasal cannula tubing to the nipple of the regulator.
6. Open the flowmeter control. Set the oxygen flow rate at the desired liters per minute.
7. With the oxygen flowing, apply the oxygen mask or nasal cannula to the patient.

TERMINATING OXYGEN THERAPY

Follow these steps to terminate oxygen administration:

1. Remove the mask or cannula from the patient.
2. Turn off the oxygen regulator flowmeter control, then turn off the cylinder valve.
3. Open the regulator valve to allow the oxygen trapped in the regulator to escape until the pressure gauge reads zero. Turn the regulator flowmeter control completely off.

TRANSFERRING THE OXYGEN SOURCE: PORTABLE TO ON-BOARD

When switching over from a portable oxygen tank to the on-board oxygen source, do not disconnect the oxygen tubing from the regulator while the mask is still on the patient's face. Instead, remove the mask from the patient's face before attempting to switch over. The oxygen tubing can easily become caught in sheets, blankets, straps, or other equipment and may require a few minutes to untangle. During this time, if no oxygen is flowing to the mask, the patient's tidal volume and blood oxygen content will be drastically reduced. Do not inadvertently cause the patient to become hypoxic while switching oxygen sources. Once the oxygen has been reconnected and is flowing, reapply the mask to the patient's face.

INITIATING OXYGEN ADMINISTRATION

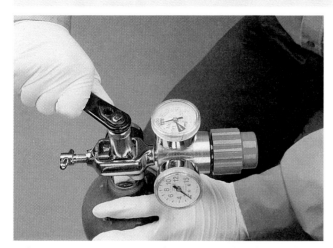

Figure 7-27e Open the main cylinder valve to check the pressure.

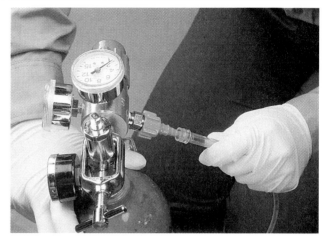

Figure 7-27f Attach the oxygen-delivery device to the regulator.

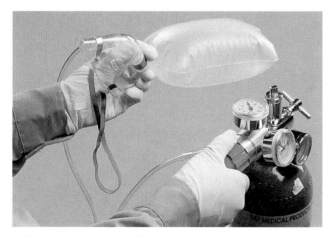

Figure 7-27g Adjust the flowmeter to the appropriate liter flow.

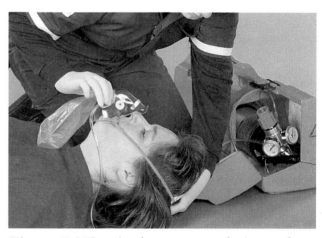

Figure 7-27h Apply an oxygen device to the patient.

OXYGEN DELIVERY EQUIPMENT

A variety of oxygen delivery devices can be used to deliver supplemental oxygen to the patient. The two primary devices used in the prehospital setting are the nonrebreather mask and the nasal cannula. Other devices that you may encounter are the simple face mask, the partial rebreather mask, and the Venturi mask.

NONREBREATHER MASK

The preferred method for delivering oxygen in the prehospital setting is with a **nonrebreather mask** (Figures 7-28a to b). This device has an oxygen reservoir bag attached to the mask with a one-way valve between them that prevents the patient's exhaled air from mixing with the oxygen in the reser-voir. The mask also has rubber washers that cover the exhalation ports. This allows air to escape on exhalation but restricts air to flow in the exhalation ports during inhalation. With each inhalation, the patient draws in the contents of the reservoir bag, which is 100 percent oxygen. Because some ambient air is inhaled from around the edges of the mask, the oxygen concentration actually delivered is usually around 90 percent.

The flow from the oxygen cylinder should be set at a rate that prevents the reservoir bag from collapsing when the patient inhales. Most typically, this is 15 lpm. Inflate the reservoir bag completely before applying it to the patient.

Various size nonrebreather masks are available for infants, children, and adults. Select the correct size mask to ensure that maximum oxygen concentration is being delivered.

THE NONREBREATHER MASK

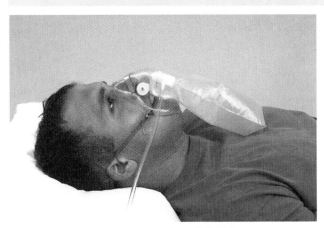

Figure 7-28a   Nonrebreather mask.

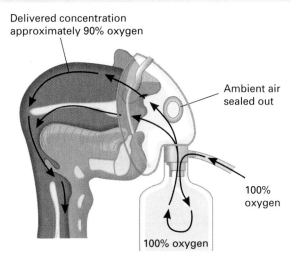

Figure 7-28b   Cutaway view of nonrebreather mask.

Most adult patients tolerate the nonrebreather mask well. However, it is restrictive and not tolerated well by infants, children, and some adults. Some patients feel as if they cannot breathe adequately with the device on. You may need to coach the patient to breathe at a normal rate and depth and provide reassurance that they are getting a sufficient amount of oxygen and air. If an infant or small child does not tolerate the mask, either you, a parent, or someone else familiar with the child can hold the mask close to his face, enriching the air he inspires.

Many patients who have been injured or are suffering medical illnesses, especially those who are cyanotic, cool, clammy, or short of breath need supplemental oxygen. Concerns about the dangers of giving too much oxygen to patients with a history of chronic obstructive pulmonary disease (COPD) or to infants and children have been shown to be invalid for short-term oxygen use in the prehospital setting. Administer high concentrations of oxygen to any patient you suspect is in need of oxygen therapy, regardless of whether he is an infant, a child, or an adult with a history of COPD, unless otherwise instructed by medical direction. If you are ever in doubt, consult medical direction.

Applying the Nonrebreather Mask   To apply the nonrebreather mask:

1. Explain to the patient that you are going to apply oxygen through a mask. Reassure him that he will be getting an increased amount of oxygen and instruct him to breathe normally.
2. Select the appropriate-sized mask. Prepare the oxygen tank and set the regulator at 15 lpm. Connect the nonrebreather tubing to the regula-

tor. Fill the reservoir bag completely. You may need to press down on the rubber valve gasket found covering the one-way valve between the mask and the reservoir. This will cause the reservoir bag to fill much faster.
3. Once the reservoir is completely inflated, fit the mask to the patient's face. Bring the elastic strap around the back of the head and secure it. Form the soft metal piece at the top of the mask to conform with the nose.
4. Constantly monitor the reservoir bag to ensure that it remains filled during inhalation.

NASAL CANNULA

An alternative oxygen delivery device is a **nasal cannula.** It is not a preferred method in the prehospital setting because it provides a very limited oxygen concentration. The main indication for its use is a patient who is not able to tolerate a nonrebreather mask, despite coaching and reassurance from the EMT-B.

The nasal cannula consists of two soft plastic tips, commonly referred to as nasal prongs, that are connected by thin tubing to the main oxygen source (Figures 7-29a to b). The nasal prongs are inserted a short distance into the nostrils. The nasal cannula is a "low-flow" system that does not supply enough oxygen to provide the entire tidal volume during inspiration. Therefore, a large portion of the patient's inhalation consists of ambient air that is mixed with the oxygen supplied by the nasal cannula. This significantly reduces the concentration of oxygen delivered by the device. As a general rule, for every liter per minute of flow delivered, the oxygen concentration the patient inhales increases by 4 percent. **The liter**

THE NASAL CANNULA

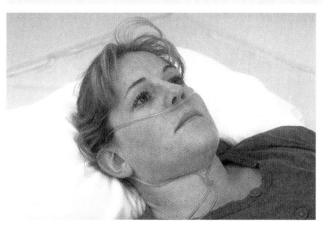

Figure 7-29a   Nasal cannula.

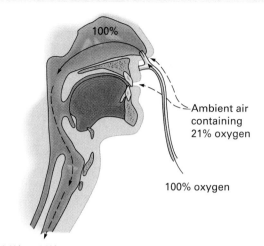

Figure 7-29b   Cutaway view of nasal cannula.

flow for the nasal cannula should be set at no less than 1 lpm and no greater than 6 lpm. Thus, the delivered oxygen concentration ranges from 24 to 44 percent.

Applying the Nasal Cannula   Follow these procedures when using the nasal cannula:

1. Explain to the patient that the oxygen will be delivered through the prongs that will fit in each nostril. Instruct the patient to breath normally while the prongs are in place.
2. Prepare the oxygen tank and regulator. Connect the nasal cannula tubing to the regulator and set the liter flow between 4 and 6 lpm or according to your local protocol or medical direction.
3. Insert the two prongs of the cannula into the patient's nostrils with the tab facing down. Make sure that the prongs curve downward.
4. Position the tubing over and behind each ear. Gently secure it by sliding the adjuster underneath the chin. Do not make the tubing too tight. If an elastic strap is used, adjust it so that it is secure and comfortable.
5. Check the cannula position periodically to ensure that it has not dislodged.

OTHER OXYGEN DELIVERY DEVICES

The following devices can be used to deliver oxygen to the patient. **Because they do not deliver as high a concentration of oxygen as the nonrebreather mask, they are not recommended for use by the EMT-B in the prehospital environment.** However, you may encounter these devices being used by first responders or other health care professionals. There-fore, you should be familiar with their design and operation.

Simple Face Mask   A simple face mask has no reservoir and can deliver up to 60 percent oxygen, depending on the patient's tidal volume and the oxygen flow rate. Exhaled air exits through the holes on each side of the mask. Air is drawn in through the holes in the side of the mask diluting the oxygen concentration being delivered. The oxygen flow rate is usually set at 10 lpm but must not be set at less than 6 lpm. Because it does not deliver as high a concentration of oxygen as the nonrebreather mask, it is not recommended for prehospital use.

Partial Rebreather Mask   The partial rebreather mask looks very similar to the nonrebreather mask but is equipped with a two-way valve that allows the patient to rebreathe about one-third of his exhaled air (Figure 7-30). Since the initial portion of exhaled air is principally from the patient's *deadspace,* areas of the respiratory system where gas exchange does not occur, it contains mostly oxygen-enriched air from the previous inhalation. The flow rate is typically set at 10 lpm but should be no less than 6 lpm. Partial rebreather masks can provide oxygen concentrations of between 35 and 60 percent.

Venturi Mask   The Venturi mask is a low-flow oxygen system that provides precise concentrations of oxygen through an entrainment valve connected to the face mask (Figure 7-31). The entrainment valve can be changed to deliver precise oxygen concentrations at preset flow rates. This mask is commonly used for a patient with a history of chronic obstructive pulmonary disease because of its ability to deliver a precise concentration of oxygen.

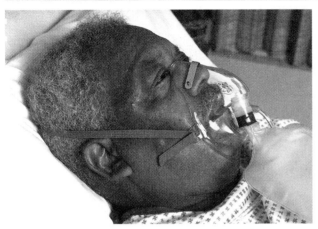

Figure 7-30   Partial rebreather mask.

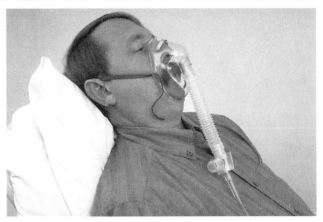

Figure 7-31   Venturi mask.

SPECIAL CONSIDERATIONS IN AIRWAY MANAGEMENT AND VENTILATION

You will sometimes encounter patients or emergency situations that will require you to alter or adjust your technique when controlling the airway or providing artificial ventilation. It is necessary for you to recognize these special situations and to be prepared to provide the appropriate intervention to ensure adequate airway control, ventilation, and oxygenation.

A PATIENT WITH A STOMA OR TRACHEOSTOMY TUBE

A **stoma** is a surgical opening in the front of the neck that may be permanent or temporary.

One reason for the presence of a stoma in the patient's neck is that a **tracheostomy** has been performed. During a tracheostomy, a stoma is created by cutting through the skin and into the trachea to relieve an obstruction higher in the trachea or to serve in place of an endotracheal tube (a tube through the mouth and into the trachea) that has been in place for a number of hours or days. Often, a **tracheostomy tube**—a curved hollow tube made of rubber, plastic, or metal—is inserted into the stoma to help hold it open. The patient may be breathing completely through the stoma and tube or may still be getting some air through the mouth and nose, around whatever blockage exists in the trachea. A tracheostomy is usually temporary and will eventually be closed and allowed to heal.

Another reason for the presence of a stoma is a **laryngectomy.** In a laryngectomy, all or part of the patient's larynx has been removed. In a *total laryngectomy,* there is no longer any connection of the trachea to the mouth and nose. The trachea is disconnected

from the pharynx, brought forward, and connected to the stoma in the neck. This alters the airway so that the patient breathes completely through the stoma. In a *partial laryngectomy,* some of the tracheal connection to the mouth and nose remains so that the patient may be getting some air through the stoma and some through the mouth and nose (Figure 7-32). With a laryngectomy, the stoma is permanent.

When you encounter a patient with a stoma (with or without a tube in the stoma), it will probably not be immediately obvious whether the patient is able to take in any air through the mouth and nose or can get air only through the stoma, unless a family member is able to tell you. The procedures described below take this into account.

BAG-VALVE-MASK-TO-TRACHEOSTOMY-TUBE VENTILATION

The bag-valve device is designed so that it can connect directly to the tracheostomy tube to provide positive pressure ventilation (Figure 7-33). When ventilating through the tracheostomy tube, it may be necessary to seal the patient's mouth and nose to prevent air from escaping. If this is not done, ineffective ventilation may result, with inadequate tidal volumes delivered to the patient.

If you are unable to ventilate through the tube, first suction it using a soft suction catheter. If you are still unable to ventilate, attempt to ventilate through the mouth and nose while sealing the stoma; this may improve the ability to ventilate or may clear the obstruction preventing ventilation through the tracheostomy tube.

BAG-VALVE-MASK-TO-STOMA VENTILATION

The permanent stoma of a laryngectomy patient is usually at the base of the neck with no tube inserted. Remember that a total laryngectomy patient has no

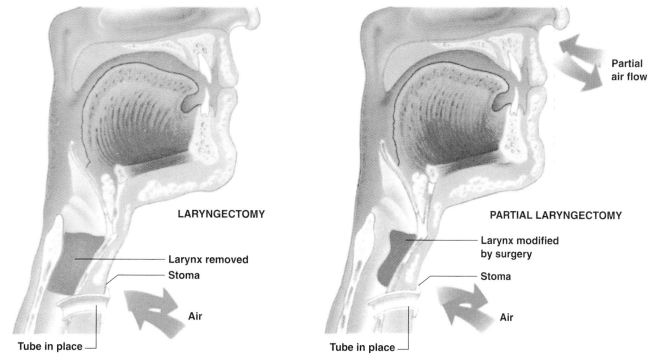

LARYNGECTOMY

Larynx removed
Stoma
Air
Tube in place

PARTIAL LARYNGECTOMY

Partial air flow

Larynx modified by surgery
Stoma
Air
Tube in place

Figure 7-32 The neck breather's airway has been changed by surgery.

air flow from the mouth and nose, but a partial laryngectomy patient may still have some air flow from the mouth and nose. To perform artificial ventilation with a bag-valve mask to the stoma, follow these guidelines:

1. Remove all coverings (e.g., scarves and ties) from the area of the stoma.
2. Clear the stoma of any foreign matter. Suction the stoma by passing a sterile soft suction catheter through the stoma and into the trachea

no more than 3 to 5 inches. Suction enough to partially open the airway.
3. **You will not need to perform a head-tilt, chin-lift or jaw-thrust maneuver on a patient with a stoma.** Keep the patient's head straight and the shoulders slightly elevated.
4. Select a mask, most often a child or infant mask, that fits securely over the stoma and can be sealed against the neck. Hold the mask seal with your hand and squeeze the bag delivering the ventilation over a 2-second period. Watch for adequate chest rise and fall. Feel to be sure that the air is escaping back through the stoma during exhalation.
5. If the chest does not rise, suspect a partial laryngectomy. Seal the nose and mouth with one hand so that air will not leak out of the mouth and nose. Pinch off the nose between the third and fourth fingers; seal the lips with the palm of the hand; place the thumb under the chin, and press upward and backward. Repeat the ventilation process.

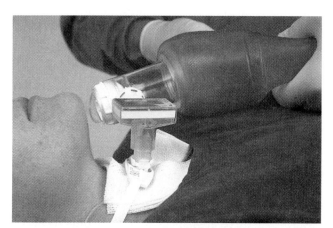

Figure 7-33 Artificial ventilation can be accomplished in the patient with a tracheostomy tube by attaching the bag-valve-mask device directly to the tube.

MOUTH-TO-STOMA VENTILATION

When performing mouth-to-stoma ventilation, follow the basic procedure as in bag-valve-mask-to-stoma ventilation. However, instead of placing a mask over the stoma, you will form a tight seal with your mouth over the stoma. Then, blow into the stoma until the patient's chest rises. Remove your mouth from around the stoma to allow for exhalation, which should occur passively when you stop ventilating. Local protocols may direct or permit ventilating through a child-size pocket mask placed over the stoma as a body substance isolation precaution.

INFANTS AND CHILDREN

Keep the following special considerations in mind when establishing and controlling the airway and providing artificial ventilation in infants and children:

- When establishing an airway by head-tilt, chin-lift, place the infant's head in a neutral position without hyperextension. The child's head should be placed in a neutral position then only slightly extended. Because of immature development of the airways, hyperextension may actually produce an airway obstruction. Because of the large size of the head, it may be necessary to elevate the upper chest of an infant or small child by placing padding under the shoulders to achieve an adequate airway.
- When providing positive pressure ventilation, regardless of the device or technique used, it is necessary to avoid excessive ventilation volumes and pressures. Excesses in these areas will lead to gastric distention, a common problem while ventilating infants and children. Gastric distention can impede lung inflation, reducing the ventilation volume being delivered, or it can cause the patient to vomit and possibly aspirate the vomitus. Also, excessive volumes can cause lung rupture and injury. The least volume that causes the chest to rise is adequate.
- Use a bag-valve-mask device without a pop-off valve. If a pop-off valve is present, disable it by placing it in a closed or off position. Because of the smaller airways and higher resistance in infants and children, a pop-off valve may unnecessarily vent air and lead to ineffective ventilation.
- Insert an oropharyngeal or nasopharyngeal airway if the airway cannot be maintained with a head-tilt, chin-lift or jaw-thrust maneuver alone or if prolonged ventilation is necessary.

PATIENTS WITH FACIAL INJURIES

The blood supply to the face is extremely rich; this can lead to two major complications with facial injuries.

1. Blunt injury can cause excessive swelling that may partially or completely occlude the airway. It may be necessary to insert an oral or nasal airway adjunct to establish and maintain the airway.

Also, positive pressure ventilation may be needed to force ventilation past the swollen airway.

2. Bleeding into the pharynx may be severe and can cause problems with airway management. Frequent or constant suctioning may be necessary.

FOREIGN BODY AIRWAY OBSTRUCTION

You may encounter a responsive or unresponsive patient with a known upper airway foreign body obstruction. It is also possible that an unresponsive patient may have a foreign body obstruction that is only detected after unsuccessful attempts at positive pressure ventilation. In these events, it is necessary to follow the procedure for foreign body airway obstruction to establish a patent airway. Refer to Appendix 1 to review the techniques of managing a foreign body airway obstruction.

If the patient is responsive and choking but is still able to move air when inhaling and exhaling, instruct him to cough. Do not perform abdominal thrusts. Place the patient on high-flow oxygen and begin transport. If the airway becomes completely occluded or the patient becomes unresponsive at any time, begin the series of abdominal thrusts as taught in Appendix 1.

If the airway is completely occluded and there is no air movement, perform three cycles of the foreign body airway obstruction maneuver. If the obstruction is not relieved, transport the patient expeditiously and continue with the foreign body airway obstruction cycles en route to the hospital until the obstruction is relieved.

Once the obstruction is relieved, closely assess the breathing status of the patient and his pulse. If the breathing is inadequate or absent, begin positive pressure ventilation with supplemental oxygen. If no pulse is present, apply the AED (see Chapter 16, "Automated External Defibrillation") or, if the AED is not available, begin CPR.

DENTAL APPLIANCES

If the patient has dentures that are secure in the mouth, leave them in place. It is much easier to establish a tight mask seal with the dentures in place. If the dentures are extremely loose, remove them so they do not dislodge and occlude the airway. Partial dentures (plates) may also become dislodged and occlude the airway. If the partial plate is loose, remove it. It is necessary to reassess the mouth frequently in patients who have dentures or partial dentures to ensure that these appliances have not come loose.

CASE STUDY FOLLOW-UP

SCENE SIZE-UP

You and your partner have been dispatched to the Twighlight Bar for an unresponsive male patient. Because you recognize the bar as one that frequently is the site of fights, stabbings, and shootings, you approach the scene very cautiously. You contact dispatch to inquire as to whether the unresponsive patient was involved in some type of altercation. Dispatch informs you that the patient is thought to be unresponsive because of drinking heavily.

As you enter the bar, it is very dark and hard to see. You turn on your flashlight and weave your way around the patrons, tables, and bar stools. You continuously scan the scene for any indication of hazards to you and your partner. You finally make your way to the bar and ask the bartender, "Where is the unresponsive patient?" The bartender says, "Oh, he's in the john." You ask what happened. He replies, "This kid was in here drinking all morning and afternoon. He stumbled to the bathroom. One of the other guys found him passed out in there."

You proceed to the bathroom and cautiously open the door, continuously scanning the scene for any signs of a hazard. You find a male patient about 30 years of age on the floor lying in a puddle of vomit. The scene does not reveal any overt signs of a mechanism of injury, but you still are unsure why the patient is unresponsive. No one at the scene knows his name or has ever seen him before.

PATIENT ASSESSMENT

You instruct your partner to take in-line stabilization. You very quickly inspect and palpate the back, and on the count of three, you log roll the patient into a supine position on a backboard. You immediately suction the remaining vomitus out of the mouth then perform a jaw-thrust maneuver. The patient is not responsive, even to a painful pinch, and has no gag reflex, so you are able to insert an oropharyngeal airway without incident.

The breathing rate is approximately 8 per minute with minimal chest rise on inspiration. The breathing is inadequate, so you begin positive pressure ventilation with a bag-valve mask and supplemental oxygen. There are only two of you to work on the patient, so your partner holds in-line stabilization with her knees and thighs, maintains the jaw thrust and seals the mask to the patient's face with one hand, and squeezes the bag against her side with the other. While she is doing this, you call for a back-up and continue with the initial assessment, which reveals a radial pulse that is slow and weak at a rate of about 55 per minute. The skin is pale, cool, and cyanotic. Because the patient is unresponsive and has no gag reflex, he is considered a priority for transport.

Your partner maintains in-line stabilization and continues to ventilate the patient. You quickly begin a physical exam to check the patient's body, starting at the head, for any evidence of injury. There are no signs of trauma to the head or neck. You palpate the posterior cervical region and apply a cervical spinal immobilization collar. You continue by checking the chest, abdomen, pelvis, and extremities (having checked the posterior body) and find no signs of trauma. You obtain a set of baseline vital signs.

Since the patient is unresponsive and there were no witnesses, except the bartender who reported his prolonged drinking, there is no way to get any additional history on the patient.

As you are completing the vital signs, your back-up crew arrives, bringing in the stretcher. You completely immobilize the patient to the backboard. One newly-arrived EMT-B establishes a seal on the bag-valve mask and your partner begins two-handed ventilation. You move the patient into the ambulance and begin transport.

En route to the hospital, you pinch the patient's hand and there is still no response. You interrupt ventilation for about 2 seconds to ensure that the airway is clear of vomitus and secretions. Ventilation is continued and the oxygen source is switched over to the on-board tank. You take another set of vital signs and continue with ventilation, monitoring the airway and breathing.

The patient begins to vomit, and you immediately begin to suction as your partner and the other EMT-B tilt the board, with the patient firmly secured to it, up on its side to help drain the vomitus from the mouth. Once the vomitus is cleared, you continue ventilation. You record the baseline vitals and contact the hospital.

Upon arrival at the hospital, you help transfer the patient to the hospital bed. You report your assessment findings and emergency care to the physician. Once your prehospital care report is completed and the unit is cleaned and restocked, you clear and mark back into service.

CHAPTER REVIEW

TERMS AND CONCEPTS

You may wish to review the following terms and concepts included in this chapter.

Adam's apple—see *thyroid cartilage.*

agonal respirations—gasping type respirations that have no pattern and occur very infrequently; a sign of impending cardiac or respiratory arrest.

alveoli—small air sacs in the lungs that fill with air on inspiration and are the point of gas exchange with the pulmonary capillaries.

automatic transport ventilator (ATV)—a positive pressure ventilation device that delivers ventilations automatically.

bag-valve-mask device (BVM)—a positive pressure ventilation device that consists of a bag with a nonrebreather valve and a mask. The bag-valve device is connected to the mask or other airway. The bag is squeezed to deliver a ventilation to the patient.

bilaterally—on both sides.

bradypnea—a breathing rate that is slower than the normal rate.

bronchi—branches of the respiratory tract from the trachea into the lungs.

bronchiole—smaller branches of the respiratory tract that continue to branch and get smaller. They eventually lead into alveolar sacs.

cricoid cartilage—the most inferior portion of the larynx and only full cartilaginous ring of the upper airway. It is felt immediately below the thyroid cartilage.

crossed-finger technique—a technique in which the thumb and index finger are crossed with the thumb on the lower incisors and the index finger on the upper incisors. The fingers are moved in a snapping or scissor motion to open the mouth.

crowing—a sound similar to that of a cawing crow that indicates that the muscles around the larynx are in spasm and beginning to narrow the opening into the trachea.

cyanosis—a bluish color of the skin and mucous membranes that indicates poor oxygenation of tissue.

deoxygenated—containing low amounts of oxygen, as with venous blood.

diaphragm—the major muscle of respiration that separates the chest cavity from the abdominal cavity.

epiglottis—a small flap of cartilaginous tissue that acts as a valve and closes over the trachea during swallowing.

esophagus—a tubular structure that serves as a passageway for food and liquids to enter the stomach.

exhalation—the passive process of breathing air out of the lungs. It is also known as expiration.

expiration—the passive process of breathing air out of the lungs. It is also known as exhalation.

flow-restricted, oxygen-powered ventilation device (FROPVD)—a device that consists of a ventilation valve and trigger or button and is driven directly by oxygen. It is used to provide positive pressure ventilation.

French catheter—see *soft catheter.*

gastric distention—inflation of the stomach.

gurgling—a gargling sound that indicates a fluid is in the mouth or pharynx.

hard catheter—see *rigid catheter.*

head-tilt, chin-lift maneuver—a manual technique used to open the airway. The head is tilted back by one hand. The tips of the fingers of the other hand are placed under the chin and used to lift it up and forward.

hemoglobin—a complex protein molecule found on the surface of the red blood cell that is responsible for carrying a majority of oxygen in the blood.

high-pressure regulator—a one-gauge regulator that is used to power the flow-restricted, oxygen-powered ventilation device. The flow rate cannot be adjusted.

hypoperfusion—the insufficient supply of oxygen and other nutrients to some of the body's cells that results from inadequate circulation of blood. Also called shock.

hypoxia—a reduction of oxygen delivery to the tissues.

inhalation—the active process of breathing air into the lungs. It is also known as inspiration.

inspiration—the active process of breathing air into the lungs. It is also known as inhalation.

intercostal muscles—the muscles between the ribs.

jaw-thrust maneuver—a manual technique used to open the airway in the patient with a suspected spinal injury. The fingers are placed at the angles of the jaw and used to lift the jaw up and forward.

laryngectomy—a surgical procedure in which a patient's larynx is removed. A stoma is created for the patient to breathe through.

larynx—the part of the air passage that connects the pharynx with the trachea. Also, it is considered the organ of voice since it contains the vocal cords.

mucous membrane—a thin layer of tissue that lines various structures within the body.

nasal airway—a nasopharyngeal airway.

nasal cannula—an oxygen delivery device that consists of two prongs that are inserted into the nose of the patient. The oxygen concentration delivered is from 24 to 44 percent.

nasopharyngeal airway—a curved, hollow rubber tube with a flange or flare at the top end and a bevel at the distal end that is inserted into the nose. It fits in the nasopharynx and extends into the pharynx providing a passage for air.

nasopharynx—the portion of the pharynx that extends from the nostrils to the soft palate.

nonrebreather mask—an oxygen delivery device that consists of a reservoir and one-way valve. It can deliver up to 100 percent oxygen to the patient.

oral airway—an oropharyngeal airway.

oropharyngeal airway—a semicircular hard plastic device that is inserted in the mouth and holds the tongue away from the back of the pharynx.

oropharynx—a portion of the pharynx that extends from the mouth to the oral cavity at the base of the tongue.

oxygenated—containing high amounts of oxygen, as with arterial blood.

oxygenation—the process by which the blood and the cells become saturated with oxygen.

oxygen humidifier—a container that is filled with sterile water and connected to the oxygen regulator to add moisture to the dry oxygen prior to being delivered to the patient.

parietal pleura—the outermost pleural layer that adheres to the chest wall.

patent airway—an airway that is open and clear of any obstructions.

pharynx—the common passageway for the respiratory and digestive tract; the throat.

pleura—two layers of connective tissue that surround the lungs.

pleural space—a small space between the visceral and parietal pleura that is at negative pressure and filled with serous fluid.

pocket mask—a plastic mask placed over the patient's nose and mouth through which ventilations can be delivered.

positive pressure ventilation (PPV)—method of aiding a patient whose breathing is inadequate by forcing air into his lungs.

respiration—the exchange of oxygen and carbon dioxide that takes place during inhalation and exhalation.

retractions—depressions seen in the neck, above the clavicles, between the ribs, or below the rib cage from excessive muscle use during breathing. It is an indication of respiratory distress.

rigid catheter—a rigid plastic tube that is part of a suctioning system, commonly referred to as a "tonsil tip" or "tonsil sucker."

serous fluid—fluid that acts as a lubricant to reduce the friction between the parietal and visceral pleura.

snoring—a sound that is heard when the base of the tongue or relaxed tissues in the pharynx partially block the upper airway; also called a *sonorous* sound.

soft catheter—flexible tubing that is part of a suctioning system, the "French" catheter.

stoma—a surgical opening into the neck and trachea; see also *tracheostomy.*

stridor—a harsh, high-pitched sound heard on inspiration that indicates swelling of the larynx.

tachypnea—a breathing rate that is faster than the normal rate.

therapy regulator—a device that controls the flow and pressure of oxygen from the tank to allow for a consistent delivery of oxygen by liters per minute.

thyroid cartilage—the bulky cartilage that forms the anterior portion of the larynx; the Adam's Apple.

tidal volume—the volume of air breathed in and out in one respiration.

tonsil tip or tonsil sucker—see *rigid catheter.*

trachea—a tubular structure that serves as the passageway for air to enter into the lungs; the windpipe.

tracheostomy—a surgical opening into the trachea in which a tube is inserted for the patient to breathe through; see also *stoma.*

tracheostomy tube—a hollow tube that is inserted into a tracheostomy to allow the patient to breathe.

ventilation—the passage of air into and out of the lungs.

visceral pleura—innermost layer of the pleura that covers the lung.

REVIEW QUESTIONS

1. Describe the two manual methods used to open an airway and explain the circumstances in which each should be used.
2. Name the two airway adjuncts that can be inserted to assist in establishing and maintaining an open airway and explain the circumstances in which each should be used.
3. Outline the assessment techniques you would use to determine if the patient's breathing is adequate or inadequate.
4. Name the signs of adequate breathing.
5. Name the signs of inadequate breathing.
6. Name, in order of preference, the recommended methods that the EMT-B can use to artificially ventilate the patient.
7. Explain the difference in the technique for ventilation of a patient with and without a suspected spinal injury.
8. List the indications that the patient is being ventilated adequately.
9. Describe the appropriate procedure for initiating oxygen administration.
10. Describe the appropriate procedure for terminating oxygen administration.

CHAPTER 8

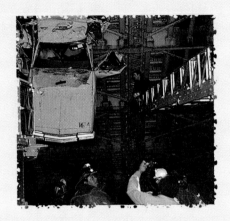

Scene Size-up

INTRODUCTION

The prehospital setting is an extremely uncontrolled environment. An EMT-Basic who does not pay close attention to the characteristics of the scene to which he has been dispatched, who fails to follow basic guidelines before entering a scene, and who fails to follow his intuition when things do not seem right runs the risk of serious injury. Many subtle hazards confront EMT-Bs at the scenes of calls. With good sense developed through experience and study, it becomes easier to recognize such hazards. But experience should never lead to complacency and a letting down of your guard. The costs of failing to recognize the hazards of an unstable scene can be high for yourself, your partners, and your patients. It is imperative that you identify and pay close attention to the scene size-up characteristics on every call, not just the ones that sound bad. Doing so can save your life.

OBJECTIVES

Numbered objectives are from the United States Department of Transportation 1994 EMT-Basic National Standard Curriculum. Asterisked objectives, if any, pertain to material that is supplemental to the DOT curriculum.

COGNITIVE

3-1.1 Recognize hazards/potential hazards. (pp. 129–138)

3-1.2 Describe common hazards found at the scene of a trauma and a medical patient. (pp. 129–138)

3-1.3 Determine if the scene is safe to enter. (pp. 129–138)

3-1.4 Discuss common mechanisms of injury/nature of illness. (pp. 139–141)

3-1.5 Discuss the reason for identifying the total number of patients at the scene. (p. 141)

3.1-6 Explain the reason for identifying the need for additional help or assistance. (pp. 131–137, 141)

* Explain how to gain scene control. (pp. 141–142)

* Explain how to establish rapport with the patient. (pp. 141–143)

AFFECTIVE

3-1.7 Explain the rationale for crew members to evaluate scene safety prior to entering. (pp. 128, 129)

3-1.8 Serve as a model for others explaining how patient situations affect your evaluation of mechanism of injury or illness. (pp. 139–141)

PSYCHOMOTOR

3-1.9 Observe various scenarios and identify potential hazards.

Objectives 3-1.4, 5, 6, and 8 are also addressed in Chapter 9, "Patient Assessment."

CASE STUDY

THE DISPATCH

EMS Unit 104—respond to an emergency at 68 Chicago Avenue—unknown problem—time out 2316 hours.

ON ARRIVAL

As you approach the street, you shut off the siren and the emergency lights to reduce the attention that you will draw. Your partner, EMT-B McKeown, is identi-

fying the addresses out loud, "56, 58, 64, 66." As she shines a spotlight on a run-down house with a front door standing open, you can barely see the number 68. Your partner calls out, "Hey, where are the lights? The whole house is pitch black."

How would you proceed at this scene?

During this chapter you will learn about the special considerations of scene size-up. Later, we will return to this case and apply the procedures you have studied.

The **scene size-up** is the EMT-B's initial evaluation of a scene to which he has been called. You have three basic goals during scene size-up. The first is to identify possible hazards at the scene and ensure the safety of yourself and other members of your team, the patient, and the bystanders. Next, you should identify what led to your being called to the scene—either an injury or a medical problem; this identification will determine the steps you follow in patient assessment and emergency care. Your final goal is to determine whether any factors such as the number of

patients or unusual characteristics of the scene might require a call for additional assistance.

DETERMINE SCENE SAFETY

The first goal of EMT-Bs upon arrival at a scene to which they have been dispatched is **scene safety.** This means the assessment of a scene to ensure the well-being of the EMT-Bs, their patient or patients, and any bystanders.

The process of ensuring scene safety is dynamic and ongoing. It is not something that is done quickly on arrival at the scene and then forgotten. The EMT-B must adjust his actions and precautions as additional information becomes available. Information gained from assessment of the scene is applied throughout the response—through the encounter with the patient, treatment, transportation, and ultimately, delivery of the patient to the hospital. You must think *scene safety* on every call, whether the scene is a street corner riot or the bedroom of an elderly patient who has fallen. Be alert at all times.

Scene safety requires that the EMT-B exercise leadership and take control of the scene. If he fails to do so, the scene will control the EMT-B. Someone has to be in charge. That "someone" might become the patient, a family member, or a crowd of bystanders if the EMT-B fails to take charge.

Sleeplessness, preoccupation with other problems, apathy, and overconfidence can lead an EMT-B to shortcut or ignore the principles of scene safety. Don't let this happen to you. The consequences can be costly for the patient, your partners, and you.

OBTAIN DISPATCH INFORMATION

The process of ensuring scene safety should begin well before the arrival of EMT-Bs at the actual scene. It should start upon receipt of the call from the dispatcher. The dispatch call can help you begin to visualize the body substance isolation protection and the gear that you will need at the scene.

However, the dispatch information is only a starting point. It is critical to emergency that dispatchers usually do not have complete and accurate information to work with. The person calling to report an accident may have hung up before giving details. The person calling may fail to recognize a medical condition that would require increased precautions.

Be aware, too, that callers at times may deliberately give inaccurate information. For example, a caller may report chest pains when the problem actually is a gunshot wound. If the caller had reported the facts, it is likely that law enforcement personnel as well as EMTs would have been dispatched, something the caller wished to avoid.

Dispatch information can have other, unintended effects on EMT-Bs. Consider the following sets of calls:

Medic 102, respond to a call at 223 Garfield Street, reports of shots fired, man down in the street.
Medic 107, caller now reports wires down and arcing at the accident scene. Fire and power companies en route. Use caution.
Medic 101, proceed to I-80 at the scales. State Patrol reports accident with multiple injuries involving tanker truck. Be advised, tanker is leaking unknown product.

Calls of this nature automatically inspire the EMT-B to be cautious. They highlight an obvious risk that must be dealt with. With such calls, EMT-Bs—from those on their first run to seasoned veterans—automatically begin to think of their safety at the scene. Such calls indicate that assistance from police, fire, power company, additional medical personnel, or other resources will be necessary. The reaction to the following calls, however, may be different.

Medic 105, respond to 6776 Quail Hollow Drive for a 67-year-old male with chest pains.
Medic 101, you have an unknown problem at Dr. Smith's office, 2225 Greenbriar Drive.

Calls such as these appear to be routine. The voice of the dispatcher lacks the urgency that might be displayed in the earlier types of calls. The routine nature of these calls may also lull the responding EMT-Bs into a lesser state of readiness. Ironically, these "routine" calls may present a greater threat than the "major" incidents first discussed. The patient may have been involved in a domestic dispute. Or family members may become hostile during the call. Or the patient may be suffering from an infectious disease that can be transmitted to the EMT-Bs. Or the patient may have inhaled toxic fumes that are still present and dangerous at the scene. Or, as noted above, the "chest pain" patient may actually have a gunshot wound. If the EMT-Bs don't consider scene safety on the way to a call, they will expose themselves to increased danger and possible injury.

Remember, use the dispatch information to prepare for the scene, but remain alert to the possibility of very different circumstances upon your arrival.

TAKE BODY SUBSTANCE ISOLATION PRECAUTIONS

The first goal of the scene size-up is to ensure the safety of the responding EMT-Bs. As you learned in Chapter 2, "The Well-being of the EMT-B," you must consider contact with all body fluids to be a true safety hazard. Appropriate body substance isolation precautions will definitely reduce your risks of contracting an infectious disease in the prehospital setting. What follows are some key points to remember about body substance isolation as you prepare for and perform the scene size-up.

Because the prehospital setting is so uncontrolled, unexpected exposures to blood and body fluids may often occur. *Gloves must be considered standard protective equipment.* Wear gloves for every patient contact. The amount of additional BSI protection you will need will vary according to the circumstances of the contact.

The call from dispatch can help you begin to plan your body substance isolation precautions. A report of a multiple-car accident on an interstate highway should indicate a high probability of exposure to blood and body fluids. In such circumstances, in addition to gloves you might need protective eyewear, a mask, and a gown. If the dispatch information alerts you to a patient with TB, or to a patient in an institutional setting such as a nursing home where such infections are common, you should wear gloves, eyewear, and a HEPA respirator.

As indicated, however, dispatch information can be incomplete or inaccurate. Remember the "chest pain" patient actually suffering from a gunshot wound. You will have to make your own assessment of the scene and of the need for additional BSI protection.

Do not be caught in a situation where you are at high risk of exposure with minimal protection because of a hasty approach to the patient and a lack of attention to the scene characteristics. For example, if you encounter a patient who coughs or complains of a chronic cough and has a recent history of fever, chills with night sweats, weight loss, or blood-tinged sputum, you should treat him as if he has TB even if

that was not the original complaint that brought you to the scene; a high-efficiency particulate air (HEPA) respirator should be worn along with gloves and eyewear. In calls involving drug users or suspected drug users, gloves, eyewear, and sometimes masks and gowns must be worn to protect against the possibility of HBV and HIV infection.

 ## CONSIDER SCENE CHARACTERISTICS

Personal protection of the EMT-Basic is of primary importance. An injured or helpless EMT-B cannot provide emergency care to a patient. In addition, attention and resources may be diverted from the patient to the injured EMT-B, risking further compromise to the patient.

You must study the scene carefully and determine if it is safe to approach the patient. This determination must be made on all responses, but different scenes will present different characteristics to consider (Figures 8-1a to d). Your final determination must be tai-

SCENE CHARACTERISTICS

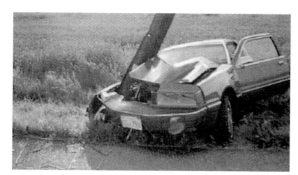

Figure 8-1a   Motor vehicle strikes utility pole.

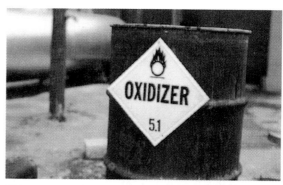

Figure 8-1b   Hazardous materials.

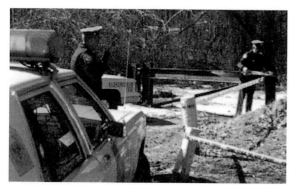

Figure 8-1c   Crime scene.

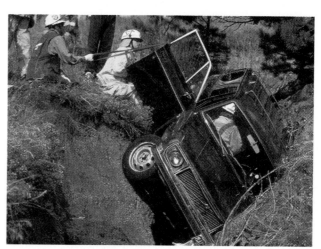

Figure 8-1d   Motor vehicle in ditch. (Howard M. Paul/Emergency! Stock)

lored to the specific scene, keeping these overriding principles in mind:

- Do not enter unstable accident scenes.
- Take extra precautions at crime scenes, suspected crime scenes, and scenes involving volatile crowd situations; wait for the arrival of police or, if a scene turns threatening, retreat and wait for the police.
- Be sure to bring your portable radio with you when you leave the ambulance so that you can contact dispatch or medical direction from the scene for needed resources or advice.
- Call for help from the appropriate agencies—police, fire department, rescue squad, utility company, water rescue squad, hazmat team, or other—if a scene is outside your area of training or expertise.
- Remove yourself if a scene turns hazardous.

Scenes you are likely to encounter and points to consider before entering those scenes are discussed below.

Crash Scenes

At a crash scene, the EMT-B's attention is drawn naturally and immediately to the patient or patients. But before approaching the patients, the EMT-B must assess the *total* scene. This includes the areas to the left, right, front, back, top, and bottom of the vehicles involved. The boundaries of the accident scene can be limited to a single vehicle or can extend for hundreds of feet in multiple-vehicle or high-speed crashes. When assessing a crash scene, pay particular attention to the points listed below. For more detailed information on crash scenes, see Chapter 41, "Gaining Access and Extrication."

- Is the vehicle stable?
- If not, can you safely make it stable or are additional personnel and equipment necessary?
- Are power lines involved?
  - *Consider all power lines to be energized until a power company representative tells you they are not.*
  - Power lines can be on the car, under the car, or touching a guardrail or wire fence that the car is in contact with.
  - The lines may be lying on wet ground and energizing a large area.
- Does jagged metal or broken glass pose a threat?
  - Can such material be avoided, covered, or otherwise isolated to minimize the threat?
- Is there fuel leaking and, if so, is there an ignition source nearby?
- Is there fire?
  - If so, has the fire department been called?
  - If rescue is possible, do not approach a burning vehicle directly from the front or the rear, where

fire or explosion hazards are greatest, but from the side.
- Are there hazardous materials involved?

Other Rescue Scenes

Some rescue scenes require specialized training and equipment. The EMT-B must be prepared to call upon additional specialized resources to assure not only his own well-being but also the successful rescue of the patient. *It is the EMT-B's duty to ensure that adequate numbers of appropriately trained and equipped personnel are summoned if necessary to handle special rescues.* Examples of rescue scenes where specialized training and equipment must be considered include the following:

- Heights (rooftops, trees, catwalks, construction areas)
- Underground areas (caves, manholes, trenches, excavations)
- Collapses/cave-ins (buildings, construction sites, excavations)
- Storage tanks/vats (regardless of contents)
- Silos/bins (suffocation hazards, regardless of contents)
- Farm equipment (This might include equipment such as combines, corn pickers, or augers. See Chapter 37, "Agricultural and Industrial Emergencies.")

Some special situations that EMT-Bs might frequently encounter include those described below.

Unstable Surfaces and Slopes Victims of injury or illness may be encountered on unstable surfaces or slopes. Such surfaces create additional difficulties and hazards and can greatly complicate treatment and transport of the patient (Figure 8-2). Access to patients in such circumstances may require the use of ropes. If you are not trained in the proper use of ropes in such situations, summon or wait for a trained rescue crew. If you have been properly trained, keep the following points in mind:

- Remember to secure the patient to the hillside to prevent him from sliding downslope during assessment, treatment, and stabilization.
- Be sure that vehicles that have gone over embankments have been secured to prevent them from sliding and carrying occupants and EMS personnel away.
- Beware of loose rocks and stones that may be knocked down to your position by rescuers working above.

Ice The presence of ice can complicate any scene, making what would normally be a simple rescue hazardous. Keep the following points in mind:

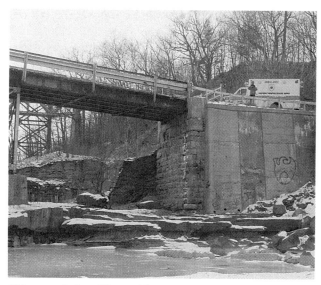

Figure 8-2 Unstable environments can pose a threat to the EMT-B.

- Apply sand, salt, or gravel to walks, steps, and roadways where you will be working or over which you will be moving a patient.
- Avoid walking onto frozen ponds, lakes, or other bodies of water if the safety and thickness of the ice is unknown. In these cases, notify rescue teams who are trained and equipped for ice rescue.
- If the ice surface is known to be safe, a tarp, rug, or other portable non-skid surface should be brought to the patient's side to provide a safe surface from which to stabilize, treat, and prepare the patient for transport.

Water Drownings are common reasons for the dispatch of an EMT team. But water can also be a factor in other types of calls. Always proceed with caution in situations where water is a factor. See Chapter 25, "Drowning, Near-Drowning, and Diving Emergencies," for more details. If you are faced with a situation beyond your capacity to handle, summon and wait for backup from those with proper training and equipment.

- *Swimming pools*—The comparatively controlled environment of a swimming pool presents a major challenge for rescue of a patient. The patient will be visible but, to the EMT-B who is untrained in water rescue, retrieving the patient will be very difficult and should never be attempted alone. The EMT-B's partner should be close at hand to lend assistance, preferably from the pool's edge. A personal flotation device (life jacket) and a line or pole to assist the rescuer and patient to the pool's edge should be used.
- *Open water*—Rescue in open water is a specialized technique which requires training and equipment. The EMT-B must ensure that adequate re-

sources are summoned to open-water scenes where people have been reported as drowned or missing. If the EMT-B goes out into the water, he must wear a personal flotation device. Under no circumstances should an EMT-B wear boots or heavy clothing that can pull him under if he goes into the water.

- *Moving water*—Rescue in moving water such as rivers, streams, or creeks presents all the problems of open-water rescue further complicated by the force of the current. Often, the current will make swimming difficult if not impossible. Patients and rescuers alike can easily be swept away, even in shallow water, if the current is strong enough. Never wade or walk into moving water in an attempt to effect a rescue without adequate training and equipment. Flooded streams, creeks, and drainage ditches as well as rivers have swept many well-meaning, but untrained rescuers to their deaths. Whitewater or moving-water rescues involve specialized techniques and equipment and extensive training. The EMT-B must ensure that adequate resources are summoned to reports of a drowning or of a person caught in moving water.

Toxic Substances and Low-Oxygen Areas The EMT-Basic must be alert to the possible presence of toxic substances or areas of low oxygen during the scene size-up. Some scenes, such as an accident involving a tanker truck, will present obvious hazards. At other scenes, the hazard may not be as obvious. For example, a call to aid someone who fell in his kitchen might present a toxic hazard if, during the fall, the person knocked over and spilled bleach and ammonia. The combination of the two creates chloramine gas, a lung irritant.

Often, the caller requesting assistance will be unaware that a toxic environment exists. It is your responsibility during the initial scene size-up to determine if the environment is safe. Suspect the presence of toxic substances or an oxygen-depleted atmosphere in the following circumstances:

- *A spill, leak, or fire*—Scenes that involve highly visible incidents such as tanker spills, pipeline ruptures, and heavy smoke conditions should automatically alert you to call upon specialized assistance to control the situation.
- *A confined space*—Caves, wells, tankers, vats, manholes, sewers, culverts, underground utility vaults, silos, and other confined spaces are areas where the EMT-B must exercise extreme caution. Such areas are frequently very low in oxygen and/or high in toxic substances such as methane. Entry into a confined space to effect a rescue should be made with appropriate self-contained breathing apparatus (SCBA) in place. Many well-meaning rescuers have failed to recognize the risk of confined-space entry

and have themselves become victims along with the patients they planned to rescue.

- *Multiple patients with similar symptoms*—A toxic environment will generally cause all people within it to suffer from similar symptoms. Therefore, the EMT-B called to a residence in which all occupants, including pets, exhibit similar signs and symptoms must assume that the environment is toxic until it is proven not to be. Faulty furnaces cause such problems every winter. The EMT-B encountering this situation during the winter months should be prepared to consider the possibility of carbon monoxide poisoning. A blocked flue on a gas hot-water tank can produce the same problem in a closed, air-conditioned residence at the peak of summer.

The EMT-B must be alert to the possibility of encountering such situations on every call. If the EMT-B is not trained to make the environment safe in such situations, he must contact specialized rescue or fire units who can.

You will learn more about the dangers of these situations and how to cope with them in Chapter 21, "Poisoning Emergencies," Chapter 37, "Agricultural and Industrial Emergencies," and Chapter 42, "Hazardous Materials Emergencies."

CRIME SCENES

Chances are good that, as an EMT-B, you will respond to crime scenes almost as frequently as you will to motor vehicle crashes. Firearms are second only to motor vehicle crashes as a cause of death by trauma. Crime scenes require special attention to ensure the personal protection of the EMT-Basic. Review material about crime scenes in Chapter 2, "The Well-Being of the EMT-Basic," for additional information.

Remember that ensuring your own safety is the first step in scene size-up. If you are sent to the scene of a crime, wait for the police to arrive and secure the scene before you attempt to enter. *Do not enter a known crime scene unless it has been secured by police.*

However, there will be times when you are sent to scenes at which no crime has been reported but where you suspect that a crime might be involved. A report of an injury at a bar late at night might be one such circumstance. A call to an area with a high crime rate might be another. Be alert to the possibility of danger on such calls. Remember that a dispatcher may not know that the scene to which he is directing you is, in fact, a crime scene. While you are en route to such a scene, check to see if police have also been called. If they have not, request their support. *If you arrive at such a scene and feel uneasy or suspect that a threat might exist, do not enter the scene.* Wait for police backup.

On calls to known or possible crime scenes, take the precautions that follow.

Arriving at the Scene While still several blocks from the scene, turn off the siren and emergency lights. By arriving discreetly, you will draw less attention to the scene and minimize the chances of drawing a crowd. This will give you better conditions in which to perform the scene size-up. If the scene appears too hostile or threatening, do not stop but drive on and await police backup in a secure area.

It is a prudent practice to anticipate the address and to park two to three houses away from the scene. This affords you an additional opportunity to study the scene before becoming involved in it.

At crime scenes in which guns might be involved, parking in such a position will usually put you outside the *killing zone*. This is defined as the area controlled by hostile fire. If someone inside the house has a gun, an area about 120 degrees in front of the house is at least partially exposed to hostile fire. This area can be much larger depending on the location of the house—for example, one on a corner lot—and on the mobility of the person with the gun. The killing zone is not static and is always subject to change.

Studying the Crowd If a crowd has gathered before your arrival, assess the crowd. Be aware that the size of the crowd is less important than its mood. Is the scene chaotic? If so, do not allow yourself to be pulled into the chaos. Is the scene hysterical? Again, do not be pulled in. Does the crowd seem hostile to your presence? If it does, your options include retreating until appropriate backup arrives or taking the patient and leaving.

Approaching the Scene When you have completed your initial evaluation and see no immediate danger, leave the ambulance to approach the scene. Be alert, however, to the possibility that the scene could suddenly turn dangerous. Be prepared to retreat if it does. When approaching the scene, follow these procedures:

- Walk on the grass, not the sidewalk, for a quieter, less obvious approach.
- If you are using a flashlight, hold it beside, not in front of, your body—so that you don't make your body a possible target (Figure 8-3).
- If you are walking with a partner, walk single-file. The last person in line should carry the jump kit (Figure 8-4). This will leave the person or persons at the front of the line unencumbered and better able to react to any problems that may be encountered.
- Only the first person in line should carry a flashlight, because anyone with a flashlight behind the first person will back-light those in front.
- As you approach the scene, make a mental map of possible places of concealment (objects, such as shrubbery, that will hide you) and cover (objects,

such as trees, that will both hide you and stop bullets). Keep illuminating or scanning dark or shadowed areas for movement as you approach a house.

- Take a moment to look at windows and corners. If you need to take a longer look, change positions to make it harder for a hostile person to get a fix on you.
- Stand to the side of a door when you knock on it; never in front of it—to avoid being a target for someone shooting, springing out, or reaching to grab at you through the door (Figure 8-5). Standing to the knob side prevents a door that opens outward from blocking you. If the door opens inward, the person opening it will most likely be looking toward the hinge side, letting you see him before he sees you.
- As soon as the door is open, assess the situation before you decide whether to retreat and call for reinforcement or to have your partner move the ambulance up to the front of the building. As you enter, leave doors open behind you to ensure an escape route. Likewise, never appear to block the patient's route of escape.

At the Patient's Side Once you are at the patient's side, your first priority remains protecting yourself and your partner. The next priority is to protect and

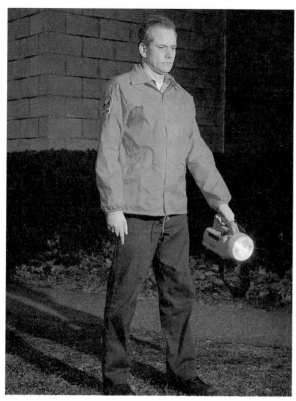

Figure 8-3 Hold a flashlight out and to the side of your body.

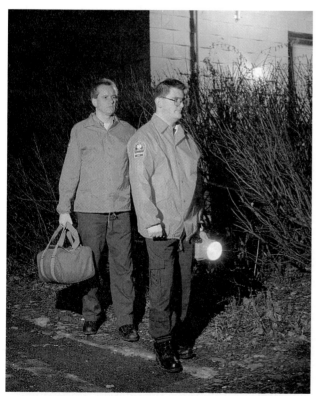

Figure 8-4 Walk single file to a potentially unstable scene.

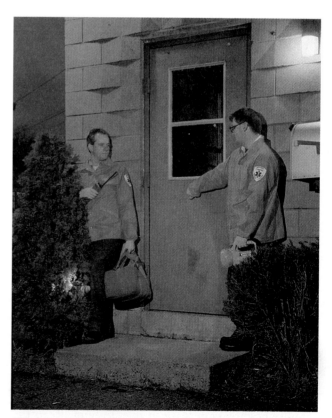

Figure 8-5 Stand to the side of the door when knocking. Do not stand directly in front of a door or window.

treat the patient. If you reach a patient and discover that a crime is, in fact, involved in the situation, be aware that a perpetrator may still be on the scene and police intervention will be necessary. Ensure that the police have been called and follow local protocols. Be ready to retreat from the scene.

When you are assisting a patient at a properly secured crime scene, follow these procedures:

- Do not allow bystanders to touch or disturb the patient or his immediate surroundings.
- Introduce yourself to the patient carefully and say that you are there to help him. Crime victims are often confused and fearful of contact with strangers.
- Be alert to the possibility that the patient at the crime scene may be not simply a victim but also a perpetrator. Always keep track of the patient's hands in a hostile situation. Be prepared for the possibility that such a patient may suddenly reach for a weapon.
- Have one EMT-B keep a constant watch on the bystanders and the surrounding area while you work on the patient—to alert you if a scene begins to turn dangerous.
- *Remember as you work on the patient that your task is to render medical assistance and to save his life, not to aid in the solving of a crime.* Be as considerate of police requests as possible, but keep your primary task in mind.
- Where appropriate, assist police in collecting and recording anything on the patient, such as blood, hair, seminal fluid, gunpowder residue, or clothing fibers, that may indicate a crime. Follow local protocol.
- Take extreme care not to disturb any evidence that is not directly on the patient's body (footprints, soil, broken glass, tire tracks, and so on).
- Never touch or move suspected weapons unless it is absolutely necessary for treating the patient's injuries. Many guns found are loaded and extremely dangerous to handle because of the possibility of accidental discharge. Such a gun in the hands of an untrained person could pose an extreme hazard to you, your partner, the patient, and bystanders. If you do touch a weapon, do not disturb any fingerprints that may be on it. Pick up a gun by the edge of the grip, and use gauze pads to pick up a knife at the very edge of the blade.
- Wear gloves throughout treatment to avoid leaving your own fingerprints at the crime scene.
- If you need to tear or cut away clothing to expose a wound, make sure that you do not cut through a bullet hole or knife slash in the clothing. Keep the clothing and submit it as evidence to the police.
- If the patient was strangled or tied with a rope or other material, cut at a point away from the knot

instead of untying it—the knot can be used as evidence and may help identify the perpetrator.
- If the patient is responsive, do not burden him with questions about the crime. Treat his injuries and transport him.
- Realize that the patient will probably show extremes of emotion and be prepared to handle them.
- Document who is at the crime scene when you arrive.
- If a patient is obviously dead when you arrive, do nothing and disturb nothing. Summon the police, if they have not already been called, and wait for their arrival. However, remember that you must provide basic life support and other appropriate care, as you would for any patient, unless injuries are so extreme or the patient has obviously been dead for so long that resuscitation is out of the question.

BARROOM SCENES

Barrooms can quickly become places of danger for EMTs responding to a call. The presence of people consuming alcohol makes any situation volatile and unpredictable. The problems are compounded in a barroom, where patrons often know each other and their actions may be affected by long-standing friendships or feuds about which you have no knowledge. In such circumstances, violence can easily erupt, even in what appears to be a routine situation.

Simply entering a barroom can present a special challenge to the EMT-B. Barrooms are often dark places. If you receive a call to one during daylight hours, your eyes can require up to thirty minutes to adjust from bright sunlight to low-light vision. By wearing sunglasses while outside, you can shorten the time of adjustment considerably. You might also keep one eye closed while still outside; this will give the closed eye a marked head start on accommodating to the low light inside the bar.

You will sometimes respond to barroom calls where none of the patrons will be able to tell you what happened to an injured person; all of them, however, will offer advice on medical treatment. Be patient in such situations. It is critical that you do not antagonize the patrons. A routine question or comment can easily be misunderstood by an inebriated patient or bystander and lead to a violent confrontation.

While working at a barroom call, have your partner stand and survey the patrons at all times. Do not turn your back on the people in the bar. Don't reply to verbal threats, but never ignore them, either. It only takes an instant for verbal abuse to turn into a physical assault. If the situation becomes threatening, retreat temporarily and call for police support.

CAR PASSENGERS

Approaching people in vehicles is another seemingly routine situation that can hold unexpected danger for the EMT-B. The EMT-B's uniform or the emergency lights on the ambulance may be misinterpreted as "the police" by the occupants of a vehicle, who may be intoxicated on alcohol and/or drugs. You should plan the approach to a parked vehicle carefully, following these steps:

- Park the ambulance at least one car-length behind the vehicle. Park with your wheels turned slightly to the left, so that if you have to back up you will not go any deeper into the shoulder of the road.
- Align your headlights in the middle of the trunk of the vehicle, and turn them to high beam. Try to reflect your beams off the rear-view mirror, illuminating the car's interior and also making your approach more difficult for the occupants of the car to see.
- While still in the ambulance, write down the license number of the vehicle and leave it at the radio.
- Note how many people are in the vehicle, their positions, and the driver's apparent condition. Be very wary around tinted windows.
- As you approach the vehicle, be alert to the possibility of other unseen occupants. Check to see if the trunk is locked, and look on the rear seat and the floor as you pass.
- Have your partner open the passenger door a split second before you open the driver's door; if you are alone, wait for help to arrive.
- Keep behind the center post. Carry an object, such as a report book or bag, that you can throw at the occupant's face if he becomes violent.
- If you have to retreat, immediately get into your vehicle and back up rapidly. Move 100 to 150 yards to clear the killing zone.

PROTECT THE PATIENT

Ensuring the safety of the patient is an important part of the scene size-up. Accidents and sudden medical emergencies frequently occur in public places or outdoors, away from the patient's home. Such emergencies expose the patient to a wide range of environmental factors that can cause him discomfort and also contribute to the deterioration of his condition (see Chapter 24, "Environmental Emergencies"). Emergencies can also expose a patient to the curiosity of the public, a situation some may find highly stressful. The EMT-B must have a keen awareness of how such factors affect his patient and be prepared to do what is necessary to change them in order to ensure the safety and comfort of his patient.

A victim of a fall onto a sidewalk on a hot sunny day, for example, can experience extreme discomfort, even burns, from the hot sidewalk. By placing the patient on a backboard as quickly as possible, you can make the patient much more comfortable and may prevent additional injury.

Conversely, the victim of a fall in a wet, slushy parking lot in mid-winter faces the risk of hypothermia. This is a potentially life-threatening condition in which the body temperature falls below normal. Providing such a patient with just a blanket is not enough. Major heat loss will occur through the patient's wet clothing and through the cold, wet surface on which he is lying. Placing such a patient on a backboard as soon as possible will slow heat loss and make him more comfortable. Also, with the patient on a backboard, he may be loaded into the ambulance for the balance of assessment and treatment, minimizing exposure to the elements.

Shade a patient's face from either the sun or precipitation. This will make him more comfortable and allow you to complete the assessment more easily.

You can easily protect a patient from the public's gaze in a way that will also assist you in crowd control. Ask several bystanders to turn their backs to the patient while holding up unfolded bed sheets at shoulder level. The patient appreciates the privacy provided. The bystanders also become involved in the patient's care and thus become easier to manage. Such a technique is usually far more effective than sternly telling the crowd to "step back."

PROTECT BYSTANDERS

Emergencies do draw crowds. Your attention as an EMT-B must be directed toward the patient. However, the crowd is part of the scene and making sure the bystanders are safe is one of your responsibilities during scene size-up.

Keeping the crowd out of the way can be as big a challenge as treating the patient. In cases of spills, leaks, fires, or heavy smoke, bystanders must be kept back through the use of roadblocks, detours, police lines, and public address systems advising bystanders of the risk. In such situations, bystanders who do not disperse should be dealt with by the police.

The hazards to the bystanders in smaller-scale emergencies are less dramatic but equally important. A one-car crash can down potentially deadly electrical wires. It can also scatter sharp glass and metal that can cut unwary bystanders. A bleeding patient injured in a fall can spread bloodborne pathogens to onlookers who get too close.

The easiest way of protecting bystanders is to prevent them from getting too close to the scene. The most effective way of doing this, as noted above, is to involve crowd members in crowd control. Giving a 50-foot length of rope to appropriately instructed bystanders who are willing to assist you and are not hostile is a good way of creating a barrier between the EMT-Bs working on the patient and the crowd. The barrier can also keep access to the ambulance clear. This technique acknowledges the concern of onlookers for the patient and involves them in ensuring that proper care is provided. Such utilization of resources at the scene of an emergency is a sign of an efficient EMT-B.

CONTROL THE SCENE

At a scene, it is the responsibility of the EMT-B to provide for the safety of himself and his partners, his patient, and any bystanders. To carry out these responsibilities, the EMT-B must sometimes take action to create a workable environment. This can be done through a variety of measures that range from providing more light, to eliminating noise, to moving the patient.

The prudent EMT-B will improve the environment subtly, avoiding a disruption of the scene. For example, a television set may be a source of noise, but turning it off may also eliminate the only source of light in a room. Therefore, if the television's noise is the interfering factor, turn it down rather than off, or ask that it be turned down. Below is a list of basic measures that you might consider adopting to improve working conditions at a scene.

- *Provide light.* Make it a point to have a good flashlight and keep it handy day and night.
- *Consider moving furniture* that interferes with access to the patient. This should be done after advising the patient or the bystanders of your intentions. In a residence, you must remember that, in spite of the emergency, you are a guest in the home and should demonstrate a proper level of respect toward the owners or occupants. If furniture is moved, it should be moved carefully to avoid any impression of ransacking the room. If possible, attempt to return furniture to its original position before leaving the scene.
- *Consider moving the patient* to an area more conducive to patient care. Attempting to resuscitate a patient in a cramped bathroom would generally make little sense when, by moving the patient five feet to the bedroom, you would have plenty of space in which to work. However, whenever an injury is suspected, the patient must be properly immobilized to a backboard before any movement is attempted. Always adapt your actions to the prevailing circumstances.
- *Maintain an escape route* and keep it open when a scene is tense or danger exists. If operating outdoors, try to position the ambulance in such a way that the crowd will not get between you and the patient and the ambulance. When working indoors, consider asking bystanders to keep all doors along the route to the ambulance open. Do not allow yourself to be cornered. If all else fails, remember that windows may be a good emergency escape route.
- *Pay attention to bystanders.* If the mood of a crowd turns ugly, you, your partners, and your patient may be in danger. Remember that a concerned crowd poses far less of a threat than an unruly crowd. Consider involving bystanders in crowd control. If the bystanders are parents or relatives of the patient, a continuing explanation of the measures you are taking will be appropriate.
- *Control the scene* or the scene will control you. Stay in control and anticipate things that will happen before they occur. Initiate action rather than respond to the actions of others at the scene.
- *Stay calm.* Other team members, the patient, and the bystanders will respond more positively.
- *Use tact and diplomacy.* A compassionate, understanding tone may produce more positive results than a harsh, demanding one.
- *Be flexible.* Have a Plan A to deal with the situation you are facing, but remain ready to shift to Plans B, C, or D if conditions indicate that Plan A won't work.
- *Be open-minded* about the situations, circumstances, and conditions you encounter on the job. Prehospital care involves working with people of a variety of ages, races, religions, and backgrounds. Many people have ways of life quite different from yours, some of them ways that you would not choose to follow. Remember that you have been called to assess, treat, and transport patients, not to judge them.
- *Be alert* to yourself, your partners, your patient, and your surroundings.
- *Be compassionate* toward the people you have been called upon to serve. Treat all people the way you would wish to have your loved ones treated in their time of need; someday you, too, may be in need.

DETERMINE THE NATURE OF THE PROBLEM

Once scene safety has been ensured, the next step in the scene size-up is determining the nature of the patient's problem that brought you to the scene. There are two basic categories of problems—trauma and medical. Which category a patient falls into will determine how you proceed with your continuing assessment and treatment of the patient.

Trauma is a physical injury or wound caused by external force or violence. Injuries caused by blunt, penetrating, or blast forces are examples of trauma, as are burns. Such injuries are typically to the skin, muscle, bone, ligaments, tendons, vessels, or organs.

A **medical problem** is a problem brought on by illness or by substances or conditions that affect the function of the body. A heart attack, a drug overdose, and a case of heat stroke are three examples of medical conditions that you may have to confront.

In prehospital care, the EMT-B first looks for evidence of an injury. If the possibility of injury is ruled out, the EMT-B may assume that the patient has a medical problem.

The dispatch information that starts you out on a call will often provide information that can be helpful in categorizing a patient. But, as you have seen, that information can be incomplete or inaccurate. You will have to be alert during the scene size-up for physical clues or other information that will help you understand the nature of the problem.

As always, you should remain open-minded and flexible as you try to determine the nature of the problem. Sometimes a patient will not fit neatly into one category or the other. For example, you may encounter a diabetic suffering from an altered mental status from failure to take his insulin who, as a result, has fallen down a flight of stairs. This patient is suffering from both trauma and a medical condition. When in doubt, treat the patient as a victim of trauma as this will mandate attention to possible spinal injury.

DETERMINE THE MECHANISM OF INJURY

When arriving on the scene of a suspected trauma, you will be looking for the **mechanism of injury (MOI).** Mechanism of injury refers to how the patient was injured. It includes the strength, direction, and nature of the forces that caused the injury. The mechanism of injury is the basis for your **index of suspicion.** The index of suspicion is the degree of your anticipation that the patient has been injured, or has been injured in a specific way, based on your knowledge that certain mechanisms usually produce certain types of injuries.

Identification of the mechanism of injury in a trauma patient may begin with the dispatch information. Dispatch to an automobile crash, a shooting, a fall, or a stabbing will provide some preliminary information as to the mechanism of injury. Once you arrive at the scene, however, it is necessary to take a much closer look at such scene characteristics as damage to the automobile, the use of restraint devices, the distance the patient fell, the type of surface the patient fell on (e.g., grass, carpet, concrete), the position in which the patient landed, the object that struck the patient, or the caliber of the gun the patient was shot with. Such characteristics will provide clues to what forces were applied to the body and the possible patterns of injury that may have resulted from them.

Common situations that should create a high index of suspicion for trauma injuries include the following:

- Falls
- Automobile crashes
- Motorcycle crashes
- Recreational vehicle crashes
- Contact sports involving intentional or unintentional collision
- Recreational sports (skiing, diving, basketball)
- Pedestrian collision with a car, bus, truck, bike or other force
- Blast injuries from an explosion
- Stabbings
- Shootings
- Burns

Chapter 28, "Mechanisms of Injury: Kinetics of Trauma," will provide more details about the nature of injuries resulting from a variety of mechanisms. The information below concerns characteristics you should look for during scene size-up in a number of common situations.

FALLS

Look for evidence of a fall when arriving on a scene. Fallen ladders, collapsed scaffolding, ropes in a tree or on buildings, trees in the immediate proximity of the patient, stairs, balconies, roofs, and windows are all common places to fall from or indicators that a fall may have occurred. When inspecting the scene of a suspected fall, you will develop a clearer idea of the types of injury the patient may have suffered if you determine the following information:

- Distance the patient fell
- Surface the patient landed on
- Body part that impacted first

AUTOMOBILE CRASHES

Automobile crashes produce some of the most lethal mechanisms of injury. Blunt forces applied to the body produce widespread injury to organs, bones, muscles, nerves, and blood vessels. The type of collision or point of impact to the vehicle commonly dictate the types of injuries to expect. Study the vehicle carefully, if possible, to identify this information. Common types of crashes include the following:

- Head-on or frontal collision
- Rear-end collision
- Side or lateral-impact collision
- Rotational impact collision
- Rollover

When approaching the scene of an automobile crash, look for evidence of both external impact to the vehicle from an outside force and internal impact to the vehicle caused by a patient's body. One EMT-B should quickly walk around all sides of the vehicle to identify the points of impact. That EMT-B should also conduct a close inspection of the passenger compartment for signs of impact that correlate with specific types of injury.

The following are significant external signs of vehicle impact to look for and document:

- Deformity to the vehicle greater than 20 inches
- Intrusion into the passenger compartment
- Displacement of a vehicle axle
- Rollover

The following are significant signs of patient impact in the passenger compartment to look for and document:

- Impact marks on the windshield caused by the patient's head
- Missing rear-view mirror
- Collapsed steering wheel
- Broken seat
- Side-door damage
- Cracked or smashed dashboard
- Deformed pedals
- Use of restraint devices and deployment of airbags

Ejection from the vehicle usually produces significant blunt or penetrating trauma. In most cases, the patient dies not from the ejection itself, but from the car rolling on top of him.

The death or significant injury of one passenger should cause you to suspect significant injury to other passengers.

MOTORCYCLE CRASHES

Try to determine and document the type of impact involved in the crash of a motorcycle. The following types of impacts are common:

- *Head-on*—The rider is propelled forward off the motorcycle.
- *Angular impact*—The rider strikes an object that produces injury.
- *Ejection*—The rider is thrown from the motorcycle and impacts the ground, the object involved in the collision, or both.
- *"Laying the bike down"*—The rider purposefully lays the bike down on its side to avoid another, potentially more serious impact.

It is important to determine and document whether the patient was wearing a helmet. The use of a helmet may prevent or reduce the severity of head injury.

RECREATIONAL VEHICLE CRASHES

Snowmobiles and all-terrain vehicles (ATVs) are commonly operated on uneven terrain, a factor that contributes to rollovers. Crush-type injuries are common. Also, snowmobiles can travel at high speed, producing severe impact upon collision with trees, rocks, or other vehicles.

With these vehicles be especially alert for "clothesline"-type injuries. In these injuries, a rider is pulled off the vehicle by a low branch, wire, rope, or other low-hanging object. Severe trauma to the neck and airway is common with this type of crash.

PENETRATING TRAUMA

Whenever you receive reports of a shooting or stabbing at the scene of a call, it is necessary to expose and assess the patient's body to confirm or rule out a gunshot or stabbing wound. With an unresponsive patient, completely expose him and look for a penetrating injury, whether or not blood is visible at the scene or around the body. Heavy coats, dark clothing, poor lighting, dark environments, or dark hair hide blood very well. You must inspect the body very carefully for open wounds. Open wounds to the chest may not produce much bleeding but can be lethal if not immediately identified and managed.

BLAST INJURIES

Explosions are another source of trauma. Gasoline, fireworks, natural gas, propane, acetylene, and grain dust in grain elevators are common causes of explosion. Look for injuries caused by the pressure wave associated with the blast, by flying debris, and by the collision that results when a patient propelled by the blast comes into contact with the ground or with other objects. Note also that burns are common at blast scenes.

DETERMINE THE NATURE OF THE ILLNESS

In a patient who is not injured but is suffering from a medical condition, you will begin to determine the **nature of illness (NOI)** during scene size-up. The patient, relatives, bystanders, or physical evidence at the scene may provide you with clues to determine what the patient is suffering from. You are not attempting to diagnose the patient's illness. You are gathering information that will narrow down the nature of the patient's complaint.

The initial information provided by the dispatcher can provide you with some preliminary clues. For example, the dispatcher may transmit, "Respond to a 77-year-old female complaining of chest pain." You can use such information to help you focus your questioning when you arrive at the scene. As usual, be alert to the possibility that information given to and relayed by the dispatcher is incomplete or inaccurate.

Once you arrive at the scene, you must determine the reason that you were called. Simply asking the patient, family members, or bystanders an open-ended question like, "What seems to be the problem today?" could provide you with the exact nature of the illness. Even if that does not happen, you might obtain at least some information that will help determine the nature of the illness.

Be aware, though, that the patient or his family may try to mislead you or to cloud the real nature of the illness. For example, use of drugs such as heroin or cocaine is illegal. Therefore, the family of a drug-overdose patient may claim they do not know why the patient is unresponsive. They may deny any drug use by the patient if directly asked. They may or may not eventually tell the truth regarding the real reason for the unresponsiveness.

Inspect the scene for clues about the illness. Look for prescription and nonprescription medications, drugs, drug paraphernalia, alcohol, and other pertinent clues. Home oxygen equipment may indicate a preexisting respiratory disease or cardiac condition; thus, you would likely suspect complaints of chest pain or difficulty breathing associated with either condition.

The physical position and condition of the patient may provide information about the illness. A tripod position—sitting up and leaning forward—may indicate respiratory distress or cardiac compromise. Patients with respiratory distress rarely lie flat unless they are completely exhausted. A patient lying very still with his legs drawn up to his chest is likely suffering from severe abdominal pain. A fruity odor emanating from the patient may indicate a diabetic condition. Look for loss of bowel or bladder control which may have resulted from a seizure or stroke.

Environmental conditions may provide clues to the nature of the illness. Extreme cold, wet and cold clothing, or a patient found outdoors in cool weather should suggest the possibility of hypothermia (low body temperature). A hot and humid environment, especially if the patient was playing a sport or performing some other strenuous activity, should suggest a possible heat emergency. Wooded areas may make you suspect snakebites or spider bites. Bites and stings from marine life are a real possibility if the patient is found at the beach. Scuba equipment should heighten your suspicion that the patient may be suffering a condition brought on while diving. If more than one person complains of similar symptoms in a tightly sealed home, consider the possibility of poisoning from carbon monoxide or some other gas.

The key to this phase of scene size-up is to study both the scene and the patient carefully as you look for clues that increase your suspicion of a particular nature of illness. Remember to write down your findings. Your report will provide emergency department personnel with valuable information that might not be otherwise available, especially if the patient is unresponsive.

DETERMINE THE NUMBER OF PATIENTS

The last major element of the scene size-up is determining the total number of patients. Sometimes this may be simple, as in the case of a single, responsive patient who has called for help because of chest pain. At other times, as in the case of a multiple-vehicle accident during a nighttime snowstorm or a suspected carbon monoxide poisoning in a multi-family dwelling, it may be more complicated.

If you discover that conditions at a scene are beyond your ability to handle, call for additional resources. Such resources may include law enforcement, fire, rescue, or utility company personnel, a hazardous materials team, or an additional basic life support unit or advanced life support team.

If, after studying the scene, you determine that there are more patients than your unit can effectively handle, initiate your local multiple-casualty plan. Follow local protocols in doing so. Such incidents will be covered in Chapter 43, "Multiple-Casualty Incidents, Triage, and Disaster Management."

Try to make any call for additional assistance before making contact with patients. Once you have made patient contact, you are likely to be completely focused on patient needs and not call for additional help.

If the number of patients surpasses your resources, begin triage and prioritization of patients. If you and your partner can manage the scene and the patients, consider spinal precautions based on the mechanism of injury, proceed with the assessment, and provide emergency care.

GAIN SCENE CONTROL AND ESTABLISH RAPPORT

When arriving on the scene, you will frequently encounter patients and family members who are frightened, injured, anxious, or in shock. In addition, you may find an angry or hostile crowd, law enforcement, or fire department personnel anxiously awaiting your arrival. You must display competence, confidence, and compassion—through your personal appearance and professional manner—in order to obtain cooperation not only from the patient but also from others at the scene.

If you do not take charge of the patient's care, someone else at the scene—whether it be a police officer, firefighter, family member, bystander, or the patient himself—will attempt to. This leads to confusion, anxiety, and irrational decision making on the part of the EMT-B.

ACHIEVE A SMOOTH TRANSITION OF CARE

When you arrive on the scene, it is important to assume a smooth transition of care from a first responder, police officer, or other individual who is providing first aid. Announce your arrival by stating, "I'm John Brady and this is Susan Kechlow. We are emergency medical technicians. Can you tell us what has happened and what care has been given?"

If the patient appears to be alert and responsive, you will have time to gain information from the first responders quickly before you make actual patient contact. This should take less than 1 minute. Do not carry on a conversation that is irrelevant to the patient, as this tends to ruin your presentation of confidence, competence, and compassion. An unresponsive or obviously injured patient needs your immediate attention. In this situation, therefore, proceed directly to the patient and obtain information from others at the scene as you begin to perform your initial assessment.

REDUCE THE PATIENT'S ANXIETY

Once you make contact with the patient, it is extremely important to attempt to reduce his anxiety and that of others at the scene. You can do this by employing the following simple techniques:

1. Bring order to the environment.
2. Introduce yourself.
3. Gain patient consent.
4. Position yourself.
5. Use communication skills.
6. Be courteous.
7. Use touch when appropriate.

BRING ORDER TO THE ENVIRONMENT

As quickly as possible, bring order to the environment by asking that televisions or radios be turned down, dogs removed from the area in which you are working, and children supervised by a family member, police officer, or first responder. Do not walk up to a television and simply turn it off while someone is watching it. No matter how serious the situation or patient appears, there are people who become ex-

tremely agitated when treated in this manner. You would be setting yourself up for a possible violent confrontation. You must explain, for example, "It is extremely important that you turn the television off so that we can hear and focus on caring for your mother." If the person refuses, ask for the sound to be turned down or remove the patient as quickly as possible from the scene.

Remember, not everyone at the scene is extremely happy to see you. Some people will become agitated and will resist your simple requests. You must remain calm and nonconfrontational and continue to focus on patient care.

INTRODUCE YOURSELF

Introduce yourself and ask for the patient's name. With older individuals, address them formally as "Mr. Jones" or "Mrs. Smith" to avoid any implication of disrespect. If time or the situation permits, you can ask, "What would you like me to call you?"

GAIN PATIENT CONSENT

Gain consent from the patient. This step is necessary before you may legally provide emergency care. You can do it simply by asking, "Is it all right for me to help you?" If the patient has an altered mental status or is unresponsive or is unable to make a rational decision, provide emergency care based on implied consent.

If the patient refuses your assistance, do not immediately pack up your equipment and pull out the refusal form, ready for the patient's signature. Many times the patient initially refuses care out of denial (a normal, and usually temporary, psychological response in which the patient cannot accept that he is ill or injured) or because he is frightened or confused. Keep talking with the patient to establish a rapport and help the patient accept the need for you to assess and treat him. If necessary, enlist the aid of a family member in convincing the patient. If the patient continues to refuse, contact medical direction for advice on how to proceed. Refer to Chapter 3, "Medical, Legal, and Ethical Issues," for further discussions on the legal implications of patient consent and refusal of emergency care.

POSITION YOURSELF

Your body position and posture are forms of nonverbal communication. Position yourself at a comfortable level in relation to the patient. If the eye levels are equal, so is the authority. If you are standing over the patient, you are in a dominant position of authority and control. This may be uncomfortable for the patient and may set the wrong tone for the scene. (At some scenes, when you need to establish control, this position is warranted.)

In the general American culture, intimate space generally starts at about 18 inches from the body. Unless you are intentionally touching your patient (see below), the patient is likely to be most comfortable if you maintain at least this distance from him during history-taking or other conversation.

Standing with your arms crossed across your chest is a closed communication posture, conveying hostility or disinterest. Instead, you want to display an openness and willingness to help.

USE COMMUNICATION SKILLS

As much as possible, maintain eye contact when talking with the patient to help establish rapport and to convey your sincere concern.

Speak calmly and deliberately to allow the patient to process the information. Raise your voice only if the patient appears to be hearing impaired. An elderly patient is not necessarily hard of hearing. Also speak in a calm and confident manner when you are communicating to your partner or others at the scene. Yelling or screaming while directing the scene and giving orders will only increase the anxiety of the patient and bystanders and exhibits a loss of control on your part.

Your body movements should be purposeful, displaying competence and confidence, and not hasty or jerky.

Most important, actively listen to what the patient is telling you. This avoids having to unnecessarily, and annoyingly, ask the same question several times. Make sure that the patient realizes you are listening by leaning forward, maintaining eye contact, and not allowing your attention to wander while the patient is talking to you.

BE COURTEOUS

The scene of an emergency is very stressful. As a result, the patient, family members, and bystanders may not be at their best. They may often seem quarrel-some, petty, rude, or hostile. As a professional, you must resist yielding to the same stresses. Try to understand why people behave as they do, and maintain a courteous manner throughout the call.

USE TOUCH WHEN APPROPRIATE

Touching the patient is a very powerful comfort measure when dealing with most people. Use eye contact to avoid the patient's perception of the touching as encroachment. Hold a hand, pat a shoulder, or lay your hand on a forearm. In order for touch to be effective, you must be sincere in your gestures, not using them as a gimmick.

MAINTAIN CONTROL

It is very difficult to conduct an assessment, gather information from the patient, and provide emergency care at a scene that is not controlled. The greater the distractions at the scene, the higher the anxiety level of the patient, family, and bystanders. Use the scene control measures described above to lessen confusion, reduce anxiety, and convey a professional attitude that the patient is in the care of capable EMT-Bs.

It is important to recognize when a scene cannot be adequately controlled. It may be impossible to gain scene control when the crowd is extremely hostile, or the family is emotionally charged or upset, threats are being made toward you, or the scene is unstable due to the risk of fire, explosion, or other hazards. You must consider your own safety when working in an uncontrolled environment. If the scene remains uncontrolled, it is best to move as rapidly as possible to remove yourself and the patient from the scene and/or to call for additional resources as needed.

CASE STUDY FOLLOW-UP

SCENE SIZE-UP

You have been dispatched to an unknown problem. As you approach the street, you shut off the siren and the emergency lights. Pulling up to the house, you notice that 68 Chicago is completely dark. No lights are noted outside or inside of the house. Your partner instructs you to proceed past the scene and park two houses up the street.

Because the house is completely dark and there appears to be no activity in or around it, you contact dispatch and inquire if they have a call-back number.

Dispatch responds, "EMS Unit 104, be advised, the call came from 71 Chicago. The patient at 68 Chicago has no phone." You look out and see that 71 Chicago is well lit. You then request, "Dispatch, can you call back the number for 71 Chicago and verify that this is a legitimate call?" A short time later dispatch contacts you, indicating that the woman at 71 Chicago said the man from 68 Chicago came to her house, said he had an emergency, and asked her to call 911. You contact dispatch and advise, "We are going to approach the scene. Please give us a radio check-up in 2 minutes."

Before leaving the ambulance, you turn on all the scene lights and focus the floodlight on the front door. You and your partner, EMT-B McKeown, exit the ambulance after agreeing that you will carry the flashlight while she brings the equipment from the ambulance. You take the lead and approach the house, holding your flashlight out in front of you and to the side. McKeown follows about eight feet behind with the jump kit. You walk up the front steps and approach the door. McKeown stays at the bottom of the steps watching the rest of the house and your back. You stand to the knob side of the door and knock. An older man opens the door and says nothing, but motions you in. You enter the house cautiously, on the alert for threats or hazards. After you are inside, McKeown enters, taking care to leave the door open behind her.

The man tells you he is Mr. Ziegler. He leads you to the living room where you find an elderly woman lying on the couch. He says, "My wife isn't feeling well," and sits in an armchair. You contact dispatch on your portable radio and indicate that you are okay and on the scene.

The room seems neat but sparsely furnished. The only light comes from a small television set. The rest of the house is completely dark. McKeown reaches for the light on the end table and Mr. Ziegler advises her, "The fuses blew. Nothing works but the TV. It's on batteries." McKeown walks over to the TV set and you tell her, "Just turn the volume down and leave the TV on. We need the light."

As you approach the patient, you notice a bottle of the medication Diabenase, used in treating diabetes, on a table next to the couch. Mrs. Ziegler looks up at you and says, "My legs are swollen. They've been like this all week."

McKeown is watching your back and the rest of the room. The scene seems secure. You note no mechanism of injury. Mrs. Ziegler appears to be suffering from a medical condition. There are no other patients to worry about at the scene. You can now begin to assess and provide treatment to the patient.

PATIENT ASSESSMENT

Having determined during scene size-up that Mrs. Ziegler is a medical patient with no signs of trauma, you proceed with the steps of patient assessment care as appropriate for a medical patient. You check for life-threatening conditions and find none: Her mental status, airway, breathing, and circulation are all normal. When you ask, "Why did you call the ambulance today?" Mrs. Ziegler states that she figured the emergency department wouldn't be busy on a Monday night. As you continue to ask questions to get her medical history, she confirms that she has diabetes controlled by Diabenase. The physical exam confirms that her legs are swollen but reveals no other problems. Her vital signs are normal.

You prepare Mrs. Ziegler for transport, positioning her on the stretcher in a sitting position, which she finds comfortable. En route to the hospital you continue to check on her condition and speak with her reassuringly. Mr. Ziegler rides along up front beside EMT-B McKeown, who is driving.

You contact the emergency department and give a brief report. You transfer Mrs. Ziegler's care to the nurse in the emergency department following an oral report. You write your prehospital report and prepare the ambulance for the next call. You contact dispatch and mark back in service.

Upon return to the emergency department on another call 3 hours later, you inquire about Mrs. Ziegler. The nurse states she was okay and released about an hour ago. The next door neighbor came to pick up Mr. and Mrs. Ziegler and take them home.

CHAPTER REVIEW

TERMS AND CONCEPTS

You may wish to review the following terms and concepts included in this chapter.

index of suspicion—an anticipation that certain types of accidents and mechanisms will produce specific types of injuries.

mechanism of injury (MOI)—factor involved in producing an injury to a patient, including the strength, direction, and nature of the forces that caused the injury.

medical problem—a problem brought on by illness or by substances or conditions that affect the working of the body.

nature of illness (NOI)—the type of medical condition or complaint a patient is suffering from.

scene safety—an assessment of the scene for safety

hazards to ensure the safety and well-being of the EMT-B, his partners, patients, and bystanders.

scene size-up—an overall assessment of the scene to which an EMT-B has been called to gain useful information that includes ensuring scene safety; determining whether a patient is suffering from trauma or a medical problem; and determining the total number of patients and whether additional resources are needed to handle them.

trauma—a physical injury or wound caused by external force or violence.

REVIEW QUESTIONS

1. Define scene size-up.
2. List three goals of the scene size-up.
3. List basic guidelines an EMT-B should follow at potentially dangerous or unstable scenes.
4. Explain the special problems an EMT-B is likely to encounter in confined areas like a cave, well, or sewer.
5. Explain how EMT-Bs should approach a house that they feel may be the scene of a crime.
6. Explain the chief determination about the nature of the patient's problem an EMT-B should make during the scene size-up.
7. Define mechanism of injury.
8. List clues to mechanism of injury that the EMT-B should be alert to at an automobile crash.
9. List clues at a scene that might indicate the nature of a patient's illness.
10. Explain why the EMT-B must determine the total number of patients at a call during the scene size-up.

CHAPTER 9

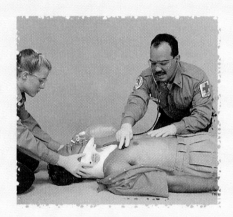

Patient Assessment

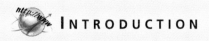 **INTRODUCTION**

As an EMT-Basic, your most important functions will be assessing the patient plus providing emergency care and transport to a medical facility. Of these functions, performing an accurate and reliable assessment will be the most important, because all of your decisions about care and transport will be based on it.

It is very important that you develop an assessment routine that is systematic. This will ensure that you assess every patient consistently and appropriately, based on the nature of that patient's illness or injury.

In this chapter, you will learn about the components of the patient assessment that you will perform on every patient you encounter during your career as an EMT-B.

CHAPTER 9 OVERVIEW

This chapter on patient assessment is divided into six parts. The chapter parts begin on the pages listed below.

CASE STUDIES

During your shift as an EMT-Basic one day, you are called to two different kinds of cases. The first call is to a patient who has been injured—a trauma patient. The second is to a patient who is suffering from a medical problem.

CALL ONE—A TRAUMA PATIENT

THE DISPATCH

EMS Unit 74—respond to Newton Drive, Greenway Apartments, Building 24. Unresponsive patient with unknown problem. Be advised police are at the scene. Time out is 1512 hours.

ON ARRIVAL

Upon arrival, you find an adult male patient lying supine at the bottom of a two-story fire-escape ladder. The police are on the scene and indicate that they were called for a domestic incident and that the neighbors heard fighting and gunshots.

How would you proceed with the assessment of this patient?

CALL TWO—A MEDICAL PATIENT

THE DISPATCH

EMS Unit 74—respond to 33 East Sassafras Street. Patient with unknown problem. Patient's daughter made the call. Time out is 1623 hours.

ON ARRIVAL

You arrive at the address, a well-kept home in a quiet neighborhood. A middle-aged woman hurries out into the driveway as you pull up.

"It's my mother," she says. "She can't seem to catch her breath."

How would you proceed with the assessment of this patient?

During this chapter, you will learn about the patient assessment procedures you will perform, as an EMT-Basic, for trauma and medical patients in a variety of situations. Later, we will return to these two cases and apply the procedures learned.

COMPONENTS OF THE PATIENT ASSESSMENT: AN OVERVIEW

When you arrive at the scene of an emergency call, you will perform certain procedures to find out what is wrong with the patient for the purpose of helping you decide what emergency medical care should be provided and how quickly the patient needs to be transported to a medical facility. These procedures are known as **patient assessment.** It is also important to keep in mind that, as the EMT at the scene, you become the eyes and ears of all emergency care personnel, since you will have access to the home environment or other emergency scene as well as to family and bystanders who will not be available to other health care providers, especially those at the hospital emergency department to whom you will transfer the care of your patient.

Patient assessment has several main purposes:

- **To determine whether the patient is injured or has a medical illness.** This determination is based on the scene size-up and general impression of the patient formed during the initial assessment.
- **To identify and manage immediately life-threatening injuries or conditions.** This is the main purpose of the initial and rapid assessments.
- **To determine priorities for further assessment and care on the scene vs. immediate transport with assessment and care continuing en route.** Priority decisions take place during initial assessment and, as appropriate, throughout the remainder of the assessment.
- **To examine the patient and gather a patient history.** This takes place during the focused history and physical exam, which is more thorough than was the initial assessment. In some situations, the focused history and physical exam is followed by the even more thorough detailed physical exam.
- **To provide further emergency care** based on findings made during the focused history and physical exam and the detailed physical exam.
- **To monitor the patient's condition,** assessing the effectiveness of the care that has been provided and adjusting care as needed. The ongoing assessment continues until the patient is transferred to the hospital staff.
- **To communicate patient information to the medical facility staff and to document the details of the call**—accurately and completely—during and at the conclusion of the call.

It is important to realize that each patient's condition or injuries are unique—even though the patient may be complaining of the same signs or symptoms as another patient that you treated previously. It is easy to develop tunnel vision and focus in on the patient's chief complaint (the reason that is stated for calling for EMS help), especially if the complaint is dramatic, without determining the entire extent of the patient's condition.

For example, if you arrive on the scene and find an elderly man who is lying in the middle of the living room floor complaining of excruciating pain to his hip with obvious deformity, it is very easy to make a quick judgment and conclude that the patient must have fallen and injured his hip. At this point, it appears that immediate immobilization of the hip, followed by transport to the hospital, is the most appropriate care for this patient.

However, it is vital that you question the patient to determine the cause of the fall. If the patient indicates that he fell as a result of tripping on the rug, the apparent hip injury is your primary concern. But suppose the patient tells you he fell because, while crossing the room, he began to suffer severe chest pain and dizziness. You realize that the patient's fall was probably caused by a medical condition, possibly a heart attack. Now the focus of the assessment and treatment has changed. You will deal first with the medical condition, which is potentially more serious than the hip injury. The hip injury, even though significant, now becomes a secondary priority.

If you had failed to recognize the medical condition and had proceeded to splint the hip at the patient's home, transport to the hospital and treatment for the potential heart attack would have been delayed, possibly with extremely serious consequences. With proper assessment and discovery of the medical problem, you would provide oxygen and transport the patient immediately—secured to a rigid backboard to provide temporary stabilization of the hip injury. Then, if time and circumstances permitted, you might splint the hip in the back of the ambulance en route to the hospital.

So you can see that it is necessary to perform a complete assessment on every patient, no matter how obvious the problem appears to be. Immediately focusing in on whatever is obvious or dramatic will often cause the EMT-B to miss injuries or conditions that are important, even potentially life threatening. No matter how significant—or how insignificant—the most obvious complaint or injury may seem, you must be suspicious that other injuries or medical conditions exist that you have not yet found.

Throughout all phases of patient assessment, respect the patient's feelings. Protect his dignity and modesty, explain what you are doing, and—without being dishonest—reassure the patient that everything is being done to help him.

For more detail on the components of patient assessment and how they are applied to different kinds of patients, see Figure 9-1. Return to this chart as you progress through the chapter to track the steps of patient assessment you are learning about.

To achieve a systematic approach to patient assessment, several components must be included. These components of the patient assessment will be discussed in Parts 1 through 6 of this chapter.

Components of Patient Assessment

1. Scene size-up
2. Initial assessment
3. Focused history and physical exam
4. Detailed physical exam
5. Ongoing assessment
6. Communication and documentation

PATIENT ASSESSMENT

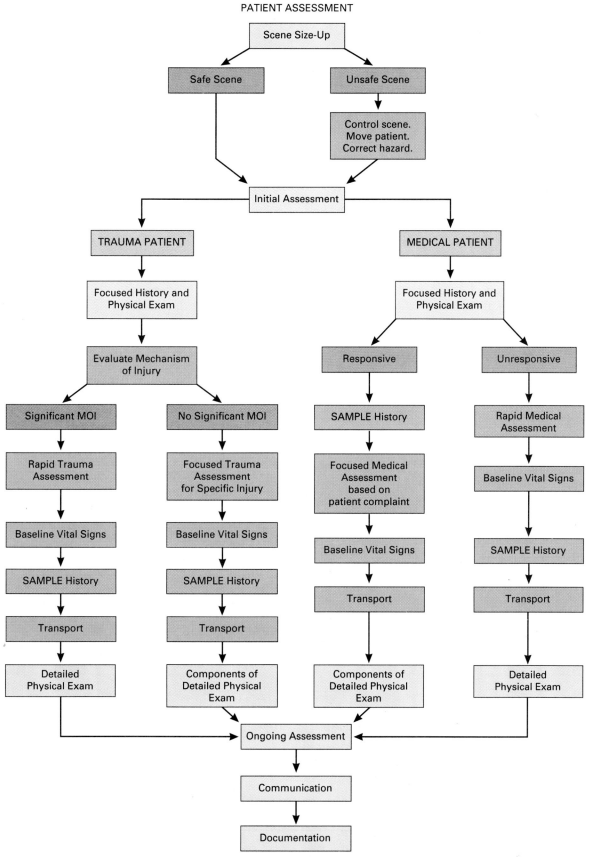

Figure 9-1   The components of patient assessment.

PART 1
SCENE SIZE-UP

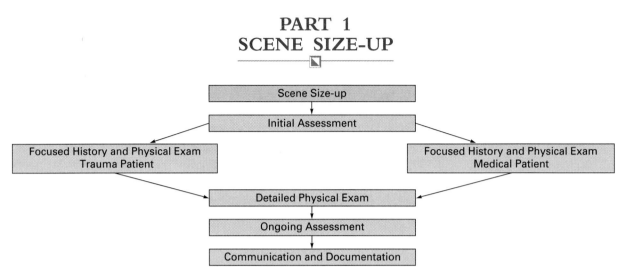

Scene size-up is the first component of patient assessment. As you learned in Chapter 8, the phases of the scene size-up are:

Steps of the Scene Size-up

1. Take necessary body substance isolation precautions.
2. Evaluate scene hazards and assure scene safety.
   – Personal protection
   – Protection of the patient
   – Protection of bystanders
3. Determine the mechanism of injury or the nature of the illness.
   – Trauma patient
   – Medical patient
4. Establish the number of patients.
5. Ascertain the need for additional resources to manage the scene or the patient(s).

The scene size-up is a dynamic process that continues throughout the entire call. Much of the scene size-up is operational, such as ensuring scene safety and ascertaining the need for additional resources. However, determining the mechanism of injury or nature of the illness and determining the number of patients actually constitute the beginning of the patient assessment process.

PART 2
INITIAL ASSESSMENT

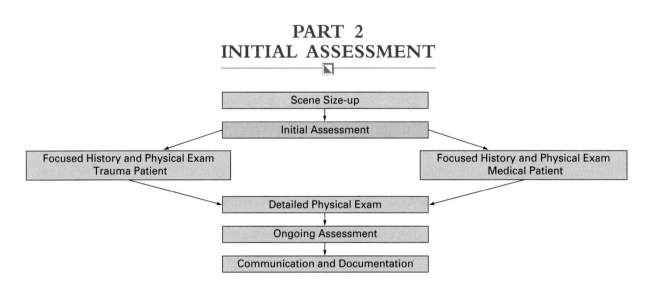

OBJECTIVES

Numbered objectives are from the United States Department of Transportation 1994 EMT-Basic National Standard Curriculum. Asterisked objectives, *if any, pertain to material that is supplemental to the DOT curriculum.*

COGNITIVE

3-2.1 Summarize the reasons for forming a general impression of the patient. (pp. 153–155)
3-2.2 Discuss methods of assessing altered mental status. (pp. 155–158)
3-2.3 Differentiate between assessing the altered mental status in the adult, child, and infant patient. (p. 156)
3-2.4 Discuss methods of assessing the airway in the adult, child, and infant patient. (pp. 158–159)
3-2.5 State reasons for management of the cervical spine once the patient has been determined to be a trauma patient. (p. 155)
3-2.6 Describe methods used for assessing if a patient is breathing. (pp. 159–160)
3-2.7 State what care should be provided to the adult, child, and infant patient with adequate breathing. (p. 161)
3-2.8 State what care should be provided to the adult, child, and infant patient without adequate breathing. (pp. 160–161)
3-2.9 Differentiate between a patient with adequate and inadequate breathing. (pp. 160–161)
3-2.10 Distinguish between methods of assessing breathing in the adult, child, and infant patient. (p. 160)
3-2.11 Compare the methods of providing airway care to the adult, child, and infant patient. (pp. 159–160)
3-2.12 Describe the methods used to obtain a pulse. (pp. 161–162)
3-2.13 Differentiate between obtaining a pulse in an adult, child, and infant patient. (p. 162)
3-2.14 Discuss the need for assessing the patient for external bleeding. (p. 162-63)

3-2.15 Describe normal and abnormal findings when assessing skin color. (p. 163)
3-2.16 Describe normal and abnormal findings when assessing skin temperature. (pp. 163–164)
3-2.17 Describe normal and abnormal findings when assessing skin condition. (p. 164)
3-2.18 Describe normal and abnormal findings when assessing skin capillary refill in the infant and child patient. (p. 164)
3-2.19 Explain the reason for prioritizing a patient for care and transport. (pp. 164–165)

AFFECTIVE

3-2.20 Explain the importance of forming a general impression of the patient. (pp. 153–155)
3-2.21 Explain the value of performing an initial assessment. (p. 151)

PSYCHOMOTOR

3-2.22 Demonstrate the techniques for assessing mental status.
3-2.23 Demonstrate the techniques for assessing the airway.
3-2.24 Demonstrate the techniques for assessing if the patient is breathing.
3-2.25 Demonstrate the techniques for assessing if the patient has a pulse.
3-2.26 Demonstrate the techniques for assessing the patient for external bleeding.
3-2.27 Demonstrate the techniques for assessing the patient's skin color, temperature, condition, and capillary refill (infants and children only).
3-2.28 Demonstrate the ability to prioritize patients.

Once you have ensured that the scene is safe and have controlled the scene, you are prepared to begin the **initial assessment**. An initial assessment is conducted on every patient, regardless of the mechanism of injury or nature of illness.

The main purpose of the initial assessment is to discover and treat immediately life-threatening conditions. During the initial assessment you will quickly form a general impression of the patient and assess the patient's mental status, airway, breathing, and circulation. *Any life-threatening condition that is identified must be treated immediately as found—before moving on to the next portion of the initial assessment.* As a result of the initial assessment, you will make decisions about priorities for further assessment, care, and transport.

The steps of the initial assessment allow a systematic approach to assessment for, and control of, life threats. It is vital that you progress through the steps in this exact sequence, and do not allow dramatic but non-life-threatening injuries or conditions to cloud your priorities. For example, a fractured humerus that is protruding through the skin is a very dramatic injury. However, the fracture will not immediately cause the death of the patient unless it is associated with major bleeding. By contrast, a patient with clotted blood in the mouth causing the airway to be blocked is in immediate danger. The blood in the mouth is not very dramatic and could easily be missed by an EMT-B who is not systematically performing the initial assessment. Systematically following the steps of the initial assessment will keep you

INITIAL ASSESSMENT

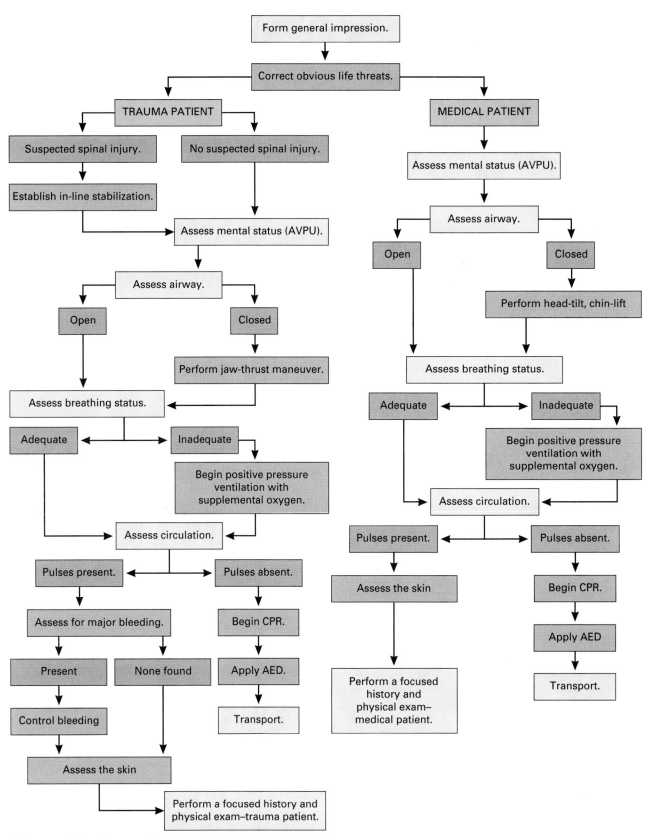

Figure 9-2 Steps of the initial assessment.

focused and allow you to identify and correct immediately life-threatening injuries or conditions.

The steps of initial assessment are conducted in the following sequence:

Steps of the Initial Assessment

1. Form a general impression of the patient.
2. Assess mental status.
3. Assess the airway.
4. Assess breathing.
5. Assess circulation.
6. Establish patient priorities.

You should be able to conduct this survey (shown in more detail in Figure 9-2) in about 60 seconds, unless confronted with life-threatening problems that must be treated immediately as found.

FORM A GENERAL IMPRESSION OF THE PATIENT

Initial assessment begins as soon as you approach the patient, allowing you, for the first time, to gain your own first-hand impression of the patient (Figure 9-3).

As you gain experience as an EMT-B, you will become more and more adept at gaining valuable information about your patient from your first impressions. For example, if this information has not already been provided to you by dispatch, first responders, or bystanders, you will immediately observe the patient's general age (for example child, adult, elderly) and sex, which may have a bearing on the patient's condition or care.

You will also often be able to gain a quick impression, just from the patient's general appearance,

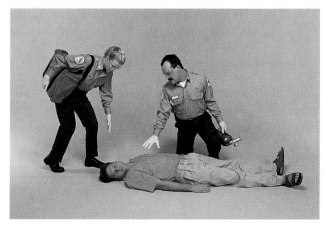

Figure 9-3   Form a general impression as you approach the patient.

TABLE 9-1

Forming a General Impression

- Estimate the patient's *age*.
- Note the patient's *sex*.
- Determine if *trauma or medical* patient.
- Obtain the patient's *chief complaint*.
- Identify (and manage) *immediate life threats*.

as to whether the patient seems well or ill or whether the patient appears to have been injured. What the patient tells you about what is wrong with him (the chief complaint) and the items or conditions you notice in the patient's immediate environment are additional elements of the general impression you form as you approach and make your first contact with the patient (Table 9-1).

If a mechanism of injury that you have identified is severe enough to cause you to suspect spinal injury, you will take immediate steps to stabilize the patient's head and spine. Often you will recognize a life-threatening problem, such as severe bleeding, right away. If you do, you will treat that condition immediately.

As you can see, although you form your general impression quickly as you approach the patient, even before you can begin a systematic assessment, the general impression can provide valuable information and often allow you to perform life-saving procedures without delay.

DETERMINE IF THE PATIENT IS INJURED OR ILL

As you form your general impression at the beginning of the initial assessment, you will categorize the patient as being injured (a trauma patient) or ill (a medical patient). In most cases, you will be confirming information already gathered from the dispatcher, scene size-up, first-responders, and bystanders. Determining whether the patient is injured or is ill is very important in the next step of assessment.

Patients who are injured have suffered from some form of trauma. There are two types of trauma, penetrating trauma and blunt-force trauma. **Penetrating trauma** is a force that pierces the skin and body tissues, often caused by gunshots and knives. You can also encounter patients who have suffered penetrating trauma from screwdrivers, ice picks, handlebars, broken glass, metal, wood, or any other sharp object.

Blunt trauma is caused by a force that impacts or is applied to the body but is not sharp enough to penetrate it. Blunt trauma usually results from blows (as in vehicle crashes, falls, and fights) or from crushing (as in a building collapse or when an extremity gets caught in machinery). Clues to the mechanism of injury may be present in the patient's immediate environment, for example a dent in the dashboard of a collision vehicle, the presence of a bloody knife, or a heavy object that appears to have fallen on the patient.

On the other hand, the patient's immediate environment may offer clues that the patient is suffering not from trauma but from a medical problem. For example, a bottle of nitroglycerin pills next to the patient may indicate that he was having chest pain prior to your arrival. Finding a patient in bed in pajamas at 2 o'clock in the afternoon may possibly indicate that he has been sick all day. A bucket or pail next to the bed may make you suspect that the patient has been vomiting. An elderly patient who is found lying on the floor of a chilly house may be suffering from hypothermia (a lowered body temperature). Information from the patient's environment can be very valuable, especially when the patient is unresponsive.

OBTAIN THE CHIEF COMPLAINT

The **chief complaint** is the patient's answer to the question "Why did you call the ambulance?" If the patient is unable to answer, the chief complaint may be the response of the family member or bystander who placed the emergency call. If no one can provide an answer to the question, the chief complaint may be what you infer from your observations of the patient.

The chief complaint may have to do with pain ("My stomach hurts"), abnormal function (slurred speech), a change in function from a normal state ("She just doesn't seem to be herself"), or an observation made by you (for example, the patient's bizarre behavior indicates a possible psychiatric problem). The chief complaint is quickly ascertained during the general-impression phase of the initial assessment.

Do not always assume that the original complaint is the true chief complaint. In a patient who is injured, you may think the chief complaint is obvious. You might suspect the pain associated with an obviously crushed and deformed leg to be the chief complaint. However, if the patient also states, "My chest is killing me," you must immediately suspect a possible chest injury or heart condition, either of which is potentially more serious than an extremity injury, and begin to focus your assessment on the patient's chest.

In the trauma patient, the EMT-B can often observe the chief complaint—for example a bleeding wound. Medical conditions, however, rarely offer such obvious and definitive external signs. So obtaining the chief complaint from a medical patient is extremely important.

It is also important to ask additional questions that refine the chief complaint. The patient's chief complaint may be abdominal pain. However, suppose that through further questioning you determine that the patient has been complaining of the same abdominal pain for the past 2 years. You must then ask, "Why did you call the ambulance *today*?" This will tend to force the patient to focus on what has changed to make him more concerned. The patient may now state, "This morning I vomited bright red blood." The chief complaint has changed; however, the abdominal pain is still an important factor to consider when assessing the patient. The chief complaint has set the tone for further assessment and emergency care.

In unresponsive patients, the chief complaint may need to be established through family, friends, or bystanders at the scene or from the environment itself. Ask, "Can you tell me what happened?" and "Was the patient complaining of anything before he became unconscious?" Do not assume that the bystander at the scene understands what unconsciousness truly means. You may need to ask, "Did the patient respond in any way when you were talking to him?"

The chief complaint, along with scene size-up, will help determine priorities for further assessment, care, and transport. The unresponsive patient who told a family member "This is the worst headache I've ever had in my life" before collapsing, or the trauma patient with a bullet wound to the chest, needs care at a hospital without delay; based on the chief complaint and general impression, you would opt for immediate transport following the initial and rapid assessments, with further assessment continuing en route. For the patient who states "I am drunk as a skunk" and exhibits all the typical signs and symptoms of intoxication, or the patient who has bleeding from a cut that can be controlled by pressure, you would proceed with assessment and emergency care on-scene before transporting the patient.

IDENTIFY IMMEDIATE LIFE THREATS

If you identify a life-threatening condition during the general impression phase, you must immediately treat it. For example, you arrive at the scene of an injury incurred during a domestic dispute. After assuring that the scene is safe, you enter. From the doorway, you spot a stab wound to the patient's left lateral chest. Since an open wound to the chest is considered to be an immediate life threat, you immediately place your gloved hand over the wound until your partner can prepare and apply the appropriate dressing. Only then do you continue with the initial assessment, watching especially for other injuries related to the stabbing.

Life threats that require immediate management as found and that you should be looking for during the initial assessment are listed in Table 9-2.

TABLE 9-2

Life Threats That Require Immediate Management as Found

- *Airway*
  - An airway that is compromised by blood, vomitus, secretions, the tongue, bone, teeth, or other substances or objects
- *Breathing*
  - Absence of breathing or inadequate breathing
  - Open wounds to the chest that may disrupt thoracic pressures
  - Injuries to the chest that do not allow for adequate chest wall expansion
- *Circulation*
  - Major bleeding

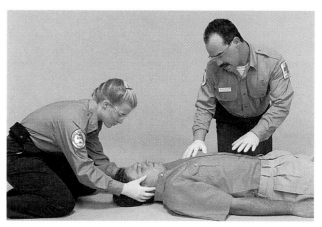

Figure 9-4   Establish in-line stabilization if spinal injury is suspected.

ESTABLISH IN-LINE STABILIZATION

If you determine or suspect that the patient has been injured, it is necessary to ask yourself if the mechanism of injury could have been significant enough to injure the spine. (Do not automatically rule out possible spinal injury in patients who are ill. Consider a diabetic patient who is found unconscious at the bottom of a stairway. You must consider the possibility that the patient fell down the steps after losing consciousness.)

If you have any suspicion that a spinal injury may exist, based solely on the mechanism of injury, you must manually stabilize the patient's spine before moving on to any other part of the assessment or care. To accomplish this, take **in-line stabilization** by bringing the patient's head into a neutral in-line position and holding it there. The procedure for accomplishing in-line stabilization (Figure 9-4) is:

1. Place one hand on each side of the patient's head.
2. Gently bring the head into a position in which the nose is lined up with the patient's navel and points 90 degrees from the direction of the spine.
3. Position the head neutrally so the head is not extended (tipped backward) or flexed (tipped forward).

Proper in-line stabilization is necessary to avoid any movement or manipulation of the vertebrae that may cause or increase the chances of spinal cord damage. It is very possible to have a stable injury of the vertebrae in which the spinal cord has not been damaged. If immediate and proper in-line stabilization is not accomplished, however, the stable injury can easily become unstable as a result of the patient moving or being moved. For example, the patient turns his head to look at you when answering a question, or you

and your partner grasp the patient by the armpits and knees to move him onto the stretcher. This could result in permanent neurologic damage, paralysis, or death.

Thus, having a high index of suspicion and recognizing the need for proper spinal stabilization is extremely important prior to and during the initial assessment.

Once in-line stabilization is established, it must be maintained, even after a cervical spinal immobilization collar (CSIC) is applied, until the patient is completely immobilized to a backboard with backboard straps and a head immobilization device.

POSITION THE PATIENT FOR ASSESSMENT

If you find the patient in a prone position (face down), it is necessary to quickly log roll him into a supine position (face up) (Figures 9-5a to c). It is not possible to properly assess the airway and breathing with the patient in a prone position. Prior to log rolling the patient, very quickly assess the posterior thorax and lumbar regions, buttocks, and posterior aspects of the lower extremities by inspecting and palpating for any major bleeding, deformities, open wounds, bruises, burns, tenderness, or swelling.

If the mechanism of injury suggests a possible spinal injury, then the patient must be log rolled only after in-line stabilization has been established.

ASSESS MENTAL STATUS

Indicate to the patient that you are an emergency medical technician and you are there to help. In the trauma patient, do this only after taking in-line stabilization to avoid any unnecessary movements by the patient. Quickly determine if the patient is awake, if he responds to a stimulus, or if he is unresponsive.

LOG-ROLLING FROM A PRONE TO A SUPINE POSITION WHEN SPINAL INJURY IS SUSPECTED

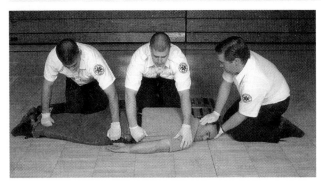

Figure 9-5a A rescuer at the patient's head establishes and maintains in-line spinal stabilization. A backboard is placed alongside the patient, and two other rescuers kneel on it. One grasps the patient's shoulder and hip. The other grasps the patient's thigh and ankle. (Carl Lee/Youngstown State University)

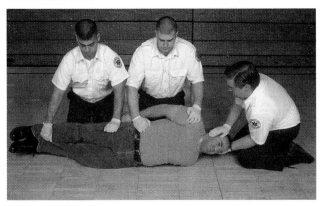

Figure 9-5b On the command of the rescuer at the head, the patient is rolled up against the thighs of the kneeling rescuers. The rescuer who is grasping the patient's thigh and ankle makes sure that the legs are slightly raised off the floor to keep them aligned with the spine as the patient is turned. (Carl Lee/Youngstown State University)

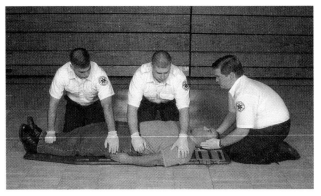

Figure 9-5c The patient is then rolled into the supine position on the backboard. In-line spinal stabilization is maintained by the rescuer at the head. (Carl Lee/Youngstown State University)

ASSESS THE LEVEL OF RESPONSIVENESS

The patient's level of responsiveness can be assessed (Figure 9-6) by using the **AVPU** mnemonic (Table 9-3).

Make adjustments in gauging the mental status of an infant or young child. Note whether the child is following movements with his eyes. Crying may replace speech as a response. For response to verbal stimulus, watch and listen for the child's reaction to a shout. The response to painful stimulus should be similar to an adult's.

ALERTNESS AND ORIENTATION

If the patient's eyes are open and he is able to speak as you approach him, you would assume that the patient is alert. However, a patient can be alert but confused or disoriented. If the patient is not alert, proceed to check his response to verbal stimulus.

RESPONSIVENESS TO VERBAL STIMULUS

If the patient opens his eyes and responds or makes an attempt to respond only when you speak to him, he is responsive to verbal stimulus. If the patient does

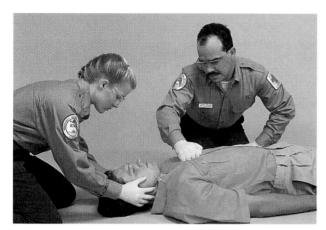

Figure 9-6 Quickly assess level of responsiveness.

TABLE 9-3
AVPU: Mnemonic for Assessment of Mental Status

A	**A**lert
V	Responds to **V**erbal Stimulus
P	Responds to **P**ainful Stimulus
U	**U**nresponsive

not speak, quickly check to determine if he will obey your commands. Instruct the patient to "squeeze my fingers" or "wiggle your toes." If the patient obeys the commands, you can assume he has a higher level of responsiveness than the patient who stares off, talks inappropriately, mumbles incomprehensibly, or does nothing at all.

RESPONSIVENESS TO PAINFUL STIMULUS

If there is no response when you speak to the patient, you should try a painful stimulus. Rubbing the sternum with your knuckles (sternal rub), pinching the earlobe or shoulder skin, applying pressure to the arch above the eye or fingernail bed, and squeezing the muscle at the base of the neck, are appropriate painful stimuli. Be sure to watch the patient's face as well as the body when applying a painful stimulus. Look for a facial grimace or other body movement.

The patient who responds to a painful stimulus typically responds with either purposeful or nonpurposeful movements. The purposeful movements are attempts made by the patient to remove the stimulus or avoid the pain. This could be as significant as the patient reaching up and grabbing your hand or as insignificant as a small movement away from the pain or a slight upward sweeping motion of the hand.

Head-injured patients or those with spinal cord injuries may respond to a painful stimulus but will not respond appropriately or normally. The patient with a spinal cord injury may only respond to pain applied above the site of the injury. Two nonpurposeful movements, having no purpose relative to the painful stimulus, are decorticate and decerebrate posturing (Figure 9-7). In **decorticate posturing,** the patient arches the back and flexes the arms inward toward the chest. In **decerebrate posturing,** the patient arches the back and extends the arms straight out parallel to the body. Both are signs of serious head injury.

UNRESPONSIVENESS

A patient who does not respond to verbal and painful stimuli is considered to be unresponsive. Unresponsive patients commonly lose their gag and cough re-

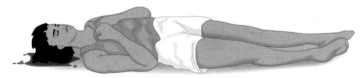

Decorticate posturing.

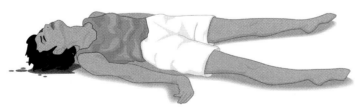

Decerebrate posturing.

Figure 9-7 Nonpurposeful movements: decorticate and decerebrate posturing.

flexes, often leading to airway compromise. Because unresponsiveness is a significant finding, the patient is considered a priority for transport.

The patient who is not alert but responds to either verbal or painful stimulus is considered to have an altered mental status. This patient is not completely unresponsive but, like the unresponsive patient, may be prone to airway compromise.

DOCUMENT THE LEVEL OF RESPONSIVENESS

It is extremely important to document the exact response to the stimulus, e.g., "The patient groaned and flexed his left arm," or "The patient made a facial grimace and grasped my hand." A patient who grabs your hand when you do a sternal rub versus a patient who has decorticate posturing indicates two significantly different levels of cerebral function. Obviously, the patient with the ability to grasp your hand has a much better level of neurologic function than the decorticate-postured patient; however, both could be placed generally into the category of responding to painful stimulus. The more specific you are regarding how the patient responds, the easier it is for others to assess for a deteriorating mental status at a later point in time.

Assessment of the patient's mental status should take you no longer than a few seconds to accomplish. Do not waste time performing an extensive neurologic exam during the initial assessment. The AVPU check is to quickly establish a baseline for mental status. A much more detailed neurologic exam will be performed later in the assessment process.

ASSESS THE AIRWAY

Once you have assessed the patient's level of responsiveness, you must immediately progress to assessment of the airway (Figure 9-8). A closed or blocked airway is an immediately life-threatening condition. Your patient will not survive without a patent airway, no matter how diligent your emergency care. You must closely assess the airway and, if it is not patent, immediately open it, using manual techniques and mechanical devices if necessary.

DETERMINE AIRWAY STATUS

The AVPU check of the patient's level of responsiveness can be used to quickly rule out a possible airway problem. A patient who is alert and responsive can be assumed to have a patent airway. Thus, the mental status check is also a helpful tool for simultaneously gathering information about airway status.

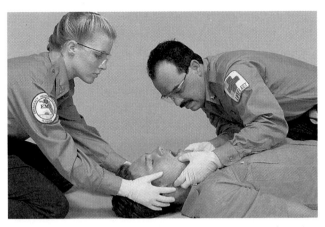

Figure 9-8 Assess the airway. To open the airway, use the jaw-thrust maneuver for a trauma patient. Use the head-tilt, chin-lift maneuver for a medical patient.

IN THE RESPONSIVE PATIENT

If the patient is alert and talking without difficulty, or if the infant or child is crying, you can assume the airway is patent and move on to the assessment of breathing. However, an alert patient who has stridor on inspiration or exhalation or who is having difficulty in speaking, gasping between words, using extremely short sentences, or not talking at all should be examined closely for a blocked or partially blocked airway or for other causes of respiratory distress. If you have any doubt that the airway is open, you should immediately take the necessary steps to open it (see below).

IN THE UNRESPONSIVE PATIENT

Unresponsive patients have a high incidence of airway occlusion due to relaxation of the muscles in the upper airway. This allows the tongue and epiglottis to fall back and partially block the lower part of the pharynx and the opening to the trachea. In this situation, use the techniques described below to open or to maintain an open airway.

OPEN THE AIRWAY

If the patient is not talking or responding normally or is unresponsive, assume that the airway is or may become closed. You must immediately open the airway and take measures to maintain the airway's patency.

The airway is opened and maintained by using, as needed, any or all of the following four techniques:

- Manual airway maneuvers to prevent the tongue and epiglottis from blocking the airway: the head-tilt, chin-lift or the jaw-thrust maneuver
- Suction and/or finger sweeps to remove blood, vomitus, food, secretions, or foreign objects

- Airway adjuncts to maintain a patent airway: the oropharyngeal airway or the nasopharyngeal airway
- Manual thrusts to the abdomen (Heimlich maneuver), or a combination of chest thrusts and back blows for infants, to force bursts of air from the lungs—used to relieve a blockage of the airway by a foreign body that cannot be relieved by any of the techniques already listed

The head-tilt, chin-lift and jaw-thrust maneuvers, suctioning techniques, and the use of airway adjuncts were taught in Chapter 7, "Airway Management, Ventilation, and Oxygen Therapy." The Heimlich maneuver and other techniques for clearing airway blockages are described in Appendix 1, "Basic Life Support."

INDICATIONS OF PARTIAL AIRWAY OCCLUSION

When you approach the patient, you may hear abnormal sounds from the upper airway. These sounds are an indication that the airway may be partially blocked. Sounds that frequently indicate partial airway occlusion are listed in Table 9-4 and discussed below.

SNORING

If a snoring (sonorous) sound is heard, it is an indication that the tongue and epiglottis are still partially blocking the airway. Use the head-tilt, chin-lift maneuver (if there is no suspicion of spinal injury) or the jaw-thrust maneuver (if spinal injury is possible) to relieve any obstruction of the airway by the tongue. If this does not correct the snoring, insert an oropharyngeal airway (for an unresponsive patient without a gag reflex). If the patient gags when inserting an oropharyngeal airway, remove it immediately, be prepared to suction, and consider insertion of a nasopharyngeal airway.

GURGLING

A gurgling sound is an indication that a liquid substance is in the airway. Immediately open the mouth and suction out the contents. If the contents are too

TABLE 9-4

Sounds That May Indicate Partial Airway Obstruction

- Snoring (sonorous)—a rough snoring-type sound on inspiration and/or exhalation
- Gurgling—a sound similar to air rushing through water on inspiration and/or exhalation
- Crowing—a sound like a cawing crow on inspiration
- Stridor—harsh, high-pitched sound on inspiration

thick to be suctioned, turn the patient on his side and sweep the mouth out with your fingers, a tongue blade, or the suction catheter itself. A patient with possible spinal injury must be log-rolled onto his side while in-line stabilization is maintained. Be cautious when placing your fingers in a patient's mouth, especially if he is unresponsive. The patient can very easily, and unintentionally, bite down and injure you significantly. Place a bite stick between the teeth if necessary to avoid a patient bite.

Do not waste time when clearing the airway. The key is to be prepared and use whatever device or technique is most readily available that clears the contents.

CROWING AND STRIDOR

Crowing and stridor are both high-pitched sounds produced on inspiration. Both are most commonly associated with the swelling or muscle spasms that result from conditions such as airway infections, allergic reactions, or burns. These conditions typically cannot be relieved by manual maneuvers, suctioning, or insertion of an airway adjunct.

Inserting anything such as an airway adjunct, suction tip, tongue blade, or fingers into the mouth or throat of a child with a suspected infection of the epiglottis can cause extremely dangerous spasm and a complete airway obstruction. (The child who complains of a sore or hoarse throat and is leaning forward with his neck jutted out and is drooling should be suspected of having a swollen epiglottis, a condition called epiglottitis.) Instead, in these cases, it may be necessary to begin positive pressure ventilation with supplemental oxygen immediately to ensure adequate movement of air past the swollen tissues. For more details on assessing respiratory illnesses, see Chapter 14, "Respiratory Emergencies."

ASSESS BREATHING

As soon as an open airway is secured, it is necessary to assess the patient's breathing status (Figure 9-9). Assess to:

- Determine if breathing is adequate or inadequate (Table 9-5).
- Determine the need for early oxygen therapy if breathing is adequate.
- Provide positive pressure ventilation with supplemental oxygen for inadequate breathing.

ASSESS RATE AND QUALITY OF BREATHING

The best method to assess breathing is by *looking, listening,* and *feeling.* When doing so, it is necessary to assess both the amount of air breathed in and out

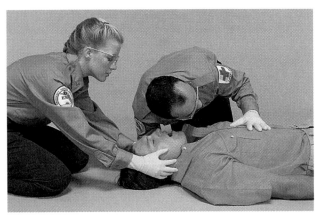

Figure 9-9   Assess breathing. If breathing is adequate and the patient requires oxygen, administer oxygen at 15 liters per minute via nonrebreather mask. If breathing is inadequate, begin positive pressure ventilation with supplemental oxygen.

(tidal volume) and the approximate respiratory rate. Remember that one respiration consists of one inhalation and one exhalation.

LOOK

Get down and place your ear and face close to the patient's nose and mouth while looking at the chest. Look for the following:

- Inadequate tidal volume—poor movement (rise and fall) of the chest wall, indicating that an inadequate amount of air is being breathed in with each respiration
- Abnormal respiratory rate—breathing that is either faster or slower than normal (Normal rates: 12 to 20 per minute for an adult, 15 to 30 per minute for a child, 25 to 50 per minute for an infant)

Also look for the following additional signs of inadequate breathing:

- Retractions—identified by a sunken-in appearance of tissues that are pulled inward on inhalation at any of these locations:
  - the suprasternal notch (above the sternum)
  - intercostal spaces (between the ribs)
  - supraclavicular spaces (above the clavicles)

- Nasal flaring—the nostrils flaring out as the patient inhales
- Excessive abdominal muscle use
- Tracheal tugging—pendulum motions of the trachea in the anterior neck during inhalation
- Cyanosis—a bluish or blue-gray tone of the skin seen early around the lips, nose, and fingernail beds indicating inadequate oxygenation

Also, quickly observe the patient's respiratory pattern. Look for:

- Asymmetrical movement of the chest wall—The chest wall should be moving symmetrically (both sides moving together), and smoothly. Unequal movement—for example, one side moving up and outward as the other moves down and inward—is an indication of a significant chest injury.

LISTEN AND FEEL

With your face down next to the patient's mouth and nose, listen for air movement and feel for escape of warm humidified air. Very little air movement is an indication of inadequate breathing.

ABSENT OR INADEQUATE BREATHING

Not all of the breathing difficulties that you may observe, or that the patient may tell you about, are immediately life threatening. A patient may be experiencing some difficulty in breathing, yet be breathing adequately to support life, at least for the time being.

During the initial assessment, you are observing for signs of absent or inadequate breathing—conditions that are immediately life threatening and that must be treated at once. Life-threatening breathing problems are:

- Absence of breathing (**apnea**)—identified by no chest wall movement and no sensation or sound of air moving in and out of the nose or mouth
- Inadequate breathing—identified by:
  - A respiratory rate less than 8 per minute or greater than 24 per minute in an unresponsive patient
  - Signs of inadequate oxygenation, such as deteriorating mental status or cyanosis
  - Signs of serious respiratory distress, including difficulty in breathing (**dyspnea**), poor chest wall

TABLE 9-5

Inadequate Breathing *vs.* Adequate Breathing

Inadequate Breathing	Adequate Breathing
Inadequate *rate* **or** inadequate *tidal volume* = inadequate breathing	Adequate *rate* **and** adequate *tidal volume* = adequate breathing

movement, retractions, nasal flaring, and/or poor air exchange from the nose and mouth

If the patient is apneic (not breathing) or is breathing inadequately, you must immediately begin positive pressure ventilation with supplemental oxygen. Any delay in treatment could lead to brain death and cardiac arrest.

As you learned in Chapter 7, "Airway Management, Ventilation, and Oxygen Therapy," positive pressure ventilation is any method that forces air and oxygen into the patient's lungs when the patient is unable to breathe adequately, or at all, on his own. It can be achieved by mouth-to-mask, bag-valve-mask device, or a flow-restricted, oxygen-powered ventilation device. Whenever positive pressure ventilation is to be performed, it is necessary to attach and deliver supplemental oxygen within the first few minutes after beginning ventilation. Also, to assure a patent airway so that the ventilations reach the patient's lungs, an oropharyngeal or nasopharyngeal airway should be inserted prior to beginning ventilation.

A patient with a breathing rate that is less than 8 per minute or greater than 24 per minute may be unresponsive and may require, as stated above, positive pressure ventilation with supplemental oxygen. If a patient with a breathing rate less than 8 per minute or greater than 24 per minute is responsive and has an adequate tidal volume, instead administer oxygen at 15 liters per minute by nonrebreather mask and continually reassess the patient for signs of inadequate breathing.

ADEQUATE BREATHING

If the chest is rising and falling adequately, you hear and feel good air exchange, the respiratory rate is greater than 8 per minute and less than 24 per minute, and no evidence of serious respiratory distress is present, assume that the patient's breathing is adequate.

If the patient with adequate breathing is responsive, but is ill or injured, administer oxygen at 15 liters per minute by nonrebreather mask.

If the patient with adequate breathing is unresponsive, with or without any additional signs of illness or injury, administer oxygen at 15 liters per minute by nonrebreather mask.

In other words, most patients will benefit from—or at least not be harmed by—oxygen. Only for alert patients without signs of significant illness or injury should oxygen therapy be omitted.

Once you have assessed and controlled any immediate life threats associated with breathing, and have begun positive pressure ventilation with supplemental oxygen or placed the patient on high flow oxygen by nonrebreather mask if necessary, you must quickly progress to assessment of the circulation.

ASSESS CIRCULATION

An assessment of the circulation includes checking the following (Table 9-6):

• Pulse
• Possible major bleeding
• Skin color, temperature, and condition
• Capillary refill in infants and children

During the initial assessment, the main purposes for checking circulation are to determine whether or not the heart is beating, there is any severe bleeding, and blood is circulating adequately (the patient possibly suffering from shock). A problem in any of these areas is life threatening and must be treated immediately.

ASSESS THE PULSE

You learned about pulses and how to assess them in Chapter 5, "Baseline Vital Signs and History Taking." During the initial assessment, you will not attempt to make a precise reading of heart rate. This will happen later, when you take the baseline vital signs during the focused history and physical exam. For now, if the patient is unresponsive you first want to ascertain whether the heart is beating. In the adult patient, if you cannot feel a radial pulse (at the wrist), immediately assess for a carotid pulse (in the neck) (Figure 9-10). The carotid pulse is typically the most prominent pulse and is the last to be lost in the patient. A pulse that is growing faint usually can be felt in the carotid artery even when it can no longer be felt in a peripheral artery. It is critical to determine if there is a pulse, no matter how weak, because it is dangerous to perform cardiopulmonary resuscitation (CPR) on a patient whose heart is still beating.

To assess for a carotid pulse, locate the thyroid cartilage (Adam's apple) and slide your fingers down the neck laterally on the same side on which you are positioned until you feel the groove between the lar-

TABLE 9-6

Initial Assessment of Circulation

Assessment of circulation during the initial assessment should occur in this sequence:

• Assess for presence or absence of *pulse*.
• Assess for possible major *bleeding*.
• Assess *skin* color, temperature, and condition.
• Assess *capillary refill* in infants and children.

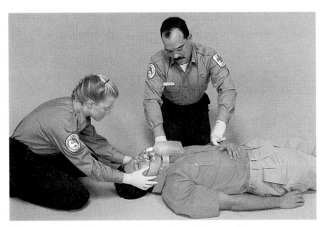

Figure 9-10   Assess pulses. If there is no radial pulse, palpate the carotid pulse. If the patient is pulseless, begin CPR and apply the automated external defibrillator as soon as it is available.

ynx and the bulk of muscles in the neck. The carotid artery is located there and should be felt with the index and middle fingers.

It is important to maintain in-line stabilization when assessing for pulses in a trauma patient. The EMT-B who is at the patient's head holding in-line stabilization can assess the carotid pulse by sliding the index and middle fingers of one hand down the neck to the correct landmark until feeling the pulse. Do not assess or compress the carotid pulses on both sides of the neck simultaneously as this may reduce circulation to and oxygenation of the brain.

As you learned in Chapter 5, in a patient who is 1 year old or less, it is necessary to palpate a brachial pulse, which is found on the lateral aspect of the upper section of the arm between the biceps and triceps muscles.

When palpating the pulses, quickly determine:

* If the pulse is present or not
* The approximate heart rate (beats per minute)
* The regularity and strength

When determining approximate heart rate, remember that a more accurate heart rate will be determined later in the patient assessment. During the initial assessment, it is most appropriate to estimate the heart rate as fast, normal, or slow.

Note heart rates that are less than 60 per minute or greater than 100 per minute. Bradycardia, a heart rate less than 60 per minute, may indicate severe hypoxia (oxygen starvation), head injury, drug overdose, heart attack, or some other medical condition. Bradycardia is an ominous sign of hypoxia in infants and children. Tachycardia, a heart rate greater than 100 per minute, may indicate anxiety, blood loss, shock, abnormal heart rhythms, heart attack, drug

overdose, early hypoxia, fever, and other medical or traumatic conditions.

The location at which you are able to palpate a pulse provides a rough estimate of systolic blood pressure. The estimated adult systolic pressure as correlated to the pulse is as follows:

* If the radial pulse is palpable, the systolic blood pressure is at least 80 mmHg.
* If the radial pulse is not palpable, but the brachial or femoral pulse is palpable, the systolic blood pressure is approximately 70 mmHg.
* If only the carotid pulse is palpable, the systolic blood pressure is approximately 60 mmHg.

If the carotid pulse is absent, begin CPR by applying chest compressions and positive pressure ventilation with supplemental oxygen. If the patient is in cardiac arrest from a medical problem and is more than 8 years of age, apply the automated external defibrillator (AED) as soon as it is available. Cardiac arrest resulting from traumatic injuries requires CPR and quick transport. Consult medical direction regarding the use of the AED in a traumatic cardiac arrest. (The AED will be covered in detail in Chapter 16, "Automated External Defibrillation.")

IDENTIFY MAJOR BLEEDING

Scan the body looking for any indication of major bleeding (Figure 9-11). If you notice large pools of blood or completely blood-soaked clothing, immediately expose the area by cutting away clothing with your scissors. Major bleeding is typically identified as bright red spurting bleeding (arterial) or dark red steady rapid bleeding (venous). If either of these types of major bleeding is present, immediately place gloved fingers or a gloved hand on the wound and

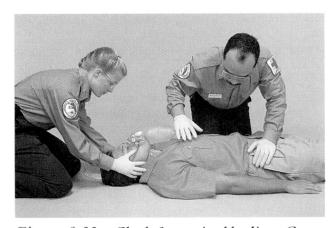

Figure 9-11   Check for major bleeding. Cut away blood-soaked clothing to expose potentially life-threatening bleeding. Control bleeding with direct pressure, then a pressure dressing.

gloved fingers or a gloved hand on the wound and apply direct pressure to control the bleeding. Apply a pressure dressing once the bleeding has been controlled. During the initial assessment, do not waste time dealing with slow, oozing capillary bleeding or other wounds that do not present with major bleeding, no matter how dramatic they may appear. The control of bleeding will be covered in detail in Chapter 29, "Bleeding and Shock."

ASSESS PERFUSION

The patient's perfusion (the sufficient supply of oxygen to the body's cells that results from adequate circulation of blood through the capillaries) can be assessed by checking the skin's color, temperature, and condition (Figure 9-12). Capillary refill is typically a more reliable indicator of perfusion status in infants and children less than 6 years of age. The assessment of skin was discussed in detail in Chapter 5, "Baseline Vital Signs and History Taking."

SKIN COLOR

The skin is normally referred to as pink, even though it doesn't have a pink color tone. In all patients, including dark-skinned patients, the color can be observed at the mucous membranes of the mouth (including the lips), the mucous membranes that line the eyelids, under the tongue, and at the nail beds. The nail bed is the least desirable place to check color because of the effects of cold temperature, some chronic medical illnesses, smoking, and other conditions that may reduce or restrict blood flow to the hands and feet.

Because the skin plays a major role in body temperature regulation, it is important to realize the ef-

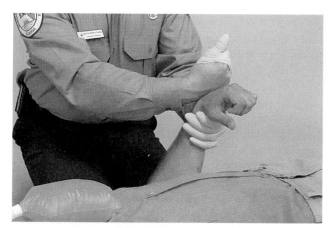

Figure 9-12 Assess perfusion by assessing color, temperature, and condition of the skin. Assess capillary refill in infants and children less than 6 years of age.

fects of the environment on the skin. You would expect a patient in a cold temperature to present with cooler and more pale-looking skin. A patient in a hot environment would typically have flushed (red), warm skin. With these exceptions, the skin colors listed below are considered to be abnormal.

- Pale or mottled—Skin that is pale or mottled typically indicates a decrease in perfusion and the onset of shock (hypoperfusion). If the patient's skin is pale or mottled, suspect that the patient is losing blood internally or externally or suffering another cause of shock.
- Cyanotic—Cyanotic, or blue-gray, skin may indicate reduced oxygenation from chest injuries, blood loss, or conditions like pneumonia or pulmonary edema that disrupt gas exchange in the lungs. It is a late sign of poor perfusion.
- Red—A flushed, or red, color usually indicates an increase in the amount of blood circulating in the blood vessels in the skin. This could indicate anaphylactic or vasogenic shock, poisonings, overdose, or some diabetic or other medical conditions. Alcohol ingestion, local inflammation, and cold exposure may also turn the skin red.
- Yellow—Liver dysfunction usually produces a yellow skin color termed jaundice. This is common in patients suffering from some form of liver disease, chronic alcoholism, or endocrine disturbance.

During the initial assessment, you are most concerned with the pale or blue colors that indicate possible shock (hypoperfusion) or inadequate oxygen intake. (See above on assessing breathing and providing positive pressure ventilation or oxygen therapy during the initial assessment if these signs are present.)

SKIN TEMPERATURE

The skin temperature is best assessed by partially taking off your gloves and placing the back of your hand or fingers on the patient's abdomen, face, or neck. The skin is normally warm to the touch but may instead be hot, cool, or cold.

- Hot skin—This may result from a hot environment or extremely elevated body core temperatures.
- Cool skin—Decreased perfusion as seen in shock, as well as exposure to cold temperatures, fright, anxiety, drug overdose, or other medical conditions that interfere with the body's ability to regulate temperature may result in cool skin.
- Cold skin—A patient with frostbite, significant cold exposure, immersion in cold water, or severe hypothermia (general cooling resulting from cold exposure) will have cold skin. The skin also may appear to be firm or stiff. This is a significant sign of frostbite or a cold-induced injury.

- Cool and clammy skin—Cool skin that is moist is referred to as cool and clammy. It may be related to blood loss, fright, nervousness, anxiety, pain, or other medical conditions. It is the most common sign of shock (hypoperfusion).

SKIN CONDITION

Skin condition refers to the amount of moisture found on the skin surface. This can simply be checked during the palpation of the skin for temperature. The skin is usually either dry or moist.

- Dry skin—A patient who is dehydrated or suffering from heat exposure or from some diabetic emergencies may have dry skin.
- Moist skin—Skin that is moist or wet to the touch, may indicate sweating in a hot environment, exercise or exertion, or fever. Moist skin may also be associated with heart attack, shock (hypoperfusion), or many other conditions.

Skin temperature, color, and condition will be discussed in more detail in the chapters dealing with specific medical conditions and injuries.

CAPILLARY REFILL

Capillary refill is a quick method to check peripheral perfusion related to shock in the infant or child under 6 years of age. Depress the nail bed, the fleshy part of the palm along the ulnar margin, forehead, or cheeks of the patient and release. If the refill of capillaries—a return of pink color—takes longer than 2 seconds, tissue perfusion is inadequate. It would be appropriate to monitor the patient closely and check for evidence of bleeding.

SHOCK (HYPOPERFUSION)

Shock (hypoperfusion) is a life-threatening condition. If your initial assessment reveals pale, cool, and clammy skin, especially if there is a significant mechanism of injury, an altered mental status, or severe bleeding, assume that the patient is in shock.

Treatment for shock needs to begin during the initial assessment and continue until the patient is transferred to the medical facility staff. Control any serious bleeding. If possible, splint any bone or joint injuries, but only if it does not delay transport. Consider elevating the patient's feet approximately 8 to 12 inches (if there is potential spine injury, raise the foot of the spine board on which the patient is immobilized; if there is potential head injury, do not elevate the feet); provide positive pressure ventilation with supplemental oxygen, if needed, or oxygen at 15 liters per minute by nonrebreather mask; keep the patient warm; and consider immediate transport with

assessment and treatment continuing en route. Treatment for shock will be covered in detail in Chapter 29, "Bleeding and Shock."

ESTABLISH PATIENT PRIORITIES

In the course of the initial assessment, you should have identified and managed any immediately life-threatening conditions related to the status of the airway, breathing, and circulation. During the initial assessment, the airway must be opened. High flow oxygen should be administered by nonrebreather mask at 15 liters per minute for any unresponsive patient or responsive patient with signs or symptoms of significant illness or injury. Inadequate breathing must be managed by positive pressure ventilation with supplemental oxygen. Any major bleeding must be controlled. If the patient is pulseless, immediately initiate CPR and apply the automated external defibrillator (AED) as soon as it is available, if appropriate. Treatment for shock (hypoperfusion) must be undertaken if the patient displays signs of shock.

At this point in the initial assessment—based on your general impression and your assessment of the patient's mental status, airway, breathing, and circulation—it is necessary to decide if the patient is a priority for rapid trauma assessment and immediate transport or if, instead, you will continue with the focused physical exam on the scene. For example, the trauma patient who is critically injured requires a rapid trauma assessment and immediate transport to the emergency department with continued assessment and treatment provided in the ambulance, whereas the injured patient who appears stable should be further assessed and treated at the scene prior to transport. The medical patient could fall into either category—rapid assessment and transport or continued on-scene assessment and stabilization—depending on the conditions found during the initial assessment.

Consider the factors listed in Table 9-7 when determining the need for rapid assessment and immediate transport.

If your priority decision is for immediate transport, you will first conduct either a quick head-to-toe assessment or a focused exam of the patient to identify any additional signs of injury or illness, and to be sure that nothing significant has been overlooked, before the patient is fully immobilized and/or secured to the stretcher. This assessment, known as the rapid trauma or rapid medical assessment, will be explained in detail on the following pages. Ordinarily, it is part of the assessment step known as the focused history and physical exam, but if the patient is to be loaded onto the ambulance for transport at the conclusion of

TABLE 9-7

Criteria for Which Rapid Transport Is Required

- A poor general impression. The patient looks ill or severely injured. Look for cyanosis, pale skin, significant blood loss, and multiple wounds or injuries to the head, chest, abdomen, pelvis, posterior thorax, or multiple extremities.
- An unresponsive patient or patient with an altered mental status who lacks a gag or cough reflex is significant, because the patient cannot protect his own airway
- A responsive patient who is not obeying commands
- Inability to establish or maintain a patent airway
- A patient experiencing difficulty in breathing or who exhibits signs of respiratory distress
- Absent or inadequate breathing for which the patient requires continuous positive pressure ventilation
- A pulseless patient
- Uncontrolled hemorrhage or severe blood loss
- A patient with pale, cool, clammy skin whom you suspect is in shock (hypoperfusion)
- A patient with an open wound to the chest or a flail segment
- Severe chest pain with a systolic blood pressure of less than 100 mmHg
- Severe pain anywhere
- Complicated childbirth
- Extremely high body temperature—above 104° F
- Signs of generalized hypothermia
- Severe allergic reaction
- Poisoning or overdose of unknown substance

the initial assessment, a rapid assessment should be conducted first. Rapid assessment techniques will be described in Part 3.

The rapid assessment can typically be accomplished in no more than 60 to 90 seconds (hence the name "rapid"). One partner can conduct the rapid assessment while the other sets up the immobilization equipment or the stretcher, so there should be no needless delay in loading the patient into the ambulance and getting transport under way.

If you have made a priority decision for rapid as-

sessment and immediate transport, consider requesting ALS (advanced life support; paramedic) intercept en route.

A decision for rapid assessment and immediate transport does not mean that a full assessment and appropriate emergency care are not conducted. However, the priority decision you make at the conclusion of the initial assessment will dictate when and where the remainder of the assessment and treatment will occur. Thus, the initial assessment sets the pace for the entire encounter with the patient.

PART 3
FOCUSED HISTORY
AND PHYSICAL EXAM

Once you have conducted the scene size-up and the initial assessment to identify and manage immediately life-threatening conditions involving the airway, breathing, and circulation, your next step is to conduct the **focused history and physical exam** to identify any additional injuries or conditions that may also be life threatening.

Further emergency care will be based on the information you gain from the focused history and physical exam. There are three major steps to the focused history and physical exam:

Steps of the Focused History and Physical Exam

- Conduct a physical exam
- Take baseline vital signs
- Obtain a SAMPLE history

The way these steps are carried out will vary according to the condition of the patient: trauma or medical, responsive or unresponsive, with a serious or a minor complaint.

For example, a patient who has lacerated his shin while operating a weed cutter does not need a complete head-to-toe exam as part of the focused history and physical exam. Your physical exam and history will deal primarily with the leg injury. Likewise, a medical patient complaining of shortness of breath does not need to have his entire body inspected and palpated. It is important to understand that not all patients will need a detailed history or a full physical exam. You must be able to tailor your assessment to the needs of the patient. However, if you have any doubt as to the significance of the mechanism of injury or the illness, err on the side of benefit to the patient and perform a complete head-to-toe exam as part of the focused history and physical exam.

The sequence of the steps of the focused history and physical exam will depend on whether the patient has suspected injuries or a medical problem and whether the patient is responsive or unresponsive. For example, history taking precedes the physical exam and vital signs for a responsive medical patient for two reasons: (1) The most significant information about a medical condition will usually be obtained from what the patient tells you, and (2) if the patient loses responsiveness, you will have lost the opportunity to get the history, whereas you can conduct the physical exam and obtain vital signs whether the patient is responsive or not.

For a trauma patient, on the other hand, the physical exam and vital signs are done before the history, because the most significant information about injuries will usually come from the physical exam. (When EMT-B partners are working together, these steps can often be done almost simultaneously, for example with one partner obtaining the history and taking vital signs while the other does the physical exam.)

Although the physical exam for a trauma patient and for a medical patient are similar, the type of information that you are assessing for may differ. For example, you will assess the lower extremities for both the trauma patient and the medical patient in most cases, including assessment of distal pulses, motor, and sensory function. However, in the trauma patient you are primarily looking for tenderness (pain in response to palpation), swelling, and deformities—in addition to weak or absent pulses, or poor motor

or sensory function—as an indication of injury. In the medical patient, you may be looking more for signs of inadequate pumping function of the heart, as in a heart attack or congestive heart failure—for example, discoloration of the lower extremities or swelling to the ankles plus poor pulses—or for poor or absent motor and sensory function as a sign of the status of the brain in a suspected stroke patient.

If you have been unable to categorize the patient as a trauma or a medical patient by the time you have completed the initial assessment, you should continue with a rapid assessment to gain additional information to appropriately categorize the patient.

As an example, suppose you are called to the scene for a "man down." When you arrive on the scene, you find a patient supine on the side of the street. Only one bystander is present who states that she found the patient lying in the street. You have no immediate clues from the dispatcher, scene, or bystander as to the emergency problem. Your general impression and initial assessment of the airway, breathing, and circulation do not provide any clear indications as to whether the patient's condition has resulted from trauma or a medical cause.

You must suspect that the patient may have been hit by a car, shot, assaulted, stabbed, fallen and hit his head, or suffered from some other mechanism of injury. However, you must also suspect that the patient could have had a heart attack or a stroke, has a low blood sugar level, or is suffering from some other medical condition. You would conduct a rapid physical exam and would continue to look for indications of both trauma and medical problems while you continue your emergency care.

EMS runs of this nature require a high index of suspicion on your part and the application of judgment and common sense to the sequence and manner in which you conduct the focused history and physical exam.

In most cases, you will have determined whether the patient is suffering from trauma or from a medical condition by the time the initial assessment has been completed. For a patient who has been injured, you will continue with the *focused history and physical exam for a trauma patient*. A patient who is suffering from a medical condition requires a *focused history and physical exam for a medical patient*.

FOCUSED HISTORY AND PHYSICAL EXAM TRAUMA PATIENT

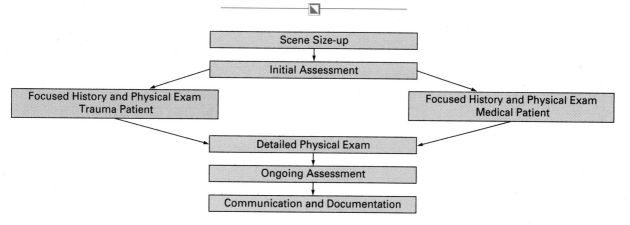

OBJECTIVES

Numbered objectives are from the United States Department of Transportation 1994 EMT-Basic National Standard Curriculum. Asterisked objectives, if any, pertain to material that is supplemental to the DOT curriculum.

COGNITIVE

3-3.1 Discuss the reasons for reconsideration concerning the mechanism of injury. (pp. 168–169)
3-3.2 State the reasons for performing a rapid trauma assessment. (p. 168)
3-3.3 Recite examples and explain why patients should receive a rapid trauma assessment. (p. 168)
3-3.4 Describe the areas included in the rapid trauma assessment and discuss what should be evaluated. (pp. 171–179)

3-3.5 Differentiate when the rapid assessment may be altered in order to provide patient care. (pp. 171, 184, 185)
3-3.6 Discuss the reason for performing a focused history and physical exam. (pp. 165–166)

AFFECTIVE

3-3.7 Recognize and respect the feelings that patients might experience during assessment. (pp. 148, 171)

PSYCHOMOTOR

3-3.8 Demonstrate the rapid trauma assessment that should be used to assess a patient based on mechanism of injury.

For the patient who has been identified as a **trauma patient**—who has an injury or injuries rather than a medical condition—perform the focused history and physical exam for a trauma patient. The focused history and physical exam for a trauma patient is generally performed in the following sequence:

1. Physical exam
2. Baseline vital signs
3. History

As mentioned earlier, if you have enough assistance, you can reduce the time that elapses before transport is initiated by performing some of these steps simultaneously. For example, while a first re-

sponder or other trained person maintains in-line stabilization, your partner might be taking vital signs and a history while you conduct the physical exam. As you and your partner work together over a period of time, you can develop efficient and effective ways of accomplishing several things at the same time.

One of two kinds of physical exam can be chosen for a trauma patient: a **rapid trauma assessment** (a rapid head-to-toe exam) or a **focused trauma assessment** (an exam that is focused on a specific injury site). These assessments will be described in detail on the following pages. Your first decision during the focused history and physical exam will be which kind of exam is most appropriate for this patient.

- A *rapid trauma assessment* followed by prompt transport, or on-scene emergency care, or . . .
- A *focused trauma assessment* followed by on-scene emergency care

Your decision regarding the kind of physical exam you will conduct for the trauma patient is based on the mechanism of injury—the force that caused the patient's injury and findings in your initial assessment. (The concept of mechanism of injury was introduced in Chapter 8, "Scene Size-up," and will be further developed in Chapter 28, "Mechanisms of Injury: Kinetics of Trauma.") You must determine whether the mechanism of injury is significant enough to cause you to suspect that the patient has been critically injured. If so, you should choose the rapid trauma assessment (the rapid head-to-toe exam) followed by prompt transport. If the mechanism of injury is not significant enough to produce critical injuries, but you suspect the patient could be suffering from injuries anywhere on the body, you should conduct a rapid trauma assessment as a basis for further on-scene emergency care. If the patient is suffering from an isolated injury that is not critical, and the mechanism of injury is minor, you should conduct a focused assessment of the injury site, followed by appropriate on-scene emergency care.

The chart below compares the two approaches to the assessment of the trauma patient.

Focused History and Physical Exam for a Trauma Patient Who Has . . .

A Significant Mechanism of Injury or Critical Findings in Initial Assessment (or for whom unknown or multiple injuries are suspected)

1. Rapid trauma assessment
   (head to toe)
2. Baseline vital signs
3. SAMPLE history

No Significant Mechanism of Injury and No Critical Finding in Initial Assessment

1. Focused trauma assessment
   (focused on the injury site)
2. Baseline vital signs
3. SAMPLE history

REEVALUATE THE MECHANISM OF INJURY

Your first step in the focused history and physical exam is to reevaluate the mechanism of injury (Figure 9-13). Remember, the mechanism of injury is directly related to the potential for critical injuries.

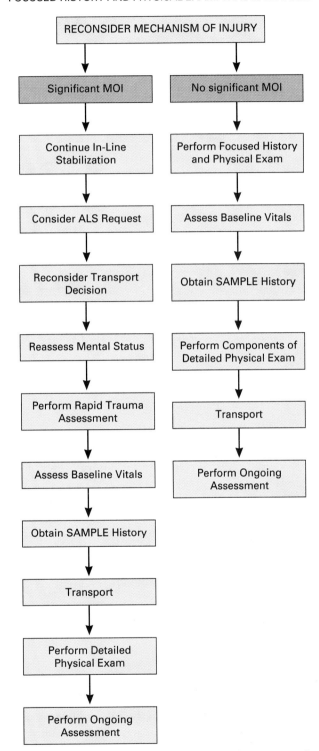

Figure 9-13 Steps of the focused history and physical exam for a trauma patient.

The more significant or severe the mechanism of injury, the greater the chance that the patient is critically injured. You must ask yourself, "Was this mechanism of injury significant enough to cause critical or multiple injuries?"

The emergency care you provide is frequently based on the findings of the scene size-up and a high index of suspicion. Most often, spinal immobilization is performed based solely on your suspicion that the patient might have suffered an injury to the spinal column. You provide the necessary emergency care for a spinal injury even though you detect no signs or symptoms of such an injury.

When there is a significant mechanism of injury—as soon as you have completed the initial assessment and management of immediately life-threatening conditions—you should proceed with a rapid trauma assessment to identify any additional serious or potentially life-threatening injuries.

SIGNIFICANT MECHANISMS OF INJURY

Mechanisms of injury that have a high incidence of producing critical trauma are:

- Ejection of the patient from a vehicle in an automobile crash
- A crash that causes death to a person in the same passenger compartment in which the patient is found
- A fall of greater than 20 feet
- Roll-over of the vehicle the patient was in
- A vehicle collision that has occurred at a high speed
- A pedestrian struck by a vehicle
- A motorcycle crash with separation of rider from motorcycle
- Blunt or penetrating trauma that results in an altered mental status, from confusion to unresponsiveness
- Penetrating injuries to the head, neck, chest, or abdomen
- Blast injuries from an explosion
- Seat-belt injuries
- Collisions in which seat belts are not worn, even if airbags have deployed
- Impact causing deformity to the steering wheel
- Collision that results in prolonged extrication

SPECIAL CONSIDERATIONS FOR INFANTS AND CHILDREN

For infants and children, significant mechanisms of injury would also include:

- A fall of greater than 10 feet
- A bicycle collision
- A vehicle collision at a medium speed
- Any vehicle collision where the infant or child was unrestrained

All other mechanisms of injury that are significant for the adult should also be considered significant in the infant and child.

Mechanism of injury is a vital component in the assessment of infants and children since they have a tendency to compensate for blood loss for a longer period of time compared to adults, then decompensate faster. (This phenomenon will be explained in Chapter 29, "Bleeding and Shock.") Consequently, an infant or child may appear to be well even though injured as severely as an adult who displays all the signs of shock. When that infant or child does deteriorate, it will happen very rapidly and perhaps too late for emergency care to save the child's life. So for the infant or child, even more than for an adult, you must rely on the mechanism of injury in your assessment. If there is a significant mechanism of injury, you must assume that the child is critically injured and in shock, even if the child looks all right, and provide treatment accordingly.

TRAUMA PATIENT WITH SIGNIFICANT MECHANISM OF INJURY OR CRITICAL FINDING

If any of the significant mechanisms of injury listed earlier are encountered at the scene, or if the patient has an altered mental status, or if you are unsure of the extent of injury to the patient, or if you cannot clearly identify the mechanism of injury, you should proceed with a rapid trauma assessment.

The rapid trauma assessment is a head-to-toe physical exam that is swiftly conducted on a patient who has suffered or may have suffered severe injuries. During the rapid trauma assessment, if the patient is responsive, he can be questioned as to symptoms and history while the exam is in progress. This will aid in identifying injuries and related problems the patient may be suffering from, such as breathing difficulty. If the patient is unresponsive, the rapid trauma assessment alone can identify a majority of the injuries.

Prior to performing the rapid trauma assessment, make sure that spinal stabilization—established during the initial assessment—is continued. Again consider requesting ALS backup, reconsider your transport decision, and reassess the patient's mental status. These steps are described in further detail below.

CONTINUE SPINAL STABILIZATION

It is necessary to maintain in-line spinal stabilization until the patient is completely immobilized to a backboard. While one EMT-B performs the rapid trauma assessment, another EMT-B or assistant should continue to hold the head and neck in a neutral in-line position until a cervical spinal immobilization collar is applied, the patient is placed on the backboard, strapped in place, and a head immobilization device is applied. Once manual spinal stabilization is established, it should never be released until immobilization is completed. Typically, complete immobilization of the patient will not be performed until the rapid assessment is completed.

CONSIDER AN ADVANCED LIFE SUPPORT REQUEST

Some trauma patients may benefit from advanced life support at the scene or while en route to the hospital. Airway trauma, an occluded airway, or any indication that air from an injured lung is trapped in the chest cavity (tension pneumothorax), causing the uninjured lung and the heart to be compressed, may be reason to consider calling for advanced life support. These are life-threatening problems in which advanced airway maneuvers or chest decompression could be life saving. These decisions should not delay transport to an appropriate facility. Follow local protocols.

RECONSIDER THE TRANSPORT DECISION

Normally, if a decision for immediate transport has not been reached at the end of the initial assessment, transport will take place after the rapid or focused trauma assessment, assessment of baseline vital signs, gathering of the SAMPLE history, and completion of appropriate emergency care based on these assessments. Throughout the focused history and physical exam, however, continually keep in mind the possibility of initiating immediate transport if evidence of critical injury or deterioration is discovered.

REASSESS MENTAL STATUS

Any deterioration in the patient's condition can have an adverse effect on the functioning of the brain and a consequent deterioration in mental status. Therefore, continuous reassessment of the patient's mental status is necessary to provide you with valuable information regarding the deterioration or improvement of the patient's condition.

Common causes of decreased mental status in trauma patients are compromised airways, inadequate breathing, blood loss, poor perfusion, poor oxygenation, and brain injuries. These commonly result from:

- Bleeding or trauma to the face, mouth, or neck
- Head injuries
- Chest injuries
- Abdominal injuries
- Bone injuries associated with blood loss

A patient who is already unresponsive upon your arrival at the scene should be considered to be seriously injured. If a responsive patient's mental status shows signs of deteriorating, you should move rapidly through the assessment, looking for the potential cause of the unresponsiveness or deterioration of the mental status, and take steps to immediately correct the problem. To assess mental status, use the AVPU method (alert, responds to verbal stimulus, responds to painful stimulus, unresponsive) that was described in Part 2, Initial Assessment.

In an alert patient, it is necessary to assess the level of orientation. This is accomplished by asking specific questions about the time, place, and person/self. Ask the patient the following questions:

- Do you know what year, month, and day it is?
- Can you tell me where you are right now?
- Who is this person with you?
- What is your full name?

Determine if the patient can provide you with the year, month, day, and approximate time of day. Orientation to place is assessed by asking the patient if he can identify where he is. If he is at home, he should be able to provide you with his address. If he is in an automobile crash, he should be able to tell you where he was coming from and where he is going. If he is at the mall or store, he should be able to give the name of the mall or the store he is in. If another person is at the scene who is a friend or relative of the patient, have the patient identify him or her. If no other person is with the patient at the scene, it is somewhat difficult to assess for orientation to person. Finally, ask the patient his own full name.

If the patient correctly answers all of the questions, he is noted to be alert and oriented to time, place, and person/self. Commonly, this is documented as "alert and oriented × 3."

Orientation to time is usually the first to be lost in a deteriorating mental status. As the patient continues to progressively deteriorate, he will lose orientation to place, then person, and finally to his own self. At this point, he would not be able to identify himself or anyone else at the scene.

If the patient is not alert, determine what type of stimulus is needed to arouse the patient. As described in Part 2, Initial Assessment, first attempt verbal stimulus. If the patient does not respond to verbal stimulus, attempt painful stimulus.

The patient may respond in the following ways to a verbal stimulus:

- Responds to verbal stimulus with inappropriate words
- Responds to verbal stimulus with incomprehensible sounds, such as mumbling
- Responds with eye opening or obeying a command
- No response to verbal stimulus

The patient may respond to a painful stimulus with:

- Purposeful movements aimed at attempting to remove the stimulus, such as grabbing your hand or making a pushing-away gesture
- Nonpurposeful movements noted by decorticate or decerebrate posturing (back arched, arms pulled upward toward the chest or extended parallel to the body) that is not an attempt to remove the stimulus
- No response

It is extremely important to document precisely the alert patient's orientation or the non-alert patient's response to verbal or painful stimulus. Examples are: "The patient is alert and oriented to person and self but not time or place," or "The patient responds to painful stimulus with upward movement of the left arm only." This information provides other emergency personnel with criteria to use later to determine if the patient's mental status has improved or deteriorated.

If bystanders, relatives, or friends are present at the scene, it is extremely important to determine from them if the patient suffered an altered mental status, lost orientation, or became unresponsive at any time prior to your arrival. If the patient is unresponsive, determine if the patient was responding and oriented at any time after the incident but prior to your arrival. It is also very important to note if the patient lost responsiveness, awoke for a period of time, then became unresponsive again. Most of these are reliable indicators of possible head injury. Patients with these patterns of responsiveness and loss of responsiveness need very close monitoring.

Critical Findings: Trauma Patient

Critical Finding: Deteriorating mental status associated with severe head injury
Intervention: If possible, hyperventilate at a rate of 20 ventilations per minute with a bag-valve-mask device connected to supplemental oxygen. If it is not possible to ventilate, apply a nonrebreather mask at 15 liters per minute. (See note on p. 215.)

PERFORM A RAPID TRAUMA ASSESSMENT

When performing the rapid trauma assessment, it is necessary to inspect and palpate the patient to identify signs and symptoms of potential injuries. Also, auscultation could reveal a collapsed lung and potential life-threatening chest injuries.

DCAP-BTLS (pronounced "dee-cap, b-t-l-s") is a mnemonic to help you remember some of the chief signs and symptoms you are looking and feeling for during the rapid trauma assessment of each major body area. It stands for deformities, contusions, abra-

sions, punctures and penetrations, burns, tenderness, lacerations, and swelling.

- *Inspect (look) for:* deformities, contusions (bruises), abrasions, punctures, penetrating wounds, burns, lacerations, swelling, unusual chest wall movements, angulated extremities, bleeding, discoloration, open wounds, significant bleeding.
- *Palpate (feel) for:* tenderness, deformities, swelling, masses, muscle spasms, skin temperature, pulsations. When palpating for **tenderness** (pain on pressure) in the unresponsive patient, it is important to watch the patient's face for grimacing. This provides a good indication that tenderness is present without the patient being able to tell you.
- *Auscultate (listen with a stethoscope) for:* presence and equality of breath sounds.
- *Listen for:* sucking sounds, gurgling, stridor (high-pitched sound of the upper airway) and crepitation (grating sound heard when broken bone ends rub against each other, or a crackling sound caused by air under the skin).
- *Use your sense of smell* to detect any unusual odors on the patient's breath, body, or clothing, such as alcohol, feces, or urine.

As you conduct the rapid trauma assessment, talk calmly to the patient, even if he may appear to be unresponsive. Don't distress the patient by describing wounds and injuries, but rather indicate what areas you are going to assess. In the responsive patient and if the condition permits, ask any relevant questions about the area to be assessed prior to examining it. If you assess the area and then ask questions, the patient will suspect that you have found something wrong.

In the rapid trauma assessment, be most concerned with identifying potentially life-threatening injuries. If you find any injuries that are potentially life-threatening, you must manage them immediately to avoid further deterioration of the patient. Each situation is different and will dictate how you proceed.

Be careful not to move the patient unnecessarily to avoid aggravating any neck or spinal injury that might exist. Do not manipulate the patient in order to attempt to remove clothing. If necessary, expose the areas to be examined by cutting the clothing off the patient. In patients with a significant mechanism of injury or for whom serious trauma is a possibility, it is very important to completely expose the patient to look for additional injuries.

For example, suppose that you arrive on the scene of a shooting and find a patient with a gunshot wound to the left upper thigh. It appears the bullet fractured the femur. Because the femur fracture is so painful, the patient is only complaining of that injury. You focus in on the femur fracture and neglect to expose the patient to look for any other injuries. It is winter and the patient has a heavy coat on. It is nighttime, and the patient has dark clothing on. Therefore, it is difficult to see blood. The patient was shot with a .22 caliber gun, which is very small. En route to the hospital, the patient begins to complain of severe breathing difficulty. You finally become suspicious and expose the chest to find a gunshot wound of the anterior chest. You missed a life-threatening injury in this patient. If you had quickly exposed the chest during your assessment, you would have found the injury.

When exposing the patient, keep modesty and environmental conditions in mind. Do not completely expose the patient in front of a crowd or television camera. Cover the patient with a sheet to protect the modesty of any patient, male or female, young or old. Also, do not inadvertently induce hypothermia by exposing the patient to the cold. Consider moving into the ambulance before completely exposing the patient.

As described below, the rapid trauma assessment is performed in a systematic sequence to ensure that all major body areas are inspected and palpated (Figures 9-14 to 9-20).

ASSESS THE HEAD

When examining the head, it is necessary to quickly examine the skull, scalp, face, ears, pupils, nose, and mouth. *The exam is not detailed unless an injury is found or suspected in that particular area. A more detailed exam of each area will be conducted at a later time.* You are primarily concerned with identifying a possible head injury by examining the scalp, skull, pupils, and ears. Also, you must quickly reassess the nose and mouth for potential obstructions of the airway.

Scalp and Skull   Inspect the scalp and skull (Figure 9-14a) for any obvious deformities, contusions, abrasions, punctures, burns, lacerations, swelling, depressions, protrusions, impaled objects, or bleeding. Palpate for any crepitation, depressions, protrusions, swelling, bloody areas, instability, or lack of symmetry. Also, listen for any sounds the patient makes and look for flinching or grimacing that reveals any tenderness the patient experiences when you are palpating. If you discover burns or the patient's hair is singed, suspect that the patient was involved in a fire and pay particular attention to the airway.

Palpate the scalp and skull by cupping your hands and moving from the frontal region to the back of the skull. Do not poke with your fingers, since you may aggravate a depressed skull fracture by pushing the bony ends into the brain. Be careful not to move the head or neck when palpating in the suspected spine-injured patient.

In a dark environment, it is difficult to see blood in the hair. Thus, when assessing the head, it is necessary to periodically look at your gloves for evidence of blood. Also, pay attention to areas that feel warm during the exam as this usually indicates leakage of blood or **cerebrospinal fluid (CSF),** a clear fluid that surrounds and cushions the brain and the spinal cord. Leakage of cerebrospinal fluid is evidence of a skull fracture.

Avoid unnecessary pressure to any areas of the skull that appear unstable, depressed, or deformed. Refrain from palpating the depressed or deformed area to avoid further injury. If an impaled object is found in the skull, stabilize it in place with bulky dressings. Do not remove or move the object. (Management of impaled objects will be discussed in detail in Chapter 30, "Soft Tissue Injuries," and Chapter 35, "Eye, Face, and Neck Injuries.") Abnormalities to the skull, especially with an altered mental status, are a clear indication of head injury. This is a critical injury that requires prompt attention and transport. If the patient requires positive pressure ventilation and shows significant signs of head injury, begin to hyperventilate the patient at a rate of 20 per minute with a bag-valve mask connected to supplemental oxygen. If the patient is breathing adequately, apply oxygen via a nonrebreather mask at 15 liters per minute.

Even though prompt transport is key in treatment of the head-injured patient, it is vital to continue with the exam to identify any other potential injuries that need immediate attention. For example, the patient could die from an open wound to the chest that you missed because of failure to continue with the exam.

If the patient is wearing a hairpiece or a wig, do not attempt to remove it. It may be held in place with permanent adhesive or tape. Feel gently through the netting to assess for bleeding, swelling, or deformity. Do not reach under the wig.

Face   Inspect the face (Figure 9-14b), looking for any evidence of trauma and bleeding that may be obstructing the airway. Look for deformities, contusions, abrasions, penetrating wounds, lacerations, or swelling. Palpate for deformities, instability, and swelling.

Of particular concern is trauma to the mid-face region. This is a common injury from blunt forces being applied to the area between the lower lip and the bridge of the nose. A patient who strikes his face on the dashboard in an automobile crash commonly suffers trauma to the mid-face. Also, blows to the face from punches, kicks, baseball bats, or other objects will cause significant trauma.

If trauma to the face is found, carefully assess the airway for possible occlusion. Many times the bones of the face are pushed posteriorly into the airway causing a blockage. Bleeding, which is common with

THE RAPID TRAUMA ASSESSMENT

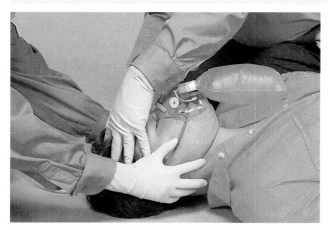

Figure 9-14a   Inspect and palpate the scalp and skull.

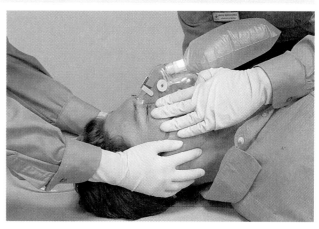

Figure 9-14b   Inspect and palpate the face, including ears, pupils, nose, and mouth. Pay particular attention to injuries that could block the airway with blood, bone, teeth, or tissue.

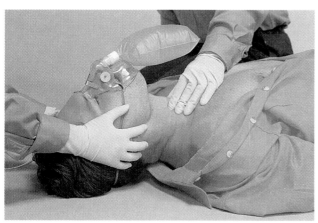

Figure 9-15a   Inspect the neck for tracheal deviation, tracheal tugging, jugular vein distention, subcutaneous emphysema, and large lacerations or punctures.

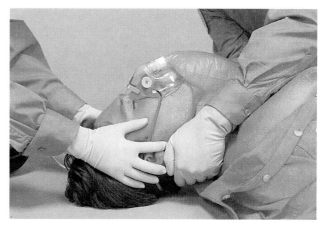

Figure 9-15b   Palpate both the anterior and posterior aspects of the neck. Note posterior muscle spasms that may indicate injury to the cervical spine.

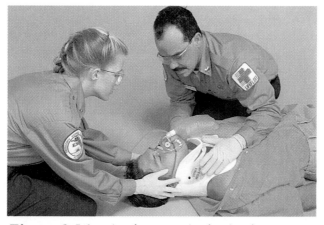

Figure 9-16   Apply a cervical spinal-immobilization collar (CSIC).

(Continued on the next page.)

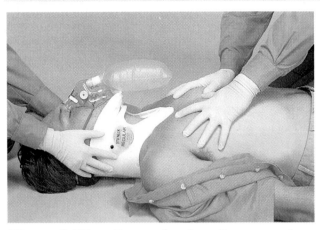

Figure 9-17a Expose the chest. Inspect and palpate for open wounds, flail segments, muscle retractions, and asymmetrical chest movement.

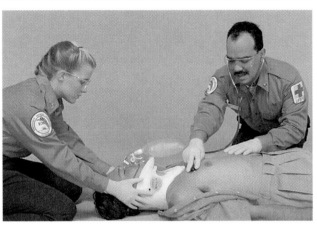

Figure 9-17b Perform a quick four-point auscultation of the chest to listen for the presence and equality of breath sounds.

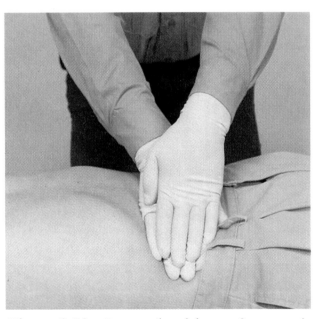

Figure 9-18 Inspect the abdomen for any evidence of trauma or distention. Palpate for tenderness and rigidity.

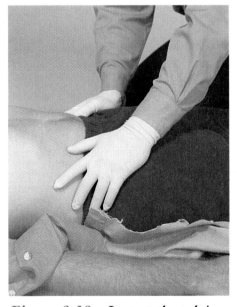

Figure 9-19 Inspect the pelvis for evidence of trauma. If the patient complains of pain or there is obvious deformity, do not palpate.

injuries to the face, may also occlude the airway or increase the risk of **aspiration** of the blood (the patient breathing the blood into the lungs). Insertion of an oropharyngeal airway and constant suction may be necessary to maintain a patent airway. Do not use a nasopharyngeal airway when injuries to the mid-face are present. The airway may be improperly placed due to a fracture to the nasal structures.

When inspecting the face, in addition to looking for burns to the skin, look for singed or burned nasal hair, eyebrows, and facial hair. This would indicate

that the patient has potentially suffered an upper airway burn. Reassess the airway for stridor and adequate air movement. If stridor is present, begin positive pressure ventilation with supplemental oxygen.

Ears   Quickly look inside the ears with a flashlight. Inspect for leakage of blood, cerebrospinal fluid, or other fluid, which are signs of a possible head injury.

Pupils   Assess the patient's pupils by opening the eyes and shining a flashlight into each eye, checking for equality of pupil size and reactivity. The pupils are

THE RAPID TRAUMA ASSESSMENT

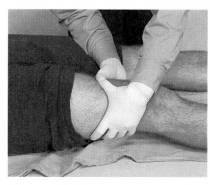

Figure 9-20a   Inspect and palpate each lower extremity.

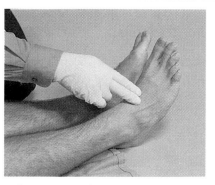

Figure 9-20b   Assess pedal pulses.

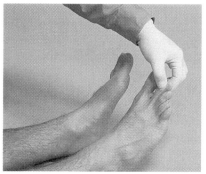

Figure 9-20c   Assess motor and sensory function in each foot.

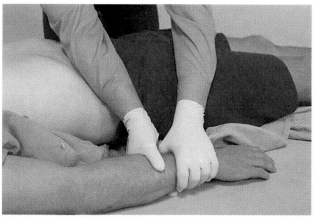

Figure 9-20d   Inspect and palpate each upper extremity.

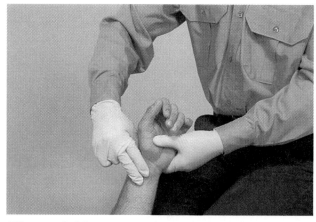

Figure 9-20e   Assess distal pulse, motor, and sensory function in each upper extremity.

Conclude the rapid trauma assessment by rolling the patient onto his side (maintaining in-line spinal stabilization) to inspect and palpate the posterior body.

normally equal in size and constrict briskly to light. Unequal pupils or pupils that do not respond to light usually indicate a severe head injury. Poor tissue perfusion and hypoxia (inadequate oxygen supply) will cause the pupils to respond sluggishly.

Note that if a patient has unequal pupils but is alert and oriented, the unequal pupils are probably not from a head injury. You need to suspect a possible eye injury, effect of eye medications, or some other condition. It is worthwhile to note that approximately 6 to 10 percent of the population normally have unequal pupils.

Nose   Inspect the nose for evidence of bleeding and leakage of cerebrospinal fluid. Suction the nose clear of blood if it is draining posteriorly into the na-

sopharynx. Your major concern with the nose is bleeding into the airway causing occlusion or possible aspiration. Also, check the nose for burned nasal hair or carbonaceous (charcoal black) discharge. This indicates likely inhalation of smoke and a possible upper airway burn.

Mouth   Your major concern when inspecting the inside of the mouth is to reassess the patency of the airway. Inspect for any bleeding, bone fragments, or dislodged teeth that may need to be suctioned or removed by finger sweeps. Also, inspect for swelling, lacerations to the tongue, and tissue damage that is causing or may cause possible obstruction.

When inspecting inside the mouth, look at the color of the mucous membranes. The mucous membranes are normally pink in color. Cyanotic membranes indicate hypoxia and pale membranes indicate poor tissue perfusion, possibly from blood loss.

If the patient is being ventilated, have the EMT-B performing the ventilation hyperventilate the patient, then stop to allow you to quickly inspect the inside of the mouth. Do not interrupt ventilation for more than 30 seconds. Once you have completed the inspection, have the EMT-B hyperventilate for one minute before resuming a normal ventilatory rate of 12 per minute.

Critical Findings: The Head

Critical Finding: Unequal pupils with deteriorating mental status, usually indicating severe head injury
Intervention: Begin hyperventilation at a rate of 20 per minute with supplemental oxygen. (See note on p. 215.)
Critical Finding: Blood, secretions, vomitus, or debris in the mouth
Intervention: Suction out the mouth or clear large debris with finger sweeps.

ASSESS THE NECK

Inspect the anterior neck (Figure 9-15a) for deformities, contusions, abrasions, punctures, burns, lacerations, and swelling. A large collection of blood under the skin in the neck might actually occlude the airway by compressing the trachea. Any large puncture wound or laceration to the neck must be immediately covered with an occlusive dressing (one that will not allow air through) and taped on all four sides. This is to prevent the possibility of air being sucked into a large vein and causing an air embolus. (Neck injuries will be discussed in detail in Chapter 35, "Eye, Face, and Neck Injuries.")

Inspect the neck for evidence of subcutaneous emphysema. Subcutaneous emphysema is air trapped under the lower layer of the skin. It appears as if the skin is bloated or inflated. Air leaking from the trachea, bronchus, bronchiole, lung, or esophagus will commonly collect in the neck. Thus, subcutaneous emphysema is a good indicator of a significant chest injury. It may be easier to find subcutaneous emphysema when palpating. It feels like bubble package wrap. Crepitation (a crackling sound) when palpating is an indication of air trapped under the skin.

Look at the trachea to determine if it is midline. A trachea shifted to one side is a late indication of a significant amount of air trapped in the pleural space of the chest cavity, the result of a severe lung or chest injury. The trachea will deviate away from the injured side. Also, look for a pendulum motion of the trachea called tracheal tugging. This usually indicates an airway obstruction on the side the trachea moves toward.

Assess the jugular veins for distention. Normally, the jugular veins are slightly engorged in a patient who is lying supine. With the patient at a 45 degree angle however, the neck veins should be flat. If the patient has neck veins that are flat in a supine position, it may indicate a decreased blood volume from bleeding. If the neck veins are engorged more than two-thirds the distance from the base of the neck to the angle of the jaw, they are considered to be distended. In trauma, jugular vein distention (JVD) is a sign of a serious injury to the chest, lungs, or heart.

Inspect the posterior portion of the neck (Figure 9-15b) for evidence of trauma. Look for deformity, contusions, and swelling. If in-line stabilization is being maintained, do not have it released to inspect or palpate. Inspection is difficult to accomplish with in-line stabilization. You may only be able to gently palpate the posterior cervical region for any deformities, tenderness, or muscle spasms. Do not move the head or neck to palpate. It is better to skip the inspection than to jeopardize the in-line stabilization and cause further injury.

Muscle spasms in the posterior cervical region are important to note. Muscle spasms occur in cervical injuries as a protective reflex, an attempt to maintain support. Thus, a patient complaining of muscle spasms anywhere along the vertebral (spinal) column who has a mechanism of injury consistent with vertebral injury, needs spinal immobilization.

Inspect the larynx for evidence of deformity and swelling. Injuries to the larynx from steering wheels, clotheslines, kicks, punches, and other blunt trauma could cause serious airway occlusion. With larynx injuries, the patient is typically hoarse or cannot speak, is showing signs of respiratory distress, and may be coughing up blood. Oropharyngeal or nasopharyngeal airways are of no use in an isolated laryngeal injury because they do not reach to the depth of the injury. If the patient is unable to breathe adequately, you must provide positive pressure ventilation with supplemental oxygen. If the patient is able to breathe adequately, apply oxygen via a nonrebreather mask at 15 liters per minute.

The patient may have a stoma, which is a surgical opening at the base of the throat. The stoma usually has a plastic or metal tube in the opening. The patient breathes through this opening. Therefore, make sure the tube is not occluded by blood, mucus, or other secretions.

Critical Findings: The Neck

Critical Finding: Jugular vein distention
Intervention: Suspect a serious injury to the chest or heart (tension pneumothorax or pericardial tamponade). Consider prompt transport and apply oxygen via a nonrebreather mask at 15 liters per minute

or positive pressure ventilation if necessary. Consider ALS intercept.

Critical Finding: Tracheal deviation

Intervention: Suspect a serious chest injury (tension pneumothorax). Consider prompt transport and apply oxygen via a nonrebreather mask at 15 liters per minute or positive pressure ventilation if necessary Also, consider a request for advanced life support.

Critical Finding: Tracheal tugging

Intervention: Suspect airway blockage. Take all steps to open the airway. If the airway is blocked as a result of trauma, apply positive pressure ventilation with supplemental oxygen and consider prompt transport and ALS support.

APPLY A CERVICAL SPINAL IMMOBILIZATION COLLAR

If the patient is suspected of having a possible spinal injury, a cervical spinal immobilization collar (CSIC) must be applied as soon as assessment of the neck is completed (Figure 9-16). The person who is maintaining in-line spinal stabilization continues to do so while the CSIC is sized and applied. It is very important not to move or manipulate the head or neck while applying the CSIC. At no time should in-line spinal stabilization be let go before, during, or after application of the CSIC. Even after the CSIC is properly applied, in-line spinal stabilization must be maintained until the patient is completely immobilized to a backboard with straps and a cervical spinal immobilization device. See Chapter 34, "Injuries to the Spine," for the proper techniques of measuring and applying the CSIC and providing immobilization.

ASSESS THE CHEST

In order for the chest to be properly examined, it is necessary to expose it (Figure 9-17a). Cut the clothing from the patient. Inspect the chest anteriorly, laterally, and in the axillary regions for open wounds. Any open wound to the chest must be immediately covered with your gloved hand. Then apply an occlusive dressing taped on three sides over the wound. The dressing will prevent air from entering the thorax (pleural space) and worsening the chest injury. The loose side will allow air to escape during exhalation, relieving the possible build-up of air in the chest.

Also inspect the chest for evidence of deformities, contusions, abrasions, burns, lacerations, swelling, and lack of symmetry. Look for segments of the chest that are moving in a **paradoxical motion**. Paradoxical motion occurs when a section of the chest that sinks inward upon inhalation while the rest of the chest is moving outward, and upon exhalation bulges outward while the rest of the chest is moving inward.

This type of motion may be seen when two or more adjacent ribs are fractured in two or more places. This is termed a **flail segment.** A flail segment interferes with the effectiveness of chest wall movement, thus reducing the adequacy of breathing and oxygenation. Since this is a life-threatening injury, you must immediately place your hand over the section to stabilize it in an inward position. Then place the patient's arm, a pillow, or bulky dressings or towels taped in position over the site of injury. A flail segment is usually accompanied by a severe contusion (bruise) to the lung, causing hypoxia. Closely monitor the patient's breathing status. If the patient's breathing is inadequate, positive pressure ventilation with supplemental oxygen must be initiated.

Determine if the patient is in respiratory distress by inspecting the muscles between the ribs (intercostal muscles) and above the suprasternal notch (the notch where the clavicles come together above the sternum). If the muscles are retracted inward during inhalation, it is very likely that the patient is having a difficult time breathing. Also look for flaring at the nostrils and excessive use of the abdominal muscles. If you suspect the patient is in respiratory distress, begin positive pressure ventilation with supplemental oxygen.

Quickly palpate the chest to confirm the findings of inspection. Check for symmetry of chest movement by placing the tips of your thumbs on the xiphoid process (the lower tip of the sternum) and spreading your hands over the lower rib cage. Both hands should move an equal distance with each breath. Apply slight pressure downward and inward on the rib cage. It may be easier to palpate for paradoxical motion in the chest wall rather than to see it on inspection, since muscle spasms usually keep the segment from moving dramatically. Also palpate for tenderness, subcutaneous emphysema, crepitation, and instability.

Use a stethoscope to auscultate for breath sounds (Figure 9-17b). It is necessary to listen to the breath sounds in the apices (top portions) and bases (bottom portions) of the lungs, comparing the left to the right side at each level. To assess each apex of the lung, place the stethoscope at the second intercostal space at the midclavicular line. Listen to each base at the fourth or fifth intercostal space in the midaxillary line. Listen during both inspiration and exhalation.

When listening to breath sounds, determine if the sounds are present and equal on both sides. Absent or diminished breath sounds on one side may indicate a serious lung or chest injury or bronchial obstruction.

If the breath sounds are absent or severely diminished, quickly reinspect the position of the trachea and the jugular veins for distention. If the trachea is deviated away from the side of the absent breath sounds and the jugular veins are distended, you should suspect the patient is suffering from a severe build-up of air in the chest cavity. This is a critical condition that could lead to immediate death. If an occlusive dressing is in place over an open chest wound, lift it off the wound for a few seconds during exhalation to allow any trapped air to escape, then re-seal it. Begin to prepare the patient for prompt transport and consider ALS intercept.

During your examination of the chest, reassess the patient's adequacy of breathing by looking at the depth of rise and fall of the chest wall, listening and feeling for air movement, and auscultating for adequate and full breath sounds. If the breathing appears to be inadequate at any time, begin positive pressure ventilation with supplemental oxygen.

Critical Findings: The Chest

Critical Finding: Open wound to the chest
Intervention: Seal the open wound immediately with your gloved hand then apply an occlusive dressing taped on three sides.
Critical Finding: Flail segment with paradoxical motion
Intervention: Stabilize the flail segment with your hand or the patient's arm until bulky dressings or a towel can be taped in place over the unstable area. Consider positive pressure ventilation.
Critical Finding: Absent or severely decreased breath sounds
Intervention: Begin positive pressure ventilation with supplemental oxygen. Look for deviated trachea or jugular vein distention, signs of air in the chest cavity. If this condition is suspected, consider requesting ALS. If an occlusive dressing is in place over an open chest wound, lift it off the wound for a few seconds during exhalation to allow any trapped air to escape, then reseal it.
Critical Finding: Poor chest wall movement with inadequate breathing
Intervention: Begin positive pressure ventilation with supplemental oxygen.
Critical Finding: Apnea (absence of breathing)
Intervention: Begin positive pressure ventilation with supplemental oxygen.

All of the above critical findings require immediate intervention and prompt transport to the emergency department.

ASSESS THE ABDOMEN

Inspect the abdomen (Figure 9-18) for evidence of deformities, contusions, abrasions, penetrations, burns, and lacerations. These signs could indicate trauma to the abdomen and the possibility of underlying abdominal organ injury. Abdominal distention, in which the abdomen appears to be abnormally large or swollen, is an indication that a significant amount of blood has been lost in the abdominal cavity. This is a sign of a critical abdominal injury that requires prompt transport.

While inspecting the abdomen, look for discoloration around the umbilicus (navel) and in the flank areas (sides). This is a sign that blood has collected in the abdomen. Usually this is not seen until several hours after the injury.

Palpate each of the four quadrants of the abdomen with the pads of your fingers by placing one hand on top of the other and rolling the hands across the quadrant. Each quadrant should be quickly palpated once for tenderness, guarding (spasm of the abdominal muscles), and rigidity (hardness or stiffness from the contraction of the abdominal muscles). To get the most reliable exam, first palpate areas farthest from the pain.

Tenderness is a pain response elicited when the abdomen is palpated. If the patient is unresponsive, watch his face for a grimace while palpating. This would indicate pain on palpation. Also when palpating, feel if the abdomen is firm or soft. A firm or rigid abdomen is due to guarding. This is an indication of organ injury or irritation of the abdominal lining. A soft abdomen is a normal finding.

Critical Findings: The Abdomen

Critical Finding: Tender, distended, or rigid abdomen
Intervention: Provide oxygen by nonrebreather mask at 15 lpm and prompt transport.

ASSESS THE PELVIS

Inspect the pelvis (Figure 9-19) for any evidence of trauma: deformities, contusions, abrasions, penetrations, burns, lacerations, or swelling. If the patient is complaining of pain or has obvious deformity to the pelvic region, you should suspect a pelvic injury. Do not palpate the pelvis if an injury is suspected.

If the patient is not complaining of any pain in the pelvic region, or no deformities are noted, place each hand on the iliac crest and gently compress the pelvis inward and downward. Note any instability, crepitation, tenderness, or deformity.

Critical Findings: The Pelvis

Critical Finding: Tender, deformed, or unstable pelvis
Intervention: Immobilize the pelvis with the pneumatic anti-shock garment or another acceptable immobilization device, place the patient on a backboard, and consider prompt transport.

ASSESS THE EXTREMITIES

Assess first the lower, then the upper extremities (Figures 9-20a to e). Inspect and palpate the extremities for deformities, contusions, abrasions, penetrations, burns, tenderness, lacerations, and swelling. Trauma to the extremities rarely produces life-threatening injuries. Major bleeding will be your major concern. Since bone and joint injuries are usually not life threatening, splinting in the critical patient must be conducted en route to the hospital and not at the scene. Too much time is lost when splints are applied at the scene of the incident.

Following inspection and palpation, check for "PMS"—distal pulses, motor function, and sensation.

- Pulses—Check distal pulses in all extremities. In the lower extremities, check the dorsalis pedis pulse. This is the pulse that is located on the top of the foot approximately midway between the toes and the ankle on the big toe side. Another distal pulse that could be assessed in the lower extremities is the posterior tibial pulse. This pulse is located behind the medial malleolus, the knob at the inner side of the ankle.

  When assessing for either pulse, it is necessary to bare the area where the pulse is to be felt. In the upper extremities, assess for a radial pulse. The radial pulse is located on the thumb side near the anterior base of the wrist.

  Determine if pulses are present in each extremity. Also, compare the strength of the pulses of each extremity. Absent or weak pulses could indicate poor perfusion from shock, a pinched or damaged artery from a bone injury, or a blood clot blocking circulation. When feeling for the pulse, also note the patient's skin color, temperature, and condition in each extremity as an indication of perfusion.

- Motor Function—If the patient is able to obey commands, ask the patient to wiggle his toes and squeeze your fingers. Simply determine if the patient can move his fingers and toes.

- Sensation—In a responsive patient, touch the finger on one hand and ask the patient to identify what finger you are touching. Then pinch the hand and ask the patient to identify the extremity with pain. (It is important to test both light touch and pain, since each of these stimuli is carried by a different nerve tract in the spinal cord.) Repeat this procedure on the other hand and then each foot, using the toes.

  If the patient is unresponsive, pinch the hand or foot and watch the response. It is important in the unresponsive patient to note the motor response associated with the painful stimulus applied to the extremity. Also, be sure to watch the patient's face for a grimace, a positive response to the pinch indicating intact sensitivity to pain.

Bilateral injury to the femurs is an exception to the rule that bone and joint injuries are not life-threatening. Injury to the femur could result in severe bleeding within the bone and around the muscle and tissue in the leg. Therefore, injury to both femurs is considered critical. If both thighs are discovered to be painful, swollen, or deformed, immobilize the patient on a backboard and initiate prompt transport. Perform traction splinting en route if possible.

Critical Findings: The Extremities

Critical Finding: Life-threatening bleeding
Intervention: Provide direct pressure and pressure dressing.
Critical Finding: Bilateral femur injuries
Intervention: Stabilize on backboard and promptly transport. Consider traction splints en route.

ASSESS THE POSTERIOR BODY

With in-line spinal stabilization being maintained, the patient will be rolled to inspect and palpate the posterior aspect of the body. With the patient rolled on his side, quickly inspect the posterior thorax, lumbar region, buttocks, and backs of the legs. Look for deformities, contusions, abrasions, punctures, burns, lacerations, swelling, or any other evidence of injury. Any open wound to the posterior thorax must be covered with an occlusive dressing.

If the patient is not complaining of pain in the area of the thoracic or lumbar vertebrae, palpate the vertebral column for any deformity and tenderness. Be extremely careful not to move the patient or cause excessive pain when palpating. This may jeopardize the in-line stabilization. If the patient is complaining of pain, assume that a spinal injury exists. Provide complete spinal immobilization.

With the patient on his side, place a backboard alongside him and roll him back down onto the backboard. Continue in-line stabilization until the patient is completely secured to the backboard.

Critical Findings: The Posterior Body

Critical Finding: Open wound to the posterior thorax
Intervention: Immediately occlude with your gloved hand. Dress with an occlusive dressing taped on three sides.
Critical Finding: Life-threatening bleeding
Intervention: Apply direct pressure and a pressure dressing.

Assess Baseline Vital Signs

In the focused history and physical exam for a trauma patient, vital sign assessment follows the rapid trauma assessment and precedes the SAMPLE history. Remember, however, that if you have enough assistance and can be sure that in-line stabilization is being maintained by a trained person, these steps may overlap. For example, one EMT-B may be able to get vital sign measurements while the other is conducting the rapid trauma assessment, or vital signs and history may be taken at the same time.

The methods for assessing the vital signs were discussed in Chapter 5, "Baseline Vital Signs and History Taking." The vital signs are reviewed briefly below with notes about vital sign assessment for the trauma patient with a significant mechanism of injury.

- Breathing—Assess both the rate and quality of breathing. Determine the quality of breathing as being normal, shallow, labored, deep, or noisy. (Review Table 9-5 on page 160 regarding adequate and inadequate breathing.)
- Pulse—Assess the radial pulse in the adult and child patient and the brachial pulse in an infant less than 1 year of age. If the radial pulse is not present, assess the carotid pulse. If there is a carotid pulse but no radial pulse (typically with a systolic blood pressure less than 80 mmHg), or if the radial pulse is weak and rapid, the patient is likely to be suffering from shock (hypoperfusion).
- Skin—The skin is assessed to determine the perfusion status of the patient. Inspect for pale or cyanotic nail beds and pale skin, oral mucosa, and conjunctiva. Feel the skin with the back of the hand for the temperature and condition. Pale, cool, clammy skin is a strong indication of poor tissue perfusion. A trauma patient with tachycardia (rapid pulse) and pale, cool, clammy skin should be assumed to be in shock.

  Assess for capillary refill in infants and children less than 6 years of age. Normal capillary refill is usually less than 2 seconds. A capillary refill of greater than 2 seconds may indicate poor tissue perfusion and shock. Cold exposure and other conditions may lengthen the capillary refill time, making it a less reliable sign of shock.
- Pupils—Quickly assess the pupils for size and reactivity by shining a light into the patient's eyes. Poor perfusion could cause the pupils to dilate and respond sluggishly to light, so this sign may be considered along with other indicators of shock. Head injury may cause the pupils to become unequal and unresponsive to light.
- Blood pressure—Take the blood pressure by auscultation. Determine the systolic and diastolic pressure. Two signs of serious blood loss and shock are narrow pulse pressure (the difference between the

systolic and diastolic pressures) and hypotension (low blood pressure). Typically, in an adult, a systolic pressure less than 100 mmHg is considered low and a pulse pressure less than 30 mmHg is considered narrow. If the blood pressure cannot be auscultated because of excessive noise at the scene, use the palpation method. Since palpation provides only the systolic pressure, pulse pressure cannot be determined by this method.

The vital signs should be reassessed and recorded every 5 minutes in the unstable patient. In the stable patient, the vitals should be reassessed and recorded a minimum of every 15 minutes. Consider any trauma patient with a significant mechanism of injury to be unstable and assess vital signs every 5 minutes.

Critical Findings: Baseline Vital Signs

Critical Finding: Inadequate breathing rate and/or depth
Intervention: Immediately begin positive pressure ventilation with supplemental oxygen.
Critical Finding: Absent pulses
Intervention: If the carotid pulse is absent, initiate CPR and automated external defibrillation (AED) as soon as it is available.
Critical Finding: Cool, clammy, pale skin with weak, rapid pulses
Intervention: Suspect shock. Apply oxygen via a nonrebreather mask at 15 liters per minute or positive pressure ventilation with supplemental oxygen if needed. Control severe bleeding, elevate the foot end of the backboard to which the patient is immobilized 8 to 12 inches, keep the patient warm, consider prompt transport, and splint bone or joint injuries en route if possible.
Critical Finding: Unequal pupils
Intervention: If associated with an altered mental status, consider severe head injury. Begin hyperventilation at 20 per minute. (See note on p. 215.)
Critical Finding: Hypotension/narrow pulse pressure
Intervention: Suspect shock. Apply oxygen at 15 lpm via a nonrebreather mask and consider prompt transport.

Obtain a SAMPLE History

In the focused history and physical exam for a trauma patient, the SAMPLE history follows the rapid trauma assessment and vital signs measurements. With two EMT-Bs working together, the SAMPLE history can be conducted while the rapid trauma assessment and vital signs are being assessed, or—if the patient is responsive—the SAMPLE history can be taken en route to the hospital. If the patient is unresponsive, you must attempt to get as much of the history as possible from family members or bystanders prior to leaving the scene.

History taking and questioning should not interfere with any assessment or treatment of life-threatening injuries or conditions or delay transport of a critically injured patient.

Methods of obtaining a SAMPLE history were covered in Chapter 5, "Baseline Vital Signs and History Taking." The elements of the SAMPLE history are reviewed briefly below with notes about their relevance for the trauma patient with a significant mechanism of injury.

- Signs—*During your assessment, you are continuously inspecting for signs of trauma.* Deformities, contusions, abrasions, punctures, burns, lacerations, and swelling, as well as indication of pain on palpation (tenderness) are all signs of blunt or penetrating trauma. It is important to correlate the sign with the mechanism of injury to focus your index of suspicion on specific possible injuries.

- Symptoms—*How do you feel? Do you hurt anywhere? What symptoms are you experiencing? (If the patient is unresponsive, ask bystanders if he complained of pain or any other symptoms before losing consciousness.)* The patient may be complaining of pain, lightheadedness, weakness, dizziness, dyspnea, numbness, tingling, nausea, or many other symptoms associated with trauma. Any complaints of dyspnea, severe headache, chest pain, or abdominal pain should cause you to closely examine the related area for life-threatening injuries. For example, a patient who is complaining of dyspnea should be examined closely for possible life-threatening chest injuries such as a flail segment, open chest wound, or air in the chest cavity. Symptoms are gathered throughout assessment. Signs, symptoms, and mechanism of injury are the basis for emergency care provided to trauma patients.

- Allergies—*Do you have any allergies? Are you allergic to any medications?* For the trauma patient, gather information on allergies to medications that may be important for the medical facility staff to know about. Look for a medical tag that may identify an allergy.

- Medications—*Have you currently been taking any medications?* In the trauma patient, it is not extremely important to gather extensive information regarding the prescription or over-the-counter medications the patient is currently taking. However, this information may help to provide a medical history in the unresponsive trauma patient, and some medications may alter the signs and symptoms expected in some conditions or may cause the patient to decompensate (succumb to shock) faster. For example, beta blocker drugs are frequently taken to control hypertension and heart rhythms.

This drug will slow the heart rate. A patient who is on a beta blocker and is in shock may not have the classic signs of shock, such as tachycardia or clammy skin.

Gather whatever information about medications you can, but do not expend any extra time at the scene to determine the patient's medications. This information is not vital for the trauma patient.

- Pertinent Past Medical History—*Have you had any recent illnesses? Have you been seeing a doctor for any condition?* Quickly determine the medical history from the patient or, if the patient is unresponsive, from a family member. A patient with an existing medical condition may decompensate faster and exhibit altered signs and symptoms related to the past medical or surgical condition. Ask quickly about any past medical problems, trauma, or surgeries. Also, inspect the neck and extremities for a medical identification tag.

- Last Oral Intake—*When did you last eat or drink anything?* Find out from the patient or family member or knowledgeable bystander the last time the patient ate solid food or drank any liquids. Also, if possible, determine the approximate amount. This information is important to the hospital staff if the patient needs anesthesia for surgery.

- Events Leading to the Injury—*How did the incident happen?* Asking the trauma patient how the accident or injuries occurred can provide information about the mechanism of injury. Information from the patient or bystanders may shed additional light on the mechanism of injury, for example the height from which the patient fell. It is also important to determine why an accident occurred. Did the patient get dizzy and swerve off the road? Was the patient having chest pain that caused him to fall down the stairs? Did the patient lose consciousness before wrecking the car? A patient in an automobile crash who tells you that he was driving 90 mph down the road because he was shot in the abdomen and was trying to get to the hospital has a clear mechanism of injury that provides you with suspicions of other injuries. Knowing what events lead up to the accident or incident could also be helpful in determining if an illness exists in addition to the trauma.

PREPARE THE PATIENT FOR TRANSPORT

Normally, the critical trauma patient is prepared for transport simultaneously as the rapid trauma assessment is being conducted. Other EMT-Bs and first-responder personnel should be preparing the backboard, head immobilization device, and stretcher. Following or simultaneously with assessment of the vital signs, the patient is secured to the backboard with straps. The head is immobilized with a head immobilization device or blanket rolls and tape (Figure 9-21). The patient should then be transported to the cot and into the ambulance. (The SAMPLE history can be taken during this process or delayed to be taken in the ambulance.) Techniques for immobilization and transfer of the patient to the ambulance will be covered in detail in Chapter 34, "Injuries to the Spine," and Chapter 39, "Moving Patients."

Once the patient is completely immobilized, transport should not be delayed. Review Table 9-7 on page 165 for factors to consider as part of a decision for prompt transport. Bear in mind that prompt transport is key in survival of the critically injured patient.

PROVIDE EMERGENCY CARE

In addition to the interventions mentioned for each critical finding listed above, the information that follows provides overall advice about emergency care based on the focused history and physical exam for the trauma patient with a significant mechanism of injury.

The focused history and physical exam for the trauma patient with a significant mechanism of injury should be conducted in a period of about 2 to 2½ minutes. This includes the rapid trauma assessment, baseline vital signs, and SAMPLE history. For this kind of patient, who is likely to be in critical condition, the rapid trauma assessment should identify any immediately life-threatening injuries and conditions that may have been missed during, or developed since, the initial assessment, as well as any other less severe injuries or problems the patient may have.

A decision to rapidly transport the patient is made based upon the findings of the rapid trauma assessment. Any of the critical findings summarized in Table 9-7 is an indication for prompt transport, with further treatment and continued assessment to take

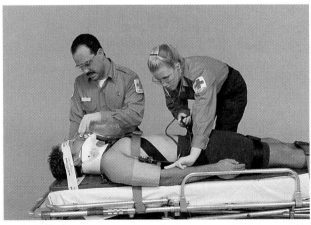

Figure 9-21 *Prepare the patient for transport.*

place en route to the hospital. *However, life-threatening injuries and conditions must be appropriately managed as found at the scene prior to transport.* Remember that, in critical patients, splinting for suspected bone or joint injuries is not done at the scene because these injuries are not life threatening.

During transport, the life threats are reassessed while further evaluating the patient and providing care, as possible, for additional conditions or injuries that are not immediately life threatening.

If the patient's condition is stable, emergency treatment for non-life-threatening conditions or injuries that have been identified may be completed at the scene before transport. However, in a trauma patient with a significant mechanism of injury, a decision to transport rapidly is likely.

En route to the hospital, your priority is to continuously reassess the components of the initial assessment—mental status, airway, breathing, and circulation—plus vital signs and components of the rapid trauma assessment focused on the patient's injuries. You will also reassess the effectiveness of your interventions. This is known as an ongoing assessment and will be described in detail in Part 5 of this chapter.

A detailed physical exam (similar to a repetition of the entire rapid trauma assessment, but in more detail) may also be conducted en route, but only if the patient's condition and time permit. The detailed physical exam must not interfere with the provision of continued care for life-threatening injuries. The detailed physical exam will be covered in Part 4 of this chapter.

You must set priorities for management of critical injuries and conditions both at the scene and throughout the transport to the hospital. If a patient has suffered blunt trauma to the face with significant bleeding in the upper airway, the EMT-B caring for the patient in the back of the ambulance is most concerned with maintaining a patent airway. This can only be done with continuous suction. In addition, the EMT-B must reassess the breathing and perfusion status and reassess vital signs. Management of the airway takes precedence over any other condition and over any additional assessment.

TRAUMA SCORE

A trauma score is a numerical way to identify the severity of trauma. Many EMS systems use the scoring system as a means to communicate the severity of the patient to the receiving facility. You should be familiar with the trauma scoring system used in your region and be familiar with the elements of that scoring system.

The Revised Trauma Score (Table 9-8), which includes the Glasgow Coma Scale, is one type of scor-

TABLE 9-8

The Revised Trauma Score with Glasgow Coma Scale

BRIEF NEUROLOGICAL EVALUATION	
A—**Alert** V—Responds to **Verbal** stimuli	P—Responds to **Painful** stimuli U—**Unresponsive**

REVISED TRAUMA INDEX

TRAUMA SCORE OPERATIONAL DEFINITIONS

Respiratory Rate

Number of respirations in 15 seconds; multiply by 4

Systolic Blood Pressure

Systolic cuff pressure, either arm—auscultate or palpate
No pulse—no carotid pulse

Best Verbal Response

Arouse patient with voice or painful stimulus

Best Motor Response

Response to command or painful stimulus

Projected estimate of survival for each value of the Trauma Score based on results from 1,509 patients with blunt or penetrating injury[2]

Trauma Score	Percentage Survival
12	99
11	97
10	88
9	77
8	67
7	64
6	63
5	46
4	33
3	33
2	29
1	25
0	4

REVISED TRAUMA SCORE

The Trauma Score is a numerical grading system for estimating the severity of injury.[1] The score is composed of the Glasgow Coma Scale (reduced to approximately one-third total value) and measurements of cardiopulmonary function. Each parameter is given a number (high for normal and low for impaired function). Severity of injury is estimated by summing the numbers. The lowest score is 1 and the highest score is 12.

Respiratory Rate	10-29/min	4
	29/min	3
	6-9/min	2
	1-5/min	1
	None (0/min)	0
Systolic Blood Pressure	> 89 mmHg	4
	76-88 mmHg	3
	50-75 mmHg	2
	1-49 mmHg	1
	No Pulse or 0 SBP (Systolic Blood Pressure)	0

Trauma Scale Total

GLASGOW COMA SCALE

			Total Glasgow Coma Scale Points
Eye Opening	Spontaneous	4	
	To Voice	3	
	To Pain	2	
	None	0	
Verbal Response	Oriented	5	13–15 = 4
	Confused	4	9–12 = 3
	Inappropriate Words	3	6–8 = 2
	Incomprehensible Words	2	4–5 = 1
	None	1	<3 = 0
Motor Response	Obeys Command	6	
	Localized Pain	5	
	Withdraw Pain	4	
	Flexion (pain)	3	
	Extension (pain)	2	
	None	1	

Glasgow Coma Scale Total

Total Trauma Score (Trauma Scale + GCS)   1–12

Source: "A Revision of the Trauma Score," *The Journal of Trauma.* 29(5): 1989, pp. 623–29.
[1]Champion, H. R., Sacco, W. J., Carnazzo, A. J., et al. "Trauma Score," *Crit. Care Med.* 9(9): 1981, pp. 672–76.
[2]Endorsed by the American Trauma Society.

ing system used. A number is assigned to each parameter being assessed. The numbers from each subset are totaled and a score is derived for that particular patient. The lower the score, the more severe the patient's condition.

The major components of the trauma score are:

- Respiratory rate
- Systolic blood pressure
- Glasgow Coma Score (GCS)

It is important to report and document the findings of the Revised Trauma Score. This information is extremely useful to the receiving facility for purposes of reassessment.

TRAUMA PATIENT WITH NO SIGNIFICANT MECHANISM OF INJURY OR CRITICAL FINDING

On the prior pages, we discussed how to conduct the focused history and physical exam when you have determined that the patient has a significant mechanism of injury. Here we will discuss the trauma patient whose mechanism of injury is not significant, who is alert and oriented, and for whom no critical findings are present. If in doubt, err to benefit the patient and consider the mechanism of injury to be significant to avoid missing injuries.

PERFORM A FOCUSED TRAUMA ASSESSMENT

Consider a patient whose injury is a laceration to one finger that resulted from a slip of the knife while cutting a tomato. The finger may be bleeding profusely, but the mechanism of injury is not significant—that is, it is a mechanism that does not lead you to suspect additional injuries or problems.

For this patient, a complete head-to-toe rapid trauma assessment is not necessary or appropriate. Instead, you conduct a focused trauma assessment— an exam that focuses primarily on the injury site, in this case the injured finger. You use the same techniques as in a rapid trauma assessment—quickly inspecting and palpating for deformities, contusions, abrasions, punctures, burns, tenderness, lacerations, and swelling— but you assess just the specific localized site of the injury. For the patient with the cut finger, you have already controlled the bleeding as part of the initial assessment, and now you conduct the focused assessment to ensure that there is no further injury to the patient's hand or arm, such as a burn or a bone or joint injury.

Another example is a suspected bone or joint injury. Earlier, it was stated that injuries to the extremities are seldom life threatening, and that complete assessment and treatment of such injuries for a critical trauma patient would not take place at the scene. Instead, treatment would be carried out in the ambulance en route to the hospital if time and care of the patient's more serious problems permit. However, for the patient who has no significant mechanism of injury but presents with indications of a possible fracture or other injury to a bone or joint, full assessment and splinting of the injured extremity would be carried out at the scene before transport to the hospital.

For instance, a high school student is playing volleyball and jumps up for the ball. She lands on the lateral aspect of her right ankle with her leg in a twisted position. You are called to the scene. The patient is complaining of severe pain to her ankle. You perform a scene size-up and brief initial assessment and determine that no significant mechanism of injury has occurred and no critical injuries exist. You would immediately focus in on the ankle injury and inspect and palpate the entire extremity. Then you would immobilize the ankle while still at the scene.

To assess an upper or lower extremity when a bone or joint injury is suspected, inspect for deformity (such as angulation to a bone where no joint exists), contusions, abrasions, punctures, burns, lacerations, and swelling. Palpate by placing your hands around the entire extremity so that the thumbs come together on the anterior surface and the little fingers are on the posterior surface. Your thumbs and fingers should never lose contact with the extremity during the palpation. Begin at the most proximal point (closest to the heart) and palpate to the most distal point (farthest from the heart), noting any deformity, swelling, tenderness, or crepitation.

Following inspection and palpation, check the distal pulses, motor function, and sensation. Always assess distal pulses, motor function, and sensation both before the injury is splinted (to detect any impairment of function caused by the injury) and after the injury is splinted (to detect any improvement or deterioration of function resulting from the intervention). Be sure to document this assessment on the prehospital care report.

OBTAIN BASELINE VITAL SIGNS AND SAMPLE HISTORY

Once the focused trauma assessment is completed on a patient with no life-threatening injuries, it is necessary to assess the baseline vital signs and obtain the SAMPLE history. Then provide emergency care for the injuries found and prepare the patient for transport. While en route to the hospital, reassess the airway, breathing, and perfusion, reassess vital signs, and check the effectiveness of the emergency care provided.

SOMETIMES PERFORM A RAPID TRAUMA ASSESSMENT

Although the focused trauma assessment is usually appropriate for a trauma patient with no significant mechanism of injury, occasionally it will be wise to conduct a full head-to-toe rapid trauma assessment.

One such instance would be when you undertake a focused trauma assessment in a patient with no significant mechanism of injury but you develop a suspicion that more injuries may exist than what the patient is complaining of, or the patient begins to deteriorate. In this case, immediately conduct a complete rapid trauma assessment.

Another instance would be when you are conducting a focused trauma assessment on a patient and you make a critical finding. Immediately perform a rapid trauma assessment and consider prompt transport. For example, you arrive on the scene and find a patient lying on the kitchen floor complaining of pain to his left hip. He says that he slipped on some water and fell. The mechanism of injury is not significant, and the initial assessment does not reveal any critical findings. Therefore, you decide to perform a focused trauma assessment on the left hip area, extending to the pelvis and both lower extremities. When you begin to palpate the pelvis, the patient complains of severe pain and you feel instability and crepitation. A pelvic injury is considered a critical finding, so you quickly conduct a rapid trauma assessment, assess baseline vitals, and prepare the patient for immediate transport. En route, you reassess airway, breathing, and perfusion, reassess vital signs, complete the SAMPLE history, and perform a detailed exam of the abdomen, pelvis, and lower extremities.

Another kind of patient with no significant mechanism of injury and no critical findings, who nevertheless must have a complete rapid trauma assessment and a detailed exam en route to the hospital, is the patient suffering from multiple injuries each of which, by itself, would not be considered critical. The patient may have multiple minor soft tissue injuries. Or the patient may have suspected multiple fractures to the extremities. In either situation, the multiple injuries may indicate a more significant mechanism of injury than was first suspected. The multiple injuries may also, cumulatively, be causing significant internal or external blood loss and shock. For this patient, it is necessary to perform a head-to-toe assessment and, if these are critical findings, consider prompt transport.

Remember: If any question exists in your mind as to what assessment to perform on a patient—the limited focused trauma assessment versus the complete rapid trauma assessment—err to benefit the patient and conduct the rapid trauma assessment.

FOCUSED HISTORY AND PHYSICAL EXAM
MEDICAL PATIENT

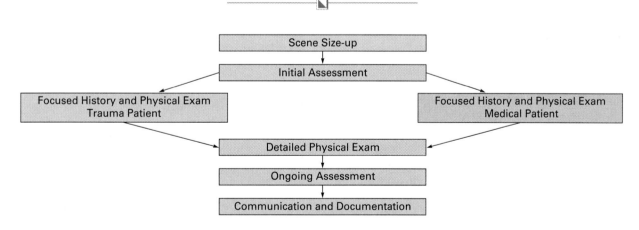

OBJECTIVES

Numbered objectives are from the United States Department of Transportation 1994 EMT-Basic National Standard Curriculum. Asterisked objectives, if any, pertain to material that is supplemental to the DOT curriculum.

COGNITIVE

3-4.1   Describe the unique needs for assessing an individual with a specific chief complaint with no known prior history. (pp. 186–194)

3-4.2 Differentiate between the history and physical exam that are performed for responsive patients with no known prior history and responsive patients with a known prior history. (pp. 192–194)
3-4.3 Describe the needs for assessing an individual who is unresponsive. (pp. 186–192)
3-4.4 Differentiate between the assessment that is performed for a patient who is unresponsive or has an altered mental status and other medical patients requiring assessment. (pp. 186–194)

AFFECTIVE

3-4.5 Attend to the feelings that these patients might be experiencing. (p. 148)

PSYCHOMOTOR

3-4.6 Demonstrate the patient assessment skills that should be used to assist a patient who is responsive with no known history.
3-4.7 Demonstrate the patient assessment skills that should be used to assist a patient who is unresponsive or has an altered mental status.

A medical patient is one who has not suffered from any type of injury or trauma, but instead is experiencing signs and symptoms related to a disease process or condition affecting the body's organs or systems.

As was true for the trauma patient, you will perform the focused history and physical exam on the medical patient (Figure 9-22) immediately following the initial assessment. Life-threatening conditions of the airway, breathing, and circulation will have already been managed as part of the initial assessment. Further emergency care will be based on your findings from the focused history and physical exam.

First, you will categorize the medical patient as either responsive or unresponsive. There are two key differences in the way you will conduct the focused history and physical exam for the responsive medical patient vs. the unresponsive medical patient.

The first difference is in the sequence of steps. For the responsive medical patient, you will gather the history from the patient first, then conduct the physical exam and obtain the vital signs. The history comes first for the responsive medical patient for two reasons: first, the most valuable information on a medical condition in the prehospital setting usually comes from what the patient can tell you about how he feels; secondly, it is important to get information from the patient before he, possibly, becomes unresponsive. For the patient who is already unresponsive when you arrive on the scene, the physical exam and vital signs will come before the history, which will need to be gathered, to the extent possible, from family members or bystanders.

The second difference is in the kind of physical exam you will conduct. For the responsive medical patient, you will conduct a **focused medical assessment**—an exam that is focused on the patient's chief complaint, signs, and symptoms. For the unresponsive medical patient, you will conduct a **rapid medical assessment**—a quick head-to-toe assessment that

will be very similar to the rapid trauma assessment. You will be looking for signs relating to the patient's medical condition as well as for any signs of possible trauma that may have been missed earlier.

As the chart below reveals, the focused history and physical exam for an unresponsive medical patient is very similar to the focused history and physical exam for a trauma patient with significant mechanism of injury because, in both instances, you first need to examine the whole body for information the patient cannot tell you about. The focused history and physical exam for a responsive medical patient (the majority of your medical calls) begins with the SAMPLE history, followed by a physical exam focused on the patient's chief complaint, signs, and symptoms.

Focused History and Physical Exam for a Medical Patient Who Is . . .

Unresponsive
1. Rapid medical assessment (head to toe)
2. Baseline vital signs
3. SAMPLE history

Responsive
1. SAMPLE history
2. Focused medical assessment (focused on the chief complaint, signs, and symptoms)
3. Baseline vital signs

UNRESPONSIVE MEDICAL PATIENT

Unresponsiveness in a medical patient should be considered as being critical. A rapid medical assessment must be performed, followed by prompt transport,

---

FOCUSED HISTORY AND PHYSICAL EXAM: MEDICAL PATIEN

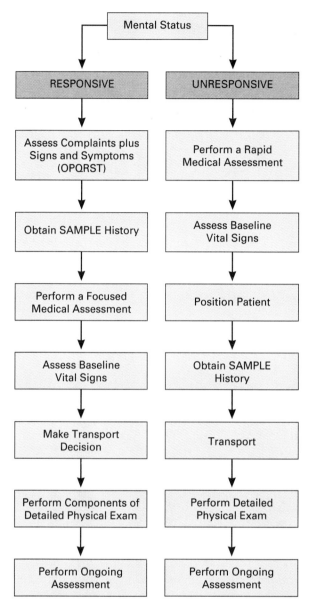

Figure 9-22 Steps of the focused history and physical exam for a medical patient.

continued assessment, and emergency care en route to the hospital.

Attempt to gain as much information from the scene as possible. Note the patient's medications, both prescribed and over-the-counter; any evidence of drugs or alcohol; signs that the patient may have been sick for a period of time; and the condition of the place in which the patient was found. Also, look at how the patient is dressed, where he was found, and what he may have been doing prior to the emergency. If you walk into the scene and find an oxygen tank or concentrator in the living room, you are likely to suspect that the patient may have a history of emphysema, chronic bronchitis, or some other type of respiratory condition. A patient in a hospital-type bed usually has a chronic illness or severe debilitating disease.

Also make use of other sources of information. Question bystanders, family members, or other relatives or friends. The patient may have been complaining of symptoms prior to the unresponsiveness. Look for a medical identification tag on the patient as evidence of a chronic illness.

Critical Findings: Medical Patient

Critical Finding: Unresponsiveness (or otherwise altered mental status)
Intervention: Ensure an adequate airway. Apply oxygen by nonrebreather mask at 15 lpm or begin positive pressure ventilation if necessary.

PERFORM A RAPID MEDICAL ASSESSMENT

Perform a rapid medical assessment on the unresponsive patient to determine the possible nature of the medical illness. The patient's airway, breathing, and perfusion status will have been assessed and managed during the initial assessment. As you perform the rapid medical assessment, reassess the airway, breathing, and circulation status and manage these or any additional life-threatening problems immediately as found.

Like the rapid trauma assessment, the rapid medical assessment should be conducted systematically, beginning at the head and covering all major portions of the body (Figures 9-23 to 9-28). The techniques of inspection, palpation, and auscultation are used to search for any signs of abnormality or dysfunction.

ASSESS THE HEAD

Inspect the head for any evidence of trauma (Figure 9-23). You may not initially expect to find trauma, due to a lack of mechanism of injury; however, the patient may have fallen several hours, days, or even weeks prior to the onset of the signs, symptoms, or unresponsiveness. Inspect for contusions, lacerations, depressions, abrasions, and punctures. Palpate the head for any deformities.

Quickly inspect inside the mouth for bleeding, secretions, or vomitus. Reassess the airway and ensure that it is patent. Inspect the nose and ears for fluid discharge or blood. Quickly inspect the pupils for equality, size, and reactivity. Unequal pupils may indicate a stroke (cerebrovascular accident or CVA) or possible head injury. Pupil size and reactivity may provide evidence of drug overdose, poisoning, oxygen starvation, or adverse environmental conditions.

THE RAPID MEDICAL ASSESSMENT

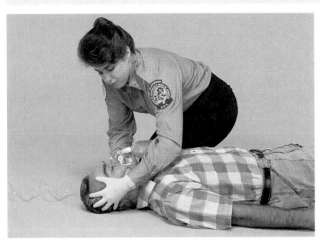

Figure 9-23   Inspect and palpate the head.

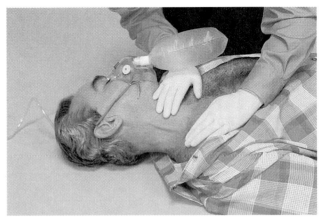

Figure 9-24   Inspect the neck for jugular vein distention, excessive neck muscle use when the patient inhales, medical identification tag, or tracheostomy tube.

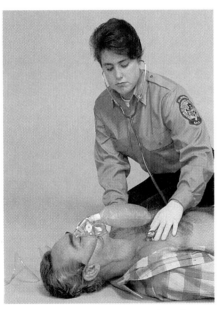

Figure 9-25   Inspect the chest for adequate rise and fall, muscle retractions, and symmetry. Auscultate the breath sounds.

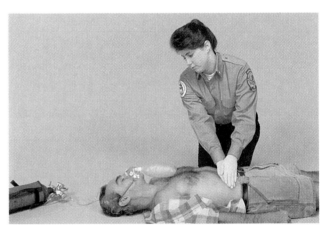

Figure 9-26   Inspect the abdomen for scars, discoloration, or distention. Palpate for tenderness, rigidity, distention, and pulsating masses.

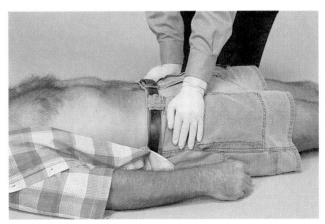

Figure 9-27   Inspect and palpate the pelvic region.

THE RAPID MEDICAL ASSESSMENT continued

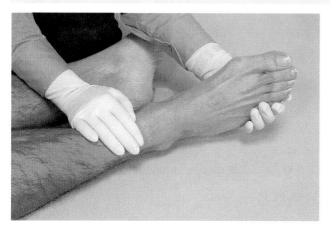

Figure 9-28a   Assess the upper and lower extremities for swelling and discoloration. Look for a medical identification tag around the wrist or ankle.

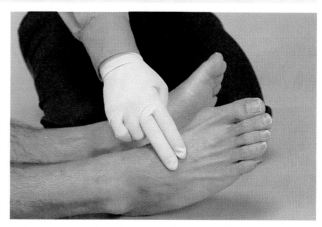

Figure 9-28b   Assess pulses in all four extremities.

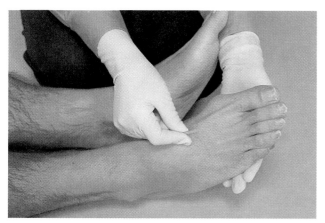

Figure 9-28c   Assess motor and sensory function in all four extremities.

Conclude the rapid medical assessment by inspecting and palpating the posterior body.

ASSESS THE NECK

Inspect the neck for jugular vein distention (Figure 9-24). In the medical patient, JVD may be a sign of right-sided heart failure or late left-sided heart failure. You might find JVD associated with complaints of chest pain, dyspnea, inability to breathe while lying flat, or severe fatigue and weakness.

Also inspect the neck for excessive accessory muscle use. If the muscles in the neck bulge and become very prominent during inhalation, respiratory distress should be suspected. Reassess the adequacy of breathing.

While inspecting the neck, look for a medical identification necklace with pertinent medical information about the patient inscribed on the back. This may provide you with an indication of the patient's condition.

Check for a tracheostomy tube at the base of the neck. Because the patient breathes through this tube, secretions and mucus could block the tube, causing an airway obstruction.

ASSESS THE CHEST

Inspect the chest for adequate rise and fall, retraction of the intercostal muscles, and symmetrical movement (Figure 9-25). An inward pulling of the muscles between the ribs during inhalation indicates respiratory distress. In an unresponsive patient, you should begin positive pressure ventilation with supplemental oxygen if retractions are noted.

Quickly auscultate the breath sounds at the second intercostal space at the midclavicular line and at the fourth or fifth intercostal space at the midaxillary line.

Compare the breath sounds from side to side. Determine if the breath sounds are present or absent, equal or unequal, clear or noisy.

ASSESS THE ABDOMEN

Inspect the abdomen for any abnormal distention or discoloration (Figure 9-26). Look for evidence of scars from previous surgeries. Palpate for tenderness, distention, rigidity, or pulsating masses. A rigid, distended, or tender abdomen is a sign of possible internal bleeding. An aortic aneurysm, which is a weakened area of the abdominal aorta, may produce a palpable pulsating mass in the midline of the abdomen.

ASSESS THE PELVIC REGION

Inspect and palpate the pelvic region for any distention and tenderness (Figure 9-27). This is most significant in the female patient of child-bearing age who could be suffering from an ectopic pregnancy. If a female patient complains of abdominal pain, usually isolated to the lower quadrants, has a history of a missed menstrual period, and is exhibiting signs and symptoms of poor perfusion, suspect an ectopic pregnancy. This is a surgical emergency that requires prompt transport.

ASSESS THE EXTREMITIES

Note any excessive peripheral edema (swelling around the hands, feet, and ankles). Excessive edema could indicate congestive heart failure, fluid overload, or a clot blocking a vein in that extremity (Figure 9-28a). Also assess the extremities for pulses, motor function, and sensation (Figures 9-28b and c). In the unresponsive patient, assess the radial and dorsalis pedis pulses. Check motor function and sensation by pinching the hands and feet. Note the response of the patient. Look for a medical identification tag around the wrist or ankle.

ASSESS THE POSTERIOR BODY

Inspect and palpate the back for discoloration, edema, and tenderness. Edema to the sacral region may be from fluid collection associated with congestive heart failure.

ASSESS BASELINE VITAL SIGNS

In the focused history and physical exam for an unresponsive medical patient, vital sign assessment follows the rapid medical assessment and precedes the SAMPLE history. Remember, however, that with EMT-B partners working together, some of these steps can be done simultaneously.

The methods for assessing the vital signs were discussed in Chapter 5. The vital signs are reviewed briefly below with notes about vital sign assessment for the unresponsive medical patient.

- Breathing—Tachypnea (rapid breathing) may indicate a central nervous system disorder, respiratory distress, cardiac problem, anxiety, poisoning, overdose, high blood sugar level, abdominal disorder, or a pulmonary problem. Abnormal respiratory patterns may be seen in patients with central nervous system disorders like stroke, poisoning, overdose, and diabetic emergencies.
- Pulse
- Skin
- Pupils—Pupillary signs are very important to document in the unresponsive patient. Note the size, equality, and reactivity to light.
- Blood pressure

The vital signs should be reassessed and recorded every 5 minutes in the unresponsive medical patient.

Critical Findings: Baseline Vital Signs
Critical Finding: Inadequate breathing rate and/or depth **Intervention:** Immediately begin positive pressure ventilation with supplemental oxygen. **Critical Finding:** Absent pulses **Intervention:** If the carotid pulse is absent, initiate CPR and automated external defibrillation (AED) as soon as it is available. **Critical Finding:** Cool, clammy, pale skin with weak, rapid pulses **Intervention:** Suspect shock. Apply oxygen via a nonrebreather mask at 15 liters per minute or positive pressure ventilation with supplemental oxygen if needed. Elevate the patient's feet 8 to 12 inches (elevate the foot of the backboard if trauma is suspected), keep the patient warm, and consider prompt transport. **Critical Finding:** Unequal pupils **Intervention:** If associated with an altered mental status, consider stroke or severe head injury. Begin hyperventilation at 20 per minute. (See note on p. 215.) **Critical Finding:** Hypotension (low blood pressure) **Intervention:** Suspect shock. Apply oxygen via a nonrebreather mask and consider prompt transport. **Critical Finding:** Chest pain (complaint may be reported by family member or bystander if patient is unresponsive) with systolic blood pressure less than 100 mmHg **Intervention:** Apply oxygen by nonrebreather mask at 15 lpm or begin positive pressure ventilation if necessary. Transport immediately.

POSITION THE PATIENT

Unresponsive patients most typically cannot protect their own airway. Secretions, mucus, blood, or vomitus can easily be aspirated into the lungs. To avoid the potential for aspiration, place the patient in the *recovery position* also known as the *coma position*—a left lateral recumbent position—as you prepare the patient for transport (Figure 9-29). In this position, the secretions, blood, mucus, or vomitus will flow out of the mouth and not into the patient's lungs. You must still have a suction device available to assist with clearing the airway if necessary.

OBTAIN A SAMPLE HISTORY

Methods of obtaining a SAMPLE history were covered in Chapter 5, "Baseline Vital Signs and History Taking." For the unresponsive patient, it is necessary to gain as much information as possible from the family members, friends, and bystanders at the scene (Figure 9-30).

- Signs—*Signs will be revealed in the physical exam and vital signs assessment.* As you conduct your rapid medical assessment and find specific signs, it may be necessary to ask the people at the scene relevant questions regarding the complaints of the patient. For example, if you find unequal pupils, it would be appropriate to ask those at the scene: *Was the patient complaining of a headache, weakness, numbness, or paralysis in the extremities?*
- Symptoms—*Was the patient complaining of any symptoms prior to becoming unresponsive?* Was the patient complaining of:
  – shortness of breath?

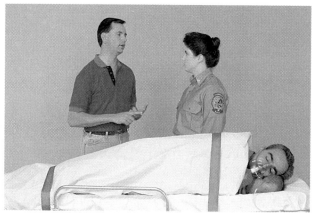

Figure 9-30   Prepare the patient for transport. Obtain a SAMPLE history from bystanders, family, or friends of the unresponsive patient.

  – chest pain?
  – severe headache?
  – lightheadedness, dizziness, or faintness?
  – severe itching?
  – feeling excessively cold or hot?
  – abdominal pain or pain in the lumbar region?
    If the patient was complaining of a particular symptom, try to determine from those at the scene:
  – Was the onset sudden or gradual?
  – Did anything provoke the symptom?
  – How severe was the symptom?
  – How long was the patient complaining of the symptom?
  – Where exactly was the symptom felt?
  – Was anything done or taken to relieve the symptom?
- Allergies—*Does the patient have any known allergies?* The patient may have a medical identification tag that identifies his allergies.
- Medications—*What medications has the patient been taking?* Have someone gather the medications the patient takes. These will provide information about the patient's past medical history. If no family members are at the scene, have your partner look around the kitchen, bathroom, and bedroom for medications, both prescription and over-the-counter medications (Figure 9-31). If the patient is suspected of being a diabetic, look in the refrigerator for insulin.
- Pertinent Past Medical History—*Does the patient have any preexisting medical condition?* Ask if the patient has ever been hospitalized or is seeing a physician. If so, for what condition? If the patient was hospitalized for the condition, ask how recently and for how long. This should provide some indication of the severity of the illness and may provide an indication as to why the patient is unresponsive.

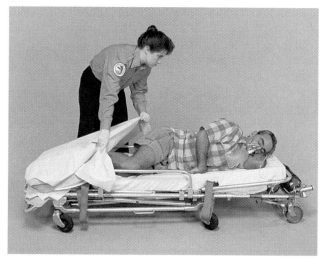

Figure 9-29   Position the unresponsive medical patient in the recovery position to protect the airway and prevent aspiration of secretions, blood, or vomitus.

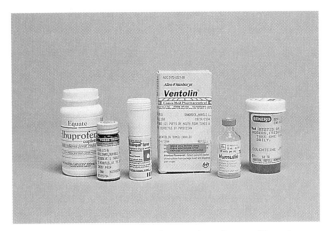

Figure 9-31 Check the patient's medications. Look for both prescription and over-the-counter medications. Check the refrigerator for insulin if the patient is unresponsive with an unknown medical history.

- Last Oral Intake—*When did the patient last eat or drink anything?* It is of extreme importance to determine when the diabetic patient most recently had a meal or last had anything to eat or drink. Attempt to determine how long after the meal the signs and symptoms occurred. Gastrointestinal disorders, anaphylaxis, and diabetic emergencies are often associated with eating. Also, if the patient will require surgery, the anesthetist will need this information.
- Events Leading to the Present Illness—*What was the patient doing prior to the onset of the unresponsiveness? What were his signs or symptoms?* This is useful in trying to rule out trauma as the cause for the unresponsiveness.

PROVIDE EMERGENCY CARE

Following the focused history and physical exam, you will provide emergency care based on the signs, symptoms, and history gathered. All unresponsive patients must receive oxygen via a nonrebreather mask at 15 liters per minute or positive pressure ventilation with supplemental oxygen, if needed.

MAKE A TRANSPORT DECISION

Any unresponsive medical patient is considered to be in critical condition and should be transported promptly. However, life-threatening injuries and conditions must be appropriately managed at the scene prior to transport.

During transport, closely monitor the airway, breathing, and circulation status. If time permits, perform a detailed physical exam. Reassess vital signs every 5 minutes. Following any intervention that you provide, check for a change in the patient's condi-

tion. If at any time the patient regains responsiveness, perform a rapid assessment and reevaluate the SAMPLE history.

RESPONSIVE MEDICAL PATIENT

In the responsive medical patient, closely assess the history of the present illness. You do this mainly by asking the patient a series of questions. With the responsive medical patient, you can add a group of questions called the OPQRST questions to the SAMPLE history to gain as complete a picture as possible of the illness the patient is experiencing. The manner in which you conduct the rest of the focused history and physical exam and provide emergency care will be based on the information you gather from the OPQRST and SAMPLE questions.

ASSESS PATIENT COMPLAINTS: OPQRST

OPQRST is a mnemonic for remembering the questions to ask when assessing the patient's chief complaint or major symptoms such as pain, that the patient can tell you about. Your questions should determine the onset, provocation/palliation, quality, radiation, severity, and time of the complaint.

- Onset—*When and how did the symptom begin?* Ask the patient if the onset was sudden or gradual. Also determine if the onset was associated with a particular activity. For example, you arrive on the scene and find a patient complaining of chest pain. The patient states the onset of the chest pain was sudden. You then ask, "What were you doing when the chest pain started?" The patient replies, "I was playing tennis at the time." Based on this response, you would document the onset of chest pain as being associated with strenuous activity.
- Provocation/palliation—*What makes the symptom worse? What makes it better?* A patient complaining of chest pain may tell you that walking up the steps made the pain much worse, or a patient complaining of dyspnea states, "When I lie flat in bed I can't breathe." Determine if the patient has taken any medication to attempt to relieve the symptoms. A patient complaining of abdominal pain may have taken an antacid. If something was taken, determine if the symptoms were relieved, made worse, or remained the same.
- Quality—*How would you describe the pain?* Quality is most often associated with a complaint of pain. Ask the patient to describe the pain. Most often, pain is described as crushing, aching, dull, stabbing, knifelike, crampy, gnawing, burning, or tear-

ing. Do not lead the patient by asking, "Is the pain sharp or dull?" Ask an open-ended question such as, "What does the pain feel like?"

The quality of pain, with other signs and symptoms, usually helps to determine what organ system is involved. For example, dull, aching, tight, pressure-type chest pain is usually associated with a cardiac problem; conditions involving the lung or chest wall muscles or nerves usually produce a sharper knifelike pain.

- Radiation—*Where do you feel the pain? Where does the pain go?* Prior to asking about radiation, it is necessary to determine the exact location of the pain. Ask the patient to point to the pain with one finger. The pain is localized if he can isolate it to one area. Generalized pain cannot be localized and is spread over a general area. From the point of the initial pain, ask if the pain extends, moves, or radiates. Commonly, pain associated with the heart radiates to the arms, neck, and back. Pain associated with an aortic aneurysm (a weakened and ballooned segment of the wall of the aorta) commonly radiates to the back in the lumbar region. Kidney stones commonly produce pain in the flank area (side) that radiates down along the groin.
- Severity—*How bad is the symptom?* Have the patient rate the pain on a scale of 1 to 10 with 10 being the most severe. Have the patient compare the pain with a previous condition they may have suffered that involved pain. The patient's appearance should give you some indication as to the severity of the pain. Is the patient squirming about in pain or easily distracted from the pain?
- Time—*How long have you had the symptom?* Determine if the symptom has been present for minutes, hours, days, weeks, months, or years. If you get called to the scene and find a patient complaining of a symptom that has been present for more than a day, ask the patient, "Why did you call us today?" If the symptoms have been present for a few hours or more, ask the patient, "Was there any change in the symptoms that caused you to call?" Most times the patient will call EMS when the pain gets worse, changes in quality, or if other associated signs or symptoms occur. Do not assume that a patient suffering pain or some other symptom accesses EMS immediately. The length of time the symptoms are present is important to document.

Obtain a SAMPLE History

You will have gained information about the patient's symptoms in response to the OPQRST questions. Information about the patient's signs will be gained during the physical exam and vital signs measurements. To complete the SAMPLE history, determine the patient's allergies, medications, pertinent past medical history, last oral intake, and events leading to

the present illness, as described earlier for the unresponsive medical patient.

Perform a Focused Medical Assessment

For the responsive medical patient, the physical exam comes after the SAMPLE history. This will be a focused exam, not the head-to-toe rapid assessment required for an unresponsive patient. The responsive patient's complaints should direct you to the appropriate areas for assessment. For example, if a patient is complaining of nontraumatic chest pain, possibly related to a heart problem, you would focus the assessment on the neck, chest, abdomen, and extremities. However, if the patient's signs and symptoms are not specific enough to make a decision about what areas to focus on—for example, a complaint such as "I just don't feel well"—you should perform a complete head-to-toe rapid medical assessment. The rapid medical assessment components will be the same as for the unresponsive medical patient.

Assess Baseline Vital Signs

Obtain the breathing rate and quality; pulse rate and quality; skin temperature, color, and condition; capillary refill in infants and children less than 6; pupil size and reactivity; and blood pressure.

Critical findings and interventions would be the same as those that were listed for the unresponsive medical patient.

Provide Emergency Care

Emergency care provided to the patient will be based on the information gathered from the focused or rapid medical assessment and in consultation with medical direction. General care involves maintaining a patent airway, administering high flow oxygen, and assisting breathing if necessary.

Make a Transport Decision

For a patient whose condition is not critical, the patient can be prepared for transport following the focused history and physical exam and provision of any required emergency care at the scene. If the patient's condition is critical, this procedure can be expedited by having one EMT-B partner begin preparing the patient for transport while the other is completing the assessment. Once on-scene management of life-threatening conditions has been accomplished—such as ensuring a patent airway or providing positive pressure ventilation with supplemental oxygen if breathing is inadequate—the critical medical patient should be transported promptly with additional assessment and emergency care provided en route. Review Table 9-7 on page 165 for criteria for which immediate transport is required. Prompt transport is the key to the survival of the critical patient.

During transport, reassess the airway, breathing, and pulses. The vital signs will be taken every 5 minutes in the critical patient and every 15 minutes in the noncritical patient. For any unresponsive patient or patient whose signs and symptoms are too general to pinpoint, a detailed physical exam should be conducted if time and the patient's condition permit. On any patient, it is necessary to assess the effectiveness of the interventions provided. For example, make sure that a nonrebreather mask is securely placed and that oxygen is flowing adequately. You should develop a pattern:

1. Assess
2. Intervene
3. Reassess

In the medical patient, you must rely heavily on the complaints of the patient and the signs and symptoms found during the focused or rapid medical assessment to proceed with emergency care. You are not required to diagnose a medical condition or disease process but rather to recognize significant signs and symptoms and, based on these findings, provide care to manage life threats. Whenever you are in doubt or whenever local protocols require it, consult with medical direction prior to providing care.

PART 4
DETAILED PHYSICAL EXAM

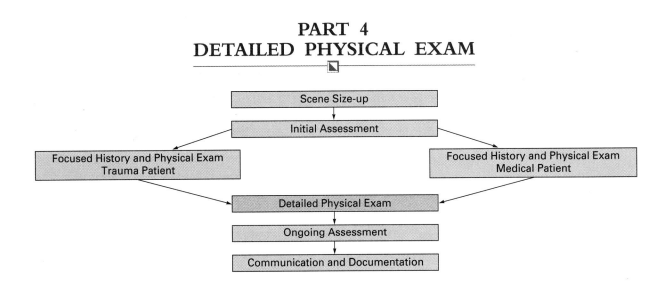

OBJECTIVES

Numbered objectives are from the United States Department of Transportation 1994 EMT-Basic National Standard Curriculum. Asterisked objectives, if any, pertain to material that is supplemental to the DOT curriculum.

COGNITIVE

3-5.1 Discuss the components of the detailed physical exam. (p. 196)
3-5.2 State the areas of the body that are evaluated during the detailed physical exam. (pp. 196–206)
3-5.3 Explain what additional care should be provided while performing the detailed physical exam. (p. 195)

3-5.4 Distinguish between the detailed physical exam that is performed on a trauma patient and that of the medical patient. (pp. 195–206)

AFFECTIVE

3-5.5 Explain the rationale for the feelings that these patients might be experiencing. (pp. 148, 196, 205)

PSYCHOMOTOR

3-5.6 Demonstrate the skills involved in performing the detailed physical exam.

The purpose of the detailed physical exam is to identify all other non-life-threatening injuries and to provide care required for those injuries or conditions.

WHEN TO PERFORM A DETAILED PHYSICAL EXAM

The **detailed physical exam** (Figure 9-32) is performed following the focused history and physical exam and only after all life-threatening injuries and conditions have been effectively managed. The exam is much more detailed than the rapid assessment, so it takes more time to complete. The exam should only be conducted if the patient's condition allows the attention of the EMT-B to be diverted from ongoing critical care.

Time is also a factor to consider. Most often, the detailed physical exam is performed in the back of the ambulance while en route to the hospital. It may be performed at the scene if ambulance response is delayed (for example, when you are serving as a first response unit that does not transport and awaiting ambulance arrival, or when you are providing emergency care when off duty, or when there are multiple patients, some of whom are awaiting additional ambulances). In a patient not considered to be critically ill or injured, it is acceptable to perform the detailed exam at the scene in order to gain additional information about the patient's condition prior to transport. If there is any question as to when the exam should be conducted, it is better to err to benefit the patient and conduct the exam en route.

If the patient is considered critically injured or ill, you must devote whatever time is necessary to monitor and care for life-threatening conditions. There must be ongoing attention to the airway, breathing, and circulation. Vital signs must be taken every 5 minutes for the critical patient. All of this may mean that there is not time to perform a detailed assessment to search for additional non-life-threatening problems.

You will conduct the detailed physical exam only if you have the time available and the patient's condition allows it.

HOW TO PERFORM A DETAILED PHYSICAL EXAM

The detailed physical exam is patient- and injury-specific. An unresponsive patient requires a complete detailed exam. So does a responsive patient with multiple trauma or a significant mechanism of injury. Any patient on whom you performed a complete head-to-toe

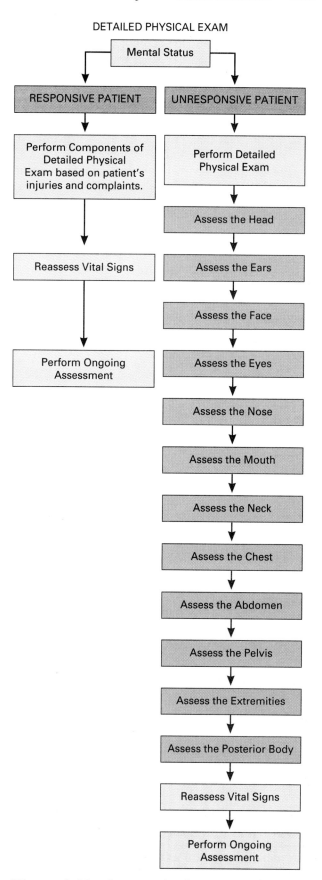

Figure 9-32   Steps of the detailed physical exam.

rapid assessment during the focused history and physical exam is a candidate for a complete detailed exam.

On the other hand, a patient who is complaining of specific symptoms and exhibiting specific signs—a patient on whom you performed a focused assessment during the focused history and physical exam—will be examined using only the necessary components of the detailed physical exam to gather additional information about the specific injury or illness.

For example, a patient with an isolated minor injury such as a lacerated foot, without a significant mechanism of injury, requires only a component of the detailed physical exam. The patient's specific injury site, the lower extremity, will be assessed further. If the injury resulted from a blunt force applied to the body, e.g., a fall, you should have a high index of suspicion and perform a complete detailed exam looking for evidence of other injuries. Use your suspicions to determine what areas of the body need further assessment.

Use the techniques of inspection, palpation, and auscultation to further identify signs, symptoms, and complaints of the patient. Any clothing that interferes with your ability to examine the patient properly should be cut on the anterior part and allowed to fall away. Take modesty into consideration and cover the patient with a sheet.

When conducting the detailed exam, the injuries will be managed as found. If you note swelling and deformity to the lower portion of the left arm, you will closely assess the area, immobilize it, and continue with the assessment. Bone injuries and soft tissue injuries such as lacerations, abrasions, and punctures are managed as found during the detailed exam.

If any doubt exists as to how extensively to assess the patient, complete the entire detailed exam. Remember, however—as stated above—the detailed physical exam should not be performed at all if it will divert attention that is required by the ongoing care of life-threatening injuries or medical conditions.

The steps of the detailed physical exam are as follows:

Steps of the Detailed Physical Exam

1. Perform the detailed physical exam.
2. Reassess the vital signs.
3. Continue emergency care.

PERFORM THE DETAILED PHYSICAL EXAM

The detailed physical exam (Figures 9-33 to 9-39) should be conducted systematically, starting at the head. The steps of the detailed physical exam are similar to those of the rapid trauma or medical assessment. However, the assessment of each part is more thorough and less hurried than during the rapid assessment, when life-threatening conditions had to be quickly discovered and managed.

ASSESS THE HEAD

Inspect the head and scalp for any deformities, contusions, abrasions, punctures, burns, lacerations, or swelling (Figure 9-33a). If conducted at the scene on the trauma patient with a spinal injury, spinal stabilization as applied during the initial assessment will be maintained. If the exam is conducted en route to the hospital, the patient will be immobilized to the backboard. Depending on the type of device used, your access to the head may be limited. Do not remove any immobilization device to further examine the head.

Palpate the entire head. Start at the parietal region (top of the head) and work your way down to the occipital region (back of the head). Palpate the temporal (side) and frontal regions of the skull. Do not poke your fingers into the scalp or skull. Cup your hands together and palpate with the palms of the hands. This will reduce the possibility of damage to the brain from inadvertently pushing in bone ends during palpation. Note any crepitation, depressions, deformities, or protrusions. Also, when palpating, note any tenderness to the head or scalp. Look at your gloved hands for evidence of blood when palpating. This is extremely useful in patients with dark hair or at night when blood is difficult to see.

Ears Inspect the ears for trauma to the external auditory canal. Look for deformities, contusions, abrasions, punctures, burns, lacerations, or swelling. Move into a position to allow you to look inside the ear with a flashlight for blood or other fluid (Figure 9-33b). A light-yellow-colored clear fluid flowing from the ear is most likely cerebrospinal fluid (CSF). Leakage of CSF usually indicates a skull fracture. If bleeding is occurring from the ear, place a loose dressing over the ear to catch the blood. Do not pack the ears or restrict the bleeding.

Look behind the ears for discoloration over the bony prominence known as the mastoid process (Figure 9-33c). Ecchymosis (black-and-blue discoloration) to the mastoid area is known as Battle's sign. This is a late sign of possible skull or head injury.

Face Inspect the entire facial region to include the eyes, nose, and mouth. Look for deformities, contusions, abrasions, punctures, burns, lacerations, or swelling. Palpate for deformity, swelling, and tenderness (Figure 9-33d). Injuries to the face are typically very dramatic and potentially life threatening. Bleeding or displacement of bone or tissue into the airway will cause an obstruction. Clear the airway with suction and insert an oropharyngeal airway if necessary

THE DETAILED PHYSICAL EXAM

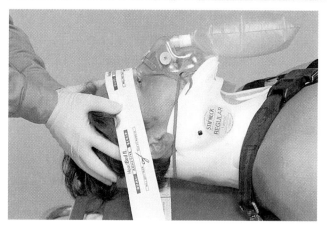

Figure 9-33a   Inspect the head for signs of trauma. Carefully palpate the skull for abnormalities.

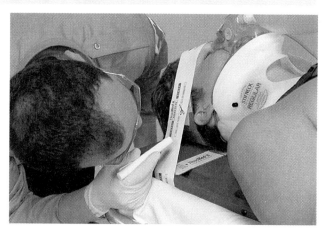

Figure 9-33b   Inspect and palpate the ear. Note any leakage of blood or fluid.

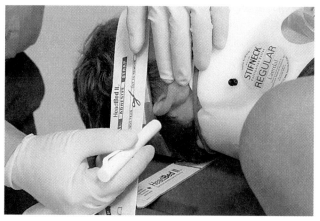

Figure 9-33c   Inspect behind the ears for any discoloration.

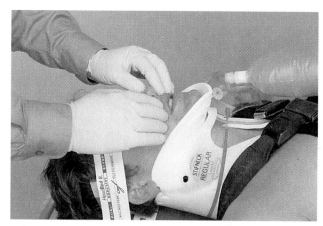

Figure 9-33d   Inspect and palpate the face. Note any deformity, instability, burns, or swelling.

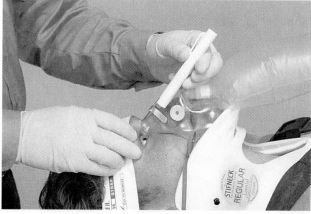

Figure 9-33e   Assess both pupils for equality of size and reactivity to light. Inspect the color of the sclerae.

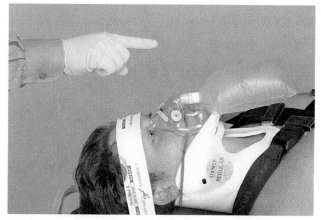

Figure 9-33f   Check eye movement by having the patient follow your finger. Note any gazes in one direction or jerky eye movements.

(Continued on the next page.)

THE DETAILED PHYSICAL EXAM continued

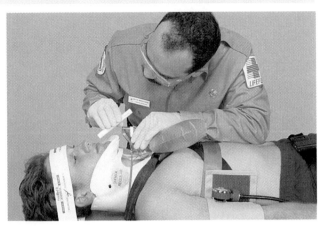

Figure 9-33g   *Inspect the conjunctiva by pulling the lower eyelid down.*

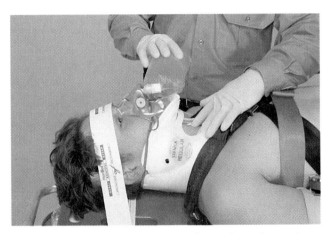

Figure 9-33h   *Inspect and palpate the nose for any signs of trauma, burns, bleeding, or fluid leakage.*

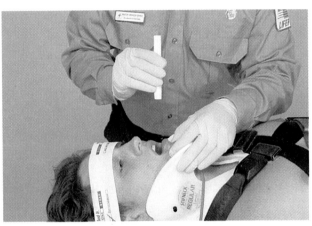

Figure 9-33i   *Inspect the inside of the mouth for signs of trauma, burns, and discoloration. Note the color of the mucous membranes. Smell the breath for any unusual odor.*

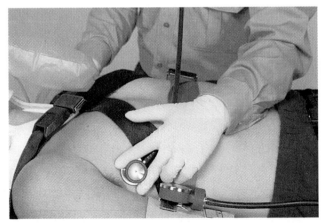

Figure 9-34   *Assess the neck for jugular vein distention, tracheal deviation, accessory muscle use, and subcutaneous emphysema.*

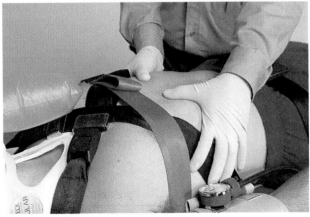

Figure 9-35a   *Inspect and palpate the entire chest. Check for symmetry of chest wall movement. Palpate the sternum, clavicles, and shoulders.*

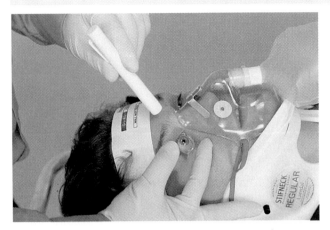

Figure 9-35b   *Auscultate breath sounds, comparing one side to the other.*

THE DETAILED PHYSICAL EXAM continued

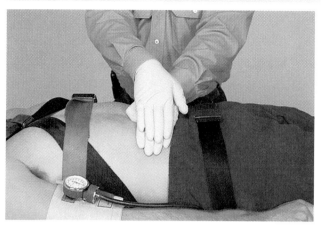

Figure 9-36 *Inspect and palpate each quadrant of the abdomen. Note any guarding, tenderness, or rigidity.*

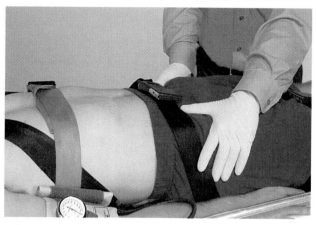

Figure 9-37 *Assess the stability of the pelvis in a patient who is unresponsive or who has no noted pain in that area.*

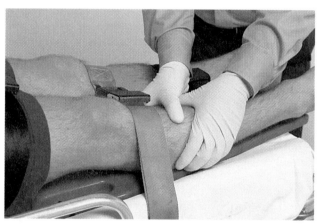

Figure 9-38a *Inspect and palpate each lower extremity. Look for signs of wounds, bleeding, deformity, swelling, and discoloration.*

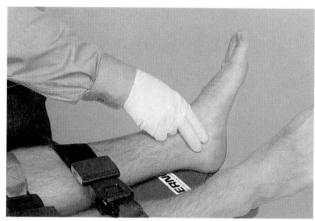

Figure 9-38b *Assess distal pulses in each lower extremity. Also note skin color, temperature, and condition.*

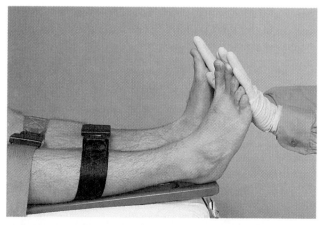

Figure 9-38c *Check motor response of both lower extremities by having the patient push both feet against your hands. Compare and note the equality of strength.*

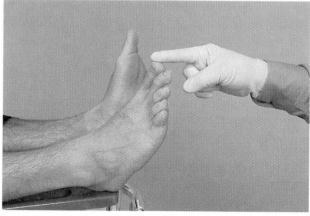

Figure 9-38d *Assess sensation by lightly touching a toe and asking the patient to identify which toe you are touching. If the patient is unresponsive, pinch the foot and note the patient's reaction.*

(Continued on the next page.)

THE DETAILED PHYSICAL EXAM continued

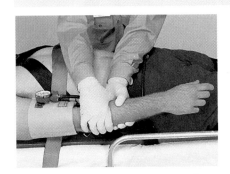

Figure 9-39a Inspect and palpate each upper extremity.

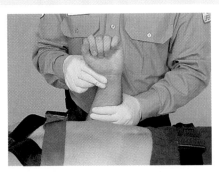

Figure 9-39b Assess the radial pulse on each upper extremity. Note skin color, temperature, and condition.

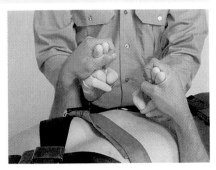

Figure 9-39c Assess motor function by having the patient grip the fingers of both your hands simultaneously. Note equality of strength. Assess sensory function by asking the patient to identify which finger you are touching. If the patient is unresponsive, pinch the hand and note the patient's reaction.

Conclude the detailed physical exam by inspecting and palpating the posterior body to the extent that immobilization of the patient allows.

and appropriate. Palpate the facial bones for deformity, instability, and crepitation. If any trauma is noted, continue to closely monitor the airway for bleeding and excessive swelling. Inspect and palpate the maxilla (upper jawbone) and mandible (lower jawbone) for any deformity or instability. The patient should be able to move the mandible without excessive pain. If the patient is unable to close his mouth, or if the teeth do not align well, the mandible is likely to be fractured or dislocated. With an injury to the maxilla or mandible, your major concern is maintaining a patent airway.

Inspect the face for singed or burnt eyebrows, nasal hair, beards, or hairline. Burns to the face should make you suspicious that the patient may be suffering from an upper airway burn. Upper airway burns frequently result in severe swelling and airway closure at the level of the larynx. If stridor (high pitched sounds on inspiration) is noted, consider positive pressure ventilation with supplemental oxygen, immediate transport, and advanced life support intervention for advanced airway management.

Eyes Inspect for deformities, contusions, abrasions, punctures, burns, lacerations, or swelling. Look especially for lacerations or trauma to the eyelids and eyeball. Do not attempt to remove foreign bodies embedded in the eye. If the patient has burns, lacerations,

or any other injuries to the eyelids, assume that the eye is also damaged. Do not force the eyelid open. Do not apply any pressure to the eye.

If the patient is unresponsive and is wearing hard contact lenses that are not properly positioned over the pupil, remove the lenses. Place them in a container with a small amount of saline, marking the container for the left and right contact. Be sure to transport the lenses with the patient. If the patient has a chemical burn to the eye, remove the contact lens to allow for adequate flushing. If the contact lens is left in place during flushing, the chemical trapped under the lens will continue to burn the eye.

Check for pupillary response (Figure 9-33e). In a dark environment, shine a light in the eye of the patient. In a bright environment, shade the eye with your hand. Both pupils should react simultaneously and equally to light being shined in either eye. This is referred to as a *consensual reflex*. While shining a light into one eye, watch the pupillary reaction of the other eye. Then shine the light a second time in the first eye and watch the pupillary reaction of that eye. Thus, the light is shined in each eye twice, first to check the response of the opposite pupil to the light, and then to check the reaction of the pupil in the eye to which the light is applied. Also, observe whether pupil response is brisk or sluggish. Under normal conditions, the pupils should respond briskly. Poor perfusion to the brain, high levels of carbon dioxide, or brain injuries may cause the pupils to respond sluggishly.

The size of the pupils is important to note. Unequal pupils usually indicate a head injury or stroke. A pupil that is large in size and not responding to light is referred to as being fixed and dilated. In cardiac arrest or severe injury to the brain both pupils may be *fixed and dilated*. Pupils that are pinpoint, or extremely constricted, and unresponsive usually indicate an injury to the brain stem or a patient under the influence of a narcotic substance.

A small portion of the population normally have unequal pupils. However, there is usually less than 1 mm difference, and their pupils remain reactive to light. Also, it is extremely important to consider the patient's level of responsiveness when determining the seriousness of the pupillary size. If the patient has unequal pupils but is completely alert and oriented, consider direct trauma to the eye, a localized nerve injury, or that the patient has used eye drops such as atropine or pilocarpine. Rely heavily on the level of responsiveness to confirm the findings of the pupils.

Check *visual acuity* (clarity of vision) by having the patient tell you how many fingers you are holding up or by reading your name tag. Hold your finger in front of the patient and have him follow it up, down, left, right, and in a circular pattern (Figure 9-33f). This checks the extraocular muscle movements. The eyes should move together *(conjugate movement)* and smoothly. Jerky eye movements *(nystagmus)* usually results from drugs or central nervous system effects. A single eye that is fixed or has a gaze in one direction *(dysconjugate gaze)* usually indicates injury to the orbit, muscles, or nerves.

Inspect the white portion of the eye, termed the *sclera,* for a redness or a yellow color. Yellow sclerae, known as *icterus,* is an indication of possible liver damage or failure. Pull the bottom part of the eye down and check the conjunctiva (Figure 9-33g). Poor perfusion, as in shock, causes the conjunctiva to appear pale. Extremely red conjunctivae with reddened sclerae is typically caused by eye irritation.

Blood in the anterior eye is a sign that the eye or the head has received a forceful blow. Inspect the eye by shining a light from the side to detect a reddish discoloration that is diffuse in a supine patient or that forms a crescent shape along the lower portion of the eye in an upright patient.

Nose Inspect the nose for deformities, contusions, abrasions, punctures, burns, lacerations, or swelling (Figure 9-33h). Look for fluid or blood drainage, nasal flaring, and singed nasal hair. Bleeding from the anterior nose is usually easily controlled by pinching the nostrils together. However some patients, especially the elderly with a history of high blood pres-

sure, experience severe posterior nosebleeds in which the bleeding is very difficult to control. Many times, the patient swallows large amounts of blood, becomes nauseated, and vomits. The vomitus contains blood and may easily be incorrectly assessed as internal bleeding in the stomach. The patient could lose a large volume of blood from the nosebleed.

Leakage of cerebrospinal fluid indicates a skull fracture which may have an associated brain injury. Singed nasal hair should increase your suspicion that the patient has been involved in a fire and possibly has an upper airway burn.

Nasal flaring, which is identified by the nares (nostrils) opening wide during inspiration, is a sign of respiratory distress. Reassess the patient closely for other evidence of airway or breathing problems.

Palpate the nose for deformity, swelling, or instability. Your major concern with an injury to the nose is possible bleeding into the airway. Be prepared to suction the airway.

Mouth Open the mouth and inspect for deformities, contusions, abrasions, punctures, burns, lacerations, or swelling (Figure 9-33i). Look for loose or missing teeth, loose or missing dentures, and discoloration of the mucosa (lining). Loose dentures should be removed in unresponsive patients so they do not fall back into the throat and become an airway obstruction. Remove any objects by suction or, if too large to suction, with your fingers. Inspect the tongue for lacerations and swelling, a possible sign that the patient has had a seizure (biting the tongue is common during seizures). Look for discoloration. Cyanosis (bluish color) of the mucosa indicates inadequate oxygenation. A pale tongue may indicate poor perfusion and shock. Any burns or extremely white areas may be caused by ingestion of a chemical poison.

Place your face close to the patient's nose and mouth and smell for any unusual odors. An alcohol odor may make you suspect alcohol intoxication as a reason for an altered mental status. It is necessary always to be suspicious that the patient's condition is from some cause other than alcohol. Look for other evidence of trauma or medical illness. A fruity odor on the breath may indicate a diabetic patient with an abnormally high blood sugar level. Also, smell for other unusual odors like rubbing alcohol, cologne, cleaners, and solvents. A desperate alcoholic may drink cologne or cough syrup because of the alcohol content. Children may accidentally ingest cleaners or solvents. Antifreeze may be ingested by teenagers as a means to get drunk.

Look for black sputum and burns inside of the mouth if the patient was involved in a fire. Suspect upper airway burns and be prepared to aggressively manage the airway and breathing if burning to the mouth or face is noted.

The mouth may provide some signs as to the oxygenation, breathing, or perfusion status. However, your chief concern is to ensure that the mouth is clear of potential airway obstructions.

ASSESS THE NECK

Inspect the neck much more closely than you did during the rapid assessment (Figure 9-34). Look for deformities, contusions, abrasions, punctures, burns, lacerations, or swelling. Large lacerations of the neck must be covered with an occlusive dressing to prevent air being sucked into a large vein, causing an air embolus. With any trauma to the neck, you should suspect possible cervical spinal injury and provide in-line spinal stabilization, if it has not already been applied. If a cervical spinal immobilization collar is in place, you typically will not remove it to inspect or palpate the neck. Most devices are manufactured with a large hole on the anterior surface to permit reassessment of the neck for JVD, blood collecting under the skin, or tracheal deviation.

The neck may appear large or swollen. This may be due to blood collection in or around the tissues or air trapped under the skin. Because of the large vessels, bleeding in the neck could be severe. A *hematoma* (collection of blood) could compress the airway or trachea and cause obstruction. Air trapped under the skin may be better palpated than seen. If you palpate an unusual sensation of air under the skin, and feel or hear crepitation (crackling), it is a sign of *subcutaneous emphysema*. Subcutaneous emphysema (which means, simply, air under the skin) is a sign of trauma to the airway, respiratory tract, lung, or esophagus. You should closely reassess the chest for evidence of chest injury and closely monitor the breathing status.

Reassess the jugular veins for distention. The jugular veins slightly distend normally in the supine patient with a normal blood volume. If possible, the jugular veins should be assessed with the patient sitting at a 45 degree angle. If two-thirds of the jugular vein is filled or engorged from the base of the neck up toward the angle of the jaw, then jugular vein distention (JVD) is present. Do not have the trauma patient with suspected spinal injuries sit up to check the neck veins. JVD is a sign of a possible *tension pneumothorax* (air trapped in the chest cavity as a result of chest or lung injury), *pericardial tamponade* (blood filling the sac around the heart), or congestive heart failure. It is vital to reassess the effectiveness of the breathing status, pulses, perfusion, and blood pressure if JVD is noted.

Check the trachea to ensure it is midline. A shifted or deviated trachea is a late sign of tension pneumothorax. It may be easier to palpate the location of the trachea than to see it. Start at the suprasternal notch (the indention where the right and left clavicle come together at the top of the sternum) and palpate with your thumb and index finger to feel the position of the trachea. It should be midline all the way up to the larynx.

Since a tension pneumothorax is a life-threatening condition, whenever tracheal deviation is noted you must immediately reassess the breathing and perfusion status. If the trachea tugs or moves to one side during inhalation, there may be an airway obstruction in the bronchi. Reassess for adequate breathing.

Another sign to look for is excessive neck muscle use. These muscles become very prominent when a patient is having difficulty with inspiration. Check for other signs of respiratory distress and inadequate breathing and provide positive pressure ventilation with supplemental oxygen if necessary.

If a cervical spinal immobilization collar was applied, the neck would have been quickly palpated for any deformities during the rapid assessment. If a collar is not in place, palpate the anterior neck and posterior neck for deformities or spasms.

ASSESS THE CHEST

Assessment of the chest during the detailed physical exam is much more thorough than during the rapid assessment. Life-threatening injuries to the chest should have already been managed during the initial assessment and rapid assessment. This exam is to discover additional signs and symptoms of injury or medical illness.

In the trauma patient, if not already done, expose the chest completely. Inspect the chest (Figure 9-35a) for evidence of trauma including deformities, contusions, abrasions, punctures, burns, lacerations, or swelling. Watch for retractions (the muscles between the ribs pulling inward during inspiration), a sign of respiratory distress. Retractions are seen more often in infants and children than in adults.

Determine if the chest is rising and falling symmetrically (evenly on both sides) or if one side of the chest appears to remain elevated during exhalation. Asymmetrical (uneven) chest wall movement is a sign of a significant pneumothorax or flail segment. Many times it is easier to feel asymmetry than to see it. Any punctures, lacerations, or other open wounds to the chest should have been managed during either the initial assessment or the rapid trauma assessment.

Look for any segments of the chest that are moving inward during inspiration and outward during exhalation, opposite to the direction of the rest of the chest. This is referred to as paradoxical motion and is a sign of a flail segment. A flail segment is considered an immediately life-threatening injury that should have been managed, if discovered, during the initial or rapid trauma assessment. However, immediately following the blunt chest injury in which a flail segment has occurred, the muscles between the ribs will commonly spasm and keep the free rib section stabilized. Therefore, you may not see exaggerated movement of the flail segment and may not detect it during the earlier assessments. Later during the call, when you are performing the detailed exam, it may become apparent that the chest wall is moving paradoxically. Stabilization of the segment is necessary. Usually, palpation will more easily identify an unstable section. Closely palpate the sides of the chest since the most common site of a flail segment is to the lateral chest wall.

Feel the chest to confirm the findings of the inspection. Check for symmetry of respirations by placing each hand with the thumbs pointed inward toward the sternum (breastbone) over the right and left lower portion of the rib cage. Both hands should move an equal distance with each breath. Also palpate for any tenderness, instability, and crepitation (crackling or crunching sounds beneath the skin), signs of subcutaneous emphysema. Apply light pressure with both hands downward and inward, slightly compressing the rib cage. If there is any rib or muscular injury, the patient will complain of pain. If the patient is already complaining of chest pain from an injury, do not compress the chest. If you suspect possible rib fractures or chest wall injury, reassess the breathing status. Because of the pain, the patient may be purposely breathing extremely shallowly and rapidly, decreasing the adequacy of breathing.

Palpate the sternum by pushing down gently with the ulnar edge of one or both hands. A pain response may indicate rib or sternum injury.

Children's rib cages are extremely pliable and flexible. Significant blunt or compression injury may not cause any fractures to occur; however, significant injury to the internal organs may be present. Look at the mechanism of injury and have a high index of suspicion if the mechanism of injury has been significant. Continuously monitor the patient for signs and symptoms of poor perfusion, respiratory distress, and shock.

Inspect and palpate the shoulder girdle (articulation of the clavicle and shoulder), the clavicles (collarbones), and scapulae (shoulder blades) for deformity, crepitation, and tenderness. Palpate the clavicles with the pads of your fingers beginning at the sternum and moving toward the shoulder. Gently slide your hand under the back on each side to palpate each scapula. Cup your hand around the shoulder girdle and compress lightly.

If the patient is not immobilized or secured to a backboard and does not have a suspected spinal injury, roll the patient or sit the patient forward to assess the posterior thorax, looking for signs of trauma.

Inspect and palpate the entire anterior and lateral chest. Injuries could easily be missed if you do not look at the patient's sides and in the axillary region (under the armpit).

Auscultation Listen to the chest with your stethoscope to determine if the breath sounds are present or absent, equal or unequal, normal or abnormal (Figure 9-35b). Place your stethoscope just below the second rib at the midclavicular line to listen to the apices of the lungs and just below the fourth rib at the midaxillary line for breath sounds in the bases. Compare the sounds of the lobes on both sides of the chest. Absent or diminished breath sounds are a sign of air, blood, or fluid in the chest cavity or obstruction of a bronchus. Typically only one side has diminished or absent breath sounds, indicating which lung is injured.

In the medical patient, breath sounds are important to auscultate if the patient is complaining of dyspnea (shortness of breath or difficult breathing), hives and itching, or has a history of allergies, anaphylactic (severe allergic) reaction, asthma, emphysema, or chronic bronchitis.

Wheezes are prolonged, high-pitched sounds most often heard on exhalation. Wheezes indicate narrowing of the airways at the level of the bronchiole. It is important to note whether the wheezing is diffuse (throughout the lung fields) or isolated to one section of the lung. Diffuse wheezing heard in all the lung fields is usually due to narrowing or spasm of the airways associated with asthma, anaphylaxis, emphysema, or chronic bronchitis. Isolated wheezing heard in only one area of the lung is a sign of localized lung infection or obstruction.

Fluid collection in the lungs produces crackles, a sound also sometimes called rales. A harsher snoring sound heard upon auscultation, called rhonchi, is from mucus in the larger airways within the lung.

Stridor, a high-pitched sound, is from partial obstruction of the upper airway at the level of the larynx. It is usually caused by a foreign body or swelling. Closely monitor the airway and provide positive pressure ventilation with supplemental oxygen if inadequate breathing is found.

Coughing is a response to bronchial irritation. Smoke, chemicals, or other inhaled gases may cause the patient to cough. If you suspect the patient has inhaled a toxic substance such as smoke, place the patient on a nonrebreather mask at 15 lpm. If mucus is produced with the cough, which is referred to as a *productive cough*, note the color, consistency, amount, and odor. Mucus is normally white and clear. Yellow or green mucus is a sign of possible infection. Also note any blood-tinged sputum (substance produced by coughing). This may indicate lung injury, airway trauma, or a cardiac or pulmonary disease. Be sure to inspect inside the mouth for lacerations if blood is found in the sputum.

Assess the Abdomen

It is best to examine the abdomen with the patient lying flat (Figure 9-36). Notice the posture of the patient. A patient lying extremely still with his knees drawn up toward the chest and with breathing that is fast and shallow is most likely suffering from significant abdominal pain. Expose the abdomen and inspect all four anterior quadrants and the lateral aspects for obvious signs of injury such as deformities, contusions, abrasions, punctures, burns, or lacerations. Look for impaled objects or open wounds with protruding organs.

Look at the abdomen for signs of swelling or distention. The abdomen could be distended from air, fluid, or blood. If the abdomen appears to be distended, look for signs of poor perfusion and shock. A significant amount of blood must be lost in the abdomen before it distends. (Two liters of blood in the abdomen may distend the girth of the abdomen by only one inch.) Note any discoloration around the navel or in the flank areas. Bleeding in the abdomen may cause discoloration to these areas; however, this is a very late sign that takes several hours to develop.

The patient may have a colostomy or ileostomy. This is a surgical opening in the abdominal wall with a bag to hold excretions from the digestive tract. Leave the bag in place and be careful not to displace or cut it. Keep the bag covered from view to save the patient from possible embarrassment.

Ask if the patient is having any abdominal pain prior to palpating. Palpate all four quadrants of the abdomen separately using the pads of your fingers with one hand on top of the other. Roll the hands across the quadrant assessing for rigidity or stiffness, tenderness or pain, and distention. (A soft abdomen is normal.) If the patient is complaining of pain, have him point to the pain with one finger. If the patient can localize the pain in this manner, start your palpation at the point farthest away from the pain and move inward. Palpate the painful quadrant last. When palpating, listen to the patient's response. In the unresponsive patient, watch the patient's face and body movement for an indication of a painful response to palpation.

A pulsating mass in the abdomen may indicate that the abdominal aorta is weakened and bulging. If noted, this requires immediate transport to a medical facility, if transport is not already under way.

The patient may reflexively guard his abdomen by tightening the muscles. Voluntary guarding (guarding the patient is able to control) is common when you begin to assess the abdomen. Attempt to distract the patient with conversation to stop the guarding. If the abdomen remains rigid, it is a sign of *peritonitis* (inflammation or irritation of the lining of the abdomen) from blood, gastric contents, bacteria, or other substances. Taking a deep breath usually produces pain, so the patient typically breathes shallowly and fast.

Do not palpate over obvious injuries or areas of severe pain. Do not poke the abdomen. If an impaled object is present, do not remove it. Stabilize the object in place. An evisceration is when organs, most commonly the small intestines, are protruding from an open abdominal wound. Do not attempt to put the organs back into the abdominal cavity. Cover them with a moist sterile dressing and seal with a large occlusive dressing.

Assess the Pelvis

Injury to the pelvis should be sought during the rapid trauma assessment because of the potential seriousness of associated bleeding. If the patient does not complain of pain or is unresponsive, gently flex and compress the pelvis to determine instability (Figure 9-37). Pelvic injuries are considered to be critical. If you identify a painful or unstable pelvis during the detailed exam, perform a rapid assessment and consider immediate transport if not already en route to the hospital.

Expose the pelvic area and inspect for deformities, contusions, abrasions, punctures, burns, lacerations, or swelling. Do not palpate if there is obvious injury or the patient is complaining of pain to the pelvis. Note any loss of bladder control, bleeding, or *priapism*. Priapism is a persistent erection of the penis in a male patient that is a possible sign of a head or spinal cord injury.

If the patient has no pain in the pelvic region or is unresponsive, place each hand on the anterior lateral wings of the pelvis and gently compress inward and downward. Do not rock the pelvis or apply unnecessary pressure. Assess for instability, tenderness, and crepitation. Place the base of your hand on the pubic bone, located immediately above the genitalia, and apply gentle pressure backward, checking for tenderness, crepitation, and instability.

If serious trauma to the area of the genitalia is suspected, for example penetrating trauma or major bleeding, expose and inspect the area. The male genitalia are relatively vascular (having many blood vessels); therefore, injury could result in significant blood loss. The female genitalia are most susceptible to penetrating trauma. Control bleeding to the external genitalia with direct pressure. If the female patient complains of vaginal bleeding, assess for signs and symptoms of shock. To assess the amount of bleeding, ask the patient how many tampons or sanitary pads she has used since the onset of the bleeding.

Respect the patient's feelings of modesty or embarrassment. Explain what you are doing and why and protect the patient's dignity and privacy by shielding the patient from the view of others during examination.

ASSESS THE LOWER EXTREMITIES

If any injury is suspected, cut the clothing away from the patient. Inspect the lower extremities, one at a time, from the hip to the toes (Figure 9-38a). Look for deformities (e.g., angulation), contusions, abrasions, punctures, burns, lacerations, or swelling. Watch for abnormal positioning. Injuries to the hip or femur may cause the leg to shorten or rotate inward or outward.

In the medical patient, look for excessive swelling around the ankles (peripheral edema). This may be an indication of possible cardiac failure.

Palpate the extremity by placing a hand on each side of the leg with the thumbs anteriorly and touching, if possible, and the little fingers to the posterior. Begin at the level of the groin and palpate down to the feet. The hands should never lose contact with the leg. Feel for any deformities, angulation, crepitation, or depressions. Determine if the patient feels pain, tenderness, numbness, or tingling.

If an injury is suspected, remove the shoes or boots. It may be necessary to cut the laces to avoid any unnecessary manipulation of the foot or leg during removal. If injury to the ankle or foot is suspected, cut the sock away. Ski boots should not be removed unless you are specially trained to do so.

Assess the distal pulses, motor function, and sensation. Loss of these functions is a sign of possible brain, spinal cord, or extremity injury.

Pulses   Assess the dorsalis pedis pulse on the top surface of the foot or the posterior tibial pulse located behind the medial malleolus (inner ankle bone) (Figure 9-38b). Compare the equality of the pulses in the two lower extremities. While feeling the pulse, check the skin color, temperature, and condition. If the pulse is absent and the skin is pale or cyanotic and cool, expect a possible blocked artery in that lower extremity. A blocked vein causes the extremity to become flushed, warm, swollen, and painful. Pedal and tibial pulses are frequently absent in patients suffering from severe blood loss and shock.

Motor Function   Have the patient move his toes. Check for equality of strength in the lower extremities by placing your hands on the soles of both feet and having the patient push down against your hands (Figure 9-38c). Then place your hands on the anterior surface of the feet and have the patient pull up against your hands. Note any inequality in strength. Do not check equality of strength if any obvious

bone or joint injury is found in the lower extremity. Any unnecessary movement should be avoided. Unequal strength may be a sign of head, spinal, or extremity injury.

Paralysis, in which the patient is unable to move or feel the extremity, may result from head or spinal injury or a stroke. Spinal injuries usually result in *paraplegia* (paralysis involving both legs only) or *quadriplegia* (paralysis involving both arms and both legs). A stroke or head injury commonly produces *hemiplegia* (paralysis of an arm and leg on one side of the body).

Sensation   Begin by lightly touching the toe on one foot and asking the patient to identify which toe you are touching (Figure 9-38d). Then pinch the foot to elicit a pain response. Repeat the same procedure for the opposite foot. (As noted for the rapid trauma assessment, is important to test both light touch and pain, since each stimulus is carried by a different spinal cord nerve tract.) Record if the patient responds appropriately to both light touch and painful stimulus. Make sure the patient is unable to see which foot you are touching or pinching. The patient may provide the right response because he is able to see which toe you are touching instead of feeling it.

In the unresponsive patient, pinch the extremity while looking at the patient's facial expression. A facial grimace usually indicates that the patient feels the pain. Also note any movement of the extremity, especially if it is withdrawal away from the source of pain. Clearly document the response to pain in your prehospital care report.

ASSESS THE UPPER EXTREMITIES

Inspect the upper extremities from the shoulder to the finger tip (Figure 9-39a). Look for deformities (e.g., angulation), contusions, abrasions, punctures, burns, lacerations, or swelling.

Palpate the entire extremity by placing a hand on each side of the arm with the thumbs touching on the anterior surface. Start at the most proximal portion of the arm and move down to the fingertips. Feel for any deformity, crepitation, or swelling. Note any pain or tenderness the patient experiences. In the unresponsive patient, watch the patient's face for grimacing and extremity movement, e.g., withdrawing the arm from the pain when applying a painful stimulus.

Assess the distal pulses, motor function, and sensation in both upper extremities.

Pulses   Assess the radial pulse, which is located at the base of the hand at the wrist on the thumb side (Figure 9-39b). Assess the color, temperature, and condition of the hand. Radial pulses may not be felt when there is severe blood loss. It is important to evaluate the mechanism of injury, mental status, and skin if radial pulses are not present.

Motor Function   Have the patient move his fingers. Check the equality of strength in both extremities simultaneously by having the patient grip your fingers and squeeze (Figure 9-39c). Head, spinal, or extremity injuries may cause the grip strength to be unequal. Do not check grip strength in an extremity with obvious injury as this will cause unnecessary movement.

Sensation   Touch the finger of one hand and ask the patient to identify which finger you are touching, making sure the patient cannot see what you are doing. Pinch the hand and note the response. In an unresponsive patient, it is necessary to pinch the hand in an attempt to elicit a response. Watch the face for a grimace and movement of the extremity that may indicate a response to the pain. Repeat the process for the other hand. Clearly document the type of response and the type of painful stimulus in your prehospital care report.

ASSESS THE POSTERIOR BODY

If the patient is not already secured to the backboard, roll the supine patient onto his side. If a spinal injury is suspected, manual in-line spinal stabilization must be maintained at all times until the patient is completely immobilized to the backboard. Inspect the posterior thorax, lumbar area, buttocks, and lower extremities for any deformities, contusions, abrasions, punctures, burns, lacerations, or swelling.

Palpate the posterior body for deformities and tenderness. If pain or tenderness is noted around any of the vertebrae, note the location and do not palpate the area. Palpating may cause further damage. Muscle spasm around the vertebrae is a sign of vertebral injury. Be extremely cautious in handling the patient. Ensure proper in-line spinal stabilization and avoid any excessive or unnecessary movements.

If the patient is already immobilized to the backboard, do not roll him to assess the posterior body. Simply place your hand at the flank area and slide it as far under the patient as possible. Check for any obvious deformity or pain.

REASSESS VITAL SIGNS

The vital signs should be reassessed throughout the entire time you are in contact with the patient, noting any changes or trends as compared to the set of baseline vital sign measurements you recorded during the focused history and physical exam (Figure 9-40). In an unresponsive or unstable patient, take the vital signs every 5 minutes. Responsive, stable patients

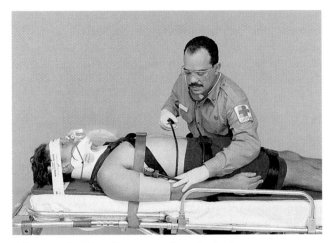

Figure 9-40   Reassess the vital signs.

should have the vital signs reassessed every 15 minutes. Set a priority for care and reassessment. In patients who need continuous supportive care, such as positive pressure ventilation, it may not be possible to reassess all the vital signs very often. Care of life threats takes precedence over the detailed exam and complete vital sign reassessment.

CONTINUE EMERGENCY CARE

Many problems you identify or suspect as a result of the detailed physical exam will be problems you, as an EMT-B, cannot directly treat, for example damage to the lungs, heart, or brain, artery blockages, or drug overdose. Remember that your chief concern is ongoing care for life-threatening problems affecting the patient's airway, breathing, and circulation and immobilization for suspected spinal injuries. The information you gather during the detailed physical exam should be used to alert you to life-threatening problems of this type as well as to any non-life-threatening conditions or injuries you can treat. Additionally, any findings you gather during the detailed physical exam should be thoroughly documented and reported to the staff of the receiving medical facility.

If at any time you are unsure as to whether the patient needs a focused approach or the complete detailed assessment, err to benefit the patient and complete the entire detailed physical exam. If you are in doubt as to the care you should provide in response to any of your findings, consult on-line medical direction.

Once the detailed assessment is complete, you would continue with the ongoing assessment of the patient. Portions of the ongoing assessment are included within the detailed physical exam, such as reassessment of the airway, breathing, and circulation status, and reassessment of the vital signs.

PART 5
ONGOING ASSESSMENT

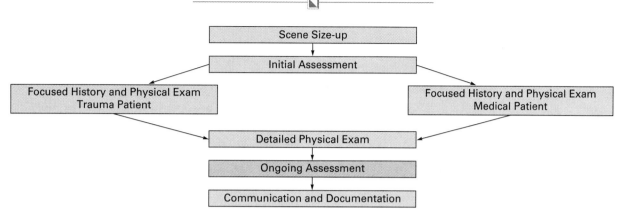

```
                    ┌─────────────────────┐
                    │   Scene Size-up      │
                    └──────────┬──────────┘
                    ┌──────────┴──────────┐
                    │  Initial Assessment │
                    └──────────┬──────────┘
        ┌──────────────────────┴──────────────────────┐
┌───────────────────────────┐           ┌───────────────────────────┐
│ Focused History and        │           │ Focused History and        │
│ Physical Exam              │           │ Physical Exam              │
│ Trauma Patient             │           │ Medical Patient            │
└───────────┬───────────────┘           └───────────────┬───────────┘
            └──────────────────┬──────────────────────────┘
                    ┌──────────┴──────────┐
                    │ Detailed Physical Exam │
                    └──────────┬──────────┘
                    ┌──────────┴──────────┐
                    │  Ongoing Assessment │
                    └──────────┬──────────┘
                    ┌──────────┴──────────────┐
                    │ Communication and Documentation │
                    └─────────────────────────┘
```

OBJECTIVES

Numbered objectives are from the United States Department of Transportation 1994 EMT-Basic National Standard Curriculum. Asterisked objectives, if any, pertain to material that is supplemental to the DOT curriculum.

COGNITIVE

3-6.1   Discuss the reasons for repeating the initial assessment as part of the ongoing assessment. (p. 209)
3-6.2   Describe the components of the ongoing assessment. (pp. 208–211)
3-6.3   Describe trending of assessment components. (p. 211)

AFFECTIVE

3-6.4   Explain the value of performing an ongoing assessment. (pp. 207–209)
3-6.5   Recognize and respect the feelings that patients might experience during assessment. (p. 148)
3-6.6   Explain the value of trending assessment components to other health professionals who assume care of the patient. (p. 211)

PSYCHOMOTOR

3-6.7   Demonstrate the skills involved in performing the ongoing assessment.

The **ongoing assessment** (Figure 9-41) is conducted following the detailed physical exam, if a detailed physical exam is performed. If the detailed physical exam is not performed, the ongoing assessment should begin immediately after the focused history and physical exam. Ongoing assessment is performed in the ambulance, continuously, until care of the patient is turned over to hospital personnel. If there is a delay in arrival of an ambulance for transport of the patient—for example when the EMT-B is performing a first response function, emergency care when off duty, or when multiple patients require dispatch of additional ambulances—ongoing assessment may begin at the scene and continue in the ambulance.

PURPOSES OF THE ONGOING ASSESSMENT

The purposes of the ongoing assessment are to determine any changes in the patient's condition and to assess the effectiveness of your emergency care. It should be performed on both the trauma and the medical patient, whether the patient is responsive or unresponsive, stable or unstable. If during the ongoing assessment you identify a critical patient condition, you should provide immediate care to correct the problem. For example, as you perform the assessment you note that the patient's breathing depth and quality have become inadequate. You would inter-

ONGOING ASSESSMENT

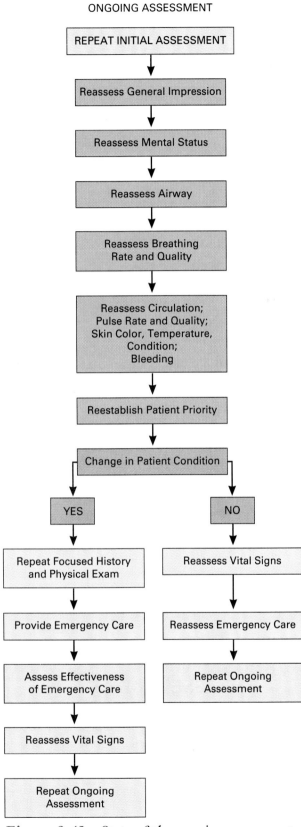

Figure 9-41 Steps of the ongoing assessment.

vene immediately to begin positive pressure ventilation with supplemental oxygen.

If this is a trauma patient, you would repeat the rapid trauma assessment looking for the possible cause of the deterioration of the patient. Does the patient now have signs of pneumothorax (air in the chest cavity, possibly from a damaged lung)? Did the occlusive dressing over an open chest wound become clotted, not allowing air to escape? Does the patient have a possible head injury? The rapid assessment should identify any signs and symptoms that may identify the possible cause of the patient's condition.

It is important to remember that the main objective is to intervene and provide the necessary emergency care for the life-threatening injuries or conditions, followed by reassessment. Remember that your routine should be as follows:

1. Assess
2. Intervene
3. Reassess

Unlike the detailed physical exam, which might not be conducted at all on some patients, the ongoing assessment must be performed on all patients.

The three basic reasons for performing an ongoing assessment are:

1. To detect any change in the patient's condition
2. To identify any missed injuries or conditions, especially those that are life threatening
3. To adjust the emergency care as needed

DETECT ANY CHANGE IN CONDITION

Rapid changes in the patient's condition can occur in the prehospital setting. Therefore, it is always necessary to look for signs and symptoms indicating deterioration as well as signs of improvement. Rapid deterioration is commonly due to continued blood loss, airway compromise, inadequate breathing, or brain injury. These areas are the focus of the ongoing assessment.

IDENTIIFY ANY MISSED INJURIES OR CONDITIONS

Many times the initial and rapid assessments are conducted in very poor environmental conditions that limit the EMT-B's ability to assess adequately. Extremely dark environments, for example, may limit your ability to see signs of injury. Noisy conditions, such as a hostile crowd or a busy highway, may interfere with your ability to hear breath sounds or patient complaints. Rain, bright sunshine, high winds, unstable vehicles, threats of explosion, smoke, or other conditions commonly reduce the effectiveness of assessment at the scene. The ongoing assessment provides the opportunity to reassess for injuries or conditions once the patient is in a more stable and favorable environment, which is most likely the patient compartment of the ambulance.

Additionally, if the patient's condition improves, he may begin to complain of other symptoms. You can then conduct a rapid assessment relevant to the areas of the new complaint, looking for additional signs of injury or illness.

ADJUST THE EMERGENCY CARE

The ongoing assessment allows you to reassess the effectiveness of the emergency care that you are providing. For example, you may have placed a nonrebreather mask with oxygen flowing at 15 liters per minute on a patient who was complaining of shortness of breath. During the reassessment, you determine that the patient's breathing depth has become extremely shallow, so you remove the nonrebreather mask and begin positive pressure ventilation with supplemental oxygen.

The steps of the ongoing assessment are as follows:

Steps of the Ongoing Assessment

1. Repeat the initial assessment.
2. Reassess and record vital signs.
3. Repeat the focused assessment for other complaints or injuries.
4. Check interventions.
5. Note trends in the patient's condition.

Repeat and record the assessment findings—particularly the components of the initial assessment and the vital signs—at least every 5 minutes in the unstable patient with critical injuries and every 15 minutes in a stable patient.

REPEAT THE INITIAL ASSESSMENT

Since the main objective of the initial assessment was to identify and manage life-threatening injuries, repetition of the initial assessment is also a key component of the ongoing assessment. It is necessary to assess the same parameters that were initially assessed.

REASSESS MENTAL STATUS

If the patient continues to talk to you throughout the entire call, reassess for any change in the speech pattern and appropriateness of his responses. A head-injured patient may continue to talk to you, but his speech pattern may become garbled and his responses inappropriate. This is a sign of continued bleeding or swelling within the skull. Also assess the patient's ability to obey commands appropriately.

If the patient is not alert or loses alertness, reassess the response based on the AVPU mnemonic. Record any change in the patient's mental status, whether it is improved or worsened.

REASSESS THE AIRWAY

If the patient is talking to you, assume the airway is patent. In the unresponsive patient, open the mouth and look inside for any evidence of blood, secretions, or vomitus. Suction the mouth if necessary. Listen for snoring sounds, gurgling, or stridor. Reassess the position of the nasopharyngeal or oropharyngeal airway if one has been inserted. Check to make sure either airway is not clogged with secretions, blood, or vomitus. If the patient is being ventilated, ask the EMT-B who is ventilating if any unusual resistance is felt. This may indicate an airway obstruction.

If the patient's condition improves and he can no longer tolerate an airway adjunct and begins to gag, remove it. Have suction available and position the patient on his side, if possible, before removing the airway. Loss of a gag or cough reflex, on the other hand, may require insertion of an airway.

REASSESS BREATHING

Look, listen, and feel for adequate breathing. If the breathing is determined to be inadequate because of poor quality or rate, begin positive pressure ventilation with supplemental oxygen. If the patient is already being ventilated, reassess effectiveness of the ventilation by looking at the rise and fall of the chest and watching for improvement in the patient's color and mental status. Also, ask the EMT-B who is ventilating if any unusual resistance is felt when squeezing the bag. If so, reevaluate the airway, the chest, the device being used for ventilation, the seal of the face mask, or the manner in which ventilation is being provided.

Apply oxygen to any patient who becomes unresponsive or has an alteration in mental status. Once oxygen is applied, continue to provide it, even if the patient's condition improves.

REASSESS CIRCULATION

REASSESS PULSE

Reassess and record the patient's pulse rate and quality. An increasing rate with poor quality may be a sign of continued bleeding. A decreasing pulse with poor quality may indicate a head injury or severe hypoxia (oxygen starvation). An increasing pulse in a patient who initially had a low rate may indicate an improvement in breathing and oxygenation. If a patient initially had an elevated pulse associated with bleeding, a decrease may indicate a reduction in the bleeding and an improvement in the patient's condition. It is important to evaluate the pulse rate in relationship to the initial findings and the injuries or medical condition.

REASSESS BLEEDING

Check the site of any major bleeding for blood seeping through the dressing and bandage, indicating the need to recontrol bleeding through elevation, pressure, and the application of additional dressings. If you detect any signs of increasing or continued blood loss, such as a decrease in perfusion or elevated pulse with poor quality, conduct a rapid assessment to detect the site of any external blood loss that you can control. Continue to treat for shock.

REASSESS SKIN

Look for skin color changes. Feel for changes in skin temperature and condition. Reassess capillary refill in infants and children. Improvements in oxygenation typically improve the color of the skin. Likewise, poor oxygenation from airway or breathing compromise will cause the skin to become cyanotic or blue-gray. As a patient continues to lose blood, the skin becomes more pale, cool, and clammy. In infants and children, capillary refill will be delayed. Continue to treat for shock.

Return of normal skin color, temperature, and condition are obvious indications of improvement.

REESTABLISH PATIENT PRIORITIES

If ongoing assessment is undertaken at the scene and deterioration of the patient's condition is noted, it may be necessary to reconsider your emergency care and transport decision. If the patient becomes a priority patient due to the injuries or conditions found, begin prompt transport and continue to provide emergency care while en route to the hospital. If there is deterioration of the patient's condition, reassess and adjust interventions as needed.

REASSESS AND RECORD VITAL SIGNS

During the ongoing assessment, reassess the breathing rate and quality, pulse rate and quality, perfusion status, pupils, and blood pressure. Record the vital signs and the time that they were taken.

REPEAT THE FOCUSED ASSESSMENT FOR OTHER COMPLAINTS

If the patient begins to complain of a symptom that was not initially identified or a change in the original symptom, complete a focused assessment for the area of the complaint. Repeat the SAMPLE history if necessary. The patient may have been initially unresponsive and unable to identify any complaints. However, due to effective care and improvement in his condition, the patient now begins to complain of symptoms of injury or medical illness. Repeat components of the physical assessment as necessary to focus on those areas or symptoms. For example, during the ongoing assessment a patient begins to complain of abdominal pain. You must reinspect and palpate the abdomen, looking for any additional signs of injury or abnormality.

CHECK INTERVENTIONS

Determine if your emergency care is adequate and your interventions are effective for the patient's condition. Assure adequacy of oxygen delivery, positive pressure ventilation, bleeding control, CPR or AED, and immobilization.

The following are some questions to ask yourself when considering adequacy of intervention:

- Have the patient's vital signs improved, or deteriorated?
- Is the patient's airway still patent?
- Is the oxygen mask and liter flow adequate? Is oxygen connected and flowing to the bag-valve-mask device?
- Has the patient's color improved with oxygen or should I consider positive pressure ventilation?
- Is the patient's chest rising and falling adequately with the ventilations?
- Are the chest compressions producing pulses? Is the rate and depth of compression adequate?
- Has a cardiac arrest patient whose heartbeat has been restored lapsed into arrest again?
- Is the AED indicating that a shock is needed (or not needed)?
- Is the pressure dressing adequately controlling the bleeding? Has the bleeding stopped or do I need to proceed to the next step in bleeding control?
- Is the patient's spine completely immobilized?
- Are bone or joint injuries adequately immobilized?

If an intervention is not effective, it may be necessary to reassess the patient's condition, look for signs of other injuries or illness, check the equipment, ensure that the equipment is being used properly, and/or select alternative methods for emergency care.

Assessment, intervention, and reassessment of the patient is the key to all emergency care provided in the prehospital environment.

NOTE TRENDS IN PATIENT CONDITION

As noted earlier, the changes for the better or worse in the patient's condition will be the basis for interventions or changes in intervention and reassessment that you will perform en route to the hospital. It is also important to document and report to the staff of the receiving facility any changes in the condition of the patient. For both the EMT-Bs and the hospital staff, it is not only the patient's condition, but the trends in the patient's condition, indicating improvement or deterioration, that are important.

PART 6
COMMUNICATION AND DOCUMENTATION

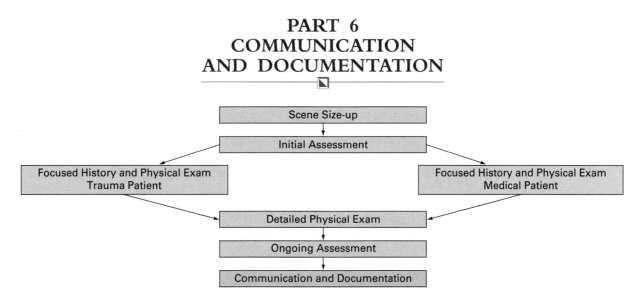

As mentioned early in this chapter, the initial information you receive about your patient comes from the dispatch. During your call you will communicate, at important points, with dispatch and with medical direction as well as with the staff of the medical facility to which you transport the patient. You must also communicate clearly with other EMS personnel, the patient, and others at the scene. A failure of clear communication—both in what others communicate to you and in what you communicate to others—can have a significant adverse effect on the quality of the assessment and care you and others provide to your patient.

In addition, a significant portion of the value of patient assessment and care is lost if what you have learned about the patient's condition and the care you have given are not clearly and adequately documented in your written reports.

The objectives for these skills will be listed and covered in detail in Chapter 11, "Communication," and Chapter 12, "Documentation."

CASE STUDY FOLLOW-UPS

During your shift as an EMT-Basic one day, you are called to two different kinds of cases. The first call is to a trauma patient. The second is to a patient who is suffering from a medical problem.

CALL ONE—A TRAUMA PATIENT
SCENE SIZE-UP

You have been dispatched to an unresponsive patient with an unknown problem. On arrival, you see an adult male supine at the bottom of a two-story fire-escape ladder. A police officer approaches the ambulance and tells you that they have been called for a reported domestic incident and gunshots. The officer motions you to park a safe distance away until the scene is secured. Moments later you see police leading a suspect from the building. The officer motions you forward and tells you the scene is safe. Anticipating that the patient may be bleeding, you already have on gloves, mask, and eyewear with side shields as you jump from the ambulance and approach the patient.

INITIAL ASSESSMENT

As you approach the patient, you notice that the shirt front and left pants leg are soaked in blood, the skin is extremely pale, and the right lower leg is severely deformed. This is obviously a trauma patient with a significant mechanism of injury—a probable fall from the fire escape and a possible gunshot wound.

Your partner immediately establishes in-line stabilization of the head and neck and performs a jaw thrust to open the airway. The patient does not respond to verbal commands; however, he moans and makes a facial grimace as you do a sternal rub.

You assess the breathing status and determine that the patient's chest is barely rising and falling and only minimal air movement can be felt or heard. You immediately instruct your partner to insert an oropharyngeal airway and begin bag-valve-mask ventilation with supplemental oxygen while maintaining in-line stabilization. A radial pulse is not palpable and the carotid pulse is extremely weak, fast, and thready. The skin is pale, cool, and clammy.

As you continue with your assessment, you quickly cut the shirt off and find a gunshot wound to the left anterior chest. You immediately place your gloved hand over the wound. You then tape the plastic package from an oxygen mask over the wound on three sides and continue to scan the anterior and lateral aspects of the chest for any other wounds.

Next you expose the area around the left thigh and find a wound with dark red bleeding at a steady flow. You apply direct pressure to control the bleeding and then immediately apply a pressure dressing.

You indicate to your partner that this is going to be a rapid patient transport.

FOCUSED HISTORY AND PHYSICAL EXAM

Now that immediate life threats are under control, you begin the rapid trauma assessment. You quickly assess the head and neck and apply a cervical spinal immobilization collar. Your partner continues in-line stabilization.

As you continue with your assessment, you find decreased breath sounds on the left side of the chest. You find no abnormalities in the abdominal or pelvic region, but the right lower extremity is swollen and deformed and the patient moans when you palpate the angulated area. With assistance from police first responders, spinal stabilization is maintained as the patient is log-rolled and the posterior thorax and lumbar region, and buttocks are exposed. No additional injuries are revealed.

While the patient is still on his side, a first responder slides the backboard next to the patient and the patient is rolled onto it and secured with straps. A head immobilization device is applied. The right lower extremity is also carefully secured to the board for stabilization.

The blood pressure is measured at a low 70/50; skin remains pale, cool, and clammy; pupils are normal in size, equal, and sluggish to respond to light; the heart rate is rapid at 136 per minute; and the spontaneous respiratory rate is only 6 per minute. You continue positive pressure ventilation with supplemental oxygen.

There is no one at the scene who knows the patient, so the only portion of the SAMPLE history you are able to gather is information about events leading to the injury. A neighbor reports hearing gunshots, seeing the patient stagger out onto the second story fire escape clutching his chest, then watching in horror as the patient pitched over the railing and fell to the pavement.

The patient is promptly loaded into the ambulance for transport with lights and siren.

DETAILED PHYSICAL EXAM

En route to the hospital, after you reassess the airway, breathing status, circulation, and vital signs, you apply a vacuum splint to the right lower leg for better immobilization.

With life threats being managed effectively, you find time to perform a detailed physical exam. The only additional problem you discover is a small laceration at the left temporal region of the patient's head to which you apply a sterile dressing and bandage.

ONGOING ASSESSMENT

Because this is a patient with critical injuries, you continuously reassess the mental status, airway, breathing, and circulation, and you take and record vital signs every 5 minutes while en route to the emergency department. You reassess the patient's injuries and check the effectiveness of interventions, making sure that positive pressure ventilation is adequate, the dressing on the chest wound is permitting escape of air on the unsecured side, the bleeding at the chest and thigh is under control, and the immobilization to the backboard and splints is secure. You radio the hospital emergency department to report patient information and to alert them to your estimated time of arrival. No change in the patient's condition has occurred and you arrive at the hospital without further incident.

You give the hospital staff your oral report on the patient, complete the written documentation, and prepare the ambulance for the next call.

CALL TWO—A MEDICAL PATIENT
SCENE SIZE-UP

Shortly after the call to the man injured in the domestic dispute, you are again dispatched to a patient with an unknown problem. This time, you arrive at a well-kept home in a quiet neighborhood and are met by a middle-aged woman who says she called EMS for her mother, who cannot catch her breath. The woman, Mrs. Colon, leads you into the house. As you enter the living room, you see an elderly woman sitting up in a chair, an oxygen tank in the corner. You conclude that your patient likely is suffering from a medical problem rather than trauma.

INITIAL ASSESSMENT

Mrs. Colon introduces you to her mother, Mrs. Ortega, and tells you that her mother is 72 years old. Mrs. Ortega is sitting up in a chair, leaning forward, with her hand on her chest. She says, "I'm glad—you came. I feel like—I can't breathe." Her remarks assure you that her mental status is alert and her airway is open. You observe that she is breathing in fast, short puffs, but with adequate rise and fall of the chest. You apply a nonrebreather mask connected to oxygen flowing at 15 lpm, explaining that this will help relieve her distress. Because she has a home supply of oxygen that she has occasionally used, she understands and welcomes the oxygen therapy. You are able to palpate a somewhat rapid radial pulse, and you note that her skin is warm, pink, and dry.

You conclude that Mrs. Ortega's condition is stable enough that transport can be delayed for a short time while you conduct the focused history and physical exam.

FOCUSED HISTORY AND PHYSICAL EXAM

You sit down on a chair next to Mrs. Ortega and begin to take the SAMPLE history. She is not experiencing pain, so most of the OPQRST questions do not apply, but she does tell you that the onset of her symptoms was gradual over this morning and afternoon and that she has been suffering from the breathing difficulty for several hours. You determine that she chronically has a difficult time breathing, but this episode was slightly worse than usual—a 5 on a scale of 1 to 10. She has no allergies that she knows of. The medications she takes, including oxygen, are related to her history of emphysema, a serious lung disease. Her last oral intake was lunch at around noon. There were no unusual events leading to the onset of the symptom.

Meanwhile, your partner has been taking and recording Mrs. Ortega's baseline vital signs. Her respirations are puffy, somewhat labored, and at a rate of 28 per minute with adequate depth. Her pulse is rapid at 100 per minute and irregular. Her skin color, temperature, and condition remain normal. Pupils are normal, equal, and reactive. Her blood pressure is 120/90.

The physical exam you conduct is focused on Mrs. Ortega's complaint. You auscultate her chest with your stethoscope and detect wheezing noises that, in fact, you can hear even without the stethoscope. The breathing sounds are present and equal on both sides.

Because Mrs. Ortega's breathing is adequate, even though difficult, you conclude that positive pressure ventilation is not needed and continue to provide high-flow oxygen by nonrebreather mask.

You place Mrs. Ortega on the wheeled stretcher and transfer her to the ambulance. You raise the head of the stretcher so that she can ride to the hospital in a sitting position, which she finds is more comfortable and helps her to breathe.

ONGOING ASSESSMENT

Mrs. Ortega's condition does not require a detailed physical exam. You perform an ongoing assessment by reassessing her mental status, airway, breathing, and circulation, and reassessing and recording her vital signs. You perform an assessment focused on her breathing problem by using your stethoscope to auscultate her chest and reconfirm that breath sounds are present and equal with wheezing sounds on both sides. You check to be sure that the nonrebreather mask is correctly placed and that the oxygen continues to flow at 15 liters per minute. Because Mrs. Ortega is a stable patient, you repeat the initial assessment and vital signs every 15 minutes en route. You radio the hospital emergency department with patient information and your estimated time of arrival.

You arrive at the hospital with no further incident, give your oral report to the receiving staff, complete written documentation, and prepare the ambulance for the next call.

CHAPTER REVIEW

TERMS AND CONCEPTS

You may wish to review the following terms and concepts included in this chapter.

apnea—the absence of breathing.

aspiration—breathing a foreign substance into the lungs.

AVPU—a mnemonic for alert, responds to verbal stimulus, responds to painful stimulus, unresponsive, to characterize levels of responsiveness.

blunt trauma—a force that impacts or is applied to the body but is not sharp enough to penetrate it, such as a blow or a crushing injury.

cerebrospinal fluid (CSF)—a clear fluid that surrounds and cushions the brain and the spinal cord. Leakage of cerebrospinal fluid is evidence of a severe head injury.

chief complaint—the patient's answer to the question "Why did you call the ambulance?"

decerebrate posturing—a posture in which the patient arches the back and extends the arms straight out parallel to the body. A sign of serious head injury.

decorticate posturing—a posture in which the patient arches the back and flexes the arms inward towards the chest. A sign of serious head injury.

detailed physical exam—a head-to-toe physical assessment for injuries and medical conditions that may follow the focused history and physical exam and is more thorough than the rapid trauma or medical assessment.

dyspnea—difficulty in breathing.

flail segment—two or more adjacent ribs that are fractured in two or more places and thus move independently from the rest of the rib cage.

focused history and physical exam—the portion of patient assessment conducted after the initial assessment, for the purpose of identifying additional serious or potentially life-threatening injuries or conditions and as a basis for further emergency care.

focused medical assessment—a physical exam that is focused on the parts of the body indicated by a responsive patient's chief complaint, signs, or symptoms.

focused trauma assessment—a physical exam that is focused on a specific injury site, performed on a responsive patient with no significant mechanism of injury.

initial assessment—the portion of patient assessment conducted immediately following scene size-up for the purpose of discovering and treating immediately life-threatening conditions. Initial assessment also includes determining whether the patient is injured or ill and making decisions about priorities for further assessment, care, and transport.

in-line stabilization—bringing the patient's head into a neutral position in which the nose is lined up with the navel and holding it there manually.

medical patient—a patient who has not suffered from any type of injury or trauma, but is experiencing signs and symptoms related to a disease process or condition affecting the body's organs or systems.

ongoing assessment—the continuous assessment that is conducted following the rapid or focused assessment, or following the detailed physical exam if one is conducted, to detect any changes in the patient's condition, to identify any missed injuries or conditions, and to adjust emergency care as needed. The initial assessment is repeated, baseline vital signs reassessed and recorded, focused assessment conducted for additional complaints, and interventions checked.

paradoxical motion—a section of the chest that moves in the opposite direction to the rest of the chest during the phases of respiration. Typically seen with a flail segment.

patient assessment—procedures performed to find out what is wrong with a patient, on which decisions about emergency medical care and transport will be based.

penetrating trauma—a force that pierces the skin and body tissues, for example a knife or gunshot wound.

rapid medical assessment—a head-to-toe physical exam that is swiftly conducted on an unresponsive medical patient or a medical patient who is suspected to also have injuries.

rapid trauma assessment—a head-to-toe physical exam that is swiftly conducted on a trauma patient who is unresponsive or who has a significant mechanism of injury.

scene size-up—an assessment of the scene for safety hazards and to determine the nature of the patient's problem and the number of patients.

tenderness—pain in response to palpation.

trauma patient—a patient who has an injury or injuries rather than a medical condition.

REVIEW QUESTIONS

1. Briefly state the purposes of patient assessment by the EMT-B.
2. List the main components of patient assessment.
3. List the three steps of the scene size-up.
4. List the six steps of the initial assessment.
5. Contrast the order of the three steps of the focused history and physical exam for a responsive medical patient with the order of the steps for an unresponsive medical patient or trauma patient. Explain why the order of the steps differs.
6. Describe the kinds of patients for whom the physical exam should be a rapid head-to-toe assessment (rapid trauma assessment or rapid medical assessment). Describe the kinds of patients for whom the physical exam should be focused on a specific site or area of complaint.
7. Name the five categories of measurements that are included in the vital signs.
8. Name the categories of information sought during history taking that the letters in OPQRST and SAMPLE represent.
9. Under what circumstances should a detailed physical exam not be performed?
10. State how often, at a minimum, during the ongoing assessment, the components of the initial assessment and the vital signs should be reassessed for the following: (a) a critical or unstable patient, and (b) a stable patient.

A NOTE ABOUT SEVERE HEAD INJURY

During this chapter, we have recommended that when a patient has signs of *severe* head injury, the patient should be hyperventilated at a rate of 20 ventilations per minute. (For patients in whom severe head injury is not suspected, the patient is ventilated at a rate of 12 per minute; hyperventilation, if indicated in the patient who does not have a suspected head injury or stroke, is performed at a rate of 24 per minute.)

The lower hyperventilation rate of 20 per minute is the current guideline in cases of possible severe head injury with herniation of the brain (the swollen brain being forced through the spinal-cord opening from the skull). Studies have shown that hyperventilation at a higher rate causes constriction of the blood vessels in the brain, resulting in reduced blood flow and an actual decrease in oxygenation of the brain—a result that is the opposite of that which is intended.

Unfortunately, it is nearly impossible for the EMT-Basic to determine whether a possible head injury is severe (involves herniation) or not. However, if signs of severe head injury are present, hyperventilation at a rate of 20/minute is recommended. The signs of severe head injury include unresponsiveness, irregular breathing patterns, increasing blood pressure, decreasing heart rate, absent motor or sensory function, abnormal posturing to painful stimuli (decorticate or decerebrate), and unequal pupils.

For a more detailed discussion of severe head injury, see Chapter 33, Injuries to the Head.

CHAPTER 10

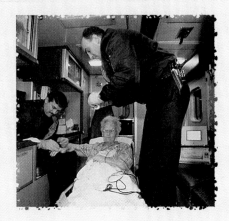

Assessment of Geriatric Patients

INTRODUCTION

Geriatric patients — those over the age of 65—differ from their younger counterparts. The elderly are at greater risk of nearly all types of injuries and illnesses. Also, they present with different signs and symptoms because of the changing physiology of the geriatric body system. Additionally, the geriatric patient often has one or more coexisting long-term conditions which can mask or change the presentation of the current emergency problem.

In the United States, people over 65 make up the fastest growing segment of the population. In fact, the majority of EMS calls involve geriatric patients. Therefore, it is important that you understand the characteristics of geriatric patients and how to tailor your assessment to their special needs.

OBJECTIVES

Numbered objectives are from the United States Department of Transportation 1994 EMT-Basic National Standard Curriculum. Asterisked objectives, if any, pertain to material that is supplemental to the DOT curriculum.

COGNITIVE

* Discuss at least four factors that contribute to the geriatric patient being at a higher risk for medical emergencies. (pp. 217–220)
* Discuss the general physiological changes in the body systems of the geriatric patient that are due to the normal aging process. (pp. 217–220)
* Discuss special considerations for assessing the geriatric patient suffering from a medical or traumatic emergency. (pp. 220–225)
* Outline the special considerations for obtaining an accurate medical history from a geriatric patient. (pp. 222–224)

* List the emergency care steps and considerations for the geriatric patient suffering either a medical or a traumatic emergency. (pp. 224–225)
* Discuss positioning, immobilization, and packaging of the elderly trauma patient with consideration of physical deformity. (p. 224)
* Recite and explain common disease processes that cause generalized complaints in the elderly. (pp. 225–232)

AFFECTIVE

* Explain why the EMT-B should use special communication skills when assessing a geriatric patient. (pp. 222–224)

PSYCHOMOTOR

* Demonstrate various immobilization techniques that would be necessary for packaging an elderly patient with degenerative skeletal deformities.

CASE STUDY

THE DISPATCH

EMS Unit 102—respond to 1700 Bentley Drive for a 72-year-old female with respiratory distress. Time out is 0813 hours.

ON ARRIVAL

As you arrive, you are met by an elderly male stating he is the patient's husband. He identifies himself as Harold Vaughn. He tells you he called for his wife, Madeline. "She hasn't been feeling well for the last three or four days. Yesterday she started having trouble catching her breath."

Mr. Vaughn asks you to hurry as you gather the equipment from the ambulance. He leads you to the back bedroom of the house where you find an elderly female sitting upright in bed, her back propped against several pillows. She smiles at you when you speak to her, and then she places her hand behind her ear as if to say "Speak louder, I can't hear you."

How would you proceed to assess and care for this patient?

During this chapter, you will learn about physiological changes, special assessment concerns, and emergency care considerations for geriatric patients. Later, we will return to the case and apply the procedures learned.

EFFECTS OF AGING ON BODY SYSTEMS

The human body changes with age. As a person ages, there are changes in cellular, organ, and system functioning. This change in physiology—which typically starts around age 30—is a normal part of aging. Al-

though people may try to slow the aging process by diet, exercise, health care, and so on, it cannot be stopped.

One trend, however, is that people are living longer with **chronic** (long-term, progressing gradually) illnesses. This means that the elderly are likely to constitute a larger and larger percentage of an EMT-B's patient volume. To further compound the picture, most elderly patients will have not one but a combination of different disease processes in varying stages of development.

Unfortunately, the aging body has fewer reserves with which to combat diseases, and this ultimately contributes to the incidence of **acute** (severe, with rapid onset) medical and traumatic emergencies. Remember, however, that while illness is common among the elderly, it is not an inevitable part of aging.

It is essential that you understand and recognize changes in geriatric body systems so that you can provide appropriate care for elderly patients (Figure 10-1). Remember that the physiological changes discussed on the following pages result from the normal aging process, not from disease progression. However, any disease or injury the patient experiences will only worsen—or be made worse by—these changes.

THE CARDIOVASCULAR SYSTEM

With age, degenerative processes affect the ability of the heart to pump blood. Calcium is progressively deposited in areas of deterioration, especially around the valves of the heart. Fibrous tissue begins to replace muscle tissue throughout the cardiovascular system. The walls of the heart become generally thickened without any increase in the size of the atrial or ventricular chambers. This process is known as **cardiac hypertrophy,** and it ultimately leads to a decrease in the amount of blood ejected by the heart's contractions (cardiac output).

The resting heart rate increases, but there are fewer electrical conducting cells ("pacemaker cells") as the heart grows older. Finally, there is a general decline in the maximum heart rate, which means that the heart rate may not increase even when there is infection, shock, or stress.

Arteries lose their elasticity (their ability to constrict and dilate easily), and this causes greater resistance against which the heart must pump. Widespread hardening of the arteries, or **arteriosclerosis,** tends to occur, which further increases the pressure the heart must pump against to maintain adequate blood flow through the vascular system.

To summarize, the heart grows weaker in strength even though it must pump against higher resistance; there may be abnormal heart rates or rhythms because of the degeneration of the conduction system; the systolic blood pressure may start to rise because of increased arterial resistance to blood flow; and the blood vessels will not react as fast (or as efficiently) in response to stimulation from the central nervous system.

THE RESPIRATORY SYSTEM

The respiratory system undergoes significant changes with aging, mainly as a result of alterations in the respiratory muscles and in the normal elasticity and recoil of the thorax. Specifically, there is a decrease in the size and strength of the muscles used for respiration, and calcium deposits begin to form where the ribs join the sternum, causing the rib cage to become less pliable. There is a progressive decrease in diffusion of oxygen and carbon dioxide across the alveolar membrane as more and more alveolar surfaces degenerate. Finally, the body becomes less sensitive to hypoxia (oxygen starvation) or to increased carbon dioxide levels in the blood and tissues.

The ability of the lungs to inhibit or resist disease and infection is also diminished. The cough and gag reflexes can both decrease, thus preventing adequate clearing of substances from the airway and allowing respiratory infections to develop more often. Dehydration, common in the elderly, increases the tendency for respiratory infection.

The net effect of these respiratory system changes in an elderly patient is that less air enters and exits the lungs, less gas exchange occurs, the lung tissue loses its elasticity, and many of the muscles used in breathing lose their strength and coordination.

THE MUSCULOSKELETAL SYSTEM

The most significant musculoskeletal change resulting from aging is a loss of minerals in the bones, which is known as **osteoporosis.** This makes the bones more brittle and susceptible to fractures and slows the healing process. The osteoporosis itself is less a problem than the resulting possible bone injury and/or immobility, which can lead to illness and death.

The disks that are located between the vertebrae of the spine start to narrow, which causes the characteristic curvature of the spine often seen in elderly patients, known as **kyphosis.** This curvature is usually most pronounced in the thoracic vertebrae and can complicate normal spinal immobilization procedures. It may be necessary to place additional padding under the patient to fill voids and create effective immobilization.

Joints begin to lose their flexibility with aging, and there is a general and progressive loss of skeletal muscle mass. In all, the elderly are more prone to falls because of general weakness and a loss in joint mobility. Unfortunately, because of the changes in bone structure, these falls commonly result in skeletal fractures that take longer to heal than in younger people and that may also cause other medical emergencies.

THE NEUROLOGICAL SYSTEM

The neurological (nervous) system also becomes impaired by the normal effects of aging. There is an actual decrease in the mass and weight of the brain and a resulting increase in the amount of cerebral spinal fluid (CSF) to occupy the extra space in the skull.

CHANGES IN THE BODY SYSTEMS OF THE ELDERLY

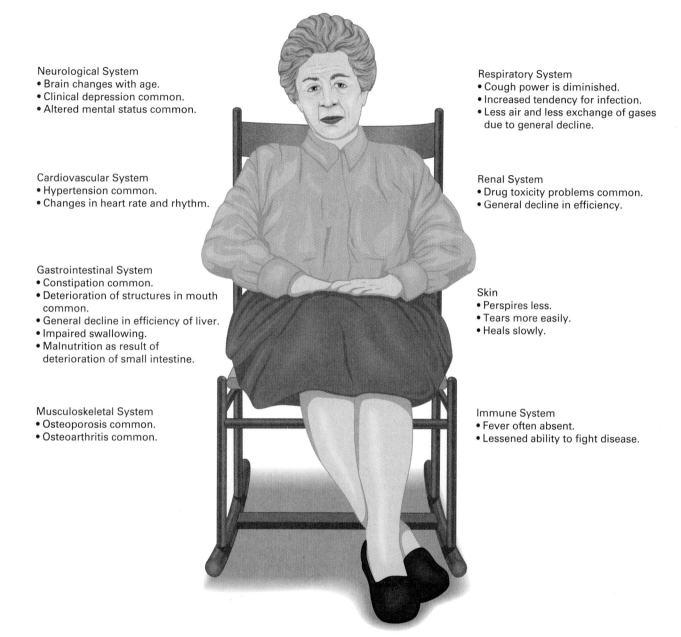

Neurological System
• Brain changes with age.
• Clinical depression common.
• Altered mental status common.

Cardiovascular System
• Hypertension common.
• Changes in heart rate and rhythm.

Gastrointestinal System
• Constipation common.
• Deterioration of structures in mouth common.
• General decline in efficiency of liver.
• Impaired swallowing.
• Malnutrition as result of deterioration of small intestine.

Musculoskeletal System
• Osteoporosis common.
• Osteoarthritis common.

Respiratory System
• Cough power is diminished.
• Increased tendency for infection.
• Less air and less exchange of gases due to general decline.

Renal System
• Drug toxicity problems common.
• General decline in efficiency.

Skin
• Perspires less.
• Tears more easily.
• Heals slowly.

Immune System
• Fever often absent.
• Lessened ability to fight disease.

Figure 10-1 Changes in the body systems of the elderly.

Nerve cells (neurons) begin to degenerate and die as early as the mid-20s, and this ultimately impedes the ability of the body to adapt rapidly to changes within and outside of the body. Nerve cell degeneration is also responsible for the slowing of reflexes. Additionally, the elderly have a harder time perceiving or sensing their body position, resulting in their becoming less and less steady on their feet. The combination of neurological degeneration and changes in the musculoskeletal system make it easy to understand why falls are so prevalent and serious in the geriatric population.

Sight diminishes (especially at night), and the ability to discern higher frequency sounds is slowly lost. Also, the geriatric patient may have difficulty in differentiating close from background noise. These neurological changes, separately or in combination, can easily cause falls or other types of injuries.

THE GASTROINTESTINAL SYSTEM

Changes in the gastrointestinal system contribute to various medical conditions including malnutrition. First, there is a reduction in the sense of taste and smell, resulting in decreased food enjoyment (possibly causing the person to stop eating regularly). There is deterioration of structures in the mouth; periodontal disease can cause loss of gum tissue and consequent tooth loss. There is a drop in salivary flow from degeneration of the salivary glands. The smooth muscle contractions of the esophagus decrease, and the opening between the esophagus and the stomach loses tone, which can result in chronic heartburn as gastric acid enters the esophagus from the stomach.

The liver decreases in size, weight, and function which decreases hepatic enzymes, causing a loss in the liver's ability to aid in digestion and metabolize certain drugs. Smooth muscle contractions (peristalsis) throughout the rest of the gastrointestinal tract are slowed; therefore, it takes much longer for food to move through the system. Because the lining of the small intestine degenerates, nutrients are not as readily absorbed, further contributing to malnutrition. Fecal impaction and constipation are common because smooth muscle contractions of the large intestine diminish. In some, degeneration of the rectal sphincter muscle can cause loss of bowel control.

THE RENAL SYSTEM

The normal aging process also affects the renal system (kidneys). The kidneys become smaller in size and weight because of a loss of the functional parts of the kidney, the nephrons. The loss of nephrons can reduce the actual weight of the kidneys by about one-third of their normal weight. The effect is a decrease in the surface area of the kidney available to filter blood. The arterial system supplying the kidneys is also subject to the changes in the cardiovascular system, which results in a drop in renal blood flow. In combination, these changes result in a lesser amount of blood per minute passing through the kidneys for filtration, in addition to the decrease in available filtration surface area.

Since the kidneys play a vital role in fluid and electrolyte balance, kidney malfunction or injury typically leads to a secondary disturbance in fluid balance and electrolyte distribution. Since many drugs (including antibiotics) are filtered out by the kidneys, it is common for the elderly to suffer from drug toxicity if they take too much medication or take it too frequently. Remember that the geriatric renal system may be functional enough to meet the demands of the body on a day-to-day basis, but as a result of acute illness or injury the elderly patient's renal system may fail.

THE INTEGUMENTARY SYSTEM

Aging results in tremendous changes in the integumentary system (the skin). The skin becomes thinner from a deterioration of the subcutaneous layer, and there is less attachment tissue between the dermis and epidermis. An elderly person's skin is much more prone to injury than the younger person's skin. Replacement cells are produced less rapidly, so wounds heal more slowly and skin is slow to replace itself. Less perspiration is produced, and the sense of touch is dulled. As the skin breaks down, there is a tendency for sores and tearing injuries to occur. This diminishes the effectiveness of the skin as a protective barrier in keeping microorganisms out of the body.

ASSESSMENT OF THE GERIATRIC PATIENT

The leading causes of illness and death in the geriatric population include heart disease, cancer, stroke, fractures, falls, respiratory diseases, pneumonia, diabetes, and misuse of drugs. The signs and symptoms of any of these problems may be masked by, or confused with, the physiological changes of aging. Is a sign or symptom the result of a present illness or injury, you may wonder, or is it the result of the normal aging process?

Also, as a result of the normal aging process, the response to illness is altered. Many medical problems present with different signs and symptoms in the elderly than in the general population. For example, a lack of chest pain in a geriatric patient who is experiencing a heart attack is common.

In general, the geriatric patient needs to be assessed and treated carefully. Any delay in recognizing health care needs and providing care may have devastating, irreversible consequences. Especially at risk are those elderly people who

- Live alone
- Are incontinent
- Are immobile
- Have been recently hospitalized
- Have been recently bereaved
- Have an altered mental status

THE SCENE SIZE-UP

Begin the scene size-up by determining if there are any safety hazards to yourself, your crew, or bystanders. As always, you should approach the patient with body substance isolation precautions taken. Since tuberculosis is prevalent in nursing homes and other extended-care facilities, wear a HEPA mask when you encounter a patient with signs or symptoms of a respiratory disorder (such as a cough) in such a facility.

Since the elderly commonly live on fixed incomes, it is not uncommon to find an elderly patient inside a house without proper heating during the winter or cooling in the summer. Remember to assess the environmental temperature (even if it means taking your arm out of your jacket in the wintertime to determine room temperature). Since the elderly patient has deteriorating compensatory mechanisms, the body's response to environmental extremes of temperature will be diminished, potentially leading to cold- or heat-related emergencies more rapidly than a younger person.

When the elderly patient shares living quarters, or lives in a extended-care facility, numerous patients may be victim to an environmental emergency (e.g., temperature extremes, toxic fumes). Determine if any additional patients are present and call for additional resources if necessary.

Part of the scene size-up is determining whether the patient is suffering from trauma or a medical problem. However, with the geriatric patient even more than with a younger patient, be alert to the fact that the cause of the emergency may be more complex than is first apparent. For example, since the geriatric patient may have numerous chronic diseases, an unresponsive patient (seemingly a medical emergency), may actually be unresponsive because he failed to eat a meal, which caused a diabetic reaction, which caused him to fall from a chair, which resulted in a head injury that is now presenting with delayed symptoms—a combined medical and trauma emergency.

There may be reliable family members or bystanders who witnessed or are aware of what happened to the patient. However, while you may make a preliminary determination of the nature of the problem during the scene size-up, maintain a high index of suspicion. Be ready to change your focus of care as you gather additional information during the initial assessment and the focused history and physical exam.

THE INITIAL ASSESSMENT

In performing the initial assessment, keep in mind the following special considerations for the geriatric patient:

- *Mental status*—The geriatric patient's mental status may be influenced by a chronic illness, the present illness or injury, prescription drugs he is taking, or relative familiarity with his surroundings. The purpose of assessing the mental status is to determine a baseline level of consciousness and the possible need for airway protection and ventilatory assistance.
- *Airway and breathing*—The elderly patient's diminished gag reflex makes him vulnerable to aspiration of fluids and food or other solids, which can be fatal. Therefore monitoring the elderly patient's airway is especially important.

  Also pay close attention to breathing patterns. If a geriatric patient is suffering acute respiratory dis-

tress, the muscles of respiration may fatigue and fail more rapidly than in a younger person. This can cause inadequate breathing (hypoventilation), which the geriatric patient tolerates even less than a younger patient. (Although it is normal for hypoxia, or oxygen deprivation, to cause an increase in respiratory rate, don't get a false sense of security if the geriatric patient's rate starts to slow. This may actually indicate respiratory failure rather than improved oxygenation.) *Be prepared to initiate positive pressure ventilation.*

- *Circulation*—Assess central and peripheral pulses, noting the rate, strength, and rhythm. Your initial pulse check should include an assessment of the radial pulse. However, since the geriatric patient is predisposed to peripheral vascular diseases, the radial pulse may be markedly diminished or absent. This is not necessarily an abnormal sign; just be sure to check other pulses if the radial pulse is weak or absent.

  While it is natural for the pulse rate of an elderly patient to be slightly higher at rest than a younger person's, you should note any irregularity to the rhythm. This could be from the degenerative processes that affect the conduction system of the heart or from a drug (or drugs) that the patient is taking. Nonetheless, an acute onset of an irregular pulse should be considered an abnormality that necessitates emergency department evaluation.

- *Skin condition and temperature*—When assessing the skin, remember that the geriatric body does not display the same signs and symptoms of dehydration as in the younger patient. Since the geriatric patient has, over all, a lower amount of body water, and because of the changes in the skin from aging, dry-looking skin may be normal. If you suspect dehydration, the best way to assess for it is to look at the mucous membranes of the eyes and in the mouth. Normal hydration status will show them to be moist. A dehydrated patient will have a dry mouth, the tongue may be furrowed, the eyes may appear to be "sunken" into the orbits, and the membranes around the eyes will also appear dry.

  Equally important is skin temperature. The geriatric patient has a depressed response to infection. Whereas you may feel unusually warm skin from a fever in a young patient, you may not feel warm skin in a geriatric patient even if he does have an infection (e.g., pneumonia, upper respiratory infection). The temperature-regulating mechanism may be depressed, leading to minimal or absent fever or even hypothermia with severe infection. (Again, this contributes to the geriatric patient's susceptibility to temperature-related emergencies.)

THE FOCUSED HISTORY AND PHYSICAL EXAM AND THE DETAILED PHYSICAL EXAM

Conduct the appropriate focused history and physical exam, followed by a detailed physical exam, based on the patient's mechanism of injury (if trauma), or chief complaint (if medical). When interviewing a geriatric patient, you may encounter characteristic challenges resulting from the general depression of the sensory organs (especially failing eyesight and diminished hearing). These special considerations are discussed below with suggestions on how best to communicate to ensure a reliable history:

- *Diminished sight or blindness*—You can expect increased patient anxiety because of an inability to see surroundings coupled with an inability to exert control over the situation. You must talk calmly and be positioned so that the patient can best see you if he has any sight at all. Explain your procedures carefully. If the patient has them, make sure he is wearing his eyeglasses.
- *Diminished hearing or deafness*—Many elderly people cannot hear high-frequency (or pitch) speech, especially consonants. Obtaining a history can be difficult if the patient cannot understand questions. Do not assume that the patient is deaf without first inquiring with the family or bystanders.

    If the patient is wearing a hearing aid, make sure that it is turned on. Do not shout, as it distorts sounds if the patient has some hearing, and it does not help if the patient is deaf. However, increasing the volume of your voice (rather than the pitch) may help with the hearing-impaired. You may also try placing your stethoscope ear pieces in the patient's ears and speaking into the diaphragm. If the patient can lip-read, speak slowly and directly toward the patient. Note-writing may help, too.

Whenever possible, verify the history with a reliable relative or friend, or seek assistance from these individuals in communicating with the patient.

FOR THE GERIATRIC TRAUMA PATIENT

Note the mechanism of injury if possible trauma is involved. Just as with younger patients, the elderly can be involved in car accidents, falls from ladders or rooftops, falls down stairs, assaults, and so on. In fact, the elderly are at a greater risk for experiencing a traumatic injury (primarily due to falls) because of a variety of factors, which we will discuss later in the chapter. Situations that may be minor in other age groups may require aggressive care in the elderly.

You will need to conduct a rapid trauma assessment whether the patient is responsive, has an altered mental status, or is unresponsive. The geriatric patient, if responsive, may not indicate that the pain he is experiencing is very severe. Again, this may be a function of the aging process. The elderly patient has a decreased sensitivity to pain; therefore the severity of pain is unreliable an as indicator of the seriousness of the injury. *You should maintain a high index of suspicion and treat any complaint of pain as a symptom of a serious injury.*

Examine the head, neck, chest, abdomen, pelvis, extremities, and posterior body. Inspect and palpate for deformities, contusions, abrasions, punctures/ penetrations, burns, tenderness, lacerations, and swelling (DCAP-BTLS).

After completing the rapid trauma assessment and before continuing with the detailed physical exam or ongoing assessment, you will assess and record baseline vital signs and then obtain a SAMPLE history from the patient, if he is responsive, or from family and bystanders. Special considerations for obtaining a SAMPLE history from the geriatric patient are detailed in the section below.

After completing the focused history and physical exam, you should perform a detailed physical exam to find any additional injuries. Remember, the elderly deteriorate much more rapidly than do young people. A minor problem may become a major one in a short period of time. Simply put, to properly treat the "entire" geriatric patient, you need to perform an "entire" physical examination.

FOR THE GERIATRIC MEDICAL PATIENT

While the mechanism of injury in a geriatric trauma patient may be easy to determine, discerning a chief complaint in a medical emergency may be more difficult. Remember again that the geriatric patient may have one or more chronic diseases or medications, which can mask or alter the presentation of signs and symptoms; or the elderly patient may not be a reliable source of information for exactly the same reasons.

Because of the aging process, the patient's memory, hearing, sight, and orientation may be diminished. This can challenge your ability, or even the patient's ability, to determine the chief complaint (what prompted the present emergency call). For example, a geriatric patient may report experiencing a headache or neck pain but forget that he fell yesterday. Compounding this, the geriatric patient typically does not have a single chief complaint. Rather, the EMT-B may find that geriatric patients present with various forms and combinations of pain, fatigue, weakness, discomfort, and so on.

Yet, even keeping in mind the above difficulties in getting the history from a geriatric patient, you should remember that not all geriatric patients are deaf, blind, or have a diminished mental status. While these problems may be more common among the elderly than among the young, they are not the rule. The best way to destroy the patient-provider relationship is to *assume* that the patient has diminished hearing, sight, or mental capabilities.

Approach the geriatric with concern and compassion and *talk to* the patient about the emergency (Figure 10-2) rather than *talking about* the patient to others, unless unavoidable. If you have some doubts about whether the patient can grasp what you are saying, you may want to make sure, subtly of course, that a family member or bystander also is hearing and noting the information. The bottom line is, don't assume the elderly patient has diminished capabilities until you have evidence (through your assessment) of it.

Finally, remember that the geriatric patient may not report everything that is wrong. One reason is that the older patient doesn't perceive pain or discomfort as readily as the younger patient. This may lead him to delay the call for an ambulance until the situation becomes critical. Or the geriatric patient may attribute his ailment to "just old age" when, really, there is a serious emergency progressing. Sometimes patients minimize their symptoms because they fear losing their independence if admitted to the hospital. (Their perception may be that old people go to the hospital to die or, at the least, to be moved on to a nursing home instead of being allowed to come home.) The EMT-B should exercise extreme caution, and use thorough history and physical assessment skills to ensure that there are no other life-threatening conditions the patient is suffering from.

In obtaining the SAMPLE history and conducting the physical examination of the geriatric medical patient, remember the following points:

- The patient may become fatigued easily.
- You should clearly explain what you are going to do before examining the elderly patient.
- The patient may minimize or deny symptoms due to fear of being bedridden or institutionalized or losing his self-sufficiency.
- Peripheral pulses may be difficult to evaluate.
- You must distinguish signs and symptoms of chronic problems or natural aging processes from the signs and symptoms of acute problems:
  - Loss of skin elasticity and mouth breathing may give the false appearance of dehydration.
  - Edema (swelling) may be caused by varicose veins, inactivity, and position rather than heart failure.

Since you should anticipate that the elderly patient may not report or fully report all complaints, elicit as much information as you can by asking questions such as these:

- Have you had any trouble breathing?
- Have you had a cough lately? (If so: Have you been coughing up anything like mucus or blood?)
- Have you had any chest pain?
- Did you get dizzy? (If so: What were you doing when this occurred?)
- Have you fainted?
- Have you had any headaches lately?
- Have you been eating and drinking normally?

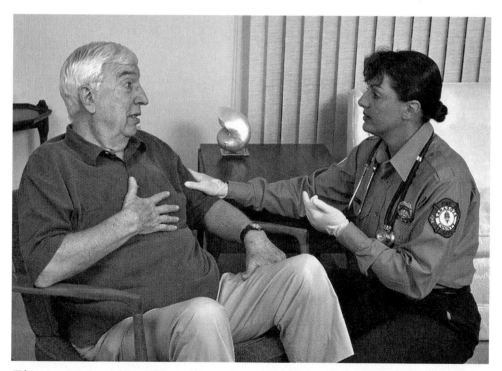

Figure 10-2   If possible, talk to the geriatric patient rather than talking about the patient to others.

- Have there been any changes in your bowel or bladder habits?
- Have you fallen lately?

While obtaining the history, it is best to address the elderly patient as "Mr." or "Mrs." or "Miss" as appropriate. Despite current misconceptions, the geriatric patient is not "set at ease" when an unknown EMT-B arrives on the scene and talks to him as if they have been friends for years. It is totally inappropriate to address the elderly patient by his first name or any other name (such as grandma, grandpa, honey, dear, or sweetie). The only exception is if the elderly patient voluntarily tells you otherwise.

As you begin the physical exam, you will notice that the geriatric patient is usually dressed in layers of clothing. This makes performing a physical exam more difficult since the manipulation necessary to remove the patient's clothing can easily fatigue the patient. In fact, it may be very tempting just to skip the physical exam rather than take the time to remove clothing. This could, however, be fatal if you miss a life-threatening injury or problem because you chose not to perform a complete physical exam.

If the patient is unresponsive or has an altered mental status because of the medical emergency, perform a rapid medical assessment of the head, neck, chest, abdomen, pelvis, extremities, and posterior body to find and treat any life threats that may be causing the alteration in mental status. Also be sure to scan the scene for any clues to the patient's problem (medicine bottles, mechanism of injury, environmental extremes, etc.). Finally, assess and record baseline vital signs.

As with geriatric trauma patients, you will perform a detailed physical exam on geriatric medical patients whether they are alert, have an altered mental status, or are unresponsive. Even the mentally competent geriatric patient may not give reliable information—for reasons discussed earlier—so the detailed physical exam will better enable you to assess for injuries, or signs of injury.

EMERGENCY MEDICAL CARE AND ONGOING ASSESSMENT

Remember, a geriatric patient can deteriorate rapidly. Therefore it is critically important to anticipate problems and to continuously reassess the patient. In the geriatric patient, the injury or failure of one body system can rapidly cause the failure of others. The following are key considerations and emergency care steps for the geriatric patient:

1. *Maintain a patent airway.* Geriatric patients often wear dentures, and if these dentures become dislodged, they can create an airway obstruction. Look in the mouth to determine if the dentures (or any other foreign object or substance) is blocking the airway. If necessary, suction and clear the airway immediately before assessing the breathing status.

2. *Insert an airway.* The geriatric patient's mental status is subject to rapid deterioration. If the patient is unable to maintain his own airway due to injury or altered mental status, insert an oropharyngeal airway. If the patient cannot tolerate an oropharyngeal airway, insert a nasopharyngeal airway.

3. *Assess and be prepared to assist ventilations.* It is vitally important to assess the geriatric patient's rate and depth of respirations. Because of the general decline in respiratory muscle strength, a minor chest injury or lung disorder can easily put the patient into respiratory failure unless proper care is initiated. If the rate or depth is inadequate, positive pressure ventilation should be initiated immediately. Be careful not to ventilate the patient with excessive pressure or volumes, which could cause lung injury.

4. *Establish and maintain oxygen therapy.* As with all patients, be sure to provide supplemental oxygen with positive pressure ventilation if the patient's breathing is inadequate. If the patient has adequate respirations, you can administer oxygen via a nonrebreather mask at 15 lpm.

5. *Position the patient.* Exercise extreme caution when preparing the patient for transport, based on the type of emergency as outlined in the following guidelines:
   - *If the emergency is medical in nature and the patient is alert and able to protect his own airway,* place the patient in a position that is comfortable for him. This is typically a Fowler's (sitting-up) position.
   - *If the patient has an altered mental status and is unable to protect his own airway,* he should be placed in a left lateral recumbent position (recovery position) to avoid aspiration.
   - *If spinal injury is suspected,* the patient needs immediate stabilization of the spine during initial assessment, followed by immobilization to a long backboard. *One limitation, however, is the geriatric patient with severe curvature of the spine due to kyphosis.* The patient with severe kyphosis could actually be injured if forced to be immobilized in the same fashion as a younger person. You may need to be creative and construct the cervical immobilization devices out of blankets to accommodate the curvature of the spine.
   - *If the patient is unresponsive,* assume a possible cervical spine injury and immobilize the patient fully as a precautionary measure.

6. *Transport.* Perform an ongoing assessment en route to the hospital, remembering that the geriatric patient's condition can rapidly deteriorate without warning.

In order to assure appropriate care, reevaluate the geriatric patient frequently. The length of time spent with the patient or the condition of the patient will assist in establishing how the ongoing assessment will be conducted and how often. Repeat and record the assessment at least every 15 minutes for a stable patient. If the patient is unstable, repeat and record at a minimum of every 5 minutes.

Overall, successful assessment and treatment of a geriatric patient will depend in a large part upon your approach, demeanor, and attitude. It can be extremely stressful to the elderly patient if you immediately start "pulling out equipment and doing things" without first gaining the cooperation of the patient. Your goal is to help lower the patient's anxiety, not increase it. Remember, what you do as an EMT-B on a regular basis (assessments, treatment, and so on) becomes routine to you. In contrast, this may be the first experience with emergency care for the patient, who has no idea what to expect. You need to explain everything that you are doing.

SPECIAL GERIATRIC ASSESSMENT FINDINGS

Because of the general decline in virtually every body system of the geriatric patient, the elderly are prone to certain traumatic and medical emergencies that can cause rapid deterioration. As stated earlier, aging may change the individual's response to illness and injury. Pain may be diminished or absent, and consequently the patient or EMT-B may underestimate the severity of the patient's condition. It is important that the EMT-B be able to recognize these emergencies and provide appropriate emergency care. Having an understanding of what is occurring physiologically in these emergencies will help in recognizing and providing prompt, appropriate care. Be alert for the findings discussed on the following pages as you assess patients over the age of 65.

ASSESSMENT FINDING: CHEST PAIN OR ABSENCE OF CHEST PAIN

HEART ATTACK

A lack of oxygen and other nutrients to the heart typically produces chest discomfort in a younger person. In contrast, due to depressed pain perception, geriatric patients may experience what is known as a **"silent heart attack."** This means that the elderly heart attack patient may have no, or very little, chest discomfort. Instead, the geriatric patient suffering a heart attack will usually present with very general complaints such as weakness or fatigue. Trouble breathing is also a common initial complaint. While one-third of the elderly victims of heart attack never experience pain, aching shoulders and indigestion are common.

The patient who chronically experiences chest pain may take nitroglycerin for the problem, so finding nitroglycerin medication at the scene will clue you in to a patient's history of heart problems. If the patient does take nitroglycerin, you may be able to assist in the administration of it with permission from medical direction (Figure 10-3). (Refer to Chapter 15, "Cardiac Emergencies," for a thorough discussion of nitroglycerin.)

Emergency care steps for a suspected heart attack—whether or not the patient's symptoms include chest pain—are to administer high flow oxygen, administer nitroglycerin as appropriate in consultation with medical direction, and transport the patient expeditiously (but cautiously) to the hospital.

CONGESTIVE HEART FAILURE (CHF)

Congestive heart failure (CHF) is another type of emergency seen typically in the geriatric patient (see Chapter 15, "Cardiac Emergencies"). It can be a chronic condition that the patient may tell you about during your history taking, or it may have an acute onset and be the cause for the elderly person summoning EMS.

Even though CHF is primarily caused by a cardiac disease, it can present differently than a heart attack does. It is caused by a heart that becomes weakened over time as a result of the changes in aging, as

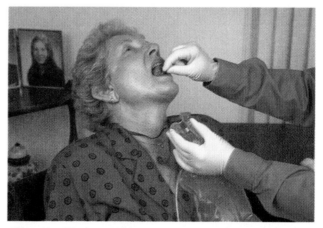

Figure 10-3 With permission from medical direction, you may be able to assist the patient suffering from chest pain in taking prescribed nitroglycerin.

well as hypertension, arteriosclerotic disease, and heart valve damage. As a result of these changes, the heart can no longer pump as effectively, and blood begins to cause a "back-up" in the periphery and lungs. Assessment findings characteristic to CHF include edema in the extremities, jugular vein distention, altered mental status, fatigue, rales or crackling upon auscultation, possible wheezing, and difficulty breathing. Emergency care steps for CHF include administering high flow oxygen, placing the patient in a Fowler's position, and expediting transport. Be sure to watch for inadequate breathing, and be prepared to ventilate.

ASSESSMENT FINDING: SHORTNESS OF BREATH

Respiratory distress can result from any of a number of conditions occurring in the geriatric patient. It can be the primary symptom of a pulmonary problem, or it can be a symptom secondary to failure of a different body system (CHF for example, can cause trouble breathing). As such, difficulty breathing or "shortness of breath" (dyspnea) is one of the more common complaints noted in the elderly (see Chapter 14, "Respiratory Emergencies"). It is important for you to realize that the elderly already have diminished respiratory function. Therefore, any additional burden can easily overwhelm the respiratory system

and lead to inadequate breathing. While shortness of breath can be caused by a number of problems, the four most common are pulmonary edema, pulmonary embolism, pneumonia, and chronic obstructive pulmonary disease (Figure 10-4).

PULMONARY EDEMA

Pulmonary edema, or fluid in the lungs, can have a gradual or sudden onset that can result in death if proper emergency care is not provided. Pulmonary edema typically results from the failure of the heart's pumping function. Causes include CHF, heart attack, or valve damage. The left ventricle starts to eject less blood than the right (the ventricles should eject the same amount of blood simultaneously) resulting in excessive pressure in the vessels in the lungs. Fluid begins to "leak" into the space between the alveoli and the capillaries, causing pulmonary edema, which results in inadequate gas exchange and respiratory distress.

Assessment findings include severe respiratory distress especially when lying down (orthopnea), altered mental status, coughing with possibly blood-tinged sputum, and other signs of CHF. As with CHF, emergency care includes administering oxygen at 15 lpm by nonrebreather mask, placing the patient in a Fowler's position, monitoring for inadequate breathing, and transporting expeditiously. It may be

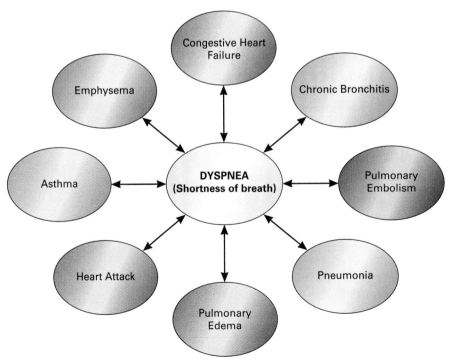

Figure 10-4 Common causes of dyspnea (shortness of breath) in the elderly patient.

necessary to perform positive pressure ventilation in severe cases.

PULMONARY EMBOLISM

Pulmonary embolism, or blockage in the arteries of the lungs, is a respiratory emergency seen more frequently in elderly than in younger patients. Pulmonary embolism may present with a very sudden onset of dyspnea, in conjunction with chest discomfort that is localized and does not radiate. This emergency usually occurs when a blood clot (embolism) breaks free from veins of the lower extremities or pelvis and is transported back through the right side of the heart. From there, the clot eventually lodges somewhere in the arteries of the lungs.

This results in poor oxygen and carbon dioxide gas exchange in the alveoli because the clot is preventing blood from flowing through the capillaries. The inadequate exchange of oxygen and carbon dioxide results in respiratory distress. The degree of respiratory distress depends on the size of the blood clot.

If a large embolism occludes more than half of the pulmonary circulation, it can rapidly cause death.

Predisposing factors to a pulmonary embolism include aging, smoking, cancer, fractures of large bones, major surgery, existing cardiovascular disease, prolonged bed rest, and trauma. Emergency care includes administering oxygen and monitoring for inadequate breathing. Provide positive pressure ventilation if necessary, and transport the patient rapidly to the hospital.

PNEUMONIA

Pneumonia is an infection of the lungs caused by a bacterium or virus. It is common in the elderly because of a diminished ability of the respiratory system to fight off infections. Of special concern is **aspiration pneumonia,** which often results from accidental aspiration of food or vomitus into the lungs. That is why preventing aspiration of foreign material is so important in the maintenance of the geriatric airway.

The elderly pneumonia victim may be insensitive to the subtle pain from pneumonia and may not exhibit the classic signs and symptoms of pneumonia that would appear in a younger patient (high fever, chills, chest pain, coughing up bloody sputum). In the elderly, watch for increased respiration rate, progressive worsening of dyspnea (breathing difficulty), congestion, with or without fever and chills, and a cough with some sputum production. The patient may also display an altered mental status.

Emergency care includes maintaining the patient's airway, administering high flow oxygen, and transporting the patient in a Fowler's position or a position of comfort.

CHRONIC OBSTRUCTIVE PULMONARY DISEASE (COPD)

Chronic obstructive pulmonary diseases (COPD) is actually a disease complex that includes a number of individual pulmonary disease processes (principally chronic bronchitis and emphysema) that result from the gradual deterioration of the pulmonary structures. (Refer to Chapter 14, "Respiratory Emergencies," for a discussion of COPD.) The effects of chronic obstructive pulmonary disease cause a disturbance in gas exchange in the lungs.

The EMT-B will typically encounter the elderly COPD patient complaining of respiratory distress and will observe the patient using accessory muscles when breathing. On arrival at the scene, the EMT-B may find the patient already on oxygen from a home oxygen unit (Figure 10-5). Emergency care includes the administration of oxygen at 15 lpm by nonrebreather mask. The EMT-B may also help relieve the respiratory distress, after consultation with medical direction, by assisting the patient with administering his prescribed metered dose inhaler.

Transport the patient in a position of comfort, which will usually be a Fowler's (sitting) position. Since the COPD patient can become easily fatigued from the effort of breathing, monitor the patient

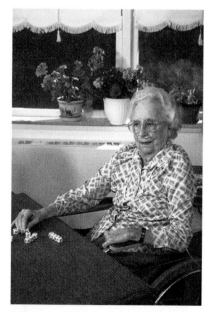

Figure 10-5 The COPD patient may use a nasal cannula with a home oxygen unit.

closely for signs of inadequate breathing. If breathing becomes inadequate, provide positive pressure ventilation with supplemental oxygen.

ASSESSMENT FINDING: ALTERED MENTAL STATUS

You will encounter many elderly patients who are alert and who respond appropriately to you and to their environment. Some, however, will be unable to remember details, while others may be routinely confused or totally unresponsive. The geriatric person presenting with altered mental status may be one of the most challenging patients you will encounter. There can be a variety of causes of altered mental status (Figure 10-6). The patient may have an altered mental status from some chronic condition (such as Alzheimer's disease), from an acute onset of the primary emergency (such as stroke), as a sign of an underlying medical illness (for example, poor perfusion of the brain when the volume of blood is depleted by severe bleeding), or even from the effect of prescription drugs.

Never assume that a patient's altered mental status is "normal" for him or that it is "senility" ("That's what happens when you get old") and risk missing an important sign of injury or illness. As you assess the patient, you will attempt to determine if the patient's mental status is, indeed, normal for him or if it represents a significant change. (Family members or others who know the patient may be able to supply this information.) Remember also that the noise of radios, a siren, or strange voices may add to the patient's confusion. Attempt to explain or reduce the noise.

While the management principles remain essentially the same regardless of the cause of the altered mental status, an understanding of common underlying causes will assist you in knowing what to look for during scene size-up and in formulating questions to ask the patient, friends, or bystanders during history taking. Following are certain types of emergencies that can cause altered mental status in an elderly patient.

STROKE

Stroke, also called *cerebral vascular accident (CVA),* is a common reason for altered mental status in the elderly patient (see Chapter 18, "Altered Speech, Sensory, or Motor Function: Stroke Emergency"). A stroke occurs when a blood vessel in the brain becomes blocked by a clot, obstructing blood flow, or ruptures and allows blood to accumulate in the brain tissue itself. Since the skull does not expand, the pressure within the brain (**intracranial pressure,** or **ICP**) sharply increases, while the nerve cells in the brain start to die or malfunction from the pressure. Also, the level of carbon dioxide in the brain increases, which causes cerebral vessels to dilate and further increases the ICP.

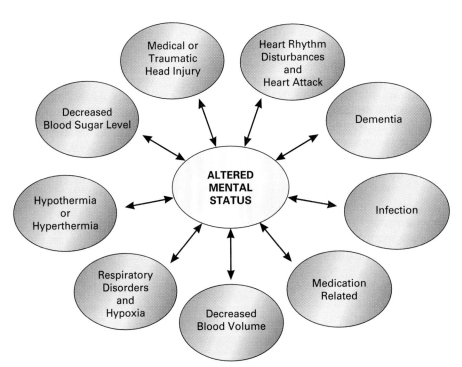

Figure 10-6 Common causes of altered mental status in the elderly patient.

The extent and location of the stroke affects the severity of the altered mental status. The patient could be simply slightly disoriented or totally unresponsive. A massive stroke can lead to death within minutes. Aside from altered mental status, you may also find the following signs and symptoms:

- Inequality of pupils
- Slurred speech
- Headache
- Memory disorders
- Alterations in the respiratory pattern
- A rapid, or abnormally slow, heart rate
- High systolic pressure (hypertension), which gradually becomes normal or hypotensive
- Possible seizures
- Nausea or vomiting
- Muscle weakness or paralysis (usually to one side of the body)
- Sensory loss

Key emergency care for a stroke centers around recognition, aggressive oxygenation, and ventilation. Your emergency care steps for stroke should also include protecting the airway and suctioning as necessary to prevent aspiration. You will transport the patient in a Fowler's position, if possible, or a lateral recumbent (recovery) position if he is unresponsive and there is no suspicion of trauma.

TRANSIENT ISCHEMIC ATTACK (TIA)

Transient ischemic attack (**TIA** or "mini stroke") is similar in presentation to a stroke, but the signs and symptoms are completely reversed within 24 hours of onset, usually sooner. No permanent neurologic dysfunction will occur with a TIA. A TIA is caused when blood supply to an area of the brain is temporarily occluded, causing a malfunction of brain tissue that is not being perfused. The malfunctioning brain tissue can cause the same signs and symptoms as stroke. Treatment steps are the same as those discussed for stroke.

SEIZURE

Seizure, a sudden and temporary alteration in the mental status caused by massive electrical discharge in a group of nerve cells in the brain, is another cause of disorientation in the elderly. (Refer to Chapter 19, "Seizures and Syncope," for a full explanation.) You may encounter the patient while he is actively seizing, or after the seizure is over and the person is still unresponsive or slow to respond (the "postictal state," or recovery period). Common causes of seizures in the elderly include cardiac arrest, low blood sugar, tumors, head trauma, stroke/TIA, infections, or electrolyte imbalance from kidney problems.

Treating an elderly seizure patient is the same as treating the younger seizure patient. Do not physically restrain the patient while he is actively seizing. Monitor the airway and suction as necessary (patients often vomit during seizures). Also, administer oxygen at 15 lpm by nonrebreather mask if breathing is adequate, or provide positive pressure ventilation if breathing is inadequate. The patient should be placed in a recovery position to help prevent aspiration if he is unresponsive and if trauma is not suspected.

SYNCOPE

Syncope (fainting) is an extremely common emergency for the elderly patient. Syncope is a temporary loss of responsiveness that usually reverses once the patient is lying down. Caused by a reduced blood flow to the brain, it can be a sign of a number of underlying diseases as well as a side effect of medications or even a reaction to strong emotion. Emergency care steps in treating a syncopal episode include ensuring an adequate airway, providing high flow oxygen by a nonrebreather mask or with positive pressure ventilation if necessary, and placing the patient in a recovery position to prevent aspiration if he is still unresponsive. Remember, if the patient suffered a fall in conjunction with the syncopal episode, he should be fully immobilized as a precautionary measure.

DRUG TOXICITY

Drug toxicity, or an adverse or toxic reaction to a drug or drugs, is a condition for which the elderly patient is more at risk than the younger patient (see Chapter 22, "Drug and Alcohol Emergencies"). The geriatric population takes approximately one-third of all prescription medications. They also buy the greatest number of over-the-counter medications. And since they tend to have a number of coexisting diseases, they are at greater risk for drug interaction from prescription medications.

Certain medications (taken individually or in conjunction with others) have a tendency to alter the patient's mental status, cause a syncopal episode, or even cause total unresponsiveness. Drug toxicity may also be caused by an error in dosing: the elderly person may take a wrong dose because of poor eyesight, confusion, forgetfulness, or a tendency to take the medication after it's no longer needed.

Treatment for a patient suffering from drug toxicity is based on figuring out not "What drug caused the problems?" but rather "How is the drug affecting the patient's airway, breathing, and circulation status?" Thus, key treatment includes airway maintenance, oxygenation, and prevention of aspiration. If possible, take all medications found on the patient or at the scene (prescription and non-prescription) to the hospital with the patient.

DEMENTIA

Dementia is a condition resulting from the malfunctioning of normal brain activity. It can be acute or chronic, but often it is irreversible. It is normal for the mental processes to undergo changes as a person ages, but approximately 15 percent of those over the age of 65 develop severe dementia which results in profound disturbances in mental functioning. The characteristic results of dementia are chronic changes, including loss of short-term memory, decline in intellectual abilities, and decline in judgment, math ability, and abstract thought. Dementia may be caused by medications, especially analgesics, sedatives, tranquilizers, and those taken to reduce blood pressure or ease the symptoms of Parkinson's disease. Other common causes of dementia in the elderly include Alzheimer's disease, brain tumors, heart disease, constipation, urinary retention, infection, depression, alcohol use, chronic pain, and other underlying diseases.

ALZHEIMER'S DISEASE

Alzheimer's disease is believed to affect more than two million Americans and be responsible for more than 100,000 deaths each year in the United States. The disease does not directly cause death, but it can cause patients to stop eating, become immobile, and eventually be subject to numerous infections. It is thought to be the most common cause of dementia in the elderly. While its cause is presently unknown, it is believed to be a disease of the nerve cells. The brain cells literally degenerate and die. Alzheimer's disease is both progressive and global in nature, involving the central nervous system. While it is commonly a disease of the elderly, it can affect people as young as 40.

The signs and symptoms of Alzheimer's disease mimic those of many other conditions. (The presence of Alzheimer's disease can be determined definitively only on examination of the brain during autopsy.) The disease causes confusion, emotional depression, irritability, and violence between lucid intervals. There is a progressive loss of appetite and a decreasing ability of the patient to care for his own needs. Eventually, the patient does not recognize loved ones; in late stages, the patient becomes childlike. Alzheimer's disease victims often attempt or commit suicide.

The treatment of patients suffering from Alzheimer's disease or another form of dementia requires special compassion from the EMT-B. Naturally, you must take necessary actions to establish and maintain the airway, breathing, and circulatory systems. But often you will be transporting these patients in a non-emergency setting. You may find the patient very uncooperative, even combative, with biting, spitting, and punching at times. It is important to remember that the uncooperativeness and aggression are symptoms of the disease, not conscious acts of aggression against you personally. You may also find yourself repeatedly informing the patient of the same thing over and over because his mind may not be able to process, let alone remember, what you are saying. Again, do not take the patient's actions or words personally.

ASSESSMENT FINDING: SIGNS OF TRAUMA OR SHOCK

Trauma is one of the leading causes of death in the geriatric population. The type of trauma seen most frequently in the elderly is blunt trauma from falls, motor vehicle crashes, and pedestrians struck by automobiles. There are numerous reasons for this, including the following:

- Altered mental status caused by a variety of conditions
- Slower reflexes
- Failing eyesight and hearing
- Activities that exceed physical limitations
- Arthritis
- Blood vessels that are less elastic and more subject to injury
- Fragile tissues, brittle bones, and stiffer joints
- General loss in muscle tone and strength

Falls are responsible for half of all accidental deaths in the elderly and are a common cause of head injuries. There are sometimes environmental reasons why the elderly fall. These may include stairways without handrails, slippery bathtubs, slipping rugs, steep steps, or improperly fitting footwear. There are also a number of medical reasons why the elderly fall. The most common are dizziness, side effects from medications, heart rhythm problems, spinal weakness, syncope, transient ischemic attacks, low blood pressure, internal bleeding, and poor vision.

Many elderly people who fall do not develop life-threatening injuries and do not die as a result of the fall. But certain injuries are common among those who fall. Make sure you assess for a hip fracture, head injuries, chest and abdominal injuries, spinal fractures, and fractures of the hand, wrist, forearm, or shoulder (caused by falling on an outstretched hand).

Head injuries are harder to detect in the elderly. As mentioned previously, the brain shrinks in size during the aging process. Even though there is additional cerebrospinal fluid surrounding the smaller brain, there is still more space in which the brain can swell in response to injury. Thus, signs of brain injury in an older person may take days or weeks to develop, and the patient may have forgotten the initial injury by the time the signs and symptoms develop.

Regardless of the type of injury incurred, whenever you assess an elderly fall victim, you should determine if the fall was preceded by dizziness, faintness, or palpitations, indicating a potential medical emergency, or resulted from slipping or tripping on something.

The effects of years of disease processes sharply diminish the ability of the geriatric body to handle the stress of trauma. Because the heart and the arteries of an elderly person don't respond well, shock progresses much more rapidly in the elderly than in any other age group. Loss of even a small amount of blood can drive an elderly person into shock. In addition, the compensatory mechanisms do not function nearly as effectively nor last as long, and the organs cannot tolerate periods of hypoperfusion (see Chapter 29, "Bleeding and Shock").

Treatment of geriatric trauma must be executed expeditiously. Stabilize the spine during the initial assessment, always administer high flow oxygen, and provide positive pressure ventilation if the patient is breathing inadequately. Regard any signs of poor perfusion (such as pale skin, tachycardia, disorientation, hypotension, or increased respiratory rate) as signs of serious trauma and transport the patient as rapidly as possible.

ASSESSMENT FINDING: ENVIRONMENTAL TEMPERATURE EXTREMES

The effects of the aging process also leave the elderly at greater risk of experiencing an emergency as a result of changes in the environmental temperature. The ability of the body to create heat when cold, or to dissipate heat when hot, may be impaired not only from the aging process but from certain diseases and medications the patient may take. Whenever you enter the scene of a geriatric emergency, you should be acutely aware of any extremes in the ambient air temperature to which the patient was subjected. Even a temperature that seems only moderately warm or cool to you may be intolerable to the elderly person.

A body temperature less than 35 degrees Celsius (95 degrees Fahrenheit), or **hypothermia,** is of special concern in an elderly patient. A number of factors make the elderly more prone to hypothermia. These factors include a smaller insulating layer of fat, reduced muscle mass, the body's metabolic rate slow-

ing with age, impaired reflexes, decreasing blood flow (especially to the extremities), and a reduced shivering response. Living on a fixed income may result in being unable to afford to keep the home adequately heated. Because of physical impairments, the elderly may not be able to move around much, so they get colder much more easily.

Treatment includes protecting the airway and maintaining normal breathing and circulatory status. Not only should you remove the patient from the cold environment, but you should also remove any wet clothes and insulate the patient in a dry blanket. Use caution when handling a severely hypothermic patient as excessive handling or moving of the patient may put the patient into a lethal heart rhythm.

Equally serious is the elderly patient suffering from a heat related disorder or an increased body temperature (**hyperthermia**). The geriatric patient's core temperature can increase more rapidly than the younger patient's, and the length of time exposed to the environmental extreme should be taken into consideration when preparing to treat the patient. To institute prehospital cooling of a hyperthermic geriatric patient, you would follow the same guidelines as for treating a younger patient. A complete discussion of the prehospital treatment for hypothermia and hyperthermia can be found in Chapter 24, "Environmental Emergencies."

ASSESSMENT FINDING: GERIATRIC ABUSE

Abuse of the elderly occurs in some care centers and other institutions, but it also can—and does—happen at home. Any elderly person is especially at risk if he is cared for by someone who is under stress from other sources. Abuse of the elderly can be physical, financial, or mental (usually involving threats or insults). At highest risk are those elderly who are bedridden, demented, incontinent, frail, or who have disturbed sleep patterns.

Signs of abuse can include bruises, bite marks, bleeding beneath the scalp (indicative of hairpulling), lacerations on the face, trauma to the ears, broken bones, deformities of the chest, cigarette burns, and rope marks. If you suspect abuse, you will want to pay particular attention to inconsistencies when you get your history from the patient and from the provider or family. Your priority is to provide emergency care for the injuries. Do not confront the family or care provider with your suspicion of abuse. Instead, if you do suspect geriatric abuse, you should make your suspicion known to the receiving hospital's staff so that they may follow up with the appropriate authorities. Follow local protocols or state laws regarding reporting of suspected abuse.

CASE STUDY FOLLOW-UP

SCENE SIZE-UP

You have been dispatched to the scene of a 72-year-old female patient complaining of difficulty in breathing. While you are walking into the house, the patient's husband, Mr. Vaughn, tells you that the patient has not been feeling well over the past few days and that yesterday she started having trouble "catching her breath." You note no particular hazards to yourself or your partner and do not see any obstacles that would make the extrication difficult. As you enter the bedroom, you note that the patient is sitting up in bed, wearing her nightgown, and you notice a bottle of nighttime cold medicine on her night stand.

INITIAL ASSESSMENT

When you introduce yourself, Mrs. Vaughn makes a motion indicating that she cannot hear you. You repeat your statement a little louder, but she still cannot hear you. You ask her husband if she has any hearing impairments, and he says that she is deaf in one ear and uses a hearing aid in the other. After assisting her in placing her hearing aid, you begin to ask her questions.

By her responses, you determine that Mrs. Vaughn is conscious with an open airway and is exchanging air adequately. She tells you that she has some trouble taking deep breaths. You immediately apply high flow oxygen via a nonrebreather mask at 15 lpm. Her radial pulse is present and strong with an approximate rate of 90 per minute. Her skin is warm, and she appears slightly flushed in color. Despite the fact that Mrs. Vaughn displays only minor respiratory distress at this time, because of her age you decide to treat her as a priority patient. Your partner leaves to get the stretcher while you continue with the focused history and physical exam.

FOCUSED HISTORY AND PHYSICAL EXAM

While waiting for your partner to return with the stretcher, you obtain more information regarding the respiratory distress complaint. In answer to the OPQRST questions, Mrs. Vaughn tells you that she was almost over a cold when she started to experience some trouble breathing and a cough which started yesterday. She complains of no other discomfort and denies any dizziness, nausea or vomiting, chest pain, or abdominal pain. On a scale of 1 to 10, she calls her breathing discomfort "about 5." Mrs. Vaughn also adds that she just took her temperature and found it to be only slightly elevated at 99.2 degrees F.

As you continue to obtain the SAMPLE history, you find that the patient is not allergic to any medications and does not take prescribed medicine for high blood pressure or any other condition, although she states that she has a medical history of hypertension and arthritis. She has not eaten nor drunk anything since last night when she started to feel worse. She reports no events that brought on the breathing difficulty other than the cough and cold.

During your focused medical exam, you determine that the patient has moist mucous membranes, that her pupils are equal and reactive to light, and note no jugular vein distention. Breath sounds reveal crackles to the right and left lung fields. The patient is not using any accessory muscles to aid respirations. You assess baseline vitals and find the blood pressure to be 130/88, the heart rate is 96 and regular, and the respirations somewhat rapid at 30 times a minute. The skin is warm and still slightly flushed.

You place her on the stretcher in a Fowler's position, which helps her to breathe, and start moving her to the ambulance.

DETAILED PHYSICAL EXAM

While en route to the hospital, you conduct a detailed physical exam because Mrs. Vaughn is a geriatric patient. You determine that there are no visible or palpable areas of injury to the head, neck, torso, or extremities, nor indications of elder abuse. You also ask her if she has experienced any injuries recently, and she denies this.

ONGOING ASSESSMENT

You perform an ongoing assessment every 15 minutes. Mrs. Vaughn states that the oxygen must be working, because she feels much better and her respiratory distress is diminishing. You notify the receiving physician of your findings, and emergency care thus far. Reassessment of the vital signs reveals a pressure of 126/86, the breathing is regular at a normal rate of 20 per minute, and the pulse is 78 per minute. After you arrive at the hospital, you give your verbal report, write the prehospital care report, and prepare the ambulance for another trip.

On the way out of the hospital, you check in on Mrs. Vaughn, and she tells you that the doctor said that she has pneumonia and will be starting antibiotics. As you leave you recall that even though she did not display the "classic" signs of pneumonia as seen in younger patients, such as high fever, chills, and chest pain, what she did display was classic to the elderly patient with pneumonia: increasing breathing difficulty, rapid respirations, and a cough. You remember that the differences are due to physiological changes as a result of aging.

CHAPTER REVIEW

TERMS AND CONCEPTS

You may wish to review the following terms and concepts included in this chapter.

acute—severe, with rapid onset.

Alzheimer's disease—disease characterized by cerebral function loss as seen with diseases that affect the brain.

arteriosclerosis—disease process that causes the loss of elasticity in the vascular walls due to thickening and hardening of the vessels.

aspiration pneumonia—inflammation of the lungs caused by the aspiration of vomitus or other foreign matter.

cardiac hypertrophy—an increase in the size of the heart from a thickening of the heart wall, without a parallel increase in the size of the cavity.

chronic—long term, progressing gradually.

chronic obstructive pulmonary disease (COPD)—umbrella term used to describe pulmonary diseases such as emphysema or chronic bronchitis.

congestive heart failure (CHF)—a cardiac disease in which the heart cannot pump blood sufficiently to meet the needs of the body.

dementia—condition resulting in the malfunctioning of normal cerebral processes.

drug toxicity—an adverse or toxic reaction to a drug or drugs.

hyperthermia—core body temperature above the normal 98.6 degrees F.

hypothermia—abnormally low core body temperature. Usually refers to body temperature under 35 degrees C (95 degrees F).

intracranial pressure (ICP)—the amount of pressure within the skull.

kyphosis—abnormal curvature of the spine evidenced by excessive convexity posterior.

osteoporosis—loss of bone minerals that results in bones becoming brittle.

pneumonia—infection of the lungs, usually from a bacterium or virus.

pulmonary edema—fluid in the lungs.

pulmonary embolism—occlusion of a pulmonary artery by a blood clot.

seizure—a sudden and temporary alteration in the mental status caused by massive electrical discharge in a group of nerve cells in the brain.

silent heart attack—a myocardial infarction (heart attack) that does not cause chest pain.

stroke—occurs when a blood vessel in the brain becomes blocked or ruptures. Also called *cerebral vascular accident (CVA)*.

syncope—a brief period of unresponsiveness due to a lack of blood flow to the brain; fainting.

transient ischemic attack (TIA)—temporary disturbance in cerebral blood flow to a portion of the brain. The difference between TIA and stroke is that the TIA will subside within 24 hours of onset.

REVIEW QUESTIONS

1. A 79-year-old male patient is crossing the street to get his mail when he is struck by a vehicle traveling at 45 miles per hour. Discuss the changes in the following body systems from the normal aging process that would increase his susceptibility to injury and the aftereffects of injury: cardiovascular system, respiratory system, and musculoskeletal system.

2. Describe communication challenges caused by sensory degeneration in an elderly patient, and outline strategies for overcoming these challenges.

3. List questions you should ask the elderly patient in order to help obtain an accurate history.

4. Explain the reasons why a detailed physical exam should always be performed on all geriatric patients, whether trauma or medical, unresponsive or alert.

5. Give emergency care guidelines for positioning and packaging the following geriatric patients: the alert medical patient, the patient with altered mental status, the patient with suspected spinal injury. Also explain procedures for immobilizing a patient with spinal curvature.

6. Discuss how an assessment finding of denial of chest pain in the geriatric patient differs from the same finding in a younger adult patient.

7. List factors that make the elderly more likely to fall.

8. List at least five possible causes of altered mental status in the geriatric patient and discuss special treatment considerations for the geriatric patient with altered mental status.

9. Explain why geriatric patients are predisposed to environmental heat or cold emergencies.

10. List signs and symptoms of geriatric abuse and discuss emergency care procedures when there is a high index of suspicion for geriatric abuse.

CHAPTER 11

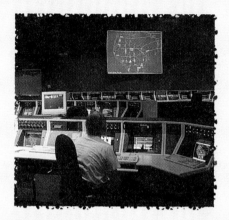

Communication

INTRODUCTION

Years ago, the job of ambulance crews was simply to transport patients to hospitals. The crews had no responsibility to provide emergency care to those patients. With such a limited role to perform, crews had no need for sophisticated communications systems.

Reliable communications systems are an essential part of EMS today. They permit EMT-Bs to reach their patients more quickly and allow hospitals to prepare appropriately for the arrival of those patients. They also link EMT-Bs in the field with doctors, enabling the EMT-Bs to provide more life-saving services than ever through contact with medical direction. For these reasons, understanding EMS communications skills and equipment is an essential part of the EMT-B's job.

OBJECTIVES

Numbered objectives are from the United States Department of Transportation 1994 EMT-Basic National Standard Curriculum. Asterisked objectives, if any, pertain to material that is supplemental to the DOT curriculum.

COGNITIVE

3-7.1 List the proper methods of initiating and terminating a radio call. (p. 240)
3-7.2 State the proper sequence for delivery of patient information. (pp. 241–242)
3-7.3 Explain the importance of effective communication of patient information in the verbal report. (p. 242)
3-7.4 Identify the essential components of the verbal report. (p. 242)
3-7.5 Describe the attributes for increasing effectiveness and efficiency of verbal communications. (pp. 242–244)
3-7.6 State legal aspects to consider in verbal communication. (pp. 238–239, 240)
3-7.7 Discuss the communication skills that should be used to interact with the patient. (pp. 242–244)
3-7.8 Discuss the communication skills that should be used to interact with the family, bystanders, individuals from other agencies while providing patient care and the difference between skills used to interact with the patient and those used to interact with others. (pp. 242–244)
3-7.9 List the correct radio procedures in the following phases of a typical call (p. 241):

- To the scene
- At the scene
- To the facility
- At the facility
- To the station
- At the station

AFFECTIVE

3-7.10 Explain the rationale for providing efficient and effective radio communications and patient reports. (p. 237)

PSYCHOMOTOR

3-7.11 Perform a simulated, organized, concise radio transmission.
3-7.12 Perform an organized, concise patient report that would be given to the staff at a receiving facility.
3-7.13 Perform a brief, organized report that would be given to an ALS provider arriving at an incident scene at which the EMT-Basic was already providing care.

CASE STUDY

THE DISPATCH

EMS Unit 2—proceed to 101 Bate Road. You have a man bleeding heavily in the driveway there. Time out is 1128 hours.

"Dispatch, this is Unit 2," your partner radios back. We copy and are responding to 101 Bate Road. Our ETA is 10 minutes. Do you have any more information on the nature of the problem?"

Dispatch replies, "Unit 2, that is negative. The caller said he was bleeding and was in the driveway. That was all."

ON ARRIVAL

Bate Road is in a semi-rural area with houses widely spaced. Because the dispatch gave little information, you approach the scene with extreme caution, realizing that some act of violence may have led to the call.

You park a short distance up the road from the house, which has an attached garage. There is one car in the driveway and only one person in sight, a man sitting on a bench next to the garage and clutching his hand. The scene appears secure, so you pull up and turn into the driveway. Your partner radios, "Unit 2 to dispatch. We are on the scene at 101 Bate Road." Dispatch responds, "Unit 2 on the scene at 1137 hours."

Because the dispatch said there was bleeding at the scene, you and your partner put on gloves and protective eyewear. Your partner grabs the jump kit and you both step out. As you walk up the driveway, you scan the scene carefully, looking for any signs of possible danger. The garage door is open, and you can see a workbench at the back of it. No one else is in sight. Meanwhile the man, who appears to be in his 40s, has gotten off the bench and is walking toward you. You note that his right hand is wrapped in a blood-soaked rag and that his shirt and pants are blood stained.

How would you proceed to assess and care for this patient? How would you use your communications skills and equipment during contact with the patient?

During this chapter, you will learn about the elements of emergency prehospital care communications and communications systems. Later, we will return to the case and apply the procedures learned.

COMPONENTS OF AN EMERGENCY COMMUNICATIONS SYSTEM

While emergency prehospital care communications systems vary considerably, many of them employ the components discussed below.

BASE STATION

The **base station** serves as a dispatch and coordination area and ideally is in contact with all other elements of the system (Figure 11-1). The base should be located on a suitable terrain, preferably a hill, and be in proximity to the hospital that serves as a medical command center. Base stations generally use relatively high power output (80 to 150 watts) and should be equipped with a suitable antenna within a short distance. The antenna plays a critical part in transmission and reception efficiency. Transmission power levels are limited by the Federal Communications Commission, and the minimum usable signal level for reception is limited by manmade noise. A good antenna system can compensate to some degree for these limitations.

MOBILE TRANSMITTER/RECEIVERS

Mobile, vehicle-based transmitter/receivers come in a variety of power ranges, and the power output determines the distance over which the signal can be transmitted effectively (Figure 11-2). A transmitter in the 75-watt range with VHF (very high frequency) will transmit for distances of 10 to 20 miles over slightly hilly terrain to base. Transmission distances are greater over water or flat terrain and are reduced in mountainous areas or where there are many tall buildings. Mobile transmitters with higher outputs have proportionally greater transmission ranges.

PORTABLE TRANSMITTER/RECEIVERS

Portable, hand-carried transmitter/receivers are useful when you must work at a distance from your vehicle but must stay in communication with the base or with one another (Figure 11-3). Such portable units may also be used by medical direction when they are stationed at a hospital that has no radio. Portable units usually have power outputs ranging from 1 to 5 watts and thus have limited range, although the signal of a hand-held transmitter may be boosted by retransmission through a repeater.

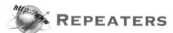 REPEATERS

Repeaters are devices that receive transmissions from a relatively low-powered source such as a mobile or portable radio and rebroadcast them at another frequency and a higher power. Repeaters make communications possible in EMS systems that cover a wide area or where the terrain makes transmission and reception of signals difficult (Figure 11-4). Repeaters can be located in emergency vehicles or at fixed sites throughout the area covered by the EMS system.

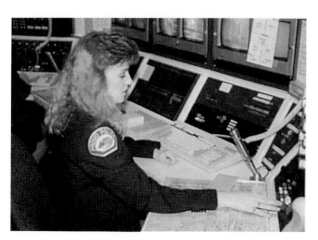

Figure 11-1   EMS communications center.

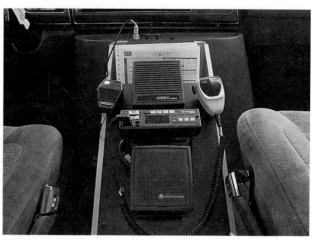

Figure 11-2   A mobile two-way radio.

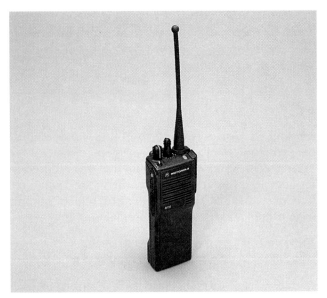

Figure 11-3   A portable hand-held radio.

DIGITAL EQUIPMENT

Technology is constantly changing the way communications are transmitted and received. Digitalized radio equipment is becoming increasingly common today. With such equipment, an **encoder** breaks down sound waves into unique digital codes, like those used in CD players, while a **decoder** recognizes and responds to only those codes. This equipment allows different mobile and base stations to operate on the same broadcast frequency, allowing more messages to be transmitted over those already crowded frequencies.

CELLULAR TELEPHONES

Some EMS communications systems are turning to another technological innovation, cellular telephones. These phones transmit and receive through the air rather than over wires (Figure 11-5). They operate in the following manner: A particular geographical service area is divided into a network of slightly overlapping geographical cells that range from 2 to 40 square miles in size. The cells are the equivalent of radio base stations. When a telephone moves beyond one cell's range, service to it is automatically picked up by another cell.

Benefits of cellular phones include excellent sound quality, availability of channels, easy maintenance, and, often, increased privacy of communications. They are often used as back-ups to an existing radio system or where the expense of establishing a radio system is too great. The major disadvantage of cellular phone systems for EMS use is that they are part of the public phone system and can easily be overwhelmed during multiple-casualty disasters.

BROADCAST REGULATIONS

The Federal Communications Commission (FCC) has jurisdiction over all radio operations in the United States, including those used by EMS systems. The FCC licenses individual base station operations, assigns radio call signs, approves equipment for use,

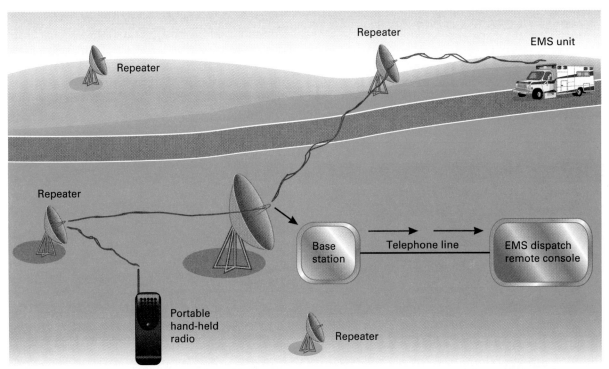

Figure 11-4   Example of an EMS communication system using repeaters.

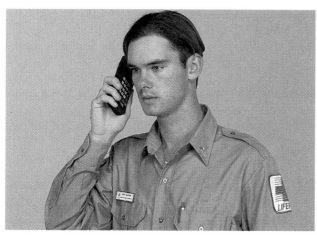

Figure 11-5   Cellular telephones are common in EMS communications.

establishes limitations for transmitter power output, and monitors field operations. The FCC has also set regulations to limit interference with emergency radio broadcasts and to bar the use of obscenity and profanity in broadcasts.

SYSTEM MAINTENANCE

Because a properly working communications system is at the heart of effective delivery of emergency medical services, regular maintenance of the system's equipment is a must. The equipment should not be mishandled or unnecessarily exposed to harsh environmental conditions. Regular cleaning with a damp cloth and a mild detergent should be part of the maintenance program.

Mobile and portable radios and telephones that operate on battery power should be checked on a daily basis. Most equipment uses rechargeable batteries. Freshly charged batteries should be inserted every day, while the removed batteries are put in the recharger. In addition, a back-up set of fully charged batteries should always be on hand.

Because communications equipment is so fragile and also so essential, your service should have some provision for backing up its communications system. Such provisions might include the availability of emergency generators at the base and repeater stations in case of power failure or the supplying of cellular phones to EMS units for use in cases of radio failure.

COMMUNICATING WITHIN THE SYSTEM

As an EMT-B, you will be expected to communicate not just with your partners and patients but also with EMS dispatch, medical direction, and medical personnel at receiving facilities (Figure 11-6). What fol-

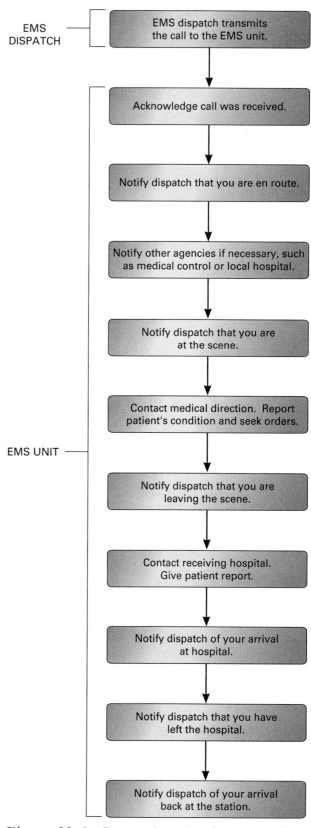

Figure 11-6   Progression of radio transmissions.

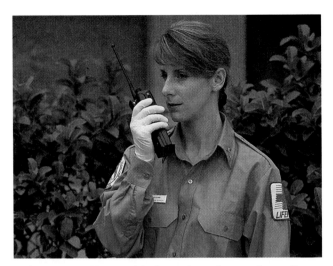

Figure 11-7   Hold the microphone about 2 inches from your lips as you speak into it.

lows are some guidelines for communication within the EMS system.

GROUND RULES FOR RADIO COMMUNICATION

Whenever you are communicating via your radio to other members of the EMS system, there are some basic ground rules to keep in mind. These rules apply to your communications with any part of the EMS system.

1. Turn on the radio and select the correct frequency. Use EMS frequencies only for EMS communication. Reduce background noise by closing your vehicle's windows.
2. Listen before transmitting. This ensures that the channel is free of any other communications and avoids interruption of someone else's transmission.
3. Push the "press to talk" (PTT) button and wait one second before speaking. This will allow time for system repeaters to operate and will ensure that the initial part of your communication is not cut off.
4. Speak with your lips about 2 to 3 inches from the microphone. Speak calmly and slowly enough to be completely understood (Figure 11-7).
5. Address the unit being called by its name and number, then identify your unit.
6. The unit being called will signal for you to begin transmission by saying "go ahead" or whatever is the standard in your system. If the unit being called responds with "stand by," that means wait to transmit until further notified.
7. Keep transmissions brief. If a transmission should take more than 30 seconds, pause for a few seconds to allow other units the chance to use the frequency for emergency transmissions.

8. Keep your transmission organized and to the point. Use plain English, avoiding slang and meaningless phrases such as "Be advised." Courtesy is assumed, so there is no need to say "Please," "Thank you," or "You're welcome." Also avoid codes and abbreviations unless their use is an accepted part of your system's communications.
9. When transmitting a number that might be confused with another (13 might be heard as 30), say the number ("thirteen"), then the individual digits that make it up ("one-three").
10. Avoid offering a diagnosis. Instead, give only the objective information (observable, verifiable information such as vital signs, chief complaint, medications the patient has) and relevant subjective information (opinions or judgments such as, "The patient appears to be in extreme pain") that you have gathered in your assessment.
11. When receiving orders or information from dispatch, medical direction, or other medical personnel, use the "echo" method. Immediately repeat the order word for word. Doing so will ensure that you have received the information accurately and understand it.
12. Always write down important information, such as addresses, orders to assist with medication, and so forth that you receive from other parts of the EMS system.
13. The airwaves are public, and scanners can pick up radio and cellular phone messages. Protect your patient's privacy by not using his name in your transmissions. Use objective, impartial language in describing the patient's condition. Do not make personalized or profane comments about the patient or his condition; such statements could be grounds for a slander suit.
14. Use "we" rather than "I" in your transmissions; an EMT-B rarely acts alone.
15. Use "affirmative" and "negative" rather than "yes" and "no" in transmissions. The latter words can be difficult to hear.
16. When you are finished, say "Over." Wait for confirmation that the other unit has received your message and does not need to have anything repeated.

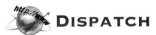 **DISPATCH**

Your first contact on a run will probably be with your EMS system's dispatch—perhaps a certified Emergency Medical Dispatcher (EMD). Dispatch is the public's point of contact with the EMS system, usually through the phone system via the 911 universal emergency telephone number or some other easy-to-remember, quick-to-dial number. It is the job of dispatch to obtain as much information as possible about an emergency, to direct the appropriate emergency service(s) to the scene, and to advise the caller on how to manage the situation until help arrives.

In many systems, dispatch records all conversations with initial callers, police, and fire personnel, EMT-B units, and receiving facilities. These communications can all become part of the legal record if a call should eventually lead to a court case. This is another reason to be sure that your radio conversations are professional, concise, and accurate.

You will also note that dispatch gives the time after most communications with you. This will help you in providing times for your written report of a run. Accurate recording of time during a run can also be critical if the run should lead to a law suit.

The information that dispatch provides to you will assist you in doing your job. But remember that dispatch coordinates the different parts of the EMS system. Dispatch also needs information from you to ensure that all those parts work together efficiently. Communicate with dispatch at the following points:

1. To acknowledge the dispatch information
2. To estimate your time of arrival at the scene while en route and to report any special road conditions, unusual delays, and so on
3. To announce your unit's arrival on the scene and to request any needed additional resources, then help coordinate the response
4. To announce the unit's departure and the destination hospital, number of patients transported (if more than one), and estimated time of arrival at the hospital
5. To announce your arrival at the hospital or another facility
6. To announce that you are "clear" and available for another assignment
7. To announce your arrival back at base

MEDICAL PERSONNEL

On a run, you may have to communicate with medical personnel at various times via your radio. The majority of these communications will be with your system's medical direction and with personnel at the facility to which you are transporting a patient.

COMMUNICATING WITH MEDICAL DIRECTION

In some EMS systems, medical direction may be at your receiving facility. In others, it will be at a separate location. You will often be expected to consult with medical direction on a run. There are cases in which medical direction may give you permission to assist in administering a patient's prescribed medication or may direct you to administer a medication from the ambulance's stock. Medical direction

may also suggest procedures that you should follow with a patient or tell you not to perform other procedures.

Radio communications between EMTs in the field and their medical direction should be organized, concise, and pertinent. For this purpose, it is helpful to have a standard format for communicating patient information over the radio. This ensures that significant information is related in a consistent manner and that nothing is omitted. When communicating with medical direction, provide the following information:

1. Your unit's identification and its level of service: BLS (Basic Life Support) or ALS (Advanced Life Support)
2. The patient's age and sex
3. The patient's chief complaint
4. A brief, pertinent history of the present illness, including scene assessment and mechanism of injury
5. Major past illnesses
6. The patient's mental status
7. The patient's baseline vital signs
8. Pertinent findings of your physical examination of the patient
9. Description of the emergency medical care you (and first responders) have given the patient
10. The patient's response to the emergency medical care

To ensure that you have communicated information accurately to medical direction and that you understand their directions completely, follow these additional guidelines:

- Be sure that the information you provide to medical direction is accurate and that you report it in a clear, understandable way. Remember that your patient's life may depend on the decisions that medical direction makes with that information.
- After receiving an order from medical direction to administer a medication or follow a procedure with a patient, repeat the order back word for word. This applies to things that medical direction tells you not to do, as well.
- If you do not understand an order from medical direction, ask that it be repeated. Then repeat it back to medical direction word for word.
- If an order from medical direction appears to be inappropriate, question the order. Possibly medical direction misunderstood something in your description of the patient's condition or misspoke in prescribing a course of action. Asking questions may prevent the administration of a harmful medication or the application of an inappropriate procedure.

COMMUNICATING WITH THE RECEIVING FACILITY

As an EMT-B, you will also be expected to communicate with medical personnel at the receiving facility to which you are transporting a patient. Staff at the facility need as much pertinent information about the incoming patient as possible to prepare for his arrival and to ensure continuity of care. Doctors and nurses may need to assign rooms and set aside equipment for your patient. If, through your communication with the receiving facility, you provide an accurate picture of your patient's condition, the correct decisions about the assignment of resources can be made at the facility.

The information the EMT-B conveys to the receiving facility is quite similar to that given to medical dispatch. When you are about to leave the scene of a call and begin transport, contact the receiving facility with this information:

1. Your unit's identification and its level of service (BLS, ALS)
2. The patient's age and sex
3. The patient's chief complaint
4. A brief, pertinent history of the present illness, including scene assessment and mechanism of injury
5. Major past illnesses
6. The patient's mental status
7. The patient's baseline vital signs
8. Pertinent findings of your physical examination of the patient
9. Description of the emergency medical care you (and first responders) have given the patient
10. The patient's response to the emergency medical care
11. Your estimated time of arrival at the facility

As you transport the patient to the receiving facility, you will reassess him and record your findings. Depending upon your local protocol, you may be expected to communicate those findings, especially if the patient's condition is deteriorating, while you are en route. Make it a routine practice to report any deterioration or improvement to the receiving facility.

THE ORAL REPORT

In any case, once you are at the facility and turning the patient over to staff there, you will deliver an oral report that takes into account your reassessment findings. That oral report should summarize the information you already broadcast to the facility, along with updated information from your ongoing assessment. Key items to include are the following:

- The patient's chief complaint
- The patient's vital signs taken en route

- Treatment given to the patient en route and his response to it
- Pertinent history not given in the earlier report to the facility

In addition to your oral reports to the receiving facility, both over the air and in person, you must also supply the facility with a copy of a written report. This document is known as the prehospital care report (PCR). You will learn more about filling out the PCR in Chapter 12, "Documentation."

INTERPERSONAL COMMUNICATIONS

When you arrive on a call, you may find the people at the scene hurt, frightened, anxious, and possibly angry and in shock. These are all high-intensity emotions that can make getting information from and delivering information to people difficult. To establish effective face-to-face communications with people in such circumstances, you should keep in mind the three Cs: competence, confidence, and compassion. If you convey these qualities, you will get better cooperation and have to deal with fewer hostile or irrational responses.

TAKING CHARGE

It will be necessary for you as an EMT-B to take charge confidently at the scene to which you have been called. Your personal appearance and professional manner from the time of your arrival throughout your stay at the scene will help communicate to bystanders and family members, as well as to the patient, that you are in charge.

If you arrive on the scene and observe that the patient is alert and that no life-threatening conditions are present, it may be appropriate to be briefed—before you make direct contact with the patient—by the first responder, whether that person is a police officer, a relative, or someone who has given first aid. This need not take more than a minute.

If the patient is unresponsive and life-threatening injuries are observed, go directly to the patient. Ask questions of the bystanders as you provide emergency care.

If a doctor is present or if fire-rescue personnel or police are also on the scene, an orderly transfer of authority must occur so that you are not simultaneously engaged in a dispute and attempting to care for the patient. Sometimes just asking a clear question like, "We're Emergency Medical Technicians. Is there anything we need to know before we provide emergency care?" will let rescue and police personnel brief you quickly and allow you to take over patient care. If a doctor is present, say, "We're certified EMTs, Doctor.

How can we help?" In any situation, the EMT-B must be the advocate for good and proper patient care and not allow secondary issues to interfere with it.

COMMUNICATING WITH THE PATIENT

Follow these guidelines when communicating with the patient:

- When you approach the patient, introduce yourself in the same manner as described above (if the patient is responsive). Ask for the patient's name. Also ask what he wishes to be called. With older people, err on the side of formality—"Mrs. Lubeck" or "Mr. Perez"—since they may consider it disrespectful for a stranger to address them by their first names. Remember to continue to use the patient's name throughout your contact with him.
- Be sure to say also, "I'm going to help you. Is that all right?" This will help in gaining consent for treatment as discussed in Chapter 3, "Medical, Legal, and Ethical Issues," and Chapter 12, "Documentation."
- Don't be surprised if a patient says, "No!" or "I'm okay!" when you ask about providing assistance. Usually he will be responding out of denial because he is simply frightened or confused. Keep talking calmly, saying something like, "Looks like an accident happened here. I can see there's something wrong with your shoulder. Does it hurt?" or "Your husband called us because he's worried about you. Would it be all right if we talked about it for a minute or two?"
- Maintain eye contact when you are speaking with the patient. Doing so helps to communicate your interest and concern. However, you should be aware that in some cultures, direct eye contact is considered rude; you may have to modify your behavior if you note that a patient is reluctant to make eye contact with you.
- Speak calmly and slowly. People who are under stress or in medical shock process information more slowly. Speak distinctly. Raise your voice only if the patient is hard of hearing or disoriented. Speak simply. Try to use language an average person will understand rather than using medical terminology, codes, and abbreviations. Try to give orders quietly. People follow emotions, and emotions can escalate quickly in tense situations.
- Think about the position you assume in relation to the patient. If your eye level is above that of the patient, you are in a dominant position, denoting authority and control. This may be intimidating to some patients, and you may find communication more effective when you are at or below the patient's eye level. If, however, a patient seems hostile or aggressive, you may find it preferable to keep your eye level above his to assert your authority.
- Be courteous. Patients and bystanders are often emotionally unstable. Explaining what you are doing, giving them choices when possible, being honest with them, and apologizing for necessary discomfort are ways of acknowledging their control in the situation. Listen when a patient asks you questions and reply as fully as you can, explaining when you cannot answer a question. Also, give the patient time to answer a question before you ask another one.
- Be sensitive to the power of touch. In American culture generally, intimate space starts at about 18 inches from the body. Eye contact is a way of allowing you into that space so that when you need to touch the person, that touch is not perceived as encroachment. Touching is an almost instinctive form of comforting another person, and it can be welcome, even from a stranger. Take a hand, pat a shoulder, smile reassuringly, or lay your hand on a forearm. Remember that you have to be comfortable doing it, too, and not just trying it as a gimmick.

SPECIAL CIRCUMSTANCES

There are some categories of patients with whom you will have to make extra efforts to establish effective communications. Remember that, even when you are having problems communicating with someone, you should remain calm, confident, and caring. The following are special communication circumstances:

- When dealing with a person who has hearing problems, be sure your lips are visible as you speak. If a patient is deaf but indicates he can communicate through American Sign Language (ASL), check to see if relatives or bystanders can interpret for you. Also consider writing notes on a pad to communicate.
- Some patients may not speak English. Again, ask if relatives or bystanders can interpret. If no one at the scene can assist, check with dispatch or medical direction to see if they have anyone who can interpret for you over the radio.
- Be prepared to take extra time in communicating with elderly people. Aging can bring with it problems with hearing and vision. Do not assume that all elderly patients have such problems, but if you detect signs of them, show understanding. Speak slowly, distinctly, and more loudly to such patients. Be sure to position yourself so that the patient can see your lips. Never appear brusque or impatient. Communicating with the elderly patient was covered in detail in Chapter 10, "Assessment of Geriatric Patients."
- Working with children also requires extra patience and effort. Having a child's parents present can aid

in communicating with the child, but be sure that the parents understand that they should remain calm and confident in front of the child. If they seem too frightened or disoriented by the situation, they will communicate those feelings to the child and complicate your ability to assist him.

- Positioning yourself close to the patient's eye level is especially important with children. A uniformed figure towering overhead can be terribly upsetting to a child. Crouch down to his level or sit on the floor if the circumstances seem to suggest it. Maintain eye contact and speak calmly. Try to explain what you are doing in simple language, without talking down to the child. Communicating with the pediatric patient will be covered in detail in Chapter 38, "Infants and Children."

ENRICHMENT

The enrichment section contains information that is valuable as background for the EMT-B but that goes substantially beyond the U.S. Department of Transportation (DOT) EMT-Basic curriculum.

RADIO CODES

Some EMS systems use radio codes, either alone or in combination with messages in plain English. Radio codes can shorten radio air time and provide clear and concise information. They can also allow transmission of information in a format not understood by the patient, family members, or bystanders. There are, however, several disadvantages to the use of codes. First, the codes are useless unless everyone in the system understands them. Second, medical information is often too complex for codes. Third, some codes are infrequently used, so valuable time may be wasted looking up a code's meaning.

Some EMS services still use the Ten-Code system (for example, "10-4" meaning "received and understood"). Published by the Associated Public Safety

Communications Officers (APCO), it is used primarily for dispatch, occasionally in EMS. Many EMS systems, however, have abandoned all codes in favor of standard English.

TIMES

U.S. Department of Transportation guidelines call for the use of accurate and synchronous clocks by EMT-Bs. As an aid to ensuring such accuracy and synchronicity, most systems use military time rather than standard A.M. and P.M. designations in radio and written reports. Military time is a very simple system and correlates with standard time as follows:

1 A.M. to 12 Noon = 0100 to 1200 hours
1 P.M. to Midnight = 1300 to 2400 hours
Examples of the military time system include the following:
1427 hours is 2:27 P.M.
0030 hours is thirty minutes after midnight.

RADIO TERMS

Radio conversations can be shortened by the use of one- or two-word phrases that are universally understood and employed. The following is a list of frequently used radio terms:

Break—afford a "pause" so that the hospital can respond or interrupt if necessary
Clear—end of transmission
Come in—requesting acknowledgment of transmission
Copy—message received and understood
ETA—estimated time of arrival
Go ahead—proceed with your message
Landline—refers to telephone communications
Over—end of message, awaiting reply
Repeat/say again—did not understand message
Spell out—asking sender to spell out phonetically words that are unclear
Stand by—please wait
10-4—acknowledging that message is received and understood

CASE STUDY FOLLOW-UP

SCENE SIZE-UP

You have been dispatched to 101 Bate Road with a report of a man bleeding. You approach the scene carefully, looking for any signs of danger. You see nothing that causes you concern, but you still exercise caution as you and your partner don gloves and protective eyewear and get out of the ambulance. As you do, a man who had been sitting next to the garage approaches you. He is holding a blood-soaked

rag around his right hand. His shirt and pants are also blood stained. The man appears pale and seems to be sweating a little.

As you start toward him, the man says, "You guys got here fast. I'm glad to see you. I feel like an idiot having to call, but no one else was home and I felt a little dizzy seeing all the blood. The bleeding's almost stopped now, though. Oh, yeah. Hi. I'm Dave Behrens."

You introduce yourselves and lead Mr. Behrens to the ambulance where he can sit down. When he's seated, you ask, "How did you injure yourself, Mr. Behrens?" He replies, "I was cutting some molding with my Sabre saw at my workbench. That's in the garage. I think the cat must have gotten in and knocked over a bottle. Anyway, it startled me. I turned to look and ran my hand into the blade. Idiot."

INITIAL ASSESSMENT

Your general impression of the patient is of a male in his mid-40s, injured, and alert. Because he responds fully to all questions you see he has no breathing problems and his airway is patent. You assess his radial pulse on the uninjured side and find it to be slightly fast, but strong. The rag wrapped around the hand he says he injured is blood soaked, but no blood appears to be dripping from the wrapping now. Because the bleeding appears to be controlled and Mr. Behrens displays no signs or symptoms of shock, he is not considered a priority for rapid transport.

FOCUSED HISTORY AND PHYSICAL EXAM

Mr. Behrens has already given you the mechanism of injury, a cut from the blade of a Sabre saw. You now expose the injury, carefully removing the greasy rag in which he has wrapped the hand. The injury is an approximately 3-inch-long laceration across the base of the palm. The wound is now bleeding only minimally. You apply a sterile dressing to the wound and bandage it in place.

You assess distal perfusion by observing skin color, which appears normal, and by feeling the injured hand, which is warm and moist. You ask Mr. Behrens if he can gently wiggle the fingers of the injured hand and he does so. You then ask him to turn his head to one side and identify the fingers on the injured hand that you touch. He does so successfully.

You and your partner obtain a set of baseline vital signs. Mr. Behrens' blood pressure is 148/86. His heart rate is 92 per minute. His respirations are 14 per minute, full and adequate. His skin is normal color, warm, and moist.

You take a SAMPLE history. It reveals the following: Mr. Behrens says the wound is causing slight pain; he has an allergy to penicillin; he is not currently taking any medications; he denies having any significant medical problems; he had a cup of coffee about 15 minutes before cutting himself; he denies that there were any strange or unusual problems prior to the accident.

You explain to Mr. Behrens that a doctor should look at and treat the cut and that you will transport him to the hospital. He refuses, however, to ride on the cot saying, "It's bad enough that I had to call you for a dumb mistake. I'm not going to go in like something from E.R." He agrees to ride on the jump seat and you secure him to it.

As you start off, you radio in a report: "Dispatch, this is Unit 2. We are en route to Columbia Memorial Hospital with a non-priority patient." Dispatch replies, "Unit 2 en route to Columbia Memorial at 1143 hours."

ONGOING ASSESSMENT

Your partner is riding in the back with Mr. Behrens. She performs the ongoing assessment. She finds that Mr. Behrens remains completely alert and oriented. Blood has not soaked through the dressing, an indication that bleeding has been controlled. She takes another set of vital signs, then radios ahead to the hospital: "Columbia Memorial, this is Craryville BLS Unit 2 en route to you with an ETA of 10 minutes. We have a 46-year-old male with a 3-inch laceration of the right hand caused by a Sabre saw. The patient is alert and oriented. The patient says he is allergic to penicillin. His vital signs are blood pressure 146/84, radial pulse 80, respirations 14 and of good quality, skin normal, warm, and moist. We have dressed and bandaged the wound. Bleeding appears to have stopped and patient acknowledges only slight pain from the wound."

Your partner continues to monitor Mr. Behrens during transport, but notes no major changes in his condition other than that he now seems completely relaxed. As you pull up to the hospital you radio this message: "Dispatch. This is Unit 2 arriving at Columbia Memorial." Dispatch acknowledges with "Unit 2 at Columbia Memorial at 1152 hours."

You and your partner assist Mr. Behrens from the ambulance and transfer him to the care of the hospital staff. Your partner says to the emergency department nurse, "This is Mr. David Behrens. He has a 3-inch laceration to the palm of his right hand from a Sabre saw. Mr. Behrens is allergic to penicillin. We applied a dressing and bandages to the wound and the bleeding appears to have stopped completely. His vitals are blood pressure 144/82, pulse 80, respirations 14, skin normal."

The nurse takes charge of Mr. Behrens while your partner fills out the prehospital care report. You begin to straighten and clean the back of the ambulance. When your partner returns, you radio, "Dispatch, this is Unit 2. We are available for assignment." Dispatch replies, "Unit 2 available for assignment at 1207 hours." You then start back to base, remembering that you will radio dispatch on your arrival there.

CHAPTER REVIEW

TERMS AND CONCEPTS

You may wish to review the following terms and concepts included in this chapter.

base station—the central dispatch and coordination area of an EMS communications system that ideally is in contact with all other elements of the system.

decoder—device that recognizes and responds to only certain codes imposed on radio broadcasts.

encoder—device that breaks down sound waves into unique digital codes for radio transmission.

repeaters—devices that receive transmissions from a relatively low-powered source such as a mobile or portable radio and rebroadcast them at another frequency and a higher power.

REVIEW QUESTIONS

1. List the standard components of an EMS communications system.
2. Explain the function of a repeater.
3. Explain legal considerations that apply to EMS communications.
4. List the points at which EMT-Bs on a run are expected to communicate with dispatch.
5. Explain the procedure that should be followed when medical direction orders an EMT-B to administer a medication or follow a designated procedure with a patient.
6. List the information that the EMT-B should provide to the receiving facility while en route with the patient.
7. List the information the EMT-B is expected to provide in the oral report when turning a patient over at a receiving facility.
8. Explain the importance of eye contact with a patient.
9. Explain the possible effects on communication with a patient of (a) the EMT-Bs body position and (b) touch.
10. Explain what measures an EMT-B might take when trying to communicate with a patient who is deaf or hearing impaired.

CHAPTER 12

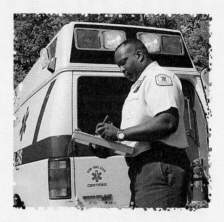

Documentation

INTRODUCTION

Assessing a patient, treating him, and transporting him to a facility where he can receive necessary medical care are the most obvious parts of the job of the EMT-Basic. But there is another function that you will have to perform as an EMT-B: the preparation of documentation for each patient you come in contact with. That documentation, in the form of written or electronically generated records, will help ensure that the patient receives the best, most appropriate care at the facility to which he is transported. The documentation you generate is important for other reasons as well, as you will learn in this chapter.

OBJECTIVES

Numbered objectives are from the United States Department of Transportation 1994 EMT-Basic National Standard Curriculum. Asterisked objectives, if any, pertain to material that is supplemental to the DOT curriculum.

COGNITIVE

3-8.1 Explain the components of the written report and list the information that should be included in the written report. (pp. 249–252)

3-8.2 Identify the various sections of the written report. (pp. 249–252)

3-8.3 Describe what information is required in each section of the prehospital care report and how it should be entered. (pp. 249–252)

3-8.4 Define the special considerations concerning patient refusal. (pp. 253–254)

3-8.5 Describe the legal implications associated with the written report. (pp. 253–255)

3-8.6 Discuss all state and/or local record and reporting requirements. (p. 255)

AFFECTIVE

3-8.7 Explain the rationale for patient care documentation. (p. 249)

3-8.8 Explain the rationale for the EMS system gathering data. (p. 249)

3-8.9 Explain the rationale for using medical terminology correctly. (p. 252)

3-8.10 Explain the rationale for using an accurate and synchronous clock so that information can be used in trending. (p. 251)

PSYCHOMOTOR

3-8.11 Complete a prehospital care report.

CASE STUDY

THE DISPATCH

EMS Unit 17—respond to 57 Vallejo Road. You have a man injured when his vehicle struck a parked car. Time out is 1321 hours.

ON ARRIVAL

You and your partner arrive at 1327 hours. As you drive up, you observe four people standing around two vehicles. As you get out of the ambulance, a woman walks over to you from the group. She says, "I called you. That's my van parked at the curb. I was in the house, heard a crash, looked out, and saw that that car had hit mine. The driver was slumped over the wheel, so I called 9-1-1 right away. When I came out of the house, though, he seemed to be all right.

He's the one in the green shirt." She indicates a man who is pacing around inspecting the damage to the two vehicles.

You and your partner walk toward the man she points to, who appears to be in his mid-30s. He looks at you and says, "Great! As if I didn't have enough trouble today, I've got to deal with you guys! Go away. I don't need any help!"

How would you proceed to assess, care for, and document this patient contact?

In this chapter, you will learn about the importance of documenting all your encounters with patients as well as the types of information that go into such documentation. Later, we will return to this case and apply what you have learned.

REASONS FOR DOCUMENTATION

The documentation you assemble as an EMT-B serves a variety of functions. It can be helpful to the patient, to the medical personnel who treat him, to the organizations that have aided him, to scientists and researchers who may never come in actual contact with the patient, and also to you.

MEDICAL USES

The prime reason for high-quality documentation is, of course, high-quality patient care. Reporting the data you have obtained during your contact with a patient and recording, simply but completely, the emergency care rendered helps ensure continuity of care for the patient throughout his need for medical attention. Your documentation gives emergency department personnel the information they need to provide the most appropriate treatment in a timely manner.

When the emergency department staff study the description of a patient's mental status as well as the vital signs that you obtained and recorded during assessment and transport, they have a baseline against which that patient's improvement or deterioration can be measured. When they read your account of the patient's complaint and the signs and symptoms you have marked down, they have a clearer idea of what course they should follow in the treatment of that patient. When they note the interventions you have or have not performed, they know more clearly what measures to take and which would duplicate earlier efforts. In addition, your documentation will provide details from sources to which hospital personnel may have no access (e.g., bystanders, family, or awake patient).

ADMINISTRATIVE USES

The documentation you provide typically becomes a part of the patient's permanent hospital record. It will be used in preparing bills and in submitting records to insurance companies.

LEGAL USES

The medical documentation you prepare may also become a legal document. A run in which you were involved may have been the result of a crime. Or the incident may have led to a lawsuit. In either case, you may have to appear in court as a witness. As such, you will refer to the documentation you generated for that run months or even years earlier. Legible, accurate, and complete documentation will be of major assistance in such cases. In addition, if you yourself are the subject of a lawsuit, your documentation may be an essential element in your defense.

EDUCATIONAL AND RESEARCH USES

Finally, your documentation provides data for researchers studying a whole range of issues. Some researchers might be scientists looking to discover positive or negative effects of certain interventions at different stages of patient contact. Others might be experts in administration studying documentation in an effort to deliver services in a more timely or cost-effective manner. Reviews of documentation are an integral part of the quality improvement process. Remedial training and continued education courses for EMT-Bs in your area may be based upon needs revealed by a study of call documentation.

THE PREHOSPITAL CARE REPORT

As you can see, the documentation you are responsible for has a variety of important uses. Because it does, you should be as careful and thorough as possible when assembling it. The major piece of documentation you must provide is the **prehospital care report (PCR)**.

The PCR can have different names in different parts of the country, such as the run report or the trip sheet. The look of the PCR can also vary, depending on the format used for it and the information required on it.

PCR FORMATS

The most traditional format for the PCR is the written report. This format usually combines check boxes and write-on lines for vital signs and other information that can be entered briefly, along with areas for writing a fuller narrative account of the patient contact (Figure 12-1).

An alternative format to the written report that is gaining wider acceptance is the computerized report. The styles of computerized reports may vary. With some, the EMT-B fills in boxes on sheets of paper and the report is scanned by a computer. In others, data is entered directly into a laptop computer.

A variation of the computerized report uses an electronic clipboard, which is a computer in the form of a clipboard (Figure 12-2). In such a "pen-based" computer system, the computer clipboard has the capability of recognizing and interpreting the user's handwriting and converting the information he enters into an electronic format.

Computerized systems offer the promise of storing more information about a patient in a more legible format than written reports. They also allow greater efficiencies in storing, retrieving, and utilizing

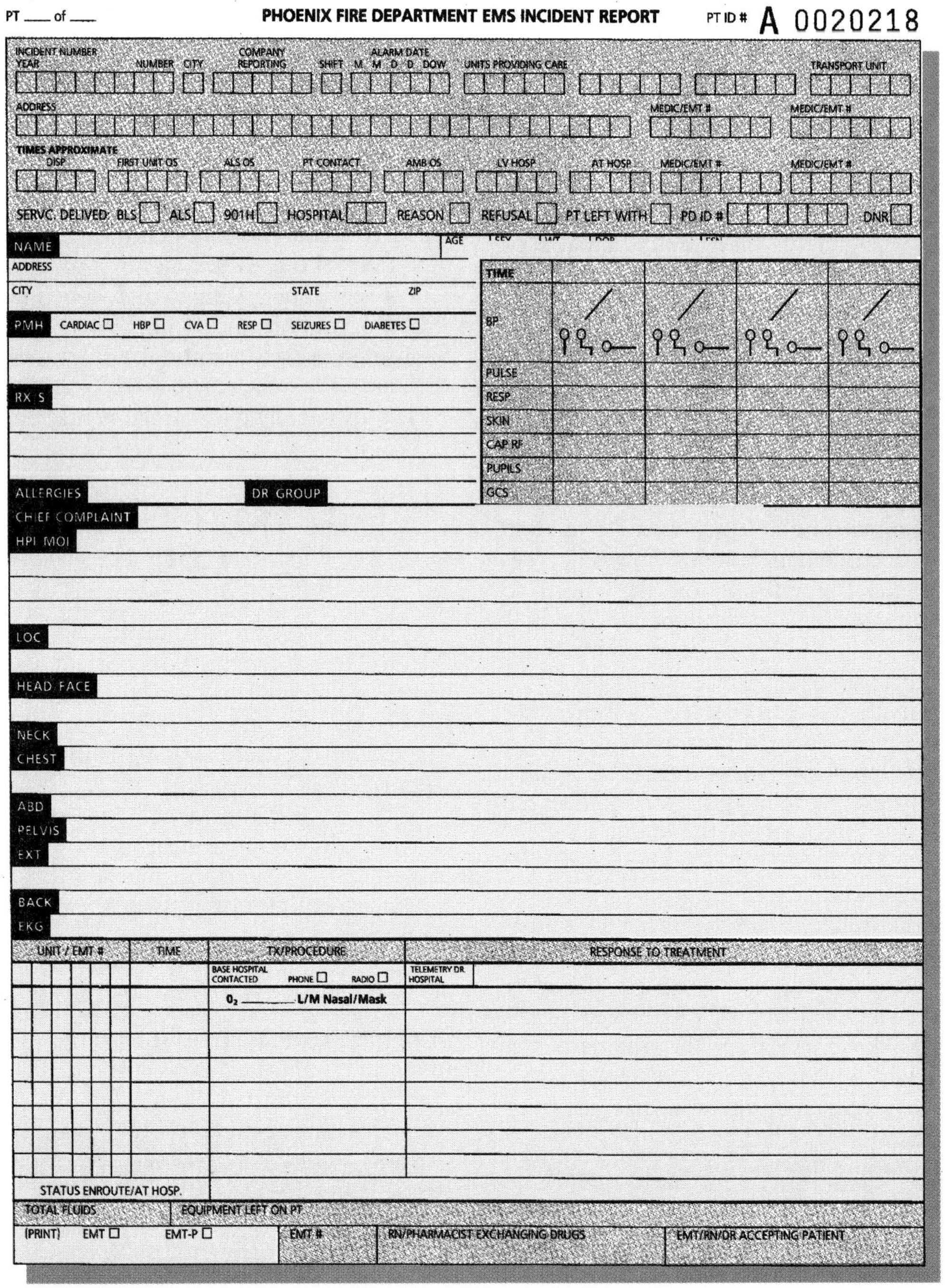
PT ___ of ___ PHOENIX FIRE DEPARTMENT EMS INCIDENT REPORT PT ID # A 0020218

INCIDENT NUMBER YEAR NUMBER CITY | COMPANY REPORTING | SHIFT | ALARM DATE M M D D DOW | UNITS PROVIDING CARE | TRANSPORT UNIT

ADDRESS | MEDIC/EMT # | MEDIC/EMT #

TIMES APPROXIMATE: DISP | FIRST UNIT OS | ALS OS | PT CONTACT | AMB OS | LV HOSP | AT HOSP | MEDIC/EMT # | MEDIC/EMT #

SERVC. DELIVED: BLS ☐ ALS ☐ 901H ☐ HOSPITAL ☐ REASON ☐ REFUSAL ☐ PT LEFT WITH ☐ PD ID # ☐ DNR ☐

NAME | AGE

ADDRESS

CITY STATE ZIP

PMH CARDIAC ☐ HBP ☐ CVA ☐ RESP ☐ SEIZURES ☐ DIABETES ☐

RX S

ALLERGIES | DR GROUP

TIME | BP | PULSE | RESP | SKIN | CAP RF | PUPILS | GCS

CHIEF COMPLAINT

HPI MOI

LOC

HEAD FACE

NECK

CHEST

ABD

PELVIS

EXT

BACK

EKG

UNIT / EMT # | TIME | TX/PROCEDURE | RESPONSE TO TREATMENT

BASE HOSPITAL CONTACTED PHONE ☐ RADIO ☐ | TELEMETRY DR HOSPITAL

O_2 ______ L/M Nasal/Mask

STATUS ENROUTE/AT HOSP.

TOTAL FLUIDS | EQUIPMENT LEFT ON PT

(PRINT) EMT ☐ EMT-P ☐ | EMT # | RN/PHARMACIST EXCHANGING DRUGS | EMT/RN/DR ACCEPTING PATIENT

Figure 12-1 Traditional types of prehospital care reports consist of a combination of check boxes, write-in spaces, and open narrative sections. The example above is from the Phoenix Fire Department Emergency Medical Services, City of Phoenix, Arizona.

data the EMT-B collects. The EMT-B's computer can be linked to diagnostic and monitoring equipment; to electronic medical records; to computer-aided dispatch (CAD); and to computer systems handling fleet management, inventory control, electronic mail, personnel, and payroll.

On a more basic level, a computerized system can check the EMT-B's spelling and use of abbreviations, ensuring a more accurate report. Such systems can also monitor data as it is input and alert the EMT-B if any necessary information has been omitted.

PCR DATA

Of course, what makes the PCR useful is the information entered on it. That information should provide a complete and accurate picture of your contact with the patient. Remember these two basic rules

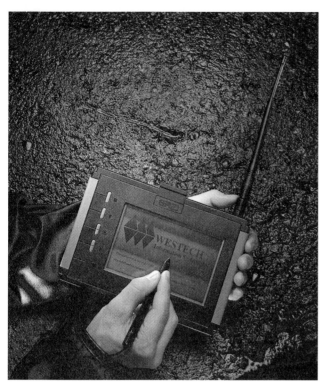

Figure 12-2   The electronic clipboard, a computer in the form of a clipboard, uses a pen-based system to record prehospital data.

when filling out any PCR: "If it wasn't written down, it wasn't done" (no one, including emergency department staff, will know it was done; and you won't be able to prove it was done, for example in a court of law) and "If it wasn't done, don't write it down" (which constitutes falsifying information).

Requirements for information on the PCR vary from system to system and state to state, but the types of information required and the sections of the PCR are generally quite similar.

The Minimum Data Set

The U.S. Department of Transportation has been making an effort to standardize the information collected on PCRs. Such standardization will, it is hoped, lead to a higher general level of patient care across the nation. It will also permit more meaningful comparison and analysis of data from various systems, which may speed the implementation of new and better methods of emergency care.

The Department of Transportation calls the information it wants on all PCRs the **minimum data set.** Below are the elements of the DOT's minimum data set.

Patient Information Gathered by the EMT-B
- Chief complaint
- Level of responsiveness (AVPU)—mental status

- Systolic blood pressure for patients greater than 3 years old
- Skin perfusion (capillary refill) for patients less than 6 years old
- Skin color and temperature
- Pulse rate
- Respiratory rate and effort

Administrative Information:
- Time the incident was reported
- Time the unit was notified
- Time of arrival at the patient
- Time the unit left the scene
- Time the unit arrived at its destination (hospital, etc.)
- Time of transfer of care

Another important element in establishing the minimum data set is the use of accurate and synchronous clocks. This means that all elements of an EMS system should use clocks or time-keeping devices that are accurately set and agree with each other. Dispatch's clock should not show one time, while the watches of the EMT-Bs show another. Accurate time-keeping helps in the gathering of accurate medical information; for example, synchronous time-keeping by dispatch and the ambulance crew makes it easier to determine how long a patient has been in cardiac arrest before CPR or defibrillation was initiated. Accurate time-keeping can also be critical if administrative issues or legal questions over quality of care arise.

Many systems already require the gathering of the information included in the DOT's minimum data set. Such information is usually arranged in the following sections on the PCR.

Administrative Information

The administrative information section of the PCR is sometimes referred to as the run data. It usually includes the administrative information listed in the minimum data set. In addition, it may also include:

- The EMS unit number and the run or call number
- Names of crew members and their levels of certification
- The address to which the unit is dispatched

Patient Data

The next major section of the PCR contains data about the patient. Most systems will require the following information:

- The patient's legal name, age, sex, birthdate
- The patient's home address
- The patient's social security number and additional insurance or billing information
- The location of the patient
- Any care given before the arrival of the EMT-Bs

Vital Signs

A third major division of the PCR documents the patient's vital signs. On many forms, boxes are provided for checking off or writing in information. This section usually includes much of the patient information called for in the DOT's minimum data set. Various systems may also require additional data.

Ideally, at least two complete sets of vital signs should be taken and recorded. It is important to note the patient's position at the time the vital signs were taken (e.g., supine, standing, sitting). It is also critical to record the times at which the vital signs were obtained.

Patient Narrative

The next part of the PCR gives more detailed information about the patient and his problem than allowed for in check boxes. This critical information will set the tone for the entire course of assessment, treatment, and documentation that will follow. This narrative section will contain the following:

- The patient's chief complaint—This should be in the patient's own words or in the words of a bystander, if the patient is unresponsive. Put such statements in quotation marks ("My leg hurts") on the report.
- The patient's SAMPLE history or a description of the mechanism of injury—This data will include an account of when the chief complaint began and how it has progressed, along with other details of the patient history.

In this section of the PCR, you will create a brief but thorough picture of the patient and his problem. Remember that you are recording details for other medical personnel to use, not presenting your own conclusions about an incident. Careful observation of the patient and the scene as well as intelligent questioning of the patient and bystanders are essential. These methods will provide both *objective* and *pertinent subjective* information for the narrative section.

Objective information is measurable or verifiable in some way. It might be a reference to the patient's pulse rate or a statement that the patient has discoloration below both eyes. A sign is an objective observation.

Subjective information is information based on an individual's perceptions or interpretations. Subjective information in the narrative section may come from either the patient or the EMT-B. For example, a patient might say, "I feel light-headed." An EMT-B might observe, "The patient seems to be in pain." A symptom is a subjective finding.

Subjective information should be *pertinent;* that is, it should relate to the medical circumstances. It should not include attempts at diagnosis. Nor should it include irrelevant observations such as, "The patient's husband offered to transport the patient."

In questioning a patient, be alert to **pertinent negatives.** These are signs or symptoms that might be expected, based on the chief complaint, but that the patient denies having. A pertinent negative might be a patient's denial of pain after an automobile crash or a lack of difficulty in breathing in a case of chest pain. By noting the absence of pertinent signs and symptoms, you will provide the medical team that takes over care of the patient a fuller picture of his condition.

The narrative should briefly document the physical assessment in the order it was performed (i.e., head, neck, chest, and so on). Include pertinent information about the scene as well as about the patient. Note, for example, the presence of bottles of medication, a suicide note, or a collapsed ladder.

Write the narrative in a simple, direct style. Do not use radio codes or nonstandard abbreviations. Table 12-1 lists common standard abbreviations.

TABLE 12-1
Commonly Accepted Abbreviations

a	before
c	with
NTG	nitroglycerin
O2	oxygen
OB	obstetrics
p	after
PE	physical exam, pulmonary edema
po	orally, by mouth
Pt	patient
q	every
QID	four times a day
R/O	rule out
RHD	rheumatic heart disease
Rx	prescription
s	without
s/s	signs/symptoms
SIDS	sudden infant death syndrome
SL	sublingual
SOB	shortness of breath
STAT	immediately
Sx	symptoms
TIA	transient ischemic attack
TID	three times a day
TKO	to keep open
Tx	treatment
X	times
y/o	years old
↑	increased
↓	decreased

Be especially careful in your use of medical terminology. Make sure you are using the proper term and that you are spelling it correctly. Look up spellings and definitions in a medical dictionary if you have any doubts. If you are still uneasy about the meaning of a term, or whether it applies to the situation you are describing, use everyday language instead. Mistakes in medical terminology can cause confusion and lead to delays or errors in treatment.

TREATMENT

The final information for entry on the PCR involves the treatment provided to the patient. This section should detail in chronological order all treatment you administer to a patient as well as indications of how the patient responded to that treatment. This information should be written in a clear narrative style, following the guidelines cited in Patient Narrative above. An emergency department physician, nurse, paramedic, or fellow EMT-B should, by reading your report, be able to learn what treatment was provided, the time it was provided, and whether the patient has improved or deteriorated since then.

LEGAL CONCERNS

As noted earlier, the PCR is a legal document. Some legal issues involving documentation are discussed below.

CONFIDENTIALITY

You must use care and discretion when handling any information about a patient. Remember that, as detailed in Chapter 3, "Medical, Legal, and Ethical Issues," confidentiality is the patient's legal right. The PCR and the information on it are considered confidential. Do not show the form or discuss the information on it with unauthorized individuals.

Follow state rules and local protocols in distributing the PCR and any additional information about a patient encounter. By law, you are generally permitted to provide confidential information about a patient to a health-care provider who needs the information in order to continue care, to the police if they request information as part of a criminal investigation, information required on a third-party billing form, or in court if required by a legal subpoena.

REFUSAL OF TREATMENT

Chapter 3, "Medical, Legal, and Ethical Issues," discussed various issues that arise when a patient refuses treatment. As noted there, any competent adult has the right to refuse treatment. But legal questions often arise after the fact about whether the patient was truly competent. For this reason, you must make extra efforts with a patient who is refusing treatment to ensure that he fully understands what he is doing. You must also document your efforts completely.

1. When you encounter a patient who refuses treatment, try to perform as much of an assessment as possible. Doing so may give you information to use in explaining what might happen if the patient continues to refuse treatment.

2. Before leaving the scene always try to make one more effort to persuade the patient to go to the hospital. Ensure that the patient can make a rational, informed decision and is not under the influence of alcohol or other mind-altering drugs, suffering from the effects of an illness or injury, and is not suicidal.

3. Inform the patient as clearly as possible why he should go to the hospital. Explain what may happen if he does not go. Discuss the possible consequences of delaying or refusing treatment.

4. If the patient still refuses treatment, discuss the situation with medical direction as directed by local protocol. Such discussion can provide two major benefits. First, the patient may consider that the doctor's opinion carries more weight than the EMT-B's; so he may change his mind and accept treatment. Second, if the patient still refuses transport, the doctor can give the EMT-B direction in providing medical assistance at the scene.

5. If the patient still refuses to accept emergency care and/or transport, document in the PCR any assessment findings you have made, any emergency medical care you have given, and the explanation you gave the patient of the consequences of failing to accept care and/or transport (including potential death). You must document that the patient is alert and oriented to time, place, and person/self so there is no question that the patient understood the information and instructions you gave him. Then have the patient sign a refusal-of-care form (Figure 12-3). You should also have a family member, police officer, or bystander sign the form as a witness. If possible, obtain witnesses' addresses in case they must be contacted.

6. If the patient refuses to sign, have a family member, police officer, or bystander sign the form verifying that the patient refused. Each section of the refusal-of-care form must be completed.

7. Before leaving the scene, you should offer alternative methods of getting care (e.g., taking a taxi to a clinic or asking a friend or family member for help in seeing a doctor).

RELEASE FROM RESPONSIBILITY

DATE _____ 19 _____ TIME _____ a.m. / p.m.

This is to certify that _____

is refusing ☐ TREATMENT ☐ TRANSPORTATION

against the advice of the attending Emergency Medical Technician and of the Phoenix Fire Department, and when applicable, the base hospital and the base hospital physician.

I acknowledge that I have been informed of the following:

1. The nature and potential of the illness or injuries.
2. The potential risks of delaying treatment and transportation, up to and including death.
3. The availability of ambulance transportation to a hospital for treatment.

Nevertheless, I assume all risks and consequences of my decision, including further physical deterioration, loss of limb, paralysis, and even death, and hereby release the attending Emergency Medical Technician and the Phoenix Fire Department, and when applicable, the base hospital and the base hospital physician from any ill effects which may result from my refusal.

Witness _____ Signed: **X** _____

Witness _____ Relationship to Patient _____

Refusal must be signed by the patient; or by the nearest relative or legal guardian in the case of a minor, or when patient is physically or mentally incompetent.

☐ Patient refuses to sign release despite efforts of attending Emergency Medical Technician to obtain such signature after informing patient of concerns listed in numbers 1, 2, and 3 above.

GUIDELINES — Patient Refusal Documentation

In addition to those items normally documented (chief complaint, history of present illness, mechanism of injury, physical assessment, etc.) the following items should be recorded, regardless of patient's cooperation:

- Mental Status (orientation, speech, etc.)
- Suspected presence of alcohol or drugs
- Patient's exact words (as much as possible) in the refusal of care OR the signing of the release form
- Circumstances or reasons (including exact words of patient, if possible) for INCOMPLETE ADVISEMENT (risk of injury, abusiveness, unruliness, risk of injury other than from patient, etc.)
- Advice given to patients' guardian(s)

Figure 12-3   Patient refusal-of-care form, Phoenix Fire Department Emergency Medical Services, City of Phoenix, Arizona.

8. Finally, explain that you or another EMT-B crew will be happy to come back if the patient changes his mind and decides to accept treatment.

FALSIFICATION

The PCR documents the nature and extent of emergency medical care an EMT-B provides. It is meant to be a thorough and accurate record. Any mistake in care must be highlighted on the PCR. In such a situation, the EMT-B might be tempted to falsify the PCR.

Such falsification of information on a PCR should never occur. When an error of omission or commission occurs, the EMT-B should not try to cover it up. Instead, he should document exactly what did or did not happen and what steps were taken (if any) to correct the situation. False information may lead to suspension or revocation of EMT-B certification or license and, potentially, to criminal charges.

More importantly, falsification of patient data will compromise patient care. Other health care providers can get an incorrect impression of the patient's condition from false assessment findings or a falsified report of treatment.

Certain areas of the PCR are more commonly falsified than others. One of those areas is vital signs. An EMT-B might, for some reason, neglect to take a set of vital signs and be tempted to make up numbers to cover his omission. Another area is treatment. An EMT-B might assist a patient in taking a medication without the approval of medical direction. Or he might have neglected to give a patient complaining of chest pain oxygen. In the former case, he might be tempted to leave out of the PCR the fact that he assisted in administration of medicine, while in the latter he might want to write in that oxygen was given. In none of these cases should the record be falsified. Although the changes might appear insignificant, they could have catastrophic results.

CORRECTING ERRORS

Even the most careful EMT-B will occasionally make errors in filling out the PCR. When such an error is discovered while the report is being written, draw a single horizontal line through the error, initial it, and write the correct information beside it (Figure 12-4).

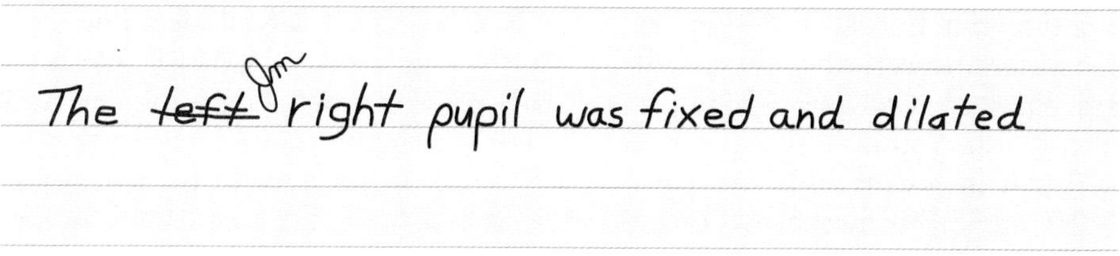

The ~~left~~ *jm* right pupil was fixed and dilated

Figure 12-4   The proper way of correcting an error in a prehospital care report is to draw a single line through the error, initial it, and write the correct information beside it.

Do not try to erase or write over the error. Such actions could be interpreted as attempts to cover up a mistake or falsify the report.

When an error is discovered after the report form is submitted, preferably using a different-color ink, draw a single horizontal line through the error. Add a note with the correct information. Initial the entry and include the date and time of the correction. If information was omitted, the EMT-B should add a note with the correct information, the date, and the EMT-B's initials. Be sure to bring such changes to the attention of those to whom the incorrect report was submitted.

SPECIAL SITUATIONS

There are certain circumstances in which the standard PCR will not be appropriate. Examples of such circumstances are discussed below.

MULTIPLE-CASUALTY INCIDENTS

During multiple-casualty incidents (MCIs) such as plane crashes or multiple-vehicle collisions, rescuers are often overwhelmed with the number of patients requiring treatment. The needs of these patients can sometimes conflict with the need for complete documentation. In these cases, there may not be enough time to complete the standard PCR before turning to the next patient.

Each EMS system has its own MCI plan. Those plans should have some means of recording important medical information and keeping that information with the patient as he is moved for treatment. Often such basic information as chief complaint, vital signs, and treatment provided is recorded on a **triage tag** that is attached to the patient. Information from the tag can be used later to complete the PCR. In MCI situations, the PCRs will usually be less detailed than those of more typical, single-patient runs. Local plans should contain guidelines for what is expected in the PCRs in those situations. More information on MCI situations will be provided in Chapter 43, "Multiple Casualty Incidents, Triage, and Disaster Management."

SPECIAL REPORTS

In some circumstances, EMT-Bs must fill out special documentation other than the usual PCR. These cases require the notification of agencies beyond the usual health care network. Such cases might include the following:

- Suspected abuse of a child or elderly person
- Possible exposure to an infectious disease (e.g., meningitis, hepatitis, TB, HIV)
- Injury to an EMS team member
- Other situations that the EMT-Basic feels might require special documentation and/or informing of another agency

State laws and local protocols usually outline the circumstances in which special reports are required and often provide a form for such reports. These special reports should be accurate, objective, and submitted in a timely manner. Always keep a copy for your own agency's records. The procedure for distribution of such reports is also set up by local protocol.

CASE STUDY FOLLOW-UP

SCENE SIZE-UP

You have been dispatched to the scene of an automobile accident. As you pull up, you observe a group of people standing by two vehicles. You note that the left front end of one vehicle that is in the street, a mid-size car, is dented in and the headlight is smashed. The right rear of the other, a minivan at the curb, is also dented and the light on that side is broken. A woman explains that the car struck her parked van while she was inside the house, and that she called 9-1-1. Your partner inspects the Taurus for signs of damage and clues to mechanism of injury sustained during the collision. You note that the man who was driving the car is in his mid-30s and has a slight bruise on the left side of his forehead. Despite this evidence of trauma, he is on his feet. He angrily says he does not want your help.

INITIAL ASSESSMENT

You remain calm and polite in spite of the driver's initial outburst. You and your partner introduce yourselves, and you say, "I understand that you've had some problems. We're certainly not here to give you any more trouble. We just want to make sure you're OK. Are you feeling all right? Do you have any pain, Mr. . . . ?"

"Makynen. Paul Makynen," he replies, appearing to grow calmer. "I'm sorry I flew off the handle, but it's been a bad day. I've been running late. I was on my way to see an important client when a dog ran out into the street. I braked and swerved. I missed it, but hit that van instead. I just bumped my forehead on the inside of the door frame. It's a little sore, I'm a little achy, but that's all. Look, I appreciate your coming out, but I'm OK, really. And I've got to get going."

You note from the patient's answer that he is alert, responsive, and is having no difficulty in breathing. However, you recall that the woman who called 9-1-1 said that right after the collision Mr. Makynen was slumped over the wheel. You ask him if he thinks he lost consciousness, however briefly. He denies it and says, "Nah, I just put my head down on the wheel because I was disgusted." You see no signs of bleeding. His skin appears to be pink and dry. Mr. Makynen refuses your partner's attempt to provide manual stabilization of his head and neck but permits you to assess his radial pulse. You find that his pulse is slightly rapid but strong and regular and that his skin is warm to the touch.

FOCUSED HISTORY AND PHYSICAL EXAM

You explain to Mr. Makynen that you would like to do a quick physical exam to check for any signs of injury. He becomes angry again and says, "Come on. I'm okay. I don't need that." You ask if you can take his blood pressure and other vital signs, and he says,

"No, no. Look, I really feel fine." He also refuses to answer any of the SAMPLE questions except to deny any pain or other symptoms. He rejects your suggestion that he be transported to the hospital.

You are not ready to give up yet. You tell Mr. Makynen that, because of the bump to the head, it would be best that he be checked by a doctor. You explain that head injuries often display no signs at first but can later develop into potentially life-threatening situations. He interrupts to say, "Fine, I'll take that chance, but I am leaving."

Your partner discreetly calls dispatch to say, "Patient is refusing emergency care and transport. We will inform you of our status shortly."

DOCUMENTATION

Meanwhile, recognizing that you are going to have no success in persuading Mr. Makynen to accept care, you explain to him that before he leaves he must sign a refusal-of-care form. You prepare the PCR and the refusal forms. On the PCR, you note the mechanism of injury, the bruise to the forehead, and your initial findings regarding his alert mental status, open airway, adequate breathing, absence of bleeding, pulse that is rapid but regular and strong, and skin color, temperature, and condition indicating adequate perfusion. You write that the patient denies pain and, although a witness reported that he was slumped over the wheel after the collision, patient denies losing consciousness.

You document that, at this point, the patient refused further care. You also note your recommendation that the patient see a doctor and your explanation of the possible consequences. You add that the patient still refused further care.

You show the PCR to Mr. Makynen and allow him to read it and the refusal form. While he is doing so, your partner explains the situation to the owner of the van and another bystander and asks them to witness the refusal. They agree and, after Mr. Makynen signs the refusal form, they also sign where you indicate.

As Mr. Makynen gets into his car, you suggest again that he see his personal physician as soon as possible. You add that if he suddenly feels dizzy or in pain, he shouldn't hesitate to call 9-1-1 for assistance.

Your partner contacts dispatch and states that the patient has refused treatment and transport. Your unit is now clear and in service.

CHAPTER REVIEW

TERMS AND CONCEPTS

You may wish to review the following terms and concepts included in this chapter.

minimum data set—the minimum information the U.S. Department of Transportation has determined should be included on all prehospital care reports.

pertinent negatives—signs or symptoms that might be expected in certain circumstances, based on the chief complaint, but are denied by the patient.

prehospital care report (PCR)—documentation of an EMT-B's contact with a patient.

triage tag—a tag containing key information about a patient that is attached to a patient during a multiple-casualty incident.

REVIEW QUESTIONS

1. Explain the various uses of the documentation that the EMT-B generates after a patient contact.
2. Describe two common formats for the prehospital care report.
3. Explain the origin and purpose of the minimum data set.
4. Explain what the phrase "accurate and synchronous clocks" means and why they are important.
5. Define pertinent negatives.
6. List the steps you should take if a patient refuses treatment.
7. Explain the meaning and importance of the following two documentation rules: "If it wasn't written down, it wasn't done" and "If it wasn't done, don't write it down."
8. Describe how errors on PCRs should be corrected.
9. Explain how a multiple casualty incident can affect EMT-B documentation.
10. Describe circumstances in which an EMT-B might be expected to file special reports with other agencies.

CHAPTER 13

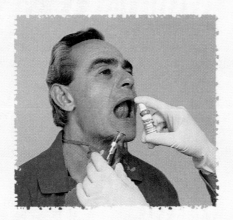

General Pharmacology

INTRODUCTION

As an EMT-Basic, you will be responsible for either administering or assisting the patient with the administration of certain medications. Only certain patients who have specific chief complaints or signs and symptoms will require medication. The medication will either be prescribed to the patient or will be carried on the EMS unit. Regardless of the source of the medication, you must attain medical direction's permission, whether as a standing order or as an on-line order, prior to administration.

Unlike a mathematician, you cannot erase your mistakes and start from scratch. Once the medication has been administered, it is not possible to extract what has been given or prevent the effects. Improper use of a medication may result in dangerous consequences for the patient. Therefore, it is vital that you be completely familiar with the medications and the proper procedures for administration.

OBJECTIVES

Numbered objectives are from the United States Department of Transportation 1994 EMT-Basic National Standard Curriculum. Asterisked objectives, if any, pertain to material that is supplemental to the DOT curriculum.

COGNITIVE

4-1.1 Identify which medications will be carried on the unit. (p. 260)

4-1.2 State the medications carried on the EMS unit by the generic name. (p. 260)

4-1.3 Identify the medications with which the EMT-Basic may assist the patient with administering. (p. 260)

4-1.4 State the medications the EMT-Basic can assist the patient with by the generic name. (p. 260)

4-1.5 Discuss the forms in which the medications may be found. (pp. 262–263)

* List and explain the various routes of drug administration used by the EMT-Basic. (pp. 261–262)

* List and describe the essential medication information that should be understood by the EMT-Basic. (pp. 263–264)

* List and describe the key steps in administering medications to a patient. (pp. 264–266)

* Describe the reassessment strategies used following medication administration. (p. 266)

* List sources that can be used to gather medication information. (p. 266)

AFFECTIVE

4-1.6 Explain the rationale for the administration of medications. (pp. 259–260)

PSYCHOMOTOR

4-1.7 Demonstrate general steps for assisting the patient with self-administration of medications.

4-1.8 Read the labels and inspect each type of medication.

CASE STUDY

THE DISPATCH

EMS Unit 202—respond to 1934 Lincoln Avenue—you have a 76-year-old male patient complaining of severe chest pain. Time out is 2136 hours.

ON ARRIVAL

The house is unlit and the surrounding area dark. You and your partner approach the house from the side, walk up onto the front porch, and stand on either side of the door. You ring the doorbell and hear a voice say, "Please help me . . . The door is open," and then, between gasps, "I'm having bad chest pain." With flashlights in hand, you and your partner decide to enter the scene very cautiously. Upon entry, you find an elderly man sitting on the hallway floor against the wall. You immediately turn on the hall light. A scan of the scene does not reveal any potential hazards. The patient is clutching his chest, complaining of severe crushing pain.

How would you proceed to assess and care for this patient—including the administration of medication?

During this chapter, you will learn about assessment and emergency care for a patient whose condition may require administration of a medication. Later, we will return to the case and apply the procedures learned.

ADMINISTERING MEDICATIONS

A **medication** is generally defined as a drug or other substance that is used as a remedy for illness. A **drug** is a chemical substance that is used to treat or prevent a disease or condition. The terms "drug" and "med-

ication" are often used interchangeably by EMTs. The study of drugs is referred to as **pharmacology.**

The EMT-Basic must take seriously the responsibility of administering medications. Medications have specific physiological effects on the cells, organs, or body systems. When the correct dose is administered appropriately, the patient's condition may improve significantly and uncomfortable symptoms may be relieved. If administered inappropriately, some drugs can cause serious side effects and deterioration in the patient's condition.

As an EMT-B, you will be administering medications under the direct order of a licensed physician. Without this order, you cannot administer any type of medication. Also, the EMT-B is only able to administer the medications identified in the local protocol, which may include all or some of the six medications covered in this chapter.

Remember that you may not administer or assist with administration of any medication other than the six medications covered in this chapter that are also identified in local protocols. For example, if you arrive on the scene and find a patient experiencing excruciating pain associated with a dislocated shoulder, and you find the patient's prescription of Percodan® at his side, it would be inappropriate for you to suggest, administer, or assist with the administration of the medication. Even though Percodan® is a pain reliever, and it might seem to "make sense" to use it to make the patient more comfortable, it is not an acceptable medication to be administered by an EMT-B.

MEDICATIONS COMMONLY ADMINISTERED BY THE EMT-B

Medications administered by the EMT-B are either carried on the EMS unit or are prescribed for the patient. The prescription medications may be found on the patient or at the scene. General steps for properly administering all of the medications mentioned below are detailed at the end of this chapter.

MEDICATIONS CARRIED ON THE EMS UNIT

The following medications may be carried on the EMS unit. Even though the EMT-B controls the administration of these medications and they are ready at hand on the ambulance, an off-line or on-line order from medical direction is still necessary.

- **Oxygen**—covered in detail in Chapter 7, "Airway Management, Ventilation, and Oxygen Therapy"
- **Oral glucose**—covered in detail in Chapter 17, "Altered Mental Status—Diabetic Emergencies"
- **Activated charcoal**—covered in detail in Chapter 21, "Poisoning Emergencies"

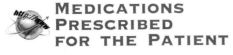

MEDICATIONS PRESCRIBED FOR THE PATIENT

Some of the medications that the EMT-B may administer or assist the patient with administering are not carried on the EMS unit. Instead, they are medications prescribed for the patient. Through good history taking, you should identify any medications the patient is currently taking.

The patient will typically have the medication in his possession; however, it may be necessary for you to locate it at the scene. For example, you arrive on the scene and find a patient who is experiencing severe chest pain. During your focused history and physical exam, you determine that the patient has a prescription for nitroglycerin tablets. The patient states that the tablets are upstairs next to the bed. You must remain with the patient while your partner, a family member, or a first responder retrieves the medication. Do not let the patient attempt to get the medication, since the activity may increase the discomfort or aggravate the medical condition.

Whether the EMT-B actually administers the medication or assists the patient in administering the medication is up to medical direction and local protocol.

The following are prescribed medications that EMT-Bs may administer or assist in administering:

- **Metered-dose inhaler** (Albuterol, Metaproterenol, Isoetharine)—covered in detail in Chapter 14, "Respiratory Emergencies"
- **Nitroglycerin**—covered in detail in Chapter 15, "Cardiac Emergencies"
- **Epinephrine**—covered in detail in Chapter 20, "Allergic Reaction"

MEDICATION NAMES

A medication, or drug, can have up to four different names: chemical, generic, trade, and official. These names are assigned during the development of the drug and are used interchangeably. The EMT-B must be most familiar with the generic and trade names. Table 13-1 lists generic and trade names and common uses for the medications the EMT-B may be allowed to administer or assist the patient with administering.

A description of the four drug names is as follows:

- *Chemical name*—The chemical name describes the drug's chemical structure. It is usually one of the first names associated with the drug.
- *Generic name*—Also referred to as the nonproprietary name, the generic name still reflects the chemical characteristic of the drug, but in a shorter form than the full chemical name. It is the name assigned to the drug before it is officially listed and is independent of the manufacturer. The generic name is listed in the U.S. Pharmacopoeia, a publication listing all drugs officially approved by the U.S. Food and Drug Administration.

TABLE 13-1

Common Generic and Trade Medication Names

Generic Name	Trade Name(s)	Used for
Oxygen emergencies,	Oxygen	a wide range of medical emergencies, traumatic and OB/gyn emergencies
Glucose, Oral	Glutose®, Insta-glucose®	altered mental status associated with diabetic history
Activated Charcoal	SuperChar™, InstaChar™, Actidose™, LiquiChar™	poisoning and overdose emergencies
Nitroglycerin	Nitrostat®	chest pain
Nitroglycerin spray	Nitrolingual Spray®	chest pain
Epinephrine	Adrenalin®	allergic reactions
Albuterol	Proventil®, Ventolin®	breathing difficulty associated with respiratory conditions
Metaproterenol	Alupent®, Metaprel®	breathing difficulty associated with respiratory conditions
Isoetharine	Bronkosol®	breathing difficulty associated with respiratory conditions
Salmeterol xinafoate	Serevent®	breathing difficulty associated with respiratory conditions
Ipratropium	Atrovent®	breathing difficulty associated with respiratory conditions

• *Trade name*—The trade name, also referred to as the brand name, is assigned when the drug is released for commercial distribution. The name is usually short, easy to recall, and may be based on the chemical name or the type of problem it is used to treat. This is the name the manufacturer uses to market the drug.

• *Official name*—Drugs meeting the requirements of the U.S. Pharmacopoeia or National Formulary are given an official name. It is commonly the generic name followed by the initials U.S.P. or N.F.

An example of the four drug names is given below for the common nitroglycerin tablet taken by many patients with chronic chest pain.

Chemical Name:	1,2,3-propanetriol trinitrate
Generic Name:	nitroglycerin tablets
Trade Name:	Nitrostat®
Official Name:	nitroglycerin tablets, U.S.P.

ROUTES OF ADMINISTRATION

The **route** describes how the medication is actually given to or taken by the patient. The route that is chosen controls how fast the medication is absorbed by the body and has its effect. Each medication administered by the EMT-B is prepared in a form that allows for the quickest and safest absorption into the body.

The following are common routes of administration of medications given by the EMT-B.

• *Sublingual*—The medication is placed under the patient's tongue. The patient does not swallow the medication. It is dissolved and absorbed across the mucous membrane in the mouth. The drug usually has a relatively quick absorption rate into the blood. The patient must be alert in order for you to administer the medication in this manner. (Medication placed into the mouth of a patient who is not alert or who is unresponsive can become lodged in the airway or aspirated into the lungs.) Only a very limited number of medications are able to be given by the sublingual route. Medications administered by the EMT-B by the sublingual route are:
  – Nitroglycerin tablets
  – Nitroglycerin spray

• *Oral*—The drug is swallowed and absorbed from the stomach or intestinal tract. The patient must be responsive and able to swallow. The patient may refuse to swallow the drug if it is unpleasant, or may vomit it. Medications administered by the EMT-B by the oral route are:
  – Activated charcoal
  – Oral glucose

• *Inhalation*—The medication is prepared as a gas or aerosol and inhaled by the patient. This method typically deposits the medication directly to the target site where the effect is needed most. The patient must be spontaneously breathing for this route to be effective. With some medications, the patient must be responsive and breathing deeply enough to move air into the lower portions of the lung in order for the drug to be properly deposited. Medications administered by the EMT-B by the inhalation route are:
  – Oxygen
  – Metered dose inhaler
  – Liquid/vaporized fixed dose nebulizer

• *Injection* (intramuscular)—The drug is injected into a muscle mass. The absorption is relatively rapid. This requires the use of a needle; therefore, it poses the danger of a needlestick injury to the EMT-B. Some discomfort is felt by the patient. Serious side effects might occur if the drug is accidentally injected into a vein. The medication can only be injected in specific muscle groups. Medication administered by the EMT-B by the intramuscular injection route is:
  – Epinephrine with the use of an auto-injector

MEDICATION FORMS

Medications come in several different forms. The form usually limits administration to one specific route. This ensures the proper administration of the medication, its correct controlled release, and also the appropriate effect on the target organ or body system. The medication form also determines the effects of the drug. Some drugs have a more local effect on specific cells or organs, whereas other drugs have a much broader, or systemic, effect on the entire body.

Common forms of medications administered by the EMT-B are:

• *Compressed powder or tablet*—A compressed powder that is shaped into a small disk or elongated shape. Nitroglycerin tablets are an example of this type of medication form (Figure 13-1).
• *Liquid for injection*—A liquid substance with no particulate matter. Because epinephrine is injected into the muscle, it is in a liquid form (Figure 13-2).

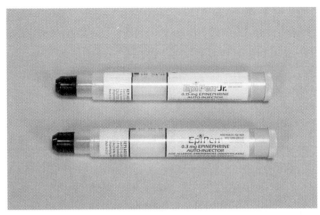

Figure 13-2   The epinephrine auto-injector may be prescribed for patients with a history of severe allergic reaction.

• *Gel*—A viscous (thick, sticky) substance that the patient swallows. Oral glucose is a gel (Figure 13-3).
• *Suspension*—Drug particles that are mixed in a suitable liquid. These mixtures do not remain mixed for long periods of time and have a tendency to separate. Suspensions must be shaken well prior to administration. Activated charcoal is a suspension (Figure 13-4).
• *Fine powder for inhalation*—This form is actually a crystalline solid that is mixed with liquid to form a suspension. A prescribed metered-dose inhaler carried by the patient for inhalation has medication in this form (Figure 13-5). Because it is a suspension, it is necessary that the canister be vigorously shaken prior to administration. The medication appears as a mist or aerosol. Each spray delivers a precise measured amount of drug to the patient.
• *Gas*—Oxygen is the medication most commonly administered by EMT-Bs. It is inhaled and has systemic effects on the cells and organs (Figure 13-6).

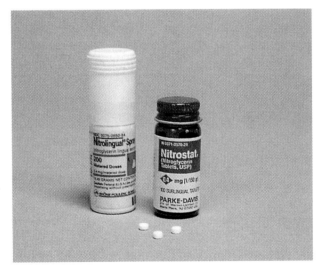

Figure 13-1   The EMT-B may assist the patient with the administration of nitroglycerin prescribed for chest pain. Two common forms are tablet and spray.

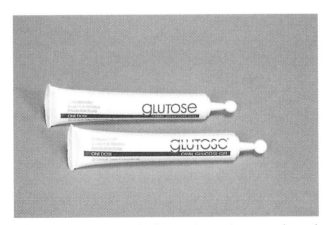

Figure 13-3   Oral glucose is a viscous gel used in diabetic emergencies. It is carried on the EMS unit.

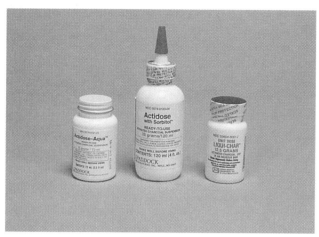

Figure 13-4   Activated charcoal comes in suspension form and is carried on the EMS unit. It is used in poisoning and overdose emergencies.

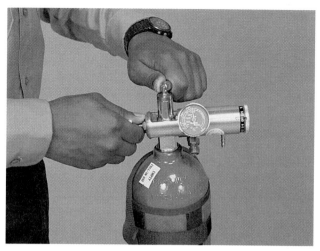

Figure 13-6   The gas oxygen is considered a medication. It is the most commonly used medication in EMS and is carried on the EMS unit.

- *Spray*—Spray droplets may be deposited under the tongue. Nitroglycerin, often in tablet form, may instead be in the form of a spray. Nitroglycerin spray is an aerosol that contains nitroglycerin in a propellant. Each spray delivers a precise metered dose.
- *Liquid/vaporized fixed-dose nebulizer*—A nebulizer is a device that uses a compressed gas, typically oxygen, that is forced into a chamber containing medication. The gas mixes with the liquid medication and forms an aerosol. The aerosol is inhaled by the patient, and the medication is directly deposited on the mucosal lining deep in the respiratory tract. By depositing the medication at the desired site, the effect is more immediate and direct than when given by other routes, and fewer systemic side effects are usually noted. The medication comes packaged in a premeasured and premixed fixed-dose container or inhaler.

ESSENTIAL MEDICATION INFORMATION

It is very important that the EMT-B understand the following terminology associated with the medications to be administered:

- Indications
- Contraindications
- Dose
- Administration
- Actions
- Side effects

We will use the example of nitroglycerin so you can see how the information applies to a medication you will actually be called upon to administer. This information is essential to ensure proper, safe, and effective medication administration.

INDICATIONS

The **indications** for a medication include the most common uses of the drug in treating a specific condition. Indications are geared toward the relief of signs, symptoms, or specific conditions—a direct therapeutic benefit derived from the administration of the drug. For example, an indication for the use of nitroglycerin would be chest pain (because nitroglycerin may relieve chest pain).

CONTRAINDICATIONS

Contraindications are situations in which the drug should not be administered because of the potential harm that could be caused to the patient. In some cases, the drug may not have any benefit to the patient

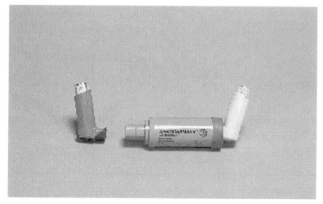

Figure 13-5   A metered-dose inhaler or a metered-dose inhaler with a spacer may be prescribed for respiratory conditions.

in improving his condition; therefore, the drug should not be given. Low blood pressure is a contraindication for the use of nitroglycerin (because nitroglycerin will lower blood pressure, possibly causing an already-low blood pressure to become dangerously low).

DOSE

The **dose** simply indicates how much of the drug should be given to the patient. It is important to distinguish between adult dosages and dosages for infants and children. It is very important that the correct dose be administered. Too much of the drug could cause serious side effects, whereas an inadequate amount of the drug may have little or no effect. For nitroglycerin, EMT-Bs are advised to administer one dose (one tablet or one spray) and repeat it in 3 to 5 minutes if there is no relief, to a maximum of 3 doses (including any doses the patient may already have taken before the ambulance arrived).

ADMINISTRATION

Administration refers to the route and form in which the drug is given. The EMT-B will administer medications sublingually, orally, by inhalation, or by injection. Nitroglycerin, for instance, is administered sublingually in tablet or spray form.

ACTIONS

The **actions,** also commonly referred to as the mechanisms of action, are the therapeutic effects the drug will have. They may simply be the desired effects or the body's physiological response to the drug. The mechanism of action provides the justification for administering a particular medication. If the action described is not or will not produce the desired effect, then the drug should not be administered. Actions of nitroglycerin include relaxation of blood vessels and decreasing workload for the heart.

SIDE EFFECTS

It is important to realize that drugs, even when given appropriately, often have actions that are not desired and that occur in addition to the desired therapeutic effects. These are referred to as **side effects.** Some side effects are unpredictable. Other side effects are predictable and are expected upon administration of certain medications. For example the desired, therapeutic actions of epinephrine are dilation of the bronchioles and constriction of the blood vessels, which will help to relieve a severe allergic reaction. However, epinephrine will also cause an increased heart rate (tachycardia). This is an undesirable side effect of epinephrine. Nitroglycerin's therapeutic effect is relief of chest pain. Side effects of nitroglycerin include

lowering of blood pressure (hypotension), headache, and pulse rate changes.

It is important that the EMT-B be aware of the potential side effects and be prepared to manage the patient and provide reassurance.

KEY STEPS IN ADMINISTERING MEDICATIONS

The following are key steps that must be followed when administering a medication to the patient.

OBTAIN AN ORDER FROM MEDICAL DIRECTION

Every medication that the EMT-B will administer, or will assist the patient with, requires an order from medical direction (Figure 13-7). The medication order may be obtained either on-line by direct communication with medical direction by phone or radio, or off-line through protocols or standing orders. Therefore, it is important to know and understand your local protocols prior to responding to any emergency call.

If you receive an on-line order from medical direction, you must verify it by restating the drug to be

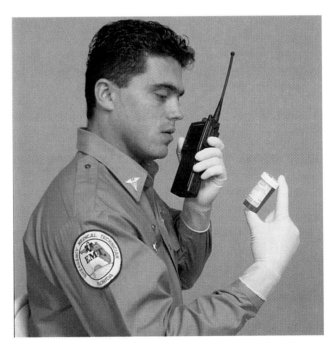

Figure 13-7 You must obtain an order from medical direction to administer medication or to assist the patient with administration of medication. Be sure the prescription is for the patient you are treating, and check the expiration date of the medication.

administered, the dose, and the route. This reduces the chances that an improper medication is inadvertently administered, the wrong dose given, or an inappropriate route is used.

It may be necessary for the EMT-B to make a judgment as to whether the patient can tolerate the administration of the medication. For example, you may have received an on-line order for the administration of oral glucose. The patient was talking incoherently when you called medical direction for the order; however, his mental status has deteriorated, and now he is only responding to painful stimuli. Obviously, administration of oral glucose may lead to aspiration in this patient. Even though the medication order exists, it is now inappropriate to administer the oral glucose to this patient. Medical direction should be contacted and made aware of the deterioration in the patient's condition. At the same time, it will be appropriate to seek further orders for emergency care from medical direction.

SELECT THE PROPER MEDICATION

Once the medication order has been received, it is the responsibility of the EMT-B to ensure that the proper medication has been selected. You must carefully read the medication label, especially in medications that are prescribed to the patient, to determine that the medication is consistent with the order. Many medications have several trade names. This may be confusing, since many trade names are very similar. (The various trade names of drugs relevant to emergency care will be identified in later chapters that discuss each particular medication.)

VERIFY THE PATIENT'S PRESCRIPTION

When the medication to be given is not carried on the EMS unit and must be obtained from the patient, it is extremely important to verify that the medication is actually prescribed for the patient and not some other individual such as a spouse, relative, or friend. Some patients may take medications that are not specifically prescribed for them. They believe that if the signs and symptoms are similar to those of someone who is taking the medication, then it is appropriate for them to take it also.

For example, you arrive on the scene of a 55-year-old female patient complaining of chest pain. Through your SAMPLE history, you determine that the patient has taken nitroglycerin in the past for similar bouts of chest pain. Your assumption is that the patient must have a prescription for nitroglycerin. However, upon inspection of the name on the prescription label, and following further questioning, you determine that the medication is actually pre-scribed for her husband. The patient has been taking the medication, not based on a physician's order, but because she recognized signs and symptoms similar to her husband's.

As you can see, it may be somewhat misleading when the patient states that he or she has been taking a medication for a condition or symptom. Therefore, to avoid medication administration errors, it is vital that the prescription label be checked and the patient's name verified. *The EMT-B should never administer medication that is not prescribed for the patient unless ordered to do so by medical direction.* For instance, in the case of the patient mentioned above, the EMT-B would not assist the patient with administration of nitroglycerin unless medical direction issued orders to administer the husband's nitroglycerin. (For a medication carried on the EMS unit—such as oxygen, oral glucose, or activated charcoal—prescription information is not relevant.)

It is important to note that some medication labels are not affixed to the medication container itself but are placed on or inside the box or other outer packaging. Nitroglycerin, epinephrine auto-injectors, and metered-dose inhalers are packaged this way. So if your patient has one of these medications, you will not be able to tell by looking at the container if the medication has been prescribed for this patient. If the outer packaging cannot be found, you must determine through careful questioning if the prescription truly belongs to the patient.

CHECK THE EXPIRATION DATE

Check the medication's expiration date. Dependent on the type of package and the medication, the expiration date is either printed on the container itself or on the prescription label.

Do not administer expired medication. Properly dispose of the medications according to your state drug or pharmacy guidelines.

CHECK FOR DISCOLORATION OR IMPURITIES

Epinephrine, or any other medication that comes in liquid form, should be inspected for any discoloration or cloudiness prior to administration. If the medication appears to be cloudy, discolored, or if any particulate material is found in the container, do not use it. Discard the medication.

VERIFY THE FORM, ROUTE, AND DOSE

Be sure the proper drug form is used for the route selected. Also, verify that the dose to be administered is correct. Check the medication label to ensure it matches the drug order received from medical direction. Some drug packages are similar but contain different doses. For example, the epinephrine auto-injector comes in adult and pediatric sizes. The packages look very similar. Without close inspection it would be easy to mistake one for the other. Administering an adult dose to a child could have detrimental effects, whereas administering a pediatric dose to an adult may have no or little effect.

The drugs are in a form that corresponds to a specific route of administration. Attempting to administer the medication by some other route may lead to ineffective action or potentially harmful side effects.

DOCUMENTATION

Once the medication has been administered, it is necessary that the EMT-B document the drug, dose, route, and time the medication was administered. Also, it is necessary to report any changes in the patient's condition. Report whether the signs or symptoms have been relieved. Also report any deterioration in the patient's condition or if side effects associated with the drug have occurred.

REASSESSMENT FOLLOWING ADMINISTRATION

Following the administration of a medication, it is necessary to perform an ongoing assessment. During the reassessment, repeat measurement of vital signs and assess for any changes in the patient's condition.

The following should be assessed and changes documented following drug administration:

- Mental status
- Patency of the airway
- Breathing rate and quality
- Pulse rate and quality
- Skin color, temperature, and condition

- Blood pressure
- Change or relief of the complaints of the patient
- Relief of signs and symptoms associated with the complaints of the patient
- Medication side effects
- Improvement or deterioration in the patient's condition following medication administration

Also during the ongoing assessment, be sure to check the adequacy of oxygen administration, whether it is being delivered by a nonrebreather mask or in conjunction with positive pressure ventilation. In addition to the medication that was administered, assess the adequacy of any other care that has been administered to manage the patient's condition. Based on the care provided, determine if improvement or deterioration in the patient's condition has occurred. Document any improvement or deterioration.

SOURCES OF MEDICATION INFORMATION

The following are sources you can use to gather more information about specific medications. These sources may also provide valuable information relevant to the patient's prescription medications:

- American Hospital Formulary Service—published by the American Society of Hospital Pharmacists
- AMA Drug Evaluation—published by the American Medical Association Department of Drugs
- Physicians' Desk Reference (PDR)—published yearly by the Medical Economics Data Production Company
- Package Inserts—information that is packaged with the particular drug
- Poison control centers
- EMS pocket drug reference guide

CASE STUDY FOLLOW-UP

SCENE SIZE-UP

You have been dispatched to the scene of an elderly male complaining of chest pain. You and your partner enter the darkened scene cautiously and find the patient sitting against the wall on the floor of the hallway. The phone is off the hook and lying next to the patient. You turn on the hallway lights and scan the scene. The scene appears to be safe. You notice a prescription bottle of nitroglycerin on the table next to the patient. He complains, "I have this crushing pain in my chest. I've never experienced pain like this be-

fore." You ask, "What is your name sir?" He responds, "Jack Brookline."

INITIAL ASSESSMENT

Your general impression is that of an elderly male patient in severe distress from chest pain. His skin is pale, sweaty, and cool to the touch. His airway is open, breathing is approximately 20 per minute and full, and the radial pulse is 80 per minute and strong. You immediately apply a nonrebreather mask to supply oxygen at 15 liters per minute.

FOCUSED HISTORY AND PHYSICAL EXAM

The SAMPLE history reveals chest pain that occurred suddenly as the patient was sleeping on the couch. Mr. Brookline was tired and was taking a nap when the pain started. It woke him from his sleep. He got up to get his nitroglycerin off the table in the hallway, but the short walk greatly intensified the pain and caused him to collapse to the floor. He describes the pain as "Crushing, like I've never experienced before." The pain does not radiate and is described as 10 on a scale of 1 to 10, with 10 being the worst. The pain began about ten minutes prior to his call to 9-1-1.

Mr. Brookline denies having any allergies and has a prescription of nitroglycerin related to his past medical history of angina, or recurring, chest pain. He states that he had a cup of coffee and a sandwich at about 6 P.M. He denies doing anything unusual today or prior to the onset of the chest pain.

You obtain a set of baseline vital signs. The blood pressure is 114/64; the radial pulse is 84 per minute and regular; the skin is pale, moist, and cool; the breathing is 20 per minute with good volume.

You ask, "Mr. Brookline, did you take any nitroglycerin before we arrived?" He states, "No, once I sat down in the hallway, I couldn't reach it."

You contact medical direction by radio for permission to administer the nitroglycerin to Mr. Brookline. You report the physical findings, SAMPLE history, and baseline vital signs. Medical direction orders, "Administer one tablet sublingually, recheck the blood pressure within 2 minutes, and reevaluate the intensity of the chest pain. If the chest pain does not subside after 5 minutes and the systolic blood pressure remains greater than 100 mmHg, administer a second tablet and reassess the blood pressure and the chest pain intensity." You repeat the order to medical direction and sign off.

You inspect the medication container, checking the medication name to make sure it is really nitroglycerin, the patient's name to make sure it is prescribed to Jack Brookline, and the expiration date to be sure the prescription is current.

You instruct, "Mr. Brookline, I need you to open your mouth and lift your tongue. I am going to place a nitroglycerin tablet under your tongue. Do not swallow the tablet and be sure to keep your mouth closed until it is completely dissolved. It may burn slightly and you may get a headache." With a gloved hand you place a nitroglycerin tablet under his tongue. You record the medication administered, dose, route, and time.

ONGOING ASSESSMENT

After 2 minutes, Mr. Brookline's blood pressure is 110/60—slightly lower than before, but still in the normal range. Mr. Brookline indicates that the pain has subsided greatly. On a scale of 1 to 10, the pain is now a 2 or a 3. His radial pulse remains strong at 82/minute, and his breathing is normal at 18/minute and of good volume. His skin is now slightly warmer, less moist, and more normal in color. You check the oxygen to ensure that it is flowing adequately.

You place Mr. Brookline on the stretcher and move him to the ambulance for transport, making sure to transport the medication along with him. You reassess the vital signs and determine that the chest pain is almost completely gone. You record the vital signs, contact the receiving medical facility, and give a report.

Upon arrival at the hospital, the Mr. Brookline is transferred without incident. He now appears to be resting comfortably and in better spirits, even managing to say a hearty, "Thanks, guys, for helping me out." You complete the necessary EMS report and prepare the unit for another call.

CHAPTER REVIEW

TERMS AND CONCEPTS

You may wish to review the following terms and concepts included in this chapter.

actions—the therapeutic (helpful) effects of a medication; for example, an action of nitroglycerin is relaxation of the blood vessels.

activated charcoal—a distilled charcoal in powder form that can absorb many times its weight in contaminants; often administered to patients who have ingested poison to adsorb the poison and help prevent its absorption by the body.

administration—the route and form by which a drug is given.

contraindications—situations in which a medication should not be used; for example, because nitroglycerin lowers blood pressure, existing low blood pressure in a patient is a contraindication for nitroglycerin.

dose—the amount of a medication that is given to a patient at one time; for example, a dose of nitroglycerin may be one tablet and a dose of epinephrine may be the contents of one auto-injector.

drug—a chemical substance that is used to treat or prevent a disease or condition.

epinephrine—a natural hormone that, when used as a medication, constricts blood vessels to improve blood pressure, reduces leakage from blood vessels, and relaxes smooth muscle in the bronchioles (causes bronchodilation); often prescribed in a single-dose auto-injector form to patients with a history of severe allergic reaction.

form—the size, shape, consistency, or appearance of a medication; for example, nitroglycerin may be in pill or spray form; oral glucose is in gel form.

indications—the common reasons for using a medication to treat a specific condition; for example, chest pain is an indication for nitroglycerin.

medication—a drug or other substance that is used as a remedy for illness.

metered dose inhaler—device consisting of a plastic container and a canister of aerosolized medication for inhalation; often prescribed for patients with respiratory problems.

nitroglycerin—medication that dilates the blood vessels, increasing blood flow and decreasing the work load of the heart; often prescribed for patients with a history of chest pain.

oral glucose—a form of sugar often given as a gel, by mouth, to help correct a glucose-insulin imbalance in patients with an altered status and a history of diabetes.

oxygen—a gaseous element required by the body's tissues and cells to sustain life; often provided as a medication to patients whose injuries or medical conditions may lead to or may be caused or exacerbated by a lack of oxygen.

pharmacology—the study of drugs.

route—the means by which a medication is given or taken; for example, sublingual (under the tongue), oral (by mouth), inhalation (breathed in), or injection (inserted by needle into a muscle or vein).

side effects—the undesired effects of a medication; for example, side effects of epinephrine are increased heart rate and anxiety.

REVIEW QUESTIONS

1. Name three medications that are carried on the EMS unit.
2. Name three medications an EMT-B may administer or assist in administering if prescribed for the patient.
3. Name four routes by which medications may be administered by the EMT-B.
4. Name several common forms of medications that may be administered by the EMT-B.
5. Define the following six terms related to medications:
   - indications
   - contraindications
   - dose
   - administration
   - actions
   - side effects
6. Describe the key steps to follow in administering a medication to a patient.
7. Describe proper reassessment following administration of a medication.

CHAPTER 14

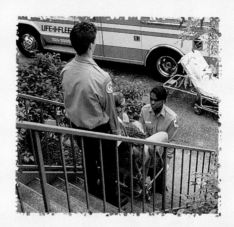

Respiratory Emergencies

INTRODUCTION

Few things are more frightening to the patient than the inability to breathe easily, and one of the most common symptoms of a respiratory emergency is shortness of breath. A number of other signs and symptoms may accompany difficulty in breathing, which is also known as respiratory distress. It is important for you to recognize the signs and symptoms of respiratory emergencies and provide immediate intervention.

OBJECTIVES

Numbered objectives are from the United States Department of Transportation 1994 EMT-Basic National Standard Curriculum. Asterisked objectives, if any, pertain to material that is supplemental to the DOT curriculum.

COGNITIVE

4-2.1 List the structure and function of the respiratory system. (p. 271)

4-2.2 State the signs and symptoms of a patient with breathing difficulty. (pp. 271–275)

4-2.3 Describe the emergency medical care of the patient with breathing difficulty. (pp. 275–280)

4-2.4 Recognize the need for medical direction to assist in the emergency medical care of the patient with breathing difficulty. (pp. 276, 277)

4-2.5 Describe the emergency medical care of the patient with breathing distress. (pp. 275–280)

4-2.6 Establish the relationship between airway management and the patient with breathing difficulty. (pp. 271–272, 276, 281–282)

4-2.7 List signs of adequate air exchange. (p. 276)

4-2.8 State the generic name, medications forms, dose, administration, action, indications and contraindications for the prescribed inhaler. (pp. 277–278)

4-2.9 Distinguish between the emergency medical care of the infant, child, and adult patient with breathing difficulty. (pp. 280–282)

4-2.10 Differentiate between upper airway obstruction and lower airway disease in the infant and child patient. (p. 282)

AFFECTIVE

4-2.11 Defend EMT-Basic treatment regimens for various respiratory emergencies. (pp. 275–280)

4-2.12 Explain the rationale for administering an inhaler. (pp. 276–280)

PSYCHOMOTOR

4-2.13 Demonstrate the emergency medical care for breathing difficulty.

4-2.14 Perform the steps in facilitating the use of an inhaler.

CASE STUDY

THE DISPATCH

EMS Unit 106—respond to 1449 Porter Avenue, Apartment 322. You have a 31-year-old female patient complaining of difficulty in breathing. Time out is 1942 hours.

ON ARRIVAL

You and your partner arrive at the scene and are greeted at the curb by the husband of the patient. As you step out of the ambulance and begin to gather your equipment, you ask, "Did you place the call for EMS, sir?" He states very nervously, " Yes. It's my wife, Anna. She can't breathe. She really doesn't look good." As you and your partner begin walking toward the apartment complex, you ask, "What is your name?" His voice breaks as he tells you, "My name is John Sanders. We've been married for only two months. Please—you've got to help my wife." You

reply, "John, we'll take good care of your wife. But, we also need you to calm down."

As you are led up narrow stairs to the third floor of the apartment complex, you scan the scene for safety hazards and note any obstacles that will make it difficult to extricate the patient from the building. Upon walking into the apartment, you note a young woman sitting upright on a kitchen chair and leaning slightly forward with her arms locked in front of her to hold her up. Before you can even introduce yourself, she begins to speak one word at a time with a gasp for breath in between. "I—can't—breathe," she complains.

How would you proceed to assess and care for this patient?

During this chapter you will learn about assessment and emergency care for a patient suffering from breathing difficulty. Later, we will return to the case and apply the procedures learned.

BREATHING DIFFICULTY

Respiratory emergencies may range from shortness of breath, or **dyspnea,** to complete **respiratory arrest,** or **apnea,** in which the patient is no longer breathing. These conditions can result from a large number of causes, but most typically they involve the respiratory tract or the lungs. Because quick intervention and appropriate emergency care could truly be life saving in a respiratory emergency, it is important for you to understand the anatomy and basic physiology of the respiratory tract and lungs and the techniques of airway management and artificial ventilation. For a review of these topics see Chapter 4, "The Human Body," and Chapter 7, "Airway Management, Ventilation, and Oxygen Therapy."

Shortness of breath, abnormal upper airway sounds, faster or slower than normal breathing rates—these and other signs and symptoms of breathing difficulty may be indications that the cells in the body are not getting an adequate supply of oxygen, a condition known as **hypoxia.** Also, these signs and symptoms may be directly related to obstructions of air flow occurring in either the upper or lower portions of the respiratory tract or from fluid or collapse in the alveoli of the lungs, causing poor gas exchange. If adequate breathing and gas exchange are not present, the lack of oxygen will cause the body cells to begin to die.

Many patients who complain of breathing difficulty suffer from a condition in which the bronchioles of the lower airway are significantly narrowed from constriction of the muscle layer, known as **bronchoconstriction** or **bronchospasm.** This causes a drastic increase in resistance to air flow in the bronchioles, making inhalation and particularly exhalation extremely difficult and producing wheezing and breathing difficulty. The patient may be prescribed a medication in aerosol form that can be inhaled during this episode of breathing difficulty. This medication, known as a **bronchodilator,** is designed to directly relax and open (dilate) the bronchioles, which results in an increase in the effectiveness of breathing and relief of the signs and symptoms.

Breathing difficulty may also be a symptom of injuries to the head, face, neck, or chest. A high index of suspicion and accurate assessment are required so no life-threatening injuries are missed. In addition, cardiac compromise, hyperventilation associated with emotional upset, and various abdominal conditions may produce difficulty in breathing.

Regardless of the cause, a complaint of breathing difficulty requires your immediate intervention. Time is critical because of the detrimental effects of low oxygen levels on all cells and organs. If a patient with inadequate breathing is not treated promptly, it is likely that he will deteriorate to respiratory arrest. Respiratory arrest can lead to cardiac arrest in minutes if not properly managed because of a lack of oxygen delivery to the heart. Whether respiratory distress is caused by trauma or a medical condition, your priorities will be to ensure a patent airway and to facilitate adequate breathing by administering oxygen.

ASSESSMENT AND CARE: BREATHING DIFFICULTY

Information provided by the dispatcher may be the first indication that a patient may be suffering from a respiratory emergency. The information that the patient is complaining of breathing difficulty should heighten your suspicion of a potential respiratory problem.

SCENE SIZE-UP

Seek clues to determine whether the breathing difficulty is due to trauma or to a medical condition. Be careful not to develop tunnel vision and miss important indications of alternative causes for the breathing difficulty that is not the result of a respiratory problem—for example a cardiac problem or an open chest wound.

Scan the scene for possible mechanisms of injury. Bystanders who indicate they heard gunshots, saw a knife, or heard loud fighting may indicate that the patient's difficulty in breathing may be trauma related. At the same time, don't forget to look for oxygen tanks, oxygen tubing, or oxygen concentrators at the scene. They usually indicate a chronic respiratory disease. Also scan the scene for alcohol, which is a common contributor to choking and upper airway obstruction and aspiration of vomitus.

INITIAL ASSESSMENT

Form a general impression and assess the mental status, airway, breathing, and circulation.

General Impression Several clues can help you form an impression of a patient who is suffering respiratory distress. These include:

• *The patient's position*—Most frequently, in severe cases of respiratory distress, patients sit upright and lean slightly forward, supporting themselves with their arms, elbows locked in place in front of them between their dangling legs, holding onto the seat. This is referred to as a **tripod position** (Figure 14-1).

The patient in a reclining or supine position could indicate two possible scenarios: (1) the patient is only in mild distress, or (2) the patient is in such severe respiratory distress that he is too

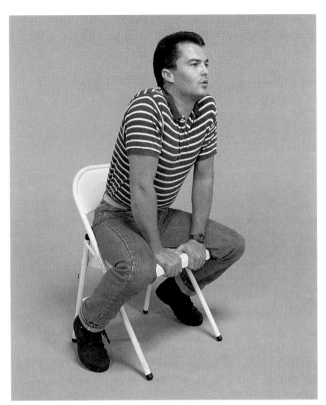

Figure 14-1   A patient in respiratory distress is commonly found in a "tripod" position.

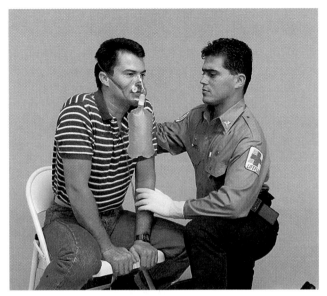

Figure 14-2   Provide oxygen by nonrebreather mask at 15 lpm to the patient who is breathing adequately but with difficulty.

exhausted from trying to breathe to hold himself up. This patient requires immediate intervention since respiratory arrest usually follows shortly after development of severe fatigue.

- *The patient's face*—An agitated or confused facial expression may indicate inadequate breathing and hypoxia.
- *The patient's speech*—Inadequate oxygenation of the brain causes an altered mental status which, in turn, can cause the patient to be disoriented or to talk incomprehensibly or mumble. If the speech is normal, assume that the airway is open and clear and the distress is minimal. If the patient is alert and makes eye contact but is unable to speak, consider a severe condition. The patient may speak one or two words and then pause to gasp for a breath. The number of words the patient can speak during one breath usually correlates with the severity of the breathing difficulty.

Mental Status   Restlessness, agitation, confusion, and unresponsiveness are frequently associated with breathing difficulty because the brain is not getting enough oxygen.

Airway   Assess the airway for any indication of a complete or partial obstruction from secretions, blood, vomitus, or a foreign body. Listen for snoring, stridor, gurgling, or crowing. Each indicates partial airway obstruction. Clear the airway with suction, manual maneuvers, and airway adjuncts as needed.

Breathing   Carefully assess the breathing. Look at the chest rise and fall, listen and feel for air flowing in and out of the mouth and nose, and quickly auscultate the lungs. Be aware of a chest that is moving up and down upon inspection but produces very little or no air movement from the mouth and nose. Efforts to breathe are being made but are not effective. This patient needs positive pressure ventilation with supplemental oxygen no matter how well the chest is rising and falling. Auscultate the breath sounds on both sides of the chest. Absent or diminished breath sounds are an indication that very little air is moving in and out of the lungs.

Determine an approximate respiratory rate. If the chest is not rising adequately with each breath, you do not hear or feel an adequate volume of air escaping on exhalation, or the rate is too slow or too fast, begin positive pressure ventilation with supplemental oxygen. Look for respiratory rates outside the normal ranges of 12–20 per minute for adults, 15–30 per minute for children, and 25–50 per minute for infants. If the patient complains of difficulty in breathing but the rate, chest rise, and exhalation volume appear to be adequate, apply oxygen via a nonrebreather mask at 15 liters per minute (Figure 14-2).

Circulation   Inspect the patient's skin and mucous membranes. Cyanosis, or bluish-gray skin, especially to the neck and chest, is an ominous sign of respiratory distress. In people with dark skin, check for cyanosis of mucous membranes under the tongue and at the lining of the mouth.

Priority Because a patient with difficulty in breathing is considered a priority patient, consider advanced life support back up and expeditious transport. In the patient with severe distress, you will want to transport as soon as possible and continue your assessment en route to the hospital. Signs that you may need to transport immediately following the initial assessment are an irregular or increased radial and carotid pulse (tachycardia) in adults and slow pulse (bradycardia) in infants and children with breathing difficulty and an altered mental status. Also, as stated earlier, cyanosis is an ominous and late sign of respiratory distress, as is a very slow respiratory rate.

FOCUSED HISTORY AND PHYSICAL EXAM

If the patient is responsive, obtain a SAMPLE history, using the OPQRST questions to evaluate the history of the present illness (Table 14-1). If the patient is unresponsive, perform a rapid trauma assessment and collect as much information as possible from the family and bystanders at the scene.

History The following questions will be particularly helpful in determining your emergency care steps for a patient with respiratory distress:

• *Does the patient have any known allergies to medications or other substances that may be related to the episode of difficulty in breathing?* For instance, some patients may experience a sudden onset of breathing difficulty when they have inhaled substances like dust, dog hair, cat hair, mold, or irritating smoke. An extreme allergic reaction (anaphylaxis), for example, to a bee sting or to something the patient has eaten, will cause swelling of the tissues of the upper airway, bronchospasm, and severe respiratory distress.

• *What medications, prescription or nonprescription, is the patient taking?* Gather them to take to the hospital. **Metered dose inhalers (MDI)** are devices that consist of a canister of aerosolized medication and a plastic container that is used to deliver a medication by inhalation. They are frequently used by patients with a chronic respiratory disease or recurring breathing problems. Occasionally you might find oral medications used specifically for respiratory problems. Common medications that might be found on the patient or at the scene are found in Table 14-2. It is important to recognize these since they might provide you with a clue that the patient has a history of respiratory problems, and also, medical direction may instruct you to administer one of them. Ask if the patient has already taken any of the medications prior to your arrival, and if so, how many times. Report this information to medical direction or the receiving hospital.

Note: Medications used by patients with chronic respiratory disease have a variety of side effects. Because many patients self-administer their medication prior to your arrival, this may confuse your assessment slightly since the signs and symptoms now exhibited may result from the medication and not necessarily from the respiratory condition. These side effects are also listed in Table 14-2.

• *Does the patient have a pre-existing respiratory or cardiac disease?*

• *Has the patient ever been hospitalized for a chronic condition that produces recurring episodes of difficulty in breathing?* If so, did he have an endotracheal tube placed down his throat to breathe or require admission to an intensive care unit? This usually indicates that the patient may have a ten-

TABLE 14-1

OPQRST for Breathing Difficulty

Use the following questions to obtain information about the difficulty in breathing:	
Onset	What were you doing when the breathing difficulty started? Did anything seem to trigger the breathing difficulty? Was the onset gradual or sudden? Was the onset accompanied by chest pain or any other symptoms? Was there a sudden onset of pain?
Provocation/ palliation	Does lying flat make the breathing difficulty worse? Does sitting up make the breathing difficulty less severe? Is there pain that occurs or increases with breathing?
Quality	Do you have more trouble breathing in or out? Is the pain sharp (knifelike) or dull?
Radiation	If there is pain associated with the breathing difficulty, does it radiate to the back, up the neck, down the arms, or to any other part of the body?
Severity	How bad is this breathing difficulty on a scale of 1 to 10, with 10 being the worst breathing difficulty you have ever experienced?
Time	When did the difficulty in breathing start? How long have you had it? If this is a recurring problem, how long does the breathing difficulty usually last? If the breathing difficulty started other than today, could you recall the exact day and time when this started?

TABLE 14-2

Medications Commonly Used for Respiratory Problems

Bronchodilators	Albuterol (Proventil®, Ventolin®) Bitolterol mesylate (Tornalate®) Ipratropium bromide (Atrovent®) Isoetharine (Bronkosol®) Metaproterenol (Metaprel®, Alupent®) Salmeterol Xinafoate (Serevent®)	Potential Side Effects: increased heart rate, nervousness, shakiness, nausea, vomiting, sleeplessness, dry mouth, and allergic skin rash
Mucolytics	Acetylcysteine (Mucomyst®)	Potential Side Effects: nausea, increased wheezing, and altered sense of taste
Steroids	Beclomethasone (Vanceril® Inhaler®, Beclovent®) Flunisolide (Aerobid®) Tri-amicinolone acetonide (Azmacort®)	Potential Side Effects: dry mouth and increased wheezing

dency to deteriorate much more rapidly and may require quicker and more aggressive intervention.

Physical Exam The physical exam will give you further information that may indicate the severity of the breathing distress and help you determine whether to simply apply high-flow oxygen by nonrebreather mask or to proceed with positive pressure ventilation with supplemental oxygen. If the patient is unresponsive, perform a rapid assessment. In the responsive patient, focus the exam in on the areas that might provide you with clues as to the severity of the condition.

The posture of the patient is very important. As the patient becomes exhausted, you will notice his posture relaxing. This is an indication that he may require artificial ventilation very shortly. Alterations in mental status, combativeness, agitation, and confusion indicate a decreasing level of oxygen getting to the brain and an increasing level of carbon dioxide. A continuous decline would be an indication of the need for aggressive emergency care to include positive pressure ventilation with supplemental oxygen.

- *Inspect the lips and around the nose and mouth* for cyanosis.
- *Assess the neck* for jugular vein distention, which might indicate an extreme increase in pressure in the chest or venous system. Inspect and palpate for an indrawing of the trachea and tracheal deviation. The trachea pulls inward during inhalation when constricted airflow is present. Tracheal deviation, which is a very late sign, is the result of an extreme amount of pressure built up on one side of the chest, collapsing the lung, and pushing the mediastinum (the tissues and organs between the lungs, including the heart) and the trachea to the opposite side. This is a sign of a life-threatening emergency.

Also inspect for retractions, or pulling of the tissue inward, involving the muscles of the neck, at the suprasternal notch, and behind the clavicles. This indicates that the patient is making an extreme effort to breathe and is another situation in which positive pressure ventilation with supplemental oxygen should be considered.

- *Inspect and palpate the chest* for retraction of the muscles between the ribs, asymmetrical chest wall movement, and also for subcutaneous emphysema, which is air trapped under the subcutaneous layer of the skin. It is felt as a crackling sensation under the fingertips. Unequal chest wall movement may be a sign that air is trapped in one side of the chest cavity and preventing adequate ventilation. Subcutaneous emphysema is a common result of trauma to the neck and chest, indicating a hole in the lung, trachea, bronchus, or esophagus. Inspect for any evidence of trauma.
- *Auscultate the lungs* to determine whether the breath sounds are equal on both sides of the chest. Diminished or absent breath sounds on one side of the chest means that the lung is not being adequately ventilated because of obstruction or collapse. If both lungs have diminished or absent breath sounds, it is an indication that the breathing is inadequate and the patient needs immediate positive pressure ventilation with supplemental oxygen.

Wheezing is a musical whistling sound that is heard in all lung fields upon auscultation of the chest. It is caused by narrowing of the lower airways, primarily the bronchioles, from bronchospasm and edema, or swelling. Wheezing is heard primarily during exhalation. You can expect to hear it most frequently in patients with a history of asthma, but it may also be heard when fluid builds up in the lungs. These patients commonly carry medications that can be administered to reverse the bronchospasm and allow for greater air movement.

Baseline Vital Signs The systolic blood pressure may seem to drop during inhalation. This is related to a drastic increase in pressure in the chest. The heart rate may be increased (tachycardia) or decreased (bradycardia). Bradycardia in adults, infants, and children is a grave sign of extremely poor oxygenation, impending respiratory failure, and possible cardiac arrest. The skin is usually moist, pale or cyanotic, and cool (lung infections associated with breathing difficulty may produce warm, dry, or moist skin). The breathing rate is typically increased (tachypnea); however, it may become decreased as the patient becomes tired and the oxygen levels drop significantly.

Signs and Symptoms There is a wide variety of signs and symptoms that may be associated with breathing difficulty, depending on the location of the obstruction or disease process, the mental status of the patient, and the severity of the respiratory distress. A large number of respiratory conditions, including both medical illness and traumatic injuries, will cause signs and symptoms of breathing difficulty. Not all of the signs or symptoms will be present with each patient, nor will you find two cases that are exactly alike. The degree of difficulty in breathing can vary widely from minor to very severe. The key is to recognize the patient who is having difficulty in breathing, perform an accurate assessment, and manage any immediate life threats.

The common signs of breathing difficulty are:

- Shortness of breath (dyspnea)
- Restlessness and anxiety
- Increased or irregular heart rate in adults and decreased heart rates in infants and children
- Breathing rates that are faster than the normal range (tachypnea)
- Slower than normal breathing rates (bradypnea)
- Cyanosis to the core of the body is a late sign of breathing difficulty. Pale or flushed (red) skin can also be present. The skin is typically moist.
- Abnormal upper airway sounds: crowing, gurgling, snoring, and stridor
- Audible wheezing upon inhalation and exhalation. In some conditions, wheezing on exhalation will develop before wheezing on inhalation. Auscultation with a stethoscope may reveal wheezing and other abnormal sounds that cannot be heard by just listening with the ear.
- Diminished ability or inability to speak
- Retractions from the use of accessory muscles in the neck, upper chest, and between the ribs
- Excessive use of the diaphragm to breathe, producing abdominal breathing in which the abdomen is moving significantly during the breathing effort
- Shallow breathing, identified by very little chest rise and fall, and poor movement of air in and out of the mouth

- Coughing, especially if it is a productive cough, one that produces mucus
- Irregular breathing patterns
- Tripod position
- Barrel chest (Figure 14-3) indicating emphysema, a chronic respiratory condition
- Altered mental status—from disorientation to unresponsiveness
- Nasal flaring, when the nostrils widen and flare out upon inhalation
- Tracheal indrawing
- Paradoxical motion, in which an area of the chest that moves inward during inhalation and outward during exhalation—a significant sign of chest trauma; can lead to ineffective ventilation
- Indications of chest trauma (e.g., open wounds)
- Pursed-lip breathing, where the lips are puckered during exhalation

EMERGENCY MEDICAL CARE

Do not take the time to try to determine the exact cause of the breathing difficulty unless it is in the trauma patient with a possible chest injury that must be managed in addition to the breathing difficulty itself. A trauma patient complaining of difficulty in breathing requires exposure of the chest and back with close inspection for and management of life-threatening injuries. Chest injuries will be discussed in more detail in Chapter 36, "Chest, Abdomen, and Genitalia Injuries."

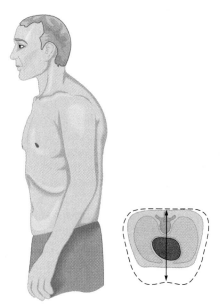

Figure 14-3 Barrel chest in an emphysema patient. The dotted line shows the increased anterior-to-posterior diameter of the chest.

Aside from the management of any chest injuries, you will use the same strategies for managing breathing difficulty no matter what its cause or underlying disease process.

A patient with breathing difficulty may deteriorate rapidly. Continuously assess the airway for possible obstruction and the breathing status for inadequacy. Have your ventilation equipment ready and be prepared to control the airway and begin positive pressure ventilation with supplemental oxygen. Delays in providing adequate ventilation can adversely effect the outcome of the patient in a short period of time. If you are ever in doubt about whether to ventilate or not, it is better to provide the positive pressure ventilation with supplemental oxygen. Waiting may cost the patient his life.

Follow the guidelines below for emergency care of the patient with breathing difficulty.

Inadequate Breathing If signs of inadequate breathing are present (poor chest rise and fall, poor volume heard and felt, diminished or absent breath sounds, or severely altered mental status):

1. *Establish an open airway.* Insert an oropharyngeal or nasopharyngeal airway if necessary to maintain the airway.
2. *Begin positive pressure ventilation with supplemental oxygen.* Check for signs of adequate ventilation (see below).
3. *Expeditiously transport* the patient to the hospital.

Adequate Breathing If the breathing is adequate (adequate chest rise and fall, good volume of air being breathed in and out, and good breath sounds bilaterally) but the patient complains of difficulty in breathing:

1. *Continue oxygen administration at 15 liters per minute via a nonrebreather mask.*
2. *Assess the baseline vital signs.*
3. *Determine if the patient has a prescribed metered dose inhaler (MDI).* If so, contact medical direction for permission to administer the medication. Assist the patient with the administration of the medication. Be sure to comply with local protocols.
4. *Complete the focused history and physical exam.*
5. *Place the patient in a position of comfort,* most typically in a Fowler's or semi-Fowler's (sitting-up) position, *and begin transport.*

ONGOING ASSESSMENT

En route to the hospital, perform an ongoing assessment to determine if your emergency care has decreased the breathing difficulty or if further intervention is necessary. Better oxygenation should improve the patient's mental status. Closely monitor the patient's airway for possible occlusion and the breathing status for signs of inadequate breathing. If the patient continues to deteriorate, it may be necessary to begin positive pressure ventilation with supplemental oxygen.

Monitor the pulse for changes in the heart rate and regularity. A decreasing heart rate in a patient who has tachycardia may indicate improvement if the mental status is also improving and the breathing difficulty subsiding. If the heart rate is declining along with the mental status, and the breathing difficulty is worsening, this is an ominous sign of impending respiratory failure. Increases in the heart rate may be seen with administration of many of the metered dose inhalers. These medications mimic the actions of the sympathetic nervous system; therefore, a slight increase in heart rate may be anticipated. This tachycardia would be expected to decrease once the condition improves and the medication begins to wear off.

Moist skin (diaphoresis) is a result of the sympathetic nervous system response in the patient with breathing difficulty. An increase in diaphoresis would correlate with a worsening condition.

Reassess and record the blood pressure. Reassess the breath sounds. Improved air movement in the lungs will produce clearer and louder breath sounds on both sides of the chest. Conversely, as the condition deteriorates, the breath sounds become diminished to absent. Note that decreased wheezing may not indicate improvement; it may actually indicate severe bronchoconstriction with less air movement.

The patient with breathing difficulty is considered a priority patient, especially if the condition does not respond to your emergency care. You should consider advanced life support back-up.

If the patient's complaint changes, repeat the focused history and physical exam. Ensure that the oxygen is applied properly and flowing adequately. Continuously assess the status of the breathing.

If positive pressure ventilation with supplemental oxygen has been initiated, continuously assess its effectiveness. Ensure that oxygen is connected and adequately flowing to the pocket mask or the reservoir of the bag-valve-mask device.

METERED DOSE INHALERS

A medication commonly prescribed for the patient with a chronic history of breathing problems is a bronchodilator that comes in a metered dose inhaler (MDI). There are a variety of bronchodilators that can be prescribed for a patient with the same types of conditions. The medication can only be administered with the approval of medical direction through on-line or off-line orders. (See Figure 14-4 for a detailed summary of the criteria and techniques for administering MDIs. See Figures 14-5a to g, which illustrate the correct method of administering medication from a metered dose inhaler.)

These bronchodilators are considered beta agonists, which mimic the effects of the sympathetic nervous system. Specifically, these drugs relax the bronchiole smooth muscle and dilate (increase the size) of the airways. This decreases the resistance in the airways and improves breathing. Most bronchodilators begin to work almost immediately and their effects may last up to 8 hours or more. Because of the swift relief they can provide, they are appropriate for prehospital administration by the EMT-B with the approval of medical direction. The most common beta-agonist bronchodilators are listed in Figure 14-4.

The bronchodilators listed above, as well as ipratropium bromide (Atrovent®) are in an aerosol form and are contained in a metered dose inhaler (MDI), also known as an "inhaler" or "puffer." This simple device consists of a metal canister and a plastic con-

METERED DOSE INHALER (MDI)

℞

Medication Name

Metered dose inhalers contain medications with a variety of generic and trade names, including the following:

Generic Name	Trade Name
Albuterol	Proventil®, Ventolin®
Metaproterenol	Metaprel®, Alupent®
Isoetharine	Bronkosol®, Bronkometer®
Bitolterol mesylate	Tornalate®
Salmeterol xinafoate	Serevent®

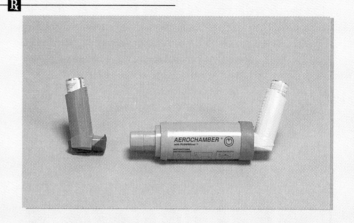

Indications

All of the following criteria must be met before an EMT-B administers a bronchodilator by MDI to a patient:

- The patient exhibits signs and symptoms of breathing difficulty.
- The patient has a physician-prescribed metered dose inhaler.
- The EMT-B has received approval from medical direction, whether on-line or off-line, to administer the medication.

Contraindications

A bronchodilator by MDI should not be given if any of the following conditions exist:

- The patient is not responsive enough to use the MDI.
- The MDI is not prescribed for the patient.
- Permission has not been granted by medical direction.
- The patient has already taken the maximum allowed dose prior to your arrival.

Medication Form

Aerosolized medication in a metered dose inhaler.

Dosage

Each time the MDI is depressed it delivers a precise dose of medication to the patient. The total number of times the medication can be administered is determined by medical direction.

Administration

To administer a bronchodilator by MDI (Figure 14-5):

1. Ensure that the medication is the patient's and is not expired. Determine if the patient is alert enough to use the inhaler and if any doses have already been administered prior to your arrival.
2. Obtain an order, either on-line or off-line, from medical direction to assist with the administration of the medication.
3. Assure that the inhaler is at room temperature or warmer. Shake the canister vigorously for at least 30 seconds.

Figure 14-4   Metered dose inhaler.

(Continued on the next page.)

METERED DOSE INHALER (MDI)

4. Remove the nonrebreather mask from the patient. Instruct the patient to take the inhaler in his hand and hold it upright. If the patient is unable to hold the device, place your index finger on the top of the metal canister and your thumb on the bottom of the plastic container.
5. Have the patient exhale fully.
6. Have the patient place his lips around the mouthpiece (opening) of the inhaler. Another technique is to have the patient open his mouth and place the inhaler 1 to 1.5 inches from the front of the lips, estimated by two finger widths.
7. Have the patient begin to slowly and deeply inhale over about 5 seconds as he or you depress the canister. Do not depress the canister before the patient begins to inhale. This would allow a majority of the medication to be lost in the air and it will not reach the lungs.
8. Remove the inhaler and coach the patient to hold his breath for 10 seconds or as long as comfortable.
9. Have the patient exhale slowly through pursed lips.
10. Replace the oxygen mask on the patient. Reassess the breathing status and baseline vital signs.
11. Reassess the patient and consult with medical direction if additional doses are needed. If an additional dose is recommended, wait at least 2 minutes between each administration or longer based on the medication being administered or medical directions order.

If using a spacer, follow the same steps with the following exceptions for steps 6 and 7 (Figure 14-6):

6. Remove the spacer cap and attach the inhaler to the spacer.
7. Depress the medication canister to fill the spacer with the medication. As soon as the canister is depressed, have the patient place his lips around the mouthpiece and inhale slowly and deeply. If the inhalation is too fast, the spacer may whistle.

Actions

Beta agonist that relaxes the bronchiole smooth muscle and dilates the lower airways. This reduces the airway resistance.

Side Effects

The side effects associated with the bronchodilator are associated with the drug action itself. The following are common side effects that the patient may complain of or that you may find in your assessment:

- tachycardia
- tremors, shakiness
- nervousness
- dry mouth
- nausea, vomiting

Reassessment

Whenever you administer a bronchodilator to a patient, you must perform an ongoing assessment. The following steps must be included:

- Reassess the vital signs.
- Question the patient about the effect of the medication on the relief of the difficulty in breathing.
- Perform a focused history and physical exam if changes in the condition or new complaints occur.
- Constantly monitor the airway and breathing status; if the breathing becomes inadequate, begin positive pressure ventilation with supplemental oxygen.
- If the medication has had no or little effect, consult medical direction to consider another dose.
- Record and document any findings during the ongoing assessment.

Figure 14-4 continued

tainer with a mouthpiece and cap. The metal canister contains the medication and fits inside the plastic container. When the canister is depressed, it delivers a precise dose of medication for the patient to inhale. The medication is directly deposited on the bronchioles at the site of bronchoconstriction. Some MDIs are connected to a device called a **spacer.** The spacer is a chamber that holds the medication until it is inhaled, thus preventing any loss of medication to the outside. This device is commonly used in patients who have difficulty using the MDI. See Figures 14-6a

to c that illustrate how to administer an MDI with a spacer to a patient with respiratory distress.

If the patient is having breathing difficulty that is not related to trauma or a chest injury, and has one of the beta agonist bronchodilators in an MDI form prescribed to him by a physician, you should contact medical direction for permission to administer the drug or follow local protocols. Instruct your patient as to what he should do even if he claims to know how to use the MDI. During the administration, you must coach the patient to breathe in slowly and deeply, hold

ADMINISTERING MEDICATION BY METERED DOSE INHALER

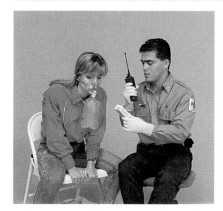

Figure 14-5a   Consult with medical direction for an order to administer the medication.

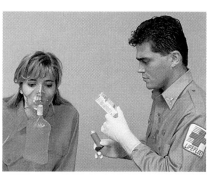

Figure 14-5b   Check to make sure the medication is for the patient, that it is the proper one to administer, and that it has not reached its expiration date.

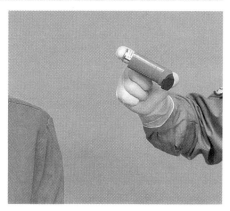

Figure 14-5c   Shake the inhaler vigorously for at least 30 seconds.

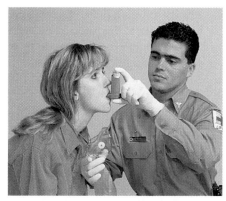

Figure 14-5d   Instruct the patient to inhale slowly and deeply for about 5 seconds. As the patient begins to inhale, depress the canister.

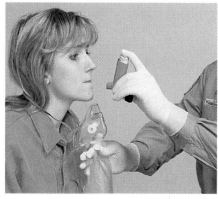

Figure 14-5e   Remove the inhaler and instruct the patient to hold the breath for 10 seconds or for as long as is comfortable.

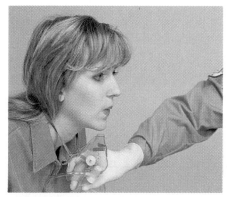

Figure 14-5f   Instruct the patient to exhale slowly through pursed lips.

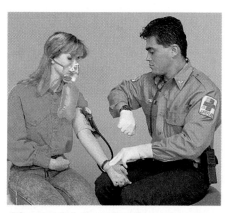

Figure 14-5g   Replace the oxygen on the patient. Reassess the breathing status and vital signs.

ADMINISTERING A METERED DOSE INHALER WITH SPACER

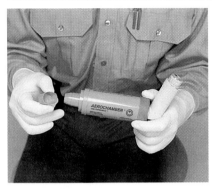

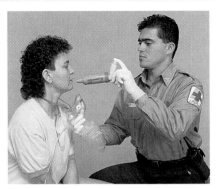

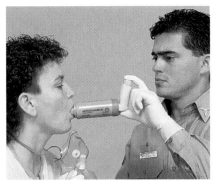

Figure 14-6a Remove the spacer cap. Attach the spacer to the inhaler mouthpiece.

Figure 14-6b Depress the medication canister to fill the spacer with medication.

Figure 14-6c Instruct the patient to inhale slowly and deeply. The spacer may whistle if the patient is inhaling too quickly.

his breath, and breathe out slowly through pursed lips. If the patient is not instructed or coached, the medication may not be effectively administered. If the patient is unable to follow the procedure, even with coaching, you may need to administer the inhaler to the patient. Table 14-3 lists a series of "dos and don'ts" for administering medication from MDIs.

BREATHING DIFFICULTY IN THE INFANT OR CHILD

A common cause of respiratory and cardiac arrest in the infant and child is a gradual deterioration of the breathing status and circulation. Either condition, if left unmanaged, will result in cardiopulmonary fail-

ure. This may be prevented if you can recognize breathing difficulty and respiratory failure early and provide the appropriate emergency care. **Respiratory failure** is defined as inadequate oxygenation of the blood and an inadequate elimination of carbon dioxide; it can lead to complete respiratory arrest. Respiratory failure may occur due to an upper airway blockage, lower airway obstruction, or lung disease, which all will cause inadequate breathing.

BREATHING DIFFICULTY IN THE INFANT OR CHILD: ASSESSMENT AND CARE

Some indication that the infant or child patient is suffering breathing difficulty may be part of the dispatch.

TABLE 14-3

MDI Administration Dos and Don'ts

When administering a metered dose inhaler, follow these tips:	
DO	Instruct the patient to breathe in slowly and deeply.
	Be sure the patient is breathing in through his mouth.
	Shake the canister for at least 30 seconds before removing the cap.
	Depress the canister as the patient begins to inhale.
	Coach the patient to hold his breath as long as possible.
	Use a spacer device if available and the patient is used to it.
DON'T	Allow the patient to breathe in too quickly.
	Allow the patient to breathe in through his nose.
	Administer the medication before shaking the canister.
	Depress the canister before the patient begins to inhale.
	Forget to coach the patient to hold his breath as long as possible.

The patient may experience a variety of side effects from the medication. The most common are an increased heart rate, tremors, and nervousness. More detailed information about bronchodilators and other side effects are listed in Figure 14-4.

SCENE SIZE-UP

During scene size-up, with the infant or child as with the adult patient, look for clues to help rule out trauma as a cause of the problem.

INITIAL ASSESSMENT

Many of the signs and symptoms of breathing difficulty can be spotted as you form your general impression during the initial assessment. Labored or noisy breathing, a child who is sitting up in a tripod position, lying limply, or unresponsive can be detected even before you approach the patient. Additional signs and symptoms will be discovered as you make contact with the infant or child to assess mental status, airway, breathing, and circulation.

FOCUSED HISTORY AND PHYSICAL EXAM

Other signs and symptoms may be noted during a focused history and physical exam. (Assessing the infant or child patient will be covered in detail in Chapter 38, "Infants and Children.") Typically, signs and symptoms of breathing difficulty will precede respiratory failure in the infant or child. This is an indication that the body is attempting to compensate for the poor oxygen and carbon dioxide exchange by increasing the work of breathing.

Early Signs of Breathing Difficulty in the Infant or Child   Because breathing difficulty may quickly proceed to respiratory failure in the infant or child, it is vital that you recognize early signs of breathing difficulty.

- Increased use of accessory muscles to breathe
- Retractions during inspiration
- Tachypnea (increased breathing rate)
- Tachycardia (increased heart rate)
- Nasal flaring
- **Grunting**—heard in infants during exhalation, indicating diseases that produce lung collapse
- Prolonged exhalation
- Frequent coughing—may be present rather than wheezing in some children
- Cyanosis to the extremities
- Anxiety

Bear in mind that retractions are much more common in the infant and child than in the adult. Also, be aware that the infant relies much more on his abdominal muscles to breathe so that the abdomen moves significantly, even during normal breathing.

Signs of Inadequate Breathing and Respiratory Failure in the Infant or Child   Signs of respiratory failure, which may be similar to those of inadequate breathing, are an indication that the cells are not receiving an adequate oxygen supply. *These signs, listed below, occur late in a respiratory emergency and are an indication that you must immediately intervene and begin positive pressure ventilation with supplemental oxygen.*

- Altered mental status—The patient may be completely unresponsive.
- Bradycardia (slow heart rate)
- Hypotension (low blood pressure)
- Extremely fast, slow, or irregular breathing pattern
- Cyanosis to the core of the body and mucous membranes—a late and inconsistent sign
- Loss of muscle tone (limp appearance)
- Diminished or absent breath sounds
- Head bobbing—bobbing of the head with each breath.
- See-saw or rocky breathing—The chest is drawn inward and the abdomen moves outward, indicating extreme inspiratory efforts.

EMERGENCY MEDICAL CARE

The emergency medical care for the infant and child is very similar to that of the adult. Your goal should be to promptly and efficiently care for the infant or child and minimize the amount of stress. An increased stress level will increase the work of breathing and the body's oxygen demand. Remember that, because of the danger that breathing difficulty will deteriorate into respiratory failure, *prompt intervention and transport is especially critical for the infant or child.*

For a child who is experiencing difficulty in breathing, take the following steps:

1. *Allow the child to assume a position of comfort* to reduce the breathing work and maintain a more patent airway. Do not remove the infant or child from his parent (or other caretaker). Allowing the parent to hold the child will reduce the apprehension and stress levels, thereby, reducing the breathing workload and oxygen demand.
2. *Apply oxygen by nonrebreather mask on a child who is sitting up in his parent's lap.* If the child does not tolerate the oxygen mask, have the parent hold it near the child's face (Figure 14-7).
3. *If at any time the infant or child's breathing becomes inadequate, remove him from the parent, establish an open airway, and begin positive pressure ventilation with supplemental oxygen.* It will be necessary to repeat the focused history and physical exam.

Just as with adults, a child may also have an MDI prescribed for respiratory problems associated with the lower airway. These children may present with audible wheezing, diminished breath sounds bilater-

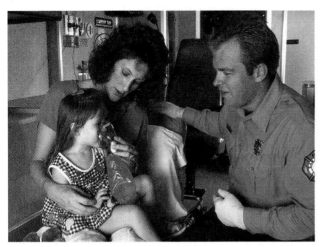

Figure 14-7 If the child does not tolerate the mask, have the parent hold the mask near the child's face.

ally, cyanosis, poor chest rise and fall, and other signs of breathing difficulty. If the child is experiencing breathing difficulty and has a prescribed inhaler, follow the same emergency care procedures for administration of the medication via MDI as for the adult.

It is important to bear in mind that the upper airway can be obstructed by foreign bodies or from swelling due to certain diseases, medical conditions, burns, or toxic inhalations. Stridor and crowing are typical sounds made when the upper airway is partially obstructed by a foreign body or swelling. If a foreign body obstruction is suspected, and the airway is completely blocked, perform foreign-body airway obstruction (FBAO) maneuvers to attempt to relieve the obstruction. Refer to Appendix 1, "Basic Life Support," and Chapter 38, "Infants and Children," to review these techniques for the infant and child. If the airway is partially blocked, place the patient on a nonrebreather mask at 15 lpm and immediately begin transport. Be alert to begin FBAO maneuvers if the partial obstruction becomes complete.

It is important to distinguish blockage caused by a foreign body in the airway from blockage caused by disease. FBAO maneuvers may involve inserting suction devices or the fingers into the airway to remove foreign materials. With some airway diseases, inserting anything into the airway will cause dangerous spasms along the airway, making the condition worse.

In one condition that can cause obstruction of an infant or child's upper airway, the epiglottis becomes extremely swollen from a localized infection. This condition is known as *epiglottitis*. The epiglottis can swell so much that it completely blocks the opening into the trachea and causes a complete airway obstruction. The child usually sits straight up, juts his neck out, and drools because he can not swallow. He typically has a history of a sore throat,

stridor, and fever. This is a life-threatening upper airway emergency. You should apply oxygen by a nonrebreather mask, place the child in a position of comfort, and begin immediate transport. Consider requesting ALS back-up. Do not inspect inside the mouth or insert anything inside the airway since it could cause the airway to spasm or completely swell shut. If the patient stops breathing or is breathing inadequately, begin positive pressure ventilation with supplemental oxygen.

Another condition, called *croup*, commonly seen in children, involves the swelling of the larynx, trachea, and bronchi. This causes breathing difficulty. The child typically does not feel well, has a sore or hoarse throat, and a fever. At night, the condition usually worsens. You might hear a hallmark sign of croup, a cough that produces a sound like a barking seal. Provide oxygen to the patient, humidified if possible, and begin transport. Usually cool night air will reduce the signs and symptoms somewhat; therefore, the condition may subside slightly after the child is taken outside during transfer to the ambulance. Inadequate breathing can result from croup, so continuously monitor the breathing status.

The *SAMPLE history* is especially important when airway blockage is suspected, since it may identify preexisting diseases that may be causing the airway closure, or events that may have led to a foreign body obstruction (for example, someone witnessed the child choking on food or saw the child put an object into his mouth, or there were small objects around the child that he could have swallowed). If the blockage was sudden and there was something around that the child could have swallowed and there is no history or other sign of disease, treat the patient for a foreign body airway obstruction. If the blockage came on gradually, the child has other signs of being ill or the child has a history of respiratory or other disease, and no one saw the child swallow anything, avoid inserting anything into the airway. Instead, provide oxygen or positive pressure ventilation with supplemental oxygen as necessary.

ONGOING ASSESSMENT

Transport any infant or child with difficulty breathing or signs of inadequate breathing or airway blockage. Provide an ongoing assessment en route, and be prepared to intervene more aggressively if the patient's condition deteriorates.

SUMMARY: ASSESSMENT AND CARE

To review assessment findings that may be associated with breathing difficulty and emergency care for breathing difficulty, see Figures 14-8 and 14-9.

✳ ASSESSMENT SUMMARY

BREATHING DIFFICULTY

The following are findings that may be associated with breathing difficulty.

SCENE SIZE-UP

Is breathing difficulty due to a medical or a traumatic cause? Look for evidence of:
  Mechanism of injury—collision, fall, guns, knives, bruising on chest
  Home or portable oxygen tanks or concentrators indicating chronic respiratory problems
  Alcohol or food that may indicate choking

INITIAL ASSESSMENT

General Impression

Position of patient:
  Tripod
  Lying flat
Facial expression:
  Agitated or confused
Speech:
  Patient may gasp for breath between words.

Mental Status

Alert to unresponsive
Restlessness
Agitation
Disorientation

Airway

Inspect for incomplete or partial obstruction
Crowing and stridor (indicate partial obstruction)
Gurgling (indicates fluid in the airway; suction required)

Breathing

Signs of inadequate breathing, including poor chest rise and fall, poor volume heard and felt, diminished or absent breath sounds
Wheezing heard on auscultation

Circulation

Tachycardia (more typical in adult with hypoxia)
Bradycardia (more typical in infant or young child with hypoxia)
Cyanosis to mucous membranes, around nose and mouth, nailbeds, chest, and neck

Status: Priority Patient

FOCUSED HISTORY AND PHYSICAL EXAM

SAMPLE History

Signs and symptoms:
  Shortness of breath
  Restlessness and anxiety
  Difficulty in breathing while lying flat
  Diaphoresis
Known allergies to medication or other substances
Medications for respiratory conditions
Home oxygen
Prescribed metered dose inhaler (MDI)
Preexisting respiratory or cardiac disease
Hospitalized for respiratory condition

Physical Exam

Head, neck and face:
  Cyanosis to face, neck, and mucous membranes
  Jugular venous distention (may indicate heart failure or lung injury [tension pneumothorax])
  Nasal flaring
  Pursed-lip breathing
Chest:
  Retractions
  Accessory muscle use
  Wheezing
  Productive cough
  Barrel chest (indicates emphysema, a chronic respiratory condition)
Abdomen:
  Use of abdominal muscles when breathing
Extremities:
  Cyanosis to fingers and nailbeds
  Pale skin
  Diaphoresis

Baseline Vital Signs

BP: normal
HR: increased in adults; slow in infants and young children
RR: increased; may decrease with greater hypoxia
Skin: cyanosis, paleness, diaphoresis
Pupils: dilated; sluggish to respond to light

Figure 14-8a   Assessment summary: breathing difficulty.

(Continued on the next page.)

EMERGENCY CARE PROTOCOL

BREATHING DIFFICULTY

1. Establish and maintain an open airway.
2. Suction secretions as necessary.
3. If breathing is inadequate, provide positive pressure ventilation with supplemental oxygen at a minimum rate of 12 ventilations/minute for an adult and 20 ventilations/minute for an infant or child.
4. If the breathing is adequate, apply a nonrebreather mask at 15 lpm.
5. If the patient has signs and symptoms of breathing difficulty and has a prescribed metered-dose inhaler, administer the beta 2 specific drug by MDI:
   - Beta 2 specific drugs mimic the sympathetic nervous system and cause bronchodilation.
   - Dose is precisely delivered by depressing canister.
   - Obtain an order from medical direction.
   - Be sure the prescription is the patient's.
   - Ensure inhaler is at room temperature.
   - Shake canister vigorously for 30 seconds.
   - Remove nonrebreather mask from the patient.
   - Have patient exhale fully.
   - Place mouthpiece of inhaler in patient's mouth and depress canister as patient slowly and deeply inhales over about 5 seconds.
   - Remove inhaler and coach patient to hold breath for about 10 seconds.
   - Have patient exhale through pused lips.
   - Replace nonrebreather mask on patient.
   - Record time and reassess patient.
   - Beta 2 side effects:
     * tachycardia
     * tremors
     * nervousness
     * dry mouth
     * nausea
6. Consider advanced life support if the condition does not improve.
7. Transport in a position of comfort.
8. Perform an ongoing assessment every 5 minutes.

Figure 14-8b Emergency care protocol: breathing difficulty.

ENRICHMENT

The enrichment section contains information that is valuable as background for the EMT-B but that goes substantially beyond the U.S. Department of Transportation (DOT) EMT-Basic curriculum.

ASSESSING BREATH SOUNDS

Auscultation of breath sounds may provide additional evidence of breathing difficulty during the focused history and physical exam. Breathing difficulty can result from a variety of conditions; therefore, being able to describe the type of breath sounds may be helpful to medical direction when asking for a medication order.

Not all patients with breathing difficulty need an aerosolized medication by MDI, even if it is prescribed to that patient. A beta agonist medication that is administered by an MDI is used to reverse bronchoconstriction. Therefore, recognizing wheezing, the abnormal breath sound that indicates bronchoconstriction, would help medical direction decide whether the MDI should be administered or not.

There are three basic types of abnormal breath sounds that you might hear upon auscultation of the lungs. These may be early indicators of impending difficulty in breathing.

- *Wheezing,* as described earlier, is a high-pitched musical whistling sound heard on inhalation and exhalation. It is an indication of bronchoconstriction. Wheezing that is diffuse, heard over all the lung fields, is a primary indication for the administration of a beta agonist medication by MDI. Wheezing is usually heard in asthma, emphysema, and chronic bronchitis. It may also be heard in pneumonia, congestive heart failure, and other conditions that may cause bronchoconstriction.
- *Rhonchi* are snoring or rattling noises heard upon auscultation. They indicate obstruction of the respiratory tract by thick secretions of mucus. This is very often heard in chronic bronchitis, emphysema, aspiration, and pneumonia.
- *Crackles,* also known as *rales,* are bubbly or crackling sounds heard during inhalation. These sounds are associated with fluid that has filled the alveoli or very small bronchioles. The bases of the lungs will reveal crackles first due to the natural tendency of fluid to be pulled downward by gravity. Crackles may indicate pulmonary edema or pneumonia.

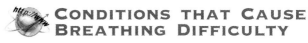

CONDITIONS THAT CAUSE BREATHING DIFFICULTY

There are many conditions that cause the patient to experience signs and symptoms of difficulty in breathing. Even though the disease processes are different,

EMERGENCY CARE ALGORITHM: BREATHING DIFFICULTY

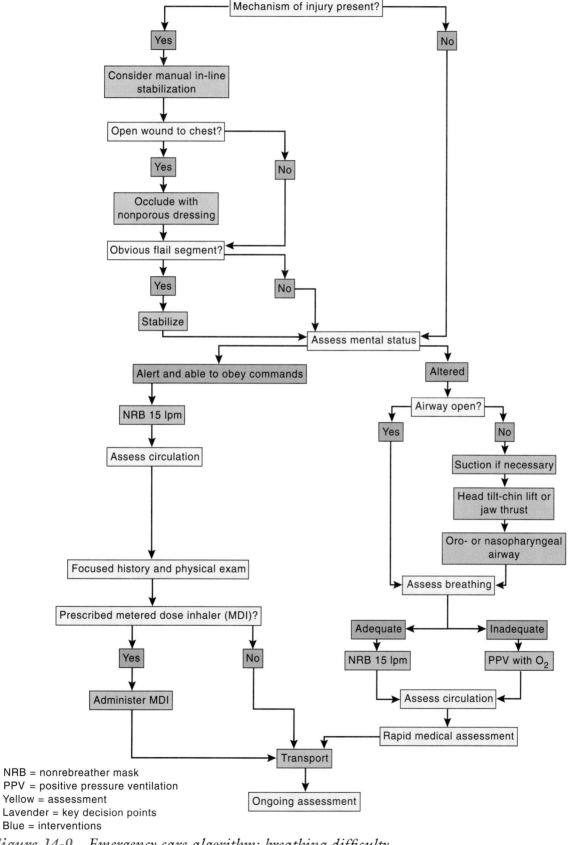

NRB = nonrebreather mask
PPV = positive pressure ventilation
Yellow = assessment
Lavender = key decision points
Blue = interventions

Figure 14-9   Emergency care algorithm: breathing difficulty.

the assessment and emergency care are basically the same. It is not your responsibility to diagnose the condition or disease causing difficulty in breathing; however, you are responsible for identifying the signs and symptoms, determining whether the breathing is adequate or inadequate, anticipating deterioration in the patient's status, and providing immediate intervention as necessary.

CHRONIC OBSTRUCTIVE PULMONARY DISEASE (COPD)

Respiratory diseases that cause obstruction to air flow in the lungs are referred to as chronic obstructive pulmonary disease (COPD). The most common con-

ditions in this disease category are emphysema and chronic bronchitis (Figure 14-10). The incidence of chronic obstructive pulmonary disease is high. These conditions are common causes of difficulty in breathing. Most patients are aware of their condition and will report it during the SAMPLE history.

Emphysema Emphysema is a permanent disease process that is characterized by destruction of the alveolar walls and distention of the alveolar sacs (air sacs). Basically, the lung tissue loses its elasticity, the alveoli become distended with trapped air, and the walls of the alveoli are destroyed. Loss of the alveolar wall reduces the surface area in contact with pulmonary capillaries. Therefore, a drastic disruption in

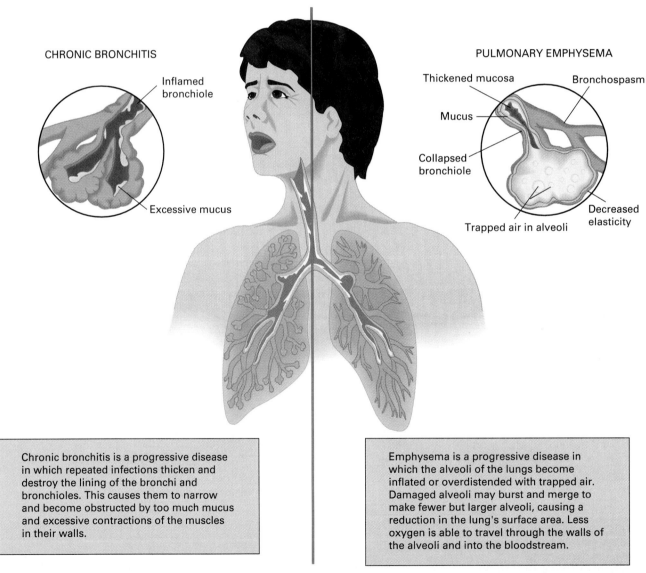

CHRONIC OBSTRUCTIVE PULMONARY DISEASE

COPD includes pulmonary emphysema and chronic bronchitis and is characterized by chronic cough or airflow obstruction or both.

CHRONIC BRONCHITIS

Inflamed bronchiole

Excessive mucus

PULMONARY EMPHYSEMA

Thickened mucosa

Bronchospasm

Mucus

Collapsed bronchiole

Trapped air in alveoli

Decreased elasticity

Chronic bronchitis is a progressive disease in which repeated infections thicken and destroy the lining of the bronchi and bronchioles. This causes them to narrow and become obstructed by too much mucus and excessive contractions of the muscles in their walls.

Emphysema is a progressive disease in which the alveoli of the lungs become inflated or overdistended with trapped air. Damaged alveoli may burst and merge to make fewer but larger alveoli, causing a reduction in the lung's surface area. Less oxygen is able to travel through the walls of the alveoli and into the bloodstream.

Figure 14-10 Chronic obstructive pulmonary disease.

gas exchange occurs and the patient becomes hypoxic and begins to retain carbon dioxide.

The distal airways also are involved in the disease process and have a greatly increased airway resistance. Breathing is extremely difficult for the emphysema patient; therefore, he uses most of his energy to breathe. The patient usually complains of extreme shortness of breath upon exertion, which may be simply walking across a room. The loss of lung elasticity and trapping of air cause the chest to increase in diameter, producing the barrel-chest appearance typical with this disease.

Signs and symptoms of emphysema are similar to those listed earlier for breathing difficulty and may include the following:

- Thin, barrel chest appearance
- Coughing, but with little sputum (material that is coughed up)
- Prolonged exhalation
- Diminished breath sounds
- Wheezing and rhonchi (rattles) on auscultation
- Pursed-lip breathing
- Extreme difficulty of breathing on exertion
- Pink complexion
- Tachypnea—breathing rate usually greater than 20 per minute
- Tachycardia (increased heart rate)
- Diaphoresis (sweating; moist skin)
- May be on home oxygen

Chronic Bronchitis   Chronic bronchitis involves inflammation, swelling, and excessive mucus production in the bronchial tree (bronchi and bronchioles). By definition, chronic bronchitis is characterized by a productive cough that persists for at least three months out of the year for at least two consecutive years. Because chronic bronchitis occurs in the bronchi and bronchioles, the alveoli are not affected. However, the alveoli do not expand fully because the air cannot get past the diseased bronchi and bronchioles. Recurrent infections leave scar tissue that further narrows the airway.

A major problem with chronic bronchitis is the swelling and thickening of the lining of the lower airways and an increase in mucus production. The airways become very narrow causing a high resistance to air movement and chronic difficulty in breathing.

Signs and symptoms of chronic bronchitis are:

- Typically overweight
- Chronic cyanotic complexion
- Difficulty in breathing, but less prominent than with emphysema
- Productive cough with sputum (material that is coughed up)
- Coarse rhonchi usually heard upon auscultation of the lungs

This patient frequently suffers from respiratory infections that lead to more acute episodes.

Emergency Medical Care   Emergency care for the emphysema and chronic bronchitis patient follows the same guidelines as for any patient suffering from difficulty in breathing. Ensuring an open airway and adequate breathing, position of comfort, and administration of supplemental oxygen are key elements in managing these patients. The patient may also have a prescribed metered dose inhaler.

COPD patients may develop a *hypoxic drive*. Normally, the body's respiratory receptors respond to carbon dioxide levels to stimulate breathing. In COPD patients, constantly high carbon dioxide levels in the blood from poor gas exchange cause the cell receptors to respond, instead, to low levels of oxygen to stimulate the breathing. Theoretically, if high concentrations of oxygen are administered to the patient, the receptors pick up the increased oxygen level in the blood and send signals to the respiratory control center to reduce or even stop breathing. This usually occurs when high concentrations of oxygen are administered over a long period of time, usually greater than 24 hours.

In the prehospital setting, since you are not typically with the patient over several hours, this is a rare event and not a major concern. Oxygen administration should take precedence over a concern about whether the hypoxic drive is going to be lost and cause the patient to stop breathing. (If this should happen, you would initiate positive pressure ventilation with supplemental oxygen, just as you would for any respiratory arrest.)

If you have categorized the COPD patient as being a high priority, if respiratory distress is evident, and if trauma, shock, cardiac compromise, or other potentially life-threatening conditions exist, high concentrations of oxygen should be delivered by a nonrebreather mask at 15 lpm. If the patient is not in significant distress or is not a priority patient, medical direction may order you to place the patient on a nasal cannula at 2 to 3 liters per minute. Since many COPD patients are on home oxygen, you may be advised to apply a nasal cannula at the same liter flow or possibly 1 lpm higher than the home oxygen setting. Follow local protocol or medical direction's order for oxygen administration in the COPD patient. *As a general rule, never withhold oxygen from any patient who requires it.*

ASTHMA

Asthma is characterized by an increased sensitivity of the lower airways to irritants that cause bronchospasm, which is a diffuse, reversible narrowing of the bronchioles. The following conditions in the asthma patient contribute to the increasing resistance to air flow and difficulty in breathing:

- Bronchospasm (constriction of the smooth muscle in the bronchioles)
- Edema (swelling) of the inner lining in the airways
- Increased secretion of mucus that causes plugging of the smaller airways

Asthma patients usually suffer acute, irregular, periodic attacks, but between the attacks usually have either no or very few signs or symptoms. A prolonged life-threatening attack that produces inadequate breathing and severe signs and symptoms is called *status asthmaticus* (Figure 14-11). Status asthmaticus is a severe asthmatic attack that does not respond to either oxygen or medication. Patients in status asthmaticus require immediate and rapid transport to the hospital. Consider requesting ALS back-up.

There are generally two different kinds of asthma. Extrinsic asthma, or "allergic" asthma, usually results from a reaction to dust, pollen, smoke, or other irritants in the air. It is typically seasonal, occurs most

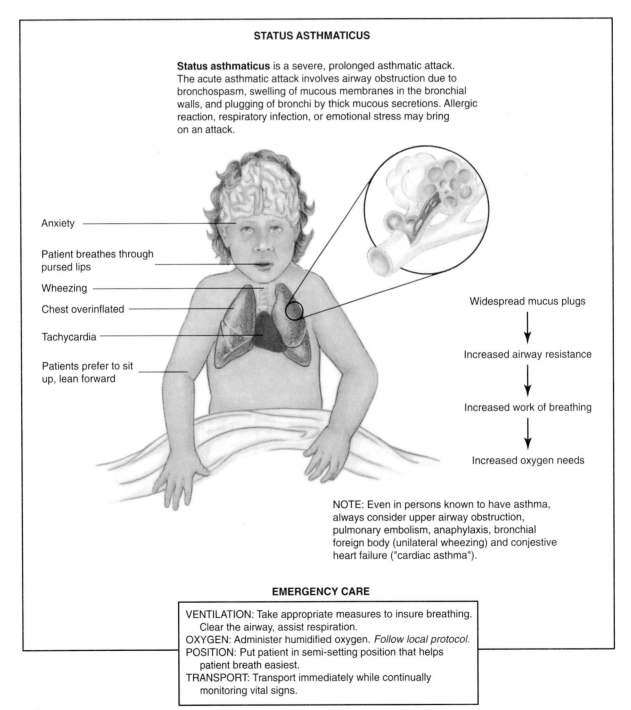

STATUS ASTHMATICUS

Status asthmaticus is a severe, prolonged asthmatic attack. The acute asthmatic attack involves airway obstruction due to bronchospasm, swelling of mucous membranes in the bronchial walls, and plugging of bronchi by thick mucous secretions. Allergic reaction, respiratory infection, or emotional stress may bring on an attack.

Anxiety

Patient breathes through pursed lips

Wheezing

Chest overinflated

Tachycardia

Patients prefer to sit up, lean forward

Widespread mucus plugs

↓

Increased airway resistance

↓

Increased work of breathing

↓

Increased oxygen needs

NOTE: Even in persons known to have asthma, always consider upper airway obstruction, pulmonary embolism, anaphylaxis, bronchial foreign body (unilateral wheezing) and conjestive heart failure ("cardiac asthma").

EMERGENCY CARE

VENTILATION: Take appropriate measures to insure breathing. Clear the airway, assist respiration.
OXYGEN: Administer humidified oxygen. *Follow local protocol.*
POSITION: Put patient in semi-setting position that helps patient breath easiest.
TRANSPORT: Transport immediately while continually monitoring vital signs.

Figure 14-11   Status asthmaticus.

often in children, and may subside after adolescence. Intrinsic, or "nonallergic," asthma is most common in adults and usually results from infection, emotional stress, or strenuous exercise.

In asthma, the smaller bronchioles have a tendency to collapse when the lungs recoil; therefore, exhalation is much more difficult and prolonged, and air becomes trapped in the alveoli. Because of this, wheezing is heard much earlier upon exhalation. The patient is forced to use energy not only to breathe in but also to eliminate the air from the lungs during exhalation. Thus, exhalation becomes an active process requiring energy that leads to increased breathing workload and eventual exhaustion. Respiratory depression or arrest may shortly follow in severe cases.

Signs and symptoms of asthma are:

- Dyspnea (shortness of breath); may progressively worsen
- Nonproductive cough
- Wheezing on auscultation
- Tachypnea (breathing faster than normal)
- Tachycardia (increased heart rate beyond normal)
- Anxiety and apprehension
- Possible fever
- Typical allergic signs and symptoms: runny nose, sneezing, red or bloodshot eyes, stuffy nose

The following signs indicate that the condition is extremely severe, the breathing is inadequate, and you should begin positive pressure ventilation with supplemental oxygen:

- Extreme fatigue or exhaustion; the patient is too tired to breathe
- Inability to speak
- Cyanosis to the core of the body
- Heart rate greater than 130 per minute
- Quiet or absent breath sounds on auscultation of the lungs

Emergency Medical Care   During the initial assessment, you would have established and maintained an airway, applied oxygen or begun positive pressure ventilation with supplemental oxygen, and assessed the adequacy of circulation. During the focused history and physical exam, it is necessary to calm the patient to reduce his workload of breathing and oxygen consumption. If the patient has a prescribed metered dose inhaler, administration of the beta agonist should provide some relief of the breathing difficulty. Transport and continuously reassess the breathing status during the ongoing assessment.

Pneumonia

Pneumonia is one of the leading causes of death in the United States. It is primarily an acute infectious disease, caused by bacteria or a virus, that affects the lower respiratory tract and causes lung inflammation and fluid- or pus-filled alveoli. This leads to poor gas exchange and eventual hypoxia. Pneumonia can also occur due to inhalation of toxic irritants or aspiration of vomitus and other substances.

The signs and symptoms of pneumonia vary with the cause and the patient's age. The patient generally appears ill and may complain of fever and severe chills. Look for the following signs and symptoms:

- Malaise and decreased appetite
- Fever
- Cough—may be productive or nonproductive
- Dyspnea
- Tachypnea and tachycardia
- Chest pain—sharp and localized and is usually made worse when breathing
- Decreased chest wall movement and shallow respirations
- The patient may splint his thorax with his arm.
- Crackles and rhonchi may be heard on auscultation.

Emergency Medical Care   The pneumonia patient is managed no differently from any patient having difficulty in breathing. Ensure adequate oxygenation and breathing. This is an acute infectious disease process that is not usually associated with severe bronchoconstriction, unless it occurs as a complication of asthma or COPD. Therefore, you would not expect the patient to have an MDI for this condition, nor would you necessarily consider its use unless indications of bronchoconstriction are present. Consult medical direction and follow your local protocol for the use of the MDI.

Pulmonary Embolism

Pulmonary embolism is a sudden blockage of blood flow through a pulmonary artery or one of its branches. The embolism is usually caused by a blood clot, but it may also be an air bubble, a fat particle, or a foreign body. The embolism prevents blood from flowing to the lung. As a result, some areas of the lung have oxygen in the alveoli but are not receiving any blood flow. This leads to a decrease in gas exchange and subsequent hypoxia, the severity of which depends on the size of the embolism or the number of alveoli affected.

Factors that commonly lead to pulmonary embolism include recent surgery, prolonged immobilization, thrombophlebitis (inflammation of the veins), certain medications (e.g., birth control pills), chronic atrial fibrillation (a heart rhythm disorder), and multiple fractures. The signs and symptoms depend on the size of the obstruction. If a clot obstructs a large artery, gas exchange will be severely impaired and signs and symptoms of respiratory distress will be evident. Suspect pulmonary embolism in any person with a sudden onset of unexplained dyspnea and stabbing-type chest pain (typically localized to a specific area of the chest) and signs of hypoxia, but who has normal breath sounds and adequate volume. Signs and symptoms of pulmonary embolism include (Figure 14-12):

- Sudden onset of unexplained dyspnea
- Signs of difficulty in breathing or respiratory distress; rapid breathing
- Sudden onset of sharp, stabbing chest pain
- Cough (may cough up blood)
- Tachypnea
- Tachycardia
- Syncope (fainting)
- Cool, moist, skin
- Restlessness, anxiety, or sense of doom
- Decrease in blood pressure (late sign)
- Cyanosis (may be severe) (late sign)
- Distended neck veins (late sign)

It is important to note that not all of the signs and symptoms will always be present. The three most common are chest pain, dyspnea (difficulty breathing), and tachypnea (rapid breathing).

Emergency Medical Care During your initial assessment, you would have opened the airway and would have initiated positive pressure ventilation with supplemental oxygen or applied oxygen by nonrebreather mask. It is important to begin oxygen administration early on and to continuously monitor the patient for signs of respiratory arrest. Immediately transport the patient.

ACUTE PULMONARY EDEMA

Acute pulmonary edema occurs when an excessive amount of fluid collects in the spaces between the alveoli and capillaries. This increase in fluid disturbs normal gas exchange and leads to hypoxia. There are two kinds of pulmonary edema: cardiogenic and non-cardiogenic. Cardiogenic pulmonary edema is typically related to an inadequate pumping function of the heart that drastically increases the pressure in the pulmonary capillaries, which forces fluid to leak into the space between the alveoli and capillaries and, eventually, into the alveoli themselves. Non-cardiogenic pulmonary edema results from destruction of the capillary bed that allows fluid to leak out. Common causes of non-cardiogenic pulmonary edema are pneumonia, aspiration of vomit, near-drowning, narcotic overdose, inhalation of smoke or other toxic gases, ascent to a high altitude, and trauma. The causes may differ, but the signs and symptoms are the same.

Signs and symptoms of pulmonary edema are:

- Dyspnea, especially on exertion
- Difficulty in breathing when lying flat

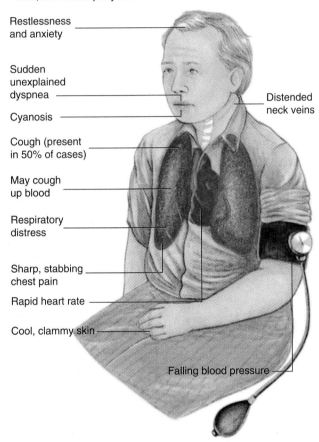

**SIGNS AND SYMPTOMS
OF PULMONARY EMBOLISM**

Pulmonary embolism is a clot or embulus that blocks a pulmonary artery. It is a serious problem accounting for 200,000 deaths per year.

Restlessness and anxiety

Sudden unexplained dyspnea

Cyanosis

Cough (present in 50% of cases)

May cough up blood

Respiratory distress

Sharp, stabbing chest pain

Rapid heart rate

Cool, clammy skin

Distended neck veins

Falling blood pressure

Figure 14-12   Signs and symptoms of pulmonary embolism.

- Frothy sputum, possibly blood-tinged (late sign)
- Tachycardia
- Anxiety, apprehension, combativeness, confusion
- Tripod position with legs dangling
- Fatigue
- Crackles and possibly wheezing on auscultation
- Cyanosis or a dusky color skin
- Pale, moist skin
- Distended neck veins
- Swollen lower extremities

Emergency Medical Care It is necessary to carefully assess the patient with pulmonary edema. If any evidence of inadequate breathing is present, you need to begin positive pressure ventilation with supplemental oxygen. If the breathing is adequate, administer oxygen via nonrebreather mask at 15 lpm and closely monitor the breathing status. Keep the patient in an upright sitting position and transport without delay.

CASE STUDY FOLLOW-UP

SCENE SIZE-UP

You have been dispatched to a 31-year-old female patient complaining of difficulty in breathing. A man nervously greets you at the curb as you gather your equipment. He indicates that the patient is his wife, Anna Sanders, who is having an extremely hard time breathing. You are lead up to the third floor of an apartment complex. You do not note any possible hazards, but are looking at how difficult the extrication might be. Upon walking into the apartment you note a young female patient sitting in a tripod position next to the kitchen table.

INITIAL ASSESSMENT

As you start to introduce yourself, the patient begins to speak, gasping for her breath after each word. With great difficulty she states, "I—can't—breathe." Based on Mrs. Sanders's facial expression and posture, she appears to be in a great deal of distress. Her airway is open and her breathing is rapid and labored at a rate of 34 per minute. There are audible wheezes when she exhales. You immediately apply oxygen via a nonrebreather mask at 15 lpm. Her radial pulse is about 110 per minute. The skin is moist and slightly pale. You recognize the patient as a priority and signal your partner to get the stretcher while you continue with the focused history and physical exam.

FOCUSED HISTORY AND PHYSICAL EXAM

You begin to evaluate the difficulty in breathing using the OPQRST mnemonic. You ask Anna questions she can answer with a nod or a shake of her head to reduce her need to respond by speaking. Some questions you direct to her husband. You ascertain that the breathing difficulty began gradually about 2 hours ago and got progressively worse. She is unable to lie down because this causes her breathing to get much worse. Sitting up is not much better, though. She has had similar episodes in the past, but none seem to have been this severe. On a scale of 1 to 10, Mrs. Sanders indicates that her difficulty in breathing is about an 8 or 9.

You continue to obtain a SAMPLE history. The primary symptom is severe difficulty in breathing. Mrs. Sanders has an allergy to penicillin. When asked about medications that she takes, Mr. Sanders brings you a prescription of Albuterol® in a metered dose inhaler. She is on no other medication. When asked if she has taken any of the Albuterol®, her husband says, "She took one puff about 15 minutes ago." She has a past medical history of asthma and suffers these attacks maybe once every 4 or 5 months. She has had nothing to eat for about 3 hours but drank a small glass of orange juice about an hour ago. She was cleaning the kitchen when the episode began.

You quickly perform a focused physical exam. You assess her neck for jugular vein distention. Inspection of her chest and abdomen reveals significant use of the abdominal muscles when exhaling. The breath sounds are diminished bilaterally and you hear wheezing even without using your stethoscope. Her fingertips are slightly cyanotic. You assess the baseline vital signs and find a blood pressure of 134/86; pulse of 118 per minute and regular; respirations at 32 per minute and labored with audible wheezing; the skin moist and slightly pale.

You contact your medical direction, Dr. Maxwell, for an order to administer the Albuterol® by MDI. You check the medication to ensure it is prescribed to Mrs. Sanders, that it is the correct medication, and that it has not expired. You report your physical findings and SAMPLE history to Dr. Maxwell. He gives you an order to administer one dose. If there is no relief of the symptoms, he instructs you to contact him for further orders. Mrs. Sanders is familiar with the MDI and its use, but she is too scared and apprehensive to use it properly. You proceed with the administration by coaching Mrs. Sanders throughout the procedure.

ONGOING ASSESSMENT

You reassess the baseline vital signs following administration of the Albuterol®. The blood pressure is 130/84, pulse rate decreases to 90 per minute, respirations are now 18 per minute and much less labored. The audible wheezes are very minimal. The skin is not as moist and both skin and fingernails begin to return to a normal color. You secure Mrs. Sanders in a Fowler's position on a stair chair, and you and your partner transport her down to a stretcher your partner has placed on the first floor.

You reassess the difficulty in breathing. Mrs. Sanders is now able to talk in complete sentences and indicates that the shortness of breath is much less severe. She is now only slightly short of breath. You continue oxygen therapy, document your findings and emergency care, and radio the hospital with a report.

Upon arrival at the hospital, you provide the nursing staff with an oral report. You write a prehospital care report form as your partner restocks the ambulance. Before leaving the hospital, you check in on Mrs. Sanders and find her to be relaxed and breathing well. She thanks you for your prompt response and emergency care. You then mark back in service and prepare for the next call.

CHAPTER REVIEW

TERMS AND CONCEPTS

You may wish to review the following terms and concepts included in this chapter.

apnea—absence of breathing; respiratory arrest.

bronchoconstriction—constriction of the smooth muscle of the bronchi and bronchioles causing a narrowing of the air passageway.

bronchodilator—a drug that relaxes the smooth muscle of the bronchi and bronchioles and reverses bronchoconstriction.

bronchospasm—spasm or constriction of the smooth muscle of the bronchi and bronchioles.

dyspnea—shortness of breath or perceived difficulty in breathing.

grunting—a sound heard in infants during exhalation when suffering from a respiratory problem that causes collapsed lungs.

hypoxia—the absence of sufficient oxygen in the body cells.

metered dose inhaler (MDI)—device consisting of a plastic container and a canister of medication that is used to inhale an aerosolized medication.

respiratory arrest—when breathing stops completely.

respiratory failure—inadequate oxygenation of the blood and elimination of carbon dioxide.

spacer—a chamber that is connected to the metered dose inhaler to collect the medication until it is inhaled.

tripod position—a position in which the patient sits upright, leans slightly forward, and supports the body with the arms in front and elbows locked. This is a common position found in respiratory distress.

REVIEW QUESTIONS

1. List the major signs and symptoms of breathing difficulty.
2. List the signs of adequate breathing.
3. List the signs of inadequate breathing.
4. List the steps of emergency care for a patient who is exhibiting signs and symptoms of breathing difficulty but is breathing adequately.
5. List the steps of emergency care for a patient who is in respiratory distress and is breathing inadequately.
6. List the signs of adequate positive pressure ventilation and the steps to take if ventilation is inadequate.
7. Explain the steps to administer a medication by MDI.
8. List the indications and contraindications for the use of a beta agonist drug.
9. Describe the early signs of breathing difficulty in the infant or child; list the signs of inadequate breathing and respiratory failure in the infant or child.
10. Explain how to distinguish airway obstruction in the infant or child patient caused by disease from airway obstruction caused by a foreign body; explain how treatment would differ for the two types of airway obstruction.

CHAPTER 15

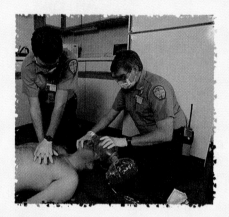

Cardiac Emergencies

INTRODUCTION

Heart disease is America's number one killer. While the EMT-Basic will occasionally be called to a patient who is in cardiac arrest, or to a patient who goes into cardiac arrest at the scene or en route to the hospital, more often the call will be to a responsive patient who has signs and symptoms—particularly chest pain—that may be caused by heart disease. The EMT-B must be prepared to treat all patients with signs and symptoms of cardiac compromise as cardiac emergencies.

OBJECTIVES

Numbered objectives are from the United States Department of Transportation 1994 EMT-Basic National Standard Curriculum. Asterisked objectives, if any, pertain to material that is supplemental to the DOT curriculum.

COGNITIVE

4-3.1 Describe the structure and function of the cardiovascular system. (pp. 295–299)

4-3.2 Describe the emergency medical care of the patient experiencing chest pain/discomfort. (pp. 301–305)

4-3.5 Define the role of the EMT-Basic in the emergency cardiac care system. (pp. 300–303)

4-3.7 Discuss the position of comfort for patients with various cardiac emergencies. (p. 301)

4-3.8 Establish the relationship between airway management and the patient with cardiovascular compromise. (p. 300)

4-3.9 Predict the relationship between the patient experiencing cardiovascular compromise and basic cardiac life support. (pp. 293, 300)

4-3.40 Recognize the need for medical direction of protocols to assist in the emergency medical care of the patient with chest pain. (pp. 301, 304, 305)

4-3.41 List the indications for the use of nitroglycerin. (p. 304)

4-3.42 State the contraindications and side effects for the use of nitroglycerin. (p. 304)

AFFECTIVE

4-3.46 Explain the rationale for administering nitroglycerin to a patient with chest pain or discomfort. (p. 301)

PSYCHOMOTOR

4-3.47 Demonstrate the assessment and emergency medical care of a patient experiencing chest pain/discomfort.

4-3.52 Perform the steps in facilitating the use of nitroglycerin for chest pain or discomfort.

4-3.53 Demonstrate the assessment and documentation of patient response to nitroglycerin.

4-3.54 Practice completing the prehospital care report for patients with cardiac emergencies.

Additional objectives from DOT Lesson 4-3 are addressed in Chapter 16, "Automated External Defibrillation."

CASE STUDY

THE DISPATCH

EMS Unit 23—respond to 321 Congress St., Reali's Restaurant. You have a 49-year-old male complaining of chest pain. Time out is 1735 hours.

ON ARRIVAL

You and your partner arrive at 1740 hours and find the patient sitting in a chair at a table clutching his chest. As you approach the patient, you note that he looks very anxious. The scene is secure and he is the only patient. You introduce your partner and yourself. Your patient gives his name as Paul Antak. He states, "I feel like someone is standing on my chest."

How would you proceed to assess and care for this patient?

During this chapter, you will learn about assessment and emergency care for a patient suffering from chest pain. Later, we will return to the case and apply the procedures learned.

CIRCULATORY SYSTEM ANATOMY AND PHYSIOLOGY

The circulatory or **cardiovascular system** has three major components: the heart, the blood vessels, and the blood.

THE HEART

The **heart** (Figure 15-1) is a four-chambered muscular pump which lies in the center of the chest. About two-thirds of it lies to the left of the **sternum,** or breastbone. The base, or top of the heart, points toward the right shoulder and the apex, or bottom, points to the left hip. The heart is about the size of an adult fist and has two major divisions, right and left. The right side receives deoxygenated blood returning from the body cells through the veins and pumps it to the lungs. The left side of the heart receives oxygenated blood from the lungs and pumps it to the body's cells through the arteries.

ATRIA

The **atria** are the two top chambers on each side of the heart. The right atrium receives blood from the body (Figure 15-2). This blood is returning from the body's cells and is depleted of oxygen. The right atrium pumps its blood to the right ventricle. The left atrium receives blood from the lungs through the **pulmonary veins.** This blood is rich in oxygen and ready to be pumped throughout the body. The left atrium pumps its blood to the left ventricle.

VENTRICLES

The **ventricles** are the bottom or lower chambers on each side of the heart. The right ventricle receives blood from the right atrium and pumps the deoxygenated blood to the lungs through the **pulmonary arteries.** In the lungs, through the alveolar/capillary exchange process, the blood is oxygenated. The left ventricle receives the oxygenated blood from the left atrium and pumps it

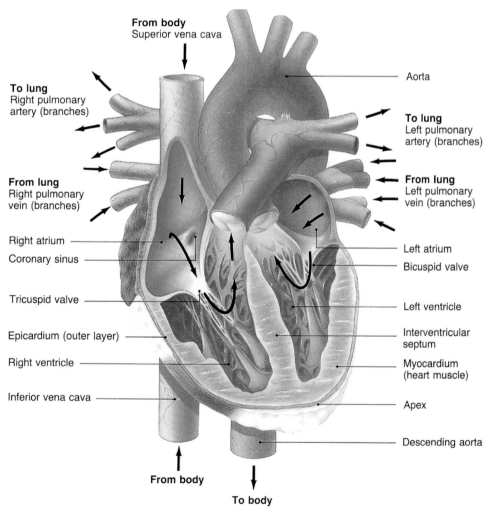

Figure 15-1 The heart.

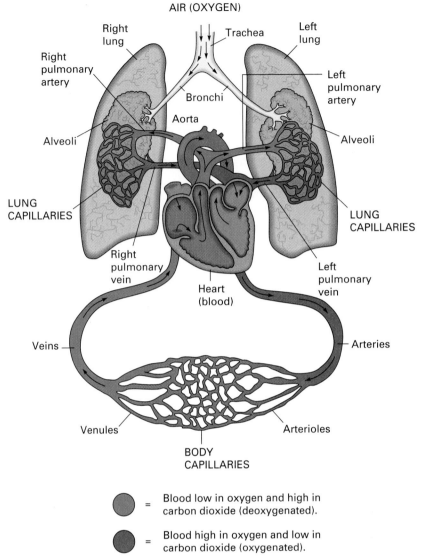

Figure 15-2   Circulation of blood through the cardiovascular system.

throughout the body. Since the left ventricle is responsible for pumping blood the greatest distance, it has the largest muscle mass of the heart and is a common site of injury associated with trauma and heart attack.

VALVES

There are four **valves** located within the heart's chambers. These valves ensure that blood flows in only one direction, preventing a backflow of blood in the system. The four valves are:

- The *tricuspid valve,* located between the right atrium and right ventricle, prevents blood from returning to the right atrium.
- The *pulmonary valve,* located at the base of the pulmonary artery, prevents blood from returning to the right ventricle from the pulmonary artery.

- The *mitral* or *bicuspid valve,* located between the left atrium and the left ventricle, prevents blood from backflowing into the left atrium.
- The *aortic* valve, located at the base of the **aorta,** the major artery of the cardiovascular system, prevents backflow of blood into the left ventricle from the aorta.

THE CARDIAC CONDUCTION SYSTEM

The heart is more than a muscle. It also contains specialized contractile tissue as well as conductive tissue, known as the **cardiac conduction system,** that allows it to generate electrical impulses. These impulses allow the heart to contract or "beat" differently than other muscles (Figure 15-3).

THE CONDUCTION SYSTEM

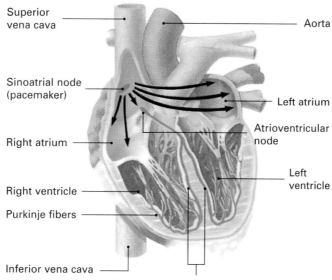

Figure 15-3 The cardiac conduction system.

The electrical impulse is generated in the right atrium at the *sinoatrial node (SA node)*. It travels through both atria, causing both to contract simultaneously, propelling blood to the ventricles. Next the impulse travels to the *atrioventricular node (AV node)*, which is the area between the atria and ventricles. The *bundle of His* then carries the impulse into the right and left ventricles to the *Purkinje fibers,* which are embedded in the ventricular muscle, causing the ventricles to contract simultaneously and propel the blood to the lungs and throughout the body.

THE BLOOD VESSELS

The blood vessels—arteries, capillaries, and veins—carry blood from the heart, to the lungs and the rest of the body, and back to the heart (Figure 15-4).

ARTERIES

The **arteries** carry blood away from the heart. Most arteries carry blood rich in oxygen and low in carbon dioxide, except for the pulmonary artery which carries oxygen-depleted blood to the lungs. Arteries are composed of three different layers containing muscle and elasticized tissue to allow for dilation or constriction depending on the system's needs. Pulsations from arteries can be felt, or palpated, when arteries lie near the body's surface, usually over bony prominences. (These "pulse points" and the taking of a pulse were discussed in Chapter 5,

"Baseline Vital Signs and History Taking.") The major arteries are:

- **Coronary arteries**—These vessels (Figure 15-5) branch off the base of the aorta and supply the heart with oxygen-rich blood.
- **Aorta**—The major artery originating from the left ventricle of the heart. It carries oxygen-rich blood to the system of arteries that branch throughout the body.
- **Pulmonary artery**—This artery originates from the right ventricle and carries blood to the lungs. It is the only artery to carry oxygen-depleted blood.
- **Carotid artery**—The major artery of the neck that supplies blood to the head and brain. Pulsations from this artery can be felt on either side of the neck.
- **Femoral artery**—The major artery of the thigh that supplies the groin and legs with blood. Pulsations from this artery can be felt in the groin area.
- **Radial artery**—The major artery of the forearm. It is palpable over the thumb side of the wrist.
- **Brachial artery**—The major artery of the upper arm. It is palpable on the inside of the arm between the elbow and shoulder. This artery is used when assessing blood pressure.
- **Posterior tibial artery**—This artery extends from the calf to the foot and is palpable behind, or posterior to, the medial malleolus (inside ankle bone).
- **Dorsalis pedis artery**—This artery is found in the foot and is palpable on the top of the foot on the great toe side.

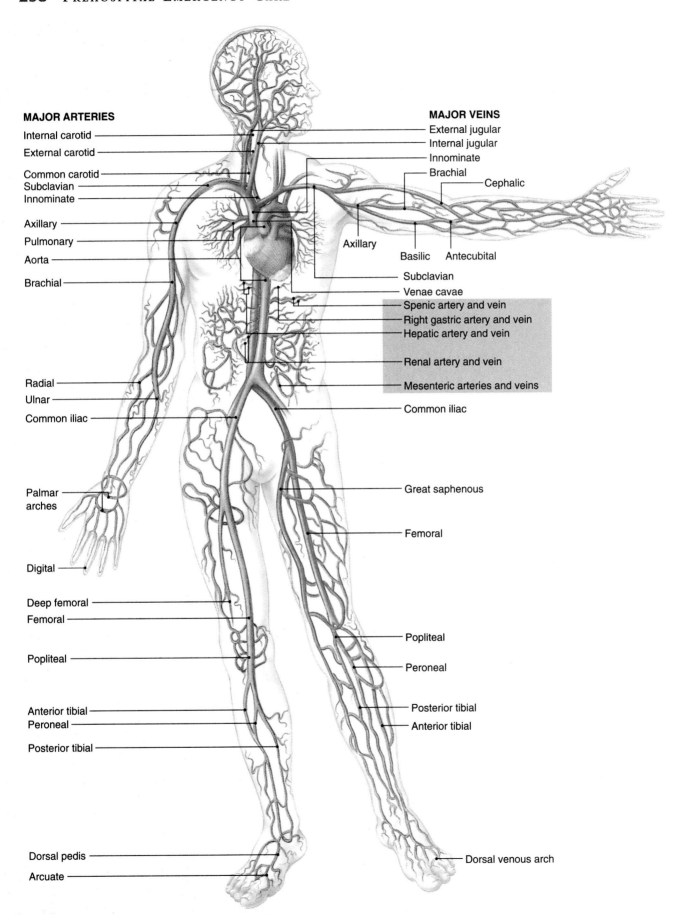

MAJOR ARTERIES

Internal carotid
External carotid
Common carotid
Subclavian
Innominate
Axillary
Pulmonary
Aorta
Brachial
Radial
Ulnar
Common iliac
Palmar arches
Digital
Deep femoral
Femoral
Popliteal
Anterior tibial
Peroneal
Posterior tibial
Dorsal pedis
Arcuate

MAJOR VEINS

External jugular
Internal jugular
Innominate
Brachial
Cephalic
Axillary
Basilic
Antecubital
Subclavian
Venae cavae
Spenic artery and vein
Right gastric artery and vein
Hepatic artery and vein
Renal artery and vein
Mesenteric arteries and veins
Common iliac
Great saphenous
Femoral
Popliteal
Peroneal
Posterior tibial
Anterior tibial
Dorsal venous arch

Figure 15-4   Major arteries and veins.

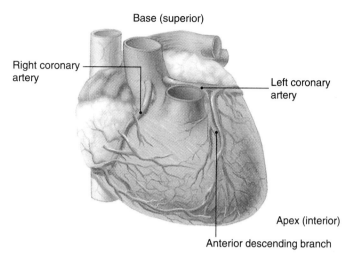

Base (superior)

Right coronary artery

Left coronary artery

Apex (interior)

Anterior descending branch

Figure 15-5   The coronary arteries.

ARTERIOLES

Arterioles are the smallest branches of the arteries leading to the capillaries. They carry blood from the arteries to the capillary beds.

CAPILLARIES

The **capillaries** are a network of tiny blood vessels connecting arterioles to venules. They are found in all parts of the body. The capillary network ensures that all body cells are nourished and their wastes removed. The one-cell-thick walls of capillaries allow oxygen and nutrients to pass from the blood into the cells and allow carbon dioxide and other waste products to pass from the cells into the blood to be carried away for exhalation and excretion from the body.

VENULES

Venules are the smallest branches of the veins. They connect the capillaries with the veins. Venules carry oxygen-depleted blood to the veins.

VEINS

Veins are the blood vessels that carry blood back to the heart. Veins usually carry oxygen-depleted blood that is high in carbon dioxide, except for the pulmonary veins, which carry oxygen-rich blood to the left atrium from the lungs. Since the blood within the veins is under less pressure than that in the arteries, there are valves located at various points within the venous system to prevent backflow of blood. The major veins are:

- **Pulmonary veins**—They carry oxygen-rich blood from the lungs to the left atrium.
- **Venae cavae**—These are the veins that carry blood back to the right atrium. There are two major divi-

sions: (1) the **superior vena cava** carries oxygen-depleted blood to the heart from the upper body; (2) the **inferior vena cava** carries oxygen-depleted blood to the heart from the lower body.

THE BLOOD

Approximately $\frac{1}{12}$ to $\frac{1}{15}$ of body weight is blood, and an average person weighing 150 pounds will have about 10 to 12 pints or approximately 5 liters of total blood volume. The components of blood include:

- **Red blood cells**—These give blood its red color, carry oxygen to the body's cells, and carry carbon dioxide away from the body's cells.
- **White blood cells**—These are part of the body's immune system, or defense against infections.
- **Plasma**—This is the serum, or fluid, that carries blood cells and nutrients to the body's cells. Plasma also carries waste products of cell metabolism away from the body's cells for excretion.
- **Platelets**—These are essential to the formation of blood clots, which are necessary to stop bleeding.

BLOOD PRESSURE

Blood pressure is defined as the pressure exerted during circulation of the blood against the arterial walls. Generally, two distinct pressures are measured using a sphygmomanometer (blood pressure cuff) and stethoscope. The **systolic pressure** represents the pressure exerted against the arterial wall during contraction of the left ventricle (systole). The **diastolic pressure** represents the pressure exerted against the arterial wall during relaxation of the left ventricle (diastole). It represents the resistance in the vessel that is determined by its size and diameter. The smaller the vessel the greater the resistance and the higher the diastolic pressure. (See Chapter 5, "Baseline Vital Signs and History Taking," for a fuller discussion of blood pressure.)

INADEQUATE CIRCULATION

A properly functioning circulatory system delivers oxygen and nutrients to the body's cells and carries away carbon dioxide and other wastes. These processes take place as blood passes through the capillaries. The delivery of oxygen and nutrients from the blood, through the thin capillary walls into the cells, and the removal of carbon dioxide and other waste products, is known as **perfusion.**

Under some conditions, blood does not circulate adequately through all the body's capillaries. The chief result of inadequate circulation is a state of profound depression of cell perfusion, called **shock (hypoperfusion)**. The cells become starved for oxygen and nutrients and become overloaded with carbon dioxide and other waste products.

Hypoperfusion can occur as a result of low blood volume (hypovolemia), insufficient pumping action of the heart (pump damage), or dilated and leaking vessels. Hypoperfusion can also result from spinal cord damage that results in massive dilation of the blood vessels, creating a system that is too large overall for the amount of available blood. A more detailed discussion of hypoperfusion, its causes, and consequences can be found in Chapter 29, "Bleeding and Shock."

CARDIAC COMPROMISE

The heart is very sensitive to a decrease in its supply of oxygen and blood. Therefore, in events that compromise cardiac function, time becomes a crucial element for patient survival. Most of the permanent damage done to the heart muscle occurs within the first few hours of the cardiac event.

Cardiac cases require prompt assessment, treatment, and transport to increase the likelihood of a positive outcome for the patient. In cardiac arrest, for example, CPR started within 4 minutes of an event is far more effective than CPR started after that time.

Likewise, prompt transport of the patient to the hospital provides a patient with access to medications such as "clot busting," or thrombolytic, drugs. The earlier these medications can be administered, the more rapidly the heart's blood supply returns, thus decreasing the extent of permanent heart damage.

ASSESSMENT AND CARE: CARDIAC COMPROMISE

Dispatch information can provide you with the first indications that a patient may be suffering from cardiac compromise. In cases in which you are directed to patients complaining of chest pain and/or difficulty in breathing, suspect the possibility of cardiac problems. Remember that any adult patient with chest pain should be treated as a cardiac emergency until proven otherwise.

SCENE SIZE-UP AND INITIAL ASSESSMENT

On arrival, perform the scene size-up to ensure that the scene is secure, and then proceed rapidly with the initial assessment.

Gather a general impression of the patient and his mental status as you approach the scene. Generally, patients experiencing cardiac emergencies fall into two categories: (1) unresponsive patients with no respiration and no pulse (cardiac arrest) and (2) responsive patients.

When you encounter an unresponsive patient with no respiration and no pulse, act immediately. For children 8 years of age or younger, begin CPR. For patients older than 8 years of age, begin CPR and apply the automated external defibrillator (AED) as soon as it is available. (A review of CPR techniques is found in Appendix 1; discussion of AED use in cases of cardiac arrest is found in Chapter 16.)

With responsive patients, first ensure adequate airway, breathing, and circulation. Note also the patient's skin color, temperature, and condition. Note the type, location, and intensity of any pain and presence of other signs or symptoms related to cardiac compromise. Apply oxygen at 15 lpm via a nonrebreather mask. Make a decision on whether early transport is needed.

FOCUSED HISTORY AND PHYSICAL EXAM

The next step is the focused history and physical exam. The type of focused history and physical exam that you will perform depends on whether the patient is responsive and able to provide a history, or if he has an altered mental status and is not able to provide any information.

SAMPLE History   If the patient is unable to answer questions, try to obtain the history from his family or from bystanders. In suspected cardiac cases, be sure to determine if nitroglycerin has been prescribed for the patient. Use the OPQRST mnemonic to obtain a description of the patient's chest pain.

- Onset: What were you doing when the pain started? What triggered it? Was onset sudden or gradual?
- Provocation/palliation: Does anything make it worse? better?
- Quality: Describe the pain. Is it sharp or dull? Pressing, squeezing, crushing, or burning?
- Radiation: Does the pain radiate to any other part of your body?

- Severity: On a scale of 1 to 10, 10 being the worst pain you have ever had, rate your current pain or discomfort. Have you had pain like this before? If so, is your current pain more or less severe?
- Time: When did the chest pain start? How long have you had it? (Try to find out the actual day and time; in some cases you may find that a patient has had the pain for one or more days.)

Physical Exam and Baseline Vital Signs You will perform a focused physical exam on the responsive patient suffering from a possible cardiac complaint such as chest pain or breathing difficulty. During the exam, assess the following:

- Pupils—Sluggish or dilated pupils may suggest hypoxia and poor perfusion.
- Oral cavity—Cyanotic mucous membranes indicate hypoxia.
- Neck—Congestive heart failure or cardiac tamponade (fluid in the sac surrounding the heart) may produce jugular venous distention.
- Chest—Auscultate for abnormal breath sounds, especially rales or crackles, which may indicate fluid in the alveoli from left ventricular heart failure.
- Lower and upper extremities—Assess for peripheral edema, suggesting heart failure, and cyanosis, indicating hypoxia.
- Posterior body—Presacral edema to the lower back would be another indicator of heart failure.

In addition to performing the focused physical exam, obtain and record the patient's vital signs.

Signs and Symptoms Signs and symptoms associated with cardiac compromise may vary widely, depending on the patient's individual response, blood loss, and degree of heart damage. Note that pain may not be the best indicator of cardiac compromise. In some cases, there is no pain associated with a cardiac event—about 20 percent of heart attacks are painless, or "silent," attacks. If pain is present, it may or may not be intensified by exertion. The pain can take many forms and is most typically described as dull, aching, burning, tightness, squeezing, or crushing.

Despite the many variables, the most common signs and symptoms of cardiac compromise are these:

- Pain or discomfort in any of the following areas: chest, neck, jaw, arm, or back; also epigastric (upper abdomen) pain that may be described as indigestion (Figure 15-6)
- Sudden onset of sweating (This may be a significant finding by itself.)
- Difficulty in breathing (dyspnea)
- Lightheadedness or dizziness
- Anxiety or irritability
- Feelings of impending doom
- Abnormal or irregular pulse rate
- Abnormal blood pressure
- Nausea and/or vomiting

EMERGENCY MEDICAL CARE

As an EMT-B, you should NOT take the time to try to diagnose the type of cardiac emergency. The treatment is the same no matter what the cause:

1. Administer oxygen at 15 lpm via a nonrebreather mask (Figure 15-7). Provide positive pressure ventilation with supplemental oxygen if breathing is inadequate.
2. Decrease the anxiety of the patient by providing calm reassurance and placing him in a position of comfort (often sitting up; let the patient tell you how he feels most comfortable).
3. Assist the patient who has prescribed nitroglycerin.
4. Consider calling for ALS (advanced life support) backup; initiate early transport.

ONGOING ASSESSMENT

Although not all patients with chest pain/discomfort or cardiac compromise will deteriorate into cardiac arrest, be ready for this possibility and closely reassess the breathing and pulse as you perform the ongoing assessment during transport. Be prepared to perform CPR and use automated external defibrillation, as appropriate, in the event that cardiac arrest does occur.

NITROGLYCERIN

While patients with known cardiac problems may be on a variety of medications, the most common will be **nitroglycerin.** Nitroglycerin is a potent vasodilator (agent that increases the diameter of blood vessels). It works in seconds to relax the muscles of the blood vessel walls. This action dilates arteries, increasing the blood flow through the coronary arteries and oxygen supply to the heart muscle and decreasing the work load of the heart.

Nitroglycerin can be either a sublingual (under-the-tongue) tablet or a sublingual spray. A paste form of nitroglycerin is also available, but it is not considered appropriate for administration by an EMT-B.

If the patient with a history of heart problems is suffering from chest pain and has nitroglycerin that has been prescribed for him by a physician, you may assist the patient in taking this medication after receiving authorization from medical direction. Because nitroglycerin lowers blood pressure, it must not be given to a patient whose systolic blood pressure is 100 mmHg or lower. If the patient is taking Viagra, *do not* administer nitroglycerin; instead contact medical direction for orders.

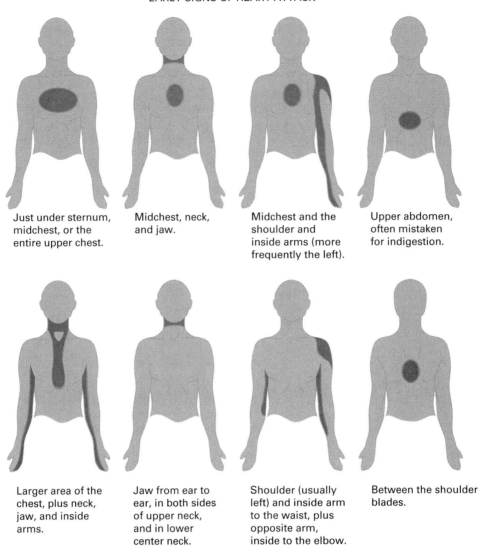

Just under sternum, midchest, or the entire upper chest.

Midchest, neck, and jaw.

Midchest and the shoulder and inside arms (more frequently the left).

Upper abdomen, often mistaken for indigestion.

Larger area of the chest, plus neck, jaw, and inside arms.

Jaw from ear to ear, in both sides of upper neck, and in lower center neck.

Shoulder (usually left) and inside arm to the waist, plus opposite arm, inside to the elbow.

Between the shoulder blades.

Figure 15-6   Typical locations and radiation of chest pain associated with cardiac emergencies.

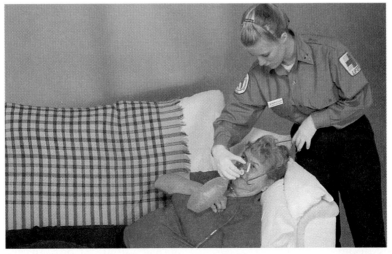

Figure 15-7   Early oxygen therapy is crucial in cardiac emergencies.

If the patient experiences no relief after one dose, another dose may be administered after 3 to 5 minutes if authorized by medical direction, to a maximum of three doses. It is important to find out if the patient has already taken one or more doses prior to your arrival to be sure that you are not inadvertently administering more than the maximum.

See Figures 15-8a to f for information on how to assist a patient with prescribed nitroglycerin. See Figure 15-9 for a detailed summary of the criteria and techniques for the administration of nitroglycerin.

SUMMARY: ASSESSMENT AND CARE

To review assessment findings that may be associated with cardiac compromise and emergency care for cardiac compromise, see Figures 15-10 and 15-11.

ENRICHMENT

The enrichment section contains information that is valuable as background for the EMT-B but that goes substantially beyond the U.S. Department of Transportation (DOT) EMT-Basic curriculum.

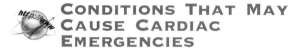 CONDITIONS THAT MAY CAUSE CARDIAC EMERGENCIES

The following is presented as enrichment information. Remember that it is not the EMT-B's function to diagnose the specific cause of the signs and symptoms the patient may be suffering. In most cases the assessment and emergency medical care given by the EMT-B, as detailed earlier in this chapter, will not change for any of these conditions.

ASSISTING A PATIENT WITH PRESCRIBED NITROGLYCERIN

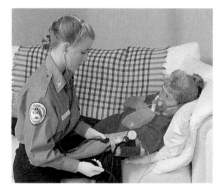

Figure 15-8a   Assess blood pressure. Systolic pressure must be greater than 100 mmHg.

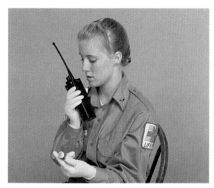

Figure 15-8b   Obtain an order from medical direction to administer the nitroglycerin.

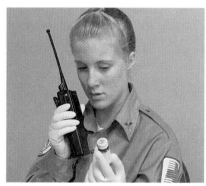

Figure 15-8c   Check the medication to ensure that it is prescribed to the patient, it is the proper medication, and it has not expired.

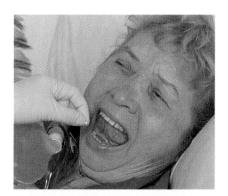

Figure 15-8d   Place the nitroglycerin tablet under the patient's tongue.

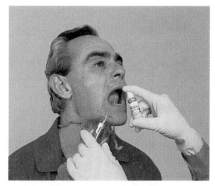

Figure 15-8e   To administer nitroglycerin spray, depress the container and deliver one spray under the tongue.

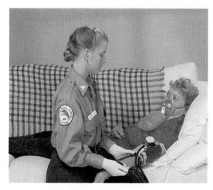

Figure 15-8f   Reassess blood pressure within 2 minutes of administering the nitroglycerin.

NITROGLYCERIN

℞

Medication Name

Nitroglycerin is the generic name. Some of the trade names of nitroglycerin are:

- Nitrostat®
- Nitrobid®
- Nitrolingual® Spray

Indications

All of the following criteria must be met before an EMT-B administers nitroglycerin to a patient:

- The patient exhibits signs or symptoms of chest pain.
- The patient has physician-prescribed nitroglycerin.
- The EMT-B has received approval from medical direction, either on-line or off-line, to give the medication.

Contraindications

Nitroglycerin should not be given if any of the following conditions exist:

- The patient's baseline blood pressure is below 100 mmHg systolic.
- The patient has a suspected head injury.
- The patient is an infant or child.
- Three doses have already been taken by the patient.
- The patient has recently taken Viagra.

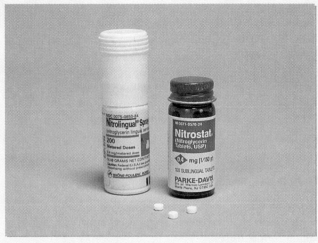

Form

Tablet, sublingual spray

Dosage

The dosage for EMT-B administration is either one tablet or one spray under the tongue. This dose may be repeated in 3 to 5 minutes if (1) the patient experiences no relief; (2) the blood pressure remains above 100 mmHg systolic; and (3) medical direction gives authorization. The total dose is three tablets or sprays, to include what the patient took prior to your arrival.

Figure 15-9 Nitroglycerin.

ANGINA PECTORIS

Angina pectoris (which means, literally, pain in the chest) is a symptom of inadequate oxygen supply to the heart muscle, or *myocardium*. It arises from a decrease in oxygen delivered to the myocardium, which is often caused by blockage of the coronary arteries, causing tissue hypoxia (ischemia). The lack of oxygen causes the pain, sometimes described as "crushing," or "squeezing," or "tightness" by the patient.

Generally, angina pectoris occurs during periods of stress, either physical or emotional. Once the stress is relieved or removed or the patient rests, the pain will usually go away. The pain is usually felt under the sternum and may radiate to the jaw, or down either arm, to the back, or to the epigastrium (upper abdomen). The pain rarely lasts more than 10 minutes, usually for 3 to 8 minutes. Many patients will be able to tell you that they have had angina as part of their past medical history and will have nitroglycerin prescribed for this condition. Prompt response of the symptoms to administered nitroglycerin is typical of angina.

The signs and symptoms of angina pectoris (Figure 15-12) are similar to those of any cardiac compromise and may include the following:

- Chest pain, pressure, or tightness
- Anxiety
- Dyspnea, or shortness of breath
- Diaphoresis, or excessive sweating
- Nausea and/or vomiting
- Complaint of indigestion pain

ACUTE MYOCARDIAL INFARCTION

Acute myocardial infarction (AMI) is the event that is commonly called a "heart attack." It occurs when there is a total and sudden occlusion, or blockage, of blood flow through a coronary artery to an area of the myocardium. This occlusion causes actual tissue

NITROGLYCERIN

℞

Administration

To administer nitroglycerin:

1. Complete the focused history and physical exam of the cardiac patient and determine that the patient has his own nitroglycerin.
2. Assess baseline vital signs to ensure that the systolic blood pressure is greater than 100 mmHg.
3. Obtain approval from medical direction, either on-line or off-line, to administer nitroglycerin.
4. Check the patient's medication to ensure that it is nitroglycerin prescribed in the patient's name and to learn the dose and route of administration.
5. Be sure that the patient is alert and responsive.
6. Check the expiration date on the nitroglycerin.
7. Ask the patient when he took his last dose of medication and what its effects were. Also, be sure that the patient understands how the medication will be administered.
8. Wear BSI gloves when handling nitroglycerin. As the patient lifts his tongue, place or spray the medication under the tongue. Alternatively, have the patient place the tablet or spray under the tongue himself.
9. Remind the patient to keep his mouth closed and not to swallow until the medication has dissolved.
10. Perform a reassessment of the patient's blood pressure in 2 minutes.
11. Record your actions, including the dosage, the

time of administration, and the patient's response.

Actions
- Dilates blood vessels.
- Decreases workload of the heart.
- Decreases cardiac oxygen demand.

Side Effects
The aim of administering nitroglycerin is to dilate blood vessels in the heart, but blood vessels in other parts of the body are dilated as well. This dilation can cause
- Headache
- A drop in blood pressure
- Changes in pulse rate as the body compensates for the changes in blood vessel size.

Reassessment
Whenever you administer nitroglycerin to a patient, you must perform a reassessment. The reassessment should include the following steps:

- Monitor blood pressure frequently during treatment and transport.
- Question the patient about the effect of the medication on relief of pain.
- Obtain approval from medical direction prior to readministration of the medication.
- Record any reassessments and findings.

Figure 15-9   continued.

death (necrosis) of the affected muscle area, and may lead to a decrease in the effectiveness of the heart's pumping ability. AMI usually occurs somewhere in the left ventricle, but it can happen anywhere in the myocardium.

The occlusion of a coronary artery generally develops over a period of time and is caused by the formation of a clot or progressive narrowing of the artery's lumen (opening) through the buildup of fatty deposits and other materials on the inner walls of the artery.

With the availability of new medications called "clot busters" and thrombolytic therapy that can be administered at a hospital, an early decision for rapid transport is more crucial than ever before. Prompt transport will allow for early intervention at the appropriate facility, thereby decreasing the possibility of more extensive damage to the myocardium.

Signs and symptoms of AMI are very similar to those of angina (Figure 15-12) and include the following:

- Chest pain radiating to jaw, arms, or back (however, AMI may not have any associated pain— "silent MI")
- Anxiety
- Dyspnea
- Sense of impending doom
- Diaphoresis
- Nausea and/or vomiting
- Lightheadedness or dizziness

CONGESTIVE HEART FAILURE

Congestive heart failure (CHF) develops when the heart is still functioning but the myocardium is damaged and can no longer pump adequately to meet the

ASSESSMENT SUMMARY

CARDIAC COMPROMISE

The following are findings that may be associated with cardiac compromise.

SCENE SIZE-UP

Look for evidence of:
   Home or portable oxygen tanks or concentrators indicating chronic respiratory problems

INITIAL ASSESSMENT

General Impression

Position of patient:
   Tripod (may indicate pulmonary edema)
Patient may have look of impending doom.
Patient may be clutching chest.

Mental Status

Alert to unresponsive
Restlessness
Agitation and irritability
Anxiety

Airway

Possibly occluded in patient with altered mental status

Breathing

Signs of inadequacy or difficulty in breathing
Abnormal sounds may be heard on auscultation (indicating heart failure)

Circulation

Tachycardia or bradycardia
Irregular
Weak peripheral pulses
Cyanosis to mucous membranes, around nose and mouth, nailbeds, chest, neck

Status: Priority Patient

FOCUSED HISTORY AND PHYSICAL EXAM

SAMPLE History

Signs and symptoms:
   Pain or pressure sensation in middle of chest that may radiate to neck, jaw, down arms
   Difficulty in breathing
   Lightheadedness or dizziness

   Anxiety and irritability
   Nausea and vomiting
Known allergies to medication or other substances
Medications for cardiac conditions
   Prescribed nitroglycerin
Pre-existing cardiac disease
Hospitalized for cardiac condition
History of past heart attack

Physical Exam

Head, neck, and face
   Cyanosis to face, neck, and mucous membranes
   Jugular venous distention (may indicate heart failure or cardiac tamponade)
   Nasal flaring
   Pupils sluggish to respond to light
Chest
   Inspect for scars indicating previous cardiac surgery
   Retractions
Abdomen
   Use of abdominal muscles when breathing
Extremities
   Cyanosis to fingers and nailbeds
   Pale skin
   Diaphoresis
   Peripheral Edema
Other Signs and Symptoms
   Nausea and vomiting
   Lightheadedness or dizziness
   Sense of impending doom

Baseline Vital Signs

BP: normal, high, or low
HR: normal, tachycardia, bradycardia, irregular
RR: increased
Skin: pale, diaphoresis, maybe cyanosis
Pupils: dilated, sluggish to respond to light

Figure 15-10a   Assessment summary: cardiac compromise.

EMERGENCY CARE PROTOCOL

CARDIAC COMPROMISE

1. Establish and maintain an open airway.
2. Suction secretions as necessary.
3. If breathing is inadequate, provide positive pressure ventilation with supplemental oxygen at a minimum rate of 12 ventilations/minute for an adult and 20 ventilations/minute for an infant or child.
4. If the breathing is adequate, apply a nonrebreather mask at 15 lpm.
5. Place patient in position of comfort.
6. If patient has signs and symptoms typical of cardiac-type chest pain and has prescribed nitroglycerin:
   - Nitroglycerin is a vasodilator and will reduce workload of the heart, dilate coronary arteries, and supply more oxygen to the heart.
   Note: DO NOT ADMINISTER NITRO-GLYCERIN IF:
   Systolic BP is less than 100 mmHg
   Patient has a suspected head injury

Patient has already taken 3 doses
Patient has recently taken Viagra (consult medical direction)
   - Obtain an order from medical direction.
   - Be sure the prescription is the patient's.
   - Wear gloves when touching nitroglycerin.
   - Remove nonrebreather mask from patient.
   - Have patient lift tongue.
   - Place nitroglycerin tablet or spray under tongue.
   - Instruct patient not to swallow.
   - Replace nonrebreather mask on patient.
   - Record time and reassess patient.
   - Side effects:
      Headache
      Decrease in blood pressure
      Changes in heart rate
7. Consider advanced life support.
8. Transport in a position of comfort.
9. Perform an ongoing assessment every 5 minutes.

Figure 15-10b Emergency care protocol: cardiac compromise.

body's demands. Usually the most significant changes that occur are an increase in heart rate (to maintain perfusion) and the enlargement of the left ventricle that results from the increased effort to pump blood.

One result of CHF is a build-up of fluid in the lungs. Because the heart cannot effectively keep up with the body's needs, there are pressure changes in the pulmonary capillaries, and fluid (mostly water) passes from the capillaries into the alveoli of the lungs. This build-up of fluid in the lungs is called pulmonary edema. There may also be a buildup of fluid throughout other parts of the body, including the neck veins and lower legs.

Signs and symptoms of CHF (Figure 15-13) may be related to an acute (sudden) event or a chronic (long-term) episode and include the following:

- Marked or severe dyspnea (patient may only be able to speak in short, one- or two-word sentences)
- Great anxiety
- Desire to sit upright
- Chest pain may or may not be present
- Distended neck veins (due to fluid backup)
- Edema, or swelling, in ankles
- Rapid, shallow respirations
- Rapid pulse
- Wheezing, crackles (rales), or fluid sounds during breathing

EMERGENCY MEDICAL CARE

The emergency treatment of patients with angina, AMI, and CHF is similar, as was detailed earlier in this chapter. It includes administering oxygen at 15 lpm via a nonrebreather mask, reassuring the patient to lessen his anxiety, assisting the patient with prescribed nitroglycerin (if authorized by medical direction), consideration of ALS backup, and early transport.

EMERGENCY CARE ALGORITHM: CARDIAC COMPROMISE

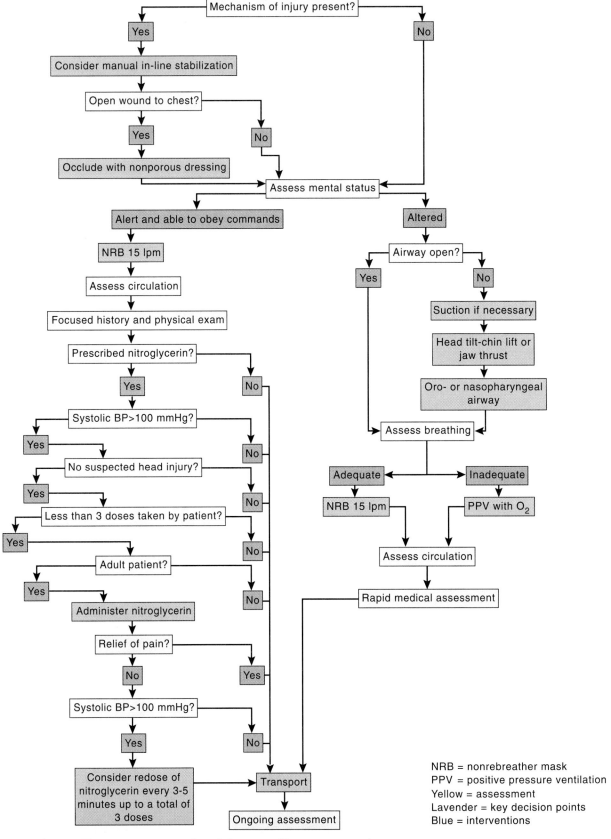

Figure 15-11   Emergency care algorithm: cardiac compromise.

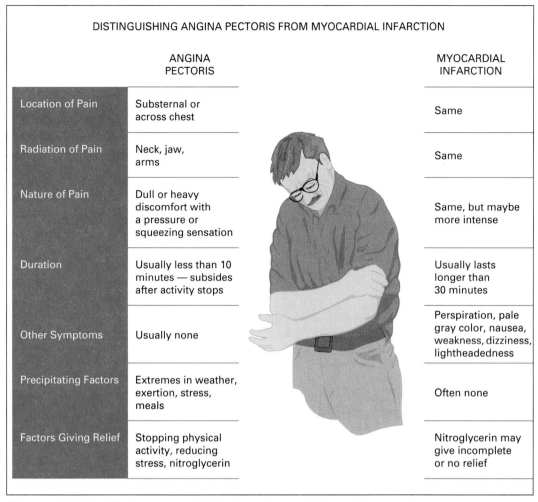

DISTINGUISHING ANGINA PECTORIS FROM MYOCARDIAL INFARCTION		
	ANGINA PECTORIS	MYOCARDIAL INFARCTION
Location of Pain	Substernal or across chest	Same
Radiation of Pain	Neck, jaw, arms	Same
Nature of Pain	Dull or heavy discomfort with a pressure or squeezing sensation	Same, but maybe more intense
Duration	Usually less than 10 minutes — subsides after activity stops	Usually lasts longer than 30 minutes
Other Symptoms	Usually none	Perspiration, pale gray color, nausea, weakness, dizziness, lightheadedness
Precipitating Factors	Extremes in weather, exertion, stress, meals	Often none
Factors Giving Relief	Stopping physical activity, reducing stress, nitroglycerin	Nitroglycerin may give incomplete or no relief

Figure 15-12   Both myocardial infarction and less serious angina can present symptoms of severe chest pain. Treat all cases of chest pain as cardiac emergencies.

SIGNS AND SYMPTOMS OF
CONGESTIVE HEART FAILURE

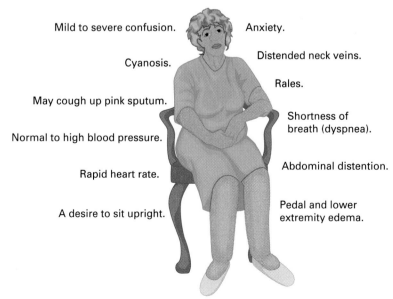

Mild to severe confusion.
Anxiety.
Cyanosis.
Distended neck veins.
Rales.
May cough up pink sputum.
Shortness of breath (dyspnea).
Normal to high blood pressure.
Abdominal distention.
Rapid heart rate.
Pedal and lower extremity edema.
A desire to sit upright.

Figure 15-13   Signs and symptoms of congestive heart failure.

CASE STUDY FOLLOW-UP

SCENE SIZE-UP

You have been dispatched to a 49-year-old male patient complaining of chest pain while eating dinner at a local restaurant. You don your gloves and grab the "jump" kit and oxygen as you leave the vehicle. You approach the patient and notice a moderately crowded dining room with several people around one particular table. There do not appear to be any hazards to your safety. You determine that there only is one patient. Upon arrival at the table you introduce your partner and yourself to the patient, who gives his name as Paul Antak.

INITIAL ASSESSMENT

After introducing yourself, you note that the patient is clutching his chest and ask, "What seems to be the problem, Mr. Antak?" The patient states, "I feel like someone is standing on my chest." The patient is responsive, alert, and oriented. His airway is open and his breathing is rapid but adequate. Your partner initiates oxygen at 15 liters per minute via a nonrebreather mask. The patient's pulse is palpable. His skin is pale, cool, and slightly moist. There are no obvious signs of any injuries or other problems. You direct your partner to get the stretcher while you continue with the focused history and physical exam.

FOCUSED HISTORY AND PHYSICAL EXAM

You begin the focused history using the OPQRST format to assess Mr. Antak's chest pain. Mr. Antak describes his pain as sudden in onset about 20 minutes ago. Nothing has made it better or worse. At first, he thought it was indigestion, but it did not go away. He describes it as a dull, squeezing pain that radiates to his left arm. He rates this as an 8 on a 1-to-10 scale of pain.

You obtain the rest of the SAMPLE history. His signs and symptoms are chest pain with some radiation to the left arm; irregular pulse; and sweaty and pale skin. He has no known allergies. He does take medication for high blood pressure, and his physician gave him nitroglycerin to take in case of severe chest pain. Mr. Antak states that, although he has the ni-

troglycerin with him, he has not taken any yet. There is no past medical history other than the high blood pressure. He was in the middle of his meal. There were no similar events prior to this incident.

You visually check the patient from head to toe and find no other obvious problems. You assess his baseline vital signs: radial pulse—irregular rate of 98; blood pressure—180/110 mmHg; breathing—28 per minute with no noisy breath sounds; skin—pinker after oxygen administration but still cool and moist.

You contact your base hospital for medical direction's approval to assist in administration of nitroglycerin. This is granted by Dr. Settler. You ask Mr. Antak for his medication container and note that it contains sublingual nitroglycerin, prescribed for him, with an expiration date of one year from today's date. Mr. Antak says he has never taken nitroglycerin before, so you explain that he may get a headache or become lightheaded from the medication. You explain that he will need to keep this tablet under his tongue and not swallow until it has dissolved completely. You ask the patient to lift his tongue and when he does, you place one tablet under the tongue.

Your partner has arrived with the stretcher as you are reassessing the blood pressure. It is now 180/100 mmHg. You place the patient on the stretcher and move him to the ambulance.

ONGOING ASSESSMENT

While en route to the hospital, you ask, "Has the pain decreased at all, Mr. Antak?" He replies that the pain has subsided and rates it at 3 on the pain scale. His skin is less sweaty and warmer. During transport you reassess vital signs, which remain stable. You check the placement of the oxygen mask and the flow of the oxygen. You radio the hospital with an update on your patient's condition and your estimated time of arrival.

Upon arrival at the hospital you give an oral report to the triage nurse and document your assessments and care. Your partner gathers the necessary supplies to ready the ambulance for the next call.

CHAPTER REVIEW

TERMS AND CONCEPTS

You may wish to review the following terms and concepts included in this chapter.

aorta—major artery that starts at the left ventricle and carries oxygen-rich blood to the body.

arteriole—smallest artery, leading to a capillary.

artery—blood vessel that carries blood away from the heart.

atrium—one of the two upper chambers of the heart.

blood pressure—the pressure exerted during circulation of the blood against the arterial walls. See also *diastolic pressure; systolic pressure.*

brachial artery—major artery of the upper arm.

capillary—tiny blood vessel connecting arterioles to venules, site of gas and nutrient exchange.

cardiac conduction system—the specialized contractile and conductive tissue of the heart that generates electrical impulses and causes the heart to beat.

cardiovascular system—system composed of the heart and blood vessels that brings oxygen and nutrients to and takes wastes away from body cells.

carotid artery—major artery in the neck.

coronary arteries—network of arteries supplying the heart with blood.

diastolic pressure—pressure exerted against the arterial walls during relaxation of the left ventricle of the heart.

dorsalis pedis artery—artery of the foot, palpable at the top of the foot on the great toe side.

femoral artery—major artery of the thigh.

heart—the four-chambered muscular organ that receives and propels blood throughout the body.

hypoperfusion—depressed delivery of oxygen and nutrients to the cells resulting from inadequate circulation of blood through the capillaries. See also *perfusion.*

nitroglycerin—medication often prescribed for patients with a history of heart problems for the relief of chest pain.

perfusion—the delivery of oxygen and nutrients to the body cells and removal of wastes by blood flowing through the capillaries.

plasma—the serum, or fluid, component of the blood.

platelet—component of the blood essential to the formation of blood clots.

posterior tibial artery—artery of the calf, palpable behind the medial ankle bone.

pulmonary artery—vessel carrying oxygen-depleted blood from the heart's right ventricle to the lungs.

pulmonary vein—vessel carrying oxygen-rich blood from the lungs to the left atrium of the heart.

radial artery—major artery of the forearm.

red blood cell—component of the blood that carries oxygen to the body's cells and carries carbon dioxide away from the body's cells.

shock—see *hypoperfusion.*

sternum—breast bone, located in the center of the chest.

systolic pressure—the pressure exerted against the arterial wall during contraction of the left ventricle of the heart.

valves—membranes located within the heart to prevent the backflow of blood in the system.

vein—vessel that carries blood toward the heart.

venae cavae—the two major veins that carries oxygen-depleted blood back to the heart: **superior vena cava** from the upper body, **inferior vena cava** from the lower body.

ventricle—one of the two lower chambers of the heart.

venule—smallest vein, leading from a capillary.

white blood cell—component of the blood that provides part of the body's immune system.

REVIEW QUESTIONS

1. Define the cardiovascular system.
2. Explain the exchange that takes place between the capillaries and the body's cells.
3. Define perfusion and shock (hypoperfusion).
4. Define blood pressure.
5. Name the procedures an EMT-B should follow in dealing with an adult patient with no pulse.
6. Name the common signs and symptoms of cardiac compromise.
7. Describe the standard emergency medical treatment for patients with signs and symptoms of cardiac compromise.
8. State how many doses of prescribed nitroglycerin an EMT-B may administer to a cardiac patient.
9. Explain under what conditions the administration of nitroglycerin is indicated.
10. Explain under what conditions administration of nitroglycerin is contraindicated.

CHAPTER 16

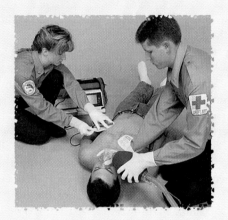

Automated External Defibrillation

INTRODUCTION

In Chapter 15, you learned how to assess and provide emergency care to patients suffering from chest pain related to various cardiac problems. Chapter 16 deals with the most serious cardiac problem of all—cardiac arrest, the complete cessation of heartbeat. Not every cardiac arrest is preceded by chest pain, nor do all patients with chest pain proceed to cardiac arrest, but for those who do, rapid intervention is vital. Without it, such patients will almost surely die. In cases of cardiac arrest, the actions of properly trained and equipped EMT-Basics can make the difference between life and death.

OBJECTIVES

Numbered objectives are from the United States Department of Transportation 1994 EMT-Basic National Standard Curriculum. Asterisked objectives, if any, pertain to material that is supplemental to the DOT curriculum.

COGNITIVE

4-3.3 List the indications for automated external defibrillation (AED). (p. 319)

4-3.4 List the contraindications for automated external defibrillation. (p. 319)

4-3.6 Explain the impact of age and weight on defibrillation. (p. 319)

4-3.10 Discuss the fundamentals of early defibrillation. (pp. 315–316)

4-3.11 Explain the rationale for early defibrillation. (pp. 315–316)

4-3.12 Explain that not all chest pain patients result in cardiac arrest and do not need to be attached to an automated external defibrillator. (pp. 312, 319)

4-3.13 Explain the importance of prehospital ACLS intervention if it is available. (p. 316)

4-3.14 Explain the importance of urgent transport to a facility with Advanced Cardiac Life Support if it is not available in the prehospital setting. (p. 325)

4-3.15 Discuss the various types of automated external defibrillators. (p. 317)

4-3.16 Differentiate between the fully automated and the semi-automated defibrillator. (p. 317)

4-3.17 Discuss the procedures that must be taken into consideration for standard operations of the various types of automated external defibrillators. (pp. 320–324)

4-3.18 State the reasons for assuring that the patient is pulseless and apneic when using the automated external defibrillator. (p. 320)

4-3.19 Discuss the circumstances which may result in inappropriate shocks. (p. 319)

4-3.20 Explain the considerations for interruption of CPR, when using the automated external defibrillator. (pp. 321, 323)

4-3.21 Discuss the advantages and disadvantages of automated external defibrillators. (pp. 316–317)

4-3.22 Summarize the speed of operation of automated external defibrillation. (p. 316)

4-3.23 Discuss the use of remote defibrillation through adhesive pads. (p. 316)

4-3.24 Discuss the special considerations for rhythm monitoring. (pp. 318–319)

4-3.25 List the steps in the operation of the automated external defibrillator. (pp. 320–324)

4-3.26 Discuss the standard of care that should be used to provide care to a patient with persistent ventricular fibrillation and no available ACLS. (pp. 324–325)

4-3.27 Discuss the standard of care that should be used to provide care to a patient with recurrent ventricular fibrillation and no available ACLS. (p. 324)

4-3.28 Differentiate between the single rescuer and multi-rescuer care with an automated external defibrillator. (p. 324)

4-3.29 Explain the reasons for pulses not being checked between shocks with an automated external defibrillator. (pp. 317, 321)

4-3.30 Discuss the importance of coordinating ACLS trained providers with personnel using automated external defibrillators. (pp. 316, 325, 329)

4-3.31 Discuss the importance of post resuscitation care. (pp. 321, 323, 324)

4-3.32 List components of post-resuscitation care. (pp. 321, 323, 324)

4-3.33 Explain the importance of frequent practice with the automated external defibrillator. (p. 326)

4-3.34 Discuss the need to complete the Automated Defibrillator: Operator's Shift Checklist. (p. 325)

4-3.35 Discuss the role of the American Heart Association in the use of automated external defibrillation. (pp. 314–316)

4-3.36 Explain the role medical direction plays in the use of automated external defibrillation. (pp. 326, 329)

4-3.37 State the reasons why a case review should be completed following the use of the automated external defibrillator. (p. 329)

4-3.38 Discuss the components that should be included in a case review. (p. 329)

4-3.39 Discuss the goal of quality improvement in automated external defibrillation. (pp. 326, 329)

4-4.43 Define the function of all controls on an automated external defibrillator, and describe event documentation and battery defibrillator maintenance. (pp. 320–324, 325)

AFFECTIVE

4-3.44 Defend the reasons for obtaining initial training in automated external defibrillation and the importance of continuing education. (pp. 315–316, 326)

4-3.45 Defend the reason for maintenance of automated external defibrillators. (p. 325)

PSYCHOMOTOR

4-3.48 Demonstrate the application and operation of the automated external defibrillator.

4-3.49 Demonstrate the maintenance of an automated external defibrillator.

4-3.50 Demonstrate the assessment and documentation of patient response to the automated external defibrillator.

4-3.51 Demonstrate the skills necessary to complete the Automated Defibrillator: Operator's Shift Checklist.

Additional objectives from DOT Lesson 4-3 are addressed in Chapter 15, "Cardiac Emergencies."

CASE STUDY

THE DISPATCH

EMS Unit 17—respond to a report of a male in his 50s with difficulty breathing at 115 Clearwater Drive. Time out is 0930 hours.

You acknowledge the call and tell dispatch that your ETA is 3 minutes. While you are en route, dispatch contacts you and advises that a bystander has called back to report that CPR is in progress at the scene. No other information was provided. Dispatch informs you that she is contacting an Advanced Life Support (ALS) unit. She is also requesting fire and police as first responders.

ON ARRIVAL

You reach 115 Clearwater at 0933 hours. A police car and Fire Engine 37 arrive moments later. As you pull up, you observe a small crowd gathered around a man lying on the ground. Kneeling beside him are a woman doing chest compressions and a man doing ventilations. The scene appears safe and no hazards are noticed. You and your partner, Claire Menzies, have put on gloves and other appropriate body substance isolation gear en route. Claire takes the jump kit and oxygen while you grab the automated external defibrillator (AED) and airway kit and start toward the patient.

As you approach the patient, one of the bystanders dashes over and tells you that the patient had been walking along the street and simply collapsed. The couple who reached him first found that he was pulseless and not breathing, so they started CPR. No one at the scene knows the patient.

How would you proceed to assess and care for this patient?

This chapter will describe the assessment and emergency medical care of a patient suffering from cardiac arrest. Later, we will return to the case and apply the procedures learned.

CARDIAC ARREST

To understand the information in this chapter, you should recall some of the information about the anatomy and physiology of the heart from Chapter 15, "Cardiac Emergencies." There you learned that the heart is a muscular organ containing specialized contractile and conductive tissues that allow it to generate electrical impulses. These impulses allow the heart to contract or "beat," pumping oxygenated blood to all parts of the body (Figure 16-1).

Cardiac arrest occurs when the heart, for any of a variety of reasons, is not pumping effectively or at all, and no pulses can be felt. The normal electrical impulses are usually absent or disrupted or the mechani-

cal response to the impulse does not occur. Instead of smooth contractions, the heart shows a different type of activity, most commonly the uncoordinated twitchings known as ventricular fibrillation. Pumping action ceases and the body's cells, without oxygenated blood, begin to die. Brain cells begin to die within 4 to 6 minutes following cardiac arrest. The patient presents as unresponsive and without pulse or respiration.

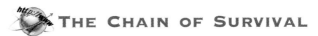 THE CHAIN OF SURVIVAL

Successfully resuscitating a cardiac arrest patient in the prehospital setting can rarely be done solely with CPR. Success, instead, depends on a sequence of events that the American Heart Association has

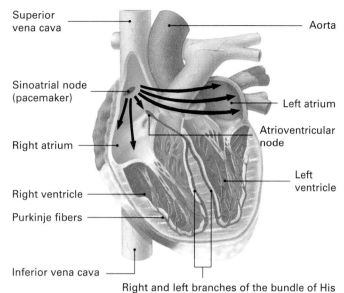

Figure 16-1   The conduction system of the heart.

termed the **chain of survival**. This chain has four links (Figure 16-2). They are as follows:

- *Early access*—Time is a critical factor for successful defibrillation and resuscitation. The quicker someone can recognize a patient in cardiac compromise or cardiac arrest and contact EMS the better the chance of patient survival. Thus, early access is influenced by two factors: 1) early recognition of a cardiac event, and 2) easy access to the EMS system. Early recognition can be achieved through public education programs, such as CPR courses for the lay person. Easy access is achieved by providing a simple access number, such as 911, to the community. In areas not serviced by 911, people must identify and dial a seven-digit number to access EMS, which usually leads to significant time delays. The extra moments it takes to find and dial the number may make the difference between successful resuscitation or not.
- *Early CPR*—Cardiopulmonary resuscitation (CPR) has been shown to significantly increase survival of out-of-hospital cardiac arrest. Thus it is important

to get trained CPR providers to the scene as quickly as possible, ideally within 2 minutes after the cardiac arrest. This can be achieved through faster response by EMS and first responders, a greater number of lay CPR providers, and by EMS communications personnel providing CPR instructions to a person at the scene of the cardiac arrest. Community-oriented CPR courses should be conducted to train as many people as possible. Recognition of a cardiac event and the proper access number should be emphasized as heavily as the actual skill of performing CPR.

- *Early defibrillation*—Defibrillation—but more important, early defibrillation—is the most critical factor in determining survival of cardiac arrest. **Defibrillation**, the procedure of sending an electrical current through the chest, is necessary to convert a heart that is in an abnormal and lethal rhythm with no pulse to a rhythm with a pulse. The time from when the patient goes into cardiac arrest to the time that the defibrillation is performed is the most essential factor in increasing the survival rates of out-of-hospital cardiac arrest patients. Most research has

Chain of Survival

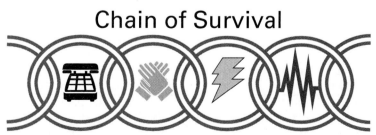

Figure 16-2   The Chain of Survival from the American Heart Association.

shown that a delay of 8 minutes until defibrillation will result in very few successful resuscitations.

Systems with response times of less than 4 minutes—or a wide network of first responders, such as fire or police personnel, who can get to the scene and defibrillate the patient within 4 minutes—have the best out-of-hospital cardiac-arrest survival rates.

- *Early advanced life support*—Advanced life support (ALS) is delivered most often by paramedics who can provide advanced cardiac life support (ACLS). In some systems, EMT-Intermediates with special training may be able to provide limited ALS.

Even though the paramedic is able to perform all of the functions of the EMT-B and also provide other advanced functions such as medication administration, endotracheal tube placement, and cardiac pacing, it is important again to recognize that time to defibrillation is the most critical factor to successful resuscitation. The role of ALS is to perform certain interventions to increase the possibility of successful defibrillation or to administer medications to keep the patient from going back into cardiac arrest.

A system that has 911 or another easily recognizable public access number, CPR performed within minutes after the arrest by first responders or laypersons, defibrillation within 4 minutes, and ALS capabilities will have better success rates for out-of-hospital cardiac arrest patients.

AUTOMATED EXTERNAL DEFIBRILLATION

If any one link in the chain of survival can be called "most important," it is early defibrillation. It is one emergency care procedure that we know works.

According to the American Heart Association (AHA), studies of communities that had initiated early defibrillation programs—even those that had no prehospital ACLS services—revealed improved survival rates of patients with cardiac arrest. These studies also verified that the earlier defibrillation took place, the better the outcome for the patient.

The AHA offers the following rationale to support the use of early defibrillation:

- The most frequent initial rhythm in sudden cardiac arrest is ventricular fibrillation.
- The most effective treatment for ventricular fibrillation is electrical defibrillation.
- The probability of successful defibrillation is directly related to the time from fibrillation to defibrillation. To be most effective, defibrillation must be administered within 4 minutes of the onset of cardiac arrest, and ALS within 8 minutes of the onset.

- Ventricular fibrillation will, within only a few minutes, degenerate into **asystole** (absence of any electrical activity in the heart). Successful resuscitation from asystole is extremely unlikely.

TYPES OF DEFIBRILLATORS

A *defibrillator* is a device that will deliver an electric shock to convert a fibrillating heart to an organized rhythm with a pulse. External defibrillators are used in emergency care—called "external" because they are applied to the outside of the chest.

There are two basic categories of external defibrillators: manual and automated. The use of manual defibrillators requires extensive training. The operator uses the machine's monitor to determine the heart's rhythm as displayed on a screen. The operator must analyze the rhythm and decide whether it is appropriate to defibrillate. He must apply the defibrillator pad or gel, hold the paddles firmly against the patient's chest, and administer the shock. **Automated external defibrillators (AEDs)** are much simpler to operate. This has made possible a much broader use of defibrillation.

With AEDs, external adhesive defibrillator pads are attached to the patient's chest. Those pads are connected by cables to the AED. The pads transmit the patient's cardiac rhythm to the AED's circuitry, where the rhythm is analyzed. If the AED determines that an electrical shock (defibrillation) is appropriate, the device delivers the shock through the cables via the pads to the patient.

ADVANTAGES OF AEDs

With the AED, the device analyzes the rhythm and indicates if a shock is required. The AED operator need only determine pulselessness and understand the steps in operating the device. Therefore, initial training and continuing education are both much simpler with AEDs than with manual defibrillators. In fact, claims have been made that it is easier to learn how to operate an AED than it is to learn proper CPR techniques.

The are several other advantages of the AED:

- *Speed of operation*—The first shock can be delivered to the patient within 1 minute of the AED's arrival at the patient's side. Clinical trials conducted by the AHA found that operators of AEDs can consistently deliver a first shock more quickly than operators of manual defibrillators.
- *Safer, more effective delivery*—Because it uses adhesive external pads, instead of the paddles that must be held against the chest during manual defibrillation, the AED allows for "hands-free" defibrillation, which is safer for EMS personnel. In addition, the adhesive pads cover a larger surface area than

the manual paddles and, therefore, deliver a more effective shock.

- *More efficient monitoring*—AEDs are manufactured with sensors that detect loose leads and false or misleading rhythm readings. The large electrodes make better contact with the patient's body and provide a better ECG tracing, even when the patient is severely diaphoretic (sweaty).

TYPES OF AEDS

In general there are two types of AEDs, fully automated and semi-automated:

- *Fully automated AEDs*—The fully automated AED (Figure 16-3a) is completely automatic. The operator attaches the device to a patient in cardiac arrest, pushes a button to turn on the power, and the device does the rest. The fully automated AED analyzes the heart rhythm and determines whether ventricular fibrillation is present. If ventricular fibrillation is detected, the AED charges up automatically and delivers the appropriate electrical shock.
- *Semi-automated AEDs*—The semi-automated AED (Figure 16-3b) requires more involvement by the operator. The operator attaches the AED to the patient in the normal manner, pushes a button to turn on the power, and initiates the heart rhythm analysis by pushing an analysis button. The AED then begins the analysis. When the analysis is complete, a computer voice synthesizer and/or display message indicates to the operator when a shock is advised. The operator must then push another button to deliver the shock. Some devices will also provide a display of the heart rhythm as it is being analyzed.

Both fully automated and semi-automated AEDs are often equipped with a variety of features that can provide a record of both the operator's use of the AED and the AED's own functions. Such devices include voice and ECG recorders and solid-state memory modules.

Most external defibrillators use a monophasic wave form in defibrillation. New technology has provided a version of the truncated exponential biphasic wave form that is currently available in one type of AED (Figure 16-3c). This type of wave form is still under intense investigation to determine if it is more effective than the traditional monophasic wave form.

Each type of AED has its own advantages and disadvantages. Any EMS unit wishing to use an AED will have to evaluate its own needs and decide on which type best meets those needs. The American Heart Association has stated that both types of AED are equally safe and effective.

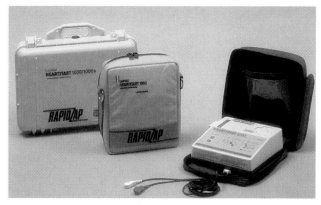

Figure 16-3a Fully automated defibrillator.

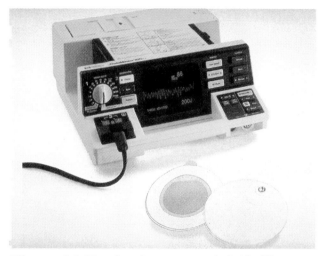

Figure 16-3b Semi-automated defibrillator. (Laerdal Medical Corporation)

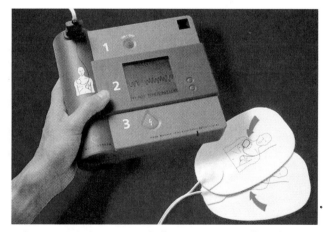

Figure 16-3c Laerdal Forerunner (bi-phasic defibrillator). (Laerdal Medical Corporation)

Whichever type of AED your service has chosen, always follow the manufacturer's directions and service recommendations as well as any local protocols for AED use.

ANALYSIS OF CARDIAC RHYTHMS

The main component of the AED is the computer microprocessor that records and analyzes whether or not a heart rhythm should be defibrillated. The rhythms for which defibrillation is appropriate are these:

- *Ventricular fibrillation*—As noted earlier, **ventricular fibrillation (VF or V-Fib)** is a disorganized cardiac rhythm that produces no pulse or cardiac output. (Figure 16-4a). It is commonly associated with advanced coronary artery disease, though it may have other causes. Somewhere between 50 to 60 percent of cardiac arrests will be in ventricular fibrillation during the first 8 minutes after becoming pulseless. V-Fib is most commonly the rhythm that AED defibrillates.

- *Ventricular Tachycardia*—**Ventricular Tachycardia (V-Tach)** is a very fast heart rhythm (Figure 16-4b) that is generated in the ventricle instead of

HEART RHYTHMS

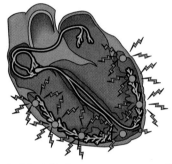

Chaotic electrical discharge as seen on an ECG tracing.

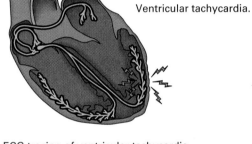

Ventricular tachycardia.

ECG tracing of ventricular tachycardia.

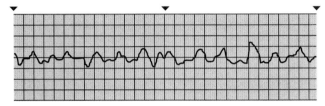

Figure 16-4a Ventricular fibrillation is associated with chaotic electrical discharge in the ventricles.

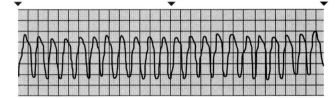

Figure 16-4b Ventricular tachycardia originates in the conduction system of the ventricle.

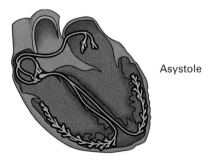

Asystole

ECG tracing of asystole

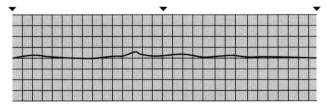

Figure 16-4c Asystole, or "flatline," is the complete absence of electrical activity in the heart.

the sinoatrial node in the atrium. Because the pumping is so rapid, the heart does not refill properly and cardiac output is sharply reduced. This rhythm can easily degenerate into ventricular fibrillation. The AED will respond to V-Tach, usually when the heart rate exceeds 180 beats a minute. However, you should be aware that some V-Tach patients remain responsive; since they are not pulseless, they are not appropriate candidates for defibrillation. The AED should ONLY be applied to patients who are *pulseless,* not breathing (apneic), and unresponsive.

The AED will detect rhythms for which no shock is indicated. They include the following:

- *Asystole*—**Asystole** is the absence of electrical activity and pumping action in the heart. This often registers on a monitoring screen as a flat or nearly flat line; hence the term "flatline" is often used for asystole (Figure 16-4c). There is no cardiac output or pulse. Chances of recovery from asystole are not good. Defibrillation is not appropriate in asystole.
- *Pulseless Electrical Activity*—In cases of **pulseless electrical activity (PEA),** the heart has a rhythm, but either the heart muscle is so weakened that it fails to pump, or the heart muscle does not respond to the electrical activity, or the circulatory system has lost so much blood that there is nothing to pump. Defibrillation is not appropriate in these rhythms.

Note that the AED is a very sensitive instrument. It can sense spontaneous patient movement, movement of the patient by others, engine vibrations if the patient is in a vehicle, and even some radio transmissions. Such "noise" interferes with the AED's analysis of the patient's heart rhythms.

For these reasons, no one should be touching the patient when the AED is analyzing the rhythm. (Nor should anyone be touching the patient during administration of AED shocks.) Always alert people to move away from the patient by saying "Clear!" in a loud voice before beginning the analysis. Also, if the patient is in the ambulance when you are using the AED, be sure that the ambulance is stopped and the motor turned off before proceeding with the analysis.

A properly maintained and operated AED will rarely deliver inappropriate shocks, but mechanical or human error can lead to them. Mechanical error is usually caused by poorly maintained or poorly charged batteries. Human error occurs when an operator misinterprets a patient's condition and uses the AED on someone not in cardiac arrest. Remember, the AED should be used ONLY on pulseless, non-breathing, unresponsive patients.

WHEN AND WHEN NOT TO USE THE AED

The AED is intended for use with adult patients in nontraumatic cardiac arrest. "Adult" in these cases means someone over 8 years of age. These patients must be unresponsive, with no breathing and no pulse. The AED is not intended for trauma patients. If such patients are in cardiac arrest, the condition very often is the result of blood loss. Defibrillation usually will not help these patients. Follow local protocols. Contact medical direction if in doubt. (See notes on p. 332 regarding cardiac arrest in children and from trauma.)

At times, you may come across situations where you cannot tell if the trauma led to cardiac arrest or vice versa. Say, for example, that you discover a man in cardiac arrest in a car that has gone off the road and hit a tree. Did the man go into cardiac arrest while driving, then swerve off and hit the tree? Or did he drive off the road for some other reason and go into cardiac arrest only after hitting the tree and sustaining other injuries? In such cases, consult medical direction and follow local protocols before deciding whether use of the AED is appropriate.

The AED is not intended for children. Children are defined here as patients under 8 years of age. Cardiac arrest in children is most often the result of hypoxia from airway or respiratory compromise. Airway management and positive pressure ventilation are emphasized more for such patients than defibrillation.

RECOGNIZING AND TREATING CARDIAC ARREST

Now that you have reviewed abnormal rhythms, basic information about defibrillation, and the AED, you can learn the procedure for defibrillation.

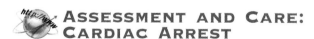 ### ASSESSMENT AND CARE: CARDIAC ARREST

Dispatch may provide information that will lead you to suspect cardiac arrest. Reports that a patient has no pulse or that first responders are performing CPR clearly indicate cardiac arrest. But also be alert to the possibility of cardiac arrest in calls to patients complaining of chest pain, difficulty in breathing, seizures, or unresponsiveness. Although not all chest pain patients will go into cardiac arrest and need the AED, remember that patients with cardiac compromise *can* rapidly deteriorate to cardiac arrest. Some patients will suffer a brief seizure immediately after going into cardiac arrest. Bring the AED from the ambulance to the patient on such calls.

SCENE SIZE-UP AND INITIAL ASSESSMENT

On arrival, take appropriate body substance isolation precautions. Ensure that the scene is secure. Then proceed rapidly with the initial assessment.

Form a general impression of the patient and his mental status as you approach. If the suspected cardiac patient is responsive, follow the procedures for assessment and care described in Chapter 15, "Cardiac Emergencies."

With unresponsive patients, open the airway and assess breathing and pulse. Those with no breathing and no pulse are in cardiac arrest. One member of the team should provide CPR while the other prepares to deliver emergency care. If first responders or bystanders are administering CPR properly when you arrive, have them stop briefly so you can do your assessment. Once you have determined that a patient is pulseless and not breathing, have them proceed with CPR while you prepare to deliver emergency care as described on the following pages.

For children younger than age 8, begin or resume CPR and transport as rapidly as possible. Contact medical direction for further orders.

For adult patients showing the signs of cardiac arrest, bystanders, first responders, or a member of the EMT-B team should begin or resume CPR. Contact dispatch and request ACLS support, if this has not already been done.

FOCUSED HISTORY AND PHYSICAL EXAM

While CPR is being done and the AED is being set up and applied, an EMT-B may be able to gather the history from bystanders or relatives. Remember, however, defibrillation should never be delayed.

Signs and Symptoms The signs and symptoms of cardiac arrest are as follows:

- No breathing (apnea)
- No pulse
- Unresponsiveness to verbal or painful stimuli

Patients who exhibit *all three* signs and symptoms should have the AED applied. (Applying a shock to a heart that is beating will cause a dangerous disruption of the heart's conduction system.) The only exceptions would be cases where trauma is suspected as the cause of cardiac arrest; in such cases, follow local protocol and consult with medical direction.

EMERGENCY MEDICAL CARE

Follow the steps listed under Performing Defibrillation to provide emergency medical care with an AED to adult victims of cardiac arrest. Remember that in caring for such patients, defibrillation should always come first. No other activities, including inserting airway devices, setting up oxygen delivery systems, or obtaining a patient history should take precedence over or delay AED application and defibrillation.

ONGOING ASSESSMENT

Defibrillation and, as needed, CPR will be performed to restore the patient's pulse (heartbeat). Once the pulse is restored, you will continue to perform an ongoing assessment en route to the hospital. As will be discussed in the following segment, a patient whose pulse has been restored may revert into cardiac arrest, so the ongoing assessment will be focused especially on monitoring the patient's pulse, breathing, and mental status.

PERFORMING DEFIBRILLATION

Ideally, at least two EMT-Bs should be available when AED operation is to be undertaken, one to operate the device and the other to perform CPR (Figure 16-5).

USING A SEMI-AUTOMATED AED

The steps below are for providing defibrillation with a semi-automated AED. A brief description of the procedure using a fully automated AED is given later in the chapter.

Note that the typical semi-automated AED has three buttons: button number 1 turns on the power,

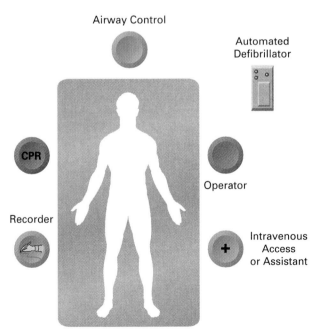

Figure 16-5 This is the preferred layout for automated defibrillation. It may not be possible in all field situations, so alternative arrangements should be tried and practiced.

button number 2 starts analysis of the patient's heart rhythms, and button number 3 delivers a shock. Visualize these three buttons as you read the following steps.

Also bear in mind, as you read the following steps, that the usual maximum total number of shocks you should deliver to the patient is six. Medical direction may approve additional shocks.

1. *Take body substance isolation precautions.* This should normally be done while en route to the scene.

2. *Perform an initial assessment of the patient* (Figure 16-6a). If bystanders or first responders have already begun CPR, instruct them to stop while you perform an assessment of the airway, breathing, and circulation.
   A. If the patient is an unresponsive adult with no breathing and no pulse, proceed with AED as below.
   B. If the patient is less than 8 years of age or is a victim of trauma, do not perform AED unless directed by local protocol and medical direction. Instead, perform CPR and transport rapidly.

3. *Begin or resume CPR while the AED is readied for operation* (Figure 16-6b). If possible, perform AED operations from the patient's left side, setting up the device by the patient's head.

4. *Attach the adhesive monitoring-defibrillation pads to the cables.*

5. *Apply the two defibrillation pads to the patient's bared chest* (Figures 16-6c and 16-7).
   A. The *sternum* pad (−) is placed on the right upper border of the sternum; the top edge should be just below the clavicle.
   B. The *apex* pad (+) should be placed over the left lower ribs at the anterior axillary line (below and to the left of the nipple).
      An alternative placement is as follows: the sternum pad (−) near the center of the patient's back and the apex pad (+) over the apex of the heart (Figure 16-8).

6. *Turn on power to the AED* (Figure 16-6d).

7. *If the AED is equipped with a tape recorder, begin your narrative,* giving your name and unit, the location and time, and the situation as you found it. Continue the narrative describing your actions and the patient's response as you carry out the steps below.

8. *Stop any ongoing CPR and say "Clear!" making sure that no one is touching the patient.* The AED machine cannot effectively analyze the heart rhythm while CPR is being performed. Also, a CPR provider in contact with the patient during delivery of a defibrillating shock could be injured. For these reasons, CPR may be interrupted for up to 90 seconds each time the AED delivers a series of three shocks.

9. *Begin analysis of the patient's heart rhythms* (Figure 16-6e). The AED will then automatically monitor and analyze the rhythm.
   A. *If the AED's analysis indicates a shock,* it provides a "Deliver Shock" message. In that case, proceed with Steps 10 to 12.
   B. *If the AED's analysis determines a non-shockable rhythm,* it gives a "No Shock" message. In that case, proceed to Step 13.

10. *If the AED indicates "Deliver Shock,"* make sure that everyone is clear of the patient by checking all personnel and stating "I'm clear, you're clear, everyone is clear." Once everyone is clear, proceed with these steps:
    A. Press the shock button to deliver the first shock (Figure 16-6f).
    B. Press the analysis button to re-analyze the patient's heart rhythm, depending on the type of device. (Some AED models do not require the operator to press a button to re-analyze the rhythm between the stacked shocks; it is done automatically. Follow the manufacturer's guidelines.)
    C. If the AED gives a "Deliver Shock" message, press the shock button to deliver a second shock.
    D. Re-analyze the rhythm.
    E. If the machine gives a "Deliver Shock" message, press the button to deliver a third shock.
       The set of three shocks you have delivered is called the "first set of three stacked shocks." The shocks are called "stacked" because they are given without any pauses to check the patient's pulse or to administer CPR.
       [Note that pulse checks should not be done during rhythm analysis. Likewise, the pulse generally will not be checked between the first and second shocks of the first set of three stacked shocks. The pulse will also not be checked between the first and second shocks of the second set—which are the fourth and fifth shocks in the full sequence of six. Performing such pulse checks can delay rhythm analysis and defibrillation.]
       If after the first or second shock in this first stack, the AED gives a "No Shock" message, proceed to Step 13 below.

11. After the first set of three stacked shocks, check the patient's pulse.
    A. *If the pulse is present,* check the breathing:
       i. If the patient is breathing adequately, deliver oxygen at 15 lpm by a nonrebreather mask and transport.

USING A SEMI-AUTOMATED AED

Ideally, at least two EMT-Bs should be present when defibrillation is to be performed with a semi-automated AED—one to operate the AED, the other to perform CPR. The AED should be placed near the patient's head, but is placed differently in these photographs to make the AED's screen and controls visible.

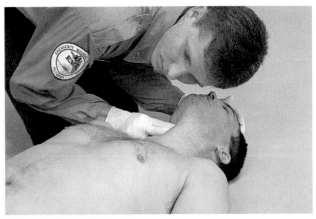

Figure 16-6a *Perform initial assessment and verify absence of pulse and breathing.*

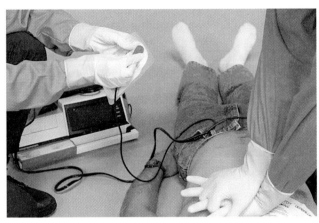

Figure 16-6b *One EMT-B should initiate CPR while the other EMT-B prepares the AED.*

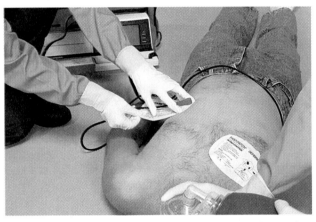

Figure 16-6c *Place the defibrillator electrodes on the patient's chest.*

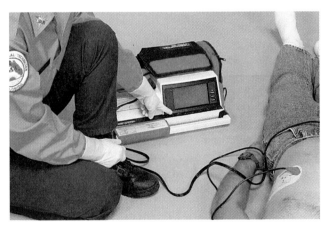

Figure 16-6d *Turn on the defibrillator and begin narrative.*

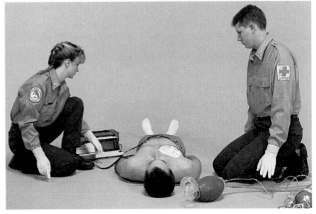

Figure 16-6e *Stop CPR and get completely clear of the patient as the AED analyzes the rhythm.*

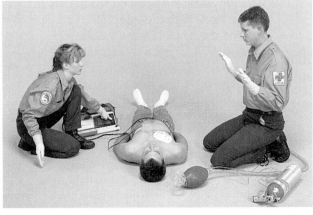

Figure 16-6f *If a shock is advised, clear all people from the patient and deliver the shock.*

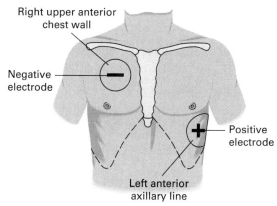

Right upper anterior
chest wall

Negative
electrode

Positive
electrode

Left anterior
axillary line

Figure 16-7   Proper placement of defib-
rillator electrodes.

ii. If the patient is not breathing adequately, provide positive pressure ventilation with supplemental oxygen and transport.

B. *If no pulse is present,* resume CPR for one minute, then re-analyze the rhythm. If indicated, provide a second set of three stacked shocks in the manner described in step 10. *If, after the first or second shock in this second stack, the AED gives a "No Shock" message, proceed to Step 13.*

You have now delivered a second set of three stacked shocks. The patient has received a total of six shocks—the maximum you can deliver without approval from medical direction.

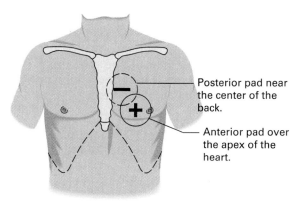

Alternate Placement
of Defibrillator Electrodes

Posterior pad near
the center of the
back.

Anterior pad over
the apex of the
heart.

Figure 16-8   An alternative placement
of defibrillator electrodes has the anterior
electrode (+) placed over the apex of the
heart and the posterior electrode (−)
placed near the center of the back, one to
two inches above the anterior pad.

12. After delivering the second set of stacked shocks, if ALS backup has not arrived, check the patient's pulse.
    A. *If the pulse is present,* check the breathing:
       i. If the patient is breathing adequately, deliver oxygen at 15 lpm by a nonrebreather mask and transport.
       ii. If the patient is not breathing adequately, provide positive pressure ventilation with supplemental oxygen and transport.
    B. *If the pulse is not present,* resume CPR and transport.

13. A "No Shock" message can mean one of three things: Either the patient you thought was pulseless has a pulse after all, the formerly pulseless patient has now regained a pulse, or the patient is pulseless but the AED is detecting a nonshockable rhythm.

    If the machine gives a "No Shock" message after any rhythm analysis, check the patient's pulse and breathing.
    A. *If the pulse is present,* check the breathing:
       i. If the patient is breathing adequately, deliver oxygen at 15 lpm by a nonrebreather mask and transport.
       ii. If the patient is not breathing adequately, provide positive pressure ventilation with supplemental oxygen and transport.
    B. *If no pulse is present,* resume CPR for one minute. Then begin another rhythm analysis.
       i. If the machine now gives a "Deliver Shock" message, deliver a shock. Remember: you may give up to a total of two sets of three stacked shocks, with the two sets separated by a pulse check and one minute of CPR.
       ii. *If the machine still gives a "No Shock" message,* resume CPR for one minute, then re-analyze the rhythm for a third time.
           a. *If the machine now gives a "Deliver Shock" message,* deliver a shock.
           b. If the machine still gives a "No Shock" message and there is no pulse, resume CPR and transport.

14. Transport after a total of two sets of stacked shocks are delivered or a total of three "No Shock" messages are received.

    Note: If V-Fib persists after six shocks, contact medical direction to request additional sets of stacked shocks with CPR between until a "No Shock" advisory is received or the patient regains a pulse.

    *Note: A patient who is in cardiac arrest and is suspected of being hypothermic (having a low body temperature) should receive only **one** set of three stacked shocks before immediate transport.*

USE OF THE AED BY A SINGLE EMT-B

There are times when only a single EMT-B is available to care for a cardiac arrest victim. If the EMT-B has immediate access to an AED, he should instead follow this sequence:

1. Perform the initial assessment.
2. Verify that the patient is unresponsive, with no breathing and no pulse.
3. Attach the AED's external monitoring/defibrillation pads.
4. Turn on the AED and begin the narration if the device is equipped with a recorder.
5. Initiate the rhythm analysis.
6. Deliver shocks as the AED indicates.
7. Leave the patient to call for help from EMS dispatch only when one of these occurs:
   – The AED gives a "No Shock" message.
   – You detect a pulse in the patient.
   – You have delivered three shocks.
   – Other help arrives.

Then, if the patient is pulseless, initiate CPR. Repeat step 5 after 1 minute of CPR.

USING A FULLY AUTOMATED AED

Procedures for using the fully automated AED are quite similar to those for using the semi-automated AED, described earlier. The major difference is that the AED itself will deliver the shock. Once the machine is connected to the patient and turned on, it also uses a voice synthesizer to give directions such as, "Stop CPR," "Stand back," and "Check breathing and pulse" to prompt you through the defibrillation process. This would include the delivery of two sets of three stacked shocks separated by a minute of CPR or checks of breathing and pulse if rhythms inappropriate for shocking are detected. Procedures for the operation of fully automated defibrillators vary, so manufacturer's instructions should be followed closely. It is important to note that, with a fully automated defibrillator, the defibrillations are delivered automatically; therefore, it is important to ensure that all EMTs and bystanders are clear of the patient.

TRANSPORTING THE CARDIAC ARREST PATIENT

If you have followed the emergency medical care procedures and operation of the AED described above and no ALS backup has appeared on the scene, you should transport the patient when any one of the following conditions applies:

- The patient regains a pulse.
- A total of two sets of stacked shocks have been delivered.

- The AED has given three consecutive "No Shock" messages (each separated by 1 minute of CPR).

The patient you transport after defibrillation will be in one of two conditions: with a pulse or without a pulse.

TRANSPORTING A PATIENT WITH A PULSE

If a patient's pulse has returned after defibrillation, do the following:

1. Check the patient's airway and provide oxygen at 15 lpm by nonrebreather mask if the patient's breathing is adequate, or provide positive pressure ventilation with supplemental oxygen if the patient's breathing is inadequate.
2. Since most cardiac arrest victims vomit, have suction ready for use and clear the airway of any obstructions or fluids.
3. Secure the patient to a stretcher and transfer him to the ambulance.
4. Consider the most efficient way of getting the patient to ACLS. Consult with dispatch and medical direction and consider rendezvousing with an ALS unit en route or awaiting arrival of the ALS unit if that will get the patient advanced care more rapidly.
5. Continue to keep the AED attached to the patient during transport. Remember to stop the emergency vehicle if you need to analyze the rhythm or deliver any shocks.
6. If you have not already done so, perform the focused history and physical exam en route.
7. Perform an ongoing assessment every 5 minutes.

Remember that patients who have been brought out of ventricular fibrillation through use of the AED have a high likelihood of slipping back into that state. Monitor these patients closely. With unresponsive patients, check the pulse every 30 seconds. Be particularly alert if a responsive patient who has been complaining of chest pain becomes unresponsive. Check for breathing and pulse. If the patient shows no pulse or breathing, then follow these steps:

1. Stop the vehicle, turning off the motor.
2. Start CPR if the AED is not immediately available.
3. When the AED is ready, stop CPR and initiate rhythm analysis.
4. Deliver as many as three shocks if indicated. Then check the pulse and resume CPR for 1 minute if there is no pulse. Deliver a second set of three shocks if indicated. If no shocks are indicated, perform CPR for 1 minute, then reanalyze until up to three "No Shock" messages have been received.
5. Continue resuscitation as per local protocol.
6. Continue transport.

Note that the "allowance" of six shocks begins again if the patient has regained a pulse, then deteriorates back into cardiac arrest. Shocks given during the previous episode of arrest are not counted in the total that may be given during any new arrest that occurs after a return of pulse. Follow local protocols.

TRANSPORTING A PATIENT WITHOUT A PULSE

If the patient has no pulse, provide CPR, contact medical direction, and follow local protocol. You will most likely transport such a patient without further defibrillation, but medical direction may instruct you to make additional attempts at defibrillation.

PROVIDING FOR ADVANCED CARDIAC LIFE SUPPORT

As an EMT-B, you can operate an AED without advanced life support (ALS) personnel on scene. With cases of cardiac arrest, however, you should keep the AHA's chain of survival in mind. The fourth link of that chain is early advanced cardiac life support (ACLS).

There are often several options for obtaining ACLS for a patient. Higher-level EMTs, such as EMT-Paramedics and some EMT-Intermediates, can provide it. If prehospital personnel are not available, other sources for ACLS might be a hospital or clinic.

Whenever you have a cardiac arrest patient, inform medical direction and request ACLS backup as soon as you can without delaying the start of defibrillation. Your system will have protocols about the transport of such patients, but medical direction, depending on the circumstances, may tell you to wait for the arrival of the ALS team, to rendezvous with them en route, or to proceed directly to a hospital or other facility. The goal is to minimize the time from the delivery of shocks to the arrival of ACLS.

SUMMARY: ASSESSMENT AND CARE

To review assessment findings that may be associated with cardiac arrest and emergency care for cardiac arrest, see Figures 16-9 and 16-10.

SPECIAL CONSIDERATIONS FOR THE AED

SAFETY CONSIDERATIONS

When you are using an AED, you are operating a device that delivers an electric shock. That shock can save the life of a cardiac arrest patient, but it can in-

jure others who come in contact with it. Such shocks are unlikely to be lethal, but they should be avoided.

Electricity can be conducted, or carried, through a variety of different substances. The human body is one of them. No one should be in contact with the patient during the AED's rhythm analysis or its delivery of defibrillating shocks. Remember to say loudly "I'm clear, you're clear, everyone's clear!" and to make sure that everyone is, in fact, clear of the patient before beginning the analysis or defibrillating.

Water is an excellent conductor of electricity. The AED should not be operated if the machine or the patient is in contact with water. It may be necessary to move a cardiac arrest victim to a dry and safe area before using the AED. You may also dry the patient (or at least his chest) before delivering a shock.

Metal is another good conductor of electricity. Be careful with patients on metal flooring, catwalks, stretchers, and other items with metal components. Ensure that no one else is directly in contact with metal that is touching the patient before you administer a shock.

If a patient has a nitroglycerin patch on his chest, remove it while wearing gloves and wipe the site with a towel or gauze pad before delivering a shock. The shock may cause the plastic in the patch to melt and ignite.

If a cardiac arrest patient has a surgically implanted pacemaker or surgically implanted defibrillator (see the Enrichment section), you can still use the AED. Just be careful not to put an AED adhesive pad directly on top of the implanted device; it is preferable to place a pad several inches from such a site.

AED MAINTENANCE

Regularly scheduled maintenance of the AED is crucial to ensuring that the machine functions properly. Follow your local protocols and manufacturer's directions when maintaining the AED.

You should be aware that AED failure is most commonly attributed to improper maintenance, especially battery failure. Operators of the AED must ensure that batteries are properly maintained and replaced on a set schedule to guarantee proper energy levels. The AED and its batteries should be checked at the beginning of each shift. Extra, fully charged batteries should always be available.

To assist in maintenance, a panel of experts has compiled a list of items in addition to batteries that must be checked regularly to ensure proper AED operation. This Operator's Shift Checklist (Figure 16-11) should be completed by EMT-Bs (or other AED operators) at the beginning of every shift. Completing the checklist will help ensure that your AED will work when you need it. Doing so will also provide documentation of your maintenance, if necessary.

ASSESSMENT SUMMARY

CARDIAC ARREST

The following are findings that indicate cardiac arrest. These findings are obtained during the initial assessment.

- Unresponsive
- Apneic (not breathing)
- Pulseless

EMERGENCY CARE PROTOCOL

CARDIAC ARREST

Note: The AED should not be used in patients under 8 years of age.

1. Take BSI precautions.
2. If no CPR in progress, assess airway, breathing, pulse. If CPR in progress, stop CPR and assess airway, breathing, pulse.
3. Second rescuer should begin or resume CPR.
4. Immediately apply the AED.
5. Start narrative of event.
6. Stop CPR and instruct to clear patient.
7. Initiate analysis of rhythm.
8. If shock advised, clear patient and deliver shock. Repeat for second and third shock only if AED advises shocks. If no shock advised, perform CPR for 1 minute.
9. Check pulse and breathing. If no pulse, continue CPR for 1 minute. Insert oropharyngeal airway, ensure oxygen is connected to ventilation device, and attempt to gather brief history from family or bystanders.
10. Reanalyze rhythm after 1 minute of CPR.
11. If shock advised, clear patient and deliver shock. Repeat for fifth and sixth shock only if AED advises shocks. If no shock advised, continue CPR for 1 minute.
12. Prepare patient for transport after two sets of three stacked shocks, after three no shock advisories, or after patient regains a pulse. Contact medical direction or follow local protocols to administer additional shocks.
13. If defibrillation is successful after a shock, assess breathing, pulse, and blood pressure. Continue positive pressure ventilation if breathing is inadequate. If breathing is adequate, apply nonrebreather mask at 15 lpm.

Figure 16-9 Assessment summary and emergency care protocol: cardiac arrest.

TRAINING AND SKILLS MAINTENANCE

In addition to ensuring that the AED functions properly when needed, EMT-Bs must also ensure that they can use the device properly when called on to do so. This can be accomplished through continuing education and skills maintenance programs. It is recommended that any AED operator refresh or practice his skills with the device every 90 days.

Operators should review incidents of AED use in the system, study any new protocols, and, most important practice working with the system's device. In addition, more information regarding updated research on AED procedures can be obtained from several sources, including EMS journals, state EMS offices, and the AHA.

MEDICAL DIRECTION AND THE AED

Medical direction must play a significant role in the provision of AED services. EMTs use AEDs under the authority of the medical director's license. Medical direction thus has a great stake in ensuring that a system's AED program functions properly. Medical direction's involvement might include the following:

- Making sure that the EMS system has all necessary links in the AHA chain of survival
- Overseeing all levels of EMTs
- Reviewing the continual competency skill review program
- Engaging in an audit and/or quality improvement program

EMERGENCY CARE ALGORITHM:
AUTOMATED EXTERNAL DEFIBRILLATION

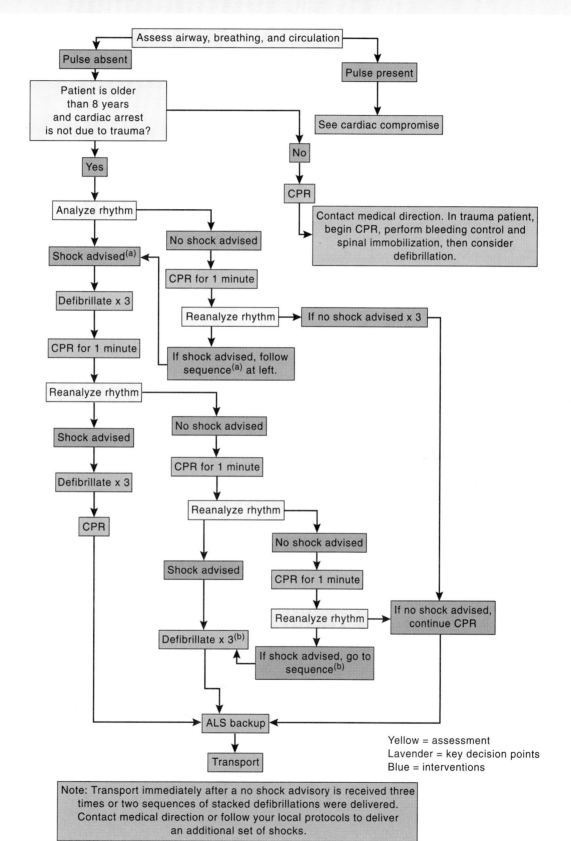

Figure 16-10   Emergency care algorithm: automatic external defibrillator.

AUTOMATED DEFIBRILLATORS: OPERATOR'S SHIFT CHECKLIST

Date: _____   Shift: _____   Location: _____

Mfr/Model No.: _____   Serial No. or Facility ID No.: _____

At the beginning of each shift, inspect the unit. Indicate whether all requirements have been met. Note any corrective actions taken. Sign the form.

	Okay as found	Corrective Action/Remarks
1. Defibrillator Unit		
Clean no spills, clear of objects on top, casing intact		
2. Cables/Connectors		
a. Inspect for cracks, broken wire, or damage b. Connectors engage securely		
3. Supplies		
a. Two sets of pads in sealed packages, within expiration date b. Hand towel c. Scissors d. Razor * e. Alcohol wipes * f. Monitoring electrodes *g. Spare charged battery *h. Adequate ECG paper *i. Manual override module, key or card *j. Cassette tape, memory module, and/or event card plus spares		
4. Power Supply		

a. Battery-powered units
  (1) Verify fully charged battery in place
  (2) Spare charged battery available
  (3) Follow appropriate battery rotation schedule per manufacturer's recommendations
b. AC/Battery backup units
  (1) Plugged into live outlet to maintain battery charge
  (2) Test on battery power and reconnect to line power		

5. Indicators/*ECG Display		
* a. Remove cassette tape, memory module, and/or event card b. Power on display c. Self-test ok * d. Monitor display functional *e. "Service" message display off *f. Battery charging; low battery light off g. Correct time displayed — set with dispatch center		
6. ECG Recorder		
a. Adequate ECG paper b. Recorder prints		
7. Charge/Display Cycle		
* a. Disconnect AC plug — battery backup units b. Attach to simulator c. Detects, charges and delivers shock for "VF" d. Responds correctly to non-shockable rhythms *e. Manual override functional f. Detach from simulator *g. Replace cassette tape, module, and/or memory card		
8. *Pacemaker		
a. Pacer output cable intact b. Pacer pads present (set of two) c. Inspect per manufacturer's operational guidelines		
☐ **Major problem(s) identified** **(OUT OF SERVICE)**		

Applicable only if the unit has this supply or capability

Signature: _____

Figure 16-11   Operator's Shift Checklist for AEDs. Courtesy of Laerdal.

As part of the quality review and improvement program, the system's medical director or a designated representative should review all incidents of AED use. Such reviews can reveal steps that might be taken to speed the entry of cardiac arrest patients into the system, to improve AED training, or to coordinate more effectively AED operation with ACLS backup. These reviews may be accomplished through the following:

- Written reports
- Review of the voice and/or ECG tapes if the system's AED is equipped with that feature
- Review of solid-state memory modules and magnetic tapes if the system's AED is so equipped

ENRICHMENT

The enrichment section contains information that is valuable as background for the EMT-B but that goes substantially beyond the U.S. Department of Transportation (DOT) EMT-Basic curriculum.

THE ELECTROCARDIOGRAM

The *electrocardiogram* (ECG or EKG) is a graphic representation of the heart's electrical activity as detected from the chest wall surface. The ECG may be displayed on a monitor screen or on a continuous strip of special graph paper that can record changes in heart activity over a period of time. (Review Figures 16-4a to c for examples of how different heart rhythms look on an ECG display.)

Each heartbeat, or mechanical contraction of the heart, has two distinct components of electrical activity: depolarization and repolarization. Depolarization is the first, in which electrical charges of the heart muscle change from positive to negative and cause heart muscle contraction. Repolarization is the second component, in which the electrical charges of the heart muscle return to a positive charge and cause relaxation of the heart muscle.

The human body acts as a conductor of electrical current. So any two points on the body may be connected with electrodes or electrical "leads" to record the heart's electrical activity. The recording or tracing of this electrical activity produces a graphic representation of depolarization and repolarization in the form of complexes or a series of waves normally occurring at regular intervals. The waves, or deflections, of a normal ECG have three portions (Figure 16-12):

- *P wave*—This is the first wave form of the ECG and represents the depolarization (contraction) of the atria.
- *QRS complex*—This is the second wave form and represents the depolarization (contraction) of the ventricles and the main contraction of the heart.
- *T wave*—This is the third wave form and represents the repolarization (relaxation) of the ventricles.

The atria also have a repolarization wave, but it is usually buried within the QRS complex.

Another portion of the ECG, the PR interval, is measured in terms of time and used for analysis of the ECG. The PR interval is calculated from the beginning of the P wave to the beginning of the QRS complex. It represents the time it takes the heart's electrical impulse to travel from the atria to the ventricles.

In a normally functioning heart, the heart's electrical impulse is generated from the sinoatrial (SA) node (see Figure 16-1). The electrical impulse then travels through the heart's conduction system, depolarizing the muscle and producing the contraction that pumps blood into the ventricles and then through the body. This electrical activity is called normal sinus rhythm. It will produce an ECG pattern of regularly spaced peaks, which occur between 60 and 100 times each minute, separated by nearly flat lines like that shown in Figure 16-12.

In some cases, the heart muscle becomes hypoxic (low in oxygen), is injured, or dies. Also, the electrical conduction system may be damaged or disturbed and may cause the improper functioning of the heart. Sometimes these conditions may produce an irritability of the heart that causes the uncoordinated firing of electrical ventricular impulses called premature ventricular complexes (PVCs). When PVCs occur in succession, they may produce ventricular tachycardia

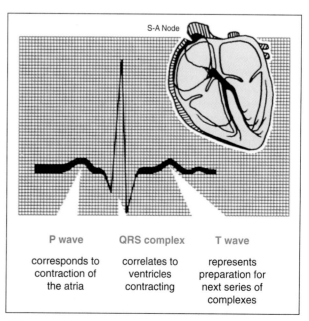

P wave	QRS complex	T wave
corresponds to contraction of the atria	correlates to ventricles contracting	represents preparation for next series of complexes

Figure 16-12 An ECG tracing of normal sinus rhythm.

(V-Tach), which shows up on an ECG as steep peaks and valleys that are very close together (Figure 16-4b). If left untreated, V-Tach can degenerate into ventricular fibrillation (V-Fib), which shows up as smaller, uneven, disorganized peaks and valleys (Figure 16-4a).

ENERGY LEVELS OF DEFIBRILLATORS

Defibrillators, automated or manual, deliver electrical current to the heart through the chest wall. Electrical current for defibrillators is measured in units called joules. Manual monophasic wave form defibrillators can deliver a range of current levels, usually from 5 or 10 joules to 360 joules. Most AEDs, whether fully automated or semi-automated, have two preset values of 200 and 360 joules programmed into the machine. Biphasic wave form defibrillators use lower energy settings for defibrillators.

CARDIAC PACEMAKERS

People whose conduction system cannot sustain a regular and effective rhythm on its own often receive surgically implanted cardiac pacemakers. These devices, powered by long-life batteries, are placed under the skin and have tiny electrodes connecting to the heart. Whenever the patient's heart rate moves outside a certain range, the device takes over the task of setting the heart's pace.

Cardiac pacemakers are usually positioned beneath one of the clavicles. They form a visible lump and can be palpated. If you detect a pacemaker in a cardiac arrest patient, you can still use the AED. However, be sure not to place an adhesive pad directly over the pacemaker.

AUTOMATIC IMPLANTABLE CARDIOVERTER DEFIBRILLATORS

As an EMT-Basic, you may encounter Automatic Implantable Cardioverter Defibrillators (AICDs) in some patients. These devices are surgically implanted and used in cases of ventricular heart rhythm disturbances that cannot be controlled by medication.

The AICD is able to monitor the heart's electrical activity and provide a shock to the heart if it detects a shockable dysrhythmia. Usually the device will deliver four to five shocks. If a patient with an AICD is responsive, he will be able to tell you if he has an AICD and when it is delivering a shock.

If you encounter a responsive cardiac patient with an AICD, allow the device to operate, stabilize the patient, and prepare him for transport. With unresponsive cardiac patients, look for surgical scars on the chest or left upper quadrant of the abdomen. Also look for medical identification tags. Treatment for the unresponsive patient with an AICD is the same as for any other unresponsive cardiac patient. However, when applying the AED's adhesive pads in such patients, do not place them directly over the implanted AICD because the device has an insulated backing that will deflect the shock.

There have been no reported injuries to EMS personnel as a result of contact with AICD patients while the device is delivering a shock. However, a slight tingling sensation may be detectable. Wearing rubber gloves may decrease this possibility.

CASE STUDY FOLLOW-UP

SCENE SIZE-UP

You and your partner, Claire Menzies, have responded to a report of a male in his 50s with breathing difficulty at 115 Clearwater Drive. En route, you receive an update that CPR is being performed at the scene. Dispatch also advises that the ALS team is being contacted and that fire and police vehicles have been sent in support.

Your ambulance and the fire and police vehicles arrive at the scene within moments of each other. There, you observe a small crowd gathered around a male patient. A man and a woman are performing CPR. There do not appear to be any hazards associated with this scene and only one patient is visible. Because the dispatcher advised of CPR in progress, you take the AED when leaving the ambulance. You

and your partner have already donned gloves and eye protection while en route.

INITIAL ASSESSMENT

Your initial assessment reveals an unresponsive man, possibly in his mid-50s, lying supine on the ground with effective bystander CPR in progress. His skin is slightly cyanotic (blue). You ask the man and woman to stop CPR while you assess the patient's pulse and breathing. As you do, Claire begins to set up the semi-automated AED. You find no carotid pulse and detect no breathing. You decide that this is a priority patient for whom defibrillation is appropriate. You direct one of the firefighters who has come to the scene to resume compressions while you ventilate the patient with a bag-valve-mask and high-flow oxygen.

EMERGENCY MEDICAL CARE

Meanwhile, your partner completes setup of the AED. She attaches the external adhesive pads to the patient's chest. She turns on the power and begins narrating an account of the case. She sharply announces "Clear the patient!" You and the firefighter move back from the patient. Claire then pushes the button to begin the rhythm analysis. As the machine charges its capacitor, a synthesized voice says "Deliver a shock." Claire checks all personnel around the patient, saying, "I'm clear, you're clear, everyone is clear." She presses the shock button and the patient jerks as the shock is delivered. She then presses the analysis button again. The AED advises that another shock is indicated and recharges. Claire delivers the second shock and again re-analyzes the rhythm. This time the machine advises "No shock."

You immediately check the carotid pulse and feel a weak one with a rate of 110. You quickly check the patient's respirations and find that he is breathing at a rate of 6 breaths per minute. You begin to assist the patient's ventilations with the bag-valve mask and high-flow oxygen. You also ask the firefighters to help you prepare the patient for transport.

Meanwhile, Claire contacts dispatch on the portable radio to find out about the ALS unit. Dispatch says that ALS Unit 2 can rendezvous with you in 3 minutes in the parking lot of the Price Slasher appliance store, which is on the way to Hahneman Hospital. Medical direction approves the plan.

You load the patient into the ambulance, keeping the AED attached to him. You request that one firefighter drive the ambulance while you and Claire assist the patient in the back. The firefighter agrees and you start off.

ONGOING ASSESSMENT

En route to the hospital, you repeat the initial assessment and are beginning to do a focused medical assessment when the patient takes two gasping breaths. You check for a carotid pulse and find none. You immediately begin CPR and tell the driver to pull over to the side of the road and turn off the engine.

You keep up CPR until the ambulance comes to a stop. When it does, you clear the patient and Claire begins another analysis of his heart rhythm. The AED advises a shock and charges up. Claire ensures that everyone is clear and presses the shock button and defibrillates the patient. When she begins the next rhythm analysis, the machine advises "No shock." You check and find a carotid pulse but discover that the patient is not breathing. You continue to use the BVM to ventilate the patient.

Claire tells the driver to resume transport. Because the patient is unresponsive, she checks his pulse every 30 seconds while carrying out the ongoing assessment. She finds that the pulse is irregular at 110 and the blood pressure is 90 by palpation. Skin color is less cyanotic than previously noted. However, the patient never regains responsiveness while en route to the hospital.

About a minute later, the driver shouts back that he sees the lights of the ALS unit in the Price Slasher lot. He pulls up next to the vehicle and one of the paramedics climbs aboard with his gear. Claire gives a brief report on the patient and what has been done for him. The paramedic tells the driver to proceed to the hospital. He instructs you to take another set of vital signs as he begins ACLS measures.

Upon arrival at the hospital, Claire and the paramedic update the emergency department physician on the patient's condition and provide him with the latest set of vital signs. Claire begins the prehospital care report. Meanwhile, you assist with the transfer of the patient to the hospital bed and retrieve the AED as the emergency department staff places the patient on their monitor/defibrillator.

Later in the day, you find out from the hospital that the patient, Frank Wong, had no prior cardiac history and suffered a heart attack while walking to a store near his home. Mr. Wong went into cardiac arrest two more times after admission to the hospital and is now in intensive care with a guarded prognosis.

CHAPTER REVIEW

TERMS AND CONCEPTS

You may wish to review the following terms and concepts included in this chapter.

asystole—a heart rhythm indicating absence of any electrical activity in the heart, also known as "flatline."

automated external defibrillator (AED)—a device that can analyze the electrical activity or rhythm of a patient's heart and deliver an electrical shock (defibrillation) if appropriate.

cardiac arrest—the cessation of cardiac function with

the patient displaying no pulse, no breathing, and un-responsiveness.

chain of survival—term used by the American Heart Association for the series of four interventions—early access, early CPR, early defibrillation, and early ACLS—that provides the best chance for successful resuscitation of a cardiac arrest victim.

defibrillation—electrical shock or current delivered to the heart through the patient's chest wall to help the heart restore a normal rhythm.

pulseless electrical activity (PEA)—a condition in which the heart generates relatively normal electrical rhythms but fails to perfuse the body adequately because of a decreased or absent cardiac output from cardiac muscle failure or blood loss.

ventricular fibrillation (VF or V-Fib)—a continuous, uncoordinated, chaotic rhythm which does not produce pulses.

ventricular tachycardia (V-Tach)—a very rapid heart rhythm which may or may not produce a pulse and is generally too fast to adequately perfuse the body's organs.

REVIEW QUESTIONS

1. List the four links in the AHA chain of survival.
2. Name and describe the heart rhythms that might benefit from defibrillation.
3. Explain the major difference between automated external defibrillation and manual defibrillation.
4. Describe patients for whom use of the AED is appropriate and those for whom it is not.
5. Explain the four general steps in AED operation.
6. Explain how delivery of CPR is coordinated with use of the AED.
7. Explain when a patient's pulse should be checked during defibrillation.
8. Assuming there is no ALS support on the scene, explain when you should transport a patient who has been receiving defibrillation.
9. Explain the basic steps to follow if a resuscitated patient goes back into cardiac arrest during transport.
10. Explain the purpose of the Operator's Shift Checklist for AEDs and when it should be filled out.

A Note about Cardiac Arrest and AED Use in Children

As noted earlier, cardiac arrest in children is more likely to be caused by hypoxia resulting from airway or respiratory compromise than from a cardiac cause. Therefore, AED use is not recommended in children; rather, efforts should be directed at restoration of an adequate airway and respiration. The 1994 DOT EMT-Basic National Standard Curriculum recommends not performing defibrillation on a patient who is less than 12 years of age or who weighs less than 90 pounds. The most current American Heart Association guidelines recommend that defibrillation be performed in patients in cardiac arrest who are greater than 8 years of age.

A Note about Cardiac Arrest and AED Use in Trauma Patients

In trauma patients, cardiac arrest is more likely to have resulted from the trauma than from an underlying cardiac cause. If a trauma patient is in cardiac arrest, begin CPR and perform bleeding control and spinal immobilization. Contact medical direction to consider use of the AED.

CHAPTER 17

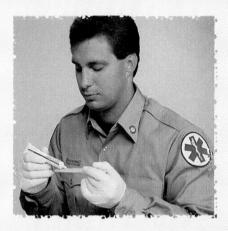

Altered Mental Status— Diabetic Emergencies

INTRODUCTION

An altered mental status is a condition in which the patient displays a change in his normal mental state that may range from disorientation to complete unresponsiveness. Significant decreases in the mental status can lead to serious airway and breathing compromise. Therefore, it is important for the EMT-Basic to recognize and provide emergency care for patients who exhibit an altered mental status.

Diabetes mellitus is a disease that frequently causes changes in the patient's mental status due to alterations in the blood sugar level. There are several million people in the United States who have been diagnosed with diabetes and, as the population ages, the incidence of diabetes is also expected to increase. Unfortunately, several million other Americans have diabetes mellitus but have yet to be diagnosed. Many times, their first indication of having the disease may be a change in mental status such as disorientation or even loss of consciousness.

Prompt recognition and appropriate emergency care of a patient who has an altered mental status, in addition to a history of diabetes that is controlled by medication, is necessary.

OBJECTIVES

Numbered objectives are from the United States Department of Transportation 1994 EMT-Basic National Standard Curriculum. Asterisked objectives, if any, pertain to material that is supplemental to the DOT curriculum.

COGNITIVE

4-4.1 Identify the patient taking diabetic medications with altered mental status and the implications of a diabetes history. (pp. 337–340)

4-4.2 State the steps in the emergency medical care of the patient taking diabetic medicine with an altered mental status and a history of diabetes. (pp. 338–340)

4-4.3 Establish the relationship between airway management and the patient with altered mental status. (pp. 335, 336, 339, 340)

4-4.4 State the generic and trade names, medication forms, dose, administration, action, and contraindications for oral glucose. (p. 341)

4-4.5 Evaluate the need for medical direction in the emergency medical care of the diabetic patient. (pp. 339, 341)

* State the steps in the emergency care of the patient with an altered mental status and an unknown history. (pp. 340–343)

AFFECTIVE

4-4.6 Explain the rationale for administering oral glucose. (p. 340)

PSYCHOMOTOR

4-4.7 Demonstrate the steps in the emergency medical care for the patient taking diabetic medicine with an altered mental status and a history of diabetes.

4-4.8 Demonstrate the steps in the administration of oral glucose.

4-4.9 Demonstrate the assessment and documentation of patient response to oral glucose.

4-4.10 Demonstrate how to complete a prehospital care report for patients with diabetic emergencies.

CASE STUDY

THE DISPATCH

EMS Unit 106—proceed to 514 Chicago Avenue— you have a 66-year-old male patient who appears to be disoriented and belligerent. Be advised, the neighbor placed the call. Time out is 1402 hours.

ON ARRIVAL

As you and your partner approach the house, a woman walks out the front door. She says, "It's Mr. Bennet. I found him in my garden next door. When I asked what he was doing, he began cursing at me.

He's always such a nice man. I can't believe how he's acting. Now he isn't making much sense when I talk to him." You proceed into the house and find the patient sitting on the edge of the couch mumbling incomprehensible words.

How would you proceed to assess and care for this patient?

During this chapter, you will learn about assessment and emergency care for a patient suffering from an altered mental status and one with a history of diabetes. Later, we will return to the case and apply the procedures learned.

ALTERED MENTAL STATUS WITH UNKNOWN HISTORY

An **altered mental status** is a significant indication of injury or illness in a patient. The alteration may range from simple disorientation to complete unconsciousness in which the patient is not responsive, even to painful stimuli. A change in the patient's mental status is an indication that the central nervous system has been affected in some manner. Causes may include trauma, where the brain is injured from a blunt force or penetrating object, or non-traumatic causes such as alterations in the patient's blood sugar level or blood oxygen level. In any patient with an altered mental status, it is vital that you manage any life-threatening injuries or conditions, recognize the mental status change, document it, and continue to monitor the patient for further deterioration.

ASSESSMENT AND CARE: ALTERED MENTAL STATUS WITH UNKNOWN HISTORY

SCENE SIZE-UP

Do a scene size-up to begin to find out why the patient has an altered mental status. Based on the dispatch information and a scan of the scene, it is important to determine if the patient has been injured or is suffering from a medical illness. For example, if you arrive on the scene and find an extension ladder next to the house and the patient lying near it, you would immediately expect that the patient has suffered some type of injury from a fall. As you are approaching the patient inspect the scene for a mechanism of injury that would be significant enough to cause an alteration in mental status. This information may be gathered from your dispatch information, the patient, the relatives, or bystanders at the scene.

If no mechanism of injury is apparent, you would then suspect that the altered mental status is a result of a medical illness. As you are approaching the patient, look for clues that may indicate the nature of the illness. Alcohol bottles, drug paraphernalia, home oxygen tanks, and chemicals may help explain the cause.

The patient's medications may provide the most valuable information to you. Have a family member gather the patient's medications while you are performing your assessment. If no family members are present, ask a first responder or police officer at the scene to look near the kitchen and bathroom sink, kitchen table, and night stand for both prescription and nonprescription medication. Since insulin, the medication taken for diabetes, must be refrigerated, be sure to instruct the individual to look for it inside the refrigerator. Once the medications have been

gathered, they should be kept with the patient. This may provide the emergency department with vital information that would otherwise not be readily available.

If more than one patient at the scene are noted to have an altered mental status, suspect that some type of hazardous gas or poison is causing the illness. Note any unusual odors. The first priority is to protect yourself so you don't become a patient also. The second priority is to move the patient out of the hazardous environment. If you do not have the proper equipment and training, call for experts to bring the patient out of the danger zone.

INITIAL ASSESSMENT

Stabilize the spine if injury is possible. Pay particular attention to the patient's airway and breathing. Severe alterations in mental status may cause the patient to lose his ability to maintain his own airway. The jaw and tongue become relaxed, fall back, and block the airway. Also, an unresponsive patient commonly has no gag or cough reflex and, therefore, is unable to keep his airway clear of secretions, blood, and vomitus.

The breathing rate and depth may be inadequate, so be prepared to perform positive pressure ventilation. All patients with altered mental status must receive high-flow oxygen therapy because ensuring an adequate supply of oxygen to the brain is important in maintaining or restoring mental function. It is also important for you to recognize that the poor breathing status or blocked airway may be the cause of the altered mental status as well as the result.

FOCUSED HISTORY AND PHYSICAL EXAM

A partner may take baseline vital signs as you begin gathering information from the patient, relatives, or bystanders regarding the patient's history. It is best to use the patient as the main historian. However, if the patient is disoriented or suffering a severely depressed mental status, he may be unable to provide the necessary answers. During your SAMPLE history, it is important to ask the following questions:

- What were the signs and symptoms the patient was complaining of prior to the alteration in the mental status?
- Did the signs and symptoms seem to get progressively worse or better?
- Does the patient have any known allergies?
- What medications, prescription and nonprescription, is the patient taking?
- What is the patient's past medical history? When was the last time he has seen a doctor for his medical condition?

- When did the patient last have something to eat or drink? What did he eat or drink? Did he take any drugs or ingest any alcohol?
- What was the patient doing prior to the onset of the altered mental status?
- Was the onset of signs and symptoms gradual or sudden?
- Did the patient suffer from a seizure, severe headache, or confusion prior to the alteration in the mental status?
- How long has the patient been sick or suffering from these signs and symptoms? When was the patient last well?

If the patient is responsive enough to provide you with an adequate history, it is necessary to focus on the areas in which the patient has a complaint, sign, or symptom. If in doubt, or if the patient is unresponsive and unable to provide you with an adequate history, perform a rapid medical assessment.

Signs and Symptoms   The signs and symptoms associated with an altered mental status will vary depending on the cause. Common signs and symptoms of altered mental status associated with trauma are:

- Obvious signs of trauma: deformity, contusions, abrasions, punctures or penetrations, burns, tenderness, lacerations, or swelling
- Abnormal respiratory pattern
- Increased or decreased heart rate
- Unequal pupils
- High or low blood pressure
- Discoloration around the eyes
- Discoloration behind the ears
- Pale, cool, moist skin
- Decorticate posturing (arms flexed, legs extended) or decerebrate posturing (arms and legs extended)

Common signs and symptoms of altered mental status associated with non-trauma or medical illness are:

- Abnormal respiratory pattern
- Dry or moist skin
- Cool or hot skin
- Pinpoint, mid-size, dilated, or unequal pupils
- Stiff neck
- Lacerations to the tongue indicating seizure activity
- High systolic blood pressure and low heart rate
- Loss of bowel or bladder control

Emergency Medical Care

If assessment has revealed an injury or set of medical signs and symptoms, perform the appropriate emergency medical care for those specific injuries or medical conditions. In addition, if the patient displays an altered mental status, provide the following care:

1. *Maintain spinal stabilization* if trauma is suspected.
2. *Maintain a patent airway.* A patient with an altered mental status may not be able to maintain his own airway. If this is the case, insert a nasopharyngeal or oropharyngeal airway adjunct to help keep the patient's airway open.
3. *Suction any secretions, vomitus, or blood.* Closely monitor the airway by frequently inspecting inside the mouth and suctioning any secretions, blood, or vomitus.
4. *Maintain oxygen therapy.* It is extremely important that the patient continuously receive a high concentration of oxygen at a high flow rate. If the patient continues to breathe adequately, maintain the oxygen therapy that was applied during the initial assessment via a nonrebreather mask at 15 lpm. If the patient is being artificially ventilated, make sure the device used to ventilate the patient is properly connected to oxygen.
5. *Be prepared to assist ventilation.* Continuously assess the breathing status. If the breathing rate or depth becomes inadequate, immediately begin positive pressure ventilation with supplemental oxygen.
6. *Position the patient.* Patients with an altered mental status should be placed in a lateral recumbent (coma or recovery) position to avoid possible aspiration. If spinal injury is suspected, the patient must be fully immobilized on a long spine board. Spine board and patient may then be rotated as a unit to place the patient on his side if necessary to clear the airway.
7. *Transport.* Any patient with an altered mental status must be transported to a medical facility for further evaluation. Consider ALS intercept according to local protocols.

Ongoing Assessment

Continuously monitor for changes in the patient's mental status, airway, breathing, and circulation. Record the vital signs and communicate your findings to the receiving medical facility. For a patient with an altered mental status, repeat the ongoing assessment every 5 minutes.

Conditions That May Cause an Altered Mental Status

There are many different medical conditions and injuries that could lead to an altered mental status. Some of the more frequent causes are listed in Table 17-1. While all of these conditions can lead to altered mental status, in this chapter we will focus on altered mental status in patients with a history of diabetes.

TABLE 17-1

Conditions That May Cause an Altered Mental Status

- Shock
- Poisoning or drug overdose
- Post seizure (the patient has suffered a seizure and is just beginning to recover)
- Infection
- Traumatic head injury
- Decreased oxygen levels due to an inadequate airway or breathing
- Alcohol intoxication
- Stroke
- Diabetes

ALTERED MENTAL STATUS WITH A HISTORY OF DIABETES

Diabetes mellitus is a disease characterized by an altered relationship between glucose and insulin. **Insulin** is a hormone secreted by the pancreas that is needed to promote the movement of glucose from the blood into the cells (Figure 17-1. **Glucose,** a simple form of sugar, is the body's main source of energy. Diabetic patients have either Type I or Type II diabetes. Type I diabetics commonly acquire the disease during childhood, do not produce any insulin, and therefore must inject insulin daily. Type II diabetics, who usually develop the disease in adulthood, typically still secrete some insulin and may control the disease by diet, exercise, oral medications or, in severe cases, insulin.

When there is a lack of insulin, glucose cannot enter the cells. Instead, it remains in the bloodstream, causing a high level of glucose in the blood, a condi-

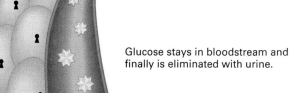

NORMAL VS. TYPE I DIABETIC USE OF GLUCOSE

NORMAL — Food is eaten. Digestion begins in the stomach. Food is broken down into glucose in the small intestine. Glucose enters the bloodstream. Insulin is released by pancreas. Glucose enters body cells with aid of insulin.

DIABETIC — Food is eaten. Digestion begins in the stomach. Food is broken down into glucose in the small intestine. Glucose enters the bloodstream. Little or no insulin is released. Glucose stays in bloodstream and finally is eliminated with urine.

Figure 17-1   Normal vs. Type I diabetic use of glucose from digestion of food.

tion known as **hyperglycemia**—from *hyper-* ("high" or "extensive"), *glyco* ("sugar" or "glucose"), and *-emia* ("blood"). Where a diabetic's insulin level is too high, the opposite effect occurs. Too much sugar enters the cells and not enough sugar remains in the blood, a condition called **hypoglycemia**—from *hypo-* ("low"), *glyco* ("sugar" or "glucose"), and *-emia* ("blood"). Both conditions can cause an altered mental status, and we will discuss them in more detail later in this chapter. In the meantime, your first consideration is how to assess and treat a patient when all you know is that he has an altered mental status and a history of diabetes controlled by medication.

ASSESSMENT AND CARE: ALTERED MENTAL STATUS WITH A HISTORY OF DIABETES

The patient with an altered mental status, who has a history of diabetes and is taking medication to control the diabetes, is assessed in the same manner as the altered mental status patient with no known history.

SCENE SIZE-UP AND INITIAL ASSESSMENT

If clues gathered during the scene size-up and initial assessment lead you to suspect that the patient may be diabetic, look for medical alert tags or medical identification that confirms a diabetic history (Figure 17-2).

INITIAL ASSESSMENT

While asking the SAMPLE history questions, remember especially to ask the "M" question about medications. It is very important that the EMT-B recognize the prescribed medications that a diabetic patient might be taking. Presence of such a medication will help to establish the history of diabetes. It is also important to document and report such a medication to

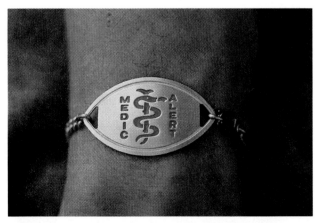

Figure 17-2 A medical identification tag may indicate that the patient is a diabetic.

hospital personnel. Medications often taken by diabetics include:

- Insulin
- Diabanese®, Glucamide®
- Orinase®
- Micronase®, Diabeta®
- Glynase®
- Tolinase®
- Glucotrol®
- Humalog®
- Rezulin®
- Glucophage®

Particularly important in the patient with a history of diabetes is to determine—from the patient, family, or bystanders—the answers to the following questions, with emphasis on the first four:

- *Did the patient take his medication the day of the episode?*
- *Did the patient eat (or skip any) regular meals on that day?*
- *Did the patient vomit after eating a meal on that day?*
- *Did the patient do any unusual exercise or physical activity on that day?*
- Was the onset of mental status alteration gradual or rapid?
- How long has the patient had the signs and symptoms?
- Are there any other signs or symptoms associated with the altered mental status?
- Is there any evidence of injury that might be the cause of the altered mental status?
- Was there any period in which the patient regained a normal mental status and then deteriorated again?
- Did the patient suffer a seizure?
- Does the patient appear to have a fever?

It's important to note that an altered mental status from hypoglycemia will typically have a sudden onset. The signs and symptoms may progress rapidly over a 5- to 30-minute period of time.

Signs and Symptoms Signs and symptoms commonly associated with a patient who has an altered mental status and has a history of diabetes that is controlled by insulin or another medication are (Figure 17-3):

- Rapid onset of an altered mental status after missing a meal, vomiting a meal, unusual exercise, or physical work
- Intoxicated appearance—from staggering or slurred speech to complete unresponsiveness
- Tachycardia (elevated heart rate)
- Cool, moist skin
- Hunger

PATIENT WITH ALTERED STATUS AND HISTORY OF DIABETES
COMMON SIGNS AND SYMPTOMS

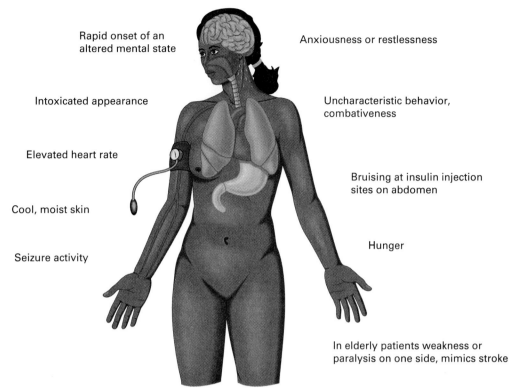

Rapid onset of an
altered mental state

Anxiousness or restlessness

Intoxicated appearance

Uncharacteristic behavior,
combativeness

Elevated heart rate

Bruising at insulin injection
sites on abdomen

Cool, moist skin

Hunger

Seizure activity

In elderly patients weakness or
paralysis on one side, mimics stroke

Figure 17-3   Common signs and symptoms of a patient with altered mental status and a history of diabetes controlled by medication.

- Seizure activity
- Uncharacteristic or bizarre behavior, combativeness
- Anxiousness or restlessness
- Bruising at insulin injection sites on the abdomen
- Elderly patients frequently suffer signs and symptoms that mimic a stroke, such as weakness or paralysis on one side of the body.

Keep in mind that some medications patients take (beta blockers) may hide the signs of hypoglycemia.

EMERGENCY MEDICAL CARE

Once you have confirmed an altered mental status and a history of diabetes controlled by medication, you will concentrate emergency care on correcting any life-threatening conditions and reversing the low blood sugar level that is likely to be the cause of the altered mental status.

1. *Establish and maintain an open airway.* If the patient's mental status is severely altered, it may be necessary to suction the airway to clear secretions or vomitus and insert an oropharyngeal or nasopharyngeal airway. Administer oxygen by nonrebreather mask at 15 liters per minute. If breathing is inadequate, assist breathing by positive pressure ventilation with supplemental oxygen.

2. *Determine if the patient is alert enough to swallow.* Oral glucose, the medication administered to the diabetic patient, is given by mouth. If the patient is unable to swallow, you risk the chance that the patient will aspirate the medication or that the thick, sticky glucose will block the airway.

3. *Administer oral glucose.* Follow protocols established by your local or state medical direction. (See the section on oral glucose, on the next pages.) *If the patient becomes unresponsive during the administration of oral glucose, remove the tongue depressor from the mouth. Immediately reassess the patient's airway, breathing, and circulation.*

4. Transport.

ONGOING ASSESSMENT

Once the oral glucose has been administered, reassessment of the patient's mental status is very important to determine if the medication has had an affect. Remember, it may take more than 20 minutes before you start seeing any improvement in the patient's mental status following the administration of oral glucose. If the patient's mental status continues to deteriorate, manage the airway and breathing. Make sure that the oxygen is flowing to the patient at the highest possible concentration. Communicate and record any changes in the patient's condition.

ORAL GLUCOSE

Oral glucose is the medication of choice in the emergency medical care of the diabetic patient with an altered mental status. Once it is administered, this heavy sugar gel raises the amount of glucose circulating in the blood. This increases the amount of glucose available to the brain. Since the brain cells need glucose to function, lowered levels alter their ability to function properly, thus a decrease in mental status. By increasing the blood glucose level, the brain receives an increased amount of glucose and is able to restore brain cell function, hence an improvement in mental status.

See Figures 17-4 and 17-5, which illustrate methods of administering or assisting a patient with oral glucose. See Figure 17-6 for a detailed summary of the criteria and techniques for administration of oral glucose.

Oral glucose may be administered only if the patient meets all of the following three criteria: (1) an altered mental status, (2) history of diabetes controlled by medication, and (3) ability to swallow. Some patients may meet one or two of these criteria, but not all three. For example, the patient may have an altered mental status and be able to swallow but have no known history of diabetes. Or the patient may have an altered mental status and a history of diabetes controlled by medication but a level of responsiveness so depressed that he cannot swallow safely.

In cases like this, in which all three criteria are not met, do not administer oral glucose. Instead, follow the emergency medical care outlined earlier in the chapter for a patient with altered mental status and an unknown history: Maintain an open airway, suction as needed, maintain oxygen therapy, be pre-

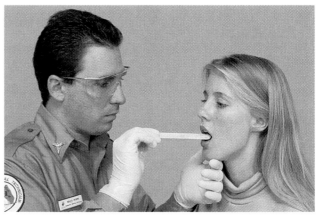

Figure 17-5 One method of administering oral glucose is to squeeze the glucose onto the end of a tongue depressor, then place the tongue depressor between the patient's cheek and gum.

pared to assist ventilations, position the patient on the side, and transport. Contact medical direction for further orders.

SUMMARY: ASSESSMENT AND CARE

To review assessment findings that may be associated with diabetic emergencies and emergency care for diabetic emergencies, see Figures 17-7 and 17-8.

ENRICHMENT

The enrichment section contains information that is valuable as background for the EMT-B but that goes substantially beyond the U.S. Department of Transportation (DOT) EMT-Basic curriculum.

CONDITIONS THAT MAY CAUSE AN ALTERED MENTAL STATUS IN THE DIABETIC PATIENT

This segment discusses two conditions that may cause altered mental status in the diabetic: hypoglycemia and hyperglycemia. Both conditions have to do with the balance of insulin and blood glucose. In diabetics, medical emergencies related to hypoglycemia are far more common than those from hyperglycemia, so the signs and symptoms listed earlier in this chapter for a patient with altered mental status and a history of diabetes are, generally, those of hypoglycemia.

The information about these two conditions that is presented here is intended as background. The EMT-B does not need to—and often cannot—diagnose whether the patient is suffering from hypoglycemia or hyperglycemia. As detailed earlier in this

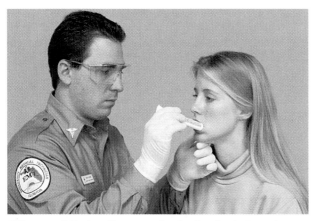

Figure 17-4 One method of administering oral glucose is to squeeze the tube of oral glucose between the patient's cheek and gum.

ORAL GLUCOSE

℞

Medication Name

Oral glucose is the generic name. Two of the trade names of oral glucose are:

* Glutose®
* Insta-glucose®

Indications

Oral glucose should be administered to a patient who meets all of the following criteria:

* An altered mental status, and . . .
* A history of diabetes controlled by medication, and . . .
* The ability to swallow the medication

Contraindications

Oral glucose should not be administered to a patient who is either:

* Unresponsive, or . . .
* Unable to swallow the medication

Form

Gel, in toothpaste-type tubes.

Dosage

Oral glucose is a viscous gel typically packaged in toothpaste-type tubes. The typical dosage is one tube.

Administration

To administer oral glucose:

1. Obtain an order from medical direction. Off-line medical direction would allow the EMT-B to administer the oral glucose without direct consultation with medical direction. An on-line order may be given by direct consultation with medical direction via phone or radio prior to the administration of the medication.
2. Assure the signs and symptoms are consistent with an altered mental status associated with a history of diabetes controlled by medication.
3. Assure that the patient is responsive, and able to swallow the medication and protect his airway. Monitor the patient's airway closely during the administration to avoid accidental blockage by or aspiration of the oral glucose.
4. There are two ways to administer the medication. One way is to hold back the patient's cheek and squeeze small portions of the contents of the tube

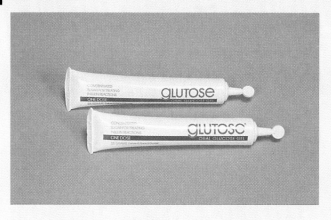

into the mouth between the cheek and gum (Figure 17-4). The other way is to place small portions of the oral glucose on a tongue depressor, pull back the cheek, and slide the tongue depressor to deposit the medication between the cheek and gum (Figure 17-5).

Whichever method you choose, do not squeeze a large amount of glucose into the patient's mouth at one time. This may cause the patient to choke or aspirate the contents. Also, lightly massage the area between the cheek and gum to disperse the gel and increase absorption.

Actions

Increases blood sugar level. Increases sugar available to the brain.

Side Effects

There are no side effects of oral glucose when administered properly. However, the thickness of the gel may cause an airway obstruction or the substance may be aspirated in the patient without a gag reflex.

Reassessment

If the patient loses responsiveness or seizes, remove the tongue depressor from the mouth. Reassessment of the patient's mental status is very important to determine if the medication has had an effect. Remember, it may take more than 20 minutes before you start seeing any improvement in the patient's mental status following the administration of oral glucose. If the patient's mental status continues to deteriorate, manage the airway and breathing. Make sure that the oxygen is flowing to the patient at the highest possible concentration. Constantly monitor the patient's airway and breathing.

Figure 17-6   Oral glucose.

ASSESSMENT SUMMARY

ALTERED MENTAL STATUS— DIABETIC EMERGENCY

The following are findings that may be associated with a diabetic emergency that presents with altered mental status.

SCENE SIZE-UP

Is altered mental status due to a medical or a traumatic cause? Look for evidence of:
Mechanism of injury
Home or portable oxygen tanks or concentrators
Alcohol and drug paraphernalia
Chemicals at or around the scene
Enclosed spaces
Improperly vented heating devices in the winter months
Medications

INITIAL ASSESSMENT

General Impression

Unusual behavior for situation
Patient may have agitated or confused facial expression

Mental Status

Alert to unresponsive
Restlessness
Agitation
Disorientation
Bizarre behavior
Aggressiveness

Airway

Secretions and vomitus
Occlusion from tongue

Breathing

Signs of inadequate breathing

Circulation

Tachycardia
Pale, cool, clammy skin

Status: Priority Patient

FOCUSED HISTORY AND PHYSICAL EXAM

SAMPLE History

Signs and symptoms:
Rapid onset of altered mental status

Intoxicated appearance
Tachycardia
Pale, cool, clammy skin
Hunger
Seizures
Bizarre behavior, restlessness, anxiety
Known allergies to medication or other substances
Medications to control diabetes:
Insulin
Diabanese®, Glucamide®
Orinase®
Micronase®, Diabeta®
Glynase®
Tolinase®
Glucotrol®
Humalog®
Rezulin®
Glucophage®
Key questions to ask: Did the patient . . .
Take his medication this day?
Eat or skip any regular meals?
Vomit after eating a meal this day?
Do any unusual exercise or physical activity this day?

Physical Exam

Head, neck, and face
Dilated pupils
Abdomen
Sensation of hunger
Extremities
Pale, cool skin
Diaphoresis
Other signs and Symptoms
Bruising at insulin injection sites
Weakness or paralysis on one side (especially elderly)

Baseline Vital Signs

BP: normal to low
HR: increased (tachycardia)
RR: may be increased, normal, or low
Skin: pale, cool, and diaphoretic
Pupils: dilated; sluggish to respond

Figure 17-7a   Assessment summary: altered mental status—diabetic emergency.

EMERGENCY CARE PROTOCOL

ALTERED MENTAL STATUS— DIABETIC EMERGENCY

1. Establish and maintain an open airway.
2. Suction secretions as necessary.
3. If breathing is inadequate, provide positive pressure ventilation with supplemental oxygen at minimum rate of 12 ventilations/minute for adult and 20 ventilations minute for infant or child.
4. If breathing is adequate, apply nonrebreather mask at 15 lpm.
5. If patient has an altered mental status with signs and symptoms of hypoglycemia, has a history of medication to control diabetes, and is alert enough to swallow, administer oral glucose.
   - Oral glucose (Glutose® or Insta-glucose®) is a concentrated sugar solution that is absorbed and raises the blood glucose level.
   - Obtain an order from medical direction.
   - Ensure patient is alert enough to swallow.
   - Squeeze contents of tube between cheek and gum or place it between cheek and gum with a tongue depressor.
   - No side effects should be seen with oral glucose.
6. Consider advanced life support.
7. Transport in lateral recumbent (coma or recovery) position.
8. Perform ongoing assessment every 5 minutes.
9. Oral glucose may take up to 20 minutes to get a response from the patient.

Figure 17-7b Emergency care protocol: altered mental status—diabetic emergency.

chapter, it is only necessary for the EMT-B to determine if the patient with altered mental status has a history of diabetes controlled by medication.

HYPOGLYCEMIA

The most common medical emergency for the diabetic patient is hypoglycemia. This condition results from the treatment of diabetes (e.g., insulin injections), or from mismanagement of the treatment regimen, and not from the diabetes itself.

An insulin-glucose imbalance can result from administration of too much insulin, or from ingestion of too little food. (The sugars in food are converted into glucose in the body.) Whatever the cause, when there is too much insulin in the blood compared to the amount of glucose, the glucose moves too rapidly out of the blood and into the cells. This results in insufficient glucose remaining in the blood for the brain to utilize.

Once brain cells are deprived of glucose, brain cell function becomes depressed. If the hypoglycemia persists for a long period of time, brain cells will eventually die. The brain is the primary organ affected in hypoglycemia; it is the first to react and the first to suffer permanent cell damage or death. Rapid recognition and emergency medical care that includes the administration of oral glucose—as outlined earlier in this chapter—is necessary to reverse this condition.

Since the most common sign of hypoglycemia is an altered mental status, and since hypoglycemia is the most common result of mismanagement of diabetes, suspect hypoglycemia in any patient who (1) displays an altered mental status and (2) has a history of diabetes and is on medication for the treatment of diabetes. During the focused history and physical exam of the patient who has an altered mental status resulting from hypoglycemia, you will most likely find one of the following:

- The patient took his insulin but did not eat a meal or skipped a meal.
- The patient took his insulin, ate a meal, but vomited after the meal.
- The patient took more insulin than is prescribed, or the dosage was accidentally injected into a vein.
- The patient took his insulin, ate a regular meal, but had an increase in physical activity level (causing sugar to be used up at a greater-than-usual rate).
- The patient's insulin dose or diet has been changed.

As noted earlier in the chapter, the most common signs and symptoms of hypoglycemia are: rapid onset of altered mental status; the appearance of intoxication; elevated heart rate; cool, moist skin; hunger; seizures; bizarre or combative behavior; anxiousness or restlessness; and, in elderly patients, weakness or paralysis that mimics stroke.

EMERGENCY CARE ALGORITHM:
ALTERED MENTAL STATUS — DIABETIC EMERGENCY

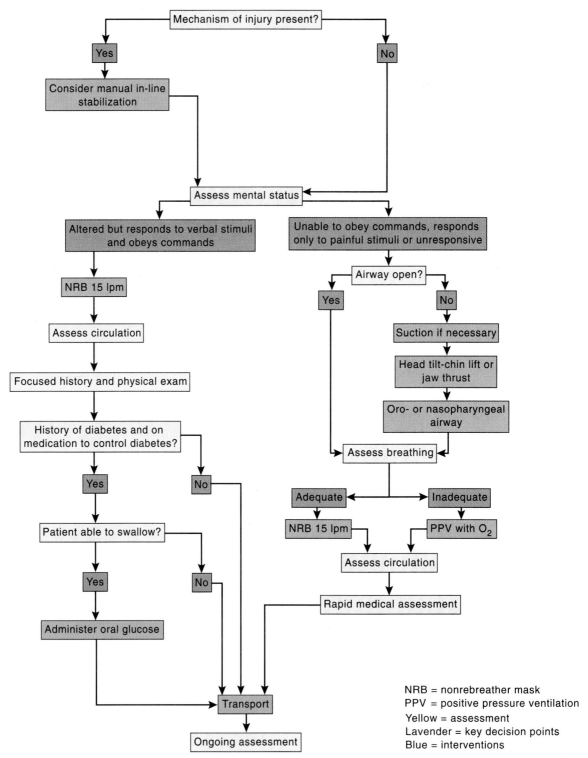

Figure 17-8   Emergency care algorithm: altered mental status—diabetic emergency.

HYPERGLYCEMIA

Another condition that the diabetic patient may exhibit—far less frequently than hypoglycemia—results from an extremely elevated blood sugar level and is known as hyperglycemia.

The hyperglycemic patient does not have enough insulin to help the glucose molecules move into the cells, so glucose begins to accumulate in the blood instead. The cells are then deprived of their primary food source and begin using fats as a source of energy.

The byproducts of fat metabolism in the cells are strong organic acids called ketones. If hyperglycemia is left untreated, the ketones not only depress cell function they also begin to destroy the cells. In addition, the high blood glucose level causes glucose to spill into the urine, promoting excessive urination and dehydration. The resulting condition is called diabetic ketoacidosis (DKA). It is characterized by acidosis (excessively acid condition of body fluids) and dehydration, which can lead to coma (deep unresponsiveness) and even death. Heart rhythm disturbances may also be evident.

Another hyperglycemic condition you may see in patients who are typically over 60 years old is hyperosmolar hyperglycemic nonketotic coma (HHNC). Unlike the DKA patient, who is not producing any insulin, the HHNC patient continues to produce and secrete a small amount of insulin. While this insulin is enough to prevent excessive ketone formation and related acidosis, it is not adequate to reduce the blood sugar level or completely supply the cells with sugar. Because of the high blood sugar level, sugar spills over into the urine causing the patient to become dehydrated. Thus the main consequence of HHNC is severe dehydration leading to an altered mental status and, commonly, coma.

During your assessment of a patient with an altered mental status, some signs and symptoms you may discover if the patient is hyperglycemic may differ from those of a hypoglycemic patient. For example, vomiting and coma are more common with hyperglycemic patients. The patient's breath may have a fruity odor, especially associated with rapid breathing. The odor comes from the formation of ketones and is a sign of DKA. Unlike the cool, moist skin of the hypoglycemic patient, the hyperglycemic's skin is warm and dry. The patient may have frequent urination and excessive thirst.

The slow onset of hyperglycemia differs from the rapid onset of hypoglycemia. In taking the history of a hyperglycemic patient, you may find that the progression of symptoms has occurred over a period as long as 12 to 48 hours. This is important information to record and communicate to the medical facility. The patient may have fever or abdominal pain. Hyperglycemic patients are more apt to have nausea or vomiting. Patients with longstanding hyperglycemia may go into coma. All of these signs and symptoms might be present in both the HHNC and the DKA patient, with the exception of fruity odor on the breath and rapid respirations, which are signs of DKA.

In addition, you might expect to find that one of the following is true of a hyperglycemic patient:

- The patient is suffering from an infection that has upset his insulin/glucose balance.
- The patient does not take insulin and the incidence of hyperglycemia may be the first indication that he has diabetes (particularly true with HHNC patients).
- The patient takes insulin for diabetes, but has taken an inadequate dose.
- The patient is on medications such as Thiazide®, Dilantin®, or steroids.
- The patient has recently undergone physical stress such as surgery or pregnancy.
- The patient has had a change in diet, has overeaten, or has increased his sugar intake.

EMERGENCY MEDICAL CARE

Remember that, as an EMT-B, you are not expected to distinguish between hypoglycemia and hyperglycemia. Although some of the signs and symptoms may differ, both conditions will produce an altered mental status, and the adult patient will usually have a history of diabetes and be taking medication for diabetes. Once you have confirmed these criteria, you will give the same treatment that was outlined earlier in this chapter for a patient with altered mental status and a history of diabetes: Establish an open airway, determine that the patient is alert enough to swallow, administer oral glucose, and transport.

You may wonder why it is acceptable to give oral glucose, a sugar gel, to a patient who may have hyperglycemia, or too much sugar in the blood. The reason oral glucose is given to all patients with an altered mental status and a history of diabetes is that most of them will have hypoglycemia, or low blood sugar. This condition can rapidly cause damage to the brain cells and must be quickly remedied by administering glucose.

If, instead, the patient is suffering from hyperglycemia, or high blood sugar, receiving extra sugar in the form of oral glucose will not do any additional harm, since it is a small amount and will not raise the blood glucose level significantly. In other words, providing glucose to the hypoglycemic patient at the emergency scene is crucial, while providing it to the hyperglycemic patient will have little effect on his condition. It would be more dangerous to decide, incorrectly, that a patient is hyperglycemic and withhold needed glucose.

If you are in doubt as to whether the patient is suffering from an emergency related to hypoglycemia or hyperglycemia, err to benefit the patient and administer oral glucose. Be sure to follow protocol and the guidelines established by your local medical direction for administering oral glucose.

If the patient has not been diagnosed as diabetic (as noted above, an incident of hyperglycemia may be the first indication of diabetes), even though the patient has an altered mental status and other signs or symptoms of a diabetic emergency, do not administer oral glucose. Instead, follow the emergency medical care outlined earlier in the chapter for a patient with altered mental status and an unknown history: Maintain an open airway, suction as needed, maintain oxygen therapy, be prepared to assist ventilations, place the patient in a lateral recumbent position, and transport. This is also the procedure to follow for the patient who is not alert enough to swallow oral glucose.

Remember that a patient who has been alert enough to swallow oral glucose may, nevertheless, deteriorate to unresponsiveness, especially if the patient is hypoglycemic. It is necessary to closely monitor the patient's airway and breathing. Be sure to perform an ongoing assessment, including reassessment of vital signs, and record and communicate any changes in the patient's condition.

CASE STUDY FOLLOW-UP

SCENE SIZE-UP

You have been dispatched to a 66-year-old male patient who was found acting oddly by his neighbor. As you approach the scene, the neighbor meets you on the front porch. She states that her neighbor, Mr. Bennet, was out earlier in her garden acting extremely strange and now is in his house on the couch talking but not making any sense. You proceed into the house with caution and find the patient in the living room. The scene appears to be in order with no sign of trauma. As you approach the patient to begin the initial assessment, you ask your partner to check the house for medications. Your partner finds digoxin near the kitchen sink and insulin in the refrigerator.

INITIAL ASSESSMENT

Your general impression is that the patient appears to be pale and perspiring profusely. As you approach you ask him his name. He responds with mumbled words. You assume the airway is open, and his breathing appears to be adequate. The respirations are at approximately 15 per minute. However, because Mr. Bennet's mental status appears to be altered, your partner places a nonrebreather mask on him at a liter flow of 15 lpm. You assess the radial pulse which is approximately 100 and strong. His skin is moist and cool.

FOCUSED HISTORY AND PHYSICAL EXAM

Since Mr. Bennet is not able to respond appropriately to your questions, you perform a rapid assessment. His pupils are equal and respond sluggishly to light. No jugular vein distention is noted to the neck. The breath sounds are equal bilaterally. His abdomen is soft and no tenderness is noted. Mr. Bennet has good pulses in all extremities. He is able to obey your commands. The grip strength is equal but weak in both upper extremities. The strength in the lower extremities is equal but weak. You find no evidence of trauma anywhere on the body. You find no medical alert identification tag.

Mr. Bennet's blood pressure is 102/60 mmHg. His heart rate is 108 per minute. Respirations are 16 per minute and of normal depth. His skin is pale, cool, and moist. You record the baseline vitals.

During the assessment, you gather a SAMPLE history. Upon questioning, the neighbor states that she found the patient out in her garden about 15 minutes prior to calling EMS. She says, "Mr. Bennet was acting strange and not himself." The neighbor thinks the patient has a heart and sugar problem. She does not know much more about him. Mr. Bennet is disoriented and does not know his name, where he is, who his neighbor is, or what day it is.

By now you are able to determine that Mr. Bennet has an altered mental status, is able to swallow adequately, has a history of diabetes, and is taking medication for the diabetes (as indicated by his neighbor's mention of "a sugar problem" and the insulin your partner found). You administer one tube of oral glucose according to standing orders from medical direction, place the patient so that he is lying on his left side on the ambulance cot, and begin transport.

ONGOING ASSESSMENT

En route to the hospital you notice that Mr. Bennet is beginning to respond more quickly to commands and questions. He can tell you his name and where he is. His airway is clear and breathing remains adequate. His pulse rate decreases to 86 per minute and his skin becomes less pale, dryer, and warmer. You reassess the baseline vital signs and record them. You check to be sure that the oxygen is still flowing at 15 lpm.

As you arrive at the hospital, Mr. Bennet is alert and oriented to person, place, and time. He has no complaints and appears in no distress. You give the hospital an oral report of the change in the patient's condition and help transfer him to the hospital bed. You and your partner complete a prehospital care report, restock the ambulance, and prepare for another call.

CHAPTER REVIEW

TERMS AND CONCEPTS

You may wish to review the following terms and concepts included in this chapter.

altered mental status—a condition in which the patient displays a change in his normal mental state ranging from disorientation to complete unresponsiveness.

diabetes mellitus—a disease in which the normal relationship between glucose and insulin is altered.

glucose—a form of sugar that is the body's basic source of energy.

hypoglycemia—low blood sugar.

hyperglycemia—high blood sugar.

insulin—a hormone secreted by the pancreas that promotes the movement of glucose into the cells.

oral glucose—a form of sugar often given as a gel, by mouth, to help correct a glucose-insulin imbalance in patient's with an altered mental status and a history of diabetes.

REVIEW QUESTIONS

1. Describe the emergency medical care for a patient with an altered mental status and no known history of diabetes.
2. Name the common signs and symptoms of a patient with an altered mental status who has a diabetic history.
3. Describe the emergency medical care for a patient who has an altered mental status and has a history of diabetes that is controlled by medication.
4. Explain why airway management is a major concern in the patient with an altered mental status.
5. Name the indications for oral glucose.
6. Name the contraindications for oral glucose.
7. Describe two methods of administering oral glucose.
8. Describe the role of medical direction in emergency care for the diabetic patient.

CHAPTER 18

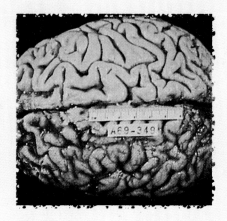

Altered Speech, Sensory, or Motor Function: Stroke Emergency

INTRODUCTION

In Chapter 17 you learned about how an altered mental status presents in patients with a diabetic history. In this chapter you will learn how to assess and treat patients who suffer a loss of speech, sensory, or motor function. This frequently occurs in patients who have suffered a stroke.

Stroke, however, is only one condition that may cause a loss of speech, sensory, or motor function. The most important thing for the EMT-B to be aware of is that, regardless of the cause, this set of signs and symptoms can lead to a compromised airway and inadequate breathing. Early recognition and expeditious transport are vital. The EMT-B must closely and continuously monitor the airway and breathing and be prepared to intervene.

OBJECTIVES

Numbered objectives are from the United States Department of Transportation 1994 EMT-Basic National Standard Curriculum. Asterisked objectives, if any, pertain to material that is supplemental to the DOT curriculum.

COGNITIVE

* Describe the assessment of the patient with an altered mental status and a loss of speech, sensory, or motor function. (pp. 349–353)

* List the common signs and symptoms of a nontraumatic brain injury. (pp. 351, 353, 355)
* Describe the emergency care for a patient with an altered mental status and a loss of speech, sensory, or motor function. (pp. 351–352, 357)
* Describe the conditions most likely to cause altered mental status with a loss of speech, sensory, or motor function. (pp. 357–358)

CASE STUDY

THE DISPATCH

EMS Unit 102—respond to 48 Delason Avenue—you have a 73-year-old female patient who has slurred speech and is unable to move her right arm or leg. Time out is 0840 hours.

ON ARRIVAL

Upon your arrival you find an elderly woman, who is not alert, lying in bed. Her husband tells you that when she woke up she was "talking funny and slurring her words." Also, he noticed that she was unable to move her right hand, arm, leg, or foot. You also note the smell of urine and feces.

How would you proceed to assess and care for this patient?

During this chapter, you will learn about assessment and emergency care for a patient suffering from, a loss of speech, sensory, or motor function, possibly as a result of a stroke. Later, we will return to the case and apply the procedures learned.

NEUROLOGIC DEFICIT RESULTING FROM NONTRAUMATIC BRAIN INJURY

The ability to be alert and aware of your surroundings, to speak, feel sensations, and move are all functions of the brain and nervous system. When the patient loses some or all of these abilities, he is experiencing a **neurologic deficit.** A neurologic deficit is defined as any deficiency in the functioning of the brain or nervous system. Altered mental status, slurred or absent speech, paralysis, weakness, and numbness are all signs and symptoms of neurologic deficit.

A neurologic deficit will alert you to the possibility of a condition that is affecting the patient's central nervous system, which is comprised of the brain and spinal cord. Thus, you must look for signs and symptoms of both traumatic and medical conditions that may be affecting the brain and/or the spinal cord. For

instance, someone whose spinal cord has been injured by a bullet and someone who has suffered a stroke may both lose the ability to feel sensation or the ability to move the arms or legs. In Chapter 33, "Injuries to the Head," and Chapter 34, "Injuries to the Spine," you will learn how to assess and care for patients with head and spinal cord injuries due to trauma (such as from a penetrating wound or a fall). In this chapter, we are primarily concerned with care for the patient with **nontraumatic brain injuries,** medical injuries to the brain that are not related to trauma.

ASSESSMENT AND CARE: LOSS OF SPEECH, SENSORY, OR MOTOR FUNCTION

SCENE SIZE-UP

The dispatch information or someone on the scene may alert you to the patient's neurologic deficit—the loss of speech, sensory, or motor function. As you arrive, scan the scene to try to determine whether the neurologic deficit is due to trauma or to a medical condition. Look for any signs that would make you suspect that the patient's head or spine has been injured. Also, scan the scene for alcohol, drugs or drug paraphernalia, and prescription or illegal drugs, which are other possible causes of altered function. Specifically, look for evidence of amphetamines, cocaine, and other stimulants since they are related to nontraumatic brain injury in young adults.

Note where the patient is found and how he is dressed. Many nontraumatic brain injuries occur at night and the patient awakens with the neurologic deficit. You would expect that a patient who is found in bed or wearing nightclothes is more likely to be suffering from a nontraumatic brain injury than from a traumatic brain injury. Another clue that the patient has suffered a nontraumatic brain injury is a bucket or ice pack next to or near the patient. This could be considered evidence that the patient has experienced nausea, vomiting, or headache, common complaints of many patients with nontraumatic brain injury.

INITIAL ASSESSMENT

Immediately inspect the patient's airway and suction any vomitus and secretions. If spinal injury is not suspected, place the patient in a lateral recumbent (recovery or coma) position. If spinal injury is suspected, perform a jaw-thrust maneuver to open the airway and provide manual in-line stabilization with the patient in a supine position. A patient with an altered neurological status may not be able to control his own airway. The tongue may block the airway. The gag reflex may be lost. In the instance of a nontraumatic brain injury, the muscles of the throat may also be paralyzed. This would prevent the patient from swallowing adequately and could lead to aspiration of secretions. Insert an oropharyngeal or nasopharyngeal airway if needed. Because the brain controls breathing rate and depth, it is very possible to find inadequate breathing or unusual breathing patterns in the patient. Provide positive pressure ventilation with supplemental oxygen if breathing is inadequate.

In the patient with a loss of speech, sensory, or motor function, you should not hastily jump to conclusions when assessing the patient's responsiveness. For instance, if you pinch the patient's right hand and he does not respond, you can't assume that he is unable to feel pain or sensation. He may be paralyzed on the right side; that is, he may be able to feel pain but be unable to move in response to the pain.

FOCUSED HISTORY AND PHYSICAL EXAM

Inspect for any evidence of trauma, especially to the head. If the patient is unresponsive, you will perform a physical exam and obtain baseline vital signs before obtaining the SAMPLE history. If the patient is responsive, you will take the history before performing the physical exam and obtaining vitals. Regardless of whether you start with the history or with the physical exam, keep in mind that paralysis or a loss of speech is very frightening to the patient. It is extremely important that you remain calm and confident and continuously reassure the patient.

The physical exam will be a rapid assessment rather than a focused exam. Inspect the face for a drooped appearance on one side, and listen for garbled sounds or slurring when the patient speaks. If you find the patient walking, note his movement and the manner in which he is walking. An abnormality, such as unsteadiness, can indicate a neurologic deficit that is affecting nervous impulses to the muscles.

When assessing the extremities, you may find a reduction in the sensory and motor function on one side of the body. The patient may lack the ability to feel your touch or to feel pain and may display weakness or paralysis. Check the grip strength in the upper extremities by having the patient grasp and squeeze your fingers. Have the patient push and pull up against your hands with his feet to assess for equality of strength in the lower extremities. Note any differences in strength between the right and left sides and the upper and lower extremities. It is important to note that loss of motor or sensory function on one side of the body is most likely due to an injury or insult to the brain, whereas loss on both sides at a certain level on the body, such as below the waist, is most likely due to a spinal cord injury.

When assessing the baseline vital signs, pay attention to the systolic and diastolic blood pressure. Carefully document both readings and repeat every 5 minutes. Hypertension (high blood pressure) may have actually caused the nontraumatic brain injury or may be a sign of increased pressure within the skull. Unequal pupils or abnormal eye movements or gaze are also significant signs of a possible brain injury (either traumatic or nontraumatic).

During your SAMPLE history, look for medical alert tags, collect the patient's prescription and nonprescription medications, and don't forget to look in the refrigerator for a vial of insulin, used to treat diabetes. Diabetics who are hypoglycemic may show signs and symptoms very similar to those of a nontraumatic-brain-injured patient, especially if the patient is elderly.

Try to gain as much information from the patient as possible. If the speech center of the brain has been affected, the patient may be unable to talk. Yet, don't assume that the patient cannot understand. Determine if the patient can respond to your commands by asking him to blink his eyes or squeeze your finger if he understands. If he is able to understand and make some type of gesture or motion, you can still obtain a history from the patient with the use of questions that can be answered "yes" and "no." For example, you may instruct the patient to blink his eyes twice for yes and once for no. Answers to the following questions will guide you in your emergency care of the patient:

- *Is there any recent history of trauma to the head?* While you may have ruled out trauma while sizing up the scene, it is important to note if the patient has suffered a head injury within the last few weeks.
- *Does the patient have a history of previous stroke?* For instance, the patient may have already lost speech, sensory, or motor function from a previous stroke. In this case the present neurologic deficit either may be the result of another stroke or may be related to some cause other than a stroke or nontraumatic brain injury.
- *Was there any seizure activity noted prior to your arrival?* If so, you should be prepared for the patient to experience a seizure again. (Seizures will be covered in Chapter 19, "Seizures and Syncope.")
- *What was the patient doing at the time of onset of the signs and symptoms?* The activity or lack of activity may point to a traumatic or nontraumatic cause.
- *Does the patient have a history of diabetes?* (Diabetes was covered in Chapter 17, "Altered Mental Status—Diabetic Emergencies.")
- *Has the patient complained of a headache? A stiff neck?* When collecting the SAMPLE history, it is especially important to note if the patient complained of a headache prior to becoming unresponsive or if the patient is currently complaining of a headache. Ask and document if the patient at any time states, "This is the worst headache I've ever had in my life," or something similar. This is consistent with some types of nontraumatic brain injury that are characterized by rapid deterioration.

The following questions are ones that will provide useful information to the hospital personnel who will be receiving the patient. If the patient's mental status is deteriorating, the hospital staff may be unable to get this information later and will need to rely on the information you are able to obtain.

- Does the patient take any oral anticoagulant drugs?
- Does the patient have a history of hypertension (high blood pressure)?
- Has the patient taken amphetamines, cocaine, or some other stimulant drug?
- Was the onset of signs and symptoms gradual or sudden?
- Did the signs and symptoms get progressively worse or better?
- Did the paralysis or weakness affect one particular part of the body first and then progress to other areas?

Signs and Symptoms   The patient can have a wide range of signs and symptoms depending on the extent and location of the nontraumatic brain injury. The following are common signs and symptoms of neurologic deficit resulting from nontraumatic brain injury (Figure 18-1):

- Altered mental status ranging from dizziness or confusion to complete unresponsiveness
- Paralysis (hemiplegia) or weakness (hemiparesis) to the face, arm, and leg on one side of the body
- Numbness or loss of sensation on one side of the body
- Speech disturbances—slurred, garbled, or incomprehensible speech to complete loss of speech
- Loss of control of the bladder or bowel
- Unequal pupils
- Loss of vision in one eye
- Double vision or other visual disturbances
- Eyes turned away from the side of the body that is paralyzed
- Nausea and vomiting
- Severe headache
- Seizure activity
- Stiff neck (late symptom)

In some types of nontraumatic brain injury, it is important to realize that the signs and symptoms may progress and the patient's condition continue to deteriorate. This is particularly true of the mental status, speech disturbance, numbness, weakness, and paralysis. For example, you may find a patient who has weakness to the right arm and leg, has slightly slurred speech, and obeys your commands. By the time you arrive at the hospital the patient is completely paralyzed on the right, is unable to speak, and is responding to only painful stimuli.

EMERGENCY MEDICAL CARE

If your assessment has revealed a traumatic injury, perform the appropriate emergency medical care for that injury. In addition, if the patient displays an altered mental status or a loss of speech, sensory, or motor function, provide the following care:

1. *Maintain a patent airway.* The patient may continue to deteriorate and the airway may become compromised. It may be necessary to insert an oropharyngeal or nasopharyngeal airway. Typically, the nasopharyngeal airway is preferred because it is better tolerated by the patient.
2. *Suction secretions and vomitus.* Since vomiting is associated with a brain injury, be prepared to remove secretions by suctioning.
3. *Be prepared to assist ventilation.* As the patient deteriorates, breathing may become inadequate. If the rate or quality of breathing is inadequate,

GENERAL SIGNS AND SYMPTOMS OF STROKE

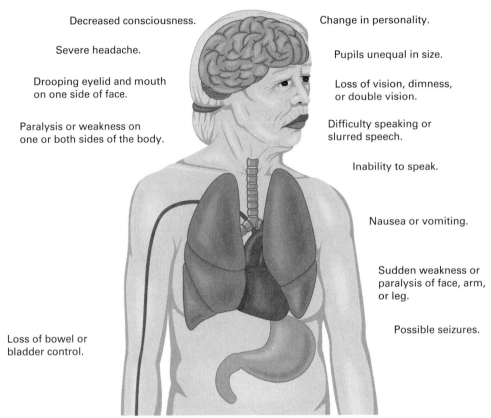

Decreased consciousness.

Severe headache.

Drooping eyelid and mouth on one side of face.

Paralysis or weakness on one or both sides of the body.

Loss of bowel or bladder control.

Change in personality.

Pupils unequal in size.

Loss of vision, dimness, or double vision.

Difficulty speaking or slurred speech.

Inability to speak.

Nausea or vomiting.

Sudden weakness or paralysis of face, arm, or leg.

Possible seizures.

Figure 18-1 Stroke (Cerebrovascular accident or CVA) and transient ischemic attack (TIA) are conditions that may result from nontraumatic brain injury. Loss of speech, sensory, or motor function and altered mental status are among the possible signs and symptoms.

begin positive pressure ventilation with supplemental oxygen. It is important to recognize early signs of respiratory failure. Inadequate breathing could drastically increase injury to the brain because of decreased oxygen flow to the brain and a build-up of carbon dioxide.

If the patient is unresponsive and breathing inadequately, consider hyperventilation at a rate of 20 ventilations per minute with the highest possible concentration of supplemental oxygen. Follow your local protocol or contact medical direction, since hyperventilation of patients with increased pressure inside the skull is considered controversial.

4. *Maintain oxygen therapy.* As long as breathing is adequate, continue oxygen therapy via a nonrebreather mask at 15 lpm. If the patient is being ventilated, continue oxygen therapy through the ventilation device.

5. *Position the patient.* If the patient is unable to protect his own airway because of a reduction in his mental status, place him in a left lateral recumbent position (Figure 18-2). Place the responsive patient in a supine position with the head and chest elevated (Figure 18-3). If spinal injury is suspected, perform a jaw-thrust maneuver to open the airway and provide manual in-line stabilization with the patient in a supine position.

6. *Protect any paralyzed extremities.* Since the patient cannot move the paralyzed extremity, it is vital that the EMT-B protect the paralyzed extremities from any injury.

7. *Transport.* It is necessary to transport any patient with an altered mental status to a medical facility for further evaluation and treatment.

During emergency care, explain your procedures—what you are doing to the patient and what the patient should expect next. Even though the patient may appear as if he cannot understand you, he may be aware of everything that is happening and be able to understand everything you are saying.

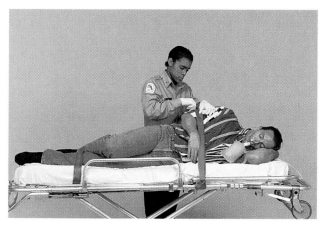

Figure 18-2   Place the unresponsive patient in a left lateral recumbent position if spinal injury is not suspected.

DETAILED PHYSICAL EXAM

If you performed a rapid assessment as part of the focused history and physical exam, it is appropriate to perform a detailed physical exam if the patient's condition and time permit. During the detailed exam, the sensory and motor function should be reassessed closely in all extremities. Document and report any changes from the earlier focused history and physical exam in the patient's speech, sensory, and motor function.

ONGOING ASSESSMENT

Perform an ongoing assessment every 5 minutes. Pay special attention to the status of the airway, breathing, circulation, and mental status. This is extremely important since many nontraumatic-brain-injured patients deteriorate rapidly and significantly. Pay particular attention to the patient's airway as the mental status changes. Repeat and record the baseline vital signs. Communicate any changes in the patient's condition to the receiving medical facility.

SUMMARY: ASSESSMENT AND CARE

To review assessment findings that may be associated with altered speech, sensory, or motor function and emergency care for a patient with these findings, see Figures 18-4 and 18-5.

STROKE AND TRANSIENT ISCHEMIC ATTACK

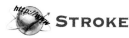 **STROKE**

Stroke (also called a **cerebrovascular accident** or **CVA**) is the most common nontraumatic brain injury that causes a loss of speech (aphasia), sensory function (anesthesia), or motor function (plegia, or paralysis; paresis, or weakness). It is also one of the most common causes of death. Stroke affects hundreds of thousands of Americans each year. More than half of stroke victims die, and many others suffer permanent neurological damage as a result of the stroke.

Stroke is also referred to as a "brain attack" because of its similiarity to a heart attack, the difference being that it affects the brain and not the heart. Also, "brain attack" communicates that it is a life-threatening condition requiring prompt recognition, emergency care, and transport.

Strokes most often affect the elderly who have a history of atherosclerosis (hardening of the arteries), heart disease, or hypertension (high blood pressure). According to the American Heart Association Council on Stroke, the most likely candidate for stroke has high blood pressure and a history of brief, intermittent stroke-like episodes called transient ischemic attacks (TIAs), which we will discuss in the next section.

The signs and symptoms of stroke are associated with the specific area of the brain that has been affected by a disruption in the blood flow. Most commonly, it involves the areas that control speech, sensation, and muscle function. The onset of the signs and symptoms is usually sudden and may be accompanied by a seizure, headache, or the inability to swallow (dysphagia). The patient may also be experiencing difficulty in breathing (dyspnea).

Paralysis is a very common sign in the stroke patient as is facial droop, in which there is a loss of facial expression on one side and the facial features droop downward. Typically, the paralysis will affect one extremity (monoplegia) or both extremities

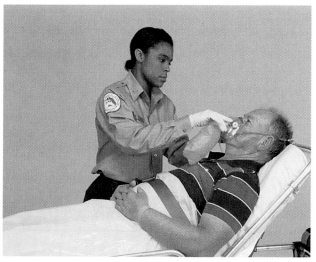

Figure 18-3   Place the responsive patient in a supine position with the head and chest elevated if spinal injury is not suspected.

ASSESSMENT SUMMARY

ALTERED SPEECH, SENSORY, OR MOTOR FUNCTION (POSSIBLE STROKE EMERGENCY)

The following are findings that may be associated with a stroke emergency that presents with altered speech, sensory, or motor function.

SCENE SIZE-UP

Is neurologic deficit due to trauma or a medical problem? Look for:
Mechanism of injury
Alcohol, drugs, or other substances that are commonly abused
Position and location of patient
Bucket or ice pack next to bed

INITIAL ASSESSMENT

General Impression

Vomitus or secretions in mouth
Slurred or incomprehensible speech
Paralysis to one side of body

Mental Status

Alert to unresponsive
Able to understand but unable to speak
Unable to understand or obey commands
Disoriented

Airway

Obstruction by tongue
Obstruction by vomitus or secretions
(Insert a nasopharyngeal or oropharyngeal airway in the unresponsive patient.)
Drooling or inability to swallow

Breathing

Shallow respirations
Irregular respirations
Absent respirations

Circulation

Heart rate may be increased or decreased.

Status: *Priority Patient*

FOCUSED HISTORY AND PHYSICAL EXAM

SAMPLE History

Signs and symptoms:
Altered mental status
Numbness or loss of sensation to one side of body
Speech disturbances (slurred, incomprehensible)
Loss of bladder and bowel control
Unequal pupils
Visual disturbances (loss of vision in one eye, blurred vision, loss of visual field)
Nausea and vomiting
Headache (severe in stroke due to hemorrhage)
Seizure
Stiff neck
Facial and eyelid droop
Ask questions regarding the following:
Anticoagulant drugs?
History of hypertension?
Abuse of amphetamines, cocaine, or other stimulant drug?
Onset gradual or sudden?
Signs and symptoms progressively get worse?
Paralysis affects one side of body first?

Physical Exam

Head, neck, and face
Eyelid droop
Facial droop
Abnormal eye movements or gaze
Extremities
Weak or paralyzed on one side
Numbness
Unequal grip strength on one side of body
Loss of sensation to one side of body

Baseline Vital Signs

BP: elevated, normal, or decreased
HR: normal or decreased
RR: normal, decreased, increased, or irregular
Skin: normal
Pupils: possibly unequal and dilated

Figure 18-4a Assessment summary: altered speech, sensory, or motor function (possible stroke).

✳ EMERGENCY CARE PROTOCOL

ALTERED SPEECH, SENSORY, OR MOTOR FUNCTION (POSSIBLE STROKE EMERGENCY)

1. Establish and maintain open airway. Insert nasopharyngeal or oropharyngeal airway if patient is unresponsive.
2. Suction secretions as necessary.
3. If breathing is inadequate, provide positive pressure ventilation with supplemental oxygen at a minimum rate of 12 ventilations/minute for an adult and 20 ventilations/minute for an infant or child.
4. If breathing is adequate, administer oxygen by nonrebreather mask at 15 lpm.
5. Place patient in lateral recumbent position, if no spinal injury suspected.
6. Transport.
7. Perform ongoing assessment every 5 minutes.

Figure 18-4b Emergency care protocol: altered speech, sensory, or motor function (possible stroke).

(hemiplegia) on one side of the body. If the stroke occurs on the left side of the brain, the damage is noticeable on the right side of the body; if the stroke occurs on the right side of the brain, the damage is evident on the left side of the body. It is extremely unusual for the paralysis to occur on both sides of the body secondary to a stroke. This is one of the factors that will help you distinguish stroke from spinal injuries, which frequently cause paralysis to both legs (paraplegia) or to all four extremities (quadriplegia). You should also note that some stroke patients experience only weakness in the arms and legs and not paralysis. Carefully monitor the patient because the weakness may progress to complete paralysis.

In stroke patients, alterations in mental status commonly range from simple confusion or dizziness to complete unresponsiveness. The speech of the patient may be slurred (dysphasia) or completely absent (aphasia). The patient may experience double or blurred vision, loss of vision in one eye, or loss of a visual field.

Since the stroke may cause an altered mental status or loss of speech, sensory, or motor function, care is the same as previously discussed. Control the airway, provide adequate oxygenation and breathing support and proper positioning, and reassess for further deterioration. Document and communicate all changes in the patient's condition to the medical facility.

Rapid transport of the stroke patient is critical because of the potential for administration of clot-dissolving drugs by the emergency department staff.

 ### TRANSIENT ISCHEMIC ATTACK (TIA)

Patients who experience **transient ischemic attack (TIA)** develop most of the same signs and symptoms as those who are experiencing a stroke. The key difference between a stroke and a TIA is that the signs and symptoms of a TIA disappear within 24 hours without causing any permanent neurologic disability. Ischemia, which refers to an oxygen deficit in the tissues, affects the brain and causes the stroke-like signs and symptoms to appear. Reversal of the ischemia leads to disappearance of the stroke-like signs and symptoms.

Most commonly, the signs and symptoms of TIAs last for approximately 5 to 10 minutes. It is unusual for them to last longer than 30 minutes. Thus, the patient may present with typical signs and symptoms of a stroke, but they progressively disappear.

For example, you arrive on the scene and find a 70-year-old male patient who responds only to verbal stimuli, has right-sided facial droopiness, slurred speech, and paralysis to the right arm and leg. You assess the patient and begin your emergency care. By the time you have loaded the patient into the ambulance 10 minutes have passed. The patient is now alert, able to move his right extremities, and speaking much more clearly, but he still complains of weakness to the right side of his body. When you arrive at the emergency department 13 minutes later, the patient has completely normal motor and sensory function in all extremities and is speaking without any difficulty. The patient has no apparent signs and complains of nothing. In fact, clear documentation by the EMT-B of the symptoms that prompted the call to EMS may be the only reliable clue to the diagnosis.

This would be typical of a TIA. In contrast, the stroke patient's signs and symptoms would have not disappeared and might have worsened. You should realize that the patient who is experiencing a TIA will be just as frightened as one who is experiencing a stroke. It is important to maintain a reassuring, optimistic and hopeful attitude in caring for TIA patients.

EMERGENCY CARE ALGORITHM:
ALTERED SPEECH, SENSORY, OR MOTOR FUNCTION
(POSSIBLE STROKE EMERGENCY)

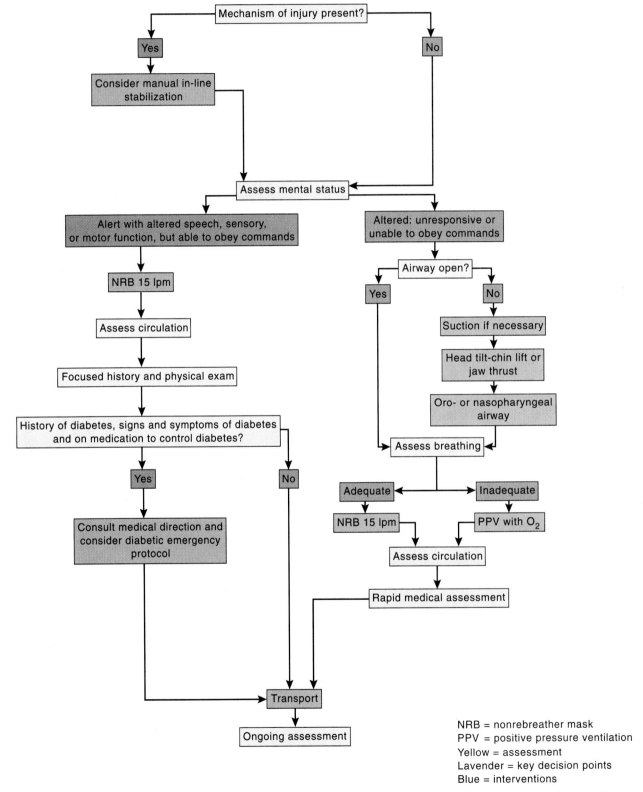

Figure 18-5 Emergency care algorithm: altered speech, sensory, or motor function (possible stroke).

TIAs are important to recognize and report. Although this incident is very frightening for patients, some may refuse emergency care and transportation to a medical facility because the signs and symptoms disappear. However, approximately one-third of those who suffer a TIA will eventually have a stroke, and many of those patients will suffer the stroke within a month after the TIA. Therefore, you must encourage the patient to seek further examination and medical care.

The emergency care for the patient suffering a TIA is the same as that discussed earlier for the patient who displays loss of speech, sensory, or motor function.

ENRICHMENT

The enrichment section contains information that is valuable as background for the EMT-B but that goes substantially beyond the U.S. Department of Transportation (DOT) EMT-Basic curriculum.

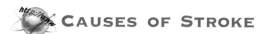 # CAUSES OF STROKE

A stroke is caused by interruption of blood flow to the brain. This occurs either by blockage of an artery that is carrying blood to a specific area within the brain or from bleeding within the brain resulting from a ruptured cerebral artery. The blockage is referred to as an *occlusive stroke* and the bleeding is referred to as a *hemorrhagic stroke* (Figure 18-6).

OCCLUSIVE STROKES

Occlusive strokes occur when the cerebral artery is blocked by a clot or other foreign matter. A clot that develops at the site of occlusion is called a *thrombus* and the process of clot formation is referred to as *thrombosis*. A clot or other matter that has traveled from another area of the body is called an embolus. When the embolus lodges in a cerebral artery and occludes it, it is known as a *cerebral embolism*.

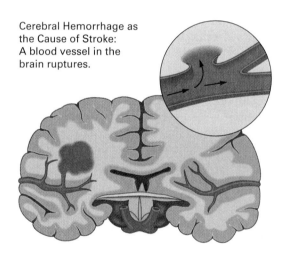
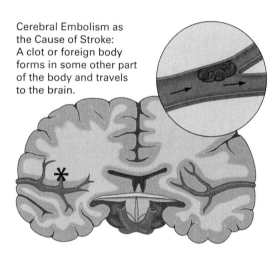
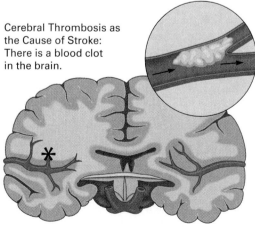
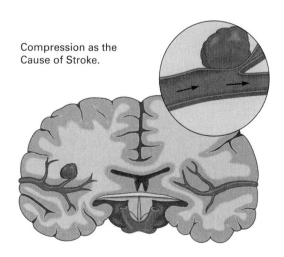

Figure 18-6   Causes of stroke.

Thrombosis As the body ages, it is common for plaque deposits to form on the inner wall of arteries and cause them to narrow, reducing the amount of blood they can carry. This process is called atherosclerosis, and the narrowed portions of the arteries are common sites for blood clot formation. Hypertension can also wear away the smooth inner lining of the artery, leaving rough areas. These areas are likely to develop plaque and are also common sites for clot or thrombus formation. When a thrombus forms inside an artery it can completely block the flow of blood through that artery to the brain. This results in the death of brain tissue, which is a stroke.

Because the narrowing and eventual occlusion of the artery occurs over a longer period of time than an embolic-type occlusion, the onset of signs and symptoms of a thrombotic-type stroke is much slower. This is the most common type of stroke. It most commonly occurs at night when the patient awakens with an altered mental status and/or a loss of speech, sensory, or motor function. Headache is not a common symptom in a thrombotic stroke.

Embolism In the stroke patient, an embolus will usually originate from the carotid artery in the neck or from the heart. The clot will travel until it becomes lodged in a small artery in the brain, blocking blood flow. The brain tissue beyond the point of blockage then begins to die from a lack of oxygen and nutrients. The embolus causing brain tissue death is most often made of clotted blood but may consist of air bubbles, tumor fragments, or fat particles.

An embolic-type stroke occurs most often when the patient is awake and active. The onset of signs and symptoms is usually much more sudden than in a thrombotic stroke, and headache, seizure activity, or brief periods of unresponsiveness are more common.

Hemorrhagic Strokes

A hemorrhagic stroke results from the rupture of an artery that causes bleeding within the brain (intracerebral) or in the space around the outer surface of the brain (subarachnoid space). People with hypertension (high blood pressure) are likely candidates for hemorrhagic stroke since ruptures are most likely to occur in arteries that have been damaged by hypertension. The constant high pressure wears away the inner surface of the artery and weakens it, leading to rupture and hemorrhage. An aneurysm, which is a weakened and dilated area within an artery wall, is a common cause of subarachnoid hemorrhages. The weakened area may be a congenital defect that has been present since birth. This is a common cause of strokes in younger, healthy adults.

The onset of signs and symptoms associated with a hemorrhagic stroke is usually very sudden and often occurs during physical activity. Headache is a very common and often very severe symptom. The patient commonly complains, "This is the worst headache I have ever had." The patient frequently presents with an altered mental status that rapidly deteriorates. Seizures and stiff neck are also common. An atypical picture without mental deterioration is also possible. Hence, any patient with sudden onset of headache must be considered serious.

CASE STUDY FOLLOW-UP

SCENE SIZE-UP

You have been dispatched to a 73-year-old female patient who was found by her husband lying in bed. As you arrive on the scene, the husband meets you at the front door, introduces himself as Mr. Stein, and leads you into the house and up to the second floor bedroom. According to her husband, the patient is unable to move the right side of her body. As you scan the scene, you notice nothing out of the ordinary. The house appears to be extremely well kept, yet the smell of urine and feces permeates the air upon entering the bedroom. You do notice bottles of prescription medications on the night stand next to the bed.

INITIAL ASSESSMENT

The patient is an elderly female who is still in her nightgown. As you approach the patient, you say "Mrs. Stein?" Mrs. Stein opens her eyes and attempts to answer. Her speech is severely slurred and her face is pulled and drooping on the right side. Her breathing is adequate at a rate of approximately 20 per minute. Your partner places a nonrebreather mask on Mrs. Stein at 15 liters per minute. Her radial pulse is strong and estimated at 70 beats per minute. Her skin is warm and dry.

FOCUSED HISTORY AND PHYSICAL EXAM

Mrs. Stein's slurred and garbled speech makes it very difficult to understand what she says. She is also not alert enough to respond appropriately to your questions, so you decide to begin with the physical exam rather than the history, and you perform a rapid assessment. Her head shows no evidence of trauma. Her pupils are equal and reactive. Her chest is rising and falling symmetrically and the breath sounds are equal bilaterally. Her abdomen is soft and no tenderness or rigidity is noted. Her pelvis is stable with no tenderness on palpation. Mrs. Stein is able to obey your commands, so you check and compare her strength in all four extremities. When asked to squeeze your fingers, she has good grip strength on the left, but grip strength on the right is absent. When asked to push up against your hands with her feet, the strength is good on the left, but again absent on the right. The posterior of her body shows no abnormalities. You find no medical alert tags.

While you are performing the rapid assessment, your partner is taking and recording Mrs. Stein's baseline vital signs. The blood pressure is 198/110 mmHg. The heart rate is 74 per minute and irregular. The respirations are 22 per minute and of normal depth. The skin is normal in color, warm, and dry.

Next, you obtain the history, primarily from Mr. Stein. He states that when his wife woke up this morning, her speech was slurred. Unlike now, however, he was still able to understand her. She complained, "I can't move my right arm or leg," and was disturbed that she had soiled the bed. Mr. Stein immediately went downstairs and called 911. He states, "It seems that she has gotten worse since I found her this way." He does not know of any known allergies his wife has. When asked if she takes any medications, he says, "She does take a water pill, a pill for her heart, and a pill for her blood pressure."

Your partner places the medications from the night stand into a paper bag to be transported with the patient. According to Mr. Stein, his wife had a heart attack 2 years ago, and she has high blood pressure. He claims that her last oral intake was a cup of coffee last night at about 10:30. He did not notice anything unusual and she did not complain of anything before going to bed or during the night.

You and your partner place Mrs. Stein on her left side on the stretcher. The oxygen is continued by a nonrebreather mask at 15 lpm. You secure Mrs. Stein to the stretcher, assuring that the paralyzed extremities are well protected, and transfer her to the ambulance.

DETAILED PHYSICAL EXAM

During the detailed physical exam, the pupils are equal and reactive. Mrs. Stein's speech remains excessively slurred and garbled. She does not respond to a deep pinch to her right hand or foot. There is no movement on the right side of her body.

ONGOING ASSESSMENT

Mrs. Stein's mental status does not change while en route to the hospital. Her airway remains open and clear. Her breathing is adequate at a rate of 22 per minute and the radial pulse is strong at a rate of 74 per minute. Her skin remains warm, dry, and a normal color. She continues to attempt to talk, but her speech remains slurred and garbled. The oxygen is flowing at 15 liters per minute. You record the vital signs and report Mrs. Stein's condition to the hospital.

Upon arrival at the emergency department, you provide an oral report of Mrs. Stein's condition as you assist in transferring her to the hospital bed. You complete your prehospital care report, restock the ambulance, notify dispatch you are in service, and prepare for another call.

Later that morning, you return to the emergency department to pick up some equipment. While there, you check on Mrs. Stein's status and learn that she has suffered a stroke and is likely to have permanent paralysis to the right side of her body.

CHAPTER REVIEW

TERMS AND CONCEPTS

You may wish to review the following terms and concepts included in this chapter.

cerebrovascular accident (CVA)—see *stroke.*
neurologic deficit—any deficiency in the nervous system's functioning.
nontraumatic brain injury—a medical injury to the brain which is not caused by external trauma. Stroke is an example of a nontraumatic brain injury.
stroke—a sudden disruption in blood flow to the

brain that results in brain cell damage. Blood flow might be blocked by a ruptured artery or a clot or other foreign matter in an artery that supplies the brain. Also called a *cerebrovascular accident (CVA).*
transient ischemic attack (TIA)—brief, intermittent episodes with stroke-like symptoms that disappear within 24 hours. TIAs are caused by an oxygen deficit in the brain tissue (ischemia) and are often a precursor to a stroke.

REVIEW QUESTIONS

1. Explain why the airway and breathing must be closely monitored in a patient with an altered mental status with a loss of speech, sensory, or motor function.
2. List several signs and symptoms of nontraumatic brain injury.
3. List the steps in the emergency care of the patient suffering from an altered mental status with a loss of speech, sensory, or motor function.
4. Compare and contrast stroke and TIA with regard to signs and symptoms, how they progress, and emergency medical care.

CHAPTER 19

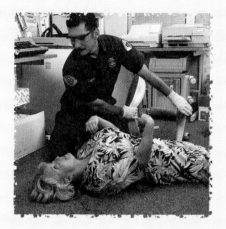

Seizures and Syncope

INTRODUCTION

A seizure is a sudden discharge of electrical activity in the brain, which can lead to unusual manifestations, from staring spells to gross muscle spasm. Most (but not all) seizure activity is accompanied by an altered mental status. Many seizures are self-limiting and last only 2 to 3 minutes. Most often, the seizure will have stopped by the time EMS arrives on the scene. Frequently, emergency care will consist of assisting the patient during recovery and transporting him to the hospital.

Although seizures can be quite dramatic and frightening to observe, they are often not dangerous in themselves. However, the seizing patient can injure himself by falling or thrashing around and the patient's airway can be compromised. Also, it is important for the EMT-Basic to recognize that some seizures are prolonged and are associated with life-threatening conditions or injuries. Your prompt intervention in the prolonged seizure may be life saving.

OBJECTIVES

Numbered objectives are from the United States Department of Transportation 1994 EMT-Basic National Standard Curriculum. Asterisked objectives, if any, pertain to material that is supplemental to the DOT curriculum.

COGNITIVE

* Explain the assessment and emergency care for a seizing patient. (p. 363)

* Recognize the common signs and symptoms of a generalized seizure. (p. 366)
* Recognize signs and symptoms of status epilepticus. (p. 364)
* Identify various conditions that cause seizures. (pp. 362–363)
* Recognize the common signs and symptoms of syncope. (p. 369)
* Differentiate between syncope and seizures. (p. 369)

CASE STUDY

THE DISPATCH

EMS Unit 106—respond to the Southern Park Mall, main concourse, for a 23-year-old female patient who is seizing. Time out is 1717 hours.

ON ARRIVAL

You and your partner arrive on the scene within 2 minutes after the alert. A fire department first responder indicates that the scene is clear of safety hazards and directs you to the location of the patient. As you weave through the shoppers with your equipment and the stretcher, you notice that the mall is unusually crowded because of a holiday craft fair. A large crowd surrounds the patient. You find her supine and actively seizing. A fire department first responder is cradling her head to protect it. Her sister is at her side holding her hand while providing the fire department with information.

How would you proceed to assess and care for this patient?

During this chapter you will learn special considerations of assessment and emergency care for a patient experiencing a seizure. Later we will return to the case and apply the procedures learned.

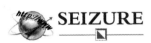 SEIZURE

A **seizure** is a sudden and temporary alteration in brain function caused by massive electrical discharge in a group of nerve cells in the brain. The abnormal electrical discharge typically produces changes in mental activity and behavior ranging from brief trancelike periods of inattention to unresponsiveness and the jerky muscle spasms known as a **convulsion**. A seizure is not a disease in itself but rather a sign of an underlying defect, injury, or disease. A common cause of seizures is **epilepsy**, a chronic brain disorder characterized by recurrent seizures.

Those who have not seen a seizing person before might easily mistake a seizure—or a phase of a seizure—for a heart attack, a behavioral disturbance, or simply daydreaming or lack of attention. What does a seizure "look" like?

The most common type of epileptic seizure, the **generalized tonic-clonic seizure**, is often called a *grand mal seizure*. Because these seizures rarely last more than a few minutes, the patient may be in a **postictal state** by the time you arrive on the scene. The postictal state follows the seizure and is the recovery period for the patient. During this period, the patient may be unresponsive, extremely sleepy, weak, and disoriented. Because such a large number of muscles were contracting during the seizure, he will feel extremely tired. He will slowly but progressively regain complete responsiveness and orientation. This phase may last up to 30 minutes.

Epilepsy is only one cause of seizures. Seizures may also result from injuries or medical conditions other than epilepsy (Table 19-1) and may last much longer than the typical epileptic seizure. Seizure activity that is related to an injury or a medical condi-

TABLE 19-1

Common Causes of Seizures

- High fever
- Infection
- Poisoning
- Hypoglycemia (low blood sugar)
- Hyperglycemia (high blood sugar)
- Head injury
- Shock
- Hypoxia
- Stroke
- Drug or alcohol withdrawal
- Dysrhythmias
- Hypertension (high blood pressure)
- Pregnancy complications (eclampsia)
- Idiopathic (unknown cause)

tion may be an ominous sign of brain injury, even permanent brain damage. It is imperative that you not develop "tunnel vision" and assume that any seizure is caused by epilepsy. If the patient who suffers a seizure has no known history of a seizure disorder, you should suspect some medical or traumatic cause of the seizure other than epilepsy. During the scene size-up and the remainder of assessment, be alert for any clues to a cause other than epilepsy—for example, an injury that must be managed. Also be aware that a heart attack, stroke, or other medical condition may be confused with a seizure or may produce a seizure.

It is also imperative for you to assess and manage the altered mental status associated with the seizure and the postictal state. Prolonged seizures could result in significant airway and breathing compromise. Your task, as an EMT-B, is not to diagnose the type of seizure, but to assess for and manage any life-threatening conditions and provide reassurance to the patient.

ASSESSMENT AND CARE: ALTERED MENTAL STATUS AND SEIZURE

SCENE SIZE-UP

Because a seizure could be a sign of head injury, look for a mechanism of injury that may suggest blunt or penetrating injury to the head. Also, check the environment for any evidence of poisoning, such as pill bottles and syringes. Look for prescription medications that may indicate a potential history of epilepsy, diabetes, or heart disease.

The patient may no longer be seizing by the time you arrive on the scene. You may find the patient in a postictal state. Once responsive, the patient may refuse emergency care and transportation. This frequently occurs in public places where the bystanders

call EMS for the patient. The epileptic patient, however, may be accustomed to the seizure activity and does not necessarily want or need emergency care. If this is the case, you might encourage him to go to the hospital for a check-up if the seizure was abnormal in any way. Always begin with the assumption that the seizure patient needs emergency care.

You can't force a patient to accept transport or treatment, but you do need to document the call and follow the proper patient refusal procedure. Bear in mind that a postictal patient (one in the period of recovery from a seizure) may be confused and not in the best state of mind to refuse transport. If this is the situation, contact medical direction for further orders.

If the patient is still seizing when you arrive, you will frequently find bystanders who are attempting to restrain the patient's jerky body movements. The patient's movements should always be guided, rather than restrained, in order to prevent further injury. It may also be necessary to move objects away from the patient (Figure 19-1). Some people place spoons or other hard objects in the patient's mouth to prevent him from "swallowing his tongue." Remove these objects immediately because they can easily cause injury to the mouth, tongue, teeth, and jaw or they can break and cause an airway obstruction. It is common for the patient to bite his tongue during the seizure; therefore, you may notice small amounts of blood around his mouth. The smell or sight of urine and feces may also be noted.

Because seizure activity may mimic a heart attack and can result in short periods of apnea (absence of breathing), you may find a bystander performing CPR on the patient on your arrival. Quickly verify a pulse, and immediately stop any unnecessary care. It is important to note that some cardiac arrests are preceded by seizure activity because of a lack of oxygen and blood to the brain. You should proceed with

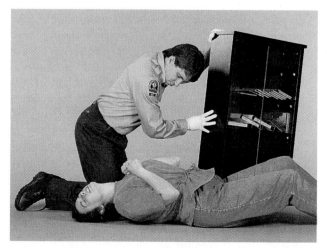

Figure 19-1   Protect the seizing patient from injury by moving furniture and objects away.

application of the AED and emergency care for cardiac arrest if no pulse is found.

Initial Assessment

Form a general impression of the patient as you begin the initial assessment. Whether you find the patient actively seizing or in a postictal state, you should consider both of these an altered mental status that warrants close assessment of the airway, breathing, and circulation. The patient who is not responding to verbal stimuli following the seizure episode, the patient who is actively seizing, or the patient who has suffered more than one consecutive seizure without an intervening period of responsiveness is at the greatest risk for airway, breathing, and circulation compromise. The postictal patient is most often confused, disoriented, weak, and exhausted, but typically has an open airway, is breathing adequately, and has adequate circulation.

When assessing patients in the postictal state:

- If the patient is talking, it indicates an open airway and adequate breathing. The heart rate is commonly elevated and the skin warm and moist. It would be appropriate to continue with the focused history and physical exam for the medical patient. If the seizure was self-limiting and typical for that patient, emergency care may not be required.

When assessing patients who are not responsive or are actively seizing:

- Especially if the seizure activity has lasted longer than 10 minutes, it is vital that you closely assess the patency of the airway and adequacy of the breathing and pulse. A patient who suffers seizures that last more than 10 minutes or seizures that occur consecutively without a period of responsiveness between them is considered to be in **status epilepticus.** *This is a dire medical emergency that requires aggressive airway management, positive pressure ventilation with supplemental oxygen, and immediate transport to a medical facility. The longer the delay in treatment, the greater the chance of the patient suffering permanent brain damage.*
- Open the airway with a jaw-thrust or head-tilt, chin-lift maneuver. It may be necessary to insert a nasopharyngeal airway. Large amounts of saliva are produced during the seizure and the tongue is commonly bitten and bleeding. Suction any secretions, vomitus, or blood from the airway (Figure 19-2). Do not place your fingers in the mouth of the seizing patient or any unresponsive patient. He can easily bite down and cause you serious injury. Do not insert an oropharyngeal airway since the patient may regain his gag reflex and vomit.
- During a seizure, the chest wall muscles contract and restrict effective breathing. The patient may appear to have an airway obstruction and may be cyan-

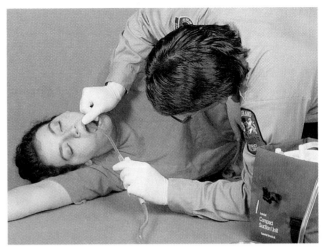

Figure 19-2   Clear the airway of secretions, blood, and vomitus.

otic. As long as the seizure does not last longer than 10 minutes or more than one seizure does not occur consecutively, this should not pose a major problem since respiration will quickly return to normal following the abnormal muscle activity. In the following circumstances, you should begin positive pressure ventilation with supplemental oxygen: The patient is severely cyanotic, the seizure has lasted for greater than 10 minutes from the time of onset (not from your arrival), or the breathing does not immediately become adequate following the episode.

- Note the skin temperature and color. High body temperatures are a common cause of seizures in infants and very young children. Hot skin may also indicate a high body temperature resulting from the excessive uncontrolled muscle movement in the adult. Cyanosis is a grave sign of inadequate oxygenation and ventilation. Provide oxygen via a nonrebreather mask at 15 liters per minute if the breathing is adequate, or, as noted above, positive pressure ventilation with supplemental oxygen if breathing is inadequate.
- Ensure the presence of a pulse if the patient is unresponsive. Initiate CPR and apply the AED if the patient is pulseless. Check for and manage any serious bleeding that may have resulted from trauma.

The seizure patient should be categorized as a priority for transport if any of the following occurs:

- The patient remains unresponsive following the seizure.
- The airway, breathing, or circulation is inadequate following the seizure activity.
- A second seizure occurs without a period of responsiveness between the seizure episodes.
- The seizure lasts longer than 10 minutes.
- The patient is pregnant, has a history of diabetes, or is injured.

- The seizure has occurred in water, such as a swimming pool or lake.
- There is evidence of head trauma leading to the seizure.

FOCUSED HISTORY AND PHYSICAL EXAM

In any of the above circumstances, immediately begin transport following the initial assessment and conduct the focused history and physical exam en route to the hospital. Perform a rapid assessment if the patient is postictal and still has an altered mental status, or if he does not have a past medical history of epilepsy or seizures. The head must be assessed for possible signs of injury (Figure 19-3). The pupils may be unequal if the brain is injured. Look for medical alert tags that might provide information about the patient.

You may find weakness on one side of the body (hemiparesis) following a seizure. This should disappear as the patient slowly becomes more responsive. If the weakness does not subside or if paralysis is present upon assessment of the motor and sensory function in the extremities, it may be an indication that a stroke or trauma is the actual cause of the seizure activity. The seizure patient usually will regain complete recovery of function soon after the postictal episode. Assess the head and extremities for injury that may have occurred as a result of the muscular activity or the fall to the ground. Some muscle contractions are so severe that a bone injury or dislocation may result. Therefore, inspect and palpate for signs of an injured extremity.

Assess and record the baseline vital signs. The respirations and heart rate may be elevated. The skin is commonly warm and moist.

Gather a SAMPLE history from the responsive patient, relatives, and bystanders. If you have decided the patient is a priority for transport, you will have to try to gather information from bystanders during the scene size-up or initial assessment or your partner will have to gather it. (Even if the patient is now responsive, he may not recall much, if anything, about how the seizure occurred or progressed.) The following are pertinent questions to ask, and the answers will be important information to pass along to the hospital staff:

- Was the patient responsive (awake) during the seizure?
- Was the muscle activity a twitching or jerking motion?
- Was the muscle activity isolated to one part of the body or generalized at the time the seizure started? (Most seizures will begin as generalized; some may start focally, then generalize.)
- When did the seizure start?
- How long did the seizure last? (Remember, however, that bystanders tend to overestimate seizure duration.)
- Did the patient experience an aura before the seizure—an unusual sensation that may precede a seizure episode by hours or only a few seconds (see signs and symptoms)?
- Did the patient hit his head or fall?
- Did the patient bite his tongue or mouth?
- Was there a loss of bowel or bladder control?
- Is there any recent history of fever, headache, or stiff neck?
- Is the patient allergic to any medications?
- What medications does the patient take? Are any to control seizures?
- Did the patient take his seizure medication as prescribed?
- Does the patient have a history of epilepsy, previous seizures, diabetes, stroke, or heart disease?
- When was the last time the patient suffered a seizure?
- Was this a typical type of seizure for him to suffer?
- When did the patient last have something to eat or drink?
- What was the patient doing immediately prior to the seizure activity? (Could there have been a fall or injury that caused the seizure, rather than the seizure causing the fall or injury?)

Initially, the postictal patient may not be able to provide you with much of a history. As he progressively improves, the questioning will be easier and the information gathered much more pertinent.

Prescription medications found at the scene or on the patient may provide you with an indication of a medical history of a seizure disorder or epilepsy (Table 19-2). It is important to be familiar with these medications since seizures can be mistaken for other disorders. For instance, some seizures produce behavioral changes that may be interpreted as the patient being drunk or under the influence of drugs. Frequently, a

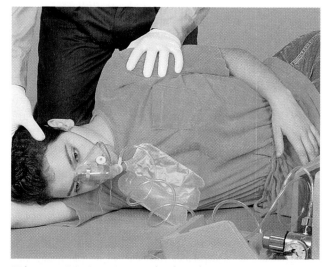

Figure 19-3   Assess the head for any sign of trauma.

TABLE 19-2

Medications Commonly Used in the Treatment of Epilepsy

Phenytoin (Dilantin®)
Phenobarbital
Ethosuximide (Zarontin®)
Carbamazepine (Tegretol®)
Valproic acid (Depakene® or Depakote®)
Primidone (Mysoline®)
Clonazepam (Clonopin®)
Clorazepate (Traxene®)
Felbamate (Felbatol®)
Nevrontin®

patient exhibiting this behavior has phenobarbital prescribed to him, which may confuse you if you are not aware that phenobarbital is used in treating epilepsy.

Signs and Symptoms   The most commonly recognized type of seizure activity is the generalized tonic-clonic (grand mal) seizure. The signs and symptoms of the generalized tonic-clonic seizure usually occur in the following four stages (Figure 19-4):

• *Aura*—The **aura** serves as a warning that a seizure is going to begin and involves some type of sensory perception by the patient. The aura may be a sound, an abnormal twitch, anxiety, dizziness, a smell or odor, an unpleasant feeling in the stomach, visual disturbance, or odd taste. Many patients will tell you that they knew they were going to seize because of the aura. However, generalized seizures do commonly occur without the preceding aura.

• *Tonic phase* (muscle rigidity)—The patient will suddenly become unresponsive and fall to the ground. This typically follows the aura. The patient's muscles become contracted and tense, and the patient exhibits extreme muscular rigidity with arching of the back.

• *Hypertonic phase*—The patient has extreme muscular rigidity with hyperextension of the back.

• *Clonic phase* (convulsion)—Muscle spasms then alternate with relaxation, producing the typical violent and jerky seizure activity of the clonic phase. During the convulsion, a loss of bowel and bladder control may result in involuntary urination and defecation. Also, the tongue, lips, or mouth may be bitten. The breathing may be shallow or absent. This phase usually lasts only 1 to 3 minutes.

• *Postictal state*—This is the recovery phase. The patient's mental status is altered and may range from complete unresponsiveness to confusion and disorientation. The mental status progressively improves

over time. The patient is exhausted and weak. A headache and temporary weakness to one side of the body (hemiparesis) may be present. The postictal phase may last from 10 to 30 minutes.

EMERGENCY MEDICAL CARE

The EMT-Basic must focus on controlling the airway and breathing in the seizing patient. Do not spend unnecessary time trying to determine the cause or type of seizure. Manage the immediate life threats and transport the patient.

1. *Position the patient.* The postictal patient should be placed in a lateral recumbent (recovery) position to protect the airway and facilitate drainage of secretions. If a spinal injury is suspected, the patient should be properly immobilized in a supine position. However, if the immobilized patient vomits, you should immediately turn the backboard and patient as a unit on the side so that the patient's airway can be cleared more easily.

2. *Maintain a patent airway.* If the patient is actively seizing or unresponsive, it may be necessary to insert a nasopharyngeal airway. Since the nasopharyngeal airway is flexible, in contrast to the rigid oropharyngeal airway, it is the airway of choice. Do not force anything into the mouth or between the teeth. You may actually do more harm by breaking the teeth. Though not necessary, a bite stick could be placed between the molars to prevent the patient from biting his tongue, lips, or mouth. Do not place your fingers in the patient's mouth or place any object between the front teeth.

   If the patient is in status epilepticus—seizing for over 10 minutes or having seizures that occur consecutively without a period of responsiveness between them—open the airway with a head-tilt, chin-lift maneuver and insert a nasopharyngeal airway. Begin positive pressure ventilation with supplemental oxygen. Immediately begin transport and continuously reassess the patient en route to the medical facility.

3. *Suction.* Suction any secretions, blood, or vomitus.

4. *Assist breathing.* If the seizures last longer than 10 minutes or the breathing status is inadequate during the postictal phase, begin positive pressure ventilation with supplemental oxygen.

5. *Prevent injury to the patient.* Move objects away from the seizing patient so he does not injure himself. Protect the head, arms, and legs. Do not restrain the patient or try to control the movements. Loosen ties, shirt collars, or other tight clothing.

6. *Maintain oxygen therapy.* Continue oxygen therapy via a nonrebreather mask at 15 liters per minute if the breathing is adequate. Ensure high

STAGES OF GENERALIZED TONIC-CLONIC (GRAND MAL) SEIZURES

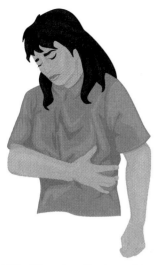

1. AURA. Often described as odd or unpleasant sensation that rises from the stomach toward chest and throat.

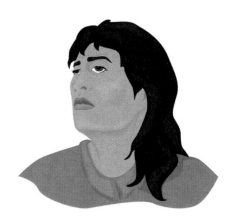

2. TONIC AND HYPERTONIC PHASE. 15 to 20 seconds of loss of consciousness followed by 5 to 15 seconds of extreme muscle rigidity.

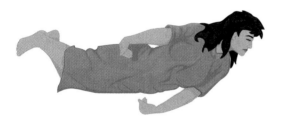

3. CLONIC PHASE. 30 seconds to 5 minutes of convulsions.

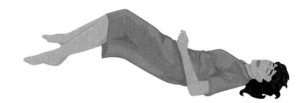

4. POSTICTAL STATE. 5 to 30 minutes to several hours of deep sleep with gradual recovery to confusion, fatigue, soreness, and headache.

Figure 19-4   A generalized tonic-clonic, or grand mal, seizure is a sign of abnormal release of electrical impulses in the brain.

flow oxygen if the patient is being artificially ventilated. Oxygen administration may actually shorten the postictal period.

7. *Transport.* You must contact medical direction or follow local protocol if confronted with a patient who refuses emergency care or transportation. Basically, if this is a normal seizure for the patient, it may not be necessary to seek additional medical treatment. However, if anything is abnormal about the seizure, more than one seizure occurred, or the seizure has lasted longer than 10 minutes, the patient must be transported for further evaluation. Follow your local protocol.

ONGOING ASSESSMENT

Be prepared to manage additional seizures. Monitor the airway, breathing, and circulation. Repeat and record the vital signs. Document and communicate any changes to the receiving medical facility.

SUMMARY: ASSESSMENT AND CARE

To review assessment findings that may be associated with seizures and emergency care for seizures, see Figures 19-5 and 19-6.

ASSESSMENT SUMMARY

SEIZURES

The following are findings that may be associated with seizures.

SCENE SIZE-UP

Is seizure due to trauma or a medical problem? Look for:

    Mechanism of injury

    Alcohol, drugs, or other substances that are commonly abused

    Position and location of patient

    Confined spaces

INITIAL ASSESSMENT

General Impression

Is patient actively seizing?

Vomitus or secretions in mouth?

Are all body parts involved in the convulsion?

Mental Status

Is patient postictal?

Alert to unresponsive

Confused or disoriented

Airway

Obstruction by tongue

Obstruction by vomitus or secretions

(In an epileptic patient who is unresponsive or actively seizing for greater than 10 minutes, insert a nasopharyngeal airway. If the patient is seizing due to a cause other than epilepsy, e.g., head injury, *immediately* insert a nasopharyngeal airway and begin positive pressure ventilation with supplemental oxygen attached to the reservoir.)

Breathing

Shallow respirations

Absent respirations

Circulation

Heart rate may be increased

Skin may be hot and moist

Cyanosis may be present

Status: Priority Patient If:

Actively seizing for greater than 10 minutes

Patient remains unresponsive between seizures

Seizure has a cause other than epilepsy (e.g., hypoxia, head injury)

Patient is pregnant

Patient remains unresponsive following seizure with no improvement

FOCUSED HISTORY AND PHYSICAL EXAM

SAMPLE History

Signs and symptoms of typical epileptic seizure:

    Aura (unusual sensation)

    Unresponsiveness

    Tonic phase (rigid muscles)

    Hypertonic phase (extremely rigid muscles with back arched)

    Tonic-clonic phase (jerky movements)

    Postictal phase (recovery period)

    Other (e.g., hyperventilation, excessive salivation, exhaustion, hemiplegia)

Signs and symptoms of seizure due to causes other than epilepsy:

    Unresponsiveness

    Jerky movements (convulsions)

    Excessive salivation

    Hot, wet skin

    Cyanosis

Ask the following questions:

    How long did seizure last?

    Did patient have an aura and know he was going to seize?

    Did patient possibly injure himself?

    Is patient allergic to any medications?

    Does patient take seizure medication?

    Did patient take his seizure medication today?

    When was the last time patient suffered a seizure?

    Was or is this seizure typical?

Physical Exam

Head, neck, and face:

    Excessive salivation

    Possible cyanosis to mucous membrane and face

    Bitten tongue

    Unequal pupils

Extremities:

    Weak or paralyzed on one side

    General weakness

    Deformities, pain, and swelling due to fractures resulting from convulsion

    Unequal grip strength on one side of body

Baseline Vital Signs

BP: increased or normal

HR: increased

RR: increased, irregular, decreased, shallow, or absent

Skin: warm to hot, moist to wet

Pupils: possibly unequal and dilated, sluggish to respond

Figure 19-5a   Assessment summary: seizures.

✳ EMERGENCY CARE PROTOCOL

SEIZURES

1. Establish and maintain open airway. Insert a nasopharyngeal airway if the epileptic patient who is unresponsive or actively seizing for greater than 5 minutes. Insert a nasopharyngeal airway *immediately* if the patient is seizing due to an etiology other than epilepsy.
2. Suction secretions as necessary.
3. If patient is actively seizing, or if breathing is inadequate in the postictal phase, provide positive pressure ventilation with supplemental oxygen at a minimum rate of 12 ventilations/minute for an adult and 20 ventilations/minute for an infant or child. Ventilations may be difficult to deliver due to resistance related to convulsions.
4. If breathing is adequate, administer oxygen by nonrebreather mask at 15 lpm.
5. Place patient in lateral recumbent position.
6. If febrile seizure in infant or child, cool with tepid water.
7. Consider advanced life support back-up if patient is actively seizing.
8. Transport.
9. Perform an ongoing assessment every 5 minutes.

Figure 19-5b   Emergency care protocol: seizures.

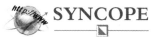

SYNCOPE

Syncope, or fainting, is a sudden and temporary loss of consciousness. It occurs when, for some reason, there is a temporary lack of blood flow to the brain and, hence, the brain is deprived of oxygen for a brief period. Some patients feel as though everything is going dark, and then they suddenly become unresponsive. Syncope usually occurs when the patient is standing up or when the patient suddenly stands up from a sitting position. The collapse that follows puts the body in a horizontal position, allowing blood circulation to the brain to improve. As a result, the patient generally recovers rapidly.

Bystanders may confuse a syncopal episode with a seizure because the patient may experience a very short period of jerky muscle movement during the episode. The difference is that with syncope:

- The episode usually begins in a standing position.
- The patient remembers feeling faint or lightheaded.
- The patient becomes responsive almost immediately after becoming supine.
- The skin is usually pale and moist.

Many patients who faint are afraid that something serious is wrong with them. Conduct an initial assessment and focused history and physical exam. Place the patient in a supine position to allow for improved blood flow to the brain, and provide reassurance. If any complaints, signs, or symptoms are present (in addition to the syncope itself), place the patient on a nonrebreather mask at 15 liters per minute. Keep the patient in a supine position and assess the vital signs. Because most patients fully recover before you even arrive at the scene, many refuse transport. Consult with medical direction or follow your local protocol in this situation. It is important that you document your assessment findings and have the patient and a witness sign a refusal form if the patient is not to be cared for or transported.

It is important to recognize that syncope could be a sign of a serious illness or injury. If the patient faints, or has an episode of syncope, and is not responding appropriately upon your arrival, consider the condition an altered mental status. Perform an initial assessment and rapid assessment and manage the patient's airway, breathing, and circulation as in any altered mental status patient. If the patient has not fallen "flat," make sure to position him in a supine position for assessment, maintaining manual stabilization of the head and spine if spinal injury is suspected.

EMERGENCY CARE ALGORITHM: SEIZURES

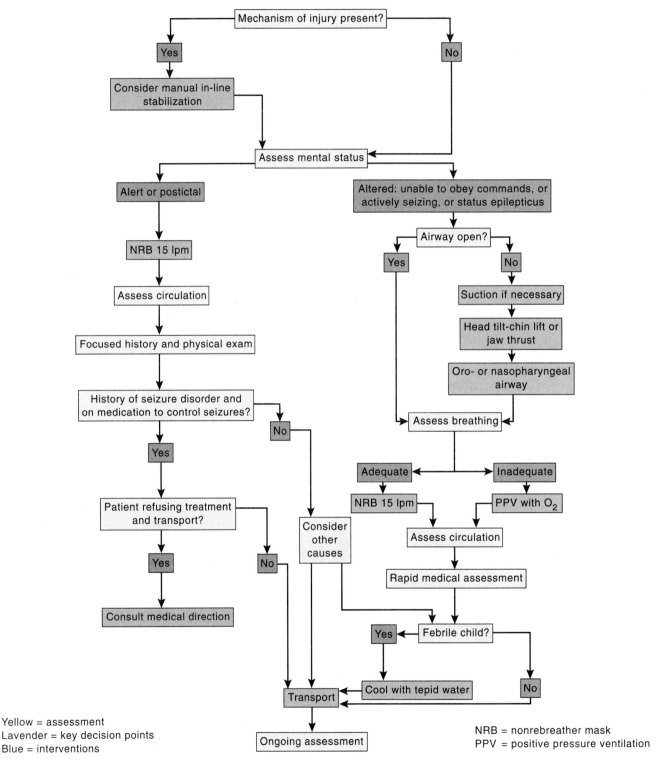

Figure 19-6   Emergency care algorithm: seizures.

ENRICHMENT

The enrichment section contains information that is valuable as background for the EMT-B but that goes substantially beyond the U.S. Department of Transportation (DOT) EMT-Basic curriculum.

TYPES OF SEIZURES

There are several types of seizures, and each has a variety of signs and symptoms. At first glance, some seizures might be mistaken for other conditions. For instance, the patient experiencing an absence seizure can be thought to be simply daydreaming, and the patient who is having a complex partial seizure could be mistaken for someone with a behavioral or psychological disturbance. So, while your treatment efforts will be focused on generalized seizure activity and managing any life threats, it's still important for you to be able to recognize the types of seizures discussed below.

GENERALIZED TONIC-CLONIC (GRAND MAL) SEIZURE

The signs and symptoms and emergency care for the most common type of seizure, the *generalized tonic-clonic seizure*, or *grand mal seizure*, were discussed earlier, in the main part of this chapter.

SIMPLE PARTIAL SEIZURE

A *simple partial seizure* is also known as a *focal motor seizure* or *Jacksonian motor seizure*. This type of seizure generally produces jerky muscle activity in one area of the body, arm, leg, or face. The patient cannot control the jerky movement but remains awake and aware of the seizure activity. The seizure activity may spread from one area of the body to another, and sometimes progresses to a generalized tonic-clonic seizure. You should document where the seizure activity began and how it progressed. This information may be extremely helpful in identifying a cause and in the long-term treatment of the patient.

Emergency Medical Care If this is a recurring problem for the patient and not a new onset, emergency care may not be necessary. Contact medical direction or follow your local protocol if the patient refuses care or transport to a medical facility. If the simple partial seizure progresses to a generalized tonic-clonic seizure, follow the emergency care guidelines given earlier in this chapter. A patient who suffers a simple partial seizure for the first time must be transported for further medical evaluation.

COMPLEX PARTIAL SEIZURE

Also known as a *psychomotor* or *temporal lobe seizure*, the *complex partial seizure* usually lasts 1 to 2 minutes. It usually starts with a blank stare, followed by a random activity such as chewing, lip smacking, or rolling the fingers as if moving a marble between them. The patient appears dazed or unaware of his surroundings and mumbles or repeats certain words or phrases. He will not respond to commands. His actions and movements are clumsy and lack direction. He may pick at his clothing, try to remove his clothes, or pick up objects. The patient may run as you approach him or appear afraid of you. Some patients will struggle with you or show abrupt personality changes, such as fits of rage.

Although the seizure will last for only a few minutes, the post-seizure confusion may last much longer. The patient will not remember what happened during the seizure.

Be alert to the possibility of this disorder, even though the patient's behavior may also cause you to suspect intoxication, drug use, mental illness, or disorderly conduct. If the patient does not recover, manage him as a patient with an altered mental status.

Emergency Medical Care Speak calmly and reassuringly. Guide the person gently away from objects that may be hazardous to him or others. Stay with the person until he is completely aware of his surroundings. Because these seizures are recurring in nature, he will most likely refuse transport. Consult medical direction or follow local protocol in this instance.

ABSENCE (PETIT MAL) SEIZURE

Absence or *petit mal seizures*, most common in children, are characterized by a blank stare, beginning and ending abruptly, and only lasting a few seconds. There maybe rapid blinking, chewing, and lack of attention. The child is unaware of what is occurring during the seizure but then quickly returns to full awareness. No emergency care is necessary for the absence seizure. If this is a first time observation of the seizure, medical evaluation should be recommended.

FEBRILE SEIZURE

Febrile seizures, caused by high fever, are most common in children between 6 months and 6 years of age. About 5 percent of children who have a fever will develop febrile seizures. These generalized seizures are often very short and may not require emergency care; however, always assume that these seizures are serious, because you won't be able to make the diagnosis. These seizures will be covered in more detail in Chapter 38, "Infants and Children."

CASE STUDY FOLLOW-UP

SCENE SIZE-UP

You have been dispatched to the mall for a 23-year-old female patient who is seizing. Your response time is only 2 minutes. The fire department first response unit is on the scene. Firefighter Wright indicates that there is a large crowd in the mall, but the scene is safe. You and your partner gather the jump kit, suction unit, a backboard, head immobilization device, and a set of cervical spinal immobilization collars, and load them onto the stretcher.

As you approach, a large crowd surrounds the patient. She is supine and actively seizing. Firefighter Demarco is cradling her head to protect it from striking the hard floor and maintaining an airway with a jaw thrust. The patient's sister is at her side holding her hand. You and your partner introduce yourself as EMTs and ask for the patient's name. The sister states, "She is my sister and she is an epileptic. Her name is Carmen Escobar." In an attempt to determine if the patient has injured herself, you ask, "Did she fall to the ground or strike anything as she began to seize?" The sister indicates that Carmen said she felt a seizure coming on, and her sister gently helped Carmen to the ground. There are no immediate indications of a mechanism of injury.

INITIAL ASSESSMENT

Your general impression of the patient is a young adult female who has a history of epilepsy. The patient is having generalized seizure activity throughout her body. Your partner assesses the airway, breathing, and circulation. The airway has been opened and is being maintained by the firefighter first responder. Carmen's breathing is irregular and shallow at approximately 18 per minute. The pulse is strong at a rate of approximately 110 per minute. Firefighter Wright places a nonrebreather mask on the patient, providing oxygen at 15 liters per minute. You ask, "How long has she been seizing?" The sister answers, "About 3 minutes." You ask, "Do you know if this is a typical type seizure for her?" She replies, "Carmen gets this unusual taste in her mouth, then goes unconscious, seizes for usually less than 5 minutes, and then becomes real tired and weak."

Carmen's seizure activity abruptly stops. You immediately reassess her airway which appears to be patent. The breathing is deep at a rate of about 20 per minute. The pulse remains strong at approximately 110 per minute. The skin is warm and moist.

Carmen makes incomprehensible sounds. You ask, "Can you tell me your name?" She mumbles, "Carmen."

FOCUSED HISTORY AND PHYSICAL EXAM

You begin by gathering a SAMPLE history. Carmen appears to be slowly regaining her orientation, so you first direct the questions to her. When she is unable to answer some questions, you then seek an answer from her sister. In your questioning, you determine that Carmen has recurring seizures as a result of her epilepsy, and that they are controlled with her medication.

She states that this seizure was normal for her condition, and she experienced nothing unusual. She states, "I had this metallic taste in my mouth, so I knew I was about to seize. I told my sister to help me to the floor. After that, I don't remember anything until I woke up and saw you here." You ask, "How do you feel right now?" Carmen responds, "I feel like I just did aerobics for about 3 hours! I'm totally exhausted, and I just feel like sleeping. I also feel so embarrassed."

She has no allergies and is on Tegretol to control the seizures. You ask, "Have you taken your medication as prescribed?" Carmen states "Yes, I took it this morning. I have about one seizure a month even with the medication." She has no other pertinent past medical history and her last intake of food or drink was about an hour prior to the episode. She was simply walking down the concourse in the mall looking at crafts when she experienced the aura and subsequent seizure.

Carmen's baseline vital signs are: breathing normal at 16 per minute; radial pulse strong at 92 per minute; skin warm, normal color, and slightly moist; pupils equal and reactive; and blood pressure 134/82 mmHg.

ONGOING ASSESSMENT

Carmen is helped up to a nearby bench. She refuses to be transported to the hospital. You contact medical direction and report the history and physical exam findings. Medical direction instructs you to document your history and physical exam findings on an EMS report form, inform the patient that you are requesting that she be transported to the medical facility, and have her and her sister sign the refusal form. The patient complies. You remove the oxygen, and quickly reassess the vital signs. Before you leave, you ask Carmen if she is feeling any abnormal symptoms. She says, "No, this is a typical seizure for me, and I'm used to it. I don't know why they called the ambulance anyway. Thanks for your help, though." "If you should suffer another seizure, be sure to contact us," you say. As you pack up your equipment, Carmen and her sister walk off into the crowd.

CHAPTER REVIEW

TERMS AND CONCEPTS

You may wish to review the following terms and concepts included in this chapter.

aura—an unusual sensory sensation that may precede a seizure episode by hours or only a few seconds.

convulsion—unresponsiveness accompanied by a generalized jerky muscle movement affecting the entire body.

epilepsy—a medical disorder characterized by recurrent seizures.

generalized tonic-clonic seizure—a common type of seizure that produces unresponsiveness and a generalized jerky muscle activity. It is also known as a grand mal seizure.

postictal state—the recovery period that follows the clonic phase of a generalized seizure. In a postictal state the patient commonly appears weak, exhausted, and disoriented and progressively improves.

seizure—a sudden and temporary alteration in the mental status caused by massive electrical discharge in a group of nerve cells in the brain. It typically results in convulsions.

status epilepticus—a seizure lasting longer than 10 minutes or seizures that occur consecutively without a period of responsiveness between them. This is a serious medical emergency that may be life threatening.

syncope—a brief period of unresponsiveness caused by a lack of blood flow to the brain; fainting.

REVIEW QUESTIONS

1. Explain why the airway is frequently compromised in the actively seizing or postictal patient.
2. List pertinent questions to ask the seizure patient, relatives, or bystanders during the SAMPLE history.
3. Name the five stages of a generalized tonic-clonic seizure and the signs and symptoms associated with each stage.
4. Describe the emergency care steps recommended for treating a generalized seizure.

5. Define *status epilepticus* and describe how you would care for a patient who is in status epilepticus.
6. List the common conditions or injuries that may cause seizures.
7. Define and describe syncope and explain how you can distinguish it from a seizure.

CHAPTER 20

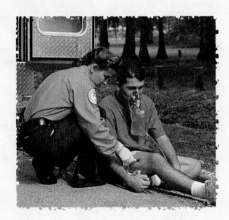

Allergic Reaction

INTRODUCTION

Allergic reactions can occur at any time and to anyone. A wide variety of substances can produce such reactions. Foods, medications, insect stings—even exercise—are common causes. An allergic reaction may be as mild as a runny nose or small skin rash or so severe that the upper airway closes, the respirations become very labored, and the blood pressure becomes dangerously low. Because the reactions are often hard to predict and their consequences potentially life-threatening, it is important for the EMT-Basic to be prepared to recognize promptly and to manage effectively severe allergic reaction in a patient. Delay in emergency care can easily lead to deterioration in the patient's condition and even to death.

OBJECTIVES

Numbered objectives are from the United States Department of Transportation 1994 EMT-Basic National Standard Curriculum. Asterisked objectives, if any, pertain to material that is supplemental to the DOT curriculum.

COGNITIVE

4-5.1 Recognize the patient experiencing an allergic reaction. (pp. 377–380)
4-5.2 Describe the emergency medical care of the patient with an allergic reaction. (pp. 380–381)
4-5.3 Establish the relationship between the patient with an allergic reaction and airway management. (pp. 377, 381)
4-5.4 Describe the mechanism of allergic response and implications for airway management. (pp. 376, 377, 381)
4-5.5 State the generic and trade names, medication forms, dose, administration, action, and contraindications for the epinephrine auto-injector. (pp. 386–387)
4-5.6 Evaluate the need for medical direction in the emergency medical care of the patient with an allergic reaction. (pp. 381, 386)

4-5.7 Differentiate between the general category of those patients having an allergic reaction and those patients having an allergic reaction and requiring immediate medical care, including immediate use of an epinephrine auto-injector. (pp. 376, 378, 379, 380)

AFFECTIVE

4-5.8 Explain the rationale for administering epinephrine using an auto-injector. (pp. 382, 386)

PSYCHOMOTOR

4-5.9 Demonstrate the emergency medical care of the patient experiencing an allergic reaction.
4-5.10 Demonstrate the use of an epinephrine auto-injector.
4-5.11 Demonstrate the assessment and documentation of the patient response to an epinephrine injection.
4-5.12 Demonstrate proper disposal of equipment.
4-5.13 Demonstrate completing a prehospital care report for patients with allergic emergencies.

CASE STUDY

THE DISPATCH

EMS Unit 204—proceed to the Veterans' Pavilion at Mill Run Park. You have a 25-year-old male patient complaining of breathing difficulty. Be advised, the Metropark Police are on the scene. Time out is 0714 hours.

ON ARRIVAL

Upon arrival, you quickly scan the scene to ensure your safety and to look for a mechanism of injury or clues to a possible nature of illness. You exit the ambulance with your emergency kit in hand and proceed to the patient. The scene appears to be safe, and no evidence of trauma is visible. The police state that they were summoned by a bicyclist who found the patient sitting by the side of the road in distress. The patient is sitting up and leaning forward. You introduce yourself and your partner and ask, "What's your name, sir?" The patient gasps out, "John Freeman—and I—feel—real bad."

How would you proceed to assess and care for this patient?

During this chapter, you will learn about assessment and emergency care for patients suffering from allergic reaction. Later, we will return to the case and apply the procedures learned.

ALLERGIC REACTION

The body has a defense mechanism, known as the **immune system,** to fight off invasion by foreign substances. Foreign substances, known as **antigens,** are recognized by the cells of the immune system and eventually destroyed.

An antigen can enter the body through the skin, the gastrointestinal tract, or the respiratory tract. When one does, it sets off an **immune response.** The immune system detects the antigen and produces **antibodies.** Antibodies are proteins that search for the antigen, combine with it, and help to destroy it. This process is known as **sensitization.** This is a normal process that occurs continuously and, most often, goes unnoticed by the person in whom it is taking place.

Most antigens that enter the body are fought off by the immune response. If, however, an **allergen** (one type of antigen) enters the body, the effect is quite different. Allergens are foreign substances, often quite common and harmless to most individuals, that cause an abnormal response by the immune system known as an **allergic reaction.** The allergic reaction is a misdirected and excessive response by the immune system to a foreign substance or an allergen. The immune system overestimates the danger of the allergen and produces an overwhelming response.

The allergen itself is usually harmless to the patient, but the response by the immune system can be life-threatening. Most allergic reactions are mild and produce nothing more than discomfort, such as itching, a runny nose, and watery eyes. However, a severe form of allergic reaction is **anaphylaxis** or **anaphylactic shock.** In anaphylaxis, the entire body is affected by the release of chemical substances by the immune system. These chemical substances produce life-threatening reactions in the airway, lungs, blood vessels, and heart. Swelling in the upper airway can cause obstruction and a reduction of air to the lungs. Bronchoconstriction and swelling in the lower airways can cause severe breathing difficulty and possible hypoxia. Blood vessels dilate and can begin to leak, decreasing the blood pressure and causing shock (hypoperfusion). Anaphylaxis is a life-threatening condition that requires prompt recognition and intervention and commonly leads to death without proper treatment.

Generally, for an allergic reaction to occur, the patient must have been sensitized by exposure to the foreign substance at least once before. In most cases, an allergic reaction cannot occur the first time an allergen is introduced into the body. (There are some drugs that can cause a severe allergic reaction the first time they are used because they resemble previous allergens.) Once sensitization occurs, the patient has produced antibodies and is primed for a possible allergic reaction. Sensitization may last for hours, days, weeks, months, or years. It may take several exposures to a foreign substance over a long period of time. For example, you may encounter a patient who has eaten crab meat for years without any noticeable reaction, but his consumption of crab on this occasion produced a severe allergic reaction and a call to you. Because of such variations in sensitization, it is very difficult to predict who is at risk of developing an allergic reaction. However, once a patient has had an anaphylactic reaction, it should be assumed that he will react in a similar fashion to an exposure to the same allergen.

CAUSES OF ALLERGIC REACTION

Allergic reactions and anaphylaxis can be triggered by a large number of substances. The most common cause is medications that are either taken orally or injected. Some cases of allergic reaction or anaphylaxis are idiopathic, which means that their causes cannot be identified. This is a difficult situation for the patient, since he does not know what substance may trigger another reaction.

An allergen may enter the body by:

- Injection—The substance is introduced directly into the body by bites, stings, needles, or infusions.
- Ingestion—The patient swallows the substance.
- Inhalation—The patient breathes the substance into his lungs.
- Contact (absorption)—The allergen is absorbed through the skin.

Injection, especially intramuscular or intravenous injection, is the route most often involved in anaphylactic reactions. Penicillin is the most common cause of allergic reactions. Some of the common causes of allergic reaction and anaphylaxis are listed below.

- *Venom* from insect bites or stings, especially of wasps, hornets, yellow jackets, and fire ants. Other bites or stings often causing reactions include those of deer flies, gnats, horse flies, mosquitoes, cockroaches, and miller moths. Snake and spider venom may also cause allergic reaction.
- *Foods,* including peanuts, nuts, milk, eggs, shellfish, whitefish, food additives, chocolate, cottonseed oil, and berries.
- *Pollen* from plants, especially ragweed and grasses.
- *Medications* (see Table 20-1), including antibiotics, local anesthetics, aspirin, seizure medications, muscle relaxants, nonsteroidal anti-inflammatory agents, and vitamins. Insulin and tetanus and diphtheria toxoids may also produce allergic reaction.
- A large number of *other substances,* such as latex in gloves and glue, can produce allergic reaction.
- *Exercise* may induce anaphylaxis when certain foods have been ingested close to the time of exercise.

TABLE 20-1

Medications That Commonly Cause Allergic Reactions

Antibiotics	Penicillin
	Tetracycline
	Cephalosporins
	Aminoglycosides
	Sulfonamides
	Amphotericin B
	Nitrofurantoin
Local Anesthetics	Procaine
	Lidocaine
	Novocain
Vitamins	Thiamine
	Folic acid

ASSESSMENT AND CARE: ALLERGIC REACTION

Because the signs and symptoms of allergic reaction are the same as those for many other medical problems, you may or may not be able to determine that the cause of the problem is an allergic reaction. However, a severe allergic reaction—anaphylaxis—should be obvious from its characteristic extreme signs and symptoms. The emergency medical treatment you will provide for these signs and symptoms is the same as you would provide no matter whether they are caused by allergic reaction or another problem.

SCENE SIZE-UP

During the scene size-up, you must be certain that your own safety is not in jeopardy, especially if the allergic reaction is a result of stings or bites. You might encounter a patient who disrupted a yellow jacket or wasp nest and was stung several times. The yellow jackets or wasps may still be at the scene and will attack once you exit the ambulance, exposing you to the risk of allergic reaction from the stings. If you detect the presence of large numbers of wasps or yellow jackets, you may have to wait until they settle or disperse before approaching the patient. It may be also necessary to warn bystanders away from the scene to prevent them from becoming patients.

Because so many different substances may cause allergic reactions, the scene size-up may not provide any obvious clues as to the nature of the illness. A response to a restaurant or a home for a patient complaining of difficulty in breathing and itching after eating may cause you to suspect a possible allergic reaction. Medications found at the scene may provide some clues. A patient at a health club, gym, or park who was exercis-

ing following ingestion of food may increase your suspicion that allergic reaction may be involved.

INITIAL ASSESSMENT

Because allergic reaction can be life-threatening, the initial assessment is an extremely important part of the patient contact. In gathering your general impression of a patient with an allergic reaction, you may note that he complains of "not feeling well" or of **malaise,** a generalized feeling of weakness or discomfort. Such a patient may display a sense of "impending doom." The patient's mental status may be anywhere on the continuum from responsive and alert, responsive but disoriented, to unresponsive.

Closely assess the airway for signs of obstruction. Stridor or crowing sounds indicate significant swelling to the upper airway. Inserting an airway adjunct may not help relieve the obstruction if the swelling is at the level of the larynx. It may be necessary to provide positive pressure ventilation to force the air past the swollen upper airway. You may also find a swollen tongue that interferes with the airway. Wheezing may be prominent upon assessment of breathing. If a patient is severely disoriented, unresponsive, or breathing inadequately, immediately begin positive pressure ventilation with supplemental oxygen. If the breathing is adequate, place the patient on a nonrebreather mask with an oxygen flow of 15 liters per minute.

Delivery of ventilations may be difficult because of the bronchoconstriction and drastically increased resistance in the lower airway. You might find it hard to squeeze the bag of the bag-valve-mask device. If a pop-off relief valve is present on the bag-valve-mask device, it may be necessary to deactivate it or to place your thumb over it in order to deliver a sufficient tidal volume of air to ventilate the patient effectively.

Management of the airway may require **endotracheal intubation,** the placement of a tube in the trachea to facilitate breathing. In some jurisdictions, this must be performed by an ALS team. In other jurisdictions, EMT-Bs will be trained to perform endotracheal intubation (see Chapter 44, "Advanced Airway Management"). If you have been properly trained to perform endotracheal intubation and have permission from medical direction, it is essential to insert an endotracheal tube if the airway is swelling shut. If you have not been trained in endotracheal intubation or have not been given permission to perform it, consider calling for advanced life support (ALS) back-up.

The pulse in a patient suffering from allergic reaction may be weak and rapid. The radial pulse may not be present because of the low blood pressure. Edema, or swelling, may be very obvious in the face, neck, lips, hands, and feet. The skin may be red and warm, or the patient's skin may be cyanotic from inadequate breathing. You may notice **hives,** raised red blotches, all over the skin. Hives are usually accompanied by severe itching. Hives and itching are the hallmark signs and symptoms of an allergic reaction.

Because of the potential seriousness of allergic reaction and its effects on the airway, lungs, blood vessels, and heart, the patient is considered a priority and should be prepared for immediate transport. If the patient exhibits signs of anaphylaxis (severe allergic reaction)—that is, respiratory distress and/or shock (hypoperfusion)—before leaving the scene, determine if the patient has a prescribed epinephrine auto-injector. Inquire of relatives or bystanders if the patient is unresponsive. If he has a prescribed epinephrine auto-injector, locate it (or them, if he has more than one) immediately.

FOCUSED HISTORY AND PHYSICAL EXAM

The focused history and physical exam should be conducted whether the patient's signs and symptoms indicate a mild or a severe allergic reaction; however if the patient exhibits signs of severe reaction, do not delay transport of the patient to complete the focused history and physical exam. Instead, perform the focused history and physical exam en route to the hospital.

History Assess the history of the present illness through the OPQRST line of questioning. Information about the onset of the reaction is especially important. What was the patient doing prior to the onset? What seemed to trigger the signs and symptoms? Such questioning may actually identify the allergen causing the reaction. Determine if anything makes the signs or symptoms better or worse. Did the patient take any medications in an attempt to relieve the symptoms?

Time can be a critical factor in dealing with patients with allergic reactions. Most anaphylactic reactions are apparent within 20 minutes after exposure to the allergen; however, reaction time can vary from seconds to hours. As a general rule, the quicker the patient develops signs and symptoms after exposure, the more severe the allergic reaction will be. Thus, if the reaction occurred within minutes after exposure, you should suspect and be prepared to manage a very severe allergic reaction.

Obtain a SAMPLE history from the patient. If he is unable to speak or is unresponsive, try to obtain as much information as possible from relatives or bystanders while preparing the patient for transport, but without delaying transport if the patient's signs and symptoms indicate severe reaction. When taking the SAMPLE history, it is important to determine the following:

Signs and Symptoms

- Are the signs and symptoms consistent with an allergic reaction?
- Do the signs and symptoms indicate a mild or a severe reaction?
- Are the signs and symptoms getting progressively worse or better?

Allergies

- Does the patient have a history of allergies to food, medications, plants, insect stings or bites, or other? Prior anaphylactic reaction? To what?

Medications

- Does the patient have a prescribed epinephrine auto-injector? (This must be determined early in the assessment for a patient with signs and symptoms of a severe reaction.)
- Has the patient taken any medications to relieve the current signs or symptoms?
- What other medication is the patient taking? Any new medications prescribed?

Pertinent Past History

- Has the patient ever suffered an allergic reaction in the past?
- How severe was the last reaction that the patient suffered?
- Does the patient have any other significant illnesses?

Last Oral Intake

- When was the last time the patient had anything to eat or drink? What did he eat or drink?
- How much food or drink did the patient consume?

Events Prior to Illness

- What was the patient doing prior to onset of the allergic reaction?
- What was the patient exposed to that may have caused the allergic reaction?
- What was the route of exposure—injection, ingestion, inhalation, or contact?

Signs and Symptoms The signs and symptoms of allergic reaction usually involve the skin, respiratory system, cardiovascular system, gastrointestinal system, central nervous system, and genitourinary system. The signs and symptoms vary with the severity of the reaction. The severe reaction known as anaphylaxis or anaphylactic shock is one that produces serious compromise of respiratory function or circulatory function (shock, or hypoperfusion) or both. Common signs and symptoms of allergic reaction, including anaphylaxis, include the following (Figure 20-1):

ALLERGIC REACTION

A grave medical emergency
Severe allergic reaction to an injected, inhaled or ingested
foreign protein can occur within minutes, even seconds.

Early signs and symptoms
• Flushing, itching. Skin rash.
• Sneezing. Watery eyes and nose.
• Airway swelling.
• Cough. "Tickle" or "lump" in the throat that cannot be cleared.
• Gastrointestinal complaints.

The signs and symptoms of an allergic reaction may swiftly lead to:

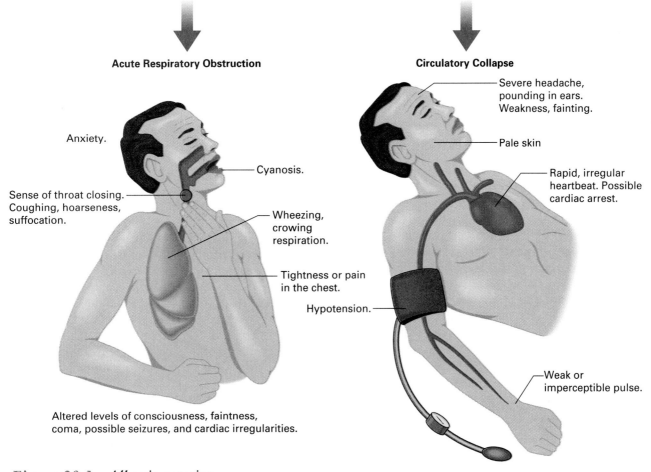

Figure 20-1   Allergic reaction.

Skin

• Warm, tingling feeling in the face, mouth, chest, feet, and hands (early symptom)
• Intense itching, especially of hands and feet (hallmark symptom)
• Hives (hallmark sign)
• Flushed or red skin

• Swelling to the face, lips, neck, hands, feet, and tongue
• Cyanosis (severe cases)

Respiratory System

• Patient complaints of a "lump in the throat"
• Tightness in the chest

- High-pitched cough
- Tachypnea (increased breathing rate)
- Labored breathing
- Noisy breathing (wheezing, stridor, or crowing)
- Impaired ability to talk or hoarseness
- Excessive amounts of coughed-up mucus
- Partially or completely occluded airway
- Difficulty in breathing

Cardiovascular System

- Tachycardia (increased heart rate)
- Hypotension (decreased blood pressure)
- Irregular pulse
- Absent radial pulse (severe shock)

Central Nervous System

- Increased anxiety
- Unresponsiveness
- Disorientation
- Restlessness
- Seizures
- Headache

Gastrointestinal System

- Nausea/vomiting
- Abdominal cramping
- Diarrhea
- Difficulty in swallowing
- Loss of bowel control

Genitourinary System

- Urgent need to urinate
- Cramping of the uterus

Generalized Signs and Symptoms

- Itchy, watery eyes
- Runny or stuffy nose
- Sense of impending doom
- Complaints of "not feeling well"
- General weakness or discomfort

The two key categories of signs and symptoms that specifically indicate anaphylaxis (severe allergic reaction) are:

- *Respiratory compromise*—airway occlusion; breathing difficulty or inadequate breathing with possible wheezing, stridor, or crowing
- *Shock (hypoperfusion)*—absent or weak pulses; rapid heartbeat; decreased blood pressure; deteriorating mental status

This patient needs immediate intervention and administration of epinephrine if possible.

Physical Exam Focus the physical exam on the patient's complaints involving the airway, breathing, and circulation. If the patient is unresponsive, con-

duct a rapid assessment. Your major concerns in both the responsive and unresponsive patient are a compromised airway, inadequate breathing, and shock (hypoperfusion). Inspection of the face and neck typically reveals a swollen appearance and hives. The lips may also be swollen and cyanotic.

Retractions and poor rise and fall of the chest may be noted upon inspection. Diffuse wheezing may be heard on auscultation of the breath sounds. Diminished breath sounds bilaterally are a sign of inadequate respiration and an indication for immediate positive pressure ventilation. The bronchoconstriction may be so severe that air movement is minimal through the bronchioles and into the lungs; therefore, wheezing or breath sounds may not be heard, especially when severe respiratory distress is evident.

The extremities should be quickly inspected for bites, stings, or injection marks. Redness may be noted around the bite or sting, providing a clue to the cause of the allergic reaction. Check pulses and skin temperature, color, and condition for indications of shock (hypoperfusion).

Baseline Vital Signs Assess the baseline vital signs, paying particular attention to the breathing, pulse, and blood pressure. The breathing rate may be beyond the normal limits. Early in an allergic reaction, you may find that the breathing rate is fast and labored. As the condition progresses and the patient begins to tire, the breathing may become slower than normal and very shallow. Wheezes may be heard without a stethoscope. The breathing may also sound noisy, with a rattling sound on inspiration and exhalation, from the excessive mucus in the larger lower airways. The pulse is rapid and may be weak. In severe cases of anaphylaxis, the radial pulse may be absent or extremely weak. The skin is usually red, dry, and warm to the touch. Hives and itching are the most common complaints, both in the mild and severe reaction. Hypotension is common in a severe reaction.

Never underestimate the severity of an allergic reaction. Because death can occur within minutes, immediate intervention is imperative. Do not mistake anaphylaxis for other conditions with similar signs and symptoms such as hyperventilation, anxiety attacks, alcohol intoxication, or hypoglycemia.

EMERGENCY MEDICAL CARE

The key to emergency care in cases of allergic reaction is for the EMT-B to distinguish between mild and severe reactions (Table 20-2). The mild reaction typically does not require aggressive intervention or administration of medication by the EMT-B. In a patient with a mild reaction, you will maintain an open airway, provide oxygen, and transport the patient as soon as possible. Your major concern is that the mild

TABLE 20-2

Differentiating between a Mild and a Severe Allergic Reaction

Sign or Symptom	Mild Reaction	Severe Reaction
Itching	Yes	Yes
Hives	Yes	Yes
Flushed skin	Localized	Widespread
Cyanosis	No	Yes
Edema	Mild to moderate	Severe
Heart rate	Normal or slightly increased	Significantly increased
Blood pressure	Normal	Decreased
Peripheral pulses	Present and normal	Very weak or absent
Mental status	Normal	Decreased to unresponsive
Breathing	Normal or slightly increased	Severely increased, or decreased with severe respiratory distress, or absent
Wheezing	No	Present in all lung fields
Stridor	No	Yes

reaction may rapidly progress to anaphylaxis, the severe reaction. Be prepared to manage the worst-case scenario and continuously reassess the patient's condition.

Patients with anaphylaxis (severe allergic reaction) require immediate and aggressive intervention by the EMT-B. Provide the following emergency care:

1. *Maintain a patent airway.* The patient may initially present with airway compromise associated with swelling of the tissues lining the larynx. Since airway adjuncts are not effective in managing the obstruction, it may be necessary to force air past the swollen tissues by positive pressure ventilation. If using a bag-valve-mask device, you may find it much harder to compress the bag to deliver the contents. It may be necessary to deactivate the popoff valve in order to deliver adequate ventilations. Inserting an oral or nasal airway in the unresponsive patient will help to prevent the tongue from occluding the airway.
2. *Suction any secretions.* In the severe allergic reaction, heavy secretions may be present. Clear the mouth of secretions by suction when necessary.
3. *Maintain oxygen therapy.* It is vital that the patient continuously receive a high concentration of oxygen. If the breathing is adequate, the oxygen should be delivered by a nonrebreather mask at 15 lpm. If the patient is being artificially ventilated, supplemental oxygen must be delivered through the ventilation delivery device.
4. *Be prepared to assist ventilation.* Patients with allergic reactions may not exhibit any respiratory distress during the length of your contact. On the other hand, a patient's condition may progress very rapidly, over minutes, or more slowly, over

hours, and eventually produce severe respiratory distress. Have your ventilation equipment ready and prepared to begin positive pressure ventilation if necessary. It is vital that you continuously reassess breathing status for signs of inadequate breathing.
5. *Administer epinephrine by a prescribed auto-injector.* In a severe reaction, obtain an order from medical direction to administer the patient's prescribed auto-injector. The order may be obtained on-line or off-line. If the patient is suffering from a mild allergic reaction and there are no signs of respiratory compromise (such as breathing difficulty, stridor, wheezing) or shock (weak pulses, decreasing mental status, or low blood pressure), do not administer epinephrine. Consult with medical direction for further orders. If an epinephrine auto-injector is not available, immediately begin transport.
6. *Consider calling for advanced life support.* Because of the potential for severe compromise to the airway, breathing, and circulation, it may be necessary to request ALS for advanced airway control and further administration of medication.
7. *Initiate early transport.* Do not unnecessarily delay transport of the patient. Continued assessment and emergency care can be done en route to the hospital.

ONGOING ASSESSMENT

The ongoing assessment is extremely important in the management of both mild and severe allergic reactions. The patient with a mild reaction should be constantly monitored for indications that the reaction is worsening and that further intervention, such as epinephrine injection or airway control, may be needed. The patient with severe allergic reaction should be reassessed to determine if the injection of epinephrine has been effective in reversing the life-threatening condition.

Regardless of the severity of the reaction, closely reassess the airway, breathing, and circulation status. Signs of deterioration are wheezing or stridor, signs of inadequate breathing, decreasing mental status, decreasing blood pressure, increasing heart rate, weak or absent radial pulses. Reassess and record the baseline vital signs and other reassessment findings.

Reassess the patient 2 minutes after the injection of epinephrine. Look for improvement in the patient's ability to breathe, improvement in his mental status, and an increase in the blood pressure. If the condition has not improved, it may be necessary to consult with medical direction about a second injection if another epinephrine auto-injector is available.

SUMMARY: ASSESSMENT AND CARE

To review assessment findings that may be associated with allergic reaction and emergency care for allergic reaction, see Figures 20-2 and 20-3.

EPINEPHRINE AUTO-INJECTOR

Epinephrine is the drug of choice for the emergency treatment of severe allergic reactions to insect stings or bites, foods, drugs, and other allergens. The drug mimics the responses of the sympathetic nervous system. It quickly constricts blood vessels to improve blood pressure, reduces the leakage from the capillaries, relaxes smooth muscle in the lungs to improve breathing and alleviates wheezing and dyspnea, stimulates the heart, and works to reverse the swelling and hives. The body's response to the drug is rapid; within seconds, the patient will begin to feel relief. However, the duration of the drug's effectiveness is short, about 10 to 20 minutes.

Epinephrine comes packaged in a disposable delivery system for self administration. A common system prescribed to patients is the EpiPen® Auto-injector. The **auto-injector** has a spring-activated, concealed needle that is designed to deliver a precise dose of epinephrine when activated.

The epinephrine auto-injector comes in two different doses (Figure 20-4). An adult EpiPen® with the yellow label delivers 0.3 mg of epinephrine. The injector for infants and children, the EpiPen Jr.® has a white label and delivers 0.15 mg of epinephrine. Because a single dose may not completely reverse

ASSESSMENT SUMMARY

ALLERGIC REACTION

The following are findings that may be associated with allergic reaction.

SCENE SIZE-UP

Ensure your own safety
Look for evidence of cause of allergic reaction:
    Injection (venom, medications)
    Ingestion (foods, medications)
    Inhalation (pollen, chemical irritants)
    Absorption (chemicals, plants)
    Location of patient may provide clues as to cause (e.g., home, physician's office, outdoors, restaurant).

INITIAL ASSESSMENT

General Impression

Feeling of impending doom
Malaise
Weakness
Discomfort

Mental Status

Alert to unresponsive
Decreasing mental status
Increased anxiety
Disorientation
Restlessness
Seizure activity

Airway

Signs of laryngeal edema (stridor, crowing)
Swollen tongue

Breathing

Inadequate ventilation
Wheezing

Circulation

Weak pulses
Tachycardia
Red, warm, dry skin
Cyanosis

Figure 20-2a   Assessment summary: allergic reaction.

(continued on the next

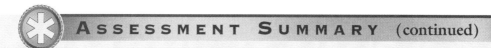

Status: Priority Patient

FOCUSED HISTORY AND PHYSICAL EXAM

SAMPLE History

Signs and Symptoms:
  Tightness in chest
  High-pitched cough
  Impaired ability to talk or hoarseness
  Urgent need to urinate
  Uterine cramping
  Hives and itching
  Red flushed skin
  Stridor or crowing respirations
  Wheezing on auscultation
  Swelling to face, hands, and feet
Ask questions regarding the following:
  Does patient have history of allergy?
  When did the exposure to the allergen occur?
  Can the allergen be identified?
  Has patient ever suffered a reaction before?
  If so, how severe was the reaction?
  Does patient have an epinephrine auto-injector?

Physical Exam

Head, neck, and face:
  Edema to face, hands, neck, and lips
  Hives
  Itching
  Warm tingling feeling

Cyanosis
Difficulty in swallowing
Itchy and watery eyes
Runny or stuffy nose
Coughed-up mucous
Headache
Chest:
  Retractions
  Accessory muscle use
  Wheezing in all lung lobes
Abdomen:
  Nausea/vomiting
  Abdominal cramping
  Diarrhea
  Loss of bowel control
Extremities:
  Warm tingling feeling in hands and feet
  Itching, especially hands and feet
  Edema (swelling) to hands and feet
  Red, warm, dry skin
  Weak or absent peripheral pulses

Baseline Vital Signs

BP: hypotension
HR: tachycardia with weak peripheral pulses
RR: tachypnea with wheezing and labored breathing
Skin: red, warm, dry, hives, itching
Pupils: normal to dilated and responsive to light

EMERGENCY CARE PROTOCOL

ALLERGIC REACTION

1. Establish and maintain open airway.
2. Suction secretions.
3. If breathing is inadequate, provide positive pressure ventilation with supplemental oxygen via reservoir at 12 to 20 ventilations/minute.
4. If breathing is adequate, administer oxygen via nonrebreather mask at 15 lpm.
5. If signs and symptoms of severe allergic reaction and respiratory distress and/or hypotension, administer epinephrine by patient's prescribed auto-injector:
   – Epinephrine is an alpha and beta drug that mimics the sympathetic nervous system and constricts blood vessels, dilates bronchioles, and increases heart rate and contractility.
   – Epinephrine adult dose: 0.3 mg
   – Epinephrine pediatric dose: 0.15 mg
     a. Obtain order from medical direction.
     b. Check medication.

c. Remove safety cap.
d. Press injector firmly against lateral thigh midway between knee and hip.
e. Hold for 10 seconds.
f. Dispose of injector in biohazard sharps container.
g. Record time and reassess patient.
– Epinephrine side effects:
  Increased heart rate
  Pale skin
  Dizziness
  Headache
  Palpitations
  Excitability and anxiousness
  Chest pain
  Nausea and vomiting
6. Consider calling advanced life support.
7. Expedite transport.
8. Perform an ongoing assessment every 5 minutes.

Figure 20-2b Emergency care protocol: allergic reaction.

EMERGENCY CARE ALGORITHM: ALLERGIC REACTION

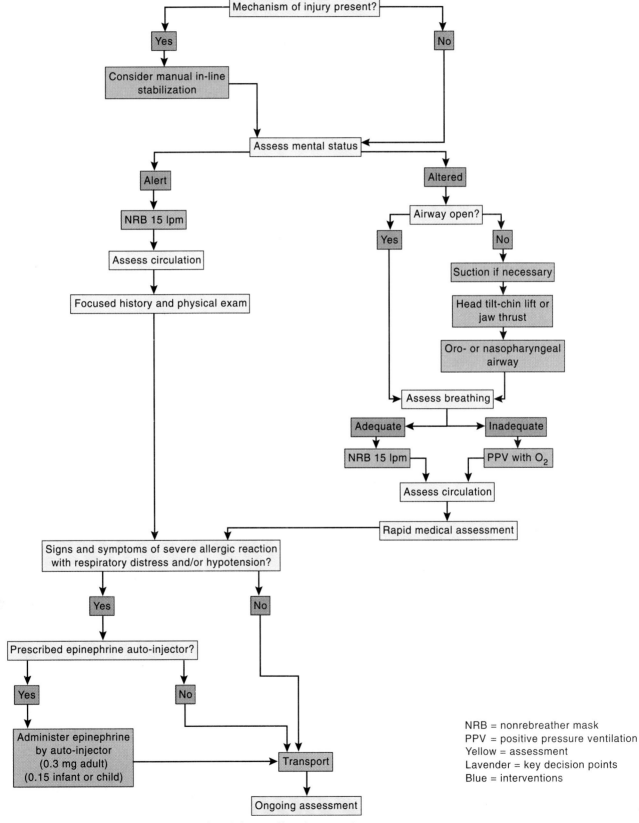

NRB = nonrebreather mask
PPV = positive pressure ventilation
Yellow = assessment
Lavender = key decision points
Blue = interventions

Figure 20-3 *Emergency care algorithm: allergic reaction.*

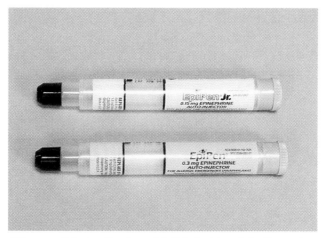

Figure 20-4   Infant/child (white label) and adult (yellow label) epinephrine auto-injectors.

ADMINISTERING AN EPINEPHRINE AUTO-INJECTOR

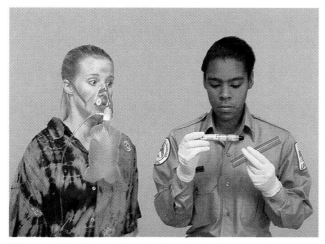

Figure 20-5a   Check the epinephrine auto-injector to ensure it is prescribed for the patient. Check the expiration date and clarity of the drug.

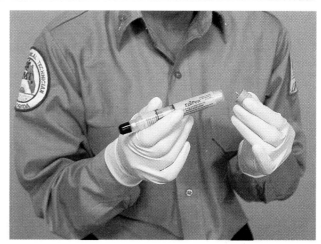

Figure 20-5b   Remove the safety cap from the auto-injector.

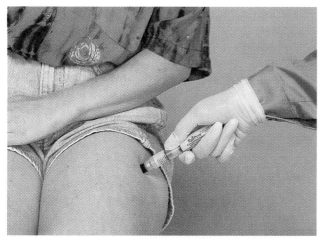

Figure 20-5c   Place the tip of the auto-injector on the lateral aspect of the thigh, midway between the waist and knee. Push the injector firmly against the thigh until it activates. Hold it in place until the medication is injected.

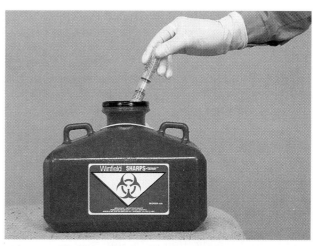

Figure 20-5d   Properly dispose of the auto-injector. Then record the time of the epinephrine injection.

Medication Name

Epinephrine is the generic name. The trade name is Adrenalin®. Trade names of epinephrine auto-injectors are EpiPen® and EpiPen Jr.®

Indications

All of the following criteria must be met before an EMT-B administers epinephrine by auto-injector to the patient:

- The patient exhibits signs and symptoms of a severe allergic reaction (anaphylaxis), including respiratory distress and/or shock (hypoperfusion).
- The medication is prescribed to the patient.
- The EMT-B has received an order from medical direction for administration, either on-line or off-line.

Contraindications

There are no contraindications for the administration of epinephrine in a life-threatening allergic reaction.

Medication Form

Epinephrine is a liquid drug contained within an auto-injector that is designed to automatically inject a precise dose when the safety cap is removed and the auto-injector is pressed firmly against the thigh.

Dosage

Both the adult and infant-and-child auto-injectors deliver a single dose of epinephrine. The adult auto-injector delivers a dose of 0.3 mg of epinephrine. The infant and child auto-injector delivers 0.15 mg of epinephrine. A single dose is administered to the patient. It may be necessary in very severe reactions to administer a second dose. Consult with medical direction or follow your local protocol for the first dose and before any additional dose beyond the first is administered.

Administration

To administer the epinephrine by auto-injector:

1. Obtain an order from medical direction either on-line or off-line.
2. Obtain the patient's prescribed auto-injector. Check the medication to be sure that:
   a. The prescription is written for the patient experiencing the allergic reaction.

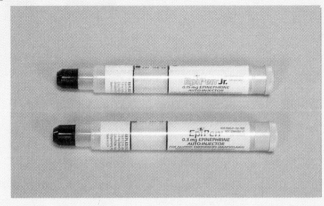

b. The medication has not expired and has not become discolored and does not contain particulates or sediments.
3. Remove the gray safety cap from the auto-injector.
4. Place the tip of the auto-injector against the lateral aspect of the patient's thigh midway between the waist and knee.
5. Push the injector firmly against the thigh until the spring-loaded needle is deployed and the medication is injected.
6. Hold the auto-injector in place until all of the medication has been injected.
7. Dispose of the auto-injector in a biohazard container designed for sharp objects. Be careful not to prick yourself since the needle will now be protruding from the end of the injector.
8. Record that epinephrine was administered, the dose, and the time of administration.

Actions

Epinephrine mimics the responses of the sympathetic nervous system. It quickly constricts blood vessels to improve blood pressure, reduces the leakage from the blood vessels, relaxes smooth muscle in the bronchioles to improve breathing and alleviate the wheezing and dyspnea, stimulates the heartbeat, and works to reverse the swelling and hives. The drug takes effect within seconds, but the duration of its effectiveness is short, about 10 to 20 minutes.

Side Effects

The patient may complain of side effects following the administration of epinephrine. Possible side effects include the following:

- Increased heart rate
- Pale skin (pallor)

Figure 20-6 Epinephrine auto-injector.

EPINEPHRINE AUTO-INJECTOR

- Dizziness
- Chest pain
- Headache
- Nausea and vomiting
- Excitability and anxiousness

Reassessment

Following the administration of epinephrine, it is necessary to reassess the patient. The reassessment should include continued evaluation of the airway, breathing, and circulatory status. Look for the following signs and symptoms that indicate the allergic reaction is worsening:

- Decreasing mental status
- Decreasing blood pressure
- Increased difficulty in breathing

If the condition is worsening, you should consider the following interventions:

- Consult with medical direction about injection of a second dose of epinephrine if a second auto-injector is available.
- Provide emergency care for shock (hypoperfusion).
- Be prepared to initiate positive pressure ventilation with supplemental oxygen if breathing becomes inadequate.
- Be prepared to initiate CPR and apply the AED if the patient becomes pulseless.

If the patient's condition improves following the administration of epinephrine, you should continue to perform ongoing assessments. Be aware that the patient may now complain of side effects from the epinephrine. Continue oxygen therapy with a nonrebreather device and treat for shock, if necessary.

Record and document your interventions and reassessment findings. The baseline vital signs should be checked and recorded every 5 minutes.

Figure 20-6   (continued).

the effects of an anaphylactic reaction, the physician may prescribe more than one injection. It is important to determine if the patient has more than one injector so that you can take it along and be prepared to deliver a second injection.

The auto-injector is simple to use. It is activated by pressing it against the patient's thigh. The pressure releases a spring-activated plunger, pushing the concealed needle into the thigh muscle and injecting a dose of the drug.

No precise location on the thigh is necessary, but the lateral portion of the thigh midway between the waist and knee is preferred. Do not inject the epinephrine into a vein or into the buttocks. It is preferable to remove clothing from the site of injection. If it is too difficult to remove the clothing or if the situation requires immediate administration, the injection can be given directly through the clothing.

See Figures 20-5a to d for an illustration of the process of administering the drug. See Figure 20-6 for a detailed summary of the criteria and techniques for administration of epinephrine.

CASE STUDY FOLLOW-UP

SCENE SIZE-UP

You have been dispatched to a 25-year-old male patient complaining of difficulty in breathing. The patient is located at the Veterans' Pavilion at Mill Run Park. The Metropark Police have been summoned by a bicyclist who found the patient in distress. The scene is safe, and you find the patient sitting on the grass. The police wave frantically for you to hurry. As you approach the patient, you introduce yourselves and ask the patient his name. He is gasping and can barely get out the name "John Freeman." He also offers that he feels "real sick."

INITIAL ASSESSMENT

Your general impression is that the patient, who is dressed in jogging clothes, appears to be having difficulty in breathing. You also note redness and hives that cover his face and neck. The patient is alert and scratching his arms and legs. John responds to questions in one- or two-word phrases with gasps for breath in between. He states, "I—can't—breathe—and—I itch—all over." You hear stridor as he inhales. Audible wheezes are heard on inhalation and exhalation. His breathing is labored at a rate of 28 per minute. Your partner immediately provides oxygen via a nonrebreather mask at 15 lpm. The radial pulse is barely palpable and is estimated at a rate of approximately 130 per minute. The skin is dry and warm to the touch.

Focused History and Physical Exam

You begin your focused history and physical exam by obtaining a SAMPLE history. You use very direct questions that require mostly yes and no answers. You determine that John has the following primary symptoms: severe breathing difficulty, itching all over his body, tightness in his throat, and lightheadedness. He indicates that he is allergic to yellow-jacket stings. He has a prescribed epinephrine auto-injector in a "fanny pack" around his waist. He suffered a similar reaction about 2 years ago, after which his family physician prescribed the auto-injector. His last reaction was so severe that he had to have an endotracheal tube and spent several days in the hospital. He states that the signs, symptoms, and intensity of this reaction are very similar to those of the last one. He last ate at breakfast—a bagel and a cup of coffee.

John states, "I was—jogging on the—trail—when I—felt a sting—in—my left leg. I—ran out of—the woods—to the road. I—felt my—throat—closing and I—began to itch badly." John estimates that it was about 3 minutes from the sting to the onset of signs and symptoms of the reaction.

Your partner is conducting a rapid medical assessment as you gather the history. He finds what appears to be the injection site. It is extremely swollen and red, and has a large area of hives surrounding it. Your partner indicates the blood pressure is low at 82/50 mmHg, the radial pulse is extremely weak and at a fast rate of 132 beats per minute. The respiratory rate is slightly high at 28 and labored. The skin is warm, dry, and red. Hives are found all over the body.

You check the epinephrine auto-injector to be sure it is John's and has not expired. You then contact medical direction at Mercy Hospital for an on-line order to administer the epinephrine. Dr. Westfield gives the order. You recheck the prescription and expiration date and look for any discoloration or sediment. You explain to John that you are going to place the auto-injector against the outer part of his thigh and that he will feel a pinch when the medication is injected. You then administer the epinephrine.

You and your partner place John in a semi-sitting position on the stretcher, maintaining oxygen therapy, and begin transport.

Ongoing Assessment

After about 2 minutes, you reassess the patient and find that the breathing is much less labored and that the wheezing has significantly decreased. John says, "Gosh, I feel much better. I can actually breathe now. I feel real nervous though, and my heart is really pounding hard. Is that normal?" You assure him that those are normal side effects from the epinephrine. Your partner indicates that the blood pressure is now higher at 112/68 mmHg, the radial pulse is much stronger now and at a slower rate of 109 per minute. The skin looks less red and the hives are beginning to disappear. You record your treatment, the time of epinephrine administration, and your reassessment findings.

A few minutes later, you again ask John about the symptoms he is currently experiencing. He says his breathing is much easier now, and he no longer feels dizzy or lightheaded. He states, "I'm still pretty itchy though!" You find upon reassessment of the vital signs that the blood pressure is now up to 124/82 mmHg and that the heart rate has decreased to 98 per minute. You contact the hospital and report the patient's condition and give an estimated time of arrival.

Upon arrival at the hospital, you give an oral report to the triage nurse. She says, "Go ahead to Room 9. Dr. Westfield is waiting for you." There, you report to Dr. Westfield the findings of the assessments before and after the epinephrine injection. As you are leaving the room, the doctor joins you for a moment and says, "You know, you've more than likely just saved this guy's life."

With a large grin on your face, you walk back to the ambulance, where your partner indicates that the unit is restocked and set for the next run. You complete your prehospital care report and notify dispatch that you are back in service.

CHAPTER REVIEW

TERMS AND CONCEPTS

You may wish to review the following terms and concepts included in this chapter.

allergen—a substance that enters the body by ingestion, injection, inhalation, or contact and triggers an allergic reaction.

allergic reaction—a misdirected and excessive response by the immune system to a foreign substance or an allergen.

anaphylactic shock—a shock (hypoperfusion) state that results from dilated and leaking blood vessels related to severe allergic reaction. It is also called anaphylaxis or anaphylactic reaction. See also *anaphylaxis.*

anaphylaxis—a severe allergic reaction that produces respiratory distress and shock (hypoperfusion). See also *anaphylactic shock.*

antibodies—special proteins produced by the immune system that search out antigens, combine with, and help to destroy them.

antigen—a foreign substance that enters the body and triggers an immune response.

auto-injector—a device with a concealed, spring-loaded needle, used for injecting a single dose of medication. An epinephrine auto-injector is often prescribed to patients with a history of anaphylactic reaction.

endotracheal intubation—placement of a tube down the trachea to facilitate air flow into the lungs and aid in breathing.

epinephrine—a medication that constricts blood vessels to improve blood pressure, reduces leakage from capillaries, and relaxes smooth muscle in the bronchioles; often prescribed in single-dose auto-injector form to patients with a history of anaphylactic reaction.

hives—raised, red blotches associated with some allergic reactions.

immune response—production of antibodies by the immune system to fight off invasion by foreign substances.

immune system—the body's defense mechanism against invasion by foreign substances.

malaise—a general feeling of weakness or discomfort.

sensitization—the process by which antibodies are produced after exposure to an antigen.

REVIEW QUESTIONS

1. Explain the meaning of *sensitization* in relation to allergic reaction.
2. List the four routes through which an allergen can be introduced into the body.
3. List the major categories of common causes of allergic reaction and give examples of each category.
4. Describe the airway complications that may occur in anaphylaxis and the appropriate management of them.
5. List the common signs and symptoms of allergic reaction and anaphylaxis in relation to the following body systems/categories: skin, respiratory system, cardiovascular system, central nervous system, gastrointestinal system, genitourinary system, generalized signs and symptoms.
6. Name the two key categories of signs and symptoms of a severe allergic reaction (anaphylaxis).
7. Describe the difference in emergency medical treatment for (a) a mild allergic reaction, and (b) a severe allergic reaction (anaphylaxis).
8. List the indications and contraindications for the epinephrine auto-injector.
9. Describe the method of administration of the epinephrine auto-injector.
10. Describe the actions and possible side effects of the epinephrine auto-injector.

CHAPTER 21

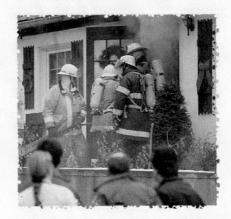

Poisoning Emergencies

INTRODUCTION

Each year in the United States, thousands of people die or become extremely ill from intentional or accidental poisoning. Most calls to poison control centers involve children, especially toddlers who get into and swallow poisonous substances while exploring their environment. Most poisonings occur at home and involve drugs, cleaning substances, and cosmetics. In addition, poisonings result from exposure to industrial chemicals, pesticides, and other substances encountered in the workplace or outdoor environment.

When EMS is promptly called, and the appropriate assessment, emergency care, and transport are provided, most cases of poisoning can have a successful outcome.

OBJECTIVES

Numbered objectives are from the United States Department of Transportation 1994 EMT-Basic National Standard Curriculum. Asterisked objectives, if any, pertain to material that is supplemental to the DOT curriculum.

COGNITIVE

4-6.1 List various ways that poisons enter the body. (p. 391)

4-6.2 List signs/symptoms associated with poisoning. (pp. 393, 398, 399, 400)

4-6.3 Discuss the emergency medical care for the patient with possible overdose. (pp. 393–395, 399–400)

4-6.4 Describe the steps in the emergency medical care for the patient with suspected poisoning. (pp. 393–395, 398, 399–400, 400–401)

4-6.5 Establish the relationship between the patient suffering from poisoning or overdose and airway management. (pp. 392, 393–394, 398, 399, 400)

4-6.6 State the generic and trade names, indications, contraindications, medication form, dose, administration, actions, side effects, and re-assessment strategies for activated charcoal. (p. 396)

4-6.7 Recognize the need for medical direction in caring for the patient with poisoning or overdose. (pp. 394, 395, 396)

AFFECTIVE

4-6.8 Explain the rationale for administering activated charcoal. (p. 395)

4-6.9 Explain the rationale for contacting medical direction early in the prehospital management of the poisoning or overdose patient. (pp. 394, 395, 396)

PSYCHOMOTOR

4-6.10 Demonstrate the steps in the emergency medical care for the patient with possible overdose.

4-6.11 Demonstrate the steps in the emergency medical care for the patient with suspected poisoning.

4-6.12 Perform the necessary steps required to provide a patient with activated charcoal.

4-6.13 Demonstrate the assessment and documentation of patient response.

4-6.14 Demonstrate proper disposal of the equipment for the administration of activated charcoal.

4-6.15 Demonstrate completing a prehospital care report for patients with a poisoning/overdose emergency.

Objectives from DOT lesson 4-6 relating to overdose are also addressed in Chapter 22, "Drug and Alcohol Emergencies."

CASE STUDY

THE DISPATCH

EMS Unit 101—proceed to 1445 Cohasset Drive—you have a 3-year-old patient with abdominal pain. Time out is 1236 hours.

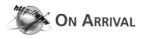 **ON ARRIVAL**

A frantic woman holding a child rushes out the door. She seems about 35 years old and identifies herself as Mrs. Horowitz. She tells you that she thinks her daughter Sophie ate the leaves of a house plant and that she has bad stomach pains.

How would you proceed to assess and care for this patient?

During this chapter, you will learn about assessment and emergency care for patients suffering from various types of poisonings. Later, we will return to the case and apply the procedures learned.

POISONS AND AIRWAY MANAGEMENT

A **poison** is any substance—liquid, solid, or gas—that impairs health or causes death by its chemical action when it enters the body or comes into contact with the skin.

Poisons may enter the body in the following ways:

- **Ingestion** by swallowing of solids or liquids
- **Inhalation** of gases, fumes, or mists
- **Injection** into the body with syringes or by bites or stings
- **Absorption** through or by contact with the skin or mucous membranes

No matter what else is done regarding poisoning treatment, if the airway and ventilations are not assured, the patient will die. Many poisons—especially those that are ingested—can also cause vomiting. Unless other injuries prevent it, keep the patient in a lateral recumbent position (on the side) to prevent aspiration, and be prepared to suction if necessary.

In poisonings, you will spend more time treating threats to the airway, breathing, and circulation caused by the poisoning than you will giving specific antidotes for the poisoning or overdose. Whether poison enters the body through ingestion, inhalation, injection, or absorption, you will be treating the patient based upon the presenting signs and symptoms rather than upon the exact substance or route by which it was taken in.

 INGESTED POISONS

In the United States alone, millions of poisonings from ingestion occur each year, and thousands of those victims die. The most common agents involved are aspirin, acetaminophen, alcohol, detergents or soaps, and petroleum distillates. More detailed information on specific alcohol and drug overdose emergencies is found in Chapter 22, "Drug and Alcohol Emergencies."

The chief causes of poisoning by ingestion are:

- Overdose of medicine
- Combining drugs and alcohol
- Storing poisons in food or drink containers
- Medicines, household cleaners, and chemicals within the reach of children
- Poisonous plants within the reach of children

The ingestion of poisonous plants is an extremely common poisoning emergency, especially in children under the age of 5. Poisonous plants are not necessarily exotic—they include common household and backyard plants, such as morning glory, rhubarb leaves, buttercup, daisy, daffodil, lily of the valley, narcissus, tulip, azalea, English ivy, mistletoe berries, iris, hyacinth, laurel, philodendron, rhododendron, wisteria, and certain parts of the tomato, potato, and petunia plants. A very high number of plant poisonings involve eating wild mushrooms.

ASSESSMENT AND CARE: INGESTED POISONS

SCENE SIZE-UP

Clues indicating that there has been an ingested poisoning can often be spotted during scene size-up. You may observe overturned or empty medicine bottles, scattered pills or capsules, recently emptied containers, spilled chemicals, spilled cleaning solvents, an overturned plant or pieces of plant, the remains of food or drink, or vomitus.

INITIAL ASSESSMENT

Even when clues at the scene and information from family members make it clear that the patient has probably swallowed something poisonous, do not skip the initial assessment. Many ingested poisons cause damage to or swelling of the airway. It is extremely important to be alert to airway swelling in any type of overdose. The swelling of the respiratory structures can occlude the airway and reduce or prohibit air exchange. Any patient who has ingested a poison that causes swelling or occlusion of the airway must be transported to the hospital as a priority patient.

FOCUSED HISTORY AND PHYSICAL EXAM

Most information about an ingested poisoning will be obtained during the focused history and physical exam. If the patient is a child, other children in the house may have also swallowed the poison, so assess all children carefully. Don't forget that children often ingest more than one poison at a time—especially if they find several bottles of pills or cleaning supplies kept in one place. Watch for the most common poisons ingested by children: plants, cleaning products kept under the kitchen sink (Figure 21-1), automotive supplies (such as windshield cleaning fluid) kept in the garage, medications (especially liquids), and toiletries (such as cologne, after-shave, and mouthwash).

Begin the focused history and physical exam by obtaining information about the patient. Getting a SAMPLE history from a poisoning victim can be difficult, and the history you do get may not be accurate; the victim may be misinformed, may be subject to a drug-induced confusion, or may be deliberately

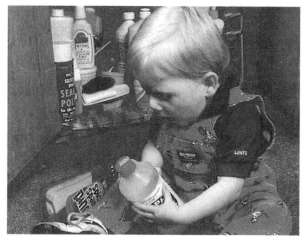

Figure 21-1　Poisoning is the number one cause of accidental death among children.

trying to deceive you. Never completely trust history in cases of intentional overdose. To manage a poisoning patient correctly, however, you need a relevant history. If the patient is unable or unwilling to communicate, you will need to question relatives or bystanders. During the SAMPLE history, it is important to ask the following questions:

- *Was any substance ingested?* The answer to this question will help in determining if activated charcoal will be administered. (Remember to ask about over-the-counter medications; these can also be very harmful.)
- *When did the patient ingest the poison?* (or) *When was the patient exposed to the poison?* This will let you determine the span of time between the exposure and the onset of symptoms. Generally the faster the onset the more serious the condition.
- *Over what time period was the substance ingested?* (or) *Over what time period was the patient exposed to the poisonous substance?* This is another indicator of the seriousness of the poisoning.
- *How much of the substance was taken?*
- *Has anyone attempted to treat the poisoning?* Someone may have tried to induce vomiting or give some type of antidote.
- *Does the patient have a psychiatric history that may suggest a possible suicide attempt?*
- *Does the patient have an underlying medical illness, allergy, chronic drug use, or addiction?*
- *How much does the patient weigh?* This is necessary to administer the proper dose of activated charcoal.

If the patient was able to provide an adequate history, conduct a focused assessment of the areas in which the patient has a complaint, sign, or symptom. If in doubt, or if the patient is unresponsive or unable to provide an adequate history, perform a rapid as-

sessment. Assess the head, neck, chest, abdomen, pelvis, extremities, and posterior body. Inspect and palpate for any deformities, contusions, abrasions, punctures or penetrations, burns, tenderness, lacerations, and swelling (DCAP-BTLS). This is especially urgent for the patient who may have suffered trauma secondary to the poisoning, or vice-versa.

Record the baseline vital signs, but realize that vitals have a limited role in establishing the degree of distress caused by a poisoning. Rather, you should use other clinical findings indicative of the seriousness of the condition (e.g., diminished mental status, fast or slow heart rate, seizures).

Signs and Symptoms　The signs and symptoms of poisoning by ingestion vary, depending on what was ingested. *A seriously poisoned person may have few or no signs or symptoms,* so don't gauge the severity of the emergency on signs and symptoms alone.

The most common signs and symptoms are listed below. See Figure 21-2 for an illustration of possible indicators of ingested poisoning in children.

- A history of ingestion
- Swelling of mucosal membranes in the mouth
- Nausea
- Vomiting
- Diarrhea
- Altered mental status
- Abdominal pain, tenderness, distention, and/or cramps
- Burns or stains around the mouth (Figure 21-3), pain in the mouth or throat, and/or pain during swallowing (corrosive poisons may corrode, burn, or destroy the tissues of the mouth, throat, and stomach)
- Unusual breath or body odors; characteristic chemical odors (such as turpentine) on the breath
- Respiratory distress
- Altered heart rate (fast or slow)
- Altered blood pressure (high or low)
- Dilated or constricted pupils
- Warm and dry or cool and moist skin

EMERGENCY MEDICAL CARE

Specific treatment for a patient who is known to have ingested a poison is as follows:

1. *Maintain the airway.* Use gloves to remove any remaining pills, tablets, capsules, or other fragments from the patient's mouth, taking care not to injure yourself. If the patient is unresponsive, maintain an open airway with an oropharyngeal or nasopharyngeal airway. Secretions may be profuse following the ingestion of certain poisons, so be prepared to suction. *Remember: a poisoning patient's status*

POSSIBLE INDICATORS OF INGESTED POISONING IN CHILDREN

PAY PARTICULAR ATTENTION TO:

The child who has swallowed a poison before.

The level of responsiveness, including any behavioral changes (clumsiness? drowsiness? coma? convulsions? mental disturbances? delirium?)

Skin and mucosa findings (color, temperature of skin, lips, mucous membranes?)

Temperature, blood pressure, pulse rate, respiratory alterations?

Paralysis?

Constriction   Dilation

The size and reaction of pupils (constriction? dilation?)

Mouth signs (burns? discoloration? dryness? excessive salivation? stains? characteristic breath odors? pain on swallowing?)

Nausea, vomiting (appearance? odor? blood present?)

Diarrhea? odor? appearance? blood present?

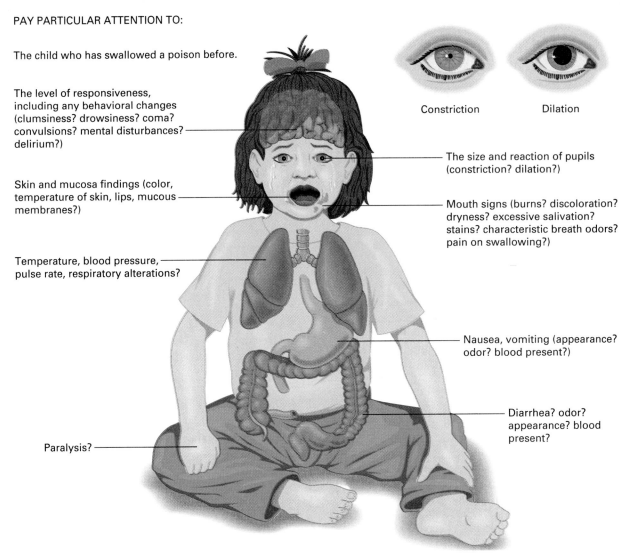

Figure 21-2   Possible indicators of ingested poisoning in children.

can change suddenly. Be prepared to protect the patient from aspiration. If possible, place the patient in the lateral recumbent position in case of vomiting.

2. *Provide oxygen or assist ventilations.* Ensure oxygenation at 15 lpm via a nonrebreather mask, or provide positive pressure ventilation with supplemental oxygen if breathing is inadequate.

3. *Prevent further injury.* If a child has handled or been poisoned by a corrosive, protect yourself while washing the child's hands and fingers and rinsing the child's mouth and lips to remove traces of the corrosive. Be careful when rinsing the mouth that the patient does not swallow the liquid. *Do not flush the mouth of an unresponsive patient as he may aspirate the fluid.*

4. *During transport, consult medical direction* or, if your protocols mandate, contact the poison control center. In most areas, you may be instructed to administer activated charcoal. Follow local protocol. Details on administering activated charcoal are found later in this chapter.

5. *Bring suspected poisons to the receiving facility.* Bring the container and all of its remaining contents, the plant portions or parts that might have been ingested, or other specimens to the receiving facility. Remember to bring all possible containers and labels. If a plant was ingested, bring the remaining roots, leaves, stems, flowers, or fruit. If the patient has vomited, bring a sample of the vomitus in a clean, closed container to the receiving facility.

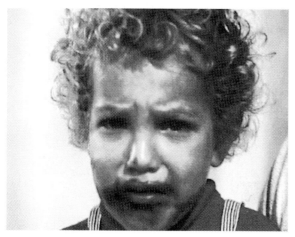

Figure 21-3   Discoloration or burns around the mouth are a sign of possible poisoning.

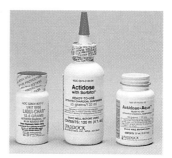

Figure 21-4   Several brands and forms of activated charcoal are available.

DETAILED PHYSICAL EXAM AND ONGOING ASSESSMENT

If injury is suspected or the patient is unresponsive, perform a detailed physical exam en route to the hospital. Provide an ongoing assessment with particular attention to the status of the patient's airway and breathing. If the patient is unstable, you should repeat the ongoing assessment every 5 minutes. Be sure to contact the receiving hospital so they can prepare for the patient's arrival.

ACTIVATED CHARCOAL

The medication of choice in the emergency medical care of ingested poisonings is **activated charcoal.** It is a special distilled charcoal treated with superheated steam. It is extremely porous and therefore can adsorb (collect onto its surfaces) many times its weight in contaminants. The adsorption of the poison by the activated charcoal inhibits the poison from being absorbed into the body. It works best when used promptly after the poisoning, but it can still be effective after several hours—as long as 4 hours after ingestion for some poisons. (Some poisons may slow the movement of ingested material through the gastrointestinal tract.)

Some of the trade names of activated charcoal (Figure 21-4) are:

- SuperChar
- InstaChar
- Actidose
- Liqui-Char

Not all brands of activated charcoal are the same; some have the ability to adsorb much more poison than others. Consult medical direction about which you should carry and use. Some activated charcoal products contain a laxative agent (cathartic) that helps speed it through the intestinal tract, further limiting any absorption of the toxin into the body.

See Figure 21-5 for a detailed summary of the criteria and techniques for administration of activated charcoal. See Figures 21-6a to c illustrating how to administer activated charcoal to a patient.

Activated charcoal should be used for a patient who has ingested poisons by mouth, upon orders from medical direction and/or the poison control center. Remember that activated charcoal should not be administered to patients who have an altered mental status because of possible aspiration, to patients who have swallowed acids or alkalis (such as hydrochloric acid, bleach, ammonia, or isolated ethanol ingestion), or to patients who are unable to swallow.

In the field, use activated charcoal that has been pre-mixed with water. The most common brands contain 12.5 grams of activated charcoal mixed with water in a plastic bottle. Activated charcoal is also available in powder form; the powder must be mixed with water before it can be administered to a patient. The use of powdered activated charcoal is discouraged in the field. Follow local protocol.

INHALED POISONS

Thousands of people also die each year in the United States from inhaling poisonous vapors and fumes, some of which are present without any sign. Most toxic inhalation occurs as a result of fire. It is critical that care be immediate, because the body absorbs inhaled poisons rapidly. The longer the exposure without treatment, the poorer the prognosis.

Common inhaled poisons include:

- Carbon monoxide
- Carbon dioxide from industrial sites, sewers, and wells

ACTIVATED CHARCOAL

Medication Name

Activated charcoal is the generic name. Some of the better-known trade names of activated charcoal are:

- SuperChar
- InstaChar
- Actidose
- Liqui-Char

Indications

Activated charcoal should be used for a patient who has ingested poisons by mouth, upon orders from medical direction.

Contraindications

Activated charcoal should not be administered to a patient who:

- Has an altered mental status (is not fully alert) because it may cause aspiration
- Has swallowed acids or alkalis (such as hydrochloric acid, bleach, ammonia, ethanol)
- Is unable to swallow

Medication Form

1. Pre-mixed in water, frequently available in a plastic bottle containing 12.5 grams of activated charcoal
2. Powder — should be avoided in the field

Dosage

Unless directed otherwise by medical direction, give both adults and children 1 gram of activated charcoal per kilogram of body weight. The usual adult dose is 25 to 50 grams. The usual dose for infants and children is 12.5 to 25 grams.

Administration

To administer activated charcoal:

1. Consult medical direction or the poison control center, according to local protocol, before administering activated charcoal to any patient. Directions that follow are general. Always follow the orders of medical direction or local protocol.
2. Shake the container of activated charcoal thoroughly; if it is too thick to shake well, remove the cap and stir it until well mixed. The activated charcoal settles to the bottom of the bottle, and needs to be evenly distributed.

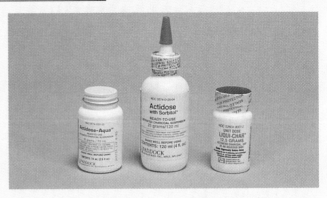

3. Activated charcoal looks like mud. The patient may be more willing to drink it if he can't see it — through a straw from a covered opaque container.
4. If the activated charcoal settles, shake or stir it again before letting the patient finish the dose.
5. Record the time and the patient response.
6. If the patient vomits, notify medical control to authorize one repeat of the dose.

Once you have given a patient activated charcoal, don't let the patient have milk, ice cream, or sherbet; these all decrease the effectiveness of activated charcoal.

Action

Activated charcoal adsorbs poisons in the stomach, prevents their absorption by the body, and enhances their elimination from the body. The ability of activated charcoal to adsorb poisons is due to a distilling process that makes it extremely porous. Activated charcoal does not bind to (is not effective for) alcohol, kerosene, gasoline, caustics, or metals, such as iron.

Side Effects

The most common side effect is blackening of the stools. Some patients, especially those who are already nauseated, may vomit. If the patient vomits, repeat the dose of activated charcoal once. Be alert for further vomiting, and transport as soon as possible. Other side effects are rare.

Reassessment

During administration assure that the patient's airway and mental status are adequate so the patient does not aspirate the medication. Check for abdominal pain or distress upon administration. Watch for possible vomiting after administration and prevent aspiration by placing the patient in a sitting or lateral recumbent position and being prepared to suction.

Figure 21-5 Activated charcoal.

ADMINISTERING ACTIVATED CHARCOAL

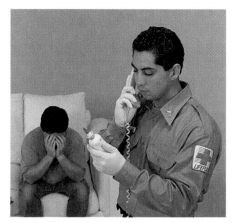

Figure 21-6a *Obtain an order from medical direction.*

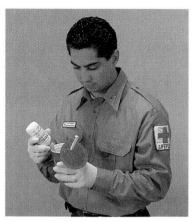

Figure 21-6b *Place the activated charcoal in a cup with a lid. A straw may also help to improve the patient's willingness to drink the charcoal.*

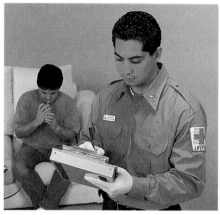

Figure 21-6c *Record the dose and time the charcoal was administered.*

- Chlorine gas (common around swimming pools)
- Fumes from liquid chemicals and sprays
- Ammonia
- Sulfur dioxide (used to make ice)
- Anesthetic gases (ether, nitrous oxide, chloroform)
- Solvents used in dry cleaning, degreasing agents, or fire extinguishers
- Industrial gases
- Incomplete combustion of natural gas
- Hydrogen sulfide (sewer gas)

ASSESSMENT AND CARE: INHALED POISONS

SCENE SIZE-UP

During the scene size-up, ensuring your safety is of prime importance. You should be acutely aware of peculiar odors or visible fumes. At the same time understand that some gases (e.g., carbon monoxide) can be odorless and colorless. Therefore, remember that the absence of odor does not guarantee safe air for breathing. You also need to ensure scene safety so that bystanders will not be injured.

If the information given by those present (or their behavior) or the presence of any hazardous materials placards at the scene indicate that toxic fumes may be present, be sure that you are wearing self-contained breathing apparatus before entering the scene. If you are not properly equipped or trained for hazardous materials rescue, call for assistance from those who are. Have those who are properly trained and equipped bring the patient or patients out of the toxic environment (Figure 21-7). Do not enter the scene unless

they tell you it is safe. As soon as you are able, determine the number of persons at the scene who may have inhaled the poison. There are likely to be more patients than the one for whom EMS was originally called. Call for additional ambulances as needed.

INITIAL ASSESSMENT

During the initial assessment of a patient who may have inhaled a poison, pay special attention to the patient's airway and breathing. Inhaled poisons may rapidly cause breathing difficulty. Be sure to properly ventilate and oxygenate your patient as appropriate. Make a decision about the patient's priority for transport.

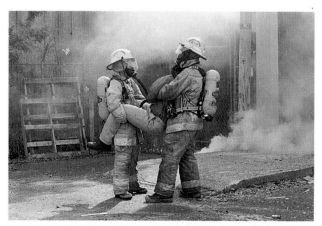

Figure 21-7 *Protect yourself. Have trained rescuers remove the patient from the toxic environment.*

FOCUSED HISTORY AND PHYSICAL EXAM

During the focused history and physical exam, get a SAMPLE history from the patient or bystanders and as much information as you can about the substance that has been inhaled. Also keep in mind that the patient may be a victim of trauma. For example, an explosion could have rendered the patient unresponsive, which caused him to inhale the poisonous fumes from the explosion itself.

Remember to ask the patient or bystanders questions about what was inhaled, when and how long it was inhaled, and what treatments might have been attempted. In addition, you should ask:

- *Does the patient have a history that suggests a possible suicide attempt?* (more common in apparently intentional carbon monoxide poisonings)
- *Did the exposure occur in an open or a confined space?*
- *How long was the patient exposed?*

If the patient is responsive enough to provide you with an adequate history, perform a focused assessment of the areas in which the patient has a complaint, sign, or symptom. If in doubt, or if the patient is unresponsive and unable to provide you with an adequate history, perform a rapid assessment. Obtain and record the patient's baseline vital signs.

Signs and Symptoms Signs and symptoms of inhaled poisoning include:

- A history of inhalation of a toxic substance
- Difficulty breathing or shortness of breath
- Chest pain or tightness; a burning sensation in the chest or throat
- Cough, stridor, wheezing, or rales
- Hoarseness
- Dizziness
- Headache, often severe
- Confusion
- Seizures
- Altered mental status, possible unresponsiveness
- Cyanosis
- Respiratory rate faster or slower than normal
- Nausea/vomiting (carbon monoxide poisoning)

Signs of respiratory tract burns include:

- Singed nasal hairs
- Soot in the sputum
- Soot in the throat

EMERGENCY MEDICAL CARE

Remember that respiratory symptoms are typically the first to appear with inhalation injuries. Specific treatment to include when treating a patient known to have inhaled poisonous gases/fumes is as follows:

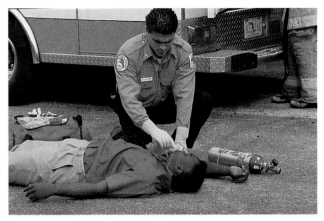

Figure 21-8 Administer oxygen to the inhaled poisoning patient.

1. *Get the patient out of the toxic environment as quickly as possible.*
2. *Have the patient lie down with the head elevated* if there are no injuries that would prevent it and no suspicion of spinal injury. Loosen all tight-fitting clothing, especially around the neck and over the chest.
3. *As soon as possible, administer oxygen by nonrebreather mask* (Figure 21-8).
4. *Start positive pressure ventilation with supplemental oxygen immediately* if the patient is not breathing or has inadequate breathing.
5. *Bring all containers, bottles, labels, or other clues about the poisoning agent to the receiving facility.*

DETAILED PHYSICAL EXAM AND ONGOING ASSESSMENT

Any time the patient is unresponsive or trauma is suspected, perform a detailed physical exam to determine if there are any other injuries that need to be managed. Provide an ongoing assessment en route to the hospital with particular attention to the patient's airway and breathing. Reassess vital signs and treat any respiratory compromise which may develop.

INJECTED POISONS

Injected poisons are those that enter the body through a break in the skin—sometimes by the intentional injection of drugs, other times by the bites or stings of animals and insects. Drugs may be injected under the skin, into the muscle, or directly into the blood stream. Information on specific drug-related emergencies is found in Chapter 22, "Drug and Alcohol Emergencies."

The most common sources of injected poisons are bites and stings. Most common are stings from bees, wasps, hornets, yellow jackets, and ants; others include the bites of spiders, ticks, marine animals (such as jellyfish, coral, anemones, and stingrays), and snakes (Figure 21-9). Injected poisons generally cause an immediate reaction at the injection site followed by a delayed systemic reaction. Of special note is the threat of anaphylactic shock following the allergic reaction to an insect bite or sting (see Chapter 20, "Allergic Reactions"). As many as 100 people in the United States die from bee stings each year. More detailed information on bites and stings is found in Chapter 24, "Environmental Emergencies."

ASSESSMENT AND CARE: INJECTED POISONS

SCENE SIZE-UP

Make note of clues such as discarded syringes or other drug paraphernalia. Consider the possibility of a bite or sting in an outdoor environment, e.g., a sting by a marine life form at a beach or by an insect at a picnic area.

INITIAL ASSESSMENT

Carefully assess the patient's airway and breathing. Assess the mental status and determine if the patient is a high priority for transport.

FOCUSED HISTORY AND PHYSICAL EXAM

During the focused history and physical exam, get a SAMPLE history from the patient or bystanders and as much information as you can about any substance that may have been injected or about the kind of insect or animal that may have inflicted a bite or sting.

Remember to ask the patient or bystanders the following questions pertaining to injected poisons:

- *Does the patient have a history of drug use?* (Bystanders and patient may be unwilling to answer this.)
- *Does the patient have a history of allergic reaction to bites or stings?*

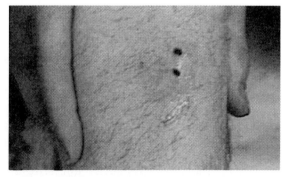

Figure 21-9   Rattlesnake bite.

- *What was the time lapse between the injection and onset of signs and symptoms?*

If the patient is responsive enough to provide you with an adequate history, perform a focused assessment of the areas in which the patient has a complaint, sign, or symptom. If in doubt, or if the patient is unresponsive, or if the patient is unable to provide you with an adequate history, perform a rapid assessment. Obtain and record the patient's baseline vital signs.

Signs and Symptoms   General signs and symptoms of toxic injection include the following:

- Weakness
- Dizziness
- Chills
- Fever
- Nausea
- Vomiting
- High or low blood pressure
- Pupillary changes
- Needle tracks
- Pain at the site of injection
- Trouble breathing
- Abnormal skin vitals (color/temperature/condition)
- Possible paralysis
- Swelling and redness at the site of injection

EMERGENCY MEDICAL CARE

Treatment for a patient known suffered to have a toxic injection is as follows:

1. *Maintain the patient's airway.* If appropriate, insert an oropharyngeal airway if the patient does not have a gag reflex. Use a nasopharyngeal airway if the patient has a depressed mental status but will not accept an oropharyngeal airway. Suction vomitus or secretions.
2. *Administer oxygen* at 15 lpm by nonrebreather mask, *or begin positive pressure ventilations with supplemental oxygen* if the patient's respirations become inadequate.
3. *Be alert for vomiting.* Position the patient in a lateral recumbent (coma or recovery) position to help prevent aspiration, and be prepared to suction if necessary.
4. *In the case of a bite or sting, protect yourself from injury and protect the patient from repeated injection.* Move the patient away from any insects that are still swarming. Bees can sting only once, then lose their stinger—but wasps, hornets, and yellow jackets can sting repeatedly.
5. *Bring all containers, bottles, labels, or other evidence of poisonous substances to the receiving facility.* If the patient was bitten or stung, try to iden-

tify the insect, reptile, or animal that caused the injury (without getting close enough to endanger yourself if it is still alive). If it is dead, bring it to the receiving facility with the patient.

DETAILED PHYSICAL EXAM AND ONGOING ASSESSMENT

If injury is suspected, perform a detailed physical exam en route to the hospital. Provide an ongoing assessment with particular attention to the airway and breathing. Monitor the patient for possible development of an anaphylactic reaction. Notify the hospital en route so they can prepare for the patient.

ABSORBED POISONS

Absorbed poisons—usually chemicals or substances from poisonous plants that enter through the skin—generally cause burns, lesions, and inflammation. The risk of exposure to a hazardous substance is increasing as more chemicals are used in farming and in everyday objects. A dog's flea collar, for example, could be dangerous to an infant if he put it in his mouth because the chemical in the flea collar could be absorbed by the mucous membranes of the mouth.

Skin reactions range from mild irritation to severe chemical burns. Absorbed poisons often cause both local and systemic reactions, which can be severe. Exposure of as little as 2.5 percent of the body surface to 100 percent hydrofluoric acid, for example, can cause death.

ASSESSMENT AND CARE: ABSORBED POISONS

SCENE SIZE-UP

Make note of any open containers of chemicals or poisonous plants in the environment. Wear gloves and other protective gear as needed to ensure that the harmful substances do not come into contact with your own skin. Call for additional help if more than one patient is injured. Patients should be removed from the dangerous area as soon as possible.

INITIAL ASSESSMENT

Carefully assess the patient's airway and breathing. Some types of absorbed poisons can cause muscle paralysis or weakness and compromise the patient's respiratory status. Or, an altered mental status secondary to the effects of the absorbed poison could cause the jaw and tongue to relax and block the airway. Inspect the patient for any poison that may still be on the person's body or clothes.

FOCUSED HISTORY AND PHYSICAL EXAM

During the focused history and physical exam, get a SAMPLE history from the patient or bystanders and as much information as you can about any substance that may have been absorbed.

If the patient is responsive enough to provide you with an adequate history, perform an assessment focused on the areas in which the patient has a complaint, sign, or symptom. If in doubt, or if the patient is unresponsive or unable to provide you with an adequate history, perform a rapid assessment. Obtain and record the patient's baseline vital signs.

Signs and Symptoms   Signs and symptoms of an absorbed poison include:

- A history of exposure to a poisonous substance
- Traces of liquid or powder on the patient's skin
- Burns
- Itching and/or irritation
- Redness
- Swelling

Signs and symptoms of contact with a poisonous plant include:

- Fluid-filled, oozing blisters
- Itching and burning
- Swelling
- Possible pain
- A rash (If the rash is scratched, secondary infections can occur.)

EMERGENCY MEDICAL CARE

If poison has been absorbed through the skin, the following specific treatment should be included:

1. *Protecting your hands with gloves, move the patient from the source of the poison and remove the patient's contaminated clothing and jewelry.*
2. *Carefully monitor the airway and respiratory status.* Apply oxygen, and provide ventilations if appropriate.
3. *Brush any dry chemicals or solid toxins from the patient's skin,* taking extreme care not to abrade the skin or spread the contamination (Figure 21-10).
4. *If the poison is liquid, irrigate all parts of the body with clean water for at least 20 minutes.* (a shower or garden hose is ideal.) Carefully check "hidden" areas, such as the nail beds, skin creases, areas between the fingers and toes, and hair. Continue irrigation en route to the receiving facility if possible. If the poison is a dry powder, brush off the substance and continue the treatment for other absorbed poisons.

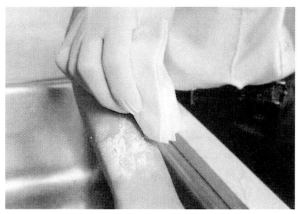

Figure 21-10   Brush dry powder off the patient. Then flush with clean water to remove poison on the surface of the skin.

If poison has been splashed into the eye:

1. *Irrigate the affected eye with clean water for at least 20 minutes* (Figure 21-11); continue irrigation while en route to the receiving facility, if possible. Position the patient so water runs away from the unaffected eye, taking care not to spread the contamination. Further details on treating chemical burns of the eye will be found in Chapter 35, "Eye, Face, and Neck Injuries."

DETAILED PHYSICAL EXAM AND ONGOING ASSESSMENT

Complete a detailed physical exam, noting any other abnormalities, and contact the receiving hospital. Provide an ongoing assessment en route to the hos-

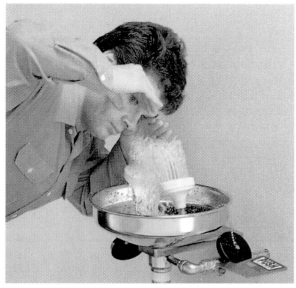

Figure 21-11   Irrigate chemical burns of the eye with clean water for at least 20 minutes.

pital with particular attention to the status of the patient's airway and breathing.

SUMMARY: ASSESSMENT AND CARE

To review assessment findings and care for poisoning emergencies, see Figures 21-12 and 21-13.

ENRICHMENT

The enrichment section contains information that is valuable as background for the EMT-B but that goes substantially beyond the U.S. Department of Transportation (DOT) EMT-Basic curriculum.

The following section provides information regarding the treatment and identification of specific poisonings you will be likely to encounter as well as information on the most valuable resources for poison treatment: poison control centers. This information is provided so that you will be better prepared to recognize and manage common forms of poisoning. You are encouraged, however, to learn about any types of poisonings that may be particular to the area in which you are providing prehospital care.

FOOD POISONING

A specific kind of ingested poison is food poisoning—caused by ingestion of food that contains bacteria or the toxins (poisons that bacteria produce). Illness can result from either the bacteria themselves or from the toxins released by the bacteria.

The incidence of food poisoning is increasing dramatically. Each year, millions of Americans develop gastrointestinal disease as a result of food poisoning. One of the most rapidly increasing sources of food poisoning is seafood. Algae ingested by fish create toxins in their tissues, which are then eaten by humans. *Ciguatera*, a very commonly reported seafood-related illness in the United States, is caused by eating tainted fish such as dolphin, sturgeon, snapper, grouper, and parrot fish, among others. Unfortunately, the toxins don't make the fish look, smell, or taste any different—and the toxins can't be killed by cooking, freezing, smoking, or drying the fish. In some cases of seafood poisoning, symptoms may spontaneously recur for a period of many years.

Because the signs and symptoms vary greatly, food poisoning can be difficult to detect. General signs and symptoms include abdominal pain, nausea and vomiting, gas, diarrhea, and loud or frequent bowel sounds. To care for a victim of food poisoning, follow the general guidelines for any ingested poison (however, activated charcoal is generally not given for

ASSESSMENT SUMMARY

POISONING EMERGENCY

The following are findings that may be associated with a poisoning emergency.

SCENE SIZE-UP

Is the poisoning due to ingestion, inhalation, injection, or absorption (contact)? Look for:
   Mechanism of injury
   Alcohol, drugs, other commonly abused substances
   Empty medicine bottles
   Spilled chemicals, cleaning solvents, other hazardous chemicals
   Pieces of plants
   Position and location of patient
   Confined spaces
   Peculiar odors
   More than one patient with similar signs and symptoms
   Drug paraphernalia
   Insects, snakes, marine life, other venomous creatures
   Powdered or liquid substance on surface of skin

INITIAL ASSESSMENT

General Impression

Burns to skin from chemical exposure
Vomitus or secretions in mouth
Stings or bites to body with areas of swelling

Mental Status

Alert to unresponsive
Confused or disoriented

Airway

Obstruction from swelling from burns to mouth, tongue, upper airway
Obstruction by vomitus or secretions
Stridor or hoarseness
Excessive salivation
Singed nasal hairs, soot in sputum and throat (carbon monoxide from fire)
(Insert an oro- or nasopharyngeal airway if necessary)

Breathing

Shallow respirations
Absent respirations
Wheezing or rales
Inadequate or excessive respiratory rates

Circulation

Heart rate may be increased or decreased
Skin may be warm, cool, moist, or dry
Cyanotic, pale, or flushed
Weak or absent peripheral pulses

Status: Priority Patient

FOCUSED HISTORY AND PHYSICAL EXAM

SAMPLE History

Signs and symptoms vary widely depending on substance ingested, inhaled, injected, or absorbed
Ask questions regarding the following:
   What substance was involved?
   When did exposure occur?
   How long was duration of exposure?
   How much was ingested, inhaled, or injected?
   Was any antidote or remedy administered?
   Any underlying medical history?
   Any psychiatric history?
   Does anyone else at the scene have similar signs and symptoms?
   Was the patient in a confined space or working with chemicals?
   Has the poison control center been consulted?

Physical Exam

Head, neck, and face:
   Excessive salivation or dry mouth
   Possible cyanosis to mucous membranes and face
   Dilated or constricted pupils
   Swelling
   Flushed, itching, hives
   Burns, discoloration, and swelling to mouth, oral cavity, tongue
   Unusual odors on breath
   Singed nasal hairs
   Soot in mouth and in sputum
Chest:
   Wheezing or rales
   Respiratory distress
Abdomen:
   Pain and tenderness on palpation
   Distention
   Cramping
   Vomiting
   Diarrhea
   Blood-tinged or bloody vomitus or stool
Extremities:
   Weakness
   Numbness
   Cyanosis
   Needle, injection, or bite marks
   Swelling, pain, or irritation at site of injection

Figure 21-12a   Assessment summary: poisoning emergency.

Burns
Liquid or powdery substances
Swelling
Flushed
Itching
Fluid filled blisters
Rash

Baseline Vital Signs

BP: increased, normal, or decreased
HR: increased, normal, or decreased; may be irregular
RR: increased, irregular, decreased, or absent
Skin: warm, cool, moist, or dry
Pupils: dilated, constricted, sluggish to respond

✳ EMERGENCY CARE PROTOCOL

POISONING EMERGENCY

1. Protect yourself from potential exposure by taking necessary BSI and safety precautions.
2. Establish and maintain open airway.
3. Suction secretions as necessary.
4. If patient is breathing inadequately, provide positive pressure ventilation with supplemental oxygen at minimum rate of 12 ventilations/minute for adult and 20 ventilations/minute for infant or child.
5. If breathing is adequate, administer oxygen by nonrebreather mask at 15 lpm.
6. Place patient in lateral recumbent position.
7. Contact poison control center and/or medical direction to proceed with treatment:

Ingested Poison

Consider activated charcoal (adsorbs poison and eliminates from GI tract): 25 to 50 grams for an adult and 12.5 to 25 grams for an infant or child.
Patient must be awake and able to swallow.
Do not administer in acid or alkali poisoning.
Avoid in alcohol, kerosene, gasoline, or metal poisoning (charcoal does not bind).
Have patient drink liquid charcoal substance; if patient vomits, administer another dose.
Side effects:
– Blackened stools and abdominal cramps, if combined with a cathartic

– Vomiting (not a result of the medication but from the taste and appearance)
Record time and amount administered to patient.

Inhaled Poison

Remove patient from environment.
Continue high concentration of oxygen by nonrebreather mask at 15 lpm or via positive pressure ventilation if patient has inadequate breathing.

Injected Poison

Scrape stinger from site.
Watch for signs and symptoms of severe allergic reaction.

Absorbed (Contact) Poisoning

Be sure to wear gloves before touching patient or his clothing.
Brush off any dry chemicals or solid toxins from skin.
Remove contaminated clothing.
Flush with large amounts of water for at least 20 minutes.
8. Consider advanced life support back-up if patient begins to seize or status has deteriorated.
9. Transport.
10. Perform ongoing assessment every 5 minutes.

Figure 21-12   continued.

food poisoning). Do not give the patient anything by mouth, and transport as soon as possible.

CARBON MONOXIDE POISONING

Of special concern is carbon monoxide poisoning by inhalation. Carbon monoxide causes thousands of deaths in the United States each year and sends thousands of persons to the hospital. Carbon monoxide poisoning is also the leading cause of death among people who inhale smoke from fires.

Carbon monoxide—formed by the incomplete combustion of gasoline, coal, kerosene, plastic, wood, or natural gas—is completely nonirritating, tasteless, colorless, and odorless. It causes a life-threatening lack of oxygen in two ways: first, it reduces the amount of oxygen carried by the bloodstream; and

EMERGENCY CARE ALGORITHM: POISONING EMERGENCY

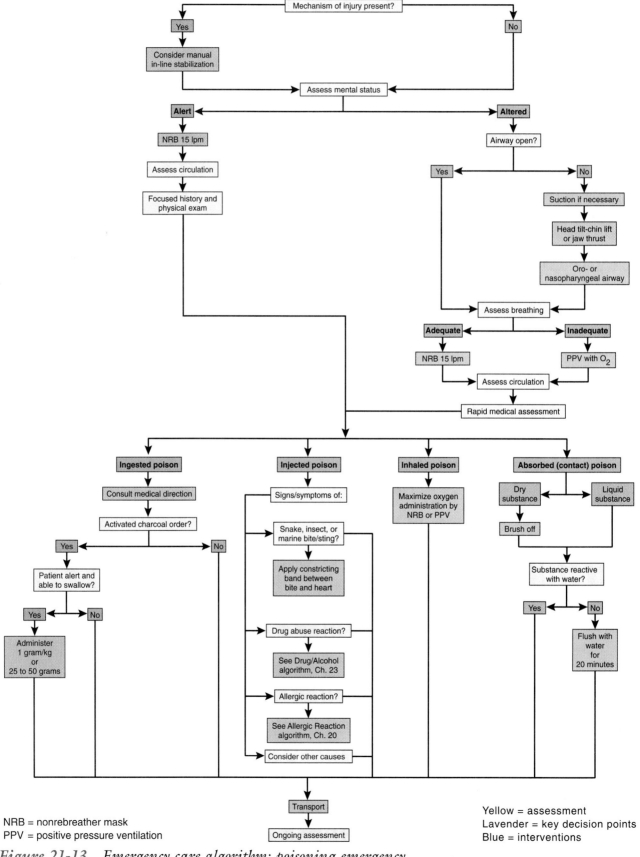

Figure 21-13 Emergency care algorithm: poisoning emergency.

second, it inhibits the ability of body cells to utilize what little oxygen is delivered. The brain, spinal cord, and heart sustain the greatest damage. Danger of carbon monoxide poisoning is increased when those exposed to this gas are in an enclosed space.

The primary sources of carbon monoxide are home-heating devices (including furnaces and wood-burning fireplaces) and automobile exhaust fumes. Other common sources are tobacco smoke, barbecue grills and charcoal briquettes, kitchen stoves, gas lamps, recreational fires, propane-powered industrial equipment, and faulty water heaters, kerosene heaters, and space heaters.

The initial symptoms of carbon monoxide poisoning are very similar to those of the flu, but there is no accompanying fever, general body aches, or swollen and tender lymph nodes. You should consider carbon monoxide poisoning whenever you encounter unexplained flu symptoms (such as headache, nausea, vomiting, and confusion)—especially if the symptoms are shared by other people in the same environment.

As the poisoning progresses, the patient may suffer temporary blindness, hearing loss, convulsions, coma, and death. In fact, one of the things that makes carbon monoxide poisoning—especially from chronic exposure—so dangerous is that it may easily be mistaken for something else. It takes only a few minutes to die from carbon monoxide poisoning. Death is so certain, in fact, that a great number of suicides are committed with automobile exhaust, which is only 7 percent carbon monoxide.

If you suspect that someone has carbon monoxide poisoning, evacuate everyone from the enclosed space—even people who apparently have no symptoms. Ideally, victims should be moved at least 150 feet from the suspected sources of the carbon monoxide into open air. All victims of carbon monoxide poisoning must receive medical care; many develop delayed neurological complications after initial recovery. Transport a carbon monoxide patient immediately with a tight-fitting nonrebreather mask at 15 l/min, even if the patient seems to have recovered. (Awakening or seeming alertness can be false signs of recovery.)

POISONOUS PLANTS

A fairly common type of absorbed poisoning comes from skin contact with a poisonous plant—usually poison ivy, poison sumac, or poison oak. Poison ivy thrives in sun and in light shade. It usually grows in the form of a trailing vine that sends out numerous kinky brown footlets that are slightly thickened at the tips. It can also grow in the form of a bush and grow to heights of 10 feet or more. You don't need direct contact with the plant in order to have a reaction from poison ivy; the poisonous element, urushiol, can be carried on animal fur, tools, and clothing. If poison ivy is burned, particles of urushiol are contained in the smoke and can be breathed in or absorbed through the skin. People with an allergy to urushiol—about 75 percent of all Americans—are likely to have severe reactions to contact with poison ivy.

Poison sumac is a tall shrub or slender tree, usually growing along swamps and ponds in wooded areas. Poison oak resembles poison ivy with one important difference: the poison oak leaves have rounded, lobed leaflets instead of leaflets that are jagged or entire. Poison oak is found mostly in the southeast and west.

Other plants that can cause mild to severe dermatitis include stinging nettle, crown of thorns, buttercup, May apple, marsh marigold, candelabra cactus, brown-eyed Susan, Shasta daisy, and chrysanthemum.

Emergency treatment includes scene safety, personal protection measures, and decontamination if any plant substance is still on the person's body. You should first ensure the airway, breathing, and circulatory status. Routine treatment for this type of absorbed poisoning is mainly supportive until arrival at the hospital. You should keep the patient from scratching the site as this may cause a break in the skin which may allow an infection to set in.

POISON CONTROL CENTERS

Poison control centers have been established across the United States and Canada to assist in the treatment of poison victims. Officials at the center can help you set priorities and formulate an effective treatment plan. Poison center officials can also provide information about any available antidote that may be appropriate for a patient. Any treatment recommended by the poison control center should be discussed with medical direction *before* it is administered to the patient.

Calls to poison control centers are toll-free, and most are staffed 24 hours a day to assist prehospital personnel as well as the public. Staffed by experienced professionals, each center is also connected to a network of nationwide consultants who can answer questions about almost any poison. In addition, information on the poison center's computer is updated every 90 days to provide the latest information on treatment options and antidotes. Finally, centers provide follow-up telephone calls, monitoring the patient's progress and making treatment suggestions until the patient is either hospitalized or no longer has the symptoms.

Be prepared to tell poison center officials the patient's approximate age and weight. Summarize the patient's condition, including level of responsiveness, level of activity, skin color, vomiting, and so on. Give as many specifics about the poison as you can. Again, any directions from a poison control center should be verified by your medical direction. Follow local protocol.

CASE STUDY FOLLOW-UP

SCENE SIZE-UP

You have been dispatched to a 3-year-old patient with abdominal pain. As you approach the patient's residence, you scan the scene, but note no safety hazards. The patient's mother runs out the door, holding the patient, and pulls on your sleeve saying "Help! I think my daughter Sophie was eating a plant, and I don't know what to do!!" You reassure the mother that you will do all you can to help. As you walk into the living room, you see an overturned plant with dirt and leaves scattered around it. Your partner gathers up some of the leaves, stems, roots, and dirt to keep with the patient and transport to the receiving facility. You have Sophie sit on her mother's lap on the couch.

INITIAL ASSESSMENT

You assess Sophie while she is on her mother's lap so as not to frighten her. Sophie is hugging her stomach and crying, so your general impression is of a child in pain with an open airway and adequate respirations. She responds appropriately to your simple questions and commands. Using gloves you sweep Sophie's mouth and remove some tiny fragments of the house plant as well as bits of dirt. You do this to help ensure that Sophie's airway remains open as well as to find evidence of what she has taken into her mouth.

As you examine her oral cavity, you notice that the mucous membranes are beginning to swell and there is some irritation in her throat. Because of the swelling, you will continue to closely monitor her airway patency. Your partner administers oxygen via a nonrebreather mask at 15 lpm. At first Sophie resists the mask, but with encouragement she accepts it.

Sophie's mother gets frightened and starts to cry, blaming herself for the poisoning. "If I would have only watched her better she'd be O.K." You reassure Mrs. Horowitz that she did the right thing by calling 911, that breathing the extra oxygen through the mask will help Sophie a lot, and that it's best for her to remain calm so that Sophie will not become frightened and so that you can treat her quickly.

FOCUSED HISTORY AND PHYSICAL EXAM

You obtain a SAMPLE history from the mother and determine that she was in the kitchen washing dishes when her daughter toddled off to the living room. About 10 minutes later she heard a crash and her daughter's scream. She ran into the living room and saw the big philodendron overturned and Sophie clutching a handful of leaves. At first she thought Sophie was hurt from the plant tipping over, but when the intensity of Sophie's crying and her complaints of "my tummy hurts" increased over the space of a half hour, she called 911. You ask if she did anything to treat Sophie and she answers that she had Sophie drink some water and spit it out into a basin to rinse her mouth. However, she adds, Sophie did not vomit.

Because you may have to administer activated charcoal, you ask Mrs. Horowitz for Sophie's weight and she tells you Sophie weighs about 35 pounds. Since the plant that overturned was in a heavy pot, you begin a rapid assessment, checking for DCAP-BTLS. You don't see any sign of trauma; however Sophie cringes in pain when you feel for tenderness in her abdomen. You place her on her side on the stretcher, in case of vomiting, while your partner records her baseline vitals. She has a radial pulse rate of 96. Her respiratory rate is 32. Her BP is 102/66, and her skin is warm and dry.

You let the mother ride in the ambulance with Sophie, and during transport you contact the poison control center as your protocol indicates. When you tell them Sophie's signs and symptoms and relate the history of ingested philodendron leaves and soil, they order you to administer activated charcoal. You follow their instructions for administering 1 gram/kg of activated charcoal or 16 grams since Sophie's weight is 35 pounds (16 kg). You prepare and administer the activated charcoal to Sophie in a plastic child's cup with a covered lid, noting the dose and time of administration.

ONGOING ASSESSMENT

You reassess Sophie's airway, breathing, and circulation and find them adequate. You also check the swelling in the oral cavity and see that the condition of the mucous membranes is not worsening. You reassess her mental status every 5 minutes without noting any change. You make sure Sophie has drunk all of the activated charcoal and reassess her abdominal pain, asking if her tummy hurts more or less or is the same. She nods when you say "same."

You arrive at the emergency department without any further change in Sophie's condition and transfer her to the staff. You and your partner complete a prehospital care report and prepare the ambulance for another call.

Two hours later, while transporting another patient, you find that Sophie was given another dose of activated charcoal by the hospital staff. Her mother tells you that the pain is subsiding and she is being held for observation but should be released soon. She thanks you for helping her daughter and seems greatly relieved.

CHAPTER REVIEW

TERMS AND CONCEPTS

You may wish to review the following terms and concepts included in this chapter.

absorption—passage of a substance through skin or mucous membranes upon contact.

activated charcoal—a distilled charcoal in powder form that can adsorb many times its weight in contaminants; often administered to patients who have ingested poison to adsorb the poison and help prevent its absorption by the body.

ingestion—swallowing.

inhalation—breathing in.

injection—forced introduction into the body through the skin, possibly into a muscle or blood vessel, usually via a syringe, bite, or sting.

poison—any substance—liquid, solid, or gas—that impairs health or causes death by its chemical action when it enters the body or comes into contact with the skin.

REVIEW QUESTIONS

1. Explain why children are frequent victims of poisoning.
2. List the four ways poisons enter the body.
3. Describe the relationship between poisoning and airway management.
4. Describe the main ways of determining if a poisoning has taken place.
5. Describe the general emergency medical care steps for a poisoning or overdose patient.
6. Give the indications, contraindications, dosage, and administration steps for the administration of activated charcoal.
7. List the general emergency care steps for an ingested poison.
8. List the general emergency care steps for inhaled poisons.
9. List the general emergency care steps for injected poisons.
10. List the general emergency care steps for absorbed poisons (a) to the skin; (b) to the eye.

CHAPTER 22

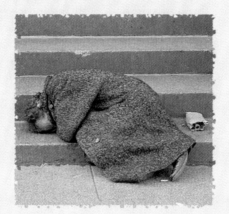

Drug and Alcohol Emergencies

INTRODUCTION

Drugs and alcohol are abused by a variety of people in a number of ways. In general, the emergency management steps you learned in Chapter 21, "Poisoning Emergencies" are applicable to treating patients in most alcohol and drug emergencies. However, the EMT-Basic needs to be aware of special problems associated with drug and alcohol emergencies. For instance, it is possible that drug and alcohol overdose patients will have injured themselves, so you may be treating them for trauma as well. You will also note that patients under the influence of, or withdrawing from, alcohol or drugs can be difficult to manage, behaving in an aggressive or even violent manner and posing threats to your own safety.

As an EMT-B, your primary concern in managing drug and alcohol emergencies will be to protect your own safety, maintain an open airway, treat for life-threatening conditions, and offer calm, nonjudgmental assistance.

OBJECTIVES

Numbered objectives are from the United States Department of Transportation 1994 EMT-Basic National Standard Curriculum. Asterisked objectives, if any, pertain to material that is supplemental to the DOT curriculum.

COGNITIVE

4-6.3 Discuss the emergency medical care for the patient with possible overdose. (pp. 413–414)
* Describe the steps in the assessment of a drug or alcohol overdose patient. (pp. 410–414)
* Explain how to determine if an emergency is drug or alcohol related. (pp. 410–413)

* List six factors that may make a drug or alcohol emergency life-threatening. (p. 412)
* Discuss the signs and symptoms that indicate a drug or alcohol emergency. (pp. 412–413)
* Discuss techniques for managing a violent drug or alcohol patient. (p. 416)

PSYCHOMOTOR

4-4.10 Demonstrate the steps in the emergency medical care for the patient with possible overdose.

Additional objectives from DOT lesson 4-4 are addressed in Chapter 21, "Poisoning Emergencies."

CASE STUDY

THE DISPATCH

EMS Unit 622—proceed to 22 Warehouse Row—police are on the scene of a minor collision with an intoxicated 30-year-old male driver who has a laceration to his head—time out 1629 hours.

ON ARRIVAL

The police officer greets you and explains that the police received a complaint from a store owner that someone seemed to be sleeping in a car. When the

store owner tried to wake the person, he started the engine and backed into a parked car. As you put on gloves and approach the patient, you note that he is responsive, arguing with the police, and has a minor laceration on his forehead.

How would you proceed to assess and care for this patient?

During this chapter, you will learn special considerations of assessment and emergency care for a patient suffering from drug or alcohol abuse. Later, we will return to the case and apply what you have learned.

DRUG AND ALCOHOL EMERGENCIES

Drug abuse is defined as the self administration of drugs (or of a single drug) in a manner that is not in accord with approved medical or social patterns. A drug or alcohol **overdose** is an emergency that involves poisoning by drugs or alcohol. In addition, a patient's **withdrawal** from alcohol or drugs—a period of abstinence from the drug or alcohol to which his body has become accustomed—can be as serious an emergency as an overdose.

Most drug overdoses you will see in the field involve habitual drug users, but drug overdose can also be the result of miscalculation, of confusion, of using more than one drug, or intent (usually from a suicide attempt).

Several major medical problems can result from any drug overdose or from sudden withdrawal from a drug. Among the most common are altered mental status, respiratory depression, internal injuries, seizures, cardiac arrest, and hyperthermia or hypothermia. The range of medical problems you may confront in a drug abuse patient is extremely wide and depends upon the type of drug taken. For example, stimulants such as cocaine will increase heart rate and blood pressure, while depressants such as barbiturates will lower them.

Table 22-1 will give you an idea of the variety of consequences of commonly used drugs. As an EMT-B, you are not expected to remember everything about each of the drug classes, but the table will help you understand the seriousness and complexity of drug and alcohol emergencies. You should remember, however, that in drug and alcohol emergencies,

TABLE 22-1

Emergency Consequences of Commonly Abused Drugs

Drug Cluster	Most Common Drug of Abuse	Consequences of Abuse
Stimulants and Appetite Depressants	Amphetamines Caffeine Cocaine Ephedrine Methylphenidate Nicotine Over-the-counter and prescription drugs	Moderate dosages cause increased alertness, mood elevation, excitation, euphoria, increased pulse rate and blood pressure, insomnia, loss of appetite. "Recreational" use of cocaine, even in small doses, can cause severe cardiac toxicity, including angina pectoris, dysrhythmias, and myocardial infarcts. Overdoses can cause agitation, violence, paranoia, increase in body temperature, hallucinations, convulsions, and possible death. Cocaine overdose can cause excitement, euphoria, rapid respiration, elevated blood pressure, cyanosis, paralysis, loss of reflexes, and can lead to circulatory failure and death. Although the degree of physical addiction is not known, sudden withdrawal can cause apathy, long periods of sleep, irritability, depression, disorientation.
Cannabis Products	Hashish Marijuana THC (tetrahydrocannabinol)	Moderate dosages cause euphoria, relaxed inhibitions, increased appetite, dry mouth, disoriented behavior. Overdoses can cause fatigue, tremors, paranoia, possible psychosis. Although the degree of physical addiction is not known, sudden withdrawal can cause insomnia, hyperactivity, and decreased appetite is occasionally reported.

Depressants— Narcotics and Opiates/Opioids	Codeine
	Heroin
	Methadone
	Morphine
	Opium
	(90% of opiate/opioid-
	    dependent abusers will have
	    a mixed overdose.)
		Moderate dosages cause euphoria, drowsiness, lethargy, respiratory depression, constricted pupils, constipation, nausea. Overdoses can cause slow and shallow breathing, clammy skin, convulsions, coma, possible death. Sudden withdrawal results in watery eyes, runny nose, yawning, restlessness, rapid pulse, elevated blood pressure, diarrhea, loss of appetite, irritability, tremors, panic, chills and sweating, cramps, nausea. Needle tracks are a sign of repeated injections.

the goals are to identify and treat the loss of vital functions caused by the drug, not the specific effects of the drug itself.

As you can see in Table 22-1, alcohol is classified as a type of drug. It is a central nervous system depressant that, in moderate doses, causes an altered mental status and, in large doses, can cause unresponsiveness or death. Alcohol is completely absorbed from the stomach and intestinal tract within 2 hours from the time it is ingested and sometimes as quickly as within 30 minutes. Once absorbed from the stomach, it is relatively quickly distributed to all body tissues. It is concentrated, however, in the blood and brain.

Habitual alcohol abusers, or alcoholics, are prone to a wide variety of illnesses ranging from cirrhosis of the liver to peritonitis. In addition to causing medical problems, alcohol intoxication is a major cause of automobile crashes. Alcohol ingestion, even in smaller doses, is also a major factor in drug overdoses, homicides, burns, drowning, non-accidental trauma, and general trauma.

In the Enrichment section later in the chapter, we will discuss some specific alcohol and drug emergencies you may encounter.

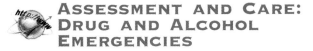

ASSESSMENT AND CARE: DRUG AND ALCOHOL EMERGENCIES

SCENE SIZE-UP

Conduct a scene size-up. First make sure that the scene is safe, since calls involving drugs or alcohol may involve physical abuse or violent acts. It may be prudent to call for police backup. (See "Managing the Violent Drug or Alcohol Patient," later in this chapter, for specific guidelines on what to do upon encountering a patient who is likely to become aggressive.)

Be very careful to note the presence of any potential weapons and not to get stuck with a drug abuser's needle, as most people who share needles also share infectious diseases. Make sure you have taken the appropriate body substance isolation (BSI)

TABLE 22-1 (CONTINUED)

Emergency Consequences of Commonly Abused Drugs

Drug Cluster	Most Common Drug of Abuse	Consequences of Abuse
Depressants— Sedatives and Tranquilizers	Alcohol Antihistamines Barbiturates Chloralhydrate Other non-barbiturate, non-benzodiazepine sedatives Over-the-counter preparations Diazepam and other benzodiazepines Other major or minor tranquilizers	Moderate dosages can result in slurred speech, drowsiness, impaired thinking, incoordination, disorientation, drunken behavior without odor of alcohol. Overdose can result in central nervous system depression, shallow respiration, cold and clammy skin, dilated pupils, weak and decreased or rapid pulse, coma, respiratory/circulatory failure, possible death. Aggressive and suicidal behavior may also occur. Sudden withdrawal results in anxiety, insomnia, tremors, delirium, convulsions, possible death.
Hallucinogens (Psychedelic Drugs)	DET (N, N-Diethyltryptamine) DMT (N, N-Dimethytryptamine) LSD (Lysergic acid diethylamide) Mescaline MDA (3, 4 Methylenedioxy-amphetamine) PCP (Phencyclidine) STP (DOM-2, 5-Dimethoxy, 4-Methylamphetamine)	Moderate dosages can result in motor disturbances, anxiety, paranoia, delusions of persecution, illusions and hallucinations, poor perception of time and distance. Overdose can result in longer, more intense "trip" episodes, psychosis or exacerbation of a pre-existing psychiatric problem, and possible death. Flashbacks can occur months or years after the original dose. PCP may also cause paralysis, violence, rage, and status epilepticus.
Inhalants	Aerosol propellants Gasoline and kerosene Glues and organic cements Lacquer and varnish thinners Lighter fluid Typing correction fluid Medical anesthetics Propane	Moderate dosages cause excitement, euphoria, feelings of drunkenness, giddiness, loss of inhibitions, aggressiveness, delusions, depression, drowsiness, headache, nausea. Overdoses can cause loss of memory, delirium, glazed eyes, slurred speech, drowsiness, hallucinations, confusion, unsteady gait, and erratic heart beat and pulse. Sudden withdrawal results in insomnia, decreased appetite, depression, irritability, and headache. Death can result from suffocation or from a phenomenon called SSD ("sudden sniffing death"), which is still poorly understood but which might follow myocardial infarction.

precautions, since alcoholics and drug abusers frequently have bloodborne and airborne diseases. Look for a mechanism of injury that could possibly have caused injury to the patient.

In addition, because drug and alcohol emergencies may mimic other medical conditions, you should inspect the area immediately around the patient (and check the patient's pockets) for evidence of drug or alcohol use—empty or partially filled pill bottles or boxes, syringes, empty liquor bottles, prescriptions, hospital discharge orders, or physician's notes that might help you identify what drug the patient has taken. Keep any such evidence with the patient since it will be useful for the staff at the poison control center or the emergency department.

INITIAL ASSESSMENT

Begin your initial assessment by forming a general impression. If a mechanism of injury was noted, take the necessary manual in-line spinal stabilization. Quickly scan the patient for any obvious life threats such as

gunshot or knife wounds to the chest, major bleeding, or an obstructed airway from vomitus, blood, or other secretions.

The mental status of the drug or alcohol abuse patient can range from extreme excitability to complete unresponsiveness, depending on the substance being abused. If the patient has an altered mental status, open the airway and closely inspect inside the mouth for secretions, vomitus, or other substances that may block the airway or could be aspirated.

Alcohol, narcotics, and other central nervous system (CNS) depressants could easily cause inadequate breathing as a result of slow or absent respiratory rates or decreased inspiratory volume. If the patient is not breathing adequately, provide positive pressure ventilation with supplemental oxygen. If the breathing is adequate, administer oxygen by a nonrebreather mask at 15 lpm.

Assess the circulation by palpating for a radial pulse. The heart rate may be decreased or rapid and weak if CNS depressants are abused, whereas the patient may have significantly increased heart rates when CNS stimulants have been taken. The skin in the CNS depressant abuse patient is usually cool, clammy, and pale because of poor perfusion related to hypotension. Assess for major external bleeding that may have occurred as a result of associated trauma.

The odor of alcohol on the patient's breath or clothing may provide a clue to alcohol abuse. However, do not confuse the fruity or acetone odor that is related to a diabetic emergency with the smell of alcohol. In addition, do not automatically decide that an altered mental status or other signs and symptoms are directly related to alcohol ingestion.

Other serious medical conditions may be present and not directly related to or caused by the alcohol. Therefore, always be suspicious that causes other than alcohol intoxication may be the cause of altered mental status and other similar signs and symptoms. As an example, the slurred speech that you assumed is due to alcohol ingestion may actually be a result of a stroke or head injury.

It is necessary to prioritize the patient at the end of the initial assessment. *The following six signs and symptoms (Figure 22-1) indicate a high priority patient:*

- Unresponsiveness
- Inadequate breathing
- Abnormal heart rate (slow, fast, weak, or irregular)
- Vomiting with an altered mental status
- Seizures
- Fever

FOCUSED HISTORY AND PHYSICAL EXAM

In the altered mental status or unresponsive patient, conduct a rapid medical assessment. Examine the patient for any evidence of trauma.

CNS depressant drugs typically cause dilated pupils, while narcotics cause pinpoint pupils. Inspect the mucous membranes inside of the mouth for evidence of cyanosis, excessive salivation, or dryness. The membranes may be swollen if volatile chemicals have been inhaled. Hallucinogens may cause the face to flush. Jugular venous distention may be found in CNS stimulant or depressant abuse if the patient has suffered heart failure. Auscultate the lungs for abnormal sounds.

The muscles in the extremities may appear very relaxed and lack any coordination if narcotics were taken. Peripheral pulses may be very weak, rapid, and irregular, if not absent. The skin may appear cool, clammy, and pale in narcotic drug abuse. Look for needle tracks on the extremities.

Get a set of baseline vital signs. The blood pressure may be low with CNS depressants and extremely high with CNS stimulants. The pulse will vary, depending on the drug, and may be elevated, slow, or irregular. The skin may be flushed, pale, or cyanotic.

Skin condition may be dry, moist, or normal. The temperature may be cool with CNS depressants and warm with CNS stimulants.

Attempt to gather a SAMPLE history from relatives, friends, or bystanders at the scene. Look for medical alert tags on the patient.

If the patient is responsive and able to answer your questions and obey your commands, gather a SAMPLE history from the patient before conducting the physical exam and gathering vital signs. During the questioning, attempt to determine what the patient has ingested, injected, inhaled, smoked, or abused in some other manner. Keep in mind that many patients will abuse more than one substance at a time, using different routes. Alcohol is commonly involved with the abuse of other drugs.

Try to establish the past medical history. Determine what prescription medications the patient is taking since these may interact with the substance being abused and worsen the condition or hide certain characteristic signs. Following the SAMPLE history, conduct a focused physical exam and establish a set of baseline vital signs.

Signs and Symptoms   The signs and symptoms can vary widely, depending on the substance or drug that was abused. Many times the patient abuses more than one substance or drug. For example, a patient may take a CNS stimulant, drink large amounts of alcohol, and then take a CNS depressant. This would produce a variety of conflicting signs and symptoms. The following are characteristic signs and symptoms based on the most common types of abused drugs and substances (review Table 22-1):

- *CNS Stimulants* excite the central nervous system. *Signs and symptoms:* Excitability, elevated mood, agitation, apprehension, uncooperativeness, tachycardia, tachypnea, dilated pupils, dry mouth, sweating, increased blood pressure, loss of appetite, lack of sleep.
- *CNS Depressants* depress the central nervous system. *Signs and symptoms:* Euphoria, drowsiness, sleepiness, decreased breathing rates and volumes, bradycardia, hypotension, dilated pupils that are sluggish to respond to light.
- *Narcotics* are CNS depressants that are derived from opium (opiates) or synthetic (opioids). *Signs and symptoms:* Bradycardia, hypotension, inadequate breathing rates and volume, cool clammy skin, lethargy, constricted pupils, nausea. Respiratory arrest can occur easily in these patients.
- *Hallucinogens,* sometimes called psychedelic drugs, cause hallucinations. *Signs and symptoms:* Motor disturbances, paranoia, anxiety, visual or auditory hallucinations, tachycardia, dilated pupils, flushed face, poor perception of time and distance.

DRUG AND ALCOHOL EMERGENCY INDICATORS

> If any of the following six danger signs are present, no matter what caused the crisis, the patient's life may be threatened and the patient is a high priority for immediate transport.

1
Unresponsiveness:
The patient cannot be awakened from what appears to be a deep sleep or coma. If awakened for a short period of time, he almost immediately relapses into unresponsiveness.

2
Respiratory difficulties:
The patient's breathing may be very weak, strong and weak in cycles, or may stop altogether. Inhalation or expiration may be noisy. If the patient's skin is bluish (cyanotic), he is almost certainly not receiving enough oxygen, but the absence of cyanosis does not necessarily mean that respiratory difficulties are not severe.

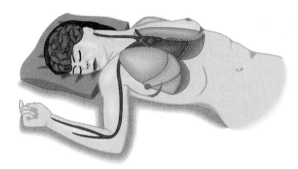

3
Fever:
As a guide it may be stated that any temperature above 100° F or 38° C falls into this category.

4
High or low pulse rate, or an irregular pulse:
Normal range for pulse rate is between 60 and 100 beats per minute for an adult; any pulse that is below or above that acceptable range indicates danger, as does a pulse that is irregular (not rhythmical).

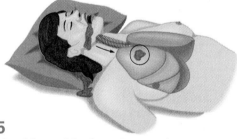

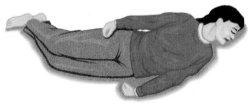

5
Vomiting with altered mental status:
If the patient vomits while not alert or unresponsive, the prime danger consists of the possibility that he may breathe vomitus back into his lungs, causing further respiratory difficulties.

6
Seizures:
Muscle rigidity, spasm, or twitching of face, trunk muscles, or extremities may indicate an impending convulsion with a series of violent muscle spasms and jerking movements.

Figure 22-1   Drug and alcohol emergency indicators.

• *Volatile Inhalants* are substances that are inhaled. *Signs and symptoms:* Excitement, euphoria, drunkenness, aggressiveness, depression, headache, drowsiness, nausea, swollen mucous membranes of the nose and mouth, glazed eyes, slurred speech, hallucinations, incoordination, erratic pulse and blood pressure, seizures.

EMERGENCY MEDICAL CARE

The emergency care provided to the drug, substance, or alcohol abuse patient is mostly supportive. Scene safety is a priority at many of these scenes. Also, close monitoring of the patient is necessary, since a rapid change in his condition may occur from the alcohol, drug, or other substance. Calming the patient may be a primary concern, since people who take stimulants or hallucinogens often become very agitated and excited. In addition to protecting yourself, protect the patient from injuring himself.

The following are steps to manage the drug, substance, or alcohol abuse patient:

1. *Establish and maintain an airway. If spinal injury is suspected, take manual in-line spinal stabilization.* Suction any substance from the mouth. If the patient is unresponsive, consider inserting an oropharyngeal or nasopharyngeal airway.
2. *Administer oxygen.* If the breathing is adequate, apply a nonrebreather mask at 15 lpm. If the breathing is inadequate, begin positive pressure ventilation with supplemental oxygen attached to the ventilation device. Closely monitor the breathing status, since many drugs may cause respiratory depression or arrest. This can occur suddenly in some cases.
3. *Position the patient.* The unresponsive patient should be placed in a lateral recumbent position to help protect the airway from aspiration.
4. *Maintain the body temperature.* Some drugs may cause an increase or decrease in the body temperature. Cover patients with decreased temperatures with a blanket and warm the back of the ambulance. If the patient's temperature is elevated, remove clothing and cool the patient accordingly.
5. *Restrain the patient only if necessary.* Use restraints according to your local protocols. Request assistance from law enforcement if necessary.

ONGOING ASSESSMENT

The ongoing assessment is extremely important in drug, substance, or alcohol abuse patients, because their condition can change so rapidly as a result of the influence of the substance. The patient may lose his gag or cough reflex and not be able to maintain his own airway. Closely monitor the airway for vomitus or secretions. The respirations may become inadequate very quickly. The heart rate and blood pressure may fluctuate, either increasing or decreasing excessively. The ongoing assessment should be conducted every 5 minutes in order to monitor the patient effectively.

SUMMARY: ASSESSMENT AND CARE

To review assessment findings that may be associated with drug and alcohol emergencies and emergency care for these emergencies, see Figures 22-2 and 22-3.

 ASSESSMENT SUMMARY

DRUG OR ALCOHOL EMERGENCY

The following are findings that may be associated with a drug or alcohol emergency.

SCENE SIZE-UP

Pay particular attention to your own safety.
Look for:
    Mechanism of injury
    Alcohol, drugs, or other commonly abused substances
    Position and location of patient
    Needles, syringes, or other drug paraphernalia

INITIAL ASSESSMENT

General Impression

Vomitus or secretions in mouth
Gunshot or knife wounds to chest
Excessively excited patient may indicate CNS stimulant drug abuse

Mental Status

Alert to unresponsive
May appear hyperactive and very nervous or excited

Airway

Obstruction by tongue
Obstruction by vomitus or secretions
(Insert naso- or oropharyngeal airway if unresponsive)
Excessive secretions may be present

Breathing

Respirations shallow or absent
Hyperventilation

Circulation

Heart rate may be increased, decreased, or normal
Irregular heart rates may be palpated
Skin color may be flushed, pale, or cyanotic
Skin temperature may be cool, normal, or warm
Skin conditions may be wet, dry, or normal

Figure 22-2a   Assessment summary: drug or alcohol emergency.

ASSESSMENT SUMMARY

Status: Priority Patient

FOCUSED HISTORY AND PHYSICAL EXAM

General Findings

CNS stimulants:
  Excitability
  Elevated mood
  Agitation
  Apprehension
  Uncooperativeness
  Tachycardia
  Tachypnea
  Dilated pupils
  Dry mouth
  Sweating
  Increased BP
  Loss of appetite
  Lack of sleep
CNS depressants:
  Euphoria
  Drowsiness
  Sleepiness
  Decreased breathing rates and volumes
  Bradycardia
  Hypotension
  Dilated pupils, sluggish to respond to light
Narcotics:
  Bradycardia
  Hypotension
  Inadequate breathing
  Cool, clammy skin
  Lethargy
  Constricted pupils
  Nausea
Hallucinogens:
  Motor disturbances
  Paranoia
  Anxiety
  Visual or auditory hallucinations
  Tachycardia
  Dilated pupils
  Flushed face
  Poor perception of time or distance
Volatile inhalants:
  Excitement
  Euphoria
  Drunkenness
  Aggressiveness
  Depression
  Headache
  Drowsiness
  Nausea
  Swollen mucous membranes of nose and mouth
  Glazed eyes
  Slurred speech
  Hallucinations
  Incoordination
  Erratic BP and pulse
Drug withdrawal:
  Anxiety and agitation
  Confusion
  Tremors
  Profuse sweating
  Increased heart rate and BP
  Hallucinations
  Nausea
  Seizures

SAMPLE History

Ask questions regarding the following:
  Did patient ingest, inhale, inject, or smoke a drug?
  What substance was abused?
  How much was taken?
  How long ago?
  Was patient given anything in attempt to reverse the drug?
  Was alcohol ingested?
  If suspected withdrawal, when was last time patient had the alcohol or drug?

Physical Exam

Head, neck, and face:
  Dilated, mid-size, or constricted pupils
  Pupils sluggish to respond to light
  Dry mouth
  Flushed face
  Swollen mucous membranes of the nose and mouth
  Glazed eyes
Extremities:
  Dry, normal, or clammy skin
  Needle marks

Baseline Vital Signs

BP: elevated, normal, or decreased
HR: normal or decreased, possibly irregular
RR: normal, decreased, increased, or irregular
Skin: normal, cool and clammy, dry, flushed
Pupils: possibly dilated, mid-size, constricted, and sluggish to respond to light

Figure 22-2a   continued.

EMERGENCY CARE PROTOCOL

DRUG OR ALCOHOL EMERGENCY

1. Establish and maintain open airway, insert nasopharyngeal or oropharyngeal airway if patient is unresponsive and has no gag or cough reflex.
2. Suction secretions as necessary.
3. If breathing is inadequate, provide positive pressure ventilation with supplemental oxygen at a minimum rate of 12 ventilations/minute for an adult and 20 ventilations/minute for an infant or child.
4. If breathing is adequate, administer oxygen by nonrebreather mask at 15 lpm.
5. Place patient in lateral recumbent position if injury is not suspected.
6. Transport.
7. Perform ongoing assessment every 5 minutes.
8. For seizures that may occur due to withdrawal, refer to the seizure emergency care protocol.

Figure 22-2b   Emergency care protocol: drug or alcohol emergency.

MANAGING A VIOLENT DRUG OR ALCOHOL PATIENT

The unusual, always unpredictable, and sometimes violent behavior of the drug or alcohol patient presents special concerns for the safety of the EMS crew, the patient, and bystanders. For more information on how to interact with and restrain a violent patient (regardless of the reason), see Chapter 26, "Behavioral Emergencies." The talk-down technique, discussed below, is useful when dealing with a patient who is experiencing a "bad trip."

THE TALK-DOWN TECHNIQUE

Emergencies associated with hallucinogens and marijuana are usually more psychological than physical. Such emergencies may present as intense anxiety or panic states ("bad trips"), depressive or paranoid reactions, mood changes, disorientation, or an inability to distinguish between reality and fantasy. Some prolonged psychotic reactions to hallucinogenic drugs have been reported, particularly with persons already psychologically disturbed.

The talk-down technique can help you reduce the patient's anxiety, panic, depression, or confusion, as follows:

1. *Make the patient feel welcome.* Remain relaxed and sympathetic. Because a patient can become suddenly hostile, have a companion with you. Be calm, but be authoritative and firm.
2. *Identify yourself clearly.* Tell the patient who you are and what you are doing to help. Be careful not to invade the patient's "personal space" until you have established rapport. Try to stay approximately 8 to 10 feet away until you sense that the patient has some trust in you. Never touch the patient until he gives you permission (Figure

22-4) or unless the patient suddenly poses a threat to safety (the patient's or someone else's). Leave yourself a way to safely exit the scene should the patient become violent.
3. *Reassure the patient that his condition is caused by the drug and will not last forever.*
4. *Help the patient verbalize what is happening to him.* Review what is going on. Ask questions. Outline the probable time schedule of events.
5. *Reiterate simple and concrete statements.* Repeat and confirm what the patient says. Orient the patient to time and place. Be absolutely clear in letting the patient know where he is, what is happening, and who is present. Help the patient identify surrounding objects that should be familiar—a process that helps with self-identification.
6. *Forewarn the patient about what will happen as the drug begins to wear off.* There may be confusion one minute, mental clarity the next. Again, help the patient understand that this is due to the drug, not to mental illness.
7. *Once the patient has been calmed, transport.*

Never use the talk-down technique for patients who you know have used PCP, because it may further agitate them. (See additional information on PCP patients under Enrichment, below.)

ENRICHMENT

The enrichment section contains information that is valuable as background for the EMT-B but that goes substantially beyond the U.S. Department of Transportation (DOT) EMT-Basic curriculum.

The drug and alcohol emergencies you encounter may be due to the effect of recently consumed alcohol or drugs, or they may be the result of the cumulative ef-

EMERGENCY CARE ALGORITHM: DRUG OR ALCOHOL EMERGENCY

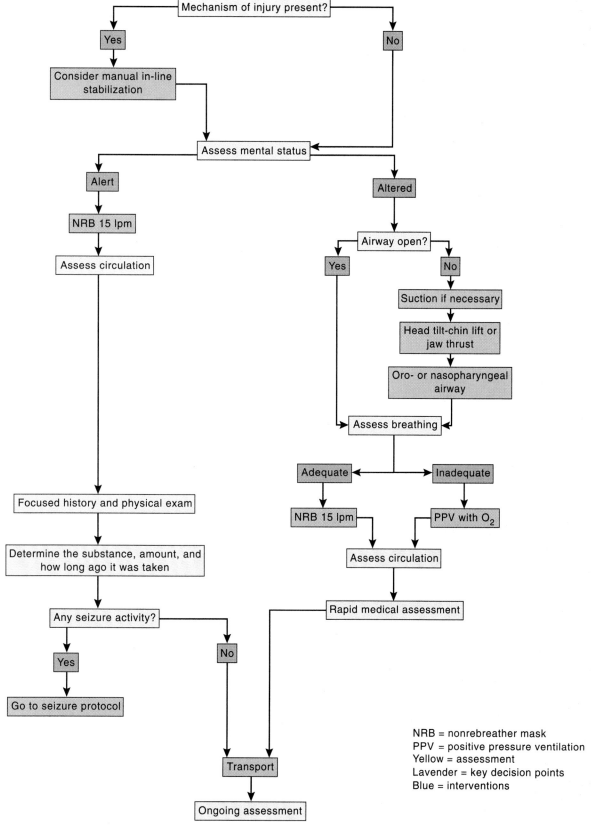

Figure 22-3   Emergency care algorithm: drug or alcohol emergency.

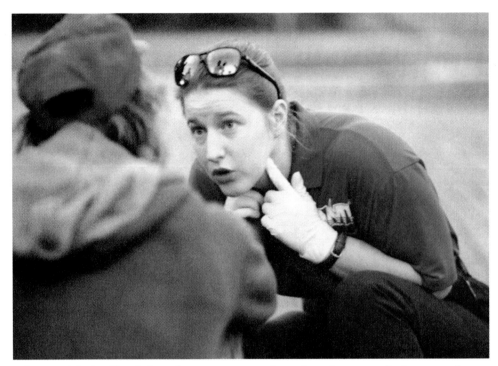

Figure 22-4   Explain who you are, and maintain a nonjudgmental attitude. (Craig Jackson/In the Dark Photgraphy)

fects of years of alcohol abuse. While it will not be necessary for you to diagnose the type of alcohol or drug emergency on the scene, it may help for you to become familiar with various conditions that are caused by consumption of too much alcohol or drugs or by habitual abuse. For instance, the alcoholic patient who has abused alcohol steadily for years may need treatment not only for acute intoxication but also for medical conditions that have been caused by alcoholism.

What follows are signs and symptoms and special considerations for managing some of the most common types of alcohol and drug emergencies.

DRUG WITHDRAWAL

A habitual drug user may develop a *tolerance* to a drug, in which larger doses are required to produce the same desired effects. This quite often leads to a physical or psychological *dependence,* in which the patient experiences a strong need to use the drug repeatedly.

The psychologically dependent person is completely preoccupied with the procurement of the drug. His behavior may be compulsive or neurotic and is geared toward acquiring another dose of the drug. There are, however, no physiologic consequences of drug withdrawal for this patient. The physically dependent drug user, on the other hand, undergoes physiological changes within the body that require the drug to be present in his system to prevent withdrawal consequences from occurring. Drugs that commonly produce physical drug dependence are narcotics, sedatives, hypnotics, barbiturates, cocaine, and marijuana.

Signs and symptoms of drug withdrawal usually begin to occur at about the time when the next drug dose is required, and they will usually peak at 48 to 72 hours after the person has stopped taking the drug.

Common Signs and Symptoms of Drug Withdrawal

- Anxiety and agitation
- Confusion
- Tremors
- Profuse sweating
- Elevated heart rate and blood pressure
- Hallucinations
- Nausea
- Abdominal cramping

It is important for you to recognize drug withdrawal as a condition that may cause seizures or a deterioration in the patient's mental status that could result in a blocked airway, inadequate breathing, or poor circulation.

THE ALCOHOLIC SYNDROME

Alcohol emergencies (Figure 22-5) are related to the alcoholic syndrome. The alcoholic syndrome usually consists of problem drinking (during which alcohol is used frequently to relieve tensions or other emotional difficulties) and true addiction (in which abstinence from drinking causes physical withdrawal symptoms).

The kind of alcohol used is irrelevant; the heavy beer or wine drinker is as much an alcoholic as the person who drinks too much hard liquor. Alcoholics may

ALCOHOL EMERGENCIES

CAUTION: Do not immediately decide that a patient with apparent alcohol on the breath is drunk. The signs may indicate an illness or injury such as epilepsy, diabetes, or head injury.

SIGNS OF INTOXICATION
• Odor of alcohol on the breath
• Swaying and unsteadiness
• Slurred speech
• Nausea and vomiting
• Flushed face
• Drowsiness
• Violent, destructive, or erratic behavior
• Self-injury, usually without realizing it

EFFECTS
• Alcohol is a depressant. It affects judgment, vision, reaction time, and coordination.
• When taken with other depressants, the result can be greater than the combined effects of the two drugs.
• In very large quantities, alcohol can paralyze the respiratory center of the brain and cause death.

MANAGEMENT
• Give the same attention as you would to any patient with an illness or injury.
• Monitor the patient's vital signs constantly. Provide life support when necessary.
• Position the patient to avoid aspiration of vomit.
• Protect the patient from hurting him- or herself.

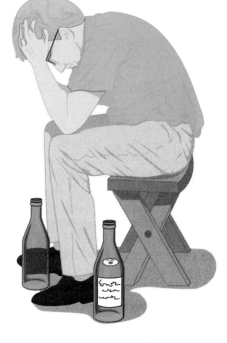

Figure 22-5 Alcohol emergencies.

abuse alcohol in many forms: Sterno, moonshine, grain alcohol, mouthwash, antifreeze, and rubbing alcohol, to name a few. Frequently, alcoholics are dependent on other drugs as well, especially those in the sedative, barbiturate, and tranquilizer categories. Some alcoholics have underlying psychiatric disorders (especially schizophrenia).

The alcoholic usually begins drinking early in the day, is more prone to drink alone or secretly, and may periodically go on prolonged binges characterized by loss of memory ("blackout periods"). Abstinence from alcohol is likely to produce withdrawal symptoms, such as tremulousness, anxiety, seizures, or delirium tremens (DTs). See the special segment on delirium tremens later.

As the alcoholic becomes more dependent on alcohol, his performance at work and relationships with friends and family are likely to deteriorate. Absences from work, emotional disturbances, and automobile collisions become more frequent.

Be aware that the signs and symptoms of disorders or injuries *unrelated to alcohol*—such as hypoxia, hypoglycemia, recent seizure activity, or head trauma—can easily be confused with the signs and symptoms of intoxication.

Also be aware that alcoholics are prone to injuries and medical conditions brought about by or related to their alcoholism. For example, alcoholics fall down often and are prone to chronic subdural hematomas. Always assess and treat an alcoholic's injuries and medical problems first, before assuming his only problem is "just being drunk."

One of the most serious disorders associated with alcoholism is *Wernicke-Korsakoff syndrome,* a chronic brain syndrome resulting from the toxic effect of alcohol on the central nervous system combined with malnutrition, which is common among alcoholics. Common signs and symptoms of the syndrome include paralysis of the eyes, dementia, hypothermia, the inability to sort fiction from reality, and eventual coma.

Alcoholics often do not eat right, and their health deteriorates. They are more prone to the following illnesses:

• Hypertension
• Altered mental status due to liver malfunction
• Cirrhosis of the liver
• Liver failure (the liver degenerates to fatty material)
• Pancreatitis (including inflammation, abscesses, and necrosis)
• Cardiomyopathy or heart muscle disease
• Peritonitis (inflammation of the abdominal lining)
• Chronic gastric ulcer
• Suppression of the bone marrow's ability to produce red and white blood cells

- Upper gastrointestinal hemorrhage due to varicose veins in the esophagus, a common cause of death among alcoholics
- Seizures
- Subdural hematoma
- Fractures of the ribs and extremities due to repeated falls
- Hypoglycemia (low blood sugar)
- Pruritus (extreme itching)

THE WITHDRAWAL SYNDROME

Withdrawal syndrome occurs after a period of abstinence from the drug or alcohol to which a person's body has become accustomed. However, it does not require that the alcoholic or drug abuser stop drinking or taking the drug completely. The withdrawal syndrome can also occur when an alcoholic's alcohol intake falls below the amount usually ingested.

Alcohol withdrawal is dose-dependent: The more the alcoholic was drinking, the more severe the syndrome will be. Alcohol withdrawal syndrome (Figure 22-6), which can mimic a number of psychiatric disorders, is characterized by the following signs and symptoms:

- Insomnia (inability to sleep)
- Muscular weakness
- Fever
- Seizures or tremors
- Disorientation, confusion, and thought-process disorders
- Hallucinations
- Anorexia (a life-threatening loss of appetite)
- Nausea and vomiting
- Hyperthermia (elevated body temperature)
- Sweating
- Rapid heartbeat

There are four general stages of alcohol withdrawal:

- *Stage 1,* which occurs within about 8 hours, is characterized by nausea, insomnia, sweating, and tremors.
- *Stage 2,* which occurs within 8 to 72 hours, is characterized by a worsening of Stage 1 symptoms plus hallucinations.
- *Stage 3,* which usually occurs within 48 hours, is characterized by major seizures.
- *Stage 4* is characterized by delirium tremens or DTs (see below).

DELIRIUM TREMENS

The last stage of alcohol withdrawal, *delirium tremens (DTs)* is a severe, life-threatening condition with a mortality rate of approximately 5 to 15 percent. DTs can occur between 1 and 14 days after the patient's last drink, most commonly within 2 to 5 days. A single episode of DTs lasts between 1 and 3 days. Multiple episodes can last as long as a month. DTs should be suspected in any patient with delirium (mental confusion) of unknown cause. Signs and symptoms of DTs are:

- Severe confusion
- Loss of memory
- Tremors
- Restlessness and irritability
- Extremely high fever
- Dilated pupils
- Profuse sweating
- Insomnia
- Elevated blood pressure
- Tachycardia
- Nausea and vomiting
- Diarrhea
- Hallucinations, mostly of a frightening nature (such as delusions of snakes, spiders, or rats)

Seizures are very common in alcoholic withdrawal, but not in DTs. However, approximately a third of all those who have seizures in early withdrawal will progress to DTs if left untreated or if treated inadequately. The treatment goals for a patient who is experiencing DTs include psychological as well as physical support (DTs can be a frightening experience).

SPECIAL CONSIDERATIONS FOR PCP AND COCAINE

The emergency consequences of commonly abused drugs were discussed in Table 22-1. Because of the unique effects of PCP and cocaine, their use requires special considerations in emergency care.

PCP

One of the most dangerous hallucinogens is phencyclidine (PCP). Known by at least forty-six names, it is also called angel dust, killer weed, supergrass, crystal cyclone, hog, elephant tranquilizer, PeaCe Pill, embalming fluid, horse tranquilizer, mintweed, mist, monkey dust, rocket fuel, goon, surfer, KW, or scuffle.

Nothing has so bewildered and amazed researchers as phencyclidine, a drug that is cheap, easy to make, easy to take, and produces horrible psychological effects (some of which can last for years). PCP is stored in body fat. If a user suddenly loses weight, the drug can be released into the bloodstream and can cause a reaction even if the drug has not been recently taken.

COCAINE

Another drug that deserves special mention is cocaine—partly because its use is so widespread, and partly because of the devastating medical complications of its use. Cocaine use in the United States has

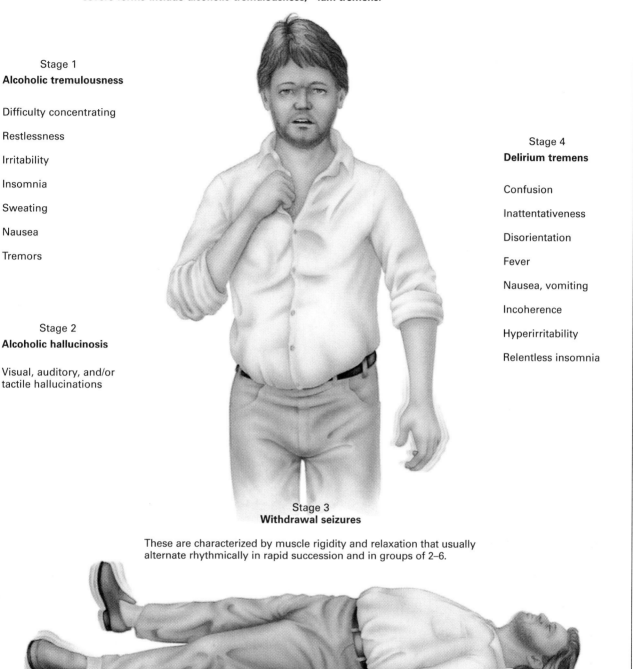

ALCOHOL WITHDRAWAL SYNDROME

Delirium tremens constitutes the most extreme form of alcohol withdrawal syndrome. Less severe forms include alcoholic tremulousness, alcoholic hallucinosis, and withdrawal seizures, which generally (but not always) precede delirium tremens.

Stage 1
Alcoholic tremulousness

Difficulty concentrating

Restlessness

Irritability

Insomnia

Sweating

Nausea

Tremors

Stage 2
Alcoholic hallucinosis

Visual, auditory, and/or tactile hallucinations

Stage 4
Delirium tremens

Confusion

Inattentativeness

Disorientation

Fever

Nausea, vomiting

Incoherence

Hyperirritability

Relentless insomnia

Stage 3
Withdrawal seizures

These are characterized by muscle rigidity and relaxation that usually alternate rhythmically in rapid succession and in groups of 2–6.

Adoption from Martin A. Alpert, M.D., "Modern Management of Delirium Tremens," Hospital Medicine, May 1990

Figure 22-6   Alcohol withdrawal.

reached epidemic proportions and is now the drug most often involved in emergency department visits.

Cocaine is inhaled through the nose, injected into the veins, and injected into the muscles. An almost-pure form of cocaine known as "crack" is smoked. Another special form of cocaine is heated and inhaled ("free based"). Cocaine is highly addictive, and an overdose can be fatal.

SIGNS AND SYMPTOMS OF PCP OR COCAINE

Physical signs and symptoms of PCP and/or cocaine usage are generally similar. Again, however, the EMT-B should remember that emergency management is supportive and not geared toward figuring out exactly what drug was used if the history is unclear. Signs of PCP and/or cocaine usage may include:

- Extreme agitation
- Involuntary horizontal and vertical movement of the eyes
- Unresponsiveness to pain
- Severe muscular rigidity
- Excessive bronchial and oral secretions (leading to choking in some cases)
- Hypertension
- Decreased urinary output
- Seizures
- Respiratory depression or arrest
- Vivid visual hallucinations
- Angina pectoris, myocardial infarction, cardiac dysrhythmias, sudden death (these can occur after even small doses, and in people who do not have pre-existing heart disease)
- Aortic dissection (a split of the wall of the aorta)
- Stroke or intracranial hemorrhage
- Severe headache, unrelated to head injury, that cannot be relieved with analgesics

- Respiratory problems, including hyperventilation, shortness of breath, rapid respiration, Cheyne-Stokes respirations (a repeating pattern of 10 to 60 seconds of apnea followed by gradually increasing then decreasing depth and frequency of respiration), and respiratory arrest
- Neurological problems, including loss of vision, headache, convulsions, tremors, dizziness, and depressed reflexes
- Psychiatric problems, including anxiety, agitation, euphoria, psychosis, paranoia, hallucinations, suicide, and depression

Before treating any suspected victim of cocaine intoxication, make certain you take body substance isolation precautions to prevent the spread of hepatitis B, HIV, and other infectious diseases. These are becoming prominent among cocaine users as intravenous use gains popularity.

EMERGENCY CARE

You will treat a cocaine or PCP overdose as you would any other drug emergency, with the following special considerations:

Your first priority in providing emergency medical care for the patient under the influence of PCP or cocaine is to protect yourself and your crew, since the patient may be combative and require restraint. Keep the patient in a quiet, nonstimulating environment.

Check quickly to determine whether there are any injuries that need attention. If there are, administer emergency medical care for those injuries as you would for any trauma patient (ensuring the airway, providing oxygen and ventilations if required, and supporting the circulatory system) before continuing with psychological care. Monitor vital signs regularly and transport the patient as quickly as possible.

CASE STUDY FOLLOW-UP

SCENE SIZE-UP

Your initial call was for a minor collision with an intoxicated 30-year-old male driver who has cut his head, according to police on the scene.

A police officer greets you and explains that the police received a complaint from the store owner that someone seemed to be sleeping in a car in front of his store. When the store owner tried to wake the person, he started the engine and backed into a parked car. As you approach the patient you put on your gloves and note he is responsive, arguing with the police and has a minor laceration on his forehead. You scan the car for any evidence of drug or alcohol use

such as medical alert tags, pill bottles, or alcohol bottles or cans but don't see any.

The scene size-up reveals no obvious hazards. There is no traffic in the lot and the police have calmed down the patient. There is only one patient, and because the mechanism of injury was a low-speed collision there is no need for additional assistance at this time.

INITIAL ASSESSMENT

Your general impression reveals an adult male in no obvious distress. His chief complaint is a laceration to the front of his forehead that has stopped bleeding freely. Due to the laceration to the head, you consider the need for spinal immobilization of the seated patient during your assessment, and you assign a partner to maintain manual stabilization of the neck as you continue to question the patient.

The patient is verbally responsive and tells you his name is Robin Lynch, but he is not quite sure where he is or what day of the week it is. You proceed to assess airway, breathing, and circulation, and find no life threats. You don't find any evidence of drugs but you do smell alcohol on his breath. You start oxygen administration at 15 lpm with a nonrebreather mask.

FOCUSED HISTORY AND PHYSICAL EXAM

A rapid trauma assessment reveals no other injuries aside from the laceration and some point tenderness in the neck. Your partner and police first responders apply a cervical spine immobilization collar and immobilize Mr. Lynch to a KED vest to prepare for extricating him to a spine board. Meanwhile, you take and record the baseline vitals, finding that he has a blood pressure of 134/88 and a heart rate of 90. His respiratory rate is 16 and his skin is warm, dry, and slightly flushed. His pupils are normal and equal in size and reactive. You proceed to ask Mr. Lynch the SAMPLE history questions. He begins sobbing and tells you he has recently started drinking heavily in response to a separation from his wife.

ONGOING ASSESSMENT

Once Mr. Lynch is prepared for transport, you reassess the motor, sensory, and circulatory function in all four extremities and then move him to the ambulance on a long spine board and stretcher. En route, you focus on reassessing the patient's mental status, monitoring vitals, preparing for vomiting, continuing oxygen administration, and contacting the hospital. In this case, since the substance abused was alcohol and there was no evidence of a mix of pills, the medical direction physician does not ask you to administer activated charcoal. Rather, you are asked to monitor Mr. Lynch's airway the entire trip in and provide emotional support.

CHAPTER REVIEW

TERMS AND CONCEPTS

You may wish to review the following terms and concepts included in this chapter.

drug abuse—self administration of drugs (or of a single drug) in a manner that is not in accord with approved medical or social patterns.

overdose—an emergency that involves poisoning by drugs or alcohol.

withdrawal—a syndrome that occurs after a period of abstinence from the alcohol or drugs to which a person's body has become accustomed.

REVIEW QUESTIONS

1. Describe how you can determine whether a patient's condition is alcohol- or drug-related.
2. Outline the special safety precautions you need to take for a drug or alcohol emergency.
3. List the six indicators that a drug or alcohol patient is a high priority for transport.
4. Explain why the signs and symptoms of alcohol- and drug-related emergencies vary so widely.
5. List the emergency care steps for an alcohol or drug emergency.

CHAPTER 23

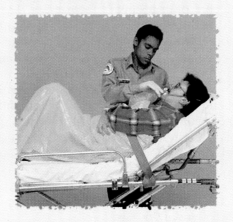

Acute Abdominal Pain

INTRODUCTION

Acute abdominal pain is a common condition you are sure to encounter during your EMS career. It can have any number of causes and may often signal a very serious medical condition. No matter what the cause, in all cases of abdominal pain it is important for you to assess for life-threatening conditions, make the patient as comfortable as possible, administer oxygen, and get the patient to the hospital quickly.

OBJECTIVES

Numbered objectives are from the United States Department of Transportation 1994 EMT-Basic National Standard Curriculum. Asterisked objectives, if any, pertain to material that is supplemental to the DOT curriculum.

COGNITIVE

* Describe the structure and function of the organs contained within the abdominal cavity. (pp. 425–426, 427)
* Define the term acute abdomen. (p. 426)
* Describe the assessment of a patient with acute abdominal pain. (pp. 428–431)

* Describe the signs and symptoms of acute abdominal pain. (p. 429)
* Discuss the appropriate emergency medical care for a patient with acute abdominal pain. (pp. 429, 431)
* Discuss possible causes of acute abdominal pain. (pp. 432–435)

PSYCHOMOTOR

* Demonstrate an assessment and examination techniques used for acute abdominal pain.
* Demonstrate appropriate emergency medical care for acute abdominal pain.

CASE STUDY

THE DISPATCH

Medic 58—respond to 7931 Rosemont Avenue, a single family dwelling, for a 16-year-old male complaining of "stomach" pain—Time out is 0945 hours.

ON ARRIVAL

Upon arrival at the address you notice a well-kept, single-floor ranch house. There are no apparent safety hazards or signs of trauma. You knock on the door and are greeted by a woman who states, "It's my son Doug. He's had a fever for the last couple of days. I thought it was the flu or something. But this morning he woke up with a bad pain in his stomach."

How would you proceed with this patient?

This chapter will describe the assessment and emergency medical care for the patient suffering from acute abdominal pain. Later we will return to this case and apply what you have learned.

ABDOMINAL STRUCTURE AND FUNCTION

The abdomen, or **abdominal cavity,** is located below the diaphragm and extends to the top of the pelvis. The abdomen contains many vital organs for digestion and excretion (Figure 23-1) including the stomach, spleen, liver, gallbladder, pancreas, small intestine, and part of the large intestine. Also, the **abdominal aorta,** a major division of the heart's primary artery, runs through the abdomen. The kidneys, while located near the abdomen, are actually located behind the lining of the abdominal cavity, or **peritoneum.** Pain in the mid-back may be caused by problems with the kidneys.

Other vital organs, such as the heart, lungs, and brain, are contained within body cavities protected by bones. However, only the upper portion of the abdominal cavity is protected by the lower ribs. The remainder of the abdomen has no bony protection. When looking at mechanisms of injury, it is easy to see why injuries to the abdomen can be very serious. Trauma to the abdomen will be discussed in Chapter 36, "Chest, Abdomen, and Genitalia Injuries."

Because you can't use bones as reference points when assessing the abdomen, it is helpful to reference the abdomen by dividing it into quarters, or quadrants, using the navel, or **umbilicus,** as the central reference point (Figure 23-2). Some organs, such as the large intestine and small intestine, are found in more than one quadrant. Remember, in naming the quadrants, that right and left are the patient's right and left.

• *Left upper quadrant (LUQ)*—contains most of the stomach, the spleen, the pancreas, and part of the large intestine. The left kidney is behind the abdominal lining.

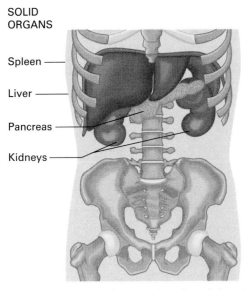

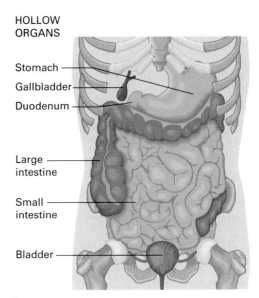

Figure 23-1   Organs in the abdominal cavity.

- *Right upper quadrant (RUQ)*—contains most of the liver, the gallbladder, and part of the large intestine. The right kidney is behind the abdominal lining.
- *Right lower quadrant (RLQ)*—contains the appendix (a worm-shaped structure extending at the beginning of the large intestine), part of the large intestine, and the female reproductive organs.
- *Left lower quadrant (LLQ)*—contains part of the large intestine and the female reproductive organs.

The function of most of the organs contained in the abdomen has to do with digestion of food and excretion of wastes. Table 23-1 provides a brief list of the organs and their functions. However, as an EMT-Basic, remember that you should not focus on determining which organ or specific illness may be causing a pa-

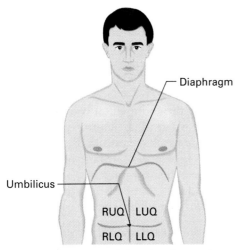

Figure 23-2   Abdominal quadrants.

tient's abdominal pain. Your priority is to recognize potential life threats related to acute abdominal pain and provide appropriate emergency medical care.

ACUTE ABDOMINAL PAIN

Acute abdominal pain, sometimes called **acute abdomen,** or **acute abdominal distress,** is a common condition. It may be severe, and it can have any number of causes. Some causes of acute abdominal pain will be obvious, but most causes will not be that apparent.

Medical texts cite approximately one hundred different causes of abdominal pain. Acute abdominal pain may arise from the cardiac, gastrointestinal, genital, urinary, reproductive, or other body systems. Pain from an abdominal condition may even be referred, or exhibited in other areas of the body (Figure 23-3). **Referred pain** is pain that is felt in a body part removed from its point of origin. Knowing about referred pain will not change the way you treat the patient, but your documentation of the location of the patient's pain will be crucial to the hospital staff.

As previously stated, it is not important that you try to isolate the exact cause of abdominal pain or distress in the prehospital setting. Rather, you should simply correctly assess and identify that the patient is suffering abdominal pain and provide suitable emergency medical care based on that symptom.

All patients with abdominal pain should be considered to have a life-threatening condition until proven otherwise. Associated signs of low blood pressure, syncope (fainting), or pale, cool, and clammy skin, coinciding with abdominal pain, are considered very serious and high priority.

TABLE 23-1

Organs of the Abdomen and Their Function

Stomach	A sac-like, stretchable pouch located below the diaphragm which receives food from the esophagus (tube-like structure from the throat). The stomach enables digestion by secreting a specialized fluid to aid in the breakdown and absorption of food.
Duodenum	The first part of the small intestine that connects to the stomach.
Small Intestine	A tube-like structure beginning at the distal end of the stomach and ending at the beginning of the large intestine. Its digestive function is to absorb nutrients from intestinal contents.
Large Intestine	A tube-like structure beginning at the distal end of the small intestine and ending at the anus. It re-absorbs fluid from intestinal contents, enabling the excretion of solid waste from the body.
Liver	A large solid organ located in the RUQ just beneath the diaphragm with a slight portion extending to the LUQ. It filters the nutrients from blood as it returns from the intestines, stores glucose (sugar) and certain vitamins, plays a part in blood clotting, filters dead red blood cells, and aids in the production of bile.
Gallbladder	A pear-shaped sac which lies on the underneath right side of the liver. The gallbladder holds bile, which aids in the digestion of fats.
Spleen	An elongated, oval, solid organ located in the LUQ behind and to the side of the stomach. It aids in the production of blood cells as well as the filtering and storage of blood.
Pancreas	A gland composed of many lobes and ducts located in both the RUQ and LUQ, just behind the stomach. It aids in digestion and regulates carbohydrate metabolism.
Kidneys	Paired organs located behind the abdominal wall lining (retroperitoneal), one on each side of the spine. The kidneys excrete urine and regulate water, electrolytes, and acid-base balance.
Bladder	A sac-like structure that acts as a reservoir for the urine received from the kidneys.

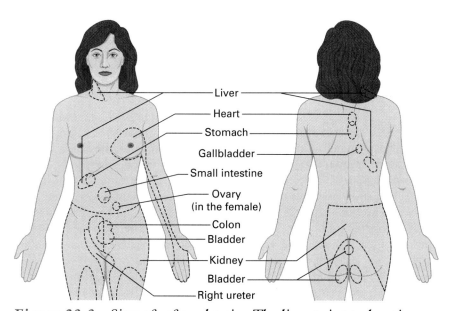

Figure 23-3   Sites of referred pain. The lines point to locations where pain may be felt when there is disease of or injury to the named organ.

Severe abdominal pain is not only very distressing to the patient, it needs to be treated as an emergency. This is especially true if the pain lasts for six hours or longer, regardless of its intensity.

ASSESSMENT AND CARE: ACUTE ABDOMINAL PAIN

SCENE SIZE-UP

Begin by looking out for any potential threats to you, the patient, or other personnel. As you approach the scene you will also want to make sure you take body substance isolation (BSI) precautions. Use face and eye protection if the patient is vomiting and splash or splatter is anticipated.

Look for any mechanism of injury to rule out trauma as the cause of the abdominal distress. For instance, you would want to be alert to any talk or evidence of knives, guns, or other items that could cause penetrating wounds to the abdomen. Also be alert to signs of blunt trauma to the abdomen—for example, any mechanism of injury indicating a fall or auto collision.

It is important to use all your senses to size-up the scene. For instance, certain types of bleeding from gastrointestinal causes will have a very distinct smell and can be determined as you arrive on the scene. Location of patients may offer clues to their condition. Many EMTs have found that patients who are experiencing abdominal bleeding are likely to faint and usually do so in the bathroom. If you find the patient in the bathroom, you might begin to suspect gastrointestinal bleeding.

INITIAL ASSESSMENT

As you approach the patient, form a general impression. A person with an acute abdomen generally appears very ill and will assume a **guarded position** with his knees drawn up and his hands clenched over his abdomen (Figure 23-4). Start by assuring that the patient has a patent airway with adequate breathing. Be alert for vomiting and possible aspiration. Assess circulation by checking the pulse for rate and regularity; checking for obvious or major bleeding; and noting skin color, temperature, and condition.

Look for signs of shock (hypoperfusion)—rapid, thready pulse; restlessness; cool, clammy skin; and as a late sign, falling blood pressure. Internal bleeding, peritonitis (inflammation or irritation of the peritoneal lining), or diarrhea are conditions that often lead to considerable fluid loss or shock.

Shock is only one indicator that this is a serious medical emergency. The patient with an acute abdomen should be categorized as a priority for transport if he meets any of the following criteria:

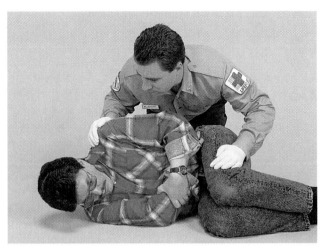

Figure 23-4   Typical "guarded" position for a patient with acute abdominal pain.

- Poor general appearance
- Unresponsive
- Responsive, not following commands
- Shock (hypoperfusion)
- Severe pain

FOCUSED HISTORY AND PHYSICAL EXAM

In any of the above circumstances, immediately begin transport following the focused history and physical exam. If the patient is responsive, first conduct the SAMPLE history. If the patient is unresponsive, conduct the SAMPLE history after the physical exam and vitals, gathering information from family or bystanders. The following are pertinent questions to ask in obtaining the SAMPLE history:

- *Ask the OPQRST questions* (onset, provocation/palliation, quality, radiation, severity, time) to get a full description of the pain, from the pain's onset and what provokes it to its severity and duration or what, if anything, makes it better. When questioning the patient about onset, make sure to note if it was sudden and abrupt. If so, it's likely that the patient has a serious medical emergency.
- *Does the patient have any known allergies* to medications, food or other substances? Is there any medical alert identification tag or information present?
- *Is the patient currently taking any medications,* either over-the-counter or physician prescribed?
- *Does the patient have any pertinent past medical history regarding the abdominal pain or distress?* Has this ever happened to the patient prior to this event and has the patient ever been hospitalized for the same type of abdominal pain? Has the patient had any abdominal surgeries or trauma?
- *When was the last time the patient had anything to eat or drink?* Did the patient ingest large quantities

of alcohol or eat very spicy food? Also ask if anyone sharing a meal with the patient is also experiencing abdominal pain.

- *Did the patient vomit,* and if so, what was the color and appearance of the vomitus? Ask if vomitus looked like coffee grounds (contains partially digested blood).
- *What was the color of the patient's last stools?* Dark and tarry stools are an indicator of gastrointestinal bleeding.
- *Was the patient doing anything prior to the onset that led to the abdominal pain or distress?* Any heavy lifting? Was the patient at rest?

The physical exam (Figures 23-5a to c) will focus on the abdomen. However, you should still assess the chest, since some abdominal complaints are associated with heart or pulmonary conditions. Also assess perfusion in all four extremities.

Perform the physical examination of the abdomen carefully and gently due to the possibility that the abdomen may be tender. Be aware that even the slightest palpation may further aggravate existing pain. Begin by inspecting the abdomen (Figure 23-5a). When beginning the exam always ask the patient to point to the area that is the most painful (Figure 23-5b) and then palpate each quadrant (Figure 23-5c), beginning with the area of the abdomen that is the least painful and farthest from the site of pain. The following are some general guidelines:

- Determine if the patient is restless or quiet and whether pain is increased upon movement.
- Inspect the abdomen to determine if it is distended (enlarged). Ask the patient if this is normal or not.
- Gently palpate the abdomen using the quadrants as landmarks. Remember to start with the least painful area first and examine the quadrant with specific pain last.
- Assess if the abdomen feels soft or rigid. If the abdomen is rigid determine if the patient can relax the abdominal muscles upon request. Note any **involuntary guarding,** an abdominal wall muscle contraction that the patient cannot control, resulting from inflammation of the peritoneum. In contrast, **voluntary guarding** is when the patient contracts the abdominal muscles, usually in anticipation of pain or an unpleasant sensation.
- Assess if the abdomen is tender or non-tender when touched.
- When palpating the abdomen note any masses that may be present. Are they pulsating?
- Ask the patient if he has any pain in other body areas.
- Document the quadrant in which any pain is located.

Obtain and document the patient's baseline vitals. Expect to find an increased respiratory rate and shallow breathing in patients with acute abdominal pain. Pay attention to blood pressure and heart rate. Decreased blood pressure, increased heart rate, and pale, cool, moist skin are indicators of shock.

Signs and Symptoms The following signs and symptoms may be associated with acute abdominal pain:

- Pain or tenderness—Can be diffuse (widespread) or localized; pain can also be crampy, sharp, aching, or knifelike.
- Anxiety and fear—Very often the patient is anxious and does not want to move for fear of aggravating or creating unbearable pain.
- Position—A patient will draw the feet up to the abdomen (guarded position) while lying on the side in order to relax the abdominal muscles. However, some patients may move about, attempting to find comfort.
- Rapid and shallow breathing—Usually to reduce movement of the diaphragm, which causes more pain
- Rapid pulse—May be from pain or shock
- Blood pressure changes—Sometimes elevated in severe pain but may be low as a late sign of shock
- Nausea, vomiting, and/or diarrhea
- Rigid abdomen—Can this be relaxed upon command?
- Distended abdomen
- Other signs and symptoms associated with shock
- Signs of internal bleeding—vomiting blood (either bright red or like coffee grounds), blood in the stool (bright red or dark and tarry, also very distinct smell)

In infants and children, suspect an acute abdominal emergency if tenderness or guarding upon palpation are present. Do not waste time with extensive exams or palpation prior to initiating transport. Excessive palpation can worsen the pain and aggravate the cause of the abdominal pain or distress.

EMERGENCY MEDICAL CARE

Follow these emergency care steps:

1. *Keep the airway patent.* Always be alert for vomiting and the potential for aspiration. It may be necessary to place the patient in the left lateral recumbent position to protect the airway. Be prepared to suction.
2. *Place the patient in the position of comfort.* If signs or symptoms of shock (hypoperfusion) are present, then place in a supine position with the feet elevated.
3. *Administer oxygen at 15 lpm via a nonrebreather mask,* if not already started during your initial assessment (Figure 23-6).
4. *NEVER GIVE ANYTHING BY MOUTH.*

EXAMINING THE PATIENT WITH ABDOMINAL PAIN

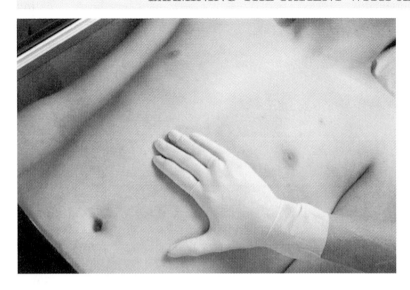

Figure 23-5a   Inspect the abdomen.

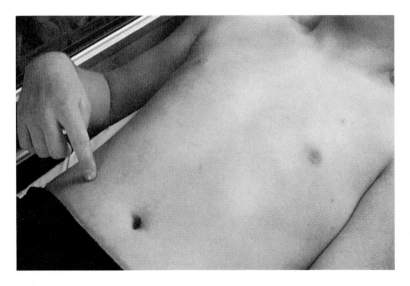

Figure 23-5b   Have the patient point to the site of pain. Palpate this quadrant last.

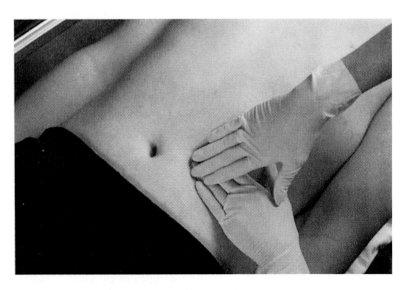

Figure 23-5c   Palpate each quadrant of the abdomen. Note any tenderness, rigidity, or masses.

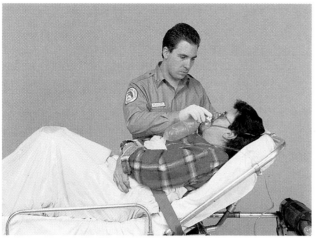

Figure 23-6 Administer oxygen and position the patient to help reduce pain.

5. *Calm and reassure the patient.*
6. *If signs and symptoms of hypoperfusion are present, treat for shock. (See Chapter 29, Bleeding and Shock.)*
7. *Initiate a quick and efficient transport.*

ONGOING ASSESSMENT

Perform an ongoing assessment during transport. Document and record all vital signs.

SUMMARY: ASSESSMENT AND CARE

To review assessment findings that may be associated with acute abdominal pain and emergency care for acute abdominal pain, see Figures 23-7 and 23-8.

 ASSESSMENT SUMMARY

ACUTE ABDOMINAL PAIN

The following are findings that may be associated with acute abdominal pain.

SCENE SIZE-UP

Pay particular attention to your own safety. Look for:
  Mechanism of injury
  Poisonous substances, especially corrosives
  Position of patient, typically "guarded," or lying very still with knees drawn up to chest
  Vomitus containing blood or displaying a coffee-ground appearance
  Dark, tarry stool or stool with blood in it
  Location; especially it patient found in bathroom

INITIAL ASSESSMENT

General Impression

Vomitus or secretions in mouth
Patient appears ill

Mental Status

Alert to altered mental status

Airway

Vomitus may cause obstruction

Breathing

Shallow and fast respirations

Circulation

Heart rate is usually increased
Skin color may be pale, cool, and clammy

Status: Priority Patient

FOCUSED HISTORY AND PHYSICAL EXAM
SAMPLE History

Signs and symptoms:
  Pain or tenderness to abdomen (crampy, sharp, aching, or knifelike)
  Rigid or distended abdomen
  Anxiety and fear
  Nausea and vomiting
  Dark tarry or bloody stool, possibly diarrhea
  Signs and symptoms of shock
Ask questions regarding the following:
  Onset of pain?
  Any unusual activity at time of onset?
  Was anything taken in an attempt to reduce the pain?
  Any history of abdominal problems?
  Was patient hospitalized for abdominal problems in the past?
  Any abdominal surgeries or history of trauma?
  Did he eat spicy food or ingest a large amount of alcohol?
  Did he vomit?
  Has his stool changed in color or consistency?
  Have his bowel habits changed? Constipation?
  Any lower back pain?

Physical Exam

Head, neck, and face:
  Pupils sluggish to respond to light

Figure 23-7a Assessment summary: acute abdominal pain. (continued on the next page)

ASSESSMENT SUMMARY

Abdomen:
  Rigid
  Pain on palpation
  Rebound tenderness
  Palpable pulsating mass (abdominal aortic aneurysm)
  Distention
  Discoloration around navel or in flank
Extremities:
  Pale, cool, clammy skin
  Reduction in peripheral pulses

Decrease in strength of femoral and pedal pulses compared to radial or brachial pulses (abdominal aortic aneurysm)

Baseline Vital Signs
BP: decreased
HR: usually elevated
RR: usually increased and shallow
Skin: normal or pale, cool, and clammy
Pupils: possibly sluggish to respond to light

EMERGENCY CARE PROTOCOL

ACUTE ABDOMINAL PAIN

1. Establish and maintain an open airway, insert a nasopharyngeal or oropharyngeal airway if patient is unresponsive and has no gag or cough reflex.
2. Suction secretions as necessary.
3. If breathing is inadequate, provide positive pressure ventilation with supplemental oxygen at a minimum rate of 12 ventilations/minute for an adult and 20 ventilations/minute for an infant or child.

4. If breathing is adequate, administer oxygen by nonrebreather mask at 15 lpm.
5. Place the patient in a position of comfort, usually with knees flexed. If patient is vomiting, place in a left lateral recumbent position only if no spinal injury is suspected.
6. Transport.
7. Perform an ongoing assessment every 5 minutes.

Figure 23-7   Emergency care protocol: acute abdominal pain.

CONDITIONS THAT MAY CAUSE ACUTE ABDOMINAL PAIN

This section will present an overview of some of the most common causes of acute abdominal pain or distress. Your familiarity with the signs and symptoms of these conditions will help you recognize life-threatening conditions. For each of these conditions, except where noted, emergency medical care is the same as outlined above for any type of abdominal pain or distress. *Definitive care for almost all of these conditions is hospitalization and possibly surgical intervention. You should never spend extended time at the scene trying to determine the exact cause for the acute abdominal pain.*

 ### APPENDICITIS

Appendicitis is an inflammation of the appendix, a small worm-shaped structure extending at the beginning of the large intestine. Appendicitis is a common cause of acute abdominal pain or distress. If left untreated, the inflammation eventually may cause the tis-

sue to die and rupture. This will result in inflammation of the abdominal lining (peritonitis) and shock. Definitive care for this condition is surgical intervention, ideally before rupture of the contents of the appendix into the peritoneal cavity.

COMMON SIGNS AND SYMPTOMS OF APPENDICITIS

• Abdominal pain or cramping—Initially this may be located around the umbilicus and diffuse. Later this pain is usually localized to the right lower quadrant medial to the iliac crest (pelvic wing), also called McBurney's point.
• Nausea and vomiting
• Low-grade fever and chills
• Lack of appetite (anorexia)
• Abdominal guarding

 ### PANCREATITIS

Pancreatitis, or inflammation of the pancreas, may cause severe pain in the middle of the upper quadrants (epigastric area) of the abdomen. It may be triggered

EMERGENCY CARE ALGORITHM: ACUTE ABDOMINAL PAIN

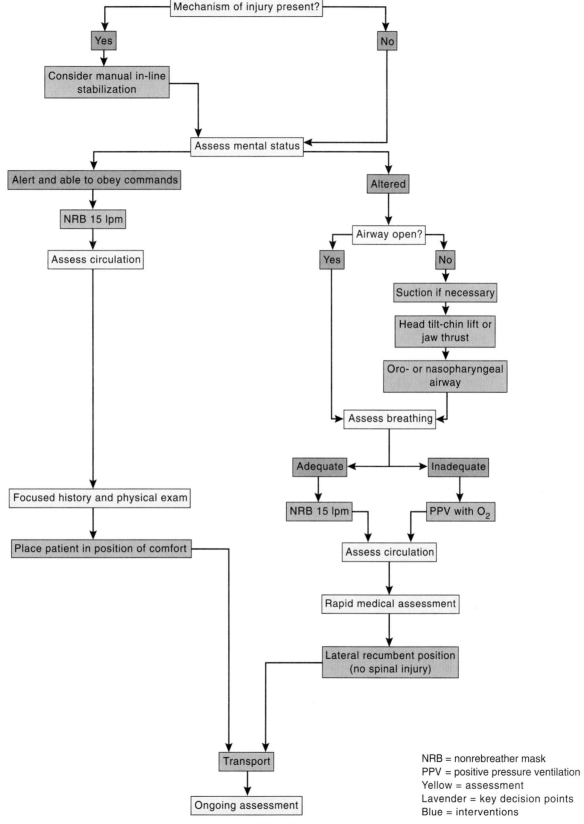

Figure 23-8   Emergency care algorithm: acute abdominal pain.

by ingestion of alcohol or large amounts of food. Note: The pancreas, like the kidneys, is a retroperitoneal structure (located behind the peritoneum).

 COMMON SIGNS AND SYMPTOMS OF PANCREATITIS

- Nausea and vomiting
- Abdominal tenderness and distention
- Severe abdominal pain with radiation from the umbilicus (navel) to the back and shoulders
- Extreme cases will have fever, rapid pulse, and signs of shock

 ## CHOLECYSTITIS

Cholecystitis, or inflammation of the gallbladder, is commonly associated with the presence of gallstones. This is a common cause of abdominal pain or distress and occurs more in women between the ages of 30 and 50 than in men. In some cases the gallstones may actually block the opening of the gallbladder to the small intestine. This blockage causes an increase in pressure inside the gallbladder causing severe pain. Definitive care for this condition is hospitalization and sometimes surgical intervention to remove the gallbladder, stones, or blockage.

COMMON SIGNS AND SYMPTOMS OF CHOLECYSTITIS

- Sudden onset of abdominal pain located from the middle of upper quadrants (epigastric area) to RUQ areas. Pain is present more commonly at night and associated with ingestion of fatty foods.
- Tenderness upon palpation of the RUQ
- Low-grade fever
- Nausea and vomiting (contents may be greenish)

 ## INTESTINAL OBSTRUCTION

Intestinal obstruction is a blockage of the inside of the intestine which interrupts normal flow of intestinal contents. This condition can be caused by several different factors such as adhesions (a sticking together of the sides of the intestines), hernia, fecal impaction or overloading, or tumors. Blockage of the small intestine is usually the result of adhesions or hernia. Blockage of the large intestine is commonly caused by tumors or impaction.

COMMON SIGNS AND SYMPTOMS OF INTESTINAL OBSTRUCTION

- Abdominal pain, moderate to severe, depending on location of obstruction—typically described as crampy

- Nausea and vomiting
- Constipation (difficulty in moving bowels)
- Abdominal distension

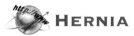 ## HERNIA

A hernia is a protrusion or thrusting forward of a portion of the intestine through an opening or weakness in the abdominal wall. Hernias are most commonly associated with increased pressure in the abdominal cavity during heavy lifting or straining, causing the peritoneum (abdominal wall lining) to be pushed into the weakness or opening.

Most hernias are not life threatening and can be easily treated. In some cases, however, they may become incarcerated or strangulated, causing the portion of the intestine to be pinched or cut off or producing obstruction.

COMMON SIGNS AND SYMPTOMS OF HERNIA

- Sudden onset of abdominal pain (usually after heavy lifting or straining)
- Fever
- Rapid pulse
- Others similar to intestinal obstruction

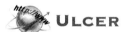 ## ULCER

Ulcers are open wounds or sores within the digestive tract, usually in the stomach or the beginning of the small intestine. Ulcers are associated with a breakdown of the lining that normally protects the intestine from the digestive fluids contained inside the digestive tract. This breakdown can cause damage to the stomach or intestine and, in some instances, massive bleeding or perforation. Patients are usually aware of their ulcers and will provide you with this information during the SAMPLE history. In some cases, the patient will take over-the-counter antacids for the condition.

COMMON SIGNS AND SYMPTOMS OF ULCER

- Sudden onset of abdominal pain in the LUQ and epigastric area, usually described as a burning or gnawing type pain before meals or during stressful events
- Nausea and vomiting (in some cases the patient may vomit blood)
- In cases of massive bleeding, signs or symptoms of shock will be present.
- Peritonitis with a rigid abdomen, in cases of perforation or bleeding

ESOPHAGEAL VARICES

Esophageal varices are a bulging, engorgement, or weakening of the blood vessels in the lining of the lower part of the esophagus. These abnormalities are common to heavy alcohol drinkers or patients with liver disease and are caused by increased pressure in the venous blood supply system of the liver, stomach, and esophagus. This condition is usually identified with painless bleeding in the digestive tract. Bleeding can be profuse, leading to shock (hypoperfusion).

COMMON SIGNS AND SYMPTOMS OF ESOPHAGEAL VARICES

- Vomiting of large amounts of bright red blood
- Absence of pain or tenderness in abdomen
- Rapid pulse
- Breathing difficulty
- Pale, cool, clammy skin
- Other signs and symptoms of shock
- Yellowing (jaundice) of the skin or sclerae of the eyes due to liver disease (may be seen in some cases)

While emergency medical care is the same as for any other abdominal pain or distress, assessment for shock is crucial. Also pay close attention to the airway and breathing status.

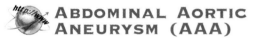

ABDOMINAL AORTIC ANEURYSM (AAA)

An abdominal aortic aneurysm is a weakened, ballooned, and enlarged area of the wall of the abdominal aorta. The aneurysm may eventually rupture. This condition is one of the most lethal causes of abdominal pain. Approximately 2 percent of the population and 20 percent of men over 50 will have an abdominal aortic aneurysm. Rupture of the aortic wall generally begins with a small tear of the inner vessel structure, which allows blood to leak between the walls of the aorta. The process continues with increasing pressure until, finally the outer wall of the aorta is damaged and blood leaks out behind the abdominal lining or into the abdominal cavity.

COMMON SIGNS AND SYMPTOMS OF AAA

- Sudden onset of severe, constant abdominal pain. May radiate to lower back, flank, or pelvis. Usually described as a "tearing" pain.
- Possible nausea and vomiting
- Mottled or spotty abdominal skin
- Pale, cool, clammy, and possibly cyanotic skin in legs due to decreased blood and perfusion
- Absent or decreased femoral or pedal pulses
- If the abdomen is soft, a pulsating abdominal mass may be felt. If the aneurysm has burst, the abdomen will be rigid and tender.

If you suspect a patient has an abdominal aortic aneurysm, you will need to palpate the abdomen very gently. Pressure or excessive movement may aggravate the aneurysm, causing it to leak or rupture. Assessment for shock is crucial. Transport without delay. If the rupture is in the process of occurring, this is a true emergency.

VOMITING AND DIARRHEA

Vomiting and diarrhea are symptoms of many of the conditions previously discussed as well as of the common stomach flu. In themselves, diarrhea and/or vomiting are rarely medical emergencies. The only cause for concern is when vomiting or diarrhea has persisted for days (or hours in the case of vomiting) and the patient has become dehydrated. For instance, infants or children who continue to vomit over a period of one day and adults who continue to vomit for several days may lose significant fluid volume and develop an electrolyte imbalance that is serious enough to cause shock, cardiac dysrhythmias, or other conditions.

When called to the scene of a patient with abdominal pain accompanied by prolonged vomiting or diarrhea, administer oxygen, treat for shock, and transport to a hospital for further treatment.

CASE STUDY FOLLOW-UP

SCENE SIZE-UP

You have been dispatched to a 16-year-old male complaining of "stomach" pain. As you approach the home, you scan the scene for any hazards or signs of trauma but find everything in order. You are greeted at the door by the boy's mother. She tells you that her son Doug has had a fever for the last couple of days and that he woke up this morning saying his "stomach hurt real bad."

INITIAL ASSESSMENT

You follow the mother into the boy's bedroom. You note that the patient is lying on his left side, curled up, and holding his stomach. Your general impression is that Doug appears ill. He speaks clearly—confirming a severe pain in his stomach—so you know that he is alert and his airway is open. His breathing is slightly rapid and his skin is flushed. His radial pulse is strong and rapid.

You tell your partner to go ahead and get the stretcher as you administer oxygen at 15 lpm via a nonrebreather.

Focused History and Physical Exam

You visually inspect the patient quickly from head to toe as you begin to ask him and his mother some questions. Using the OPQRST mnemonic, you find the following: The pain began this morning around 5 o'clock; nothing makes the pain better but lying flat makes it worse; the pain is a dull cramping and is located around the navel, radiating down to the RLQ; Doug says it is "the worst stomach pain" he has ever had; and it has been constant since early this morning.

The SAMPLE history reveals the following: Doug does not have any known allergies; his mother gave him some cold medicine before bed last night; he does not have any significant medical history; he last drank some fluid around 5:30 this morning but vomited shortly thereafter; nothing seems to have led to this condition; his mother states he has not eaten since lunch yesterday; he has had some nausea with one episode of vomiting. The vomitus was not abnormal and did not contain any blood.

While you are still asking the SAMPLE questions you begin the physical exam. You determine that the patient's abdomen is soft but tender to palpation in the RLQ with some guarding. Meanwhile your partner, who has returned with the stretcher, obtains and documents Doug's baseline vitals. His breathing is adequate but somewhat rapid and shallow with a rate of 28; his radial pulse is strong, regular, and rapid with a rate of 130. His blood pressure is 108/60. His skin is warm, dry, and flushed.

You explain to Doug that he needs to go to the hospital. You move him onto the stretcher and allow him to lie in a position that is comfortable for him. His mother elects to drive her own car to the hospital. Once in the ambulance, you prepare for suction in case Doug vomits. Meanwhile, you talk to him about how the football season has been going to help keep his mind off the pain.

Ongoing Assessment

While en route to the hospital you continually reassess Doug for any signs of shock, repeat his vital signs, and check to make sure the oxygen is working. Once at the hospital, you give a detailed report regarding Doug's condition to the triage nurse and finish writing your prehospital care report as your partner readies the ambulance for the next call.

Later, while you are at the hospital on another call, you find out that Doug has had successful surgery to remove his appendix.

CHAPTER REVIEW

TERMS AND CONCEPTS

You may wish to review the following terms and concepts included in this chapter.

abdominal aorta—a major division of the primary artery that runs through the abdomen.
abdominal cavity—the space located below the diaphragm that extends to the top of the pelvis.
acute abdomen—a sharp, severe abdominal pain with rapid onset. Acute abdomen can have a number of causes. Also called acute abdominal distress.
acute abdominal distress—See *acute abdomen*.
guarded position—a position generally assumed by

patients with acute abdominal pain with knees drawn up and hands clenched over the abdomen.
involuntary guarding—an abdominal wall muscle contraction due to inflammation of the peritoneum that the patient cannot control.
peritoneum—the lining of the abdominal cavity.
referred pain— pain that is felt in a body part removed from its point of origin.
umbilicus—the navel.
voluntary guarding—a deliberate abdominal wall muscle contraction.

REVIEW QUESTIONS

1. List the organs contained within the abdominal cavity.
2. Using the umbilicus as a reference point, name the quadrants of the abdominal cavity and the organs you would expect to find in each quadrant.
3. List the signs and symptoms of acute abdomen.
4. List the factors that would make you consider a patient who is suffering abdominal pain as a priority for transport.
5. Describe the general guidelines for conducting a physical examination of a patient with acute abdominal pain.
6. Outline the steps for emergency medical care of a patient with acute abdominal pain.

CHAPTER 24

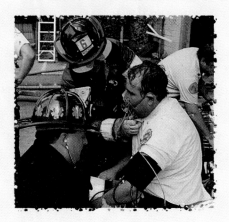

Environmental Emergencies

INTRODUCTION

A number of situations that you may face as an EMT-Basic are termed "environmental emergencies." These are conditions brought on or worsened by some element or combination of elements in the patient's natural surroundings. Such emergencies can arise from interaction with the climate, as in exposure to excessive cold or heat. They can also be brought on by contact with creatures living in the environment, as in the bites or stings of snakes or spiders.

Because environmental emergencies often occur in isolated areas that do not have ready access to a hospital emergency department, it is important for the EMT-B to learn how to assess and provide on-scene or en-route emergency medical care for patients affected by them.

OBJECTIVES

Numbered objectives are from the United States Department of Transportation 1994 EMT-Basic National Standard Curriculum. Asterisked objectives, if any, pertain to material that is supplemental to the DOT curriculum.

COGNITIVE

4-7.1 Describe the various ways that the body loses heat. (pp. 440–441)

4-7.2 List the signs and symptoms of exposure to cold. (pp. 441–452)

4-7.3 Explain the steps in providing emergency medical care to a patient exposed to cold. (pp. 448–450)

4-7.4 List the signs and symptoms of exposure to heat. (pp. 451, 455–459)

4-7.5 Explain the steps in providing emergency medical care to a patient exposed to heat. (pp. 456–458)

4-7.8 Discuss the emergency medical care of bites and stings. (p. 461–462)

PSYCHOMOTOR

4-7.9 Demonstrate the assessment and emergency medical care of a patient with exposure to cold.

4-7.10 Demonstrate the assessment and emergency medical care of a patient with exposure to heat.

4-7.12 Demonstrate completing a prehospital care report for patients with environmental emergencies.

Additional objectives from DOT Lesson 4-7 are addressed in Chapter 25, "Drowning, Near-Drowning, and Diving Emergencies."

CASE STUDY

THE DISPATCH

EMS Unit 621—proceed to 2125 Central Avenue. Police are on the scene with a disoriented elderly woman who fell in a snow bank approximately 2 hours ago. Time out is 1314 hours.

ON ARRIVAL

You arrive at the scene at 1321 hours. A police officer greets you and says his car received a call about a woman found by a neighbor behind a single-family house at 2125 Central. When they arrived, they found a 62-year-old woman who had apparently been taking out her garbage, wearing a housecoat and slippers, when she slipped and fell. She has been lying in the snow bank for at least 2 hours, according to her broken watch. The officer adds that the woman complained of pain in her left ankle from the fall. As you approach the patient, you note she is responsive and is not shivering.

How would you proceed to assess and care for this patient?

In this chapter you will learn considerations for assessing and managing patients who have suffered from environmental emergencies including exposure to heat and cold as well as bites and stings. Later, we will return to the case and apply what you have learned.

HEAT AND COLD EMERGENCIES

To understand how exposure to heat or cold can create life-threatening situations, you should have a basic understanding of how the body regulates its temperature.

REGULATION OF TEMPERATURE

The human body stubbornly defends its constant core temperature of approximately 98.6° Fahrenheit. To do this, the body attempts to balance heat production and heat loss. How does the body produce and conserve heat? The body produces heat mainly through processes of metabolism, including digestion of food. In a cool or cold environment, the body conserves heat by constricting blood vessels and sending warm blood from the surface of the skin to internal organs. Hair on the skin surface erects, thickening the layer of warm air that is trapped immediately next to the skin. Little or no perspiration is released to the skin surface (preventing cooling by evaporation), and the body produces more heat through shivering and the production of certain hormones, such as epinephrine.

How does the body cool itself? Generally, it does so by increasing the blood flow to the outer parts of the body. When the core temperature rises, blood vessels near the skin dilate. The increased blood flow near the skin helps dissipate excess heat by radiation and convection (see below). This works only if the outside air is cooler than the skin temperature. If the outside air is as warm as, or warmer than, the temperature of the skin, the body relies on dissipation of the heat through the evaporation of sweat.

WHEN HEAT LOST EXCEEDS HEAT GAINED

When the body loses more heat than it gains or produces, the result is **hypothermia,** or low body temperature. Generally, heat loss occurs through five mechanisms: radiation, convection, conduction, evaporation, and respiration (Figure 24-1). As an EMT-B, you must be aware of the ways in which heat is lost so that you can be alert to the fact that a patient may be suffering from hypothermia and so that you can protect a victim of hypothermia from further heat loss.

Radiation   The most significant mechanism of heat loss is **radiation,** which involves the transfer of heat from the surface of one object to the surface of another without physical contact. Most heat loss through radiation is from the head, hands, and feet. That is why it is so important to cover a newborn's head!

The amount of heat a person loses through radiation depends completely on environmental conditions. In a temperate climate and under normal conditions, a person loses about 60 percent of his heat production by radiation. At temperatures of 90°F, however, radiation loss will probably drop to zero. In subzero temperatures, it will drastically increase.

Convection   The process of **convection** causes cold air molecules that are in immediate contact with the skin to be warmed. The heated air molecules move away, and cooler ones take their place. Those in turn are warmed, and the process starts all over again. Anything that speeds movement of the air, such as the

MECHANISMS OF HEAT LOSS

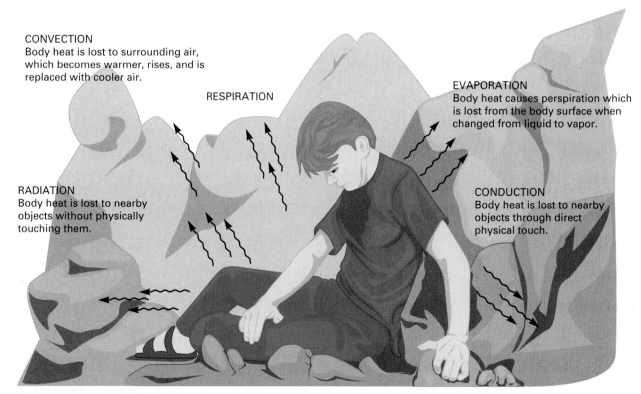

CONVECTION
Body heat is lost to surrounding air, which becomes warmer, rises, and is replaced with cooler air.

RESPIRATION

EVAPORATION
Body heat causes perspiration which is lost from the body surface when changed from liquid to vapor.

RADIATION
Body heat is lost to nearby objects without physically touching them.

CONDUCTION
Body heat is lost to nearby objects through direct physical touch.

Figure 24-1   The illustration shows a situation in which a wet, poorly dressed climber has taken shelter in a crevasse or among cold, wet rocks.

WIND-CHILL INDEX

WIND SPEED (MPH)	WHAT THE THERMOMETER READS (degrees °F.)											
	50	40	30	20	10	0	–10	–20	–30	–40	–50	–60
	WHAT IT EQUALS IN ITS EFFECT ON EXPOSED FLESH											
CALM	50	40	30	20	10	0	–10	–20	–30	–40	–50	–60
5	48	37	27	16	6	–5	–15	–26	–36	–47	–57	–68
10	40	28	16	4	–9	–21	–33	–46	–58	–70	–83	–95
15	36	22	9	–5	–18	–36	–45	–58	–72	–85	–99	–112
20	32	18	4	–10	–25	–39	–53	–67	–82	–96	–110	–121
25	30	16	0	–15	–29	–44	–59	–74	–88	–104	–118	–133
30	28	13	–2	–18	–33	–48	–63	–79	–94	–109	–125	–140
35	27	11	–4	–20	–35	–49	–67	–82	–98	–113	–129	–145
40	26	10	–6	–21	–37	–53	–69	–85	–100	–116	–132	–148
	Little danger if properly clothed				Danger of freezing exposed flesh				Great danger of freezing exposed flesh			

Source: U.S. Army

Figure 24-2   Wind-chill index.

wind, also speeds the cooling process. That is where the concept of **wind chill** comes in (Figure 24-2).

A unit of wind chill is defined as the amount of heat that would be lost in an hour from a square meter of exposed skin surface with a normal temperature of 91.4°F. In essence, the wind-chill factor combines the effects of the wind speed and environmental temperature into a number that indicates the danger of exposure. For example, on a windless day, exposed flesh will normally freeze in less than one minute at a temperature of –70°F. Because of the wind-chill factor, the same results will occur at a temperature of –20°F if there is a wind speed of between 20 and 25 mph.

Conduction   The mechanism of **conduction** causes body heat to be lost through direct contact. Water conducts heat 240 times faster than air, and conduction is the method of heat loss in **water chill.** This means that wet clothing will conduct heat away from the body at a much higher rate than dry clothing and much more rapidly than the body can produce it.

Evaporation   The process in which a liquid or solid changes to a vapor is called **evaporation.** Evaporation has a cooling effect. When body heat causes the body to perspire and the perspiration evaporates, the body surface is cooled. When air temperature equals or exceeds skin temperature, evaporation is the only way the body has of losing heat. Loss of heat by evaporation of perspiration is usually more dramatic in hot weather. In cold weather, the only loss from perspiration occurs when improper (too warm) clothing is worn.

The sweat mechanism has its limits. The normal adult can sweat only about one liter per hour and can sweat at that rate for only a few hours at a time. In addition, sweating only cools the body effectively if the relative humidity of the air is low. When the air humidity is high, the water vapor contained in the air inhibits the evaporation of moisture from the skin surface. Sweat evaporation ceases entirely when the relative humidity reaches 75 percent.

Respiration   The process of breathing also produces heat loss. A person breathes in cold air from the atmosphere and breathes out air that has been warmed inside the lungs and the airway. Some of the body's heat is carried away with the exhaled warm air.

WHEN HEAT GAINED EXCEEDS HEAT LOST

When the amount of heat the body produces or gains exceeds the amount the body loses through the processes just described, the result is **hyperthermia,** or high body temperature. At times, the body may produce more heat than needed even at moderate air temperatures. However, in most cases, hyperthermia occurs in a hot environment. Hyperthermia is most common in situations where the air temperature is high, the humidity is high, and there is little or no breeze.

EXPOSURE TO COLD

Exposure to cold can cause two kinds of emergencies. One is **generalized cold emergency,** or **generalized hypothermia,** which is an overall reduction in body temperature, affecting the entire body. The other is **local cold injury,** or damage to body tissues in a specific (local) part or parts of the body.

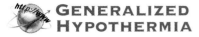

GENERALIZED HYPOTHERMIA

Generalized hypothermia results from an increase in the body's heat loss, a decrease in the body's heat production, or both. It is the most life-threatening cold injury because the severe generalized cooling affects the entire body. Mortality (death) from generalized hypothermia is as high as 87 percent.

Hypothermia can have a sudden onset, as when someone falls through ice, or a gradual onset, as from prolonged exposure to wind, cold air, or cool water.

In general, thermal control (the ability of the body to regulate its temperature) is lost once the body temperature is lowered to 95°F. Coma (deep unresponsiveness, severely depressed vital signs) occurs when the body's core temperature reaches approximately 79°F. Cases have been documented in which patients have survived after reaching a core temperature as low as 64.4°F. Death can occur within 2 hours of the first signs and symptoms (Figure 24-3).

PREDISPOSING FACTORS

Factors that put a patient at risk for generalized hypothermia include the following:

* *Cold Environment*—Extremely low temperatures are not necessary for hypothermia to occur. It can occur in temperatures as high as 65°F, depending on the wind-chill factor. Wetness, either from perspiration, immersion in water, or rain, always compounds the problem and increases the risk of hypothermia.

* *Age*—Patients who are at the extremes of age, such as infants (especially newborns) and toddlers and the elderly, are at increased risk of hypothermia. Infants and young children have a large surface area in relation to their overall size, increasing both the amount and speed of heat loss. The ability to shiver (a heat-producing mechanism) is not well developed in children and does not exist in infants because of their small muscle mass. Both the very young and very old tend to have less body fat, which also contributes to heat loss. In addition, the elderly have an impaired recognition of cold, a diminished basal metabolism, and poor constriction of blood vessels in the extremities (a heat-conserving mechanism). Also, infants and young children are unable to use adaptive behaviors, such as moving to a warm environment.

* *Medical Conditions*—Some medical conditions also increase a patient's risk of hypothermia. At increased risk are patients who have had recent surgery or who have shock, head injury, burns, generalized infection, spinal cord injuries, thyroid gland disorders, and diabetic emergencies such as hypoglycemia.

* *Drugs and Poisons*—Some drugs (including alcohol) and poisons, when ingested or injected, can increase the patient's risk of hypothermia.

STAGES OF HYPOTHERMIA

Hypothermia can occur with little warning. Initial reactions to cold exposure are shivering and "goose bumps." However, in hypothermia, these compen-

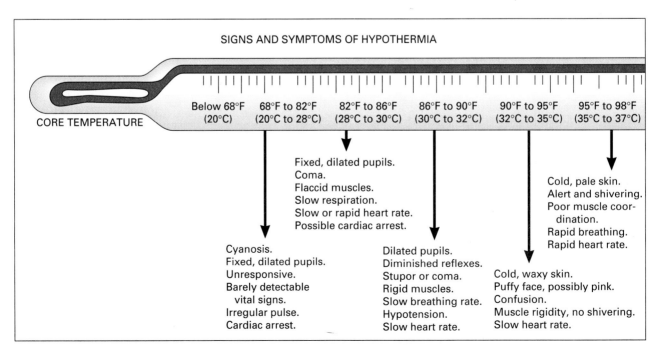

Figure 24-3   Signs and symptoms of a sinking core temperature.

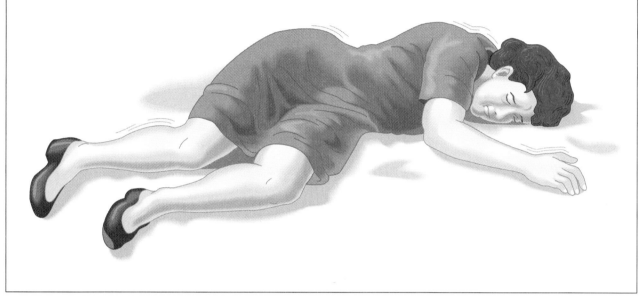

STAGES OF HYPOTHERMIA

Stage 1: **Shivering** is a response by the body to generate heat. It does not occur below a body temperature of 90°F.

Stage 2: **Apathy and decreased muscle function**. First fine motor function is affected, then gross motor functions.

Stage 3: **Decreased level of responsiveness** is accompanied by a glassy stare and possible freezing of the extremities.

Stage 4: **Decreased vital signs**, including slow pulse and slow respiration rate.

Stage 5: **Death**.

Figure 24-4   Hypothermia is an acute medical emergency requiring immediate attention.

satory mechanisms are not enough to maintain body temperature. As the core temperature drops, the body's thermal-regulating mechanism and perception become confused. A patient, even though dangerously cold, may undress, thinking he is too warm.

The five stages of hypothermia are illustrated above in Figure 24-4.

IMMERSION HYPOTHERMIA

Immersion hypothermia occurs as a result of the lowering of the body temperature from immersion in cool or cold water. The possibility of immersion hypothermia should be considered in all cases of accidental immersion you encounter. Familiarize yourself with normal spring, summer, fall, and winter river and lake temperatures in your community.

Body temperature drops to the water temperature within 10 minutes; in fact, body temperature drops 25 to 30 times faster in water than in air of the same temperature (Figure 24-5). Extra fat layers tend to insulate people from cooling. Pound per pound, adult women have greater resistance to heat loss in cold water than men. Similarly, adults can withstand

the cold longer than children, and girls have more resistance than boys. Layers of clothing can also help to insulate a patient in the water.

Contrary to the popular idea that people only die in water when the water temperature approaches freezing, death can occur within a few minutes when the water is 50°F or lower. The priority with a patient immersed in cool or cold water is getting him out of the water as rapidly as possible and then out of his wet clothes and into a warm environment.

LOCAL COLD INJURY

Local cold injury, the condition commonly called "frostbite," results from the freezing of body tissue. Such a local cold injury often accompanies generalized hypothermia; in cases where it does, emergency medical care for hypothermia always takes precedence over care for the local injury.

Local cold injury occurs when ice crystals form between the cells of the skin and then expand as they extract fluid from the cells. Circulation is obstructed, causing additional damage to the tissue. Such injuries tend to occur on the hands, feet, ears, nose, and cheeks, which are most commonly exposed to cold.

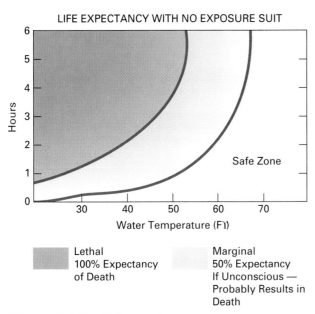

LIFE EXPECTANCY WITH NO EXPOSURE SUIT

Safe Zone

Lethal
100% Expectancy
of Death

Marginal
50% Expectancy
If Unconscious —
Probably Results in
Death

Figure 24-5 Effects of water temperature on survival in cold-water immersion.

PREDISPOSING FACTORS

Several factors can increase the likelihood of a person suffering a local cold injury. They include:

- Any kind of trauma (always check for local cold injury on people injured in cold weather)
- Extremes of age (the elderly and the newborn are most susceptible)
- Tight or tightly laced footwear
- Use of alcohol during exposure to cold
- Wet clothing
- High altitudes
- Loss of blood

STAGES OF LOCAL COLD INJURY

Local cold injuries fall into two basic categories: early or superficial injury and late or deep injury (Figure 24-6).

STAGES OF LOCAL COLD INJURY

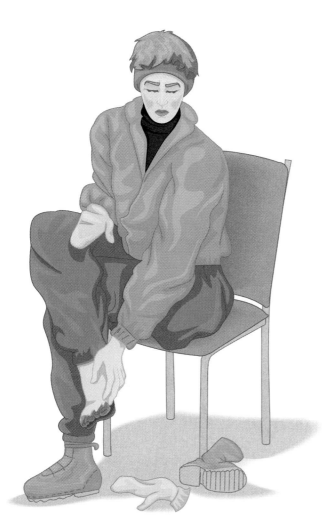

EARLY OR SUPERFICIAL COLD INJURY usually involves the tips of the ears, the nose, the cheek bones, the tips of the toes or fingers, and the chin. The patient is usually unaware of the injury. As exposure time lengthens or temperature drops, the patient will lose feeling and sensation in the affected area. The skin remains soft but cold to the touch, and normal skin color does not return after palpation. As the area rewarms, the patient may report a tingling sensation.

LATE OR DEEP COLD INJURY
involves both the skin and tissue beneath it. The skin itself is white and waxy with a firm to completely solid, frozen feeling. Swelling and blisters filled with clear or straw-colored fluid may be present. As the area thaws, it may become blotchy or mottled, with colors from white to purple to grayish-blue. Deep cold injury is an extreme emergency and can result in permanent tissue loss.

Figure 24-6 Local cold injuries may progress from early or superficial to late or deep.

- *Early or superficial cold injury* usually involves the tips of the ears, the nose, the cheek bones, the tips of the toes or fingers, and the chin. The patient is usually unaware of the injury, which commonly develops after direct contact with a cold object, cold air, or cold water. As exposure time lengthens or temperature drops, the patient will lose feeling and sensation in the affected area, and the skin may begin to turn a waxy gray or yellow color. The skin remains soft but cold to the touch, and normal skin color does not return after palpation. If the affected area is rewarmed, the patient will usually report a tingling sensation as the area thaws and circulation improves.
- *Late or deep cold injury* involves both the skin and tissue beneath it. The skin itself is white and waxy in appearance. Palpation of the affected area will reveal a firm to completely solid, frozen feeling. The injury may involve the whole hand or foot. Swelling and blisters filled with clear or straw-colored fluid may be present (Figure 24-7a). As the area thaws, it may become blotchy or mottled, with colors from white to purple to grayish-blue (Figure 24-7b). Deep cold injury is an extreme emergency and can result in permanent tissue loss.

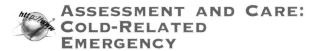

ASSESSMENT AND CARE: COLD-RELATED EMERGENCY

SCENE SIZE-UP

Your first step should be to ensure your own safety and that of your partner. Do not put yourself in danger by attempting to make rescues for which you are not properly trained or prepared.

For example, you might be called to a scene at which a skater has fallen through the ice on a pond and is partially or completely immersed when you arrive. Your first reaction would probably be to go immediately to his aid by walking out onto the ice. You must stop and consider the situation, noting that the ice is obviously unstable. Walking out onto the ice would likely make you a second hypothermia patient at best or a drowning victim at worst. Without adequate ropes and gear like ladders or boats with which to reach the patient (and training in how to use them), you should await the arrival of rescuers from the fire department or other agencies.

Also, remember that cold temperatures and high winds pose hazards for EMT-B crews. Be prepared for exposure to the cold by putting on layered clothing before leaving your station. You may get called to the scene of an automobile crash where a patient is trapped in the vehicle. The extrication time may be lengthy and you may be exposed to the cold for a prolonged period while treating the victim inside the vehicle.

Be aware that cold weather conditions can create or exacerbate unstable environments. Ice may make normally secure surfaces slippery. Snow may pile up on roofs or slopes and suddenly collapse or avalanche. Snow or sleet storms reduce visibility on roads.

Once you have taken appropriate measures to ensure your own safety at the scene, and that of your crew, consider how the characteristics of the scene may have affected the patient. Be alert for signs or evidence of how the patient interacted with the environment before your arrival. Things to look for include the following:

- *Is the patient protected from the cold environment?*
- *Is the ambient (surrounding air) temperature cool or cold?*
- *Is the wind blowing?*
- *Does it appear that the patient has been outside for a prolonged period of time?* Is he lying in a driveway, on a porch, or in a garage? Is he in a remote area where a long time might have elapsed before he

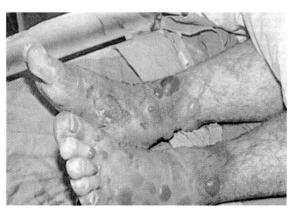

Figure 24-7a   In late or deep cold injury, the skin may appear white and waxy and feel firm to solidly frozen. Swelling and blisters may be present.

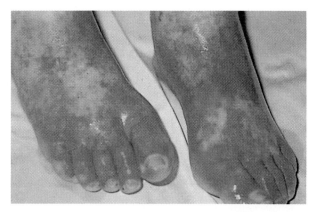

Figure 24-7b   As a late or deep cold injury thaws, it may become blotchy or mottled and colored from white to purple to grayish-blue.

was discovered? This may be particularly true with snowmobile operators, skiers, hikers, hunters, and people involved in car crashes in remote areas.

Note that hypothermia can occur after prolonged exposure when the ambient temperature goes no lower than 65°F. You may, for example, encounter a patient who has become intoxicated and fallen asleep on a park bench. The combination of the patient's alcohol consumption and his prolonged exposure, even though the temperature that night never got below 65°F, should alert you to consider the possibility of hypothermia in this case.

- *Is there any evidence that the patient's clothing is wet?* This could occur from immersion in a body of water or from rain, snow, sleet, or perspiration.
- *Is the patient properly dressed for the environment?* Finding a patient outside in the snow wearing only a bathrobe should lead you to consider the possibility of hypothermia.
- *What is the temperature inside a residence?* Hypothermia does not occur only outdoors. Many people on low or fixed incomes keep thermostats low to save on heating costs. This practice may lead to hypothermia, especially in the elderly with limited mobility.
- *Is there any evidence that a patient has ingested alcohol or has been using drugs?* These can decrease a person's ability to tolerate or compensate for heat loss.
- *Does the patient have any injury that may interfere with normal thermoregulation such as a spinal injury or a head injury?*

INITIAL ASSESSMENT

Gather a general impression of the patient. Is the patient dressed appropriately for the weather conditions? Is his posture stiff or does he appear to be rigid? The patient may be staggering or appear uncoordinated. His mental status will deteriorate with the level of hypothermia. He may appear drowsy or irrational or may be completely unresponsive in severe cases.

Closely assess the airway, especially in the unresponsive patient. It may be necessary to perform a manual maneuver to establish and maintain an open airway. Early in hypothermia, the breathing rate may be increased and of a normal depth. As the body temperature decreases, the respirations will become slow and shallow and eventually absent. Be prepared to provide positive pressure ventilation with supplemental oxygen if the breathing is inadequate. If the patient is breathing adequately, administer oxygen, warmed and humidified if possible, by a nonrebreather mask at 15 lpm. Insertion of a nasal or oral airway may precipitate a cardiac dysrhythmia in the hyperther-

mic patient. Therefore, an airway adjunct should be used only if definitely necessary in establishing and maintaining the airway.

Check the carotid and radial pulses very carefully. They may be difficult to find in the severely hypothermic patient. Early, the pulse rate may be elevated, but it will continue to decrease with a falling core body temperature. If the pulse is completely absent, begin chest compressions with artificial ventilation. The skin may appear red early in hypothermia, but as the condition worsens, the skin will change to pale, then cyanotic, then gray. As the skin continues to cool, it will become firm and cold to the touch.

The hypothermic patient is a priority for early transport. You should immediately remove the patient from the cold environment, remove any wet clothing, dry the patient thoroughly, and wrap the patient in warm blankets. Since the cold makes the heart very irritable, the patient could easily go into a cardiac dysrhythmia, especially ventricular fibrillation, so handle the patient gently.

FOCUSED HISTORY AND PHYSICAL EXAM

The focused history and physical exam should be conducted in the back of the warmed ambulance. Do not delay moving the patient out of the cold environment to conduct the exam. If the patient is responding, gather a SAMPLE history. It is important to document complaints of pain or of other symptoms. Determine if the patient is using any medications, especially drugs that might depress the central nervous system or cause blood vessels to dilate. A past medical history is important because the patient with pre-existing diseases or significant medical conditions may deteriorate much faster than the previously healthy individual. Determine the last intake of food and what the patient was doing prior to the incident. Determining how long the patient has been out in the cold is extremely important.

If a mechanism of injury consistent with trauma is suspected or the patient complains of pain to several areas of the body, perform a rapid assessment. Look for evidence of trauma to the head, neck, or spine, and immobilize the spine. Look for any other evidence of injury to the chest, abdomen, or pelvis if trauma is suspected. Significant burns may also lead to hypothermia because the skin's temperature-regulating functions have been destroyed. Feel with your hand the warmth of the abdomen to get an idea of how cold the patient actually is. When assessing the extremities, be alert for signs of local cold injuries. The patient may experience a decrease in sensation in the extremities and may exhibit lack of coordination or difficulty in movement during motor assessment.

The baseline vitals may reveal a blood pressure that decreases with a falling core body temperature.

The heart rate will initially be increased but will also fall with the temperature decrease. Respirations will be full initially with an increased rate, but will begin to decrease and become shallow as the hypothermia worsens. The skin early on will appear red, then turn pale, then cyanotic, then gray. It will be cold and firm to the touch.

If the patient is unresponsive, perform a rapid assessment and attempt to gather information for the SAMPLE history from family or bystanders.

Signs and Symptoms of Generalized Hypothermia

It is possible to measure the core body temperature only with a specialized thermometer. This measurement is not always practical in the field. Instead of using body temperature measurement, the EMT-B can rely on signs and symptoms in the assessment of generalized hypothermia.

Remember the factors predisposing people to hypothermia discussed above:

- Exposure to a cold environment
- Age (either very young or elderly)

- Pre-existing medical conditions
- Use of drugs (including alcohol) or poisons

Be especially cautious for hypothermia when treating a patient who was resuscitated outside. Sometime rescuers lose track of the time as they work on a patient in a snow bank or on an icy road. Remember that a patient in a motor vehicle is actually inside a microclimate. If the vehicle is involved in a collision, that microclimate can be disrupted, with the heat of the vehicle lost and the patient exposed to environmental conditions similar to those outside the vehicle. For the most accurate temperature assessment, place the back of your hand on the patient's abdomen beneath the clothing. A patient with generalized hypothermia will have cool abdominal skin.

Signs and symptoms of generalized hypothermia include the following (Figure 24-8):

- Decreasing mental status correlating with the degree of hypothermia:
  - Amnesia, memory lapses, and incoherence
  - Mood changes

SIGNS AND SYMPTOMS OF HYPOTHERMIA

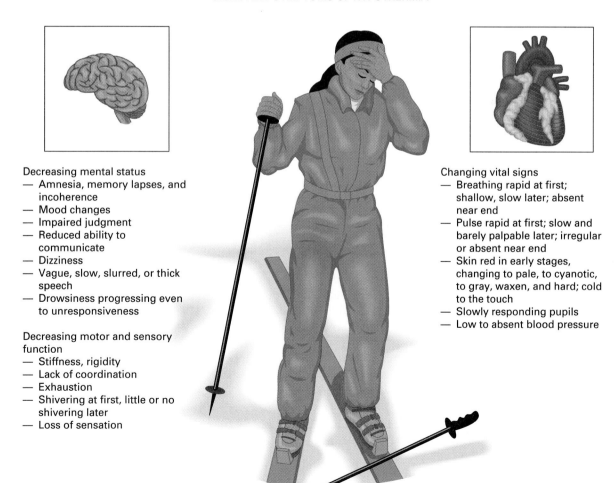

Decreasing mental status
— Amnesia, memory lapses, and incoherence
— Mood changes
— Impaired judgment
— Reduced ability to communicate
— Dizziness
— Vague, slow, slurred, or thick speech
— Drowsiness progressing even to unresponsiveness

Decreasing motor and sensory function
— Stiffness, rigidity
— Lack of coordination
— Exhaustion
— Shivering at first, little or no shivering later
— Loss of sensation

Changing vital signs
— Breathing rapid at first; shallow, slow later; absent near end
— Pulse rapid at first; slow and barely palpable later; irregular or absent near end
— Skin red in early stages, changing to pale, to cyanotic, to gray, waxen, and hard; cold to the touch
— Slowly responding pupils
— Low to absent blood pressure

Figure 24-8 Signs and symptoms of hypothermia.

  - Impaired judgment
  - Reduced ability to communicate
  - Dizziness
  - Vague, slow, slurred, or thick speech
  - Drowsiness progressing even to unresponsiveness to verbal or painful stimuli
- Decreasing motor and sensory function correlating with the degree of hypothermia:
  - Joint and/or muscle stiffness; muscle rigidity as hypothermia progresses; stiff or rigid posture
  - Lack of coordination
  - Apparent exhaustion or inability to get up after rest
  - Uncontrollable fits of shivering at first, with little or no shivering as hypothermia progresses
  - Reduced sensation or loss of sensation
- Changing vital signs
  - Respiratory changes: Rapid breathing at first; shallow and slow later; absent near the end
  - Changes in pulse: Rapid pulse at first; slow and barely palpable pulse later; irregular or absent pulse near the end
  - Changes in skin color, from red in early stages, changing to pale, then cyanotic, and finally to gray, waxen, and hard; skin that is cold to the touch
  - Slowly responding pupils, typically dilated
  - Low to absent blood pressure

EMERGENCY MEDICAL CARE FOR GENERALIZED HYPOTHERMIA

The basic principles of emergency care for generalized hypothermia are:

- Preventing further heat loss
- Rewarming the patient as quickly and safely as possible
- Staying alert for complications

The steps to follow in care are these:

1. *The top priority is to remove the patient from the cold environment and to prevent further heat loss.* Remove any wet clothing, dry the patient, and use blankets to insulate the patient from the cold. Insulate the patient from the ground up; get something underneath the patient as quickly as possible. Remember to insulate the head. Protect the patient from exposure to the wind. You can help prevent further heat loss by using warm, humidified oxygen when possible.
2. *Handle the patient extremely gently.* Rough handling can cause a cardiac dysrhythmia, especially ventricular fibrillation. (Cardiac arrest due to ventricular fibrillation is a frequent cause of death in people with severe hypothermia.) Never

allow the patient to walk or exert himself in any way. Even minor physical activity can disrupt the rhythm of the heart. Whenever possible, keep the patient in a supine position to increase blood flow to the brain. Elevate the patient's head if the patient has head or chest injuries, shortness of breath, chest pains, or needs to be transported over steep terrain.

3. *Administer oxygen via nonrebreather mask at 15 lpm* if you have not already done so as part of the initial assessment. If possible, use warm, humidified oxygen. Do not hyperventilate the patient as a patient with hypothermia has a reduced need for oxygen, and hyperventilation can cause further cardiac complications.
4. *If the patient goes into cardiac arrest, provide only one set of three defibrillation shocks if the AED is available or, if necessary, begin CPR.* Continue CPR aggressively, since prolonged survival in cases of hypothermia has been reported. Assess the hypothermic patient for 30 to 45 seconds to confirm pulselessness, because the pulse may be present but extremely slow. Only one set of three defibrillation shocks should be delivered. Further defibrillation in the hypothermia patient should be done only after consultation and orders from medical direction or based on local protocol. Respiration of only three or four breaths a minute and a pulse of five to ten beats per minute is enough to sustain life in a hypothermic patient. *If you cannot detect a pulse or respiration, but an unresponsive patient shows any movement at all, assume there is some cardiac activity and do not start defibrillation or CPR.*
5. *If the patient is alert and responding appropriately, actively rewarm him.* Note: Some experts advise active rewarming only if you are more than 30 minutes from the receiving facility: Follow medical direction and your local protocol for hypothermia treatment.

   Active rewarming is a technique of aggressively applying heat to warm the patient's body and includes these measures: wrapping the patient in warm blankets; placing heat packs or hot water bottles in the groin, armpits, and on the chest (Figure 24-9); and turning up the heat in the patient compartment of the ambulance.

   Heat should be added to the patient gradually and gently; slower is safer in such cases. *Never immerse a patient in a tub of hot water or in a hot shower.* The body temperature should not be increased more than 1°F per hour. As a general rule, keep the patient's extremities protected from cold, but do not apply heat to them; the object is to rewarm the core body, and rewarming the extremities can be danger-

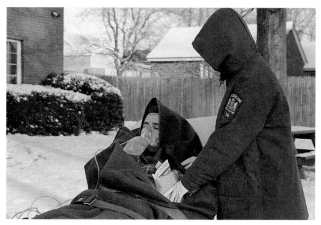

Figure 24-9   One way to actively warm the patient is to place heat packs in the groin, armpits, and on the chest. Insulate the packs to prevent burns.

ous. Check the patient often to make sure you are not burning his skin with the hot packs or water bottles.

6. *If the patient is unresponsive or is not responding appropriately, do not actively rewarm; use only passive rewarming. Seek medical direction and follow local protocol.* **Passive rewarming** is taking measures to prevent further heat loss and giving the patient's body the optimum chance to rewarm itself. Passive rewarming can include wrapping the patient in blankets and turning up the heat in the patient compartment of the ambulance (Figure 24-10). All hypothermia patients should receive passive rewarming.

7. *Do not allow the patient to eat or drink stimulants,* including tobacco, coffee, or alcohol.

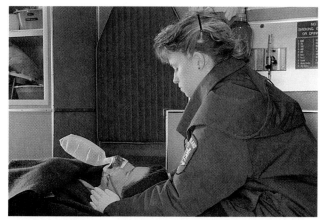

Figure 24-10   Passive rewarming includes wrapping the patient in blankets and turning up the heat in the patient compartment.

8. *Never rub or massage the patient's arms or legs.* You could force cold venous blood into the heart, resulting in cardiac irritability or arrest.

9. *Transport as quickly as possible.* The safest rewarming takes place at a medical facility, so transport is the most important factor.

EMERGENCY MEDICAL CARE FOR IMMERSION HYPOTHERMIA

In general, patients with immersion hypothermia should be treated the same as patients with generalized hypothermia with the following steps also taken:

1. *Instruct the patient to make the least effort needed to stay afloat until you reach him.* Turbulence and activity in the water decrease survival time by about 75 percent. If the patient moves or struggles, the patient will cool more quickly due to an increase in the movement of water molecules next to the skin and around the body.

2. *Lift the patient from the water in a horizontal or supine position to prevent vascular collapse.*

3. *Remove the patient's wet clothing carefully and gently.* Excessive activity can cause the heart to go into ventricular fibrillation. If it is too difficult to remove the clothing, cut it off and layer dry, warm materials around the patient.

Continue treatment as you would for a patient with generalized hypothermia.

Signs and Symptoms of Local Cold Injury   Local cold injury can be difficult to assess. While still frozen, even severely affected tissue may appear almost normal with purplish or other abnormal colors appearing only with thawing. The tissue may be completely numb when frozen but will be painful, burning, stinging, and throbbing before it freezes and as it thaws. While you may not be able to assess its severity accurately, you can almost always see a clear demarcation at the site of a local cold injury.

The signs and symptoms of early or superficial local cold injury include the following:

- Blanching of the skin (when you palpate the skin, normal color does not return)
- Loss of feeling and sensation in the injured area
- Continued softness of the skin in the injured area and in the tissue just beneath it
- Tingling sensation during any rewarming

The signs and symptoms of late or deep local cold injury include the following:

- White, waxy skin
- A firm-to-frozen feeling when the skin is palpated
- Swelling
- Blisters

- If partially or wholly thawed, the skin appears flushed with areas of purple and blanching or the skin appears mottled and cyanotic

EMERGENCY MEDICAL CARE FOR LOCAL COLD INJURY

The key to emergency care for local cold injury is never to thaw the tissue if there is any possibility of its refreezing. Always seek medical direction and follow local protocol. General guidelines for care include the following:

1. *Remove the patient immediately from the cold environment,* if possible.
2. *Never initiate thawing procedures if there is any danger of refreezing.* Keeping the tissue frozen is less dangerous than submitting it to refreezing.
3. *Administer oxygen at 15 lpm by nonrebreather mask* if you have not already done so as part of the initial assessment.
4. *Prevent further injury to the injured part.*
   If the patient has an early or superficial injury:
   - Carefully remove any jewelry or wet or restrictive clothing to prevent causing further injury. If clothing is frozen to the skin, leave it in place.
   - Immobilize the affected extremity to prevent movement and elevate.
   - Cover the affected skin with dressings or dry clothing to prevent friction or pressure.
   - Never rub or massage the affected skin.
   - Never re-expose the injured skin to the cold.
   If the patient has late or deep injury:
   - Carefully remove any jewelry or wet or restrictive clothing to prevent causing further injury. If clothing is frozen to the skin, leave it in place.
   - Cover the affected skin with dressings or dry clothing to prevent friction. Avoid pressure.
   - Do not break any blisters or treat them with salve or ointment.
   - Do not rub or massage the affected skin.
   - Never apply heat or rewarm the skin.
   - Do not allow the patient to walk on an injured extremity.

If you are in a wilderness situation or are facing an extremely long or delayed transport, you should initiate active, rapid rewarming of the injured tissue provided you will be able to keep it thawed. In such circumstances, contact medical direction or follow local protocol. Do not thaw tissue and then allow it to refreeze, as this will completely destroy the tissue. It is also a mistake to thaw frozen tissue gradually; thaw the tissue rapidly, as slow rewarming leads to tissue loss.

Rewarming frozen tissue is extremely painful for the patient, and medical control may want him to take an analgesic, such as aspirin or a nonaspirin product, to help relieve pain during the process.

To rewarm frozen tissue, follow these steps:

1. *Immerse the affected tissue in a warm water bath* (Figure 24-11). The water temperature should be just above body temperature (approximately 100° to 110°F). Never use dry heat as it is too difficult to control the temperature.
2. *Monitor the water to make sure it stays at an even temperature.* If possible, use a thermometer. (Water that is too hot can inflict a burn injury.) Keep the water warm by adding warm water. Never heat cooled water with any type of flame or electric unit.
3. *Continuously stir the water to keep heat evenly distributed and constant.*
4. *Keep the tissue in warm water until it is soft and color and sensation return to it.* The affected skin should turn a deep red or bluish color, and the skin should be soft and pliable.
5. *Dress the area with dry sterile dressings. If the affected area is a hand or foot, place dry sterile dressings between the toes and fingers. Once the skin is thawed, anything that contacts it, including water, must be sterile.*
6. *Elevate the affected extremity.*
7. *Protect against refreezing of the warmed part.*
8. *Transport as soon as possible.* ALL victims with frozen tissue require hospitalization.

DETAILED PHYSICAL EXAM

If there has been a mechanism of injury or any possibility of injury, and if time and the patient's condition permit, conduct a detailed physical exam of the cold emergency patient (whether suffering from generalized hypothermia and/or from local cold injury) to be sure that no injuries have been overlooked.

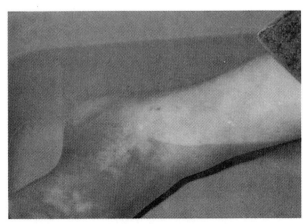

Figure 24-11   Thaw the affected area rapidly in water just above body temperature (100° to 110°F).

ONGOING ASSESSMENT

During the ongoing assessment of cold emergency patients, it is important to carefully reassess the patient's mental status. A decreasing mental status will indicate deterioration in the patient's condition. Closely monitor the airway and breathing. The breathing rate and depth may continue to decrease to a point of inadequacy where positive pressure ventilation with supplemental oxygen may be required. The pulses may also continue to decrease. Be prepared to begin CPR or to stop the ambulance to defibrillate the patient. Inspect the skin for changes in color and temperature. The patient may begin to feel sensations and pain if being rewarmed. Repeat and record the baseline vital signs every 5 minutes. Keep the patient warm and try not to re-expose him to the cold.

SUMMARY: ASSESSMENT AND CARE—COLD EMERGENCY

To review assessment findings that may be associated with a cold emergency and emergency care for a cold emergency, see Figures 24-12 and 24-13.

EXPOSURE TO HEAT

Just as exposure to cold can produce a variety of medical problems, so too can exposure to heat. Problems created by heat exposure can range from mild discomfort to life-threatening emergencies.

 HYPERTHERMIA

Heat-related emergencies are grouped under the name **hyperthermia.** They are brought on by an increase in the body's heat production or by an inability to eliminate the heat produced. Most heat injuries occur early in the summer season, before people have acclimated themselves to the season's higher temperatures. Various stages of hyperthermia are commonly called "heat cramps," "heat exhaustion," and "heat stroke."

- *Heat Cramps*—The least serious form of heat-related injury is muscle spasms, or cramps, that are thought by some researchers to result from the body losing too much salt during profuse sweating. The cramping is made worse when not enough salt is taken into the body, when calcium levels are low, or when too much water is drunk by the patient. Such cramping is occasionally caused by overexertion of muscles, inadequate stretching or warm-up, and lactic acid buildup in poorly conditioned muscles. This condition is referred to as "heat cramps."
- *Heat Exhaustion*—Extreme physical exertion in a hot, humid environment can affect even an otherwise fit individual. It can produce a disturbance of the body's blood flow, resulting in a mild state of shock. This is brought on by the pooling of blood in the vessels just below the skin, which causes blood to flow away from the major organs of the body. Due to prolonged and profuse sweating, the body loses large quantities of salt and water. When these are not adequately replaced, blood circulation diminishes, affecting the brain, heart, and lungs. This condition is referred to as "heat exhaustion." *In such cases, a patient's skin will be normal-to-cool in temperature, either pale or ashen gray in color, and sweaty.*
- *Heat Stroke*—If measures are not taken to remove the patient to a cool environment or stop the physical activity and replace lost fluid, his condition can deteriorate into the form of hyperthermia commonly called "heat stroke." This is a life-threatening medical emergency with a mortality ranging from 20 to 70 percent. It occurs when the body's heat-regulating mechanisms break down and become unable to cool the body sufficiently. The body becomes overheated, body temperature rises, and sweating ceases in about half the victims. Because no cooling takes place, the body stores increasingly more heat, the heat-producing mechanisms speed up, and eventually the brain cells are damaged, causing permanent disability or death. In such patients, the skin will be hot and red; it may be either moist or dry, since about half the victims in this stage of hyperthermia sweat while about half cease to sweat.

PREDISPOSING FACTORS

Several factors can predispose an individual to heat-related injuries. They include the following:

- *Climate*—Hot temperatures reduce the body's ability to lose heat by radiation; high humidity reduces the body's ability to lose heat by evaporation.
- *Exercise and Strenuous Activity*—They can cause the loss of more than one liter of sweat per hour.
- *Age*—Individuals at the extremes of age, such as the elderly and infants (especially newborns), have poor ability to regulate body temperature. Elderly patients often take medications that increase the risk of heat injury and may lack the mobility to escape a hot environment. Infants cannot remove their clothing if they get too hot.
- *Pre-existing Illnesses*—including the following:
  - Heart disease
  - Kidney disease
  - Cerebrovascular disease
  - Parkinson's disease
  - Thyroid gland disorders
  - Skin diseases, including eczema, scleroderma, and healed burns
  - Dehydration

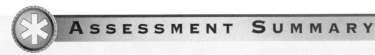

✳ ASSESSMENT SUMMARY

COLD EMERGENCY

The following are findings that may be associated with a cold emergency.

SCENE SIZE-UP

Pay particular attention to your own safety. Look for:
  Mechanism of injury
  Unstable ice
  Water hazards
  Source of cold exposure
  Ambient temperature
  Wind chill
  Wet clothing
  Alcohol or drugs
  Suspected head or spinal injury
  Exposed areas of skin

INITIAL ASSESSMENT

General Impression

Is patient dressed appropriately for weather?
Stiff posture
Staggering or incoordination
Drowsy or irrational appearance
Shivering may be apparent if body core temperature is above 90°F or absent if body core temperature is below 90°F.

Mental Status

Alert to unresponsive based on body core temperature

Airway

Potentially closed airway if mental status is altered

Breathing

Initially fast and normal depth, becoming shallow and slow as body temperature decreases

Circulation

Pulses may be difficult to find and assess
Heart rate is usually increased initially
Heart rate decreases as body temperature continues to decrease
Skin is red early, becoming pale, cyanotic and mottled as body temperature drops; skin becomes cold to touch

Status: Priority Patient if generalized cold injury (hypothermia) is suspected

FOCUSED HISTORY AND PHYSICAL EXAM

SAMPLE History

Signs and symptoms of generalized cold injury:
  Decreasing mental status

Decreasing motor and sensory function
  Changes to vital signs
Signs and symptoms of local cold injury—early or superficial:
  Blanching of skin
  Loss of feeling or sensation in injured area
  Underlying tissue remains soft
  Tingling sensation when rewarmed
Signs and symptoms of local cold injury—late or deep:
  White, waxy skin
  Underlying tissue is firm and hard to touch
  Blisters
  Swelling
  Skin purple, blanched, mottled, or cyanotic if thawed
History:
  Did patient ingest alcohol or drugs?
  Does patient have a circulatory disorder, cardiac disorder, or other medical condition?
  How long has patient been exposed to cold?

Physical Exam

Head, neck, and face:
  Pupils may be dilated, sluggish to respond to light
  Slurred speech
  Difficulty forming words and moving mouth
  Red, blanched, cyanotic, or white and waxy if exposed
Abdomen:
  Cold to touch
Extremities:
  Stiff and rigid
  Lack of coordination
  Shivering (body core temperature above 90°F)
  Reduced sensation
  Blanched skin that remains soft to touch (superficial local cold injury)
  Skin white, waxy, cyanotic, swelling, blisters, cold, and firm (deep local cold injury)

Baseline Vital Signs—Generalized Cold Injury

BP: normal early, continues to decrease, may be absent
HR: increased early; becoming decreased and barely palpable as body core temperature continues to drop
RR: initially increased, decreases as body continues to cool
Skin: red early, becoming pale, cyanotic, gray, waxy, and firm to touch late
Pupils: dilated; sluggish to respond to light

Figure 24-12a Assessment summary: cold emergency.

EMERGENCY CARE PROTOCOL

GENERALIZED COLD EMERGENCY

1. Remove patient from cold environment and remove all wet clothing. Prevent further heat loss.
2. Establish and maintain an open airway.
3. Suction secretions as necessary.
4. If breathing is inadequate, provide positive pressure ventilation with supplemental oxygen at a minimum rate of 12 ventilations/minute for an adult and 20 ventilations/minute for an infant or child.
5. If breathing is adequate, administer oxygen by nonrebreather mask at 15 lpm. If possible, deliver warm humidified oxygen.
6. If no pulse is present, apply the AED. Deliver only one set of three stacked defibrillations and

perform CPR. Contact medical direction for further orders.
7. Turn up heat to maximum in back of ambulance. Cover patient with blankets (passive rewarming).
8. If patient is alert, actively rewarm by placing hot packs under armpits, in groin area, and to chest. Also perform normal passive rewarming.
9. If patient is unresponsive or not responding appropriately, perform passive rewarming only.
10. Do not allow patient to eat or drink stimulants.
11. Do not rub or massage patient's extremities.
12. Handle patient gently to prevent stimulation of cardiac dysrhythmias; place in lateral recumbent position only if spinal injury is not suspected.
13. Transport.
14. Perform an ongoing assessment every 5 minutes.

EMERGENCY CARE PROTOCOL

LOCAL COLD INJURY

1. If you suspect a decreased body core temperature, follow the "Generalized Cold Emergency" protocol before proceeding with the "Local Cold Injury" protocol.
2. Remove patient from cold environment and remove all wet clothing; prevent further heat loss.
3. Remove jewelry, wet, or restrictive clothing. (Do not remove clothing that is frozen to the skin.)
4. Cover affected skin with dry sterile dressings.
5. For early or superficial injury:
   - Immobilize affected extremity.
   - Do not rub or massage.
   - Do not re-expose to cold.
6. For late or deep injury:
   - Do not rub or massage.
   - Do not break blisters.

   - Do not apply heat or rewarm area.
   - Do not allow patient to walk on affected extremity.
7. If required or instructed to rewarm, follow these guidelines:
   - Immerse affected tissue in warm water bath at 100 to 110°F.
   - Monitor water and stir to keep at constant temperature.
   - Keep immersed until color returns and skin and underlying tissue become soft.
   - Dress affected area.
   - Elevate involved extremity.
   - Protect against refreezing.
8. Transport.

Figure 24-12b *Emergency care protocols: generalized and local cold emergencies.*

EMERGENCY CARE ALGORITHM: COLD EMERGENCY

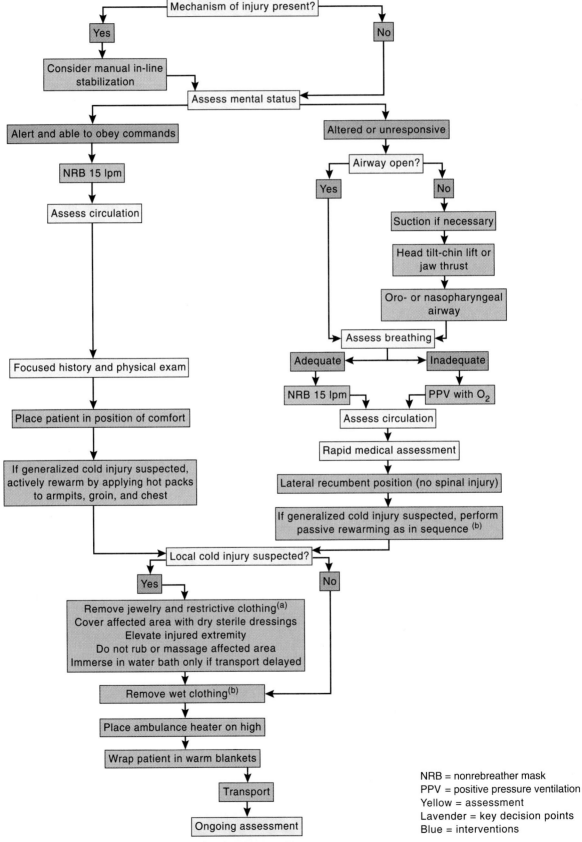

Figure 24-13 Emergency care algorithm: cold emergency.

– Obesity
– Infections or other conditions that cause fever
– Fatigue
– Diabetes
– Malnutrition
– Alcoholism
– Mental retardation
• *Certain Drugs and Medications*—including alcohol, cocaine, diuretics, barbiturates, hallucinogens, and medications that hamper sweating

ASSESSMENT AND CARE: HEAT-RELATED EMERGENCY

SCENE SIZE-UP

Scan the scene for evidence that the patient is suffering from a heat-related emergency. Probably the most important factors to consider are the ambient temperature and humidity. High temperatures, especially if greater than 90°F, and relative humidity greater than 75 percent, combine to create an environment that renders the body's cooling mechanisms less effective (Figure 24-14).

Exercise and activity are common precursors to heat-related emergencies. Look for clues to the patient's activities prior to the incident. Where is he found? If you find someone lying in a flower bed in the middle of a steamy August afternoon with gardening tools at his side, you could assume that he had been working outside in the hot sun before collapsing.

A person's clothing can also give clues to his activity. If you receive a call to assist a patient in the park in mid-July and find someone dressed in jogging shorts and running shoes, you might assume that he was exercising before the incident. You might find a patient collapsed in a cool, air-conditioned home on a summer day. If he is wearing jogging shorts and running shoes, you might at least suspect that he was outside exercising, felt ill, and returned home to call EMS. Reports of an ill or collapsed patient at an outdoor sporting event held in hot, humid weather should also make you suspect possible heat emergency.

Infants and children left in closed vehicles or in structures that are hot and poorly ventilated are prone to heat emergencies, especially if the infant or child is overdressed and too young to remove his own clothing. Elderly patients, especially those who are not mobile enough to escape their hot environments, are also very likely to become victims of a heat emergency.

Also, look for medications or drugs since these may also precipitate a heat-related emergency.

During the scene size-up, recognize your own limits and protect yourself from overexposure to the

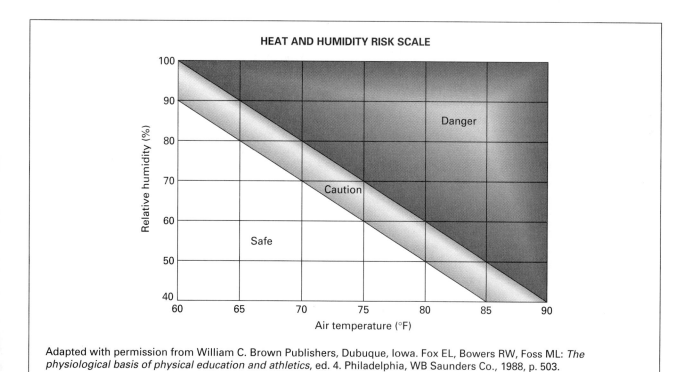

HEAT AND HUMIDITY RISK SCALE

Adapted with permission from William C. Brown Publishers, Dubuque, Iowa. Fox EL, Bowers RW, Foss ML: *The physiological basis of physical education and athletics*, ed. 4. Philadelphia, WB Saunders Co., 1988, p. 503.

Reproduced with permission from *Patient Care*, June 15, 1989. Copyright © 1989 Patient Care, Oradell, NJ. All rights reserved.

Figure 24-14   The risk of illness is increased when heat and humidity produce dangerous conditions. Lower temperatures with high humidity can also cause the body's temperature to rise.

heat. Dress appropriately and be sure to drink enough water to stay hydrated. Remember, if you are on stand-by at a public event held during the summer or if you have to walk long distances carrying heavy gear on a hot, humid day, you will be exposed to the same environmental extremes as the patients you are expected to treat.

INITIAL ASSESSMENT

While gathering a general impression of the patient, determine if he is dressed inappropriately for the hot environment. The mental status of the patients you encounter in heat emergencies may range from alert and oriented to completely unresponsive. The patient may complain of dizziness or may have fainted prior to your arrival. The mental status may deteriorate as the condition worsens.

Assess the airway and breathing. Closely monitor the airway and provide oxygen at 15 lpm by nonrebreather mask if the mental status is altered or continues to deteriorate. If the breathing is inadequate, begin positive pressure ventilation with supplemental oxygen.

The patient's radial pulse may be weak and rapid or absent, depending upon the level of dehydration. The skin may be moist and pale with a normal-to-cool temperature or hot and dry or moist. *The patient with altered mental status who has hot skin should be considered a priority patient.*

FOCUSED HISTORY AND PHYSICAL EXAM

If the patient is found in a hot environment, move him to a cool environment as quickly as possible. If the patient is responsive, gather a SAMPLE history, paying particular attention to the symptoms of which the patient complains. The OPQRST can be modified to gather further information about some of the symptoms. Pay particular attention to medications the patient may be taking, since some can contribute to the heat emergency. Be sure to determine the patient's last oral intake, especially consumption of water or other liquids. Get a description of events that preceded the incident. Conduct a focused medical assessment, targeting areas of complaint that were gathered during the SAMPLE history.

The baseline vital signs may reveal a blood pressure that is normal or low. The heart rate and respirations are typically elevated in heat emergencies. Pulses may be bounding or weak. Skin could be cool, normal, or hot to the touch and either moist or dry. *Hot skin is most alarming, since it indicates the most severe type of heat emergency.*

If the patient is unresponsive, conduct a rapid medical assessment, take baseline vital signs, and then gather the SAMPLE history from family or bystanders.

Signs and Symptoms of Generalized Hyperthermia The general signs and symptoms of heat-related injuries include the following (Figure 24-15):

- Muscle cramps
- Weakness or exhaustion
- Dizziness or faintness
- A rapid pulse that is usually strong at first, but becomes weak
- Initial deep, rapid breathing that becomes shallow and weak as damage progresses
- Headache
- Seizures
- Loss of appetite, nausea, or vomiting
- Altered mental status, possibly unresponsiveness
- The skin may be either moist and pale, with a normal-to-cool temperature, or hot and either dry or moist. *Hot skin that is either dry or moist represents a dire medical emergency.*

EMERGENCY MEDICAL CARE FOR A HEAT EMERGENCY PATIENT WITH MOIST, PALE, NORMAL-TO-COOL SKIN

For a patient whose skin is moist and pale, with normal-to-cool skin temperature, provide the following care:

1. *Move the patient to a cool place,* such as the back of an air-conditioned ambulance, away from the source of heat. If no cooler location is immediately available, at least move the patient out of the sun and into the shade.
2. *Administer oxygen at 15 lpm via a nonrebreather mask* if you have not already done so as part of the initial assessment.
3. *Remove as much of the patient's clothing as you can;* loosen what you cannot remove. The patient should be kept as comfortable as possible.
4. *Cool the patient by applying cold, wet compresses and/or by fanning lightly* (Figure 24-16). You want to help cool the patient, but make sure he does not get chilled.
5. *Place the patient in a supine position and raise his feet and legs 8 to 12 inches* to improve blood circulation to the brain.
6. *If the patient is fully responsive and is not nauseated, have him drink cool water.* Some physicians advise that the patient drink half a glassful every 15 minutes for an hour. Consult with medical direction and follow local protocol.
7. *If the patient is unresponsive or has an altered mental status or is vomiting, do NOT give fluids.*
8. Generally, a hyperthermic patient with moist, pale skin that is normal-to-cool in temperature needs *transport* when the patient:
   - Is unresponsive or has an altered mental status

SIGNS AND SYMPTOMS OF HEAT EMERGENCY

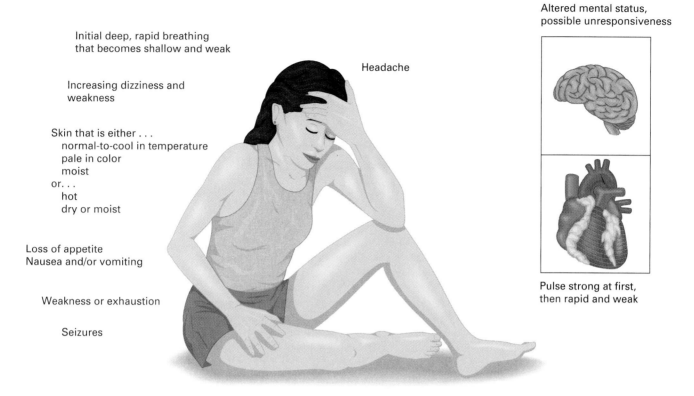

Initial deep, rapid breathing
that becomes shallow and weak

Increasing dizziness and
weakness

Skin that is either . . .
   normal-to-cool in temperature
   pale in color
   moist
or . . .
   hot
   dry or moist

Loss of appetite
Nausea and/or vomiting

Weakness or exhaustion

Seizures

Headache

Altered mental status,
possible unresponsiveness

Pulse strong at first,
then rapid and weak

Muscle cramps

Figure 24-15 Signs and symptoms of a serious heat emergency.

- Is vomiting or is nauseated and will not drink fluids
- Has a history of medical problems
- Has a temperature above 101°F
- Has a rising temperature
- Does not respond to therapy (symptoms do not improve)

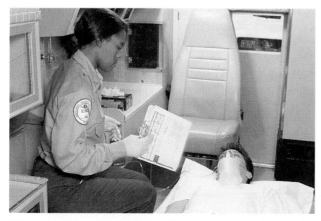

Figure 24-16 If the skin is moist, pale, and normal-to-cool, place the patient in a cool environment and fan to promote cooling.

EMERGENCY MEDICAL CARE FOR A HEAT EMERGENCY PATIENT WITH HOT SKIN, MOIST OR DRY

A patient with hot skin that is either moist or dry represents a dire medical emergency. Cooling the patient takes priority over everything other than airway, breathing, and circulatory management. Provide the following care:

1. *Remove the patient from the source of heat and place him in a cool environment,* such as an air-conditioned room or ambulance. If nothing else, move the patient out of the sun and into the shade.
2. *Remove as much of the patient's clothing as is possible or reasonable.*
3. *Administer oxygen at 15 lpm via a nonrebreather mask* if you have not already done so as part of the initial assessment.
4. *Immediately begin to cool the patient.* Generally, one method alone will not effectively cool the patient, so use a combination of the following (Figure 24-17):
   - Pour cool water over the patient's body.
   - Place cold packs in the patient's groin, at each side of the neck, in the armpits, and behind each knee to cool the large surface blood vessels.

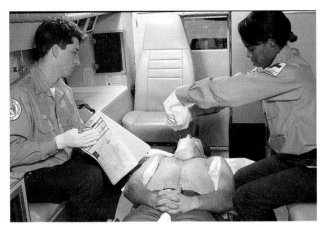

Figure 24-17   If the skin is hot and dry or moist, promote cooling by applying cool packs, fanning, and pouring cool water over the patient's body.

– Wrap a wet sheet that has been soaked in cool water around the patient.
– Fan the patient aggressively or direct an electric fan at the patient.
– Keep the patient's skin wet to promote cooling.
– Use slower cooling if the patient starts to shiver, since shivering produces heat.

5. Because the patient's entire body is involved in the heat emergency, several complications may result from the condition or from the treatment of it. *Be prepared to manage seizures or prevent the aspiration of vomitus.*

6. Transport immediately, continuing to administer oxygen and cooling methods during transport. *Always transport a hyperthermic patient with hot skin that is moist or dry.* Such a patient always needs hospital care.

 ASSESSMENT SUMMARY

HEAT EMERGENCY

The following are findings that may be associated with a heat emergency.

SCENE SIZE-UP

Pay particular attention to your own safety. Look for:
　High ambient temperatures, usually greater than 90°F
　Humidity greater than 75%
　Evidence of exercise or other activity
　Patient's clothing

INITIAL ASSESSMENT

General Impression

Is patient dressed appropriately for weather?
Excessive sweating or excessively dry skin
Dizziness or fainting

Mental Status

Alert to unresponsive based on body core temperature

Airway

Potentially closed airway if mental status is altered

Breathing

Initially fast and normal depth; becoming shallow and slow as body temperature increases

Circulation

Heart rate is usually increased initially
Pulse decreases as body temperature increases excessively

Skin may be excessively dry or wet, but may be extremely hot (heat stroke)
Skin may be moist, pale, and normal to cool (heat exhaustion)

Status: Priority patient if hot skin, whether moist or dry, or altered mental status is present

FOCUSED HISTORY AND PHYSICAL EXAM

SAMPLE History

Signs and symptoms:
　Dizziness and weakness
　Headache
　Nausea and/or vomiting
　Seizures
　Muscle cramps
　Hot, dry or moist skin
　Pale, cool, and moist skin
　Altered mental status
History:
　Did patient ingest alcohol or drugs?
　Does patient have a circulatory disorder, cardiac disorder, or other medical condition?
　How long has patient been exposed to heat?

Physical Exam

Head, neck, and face:
　Pupils may be dilated and sluggish to respond to light
　Slurred speech
　Headache

Figure 24-18a   Assessment summary: heat emergency.

ONGOING ASSESSMENT

During the ongoing assessment, reevaluate the mental status, airway, breathing, circulation, baseline vital signs, and treatment. The mental status may continue to deteriorate if the body temperature continues to rise. The mental status may improve once the patient is cooled and treatment is initiated. Closely reassess the airway and breathing. Be prepared to establish an airway and to provide positive pressure ventilation if breathing becomes inadequate, especially in patients with hot skin. Also, be prepared to manage seizures with such patients.

The pulse may continue to weaken, or the rate may increase further. Correlate changes in the pulse rate with the patient's mental status. If the pulse is decreasing and the mental status improving, it is a sign that the treatment is proving effective. If the pulse is rapidly increasing or decreasing and the patient's mental status is declining, it is a grave indication that the patient is deteriorating. Reassess and record the baseline vital signs every 5 minutes. Report your assessment to the receiving hospital.

SUMMARY: ASSESSMENT AND CARE—HEAT EMERGENCY

To review assessment findings that may be associated with a heat emergency and emergency care for a heat emergency, see Figures 24-18 and 24-19.

Extremities
    Muscle cramps
    Hot skin that is dry or moist (priority patient)
    Cool, pale, and moist skin

Baseline Vital Signs—Heat Emergency

BP: normal to decreased
HR: increased; may decrease if body core temperature becomes excessively high

RR: initially increased; may decrease if body core temperature continues to rise excessively
Skin: may be hot, dry or moist (priority patient) or cool, moist, and pale
Pupils: midsize to dilated; sluggish to respond

EMERGENCY CARE PROTOCOL

HEAT EMERGENCY

1. Remove patient from hot environment and remove clothing. Prevent further heat gain.
2. Establish and maintain an open airway; insert a nasopharyngeal or oropharyngeal airway if patient is unresponsive and has no gag or cough reflex
3. Suction secretions as necessary.
4. If breathing is inadequate, provide positive pressure ventilation with supplemental oxygen at a minimum rate of 12 ventilations/minute for an adult and 20 ventilations/minute for an infant or child.
5. If breathing is adequate, administer oxygen by nonrebreather mask at 15 lpm.
6. Turn up air conditioner to maximum in back of ambulance.
7. If skin is cool, moist, and pale (heat exhaustion), do the following:
   - Cool patient by applying cold, wet compresses; fan lightly.
   - Place patient in supine position with legs elevated 8 to 12 inches.
   - If patient is vomiting, place in lateral recumbent position.
   - If patient is responsive and not nauseated, administer water by mouth at a half glass every 15 minutes.
8. If skin is hot and dry or moist (heat stroke), do the following:
   - Pour cool water over patient.
   - Place cold packs in armpits, behind each knee, and at side of the neck.
   - Fan patient aggressively.
   - If patient shivers, slow cooling process.
   - Be prepared to manage seizures.
9. Transport.
10. Perform an ongoing assessment every 5 minutes.

Figure 24-18b   Emergency care protocol: heat emergency.

EMERGENCY CARE ALGORITHM: HEAT EMERGENCY

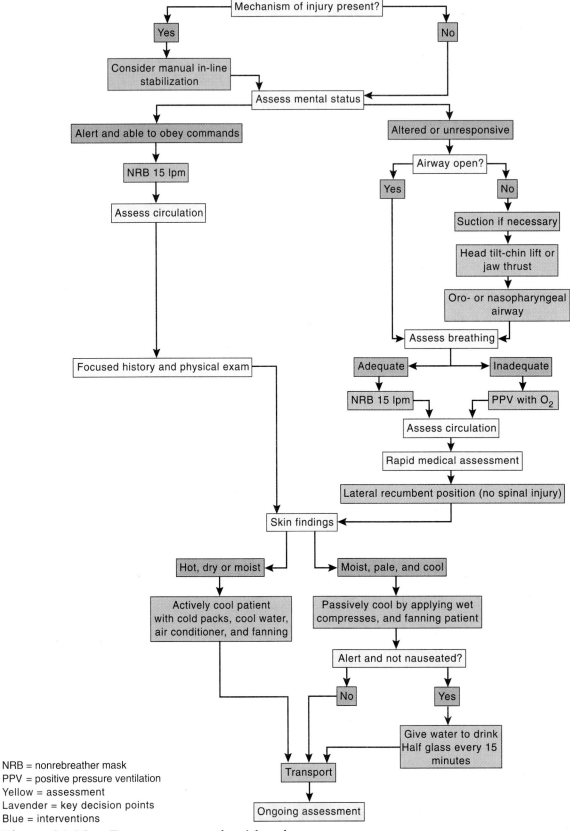

Figure 24-19   Emergency care algorithm: heat emergency.

BITES AND STINGS

◥

Many people who venture into the outdoors fear the possibility of a snakebite. But, in fact, such bites are relatively uncommon and the number of people who die from a snakebite each year is extremely small. Still, the possibility of death or crippling injury from a snakebite does exist and you should be prepared to deal with the situation if you encounter it.

Insect bites and stings are far more common, and most are considered minor. It is only when the patient has an allergic reaction and runs the risk of developing anaphylactic shock that the situation becomes an emergency. Even under those conditions, accurate recognition and prompt treatment can save lives and prevent permanent tissue damage.

ASSESSMENT AND CARE: BITES AND STINGS

SCENE SIZE-UP

Your priority during scene size-up should be to protect yourself and your partner. If your patient has been bitten or stung, you too might fall victim to bites and stings unless you exercise caution.

Rather than going directly to the patient's side, pause and look and listen for swarming bees or hornets. If they are present, you may have to wait until they disperse before approaching.

When you get to the patient's side, scan the ground around him carefully, looking for snakes, ant hills, or openings to underground yellow jacket nests. When you begin to examine the patient, be alert to the possibility that insects have become trapped in his clothing and may bite or sting when you move it.

Once your safety is assured, look around the scene for evidence of what may have bitten or stung the patient. Is an insect nest visible in a nearby tree, or under the eaves of a house, or in the ground nearby? Are there signs that the patient was engaged in activity such as clearing underbrush or gardening that might have disturbed snakes or insects? Was the patient working in a garage, basement, attic, or shed where spiders and other insects might nest? Are there dead insects on the ground around the patient?

INITIAL ASSESSMENT

During the initial assessment, gather a general impression of the patient and his mental status. If elements of the scene size-up have led you to suspect the possibility of bites or stings, be especially alert when assessing the airway and breathing. Remember that some patients have an allergic reaction to bites and stings that can lead to anaphylactic shock, an emergency that generally has a rapid and life-threatening affect on the airway and breathing.

FOCUSED HISTORY AND PHYSICAL EXAM

If you detect the signs and symptoms of anaphylactic shock listed below, continue with assessment and emergency medical care as described in Chapter 20, "Allergic Reaction." If the patient displays the more common signs and symptoms of reaction to bites and stings listed below, continue with the assessment as described in the section on injected poisons in Chapter 21, "Poisoning Emergencies." Then, provide emergency medical care as described below.

Signs and Symptoms of Anaphylactic Shock   Anaphylactic shock, a life-threatening medical emergency, may develop following bites or stings. If a patient develops signs and symptoms of this condition, perform the necessary emergency care and transport immediately. Signs and symptoms include the following:

- Hives
- Flushing
- Upper airway obstruction
- Faintness
- Dizziness
- Generalized itching
- Generalized swelling, including eyelids, lips, tongue
- Difficulty swallowing
- Shortness of breath, wheezing, or stridor
- Labored breathing
- Abdominal cramps
- Confusion
- Loss of responsiveness
- Convulsions
- Hypotension (low blood pressure)

EMERGENCY MEDICAL CARE FOR ANAPHYLACTIC SHOCK

Care for anaphylactic shock is as follows:

1. *Maintain a patent airway.* Suction secretions.
2. *Administer oxygen and support breathing.* Provide oxygen at 15 lpm by nonrebreather mask if breathing is adequate. Provide positive pressure ventilation with supplemental oxygen if breathing is or becomes inadequate.
3. *Administer epinephrine by a prescribed auto-injector* with permission from medical direction.
4. *Consider calling for advanced life support.*
5. *Initiate early transport.*

Review the complete description of signs and symptons and emergency medical care for this condition in Chapter 20, "Allergic Reaction."

Signs and Symptoms of a Bite or Sting   General signs and symptoms of bites and stings include the following:

- History of a spider or snake bite or a sting from an insect, scorpion, or marine animal

- Pain that is often immediate and severe or burning; within several hours the area may become numb
- Redness or other discoloration around the bite
- Swelling around the bite, sometimes gradually spreading
- Weakness or faintness
- Dizziness
- Chills
- Fever
- Nausea or vomiting
- Bite marks
- Stinger

EMERGENCY MEDICAL CARE FOR A BITE OR STING

General emergency medical care for bites and stings includes the following steps:

1. *If the stinger is still present, remove it by gently scraping against it* with the edge of a credit card or the edge of a knife. Scrape in the direction of the base of the stinger to avoid breaking it off below the skin. Be careful not to squeeze the stinger with tweezers, forceps, or your fingers as doing so can force additional venom from the venom sac into the wound. Make sure you remove the venom sac as it can continue to secrete venom even though the stinger is detached from the insect.
2. *Wash the area around the bite or sting* gently with a mild agent or strong soap solution. If necessary, irrigate the area with a large amount of sterile saline. Make sure contaminated saline flows away from the body. Never scrub the area.
3. *Remove any jewelry or other constricting objects* as soon as possible; ideally, before any swelling begins.
4. *Lower the injection site slightly below the level of the patient's heart.*
5. *Apply a cold pack to an insect bite or sting* to relieve pain and swelling. *Do not apply cold to snakebites or to injuries inflicted by marine animals.*
6. *Some experts advise the use of a constricting band in the treatment of snakebite.* Consult medical direction and follow local protocols.
7. *Observe the patient carefully for the signs and symptoms of an allergic reaction;* in cases of reaction, treat as described in Chapter 20, "Allergic Reaction."
8. *Keep the patient calm, limit his physical activity, and keep him warm. Transport as soon as possible.* If the patient shows any signs of allergic reaction, begin transport immediately.

ONGOING ASSESSMENT

Most important during the ongoing assessment is to monitor the patient's airway, breathing, and circulation carefully. The signs and symptoms of anaphylac-

tic shock may take minutes to several hours to develop. You should be alert to their appearance and be prepared to provide the emergency medical care for this life-threatening condition just outlined.

ENRICHMENT

The enrichment section contains information that is valuable as background for the EMT-B but that goes substantially beyond the U.S. Department of Transportation (DOT) EMT-Basic curriculum.

HEAT CRAMPS

As mentioned earlier in this chapter, one of the symptoms of a heat emergency is muscle cramping. In some patients with the mildest hyperthermia, cramping may be the only symptom. Cramping typically occurs to the muscles of the legs and abdomen.

EMERGENCY MEDICAL CARE FOR HEAT CRAMPS

To treat a patient with heat cramps:

1. *Remove the patient from the source of heat to a cool environment.* If nothing else, move the patient out of the sun and into the shade.
2. *Consult medical direction before giving the patient sips of low-concentration salt water* at the rate of half a glassful every 15 minutes. If possible, use a commercial product, such as Gatorade, with a low glucose content. Salt water is made by diluting one teaspoon of salt in one quart of water. Do not give the patient salt tablets. Follow local protocol.
3. *Apply moist towels to the patient's forehead and over the cramping muscles.* Try to gently stretch the involved muscle groups. Some experts advise massaging the involved muscles if it does not cause additional pain. Consult with medical direction and follow local protocol.
4. *Explain to the patient what happened so he can avoid a recurrence of the problem.* Advise the patient to avoid exertion for 12 hours.

Generally, you need to transport a patient with heat cramps only if the patient has other illnesses or injuries, develops other symptoms, or does not respond to your care and deteriorates.

 SNAKEBITE

About 45,000 people per year are bitten by snakes in the United States; of those, 7,000 receive bites from one of the two types of poisonous snakes: coral snakes and pit vipers (rattlesnakes, copperheads, and water moccasins). More than half the poisonous snakebites involve children, and most occur between April and October during daylight hours.

The bites of nonpoisonous snakes are not considered serious and are generally treated as minor wounds; only bites of poisonous snakes are considered medical emergencies. In only about a third of the cases of bites by poisonous snakes do the snakes inject venom into the victim. When venom is injected, symptoms generally occur immediately.

A poisonous snakebite is characterized by one or two distinct puncture wounds (Figure 24-20). The exception is the coral snake, which leaves a semicircular pattern with its teeth as it "chews" the skin. Most poisonous snakes have the following characteristics:

- Large fangs; nonpoisonous snakes have small teeth. The exception is the coral snake, a poisonous snake that does not have fangs.
- Elliptical pupils or vertical slits, much like those of a cat; nonvenomous snakes have round pupils.
- A pit between the eye and the mouth.
- A variety of different shaped blotches on backgrounds of pink, yellow, olive, tan, gray, or brown skin. The exception is the coral snake, which is ringed with red, yellow, and black.
- A triangular head that is larger than the neck.

The signs and symptoms of a pit viper bite generally occur immediately; those of a coral snake bite are usually delayed by at least 1 and as many as 8 hours. The severity of a pit viper bite, depending on how much poison was injected, is gauged by how rapidly symptoms develop (Figure 24-21). Other factors that determine the severity of a snakebite include the following:

- The location of the bite, since fatty tissue absorbs the venom more slowly than muscle tissue
- Whether pathogens (organisms or substances capable of causing disease) are present in the venom
- The patient's size and weight
- The patient's general health and condition
- How much physical activity the patient engaged in immediately following the bite, since physical activity will spread the venom

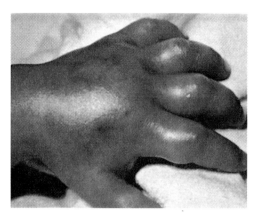

Figure 24-21   *Snake bite to the hand.*

The emergency medical care for snakebite is the same as general emergency medical care for bites and stings described earlier in the chapter.

INSECT BITES AND STINGS

Most insect bites are treated like any other wound. Generally, medical help is necessary only if the itching lasts longer than two days, signs of infection or an allergic reaction develop, or the insect is poisonous.

The normal reaction to an insect sting is a sharp, stinging pain followed immediately by an itchy, painful swelling. Redness, tenderness, and swelling at or around the sting site, even if severe, in the absence of other symptoms is considered to be a local reaction. Local reactions are rarely serious or life threatening and can be treated successfully with cold compresses.

Allergic reactions are another story: Thousands of people are allergic to the stings of bees, wasps, hornets, and yellow jackets. For those people, a sting may precipitate anaphylactic shock. This condition may cause death from within a few minutes to an hour of the sting. For more information on anaphylactic shock, see Chapter 20, "Allergic Reaction."

BLACK WIDOW SPIDER

The black widow spider is characterized by a shiny black body, thin legs, and a crimson red marking on its abdomen, usually in the shape of an hourglass or two triangles. Of the five species in the U.S., only three are black, and not all have the characteristic red marking.

The female black widow spider, larger than the male, is one of the largest spiders in the U.S. Males generally do not bite; females bite only when hungry, agitated, or protecting the egg sac. The black widow spider is usually found in dry, secluded, dimly lit areas; it has an extremely strong, funnel-shaped web.

Black widow spider bites are the leading cause of death from spider bites in the U.S. Those at highest

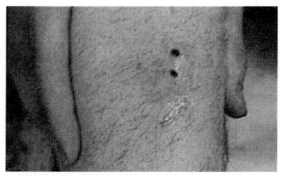

Figure 24-20   *Typical rattlesnake bite.*

risk for developing severe reactions to the bites are children under the age of 16, people over the age of 60, people with chronic illness, and anyone with hypertension.

In addition to the general signs and symptoms of bites and stings discussed below, black widow spider bites cause the following:

- A pinprick sensation at the bite site, becoming a dull ache within about 30 minutes
- Severe muscle spasms, especially in the shoulders, back, chest, and abdomen
- Rigid, boardlike abdomen

When treating victims of black widow spider bite, you should usually provide general wound care and transport.

Brown Recluse Spider

The brown recluse spider is generally brown but can range in color from yellow to dark chocolate brown. The characteristic marking is a brown, violin-shaped marking on the upper back. The bite of the brown recluse spider is a serious medical condition: The bite usually does not heal and may require surgical repair (Figure 24-22).

Unfortunately, most brown recluse spider bite victims are unaware that they have been bitten, since the bite is often painless at first. Several hours after the bite, it becomes bluish surrounded by a white periphery, then a red halo or "bull's-eye" pattern. Within 7 to 10 days, the bite becomes a large ulcer.

Scorpion

Of the three species of scorpion in the U.S. that sting and inject poisonous venom, the sting of only one is generally fatal. The severity of the sting depends on the amount of venom injected. Ninety percent of all scorpion stings occur on the hands.

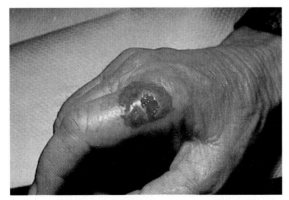

Figure 24-22 Wound from a brown recluse spider bite.

In addition to the general signs and symptoms of bites and stings, scorpion stings cause the following: a sharp pain at the injection site, drooling, poor coordination, incontinence, and seizures.

Fire Ant

Most common in the southeastern U.S., the fire ant gets its name not from its red to black color, but from the intense, fiery, burning pain its bite causes. Fire ants bite down into the skin, then sting downwardly as they pivot; the result is a characteristic circular pattern of bites. Fire ant bites produce extremely painful vesicles that are filled with fluid. At first the fluid is clear; later it becomes cloudy. Fire ant bites can also cause a large local reaction, characterized by swelling, pain, and redness that affect the entire extremity.

Tick

Tick bites are serious because ticks can carry tick fever, Rocky Mountain spotted fever, and other bacterial diseases. Lyme disease, usually transmitted by the tiny deer tick but now thought sometimes to be transmitted by the larger dog tick, can cause long-term neurologic and other complications if not identified and treated early.

Ticks are visible after they have attached themselves to the skin; they often choose warm, moist areas, such as the scalp, other hairy areas, the armpits, the groin, and skin creases. Many patients are unaware that they have been bitten by a tick.

The only appropriate prehospital treatment for tick bite is prompt removal of the tick, which can help prevent infection. To remove a tick, use tweezers and grasp the tick as close as possible to the point where it is attached to the skin. Pull firmly and steadily until the tick is dislodged. Do not twist or jerk the tick, since that may result in incomplete removal. Never pluck an embedded tick out of the skin, as you may force infected blood into the patient. Avoid squashing an engorged tick during removal, since infected blood may spread contamination. After removal, wash the bite area thoroughly with soap and water and apply an antiseptic to the area.

Marine Life Bites and Stings

There are approximately 2,000 poisonous marine animals. While most types live in temperate or tropical waters, some can be found in virtually all waters. Most poisonous marine life is not aggressive; in fact, most cases of such poisoning occur when a person swims into or steps on an animal.

There are two important differences between the bites and stings of marine animals and those of land animals. First, the venom of marine life may cause more extensive tissue damage than that of land animals. Second, venoms of aquatic organisms are destroyed by heat; so heat, not ice, should be applied to marine bites and stings.

In cases of marine life bites and stings, try to identify the animal because some very effective antivenins are available.

EMERGENCY MEDICAL CARE FOR MARINE LIFE POISONING

In general, bites and stings inflicted by marine life should be treated the same as soft-tissue injuries. However, follow these specific guidelines as needed:

- Use forceps to remove any material that sticks to the sting site on the surface of the flesh, then irrigate the wound with water.
- Do not attempt to remove spines that are embedded in joints or neurovascular structures or that are deeply embedded in skin.
- If the patient was stung by a jellyfish, coral, hydra, or anemone, carefully remove dried tentacles and pour vinegar on the affected area to denature the toxin. If meat tenderizer is available, sprinkle the area with it; doing so will help stop the stinging.
- Apply heat or soak the affected area in hot water for at least 30 minutes or throughout transport.

CASE STUDY FOLLOW-UP

SCENE SIZE-UP

Your initial call was for a disoriented elderly woman who fell into a snow bank wearing only a housecoat and slippers approximately 2 hours prior to the call. The woman has also complained of pain in her left ankle.

You pull up at 2125 Central Avenue at 1321 hours. The police radioed in the call, and their presence on the scene assures you that is secure. It is an overcast afternoon, with gusty winds. The outside temperature is 26°F. Because of information in the dispatch and the weather conditions, you are alert to the probability of generalized hypothermia as well as possible local cold injury and other injuries that might have resulted from a fall. With police on the scene to watch the ambulance, you leave its motor running and the heat turned up in the patient compartment as you get out. One officer stays with the ambulance, while another leads you to the woman.

The scene size-up reveals no obvious hazards; the patient is in the alley behind the house and there are no traffic hazards. Because there is only one patient and the mechanism of injury was a fall, there is no need for additional units.

INITIAL ASSESSMENT

You approach the woman and say to her, "Hello. My name is Sonia Weill and this is my partner, Jake Gallow. Could you tell us your name and if you're in any pain?" The woman replies, "I'm Harriet Rector. I'm cold. I want to go home. My husband fell once like this, but not for so long. He's dead now. I just want to go inside. I have to feed Fluffy. Nothing hurts. I should have taken out the garbage tomorrow. Is that

Thursday? But I hadn't taken it out yesterday. My ankle hurts. On the right. No, the left. Where's my dog?"

In spite of the fact that Mrs. Rector fell into a big, soft snow bank, your partner initiates manual in-line stabilization of her head and neck as a precaution. Your general impression is of an elderly female who is responsive but disoriented. The patient knows her name but is unclear as to the day of the week and exactly where she is. You proceed to assess airway, breathing, and circulation and find no life threats other than the cold environment. You begin oxygen therapy at 15 lpm with a nonrebreather mask and cover the patient with a blanket, making sure to roll her carefully in order to place the blanket under her also.

FOCUSED HISTORY AND PHYSICAL EXAM

Although the possibility of spine injury is small, you and Jake transfer and immobilize Mrs. Rector to a long spine board and quickly move her into the back of the warm ambulance before undertaking the focused history and physical exam. You take care to be extremely gentle in moving her.

Once Mrs. Rector is comfortably settled inside the ambulance, you continue questioning her, using the OPQRST format. You determine that her chief complaint is that her left leg hurts from the fall. You attempt to obtain a SAMPLE history, but Mrs. Rector does not respond appropriately to your questions, chiefly asking about her dog. You reassure her that you will get someone to take care of Fluffy.

You initiate a rapid trauma assessment. As you are examining the abdomen, you slide your hand inside Mrs. Rector's housecoat and place the back of your hand on her abdomen. You note that the skin there is cool to the touch, one of the signs of generalized hypothermia. The extremities exam reveals a painful, swollen left ankle. You quickly apply a splint, being sure to check motor function, sensation, and circulation before and after application of the splint.

At the same time, you check for signs of local cold injury. Mrs. Rector was able to keep her hands warm by tucking them under her armpits, but her feet, which were covered only by flimsy slippers, show signs of early superficial cold injury. She has no sensation in her toes. The skin is soft but very cold to the touch and normal skin color does not return after palpation. You have already removed the slippers and splinted the painful, swollen ankle. Now you splint the other foot as well to prevent movement and protect both feet with dry dressings.

Jake, meanwhile, has finished gathering the vital signs: they are blood pressure 102/60, heart rate 60, respiration rate 12, and skin pale, cold, and firm to the touch.

Ongoing Assessment

Once en route to the hospital, you cover Mrs. Rector in an additional warm, dry blanket. You had previously turned up the heat in the patient compartment, producing a suitable environment for passive rewarming.

Your priority is to maintain an airway and breathing and reassess vital signs and mental status. Mrs. Rector continues to speak distractedly about her dog and a number of seemingly unconnected events, indicating that her airway and breathing are adequate but her mental status is still altered. You check to be sure that the nonrebreather mask is securely sealed to her face and that the oxygen flow is adequate. Jake takes another set of vital signs: Blood pressure is still 102/60, but the heart rate has increased to 65 and the respiration rate is now 14. The skin is still cool, but it now has a mottled appearance. Mrs. Rector begins to complain that her feet tingle and hurt.

You arrive at Ellis Hospital at 1341 hours. You give your report on the case to the emergency department nurse, being sure to include the latest set of vitals taken in the ambulance and to note Mrs. Rector's new complaints about pains in her feet. Then you telephone Mrs. Rector's neighbor who agrees to take care of the dog. Before you leave the hospital, you see the emergency department physician and ask about Mrs. Rector's prognosis. She says that they've begun actively rewarming Mrs. Rector, but that it's too early to tell how she will respond.

A few weeks later, you and Jake pass by 2125 Central Avenue on your way back from a call and see Mrs. Rector out walking Fluffy. You return her wave and smile as you go by.

CHAPTER REVIEW

TERMS AND CONCEPTS

You may wish to review the following terms and concepts included in this chapter.

active rewarming—technique of aggressively applying heat to a patient to rewarm his body.
conduction—transfer of heat through direct physical touch with nearby objects.
convection—loss of body heat to the atmosphere when air passes over the body.
evaporation—conversion of a liquid or solid into a gas; evaporation of sweat is a means by which the body is cooled.
generalized cold emergency—see *generalized hypothermia*.
generalized hypothermia—an overall reduction in body temperature, affecting the entire body; also called hypothermia or generalized cold emergency.

hyperthermia—high body temperature.
hypothermia—low body temperature. See also *generalized hypothermia*.
local cold injury—damage to body tissues in a specific part of the body resulting from exposure to cold.
passive rewarming—the use of the patient's own heat production and conservation mechanisms to rewarm him, for example, simply placing the patient in a warm environment and covering him with blankets.
radiation—transfer of heat from the surface of one object to the surface of another without physical contact between the objects.
water chill—the increase in rate of cooling in the presence of water or wet clothing.
wind chill—the combined cooling effect of wind speed and environmental temperature.

REVIEW QUESTIONS

1. Name the five processes through which the body loses heat.
2. Explain the difference between hypothermia and hyperthermia.
3. List the signs and symptoms of generalized hypothermia.
4. Explain the steps in treatment of a patient suffering from a local cold injury.
5. Explain the treatment of the patient suffering from a heat emergency.
6. List conditions that would predispose a patient to experience a cold emergency.
7. List conditions that would predispose a patient to experience a heat emergency.
8. Explain the difference between active and passive rewarming.
9. List the signs and symptoms associated with bites and stings.
10. Explain the general emergency medical care for a patient suffering from a bite or sting.

CHAPTER 25

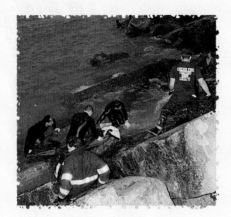

Drowning, Near-Drowning, and Diving Emergencies

INTRODUCTION

Water-related incidents make up a category of environmental emergencies posing special challenges for EMT-Basics. Patients in such incidents have often sustained life-threatening injuries. They need emergency medical care as rapidly as possible. But the circumstances in which they have received the injuries may expose medical personnel attempting to assist them to the risk of injury. Caring for patients in such circumstances requires of EMT-Bs not only emergency medical skills but also the ability to recognize and avoid or reduce potential hazards at the scene.

OBJECTIVES

Numbered objectives are from the United States Department of Transportation 1994 EMT-Basic National Standard Curriculum. Asterisked objectives, if any, pertain to material that is supplemental to the DOT curriculum.

COGNITIVE

4-7.6   Recognize the signs and symptoms of water-related emergencies. (p. 474)

4-7.7   Describe the complications of near-drowning. (pp. 470, 472, 473–474, 477)

PSYCHOMOTOR

4-7.11   Demonstrate the assessment and emergency medical care of a near-drowning patient.

4-7.12   Demonstrate completing a prehospital care report for patients with environmental emergencies.

Additional objectives from DOT Lesson 4-7 are addressed in Chapter 24, "Environmental Emergencies."

CASE STUDY

THE DISPATCH

EMS Unit 631—proceed to a possible drowning at 99 Wolf Road in the Delmar Hotel. The manager stated a 25-year-old male is in trouble in the pool. Police are en route at this time. Time out is 2132 hours.

ON ARRIVAL

Your ambulance arrives at the same time as the police unit. You are met at the hotel entrance by a frantic man who identifies himself as the manager. He leads you back to the pool, saying on the way, "I told them they couldn't have alcohol in the pool area. But they're so smart. They sneak it in anyway. Then they come running into the office, drunk, yelling for help. One of them thinks he can do a jack-knife into the shallow end. Idiots."

As you reach the pool area, you note a small crowd of young men and women on the deck. Some of them are yelling, "Come on, Robby! Get out, man! Come on!" A couple of paper bags and carry-alls are tipped over near the deck chairs, and empty beer bottles have rolled out from them. The police move the bystanders back and quiet them down.

With the scene secure, you approach the edge of the pool and observe in it a young man floating supine with the support of a hotel employee. The young man appears very scared and tells you he cannot feel his arms or legs.

How would you proceed to assess and care for this patient?

During this chapter, you will learn special considerations of assessment and care for patient in water-related emergencies. Later, we will return to the case and apply what you have learned.

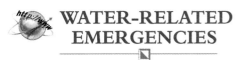

WATER-RELATED EMERGENCIES

While drownings are the type of fatality most commonly associated with water emergencies, drownings are actually responsible for only about one in twenty water-related deaths. The rest are mostly caused by diving and deep-water exploration, boating, and water skiing. Water-related deaths may also result from motor vehicle accidents. In addition to drown-ing and near-drowning, water-related accidents can cause bleeding, soft tissue injuries, and musculoskeletal injuries.

Drownings and near-drownings do not always occur in large bodies of water. An adult can drown in just a few inches of water, and an infant in even less. Recent studies indicate that one-fourth of all infants who drown do so in five-gallon buckets; others drown in bathtubs and toilets.

The statistics regarding water emergencies are especially tragic because many of the deaths could be prevented with the wearing of personal floatation devices (PFDs) when in or around water or when boating, with proper adult supervision of swimming pools, and with the provision of locked fences around pools. Prompt and proper application of basic life support techniques by bystanders could also significantly reduce deaths. A number of prevention measures are summarized in Figure 25-1.

NEAR-DROWNING AND DROWNING

Near-drowning is defined as survival, at least temporarily (24 hours), from near-suffocation due to submersion. **Drowning** is death from suffocation due to submersion. Drowning is the third leading cause of accidental death in the United States. In children under the age of 5, drowning is the leading cause of death. Among adults, alcohol intoxication is a frequent contributing factor to drowning deaths.

The poorest prognosis for near-drowning/drowning patients is among older people, those who struggle in the water, those who suffer associated injuries, those who are submerged for a long time, and those who are in warm, dirty, or brackish (salty) water. Panic on the part of a swimmer can often contribute to a drowning death (Figure 25-2).

The major causes of drowning include the following:

- Getting exhausted in the water
- Losing control and getting swept into water that is too deep
- Losing a support (such as sinking a boat)
- Getting trapped or entangled while in the water
- Using drugs or alcohol before getting into the water
- Suffering seizures while in the water
- Using poor judgment in the water
- Suffering hypothermia
- Suffering trauma
- Having a diving accident

PREVENTING NEAR–DROWNING ACCIDENTS

Three caveats apply to the vast majority of drowning and near-drowning incidents (see table).

- *Children should be under constant supervision if a lake, pool, or pail of water of any size is nearby.*
- *Water sports and alcoholic beverages never mix.*
- *Life preservers or life jackets should always be worn when boating.*

Where people drown	
Type of water or site	Drownings (%)
Salt water	1%–2%
Fresh water	98%–99%
Swimming pools Private	50%
Public	3%
Lakes, rivers, streams, storm drains	20%
Bathtubs	15%
Buckets of water	4%
Fish ponds or tanks	4%
Toilets	4%
Washing machines	1%

Adapted with permission from Orlowski JP: Drowning, near-drowning, and ice-water submersions. *Pediatr Clin North Am* 1987;34(1):77.

These and other standard water safety precautions for swimming, diving, and boating should be made clear and repeated frequently.

Effective prevention in children requires constant supervision and common sense. A young child can find and fall into water in just a minute or two — less time than anyone would realize he or she is gone unless attention is continuous — and fences are not always effective in keeping children out of places where they should not go. A fence may appear to enclose a pool completely, but the gate may not be self-closing or the lock may be broken. The vast majority of children who drown in swimming pools do so in the backyards of their own homes, usually in the later afternoon on summer weekends. And isn't it sensible to require that baby sitters know CPR?

Programs that claim to "drown–proof" or teach young children to swim are controversial, and many experts feel they provide a false sense of security. The American Academy of Pediatrics does not recommend teaching children younger than 3 years of age to swim, although some regional programs take children as young as 6 months. Drown-proofing programs fail — studies indicate that a significant number of children have submersion accidents despite their training — because the sequential patterning approach used to teach the very young child in a structured environment engenders, in effect, learned helplessness. The cues a child learns in the class or pool setting are missing in the real-life crisis.

A large number of adult drowning victims have detectable levels of blood alcohol. Swimmers should be warned about diving into shallow or unexplored water. Boating precautions should be heeded by all boaters. Seizure disorders are an important but easily overlooked risk factor in persons of all ages.

Figure 25-1   Preventing near-drowning accidents.

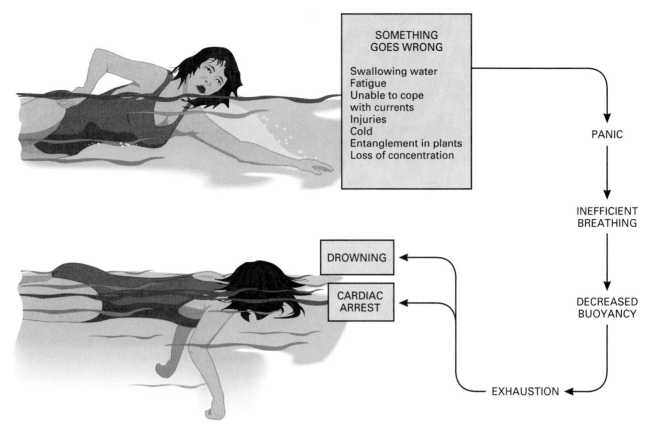

Figure 25-2   Panic can often contribute to the death of the person who loses self-control.

DIVING EMERGENCIES

Near-drownings can be additionally complicated in cases where diving is involved. In most such cases, people sustain injuries as a result of diving into a pool or other relatively shallow body of water. (Other diving emergencies, those resulting from diving in deep water with scuba gear, will be discussed in the Enrichment section later in this chapter.) Patients who dive into water from a diving board, shore, poolside, boat, or dock often sustain injuries to the head and spine and fractures of the arms, legs, and ribs.

You should always assume that a diver has sustained neck and spine injuries, even if the diver is still responsive. If the patient is still in the water, provide the care as described for a near-drowning patient under Emergency Medical Care later in this chapter. If the patient has left the water, provide care, including resuscitation if necessary, as you would for any other trauma or near-drowning patient.

SAFETY MEASURES IN WATER-RELATED EMERGENCIES

In a water-related emergency, you need to reach the patient, but you must do it with utmost concern for your own safety. Certain deep-water accidents require specialized equipment to correct medical complications, but many victims of water-related emergencies can be saved by basic life support measures, such as removing them from the water and suctioning the airway.

However, do not let your desire to provide these simple life-saving measures overwhelm your judgment. You may easily fall victim to the same hazard as the patient. Remember that water can conceal many hazards. Holes, sharp drop-offs, and underwater entanglements such as fallen trees or wire fences may not be visible from shore. In addition, currents in streams, rivers, or storm drains can easily overpower the best swimmer.

Unless a water emergency occurs in open, shallow water that has a stable, uniform bottom, *never go out into the water to attempt a rescue unless you meet all of the following criteria:*

• You are a good swimmer, *and* . . .
• You are specially trained in water rescue techniques, *and* . . .
• You are wearing a personal flotation device, *and* . . .
• You are accompanied by other rescuers.

Failure to follow these guidelines can result in your becoming a patient or a fatality also.

If the patient is responsive and close to shore, use the *reach, throw, row, go* strategy. Make sure you have firm, solid footing and can't slip into the water. Try to reach to the patient by holding out an object for him to grab. You can use an oar, branch, fishing pole, towel, shirt, or other strong object that won't break. Once the patient has grabbed the object, pull him to shore.

If the patient is responsive but too far away to grasp an object you are holding, another way of reaching him is to throw something. The best thing to throw is a rope. Any EMS unit whose territory includes bodies of water should carry 100 feet of polypropylene rope in a throw bag that can be quickly deployed. Make sure you have firm, solid footing and can't slip into the water. Tie a long rope or line to an object that floats and is heavy enough to throw (an inflatable ball, a rescue ring, a thermos jug, a picnic cooler, a capped empty plastic milk jug, or the like). Throw the object underhand to the patient. Once he has grabbed the floating object, pull him to shore (Figure 25-3).

If the patient is unresponsive or out of reach with a line, you will need either to row to him in a boat if one is immediately accessible (Figure 25-4) or to go to him by wading out or swimming or using a float board.

Never try to go to the swimmer unless you meet the safety criteria listed earlier.

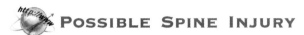

POSSIBLE SPINE INJURY

If the swimmer may have been involved in a diving accident or may have been struck by a boat, water skier, surfboard, or other object, you should suspect possible spine injury. You should also suspect spine injury in any swimmer who is unresponsive (especially one in shallow, warm water).

In the case of possible spine injury, the goal is to support the back and stabilize the head and neck as other care is given. It is important to stabilize the patient properly in the water, then to remove him carefully from the water. The American Red Cross suggests that the patient not be removed from the water until a backboard or other rigid support can be applied to the patient for stabilization (see the method outlined under Emergency Medical Care later in this chapter).

RESUSCITATION

There is a significant difference between warm-water and cold-water drowning: When a person dives into cold water (below 68° Fahrenheit), the **mammalian diving reflex** can prevent death, even after prolonged submersion.

Here's how the mammalian diving reflex works: When the face of a human, or any mammal, is submerged in cold water, breathing is inhibited, the heart rate slows, and the blood vessels throughout most of the body constrict. Blood flow to the heart and brain, however, is maintained. In this way, oxygen is sent and used only where it is needed to immediately sustain life. The colder the water, the more oxygen is diverted to the heart and brain. The diving reflex is more pronounced and cooling is more rapid in the young (whose skin surface is greater relative to their body mass). In water at or below 68°F, the body's metabolic requirements are only about half of normal. The brain and heart remain oxygenated for some time and, as a consequence, death can be significantly delayed in the cold-water submersion victim.

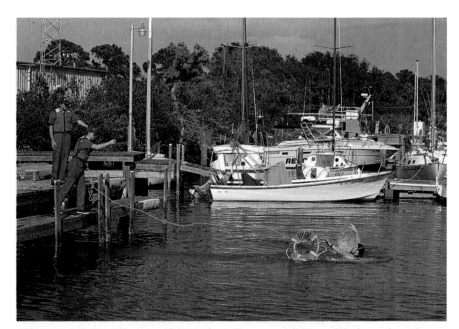

Figure 25-3 Use an object that floats and is unlikely to break tied to the end of a rope to pull the patient to shore.

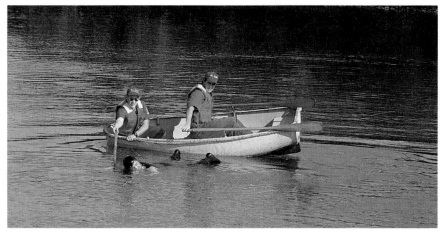

Figure 25-4   Don't become a patient yourself. Use a boat to reach an unresponsive patient.

Often, patients who have been submerged in cold water—even after 30 minutes or longer in cardiac arrest—can be resuscitated. As a guideline, you should attempt resuscitation on any pulseless, nonbreathing patient who has been submerged in cold water.

Some experts advise providing resuscitation to every drowning patient, regardless of water temperature, even those who have been in the water for a prolonged period. In other words, never assume that the patient has drowned, but rather consider him to be a near-drowning patient. *Seek medical direction and follow local protocol.*

ASSESSMENT AND CARE: WATER-RELATED EMERGENCIES

SCENE SIZE-UP

The scene size-up is especially critical in water-related emergencies. As an EMT-B, one of your first responsibilities is to ensure your safety and that of your partner; you cannot aid a patient if you yourself become a casualty.

First, study the scene and make sure that it is safe for you to enter. Anytime you are within 10 feet of water's edge you should consider wearing a PFD. If you choose to go into the water to rescue a patient, be sure you are capable of swimming and do not put yourself in danger. Make sure to take appropriate body substance isolation precautions, because drowning patients often vomit. Note any relevant mechanism of injury that could contribute to the severity of the situation such as a deep dive in a shallow pool.

Decide if you will need any additional assistance such as a dry team to work on shore and a wet team to immobilize the patient in the water. Be aware that rescues in white water or swift water require specialized techniques and training. If you are not qualified

to undertake a rescue, be prepared to contact rescue teams that are.

Survey the scene to determine the number of patients. Usually there will be just one patient, but in some circumstances, such as a car in the water or victims struck by a moving boat, there could be more. Call for any extra or expert assistance that may be required.

INITIAL ASSESSMENT

Form a general impression of the patient. Is this a responsive or unresponsive patient? Assess the level of responsiveness and document it, especially noting the reaction to painful stimuli in all four extremities because of the possibility of spinal injury.

Assess the airway, keeping in mind the potential for spinal injury. If the patient is found face down, work with a partner or partners, if possible, to carefully turn the patient over while maintaining manual in-line stabilization. Suction water, vomitus, and secretions from the airway. Insert an oral or nasal airway if the airway cannot be managed with manual maneuvers.

Check the breathing to be sure that respirations are present and adequate. Remember that patients with spinal injury often do not breathe if they have a high cervical injury. Assess for any open wounds to the chest that would seriously impede breathing. If the breathing is adequate, administer oxygen via a nonrebreather mask. If breathing is inadequate, provide positive pressure ventilation with supplemental oxygen.

Check the circulation to make sure the patient has a pulse and no life-threatening external bleeding that needs to be controlled. Assess for signs or symptoms of internal bleeding or hypoperfusion (shock). Remember that some patients rescued from the water may have internal injuries, for example from jumping off a bridge into the water.

Make a decision on the priority of the patient. Is he a high priority in need of rapid transport to a hospital or is the patient a low priority at this time? Patients with high spinal injuries affecting respirations or who are found in respiratory distress or who are unresponsive are high priority.

FOCUSED HISTORY AND PHYSICAL EXAM

Perform a rapid assessment if the patient has an altered mental status or is unresponsive. Also, look for evidence of possible injury. If the patient is alert, conduct a SAMPLE history and a focused physical exam.

Signs and Symptoms   For the water-related emergency patient, look for signs and symptoms of any of the following injuries or medical problems:

- Airway obstruction
- Absent or inadequate breathing
- Pulselessness (cardiac arrest)
- Spinal injury or head injury
- Soft tissue injuries
- Musculoskeletal injuries
- External or internal bleeding
- Shock
- Hypothermia
- Alcohol or drug abuse
- Drowning or near-drowning

Drowning or near-drowning patients may be unresponsive, not breathing, or pulseless, or they may be responsive and possibly gasping or coughing up water.

EMERGENCY MEDICAL CARE— NEAR-DROWNING

Remember that—unless otherwise directed by local protocol or medical direction—do not assume that a patient has drowned, even if he is unresponsive and without breathing or pulse and has been submerged for some time, but rather consider him to be a near-drowning patient in need of resuscitation. Follow the steps below in caring for near-drowning patients:

1. Remove the patient from the water as quickly and safely as you can. If you suspect that the patient has a spine injury, maintain in-line stabilization and then secure the patient to a backboard before removing him from the water (Figure 25-5). Follow these steps to remove a patient with a suspected spinal injury from the water.
   - If you find the patient face-down, stabilize the patient's head and neck with your arms, then roll the patient over, supporting the back and stabilizing the head and neck.
   - If the patient is not breathing, begin rescue breathing, using a pocket mask if possible.
   - Keeping the head and neck in line with the spinal column, slide a long backboard under the patient; secure the torso and legs to the backboard with straps.
   - Apply a cervical spinal immobilization collar and a head immobilization device.
   - Float the board to shore or poolside and lift the patient from the water. Bear in mind that the chest and head are heavier than the lower extremities, and this results in a tendency for the head of the backboard, and the patient immobilized to it, to slip underwater. So make sure that sufficient support is given to the head end of the backboard.

2. If you do not suspect spine injury, place the patient on his left side so that water, vomitus, and secretions can drain from the upper airway.

3. Suction as needed.

4. As rapidly as you can, establish an airway and begin positive pressure ventilations with supplemental oxygen. Water in the airway can cause resistance to ventilations. *Once you have determined that there are no foreign objects in the airway,* apply ventilations with more force until you see the patient's chest rise and fall.

5. The patient may suffer from **gastric distention,** a condition in which the stomach fills with water, enlarging the abdomen to the point that it interferes with the ability to inflate the lungs. Gastric distention can also be caused by air that is forced into the stomach during artificial ventilation when resistance along the airway or too-forceful ventilations cause air to be forced into the esophagus and stomach. When gastric distention reaches the point where it interferes with the ability to ventilate the patient, place the patient on his side. *With suction immediately available,* place your hand over the epigastric area of the abdomen and apply firm pressure to relieve the distention. This will cause regurgitation, which you must immediately manage by positioning the patient on his side (turning the backboard and patient as a unit if the patient is immobilized to a backboard) and suctioning. Remember: *Apply pressure only if the gastric distention interferes with your ability to ventilate the patient effectively.*

6. Manage any other medical or trauma conditions associated with the near-drowning event, such as soft-tissue injuries, seizure, or diabetic emergencies.

7. Transport the patient as quickly as possible, continuing resuscitative measures during transport.

Always transport a near-drowning patient, even if you think the danger has passed. A near-drowning

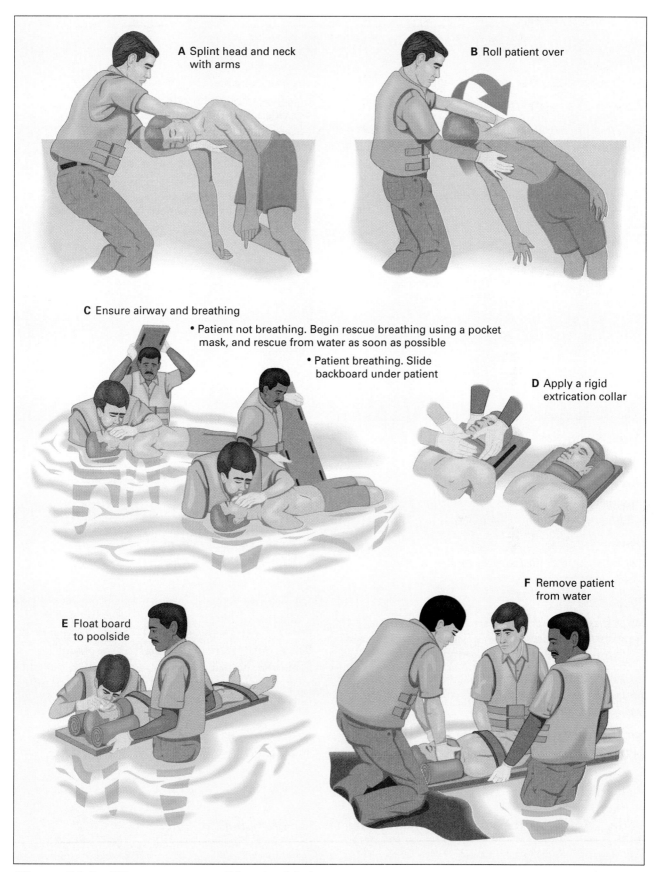

A Splint head and neck with arms

B Roll patient over

C Ensure airway and breathing

- Patient not breathing. Begin rescue breathing using a pocket mask, and rescue from water as soon as possible
  - Patient breathing. Slide backboard under patient

D Apply a rigid extrication collar

E Float board to poolside

F Remove patient from water

Figure 25-5   Water rescue, possible spinal injury.

ASSESSMENT SUMMARY

DROWNING OR NEAR-DROWNING

The following are findings that may be associated with a drowning or near-drowning emergency.

SCENE SIZE-UP

Pay particular attention to your own safety. Look for:
- Mechanism of injury
- Swift-moving water
- Water hazards
- Cold water
- Cold ambient temperature
- Alcohol or drugs
- Scuba diving equipment
- Is patient still in the water?
- Do you suspect the patient has a possible spine or head injury?

INITIAL ASSESSMENT

General Impression

Is the patient moving any extremities?

Mental Status

Alert to unresponsive

Airway

Potentially closed airway if mental status is altered
Vomiting or coughing up water

Breathing

May be adequate, inadequate, or absent
Patient may be gasping

Circulation

Pulses may be present or absent
Cyanosis may be present
Cold to touch based on water temperature

Status: Priority Patient (All near-drowning patients must be transported for further evaluation and management.)

FOCUSED HISTORY AND PHYSICAL EXAM

SAMPLE History

Signs and symptoms:
- Altered mental status
- Pulselessness
- Motor or sensory deficits
- Evidence of trauma to head or neck
- Coughing up or vomiting water

History:
- Did the patient ingest alcohol or drugs?
- Does the patient have a cardiac disorder or other medical condition?
- How long has the patient been submerged
- Did the patient dive into the water?

Physical Exam

Head, neck, and face:
- Pupils may be dilated and sluggish to respond to light
- Large amounts of water or vomitus in mouth
- Evidence of trauma to head, neck, or face
- Cyanosis
- Nasal flaring

Chest:
- Crackles in lungs on auscultation
- Decreased breath sounds
- Retractions and accessory muscle use

Abdomen:
- Distended from ingested water
- May be cold to touch if hypothermia is present

Extremities:
- Loss of sensory or motor function in spine-injured patient
- Weak or absent peripheral pulses
- Cyanosis or pallor

Baseline Vital Signs

BP: normal to decreased; may be absent or extremely difficult to obtain
HR: normal, increased, decreased, or absent
RR: normal, increased, decreased, or absent
Skin: may be pale, cyanotic, cool to cold, depending on water temperature and length of submersion
Pupils: dilated and sluggish to respond to light

Figure 25-6a   Assessment summary: drowning or near-drowning.

EMERGENCY CARE PROTOCOL

NEAR-DROWNING

1. Establish and maintain in-line spinal stabilization if spinal injury is suspected.
2. Begin positive pressure ventilation with pocket mask in the water if possible.
3. Float backboard under patient and move to shore. Remove patient on backboard while maintaining in-line spinal stabilization.
4. Establish and maintain open airway, insert nasopharyngeal or oropharyngeal airway if patient is unresponsive and has no gag or cough reflex.
5. Suction secretions as necessary.
6. If breathing is adequate, provide positive pressure ventilation with supplemental oxygen at a minimum rate of 12 ventilations/minute for an adult and 20 ventilations/minute for an infant or child.
7. If breathing is adequate, administer oxygen by nonrebreather mask at 15 lpm. If possible, deliver warm, humidified oxygen if hypothermia is suspected.
8. If no pulse, apply AED; follow AED protocol.
9. If hypothermia is suspected, follow the generalized cold injury protocol.
10. Place patient in lateral recumbent position only if spinal injury is not suspected.
11. Always transport a near-drowning patient.
12. Perform an ongoing assessment every 5 minutes.

Figure 25-6b   Emergency care protocol: near-drowning.

patient can develop complications that lead to death as long as 72 hours after the incident. Approximately 15 percent of all drowning deaths are due to secondary complications. During transport, you should keep the patient warm and continue to provide high-flow oxygen.

DETAILED PHYSICAL EXAM AND ONGOING ASSESSMENT

If time and the patient's condition permit, perform a detailed physical exam to be sure that no injuries have been overlooked.

During the ongoing assessment, be especially alert for signs the patient is deteriorating into respiratory or cardiac arrest, especially if you previously resuscitated this patient. Perform the ongoing assessment (repeating the initial assessment, repeating the focused history and physical exam, repeating vital signs, and checking interventions) every 5 minutes if the patient is unstable, every 15 minutes if the patient is stable.

SUMMARY: ASSESSMENT AND CARE

To review possible assessment findings and emergency care for a drowning or near-drowning emergency, see Figures 25-6 and 25-7.

ENRICHMENT

The enrichment section contains information that is valuable as background for the EMT-B but that goes substantially beyond the U.S. Department of Transportation (DOT) EMT-Basic curriculum.

DEEP-WATER DIVING EMERGENCIES

People who take part in scuba, or deep-water, diving may become victims of drowning or near-drowning incidents such as those described above. But the environmental extremes to which deep-water divers are exposed create some special problems.

A major complication of deep-water diving emergencies is coma, which may result from asphyxiation, head injury, heart attack, air-tank contamination, intoxication, or aspiration. It can also result from air embolism, decompression sickness, or barotrauma.

AIR EMBOLISM

An air embolism is a blocking of blood vessels by an air bubble or clusters of air bubbles. The blockage interferes with perfusion of body tissues by oxygen and nutrients normally supplied by the blood. During a dive, pressure on the diver's body increases and the volume of a gas decreases as he descends. Conversely, that pressure is lessened as the diver ascends. If the diver ascends rapidly while holding his breath, the air in the lungs expands rapidly, rupturing the alveoli and damaging adjacent blood vessels. As a result, air bubbles enter the bloodstream.

The signs and symptoms of air embolism have a rapid onset, often appearing within 15 minutes of a diver's surfacing. They included the following:

- Itchy, blotchy, or mottled skin
- Difficulty in breathing
- Dizziness
- Chest pain

EMERGENCY CARE ALGORITHM:
NEAR-DROWNING EMERGENCY

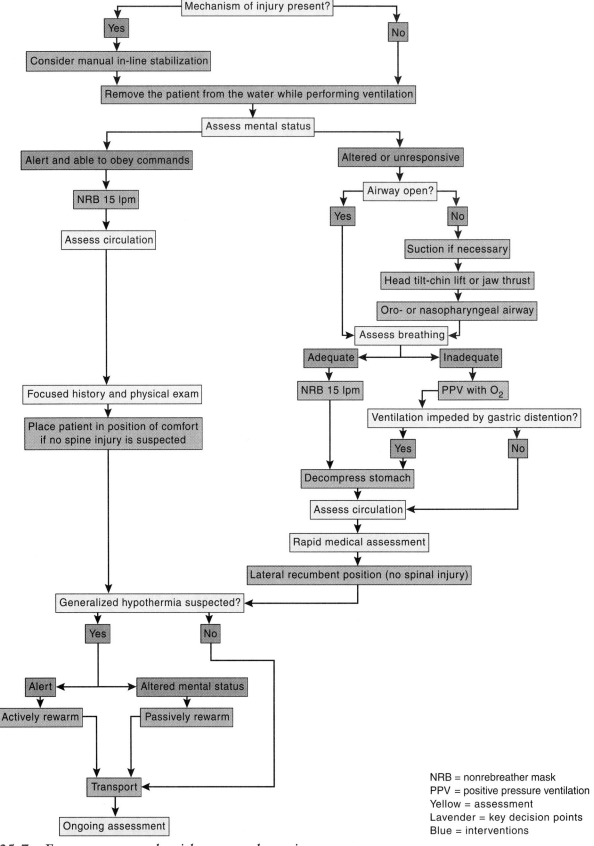

Figure 25-7   Emergency care algorithm: near-drowning emergency.

- Severe, deep aching pain in the muscles, joints, and tendons
- Blurred or distorted vision
- Partial deafness, distortion of senses
- Nausea and vomiting
- Numbness or paralysis
- Weakness or numbness on one side of the body
- Staggering gait or lack of coordination
- Frothy blood in the nose and mouth
- Swelling and crepitus in the neck
- Loss or distortion of memory
- Coma
- Cardiac or respiratory arrest
- Behavioral changes (sometimes the only sign)

DECOMPRESSION SICKNESS (BENDS)

Decompression sickness ("the bends") usually occurs when a diver ascends too quickly from a deep, prolonged dive. Gases (usually nitrogen) breathed by the diver are absorbed into the bloodstream. As the diver comes up, the nitrogen is transformed into tiny bubbles which lodge in body tissues and enter the bloodstream, causing pain and obstructing circulation.

Decompression sickness is gradual in onset and symptoms usually occur 12 to 24 hours after the dive. They include the following:

- Itchy, blotchy, or mottled skin
- Difficulty in breathing
- Dizziness
- Chest pain
- Severe, deep aching pain in the muscles, joints, and tendons
- Blurred or distorted vision
- Partial deafness, distortion of senses
- Nausea and vomiting
- Numbness or paralysis
- Staggering gait or lack of coordination
- Pitting edema (swelling of tissues that doesn't return quickly when pressed with a finger)

- A migraine-like headache
- Choking or coughing
- Inability to void the bladder
- Hallucinations

BAROTRAUMA

Sometimes called "the squeeze," barotrauma occurs during ascent or descent when air pressure in the body's air cavities (such as the sinuses or middle ear) becomes too great. As a result, tissues in the air cavities are injured; for example, the eardrum or sinus may rupture.

Divers with upper respiratory infection or allergy are at increased risk of barotrauma. Signs and symptoms of the condition include the following:

- Mild to severe pain in the affected area
- Possible discharge from the nose or ears
- Extreme dizziness
- Nausea
- Disorientation

Patients suffering from barotrauma must be cared for at a medical facility immediately to prevent permanent deafness, residual dizziness, or the inability to dive in the future.

EMERGENCY MEDICAL CARE

Follow these steps in caring for a patient who you suspect has an air embolism, decompression sickness, or barotrauma:

1. If there is no sign of neck or spine injury, position the patient on a board on his side with the head down; slant the entire body 15 degrees, head down, to force air or gas bubbles to stay in the abdomen (Figure 25-8).
2. Administer oxygen at 15 lpm by nonrebreather mask or positive pressure ventilation with supplemental oxygen as appropriate. Initiate CPR and apply the AED if needed. Oxygen is critical in

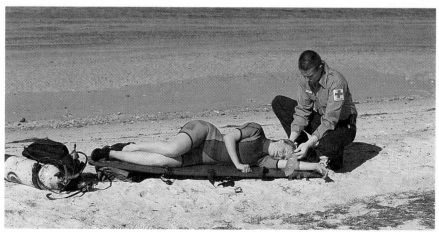

Figure 25-8   Proper positioning of a scuba-diving accident patient.

these cases because it reduces the size of nitrogen bubbles and improves circulation.

3. Transport the patient immediately. If it is a diving emergency, try to obtain the patient's diving log and transport it with him to the hospital. Contact medical direction to consider transport to a facility with a recompression chamber. Continue to provide oxygen during transport.

CASE STUDY FOLLOW-UP

SCENE SIZE-UP

Your initial call was for a possible drowning involving a 25-year-old male reported in trouble in the Delmar Hotel pool. Your unit and the police arrive at the same time. You are led to the pool by the hotel manager, who complains that the young man and his friends have been drinking. A crowd of intoxicated bystanders has gathered around the pool and are shouting comments. The police move to clear the crowd. With the only obvious hazard under control, the scene is secure and you approach the pool.

In it is a young man, floating in a supine position supported by a hotel employee. According to the manager, the man had been drinking and suddenly dove into the shallow end of the pool. He floated to the top but said he couldn't move his feet. A hotel employee jumped in and has been supporting him in a supine position in the water, keeping his head, neck, and spine in alignment.

INITIAL ASSESSMENT

Your general impression is of an adult male in no obvious distress except for his chief complaint, the inability to move his feet, which leads you to suspect a possible spinal injury. There is a lifeguard's float board propped up by the pool house. You get it while your partner grabs a cervical spinal immobilization collar, then you both slip into the pool, trying not to create unnecessary waves. Your partner takes over manual in-line stabilization from the hotel employee while you assess the airway, breathing, and pulse. The patient keeps up a stream of chatter as you assess, but his speech is somewhat disconnected and slurred. He knows his name, Robby Ash, but not exactly where he is or what day it is.

With Robby's airway and breathing adequate, and no signs of major bleeding or immediate signs of shock, you maneuver the float board into position. You immobilize his torso, then apply the collar and immobilize his head to the board. Then you gently push the board to the side of the pool. There, with the assistance of the employee and two police officers, you remove the board and Robby, as a unit, from the water and set them down on the deck. You and your partner climb out and begin to administer oxygen at 15 lpm by nonrebreather mask. Since the patient is responsive with an adequate airway and breathing, he is not a high priority for rapid transport, so you proceed to carry out the focused history and physical exam at poolside.

FOCUSED HISTORY AND PHYSICAL EXAM

A rapid trauma assessment reveals no other injuries aside from a contusion on the top of the head and some point tenderness in the neck. Because of Robby's complaint that he cannot feel his feet, you pay particular attention to the assessment of pulses and motor and sensory function in the extremities. In the upper extremities, radial pulses are present and strong. Robby cannot grip your fingers on command and cannot identify which of his fingers you are touching or pinching. In the lower extremities, pedal pulses are present. Robby cannot move his feet or toes on your command and cannot identify the location of a touch or pinch to any part of either foot.

You take a set of vital signs; they show blood pressure 112/72, a heart rate of 78, and a respiration rate of 15. The patient's overall skin color appears normal, but because of his extended time in the pool you cannot accurately assess the temperature of the skin or whether it would be wet or dry if he had not just been removed from the water. His pupils are equal in size and reactive to light.

While your partner, with the assistance of the police officers, proceeds to prepare the patient for transport, you ask the SAMPLE history questions and find out that Robby's only symptom is the lack of feeling in his feet. He has an allergy to penicillin, is taking no medications, has no pertinent past medical history, and his last solid meal was two hours ago. He has been drinking beer all night long which, he agrees, probably led him to attempt the dive into shallow water.

When your partner has finished preparing the patient, you load him into the ambulance and begin transport.

DETAILED PHYSICAL EXAM

En route, you perform the detailed physical exam, assessing the head and neck with extra care. You also carefully reassess the extremities. The upper and lower extremities still show adequate pulses. However, there is still no voluntary motor function. He does not feel anything in either hand or foot. You then move up the arms and legs, pinching at various levels, but still get no response from the patient.

ONGOING ASSESSMENT

The focus of your care en route to the hospital is to monitor Robby's ABCs and keep him warm. You take another set of vital signs: Blood pressure is still 112/72, heart rate is now 76, and respirations 15. His skin is normal color, but still feels cool and damp. You check to be sure that the nonrebreather mask is secure, oxygen is flowing adequately, and Robby is well secured to the long spine board.

Because you know Robby has been drinking heavily and probably swallowed a fair amount of pool water, you are prepared for the possibility of vomiting and have suctioning equipment ready. And, in fact,

he soon says, "I feel real sick, man." You remove the nonrebreather mask and with your partner's help, turn the board so that Robby is on his left side. You apply suction to clear his mouth and airway as he vomits. When he stops, you return him to the normal position just as you arrive at the hospital.

Upon arrival, you give an oral report to the emergency department nurse, being sure to mention the vomiting incident and the latest set of vital signs taken in the ambulance. You fill out the prehospital care report while your partner cleans up and restocks the ambulance. Before you leave the hospital, you see the emergency department doctor, who tells you that Robby has been taken upstairs for a CAT scan. He is not optimistic about the possibility that Robby will walk again.

As you pull away from the hospital, you contact dispatch and announce that you are temporarily out of service. You are going back to base so that you can change into dry uniforms.

CHAPTER REVIEW

TERMS AND CONCEPTS

You may wish to review the following terms and concepts included in this chapter.

drowning—death from suffocation due to submersion.

gastric distention—the filling of the stomach with water and/or air, causing an enlarged abdomen which makes ventilations difficult.

mammalian diving reflex—the body's natural response to submersion in cold water in which breathing is inhibited, the heart rate decreases, and blood vessels constrict in order to maintain cerebral and cardiac blood flow.

near-drowning—survival for at least 24 hours from near suffocation due to submersion.

REVIEW QUESTIONS

1. List at least five common causes of drowning.
2. Explain the conditions that must apply before an EMT-B enters the water to attempt a rescue.
3. Describe the four basic methods used in attempting to rescue a patient from the water.
4. Explain why patients who have been submerged in cold water can often be resuscitated after 30 minutes or more.
5. List the injuries and medical problems whose

signs and symptoms the EMT-B should be alert for when assessing the water-related emergency patient.
6. List the steps for removing a near-drowning patient with a possible spine injury from the water.
7. List the steps of emergency medical care for a near-drowning patient that should take place after the patient is removed from the water and, if necessary, immobilized to a spine board.

CHAPTER 26

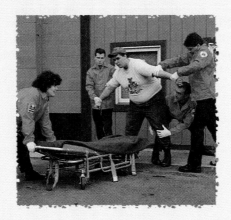

Behavioral Emergencies

INTRODUCTION

Emergency care for physical problems is tangible. You can see the wounds you bandage and touch the patient to provide treatments such as splinting bones or restoring breathing. Often, you can see immediately positive results from your efforts.

Care for behavioral emergencies is different. You cannot readily see the comfort that your words or your mere presence provide to someone who is panicked or agitated. It is hard to gauge the immediate results of your care for someone who is depressed. But the care you give patients in behavioral emergencies can just as easily save lives as the care you provide for physical problems.

OBJECTIVES

Numbered objectives are from the United States Department of Transportation 1994 EMT-Basic National Standard Curriculum. Asterisked objectives, if any, pertain to material that is supplemental to the DOT curriculum.

COGNITIVE

4-8.1   Define behavioral emergencies. (p. 484)

4-8.2   Discuss the general factors that may cause an alteration in a patient's behavior. (p. 484)

4-8.3   State the various reasons for psychological crises. (pp. 484–486)

4-8.4   Discuss the characteristics of an individual's behavior which suggest that the patient is at risk for suicide. (pp. 485–486)

4-8.5   Discuss special medical/legal considerations for managing behavioral emergencies. (pp. 494–496)

4-8.6   Discuss the special considerations for assessing a patient with behavioral problems. (pp. 488–490)

4-8.7   Discuss the general principles of an individual's behavior which suggest that he is at risk for violence. (p. 486)

4-8.8   Discuss methods to calm behavioral emergency patients. (pp. 487–488)

AFFECTIVE

4-8.9   Explain the rationale for learning how to modify your behavior toward the patient with a behavioral emergency. (p. 454)

PSYCHOMOTOR

4-8.10   Demonstrate the assessment and emergency medical care of the patient experiencing a behavioral emergency.

4-8.11   Demonstrate various techniques to safely restrain a patient with a behavioral problem.

CASE STUDY

THE DISPATCH

EMS Unit 204—proceed to 3486 East Market Street, King's Motel, Room 22. You have a woman who is cut and bleeding. No other information is available. Time out is 2235 hours.

ON ARRIVAL

You call back to dispatch and ask to arrange for the motel manager to meet you in the parking lot. You arrive at 2241 hours, position your ambulance, and turn on the scene lights. Because of the report of blood, you don appropriate body substance isolation gear. Noting nothing unusual about the scene, you and your partner gather your equipment and exit the ambulance. As you walk toward the motel, a man approaches and says, "Hi. I'm Tom Slavina, the night manager here. Sorry, guys, but I really have no idea what's going on. Your dispatcher called me and asked me to meet you, but I didn't call in a problem and I haven't seen or heard any signs of trouble."

Mr. Slavina leads you to Room 22. The door is closed and the room's drapes are drawn, but there is a light on inside. You pause, but hear no sounds coming from the room. You and your partner stand on opposite sides of the door as you prepare to knock. When you do, your knock swings the door open slightly. You now hear crying from somewhere inside the room, followed by a woman's voice saying faintly, "Please help me. I'm cut and bleeding."

You ask, "Where are you?" and the voice replies, "In the bathroom." You ask, "Is anyone else in the room with you?" The woman sobs for a moment, then gasps out, "No, there's no one here. There's never anyone here. Never. No one cares. No, there's no one."

You cautiously enter the room first, while your partner waits outside. There's no one in the room itself, but you note the closet door is open and a few garments are hanging in it. The bed is rumpled, as if someone had been lying on top of the covers. On the night table by the bed are a lamp, a phone, an opened bottle of rum, and a glass. There are a few dark stains on the carpet between the night table and the bathroom door.

You approach the bathroom and cautiously peer around the corner through the doorway. A woman is sitting on the floor in the middle of the room. Blood from a cut on her left wrist has pooled on the floor and she is holding a large, folding hunting knife in her right hand.

How would you proceed to assess and care for this patient?

In this chapter, you will learn special considerations of assessment and emergency care for a patient who has attempted or is threatening suicide as well as for patients suffering other behavioral emergencies. Later, we will return to the case study and apply what you have learned.

BEHAVIORAL PROBLEMS

Behavior is the way a person acts or performs. A person's "behavior" encompasses any or all of that person's activities and responses, especially those responses that can be observed. A **behavioral emergency** is a situation in which a person exhibits "abnormal" behavior—behavior that is unacceptable or intolerable to the patient, the family, or the community. The abnormal behavior that precipitates the emergency may be due to a psychological condition (such as a mental illness), to extremes of emotion, or even to a physical condition (such as a lack of oxygen or low blood sugar).

Patients in the midst of behavioral emergencies may display panic, agitation, and bizarre thinking and actions. Such patients can pose a danger to themselves, through suicidal or self-injurious acts, or to others, through violent acts or actions whose consequences they may be incapable of understanding.

BEHAVIORAL CHANGE

A number of factors may cause a change in a patient's behavior, among them situational stresses, medical illnesses, psychiatric problems, alcohol, or drugs. Some common reasons why behavior may change include the following:

- Low blood sugar in a diabetic, which can cause delirium, confusion, and even hallucinations
- Hypoxia (lack of oxygen)
- Inadequate blood flow to the brain
- Head trauma
- Mind-altering substances, such as alcohol, depressants, stimulants, psychedelics, and narcotics
- Psychogenic substances, which can cause psychotic thinking, depression, or panic
- Excessive cold or heat
- Infections of the brain or its coverings

As obvious as it sounds, you need to be sure you are dealing with a *behavioral,* and not a *physical,* emergency. For example, you may detect what smells like alcohol on a patient's breath. Do not simply assume the patient is intoxicated; diabetic emergencies can cause alcohol-like odors on the breath, as can Antabuse, a drug used by alcoholics to decrease alcohol dependency.

Clues that the problem may be physical rather than psychological include the following:

- The onset of symptoms was relatively sudden; most behavioral problems develop more gradually.
- If the patient has hallucinations, they are visual but not auditory.
- The patient has memory loss or impairment; in most behavioral problems, the memory remains intact and the patient is usually alert, being oriented to person, place, and time.
- The patient's pupils are dilated, constricted, or unequal, or they respond differently to light.
- The patient has excessive salivation.
- The patient is incontinent (has lost bladder or bowel control).
- The patient has unusual odors on his breath.

Remember that behavioral changes and crises often *follow* (or are a result of) physical trauma or illness. Even if all the clues point to a behavioral problem, assess the patient adequately to rule out a physical cause.

PSYCHIATRIC PROBLEMS

A number of psychiatric conditions can lead to behavioral emergencies. Among them are anxiety, phobias, depression, bipolar disorder, paranoia, and schizophrenia.

ANXIETY

Anxiety is a state of painful uneasiness about impending problems. It is characterized by agitation and restlessness and is one of the most common emotions; in fact, anxiety disorders are thought to be the most common form of mental illness. According to estimates, anxiety disorders affect approximately 13 million Americans, or about one in every ten adults. Most clinicians feel that approximately three-fourths of the cases are never correctly diagnosed because they so closely mimic other disorders.

One form of anxiety disorder is the panic attack. Patients who are panicked may show intense fear, tension, or restlessness. They often feel overwhelmed and can't concentrate. Their behavior may also cause anxiety among the people around them, so they may be surrounded by a crowd of anxious and excited people when you arrive. These patients often hyperventilate (breathe too deeply), which causes physical symptoms such as dizziness, tingling around the mouth and fingers, spasms of the hands and feet (carpal-pedal spasms), tremors, irregular heartbeat, palpitations (rapid or intense heartbeat), diarrhea, and sometimes feelings of choking, smothering, or shortness of breath. If severe, anxiety has been known to cause sudden cardiac death.

PHOBIAS

Phobias are closely related to anxiety problems. They are irrational fears of specific things, places, or situations. One of the most disabling is agoraphobia, or "fear of the marketplace," which renders its victims terrified of leaving the safety of their own homes.

Patients suffering phobias may show evidence of intense fear. Tense and restless, they often wring their hands and pace. They frequently suffer from tremors, tachycardia (rapid heartbeat), irregular heartbeat, dyspnea (difficult breathing), sweating, and diarrhea.

DEPRESSION

Depression is one of the most common psychiatric conditions. It is a condition characterized by deep feelings of sadness, worthlessness, and discouragement, feelings that often do not seem connected to the actual circumstances of the patient's life. Depression is a factor in approximately 50 percent of all suicides and may cause other psychological disorders as well.

Depressed patients often present a sad appearance and may have crying spells and listless or apathetic behavior. They feel helpless, hopeless, withdrawn, and pessimistic; they often suffer appetite loss, sleeplessness, fatigue, despondence, and severe restlessness. Believing that no one understands or cares about them or that their problems cannot be solved, they often express the desire to be left alone.

BIPOLAR DISORDER

Bipolar disorder, also known as manic-depressive disorder, causes a patient to swing to opposite sides of the mood spectrum. During one phase, he has an inflated view of himself; he may feel deliriously happy, elated, and super powerful. The manic phase alternates with normal moods and a depressive state in which the patient loses interest, feels worthless, worries, and may contemplate suicide. In either the manic or depressive stage, the patient may suffer delusions and hallucinations. Sometimes one phase may last for months; at other times, the patient may swing from one mood to another rather quickly (sometimes within hours).

PARANOIA

Paranoia is a highly exaggerated or unwarranted mistrust or suspiciousness. Paranoid patients are often hostile and uncooperative and suffer from the firmly held, but untrue, belief that someone is "out to get them."

Most paranoid patients have elaborate delusions, mostly of persecution. They tend to brood over real or imagined injuries, carry grudges, and recall wrongs done to them years earlier. They seem cold, aloof, antagonistic, hypersensitive, defensive, and argumentative. They cannot accept fault or blame, avoid intimacy, and are excitable and unpredictable, displaying outbursts of bizarre or aggressive behavior.

SCHIZOPHRENIA

Schizophrenia is the name given to a group of mental disorders. Patients with the illness suffer debilitating distortions of speech and thought, bizarre delusions, hallucinations, social withdrawal, and lack of emotional expressiveness. Rarely is schizophrenia manifest as multiple-personality disorder, as commonly believed.

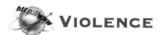 **VIOLENCE**

Patients in behavioral emergencies brought on by the conditions described above or by other circumstances sometimes express their inability to handle the pressures they are feeling through violent acts. Those acts can be directed against themselves or against others.

SUICIDE

A **suicide** attempt is any willful act designed to end one's own life. Men are more often successful at suicide, but women make three times as many attempts. More than half of all suicides are committed with firearms; among unsuccessful attempts, the most common methods are drug ingestion and wrist slashing.

Suicide is now the tenth leading cause of death in the United States among all ages and the second leading cause of death among college-age students. Many people believe that suicide is vastly underreported because of the stigma that still surrounds it.

At least half of all people who succeed at suicide have attempted it previously, and 75 percent give clear warning that they intend to kill themselves. The four most common methods of suicide, in order, are (1) self-inflicted gunshot wound, (2) hanging,

(3) poisoning by ingestion, and (4) carbon monoxide poisoning.

Many suicide victims make last-minute attempts to communicate their intentions. It is thought that most do not really want to die but use the suicide attempt as a way to get attention, to receive help, or to punish someone. Suicide attempts, however, are too often dismissed as "just trying to get attention." As an EMT-B, you must understand that the person who attempts suicide, whatever his motive, has a real problem and needs some kind of help or treatment. Remember, too, that the patient who attempts suicide unsuccessfully is at high risk of making a successful attempt later if not helped. *Every suicidal act or gesture should be taken seriously, and the patient should be transported for evaluation.*

Studies of suicides and suicide attempts have produced statistical data about those most likely to take their own lives:

- Men who are over 40 years old, single, widowed, or divorced, account for 70 percent of all suicides.
- Suicide is five times higher among people who are widowed or divorced.
- Suicide is more common among people with histories of alcoholism or drug abuse.
- Severe depression significantly increases the risk of suicide.
- Approximately 80 percent of people who succeed in committing suicide have made previous suicidal gestures or attempts.
- At highest risk are patients who have formulated a highly lethal plan and told others about it.
- An unusual gathering of articles that could be used to commit suicide (such as purchasing a gun or stockpiling a large quantity of pills) or immediate access to a suicide device may be signs of a potential suicide attempt.
- A previous history of self-destructive behavior, even if that behavior was not overtly suicidal, may indicate future attempts at suicide.
- A recent diagnosis of serious illness, especially an illness that signals a loss of independence, is sometimes a trigger to suicidal behavior.
- The recent loss of a loved one may spur a suicide attempt. Suicides also occur when a person's close emotional attachments are perceived to be in danger.
- An arrest, imprisonment, or the loss of a job are some of the general signs that the patient has lost control or is unable to manage life and is therefore at greater risk of attempting suicide.

VIOLENCE TO OTHERS

Studies show that 60 to 75 percent of all behavioral emergency patients will become assaultive or violent. The angry, violent patient may be ready to fight with anyone who approaches and will probably be difficult to control. Violence can be caused by patient mismanagement (real or perceived), psychosis, alcohol or drug intoxication, fear, panic, or head injury.

Early signs that a person may have lost control and may become violent include:

- Nervous pacing
- Shouting
- Threatening
- Cursing
- Throwing objects
- Clenched teeth and/or fists

DEALING WITH BEHAVIORAL EMERGENCIES

Dealing with patients in behavioral emergencies requires extra sensitivity on the part of the EMT-B. Remember that in such cases it is often not the tangible treatment you provide but the intangibles of your interactions with the patient that make the difference between helping the patient through the crisis or deepening it or prolonging it. The way you carry yourself around the patient and how you look at him and speak to him are of great importance in these situations.

BASIC PRINCIPLES

Keep the following basic principles in mind whenever you encounter a behavioral emergency:

- *Every person has limitations.* In a behavioral emergency, every person there, including you, is susceptible to emotional injury. Every person has a threshold, and some are able to cope with more than others.
- *Each person has a right to his feelings.* A person who is emotionally or mentally disturbed does not want to feel that way, but at that particular time, those feelings are valid and real.
- *Each person has more ability to cope with crisis than he might think.* For every manifestation of crazed emotion, some strength is probably left within.
- *Everyone feels some emotional disturbance when involved in a disaster or when injured.* You do not know what a particular physical injury might mean to a given individual. A relatively minor hand injury may seem of little consequence, but it could ruin the career or the personal fulfillment of a person who works with his hands as a profession or a hobby.
- *Emotional injury is just as real as physical injury.* Unfortunately, because physical injury is more visible, it is more often accepted as being more "real."
- *People who have been through a crisis do not just "get better."* They will probably suffer from their

pain and loss for a long time, sometimes for years. Do not expect instantaneous or automatic results; the patient probably will not realize the extent of the event until long after you leave. You're first on the scene, and your role is to provide a positive beginning to a long, difficult healing process.

- *Cultural differences have special meaning when you are called to intervene in behavioral emergencies.* Come to terms with your own feelings as you approach a situation, and take the time to understand where your patient is coming from.

TECHNIQUES FOR TREATING BEHAVIORAL EMERGENCY PATIENTS

The situations presented by behaviorally disturbed patients can be difficult. However, there are a number of techniques that you can follow that can make dealing with those situations easier for you and more helpful to the patient. These techniques include:

- *Speak in a calm, reassuring voice directly to the patient.* Explain who you are and why you are there.
- *Maintain a comfortable distance between yourself and the patient.* Many patients are threatened by physical contact. Unwanted touching could set off a violent response. After you have established some rapport with the patient, you might then ask if it is okay to touch or to get a little closer, which can be comforting to some patients (Figure 26-1).
- *Seek the patient's cooperation.* Encourage him to explain the problem. Never assume that it is impossible to communicate with a patient until you have tried, even if friends or family members insist it cannot be done. Ask questions. Use gestures to encourage the patient, such as a nod of your head, or by verbal responses, such as "I see" or "Go on," that show you are paying attention.

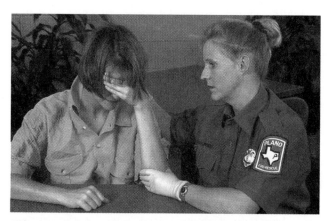

Figure 26-1 Touch may be comforting to some patients, but do not touch the patient suffering a behavioral disturbance without the patient's consent.

- *Maintain good eye contact with the patient.* There are two reasons why: First, it communicates your control and confidence. Second, the patient's eyes can reflect emotions and tell you whether the patient is terrified, confused, struggling, or in pain. Further, the eyes can telegraph intentions. If a patient is about to reach for a weapon or make a leap or a dash, his eyes may alert you.
- *Do not make any quick movements.* Act quietly and slowly; let the patient see that you're not going to make any sudden moves (which could precipitate panic or violence on his part).
- *Respond honestly to the patient's questions, but don't foster unrealistic expectations.* Instead of saying, "You have nothing to worry about," say something like, "Even with all the problems you've had, you seem to have lots of people around you who really care about you."
- *Never threaten, challenge, belittle, or argue with disturbed patients.* Many behaviorally disturbed patients will be adept at picking out your weaknesses; they may feel threatened themselves, and may try to improve their situation by belittling you. Remain kind and calm and treat the patient with respect. Remember that the patient is ill, and comments are not directed at you personally.
- *Always tell the truth; never lie to the patient.*
- *Do not "play along" with visual or auditory disturbances.* Reassure the patient that these are temporary and will clear up with treatment.
- *When you can, involve trusted family members or friends.* Some patients are calmed and reassured by the presence of these people, but others may be upset or embarrassed. Let the patient decide.
- *Be prepared to stay at the scene for a long time.* Don't rush to the hospital unless a medical emergency dictates the need for life-saving care. Instead, spend enough time to gain important clues from the environment and to avoid panicking the patient.
- *Never leave the patient alone.* All behavioral emergency patients are escape risks and violence to self or others is a distinct possibility. Once you have responded to the emergency, the patient's safety is legally your responsibility. Even if the patient pleads to be left alone for just a few minutes, firmly explain that you realize he is capable of handling things, but that you could get into trouble for leaving a patient alone. If the patient needs to go to the bathroom, first check the bathroom for potential weapons (e.g., razors, scissors). Leave the door ajar, but be discreet as you watch. Follow local protocol.
- *Avoid the use of restraint.* Enlist the support of law enforcement or those trained in the use of restraint if you decide restraint is absolutely necessary.
- *Do not force the patient to make decisions.* The patient has probably lost the ability to cope. If neces-

sary, "suggest" things that need to be done (e.g., "How about you lying back so we can take you to the hospital. OK?"

- *Encourage the patient to participate in a motor activity,* which helps reduce anxiety.
- *If the patient has attracted a crowd, do what you can to disperse it* so you can deal with the patient on a one-to-one basis. If the scene is especially hectic, remove the patient from it or remove distressing stimuli from the scene before trying to calm the patient.

ASSESSMENT AND CARE: BEHAVIORAL EMERGENCIES

Behavioral emergencies can be unpredictable, volatile situations. You must make every effort to ensure your safety before you enter such a scene and while you are at one. Remember, if you become a victim, you will not be able to help the patient.

SCENE SIZE-UP

Steps to ensure your safety should begin even before you arrive on the scene. Pay close attention to the dispatch. Does it indicate any violence or potential for violence? Check with dispatch to see whether police are on the way. Begin scene size-up immediately on arrival. Never enter a potentially violent situation without support. *If you cannot guarantee your own safety, call the police and wait for them to arrive before you leave your vehicle.*

Also be alert, if you are dispatched to the scene of a suicide or potential suicide, that you do not fall victim to a mechanism that the patient planned to use to end his own life. Running an automobile in a closed garage, blowing out a pilot light and turning on all the burners on a gas stove, and using electrical devices in water are common suicide methods that can pose risks for EMT-Bs.

Locate the patient visually before you enter the scene (Figure 26-2). You can be too easily surprised or even jumped by a patient as you enter the scene if you don't know exactly where he is. You will also be unable to observe his response to your entry if you can't see him. Again, if you can't visually locate the patient, wait for police to enter and secure the scene. Always stay between the patient and an open door so you can exit quickly should the scene deteriorate.

Never let down your guard or turn your back on the patient. Scan quickly for instruments or objects the patient might use to injure himself or others. If you see any dangerous articles, if possible discreetly move them out of the way. If the patient displays a weapon, never ignore or disregard it. Instead, in a calm and nonconfrontational way, tell the patient that you want to help but cannot do so until the weapon

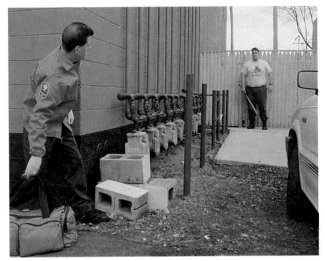

Figure 26-2   Visually locate the patient before approaching. Look for any weapons.

is released. Ask the patient to give you the weapon. If he does not, back out of the scene and call or wait for police response. Remember that any weapon can be used against the EMT-B. Stay outside the danger zone—for a knife, 22 feet; for a gun, much farther.

Early in the assessment, before you physically approach the patient, determine whether you and your partner can handle the situation alone. Even a small person who is sufficiently agitated can be very difficult to handle. If you doubt that you can handle the patient alone, call the police and wait for them to arrive.

If the scene seems secure, scan it for signs of things that may have contributed to the crisis or that the patient might have used in a suicide attempt. Be especially alert for liquor bottles, containers for pills or other medications, or any drug paraphernalia.

Remember that what appears to be a behavioral emergency can actually be caused by trauma, such as a blow to the head, or by a medical condition, such as hypoglycemia. Study the scene for clues that will help you determine the nature of the emergency. Look for a mechanism of injury or a sign of the nature of illness. If a patient has, in fact, made a suicide attempt, determining either the mechanism of injury (such as a razor blade or handgun) or the nature of illness (such as pills or carbon monoxide poisoning) will be critical.

Remember that sometimes two or more persons will make a suicide pact, that occasionally a person tries a murder-suicide (attempting to kill someone else and then himself), or that a method such as carbon monoxide poisoning may have made others ill, too. A person with a violent behavior disturbance may have injured someone else. Therefore, always determine the number of patients, not automatically assuming that there is just one. Call for additional resources as needed.

INITIAL ASSESSMENT

Gather a general impression of the patient. Assess the patient's mental status by asking specific questions that will help you measure the patient's level of responsiveness and orientation. Watch the patient's appearance, level of activity, and speech patterns. Specifically try to determine whether the patient is oriented to time, person, and place.

Pay particular attention to the patient's airway and breathing. Patients who have attempted suicide may have trouble maintaining their airway and respiration. Be prepared to provide oxygen by a nonrebreather mask at 15 lpm or positive pressure ventilation with supplemental oxygen if necessary.

If a patient has, in fact, attempted suicide, caring for his trauma or medical problem rather than his behavioral problem will be your priority. Proceed with assessment and care based on the mechanism of the suicide attempt. For example, if the patient has taken a large number of pills, or if he attempted to asphyxiate himself in his car, assess and treat him as a poisoning emergency. If he has slit his wrists, treat for bleeding and shock and soft tissue injuries. Make a priority decision regarding further assessment and transport.

FOCUSED HISTORY AND PHYSICAL EXAM

Once life threats have been managed, proceed with the focused history and physical exam. In the patient who is alert and has no significant mechanism of injury, try to obtain a SAMPLE history first. Pay particular attention to medications the patient has taken; they can help you clarify if the situation is a behavioral or medical emergency. It is also important to note carefully events leading to the emergency to help clarify if a suicide attempt is involved.

Inform the patient of what you are doing. Once you have determined what the problem is, explain it to the patient. Without frightening the patient, be honest in explaining what is going to be done to help. (Uncertainty is likely to make the patient more anxious and fearful.) Ask questions in a calm, reassuring voice. Stay polite, use good manners, show respect, and make no unsupported assumptions.

Allow the patient to tell you what happened. If you can, interview the patient in a quiet room where he has privacy. A patient may be ashamed and hesitant to talk in front of family or friends. Avoid asking questions that can be answered with a simple "yes" or "no"; the patient's method of explanation can help you during the assessment.

Show you are listening by rephrasing or repeating part of what the patient says. Look at the patient's eyes, show interest in what the patient is saying, and avoid being judgmental. Give the patient supportive information that is truthful. Acknowledge the patient's feelings. Use phrases like, "I can see that you are very depressed," or "I understand that you must feel frightened." You will have determined the patient's level of responsiveness and orientation during the initial assessment. During the focused history and physical exam, note any answers to your questions that reveal his general contact with reality, such as an auditory or visual hallucination (the patient is "hearing things" or "seeing things" that are not there).

Determine the patient's chief complaint, then perform a focused physical exam centered on those areas in which the patient has a complaint. Finally, take a set of baseline vital signs.

If the patient is unresponsive or has an otherwise severely altered mental status or a significant mechanism of injury, you should perform a rapid assessment, head to toe, to seek physical clues or signs as to whether the problem is behavioral or medical or traumatic. Obtain a set of baseline vital signs. Then try to obtain a SAMPLE history, if not from the patient himself, then from family or bystanders.

Specific tips for assessing suicidal and violent patients and preparing them for transport follow.

Suicidal Patients When performing an assessment on a patient who has attempted or threatened suicide, keep these additional guidelines in mind:

- *Injuries or medical conditions related to the suicide attempt are your primary concern.*
- *Listen carefully.*
- *Accept all the patient's complaints and feelings.* Do not underestimate what the patient may be feeling and do not dismiss what you consider to be minor.
- *Do not trust "rapid recoveries."* Transport the patient even if he seems to be "better."
- *Be specific in your actions.* Do something tangible for the patient such as arranging for a member of the clergy to meet the patient at the hospital.
- *Never show disgust or horror when you care for the patient.* Watch your body language!
- *Do not try to deny that the suicide attempt occurred.* Your denial may be perceived as condemnation of the patient's feelings.
- *Never try to shock a patient out of a suicidal act.* Never try to argue the person out if it, and never challenge the patient to go ahead.

Violent Patients When performing an assessment on a patient who has been violent or seems to offer the potential for violence, keep the following guidelines in mind:

- *Take a history.* Ask bystanders what's been going on. Has the patient been violent or threatened violence? If family members or friends are on the scene, find out if the patient has a history of violence, aggression, or combativeness.

- *Look at the patient's posture.* Anticipate violence if the patient is standing or sitting in a way that threatens anyone (including himself), if the patient's fists are clenched, or if the patient is holding anything that could be used as a weapon.
- *Listen to the patient.* Anticipate violence if the patient is yelling, cursing, arguing, or verbally threatening to hurt himself or others.
- *Monitor the patient's physical activity.* Signs of potential violence include moving toward the caregiver, carrying a heavy or threatening object, using quick or irregular movements, and having muscle tension.
- *Be firm and clear.* Give the patient instructions regarding his behavior. Clearly state the consequences of an aggressive behavior before such behavior occurs.
- *Be prepared to use restraints, but only if necessary.* See Restraining a Patient, later.

Signs and Symptoms   One or more of the signs and symptoms listed below may indicate a behavioral emergency:

- Fear—of a person or persons, an activity or a place
- Anxiety—not related to any specific person, place, or situation
- Confusion—may be preoccupied with fears or imaginary attacks
- Behavioral changes—such as radical alterations in lifestyle, values, relationships
- Anger—inappropriate anger directed at an inappropriate source; usually brief but intense and, often, destructive
- Mania—unrealistically optimistic; prone to take unwarranted risks and display poor judgment
- Depression—crying; inability to function; feelings of worthlessness or hopelessness; threats of suicide
- Withdrawal—loss of interest in people or things previously considered important
- Loss of contact with reality—hallucinations, auditory or visual
- Sleeplessness
- Loss of appetite
- Loss of sex drive
- Constipation
- Crying
- Tension
- Irritability

Emergency Medical Care

Behavioral emergencies come in many forms. A patient may be violent, raving, and threatening others or depressed and totally withdrawn. One patient may attempt to commit suicide by shooting himself while another may take pills. You must be adaptable when providing emergency care for behavioral emergencies.

Keep the following guidelines in mind when providing such care:

1. *Your safety is of utmost importance.* Be alert at all times to the possibility that the patient may become violent and do harm to you, others at the scene, or himself. Do not let yourself fall victim to the same mechanism of injury as the patient (e.g., carbon monoxide, electrocution).
2. *Assess the patient for trauma or a medical condition.* Remember that what seems to be a behavioral emergency may arise from trauma or a medical condition. Also, when patients have attempted suicide, their medical treatment has priority.
3. *Calm the patient, and stay with the patient.* Follow the guidelines above for communicating with a patient in a behavioral emergency. Never leave a suicidal patient alone. Never turn your back or drop your guard with a violent or potentially violent patient.
4. *If it's necessary to protect yourself or others, or the patient from harming himself, use restraints.* Never use restraints as a substitute for observation, and never use metal handcuffs. Use restraints only if emergency care would be dangerous or impossible without them. Enlist the aid of trained public safety personnel.
5. *Transport the patient* to a facility where he can get the physical and psychological treatment that is needed. If a patient attempted to commit suicide by drug or medication overdose, be sure to monitor airway, breathing, and circulation carefully and be prepared to assist ventilation. With such a patient, bring any drugs or medications you find at the scene to the receiving facility with the patient.

Detailed Physical Exam and Ongoing Assessment

As for any medical or trauma patient, perform a detailed physical exam en route to the hospital if the patient is unresponsive or has suffered a significant mechanism of injury and if time and the patient's condition permit—to identify any injuries or problems overlooked at the scene. Perform an ongoing assessment as warranted by the patient's condition. Monitor the patient's airway, breathing, circulation, and mental status. Repeat vital signs assessment and check any interventions, such as the security of restraints, if any. Continue to calm and reassure the patient.

Summary: Assessment and Care

To review possible assessment findings and emergency care for a behavioral emergency, see Figures 26-3 and 26-4.

✳ ASSESSMENT SUMMARY

BEHAVIORAL EMERGENCY

The following are findings that may be associated with a behavioral emergency.

SCENE SIZE-UP

Pay particular attention to your own safety. Look for:
   Mechanism of injury
   Weapons
   Hazards in attempted suicide such as a hair dryer in
      tub filled with water
   Alcohol or drugs
   Evidence of a medical condition
   Routes of escape

INITIAL ASSESSMENT

General Impression

Obvious life threats such as open wounds to chest,
   potentially self-inflicted
Posture and body language, violent or non-violent

Mental Status

Alert
Confusion or disorientation
Hyperactivity
Unresponsiveness

Airway

Potentially closed airway in attempted suicide from
   altered mental status or vomitus

Breathing

Normal
May be adequate, inadequate, or absent in attempted
   suicide

Circulation

Normal
Pulse may be increased, decreased, or absent in attempted suicide
Skin normal; may be pale, cyanotic, red, cool, or
   clammy in attempted suicide

Status: Priority Patient—if attempted suicide with life-threatening injuries or conditions

FOCUSED HISTORY AND PHYSICAL EXAM

SAMPLE History

Signs and symptoms:
   Fear
   Anxiety
   Confusion
   Anger
   Depression
   Withdrawal
   Hallucinations (auditory or visual)
   Irritability
   Excessive crying
History:
   Did patient ingest alcohol or drugs?
   Does patient want to commit suicide?
   Is patient on medications for a behavioral condition?
   Has he taken the medication as prescribed?
   Does patient have history of violence, aggression,
      or combativeness?
   Has patient had a recent tragic event?

Physical Exam

Head, neck, face:
   Pupils may be dilated, constricted, or mid-size
   Facial expression may indicate anger, depression,
      anxiety
Chest:
   Inspect for evidence of self-inflicted wounds
Abdomen:
   Inspect for evidence of self-inflicted wounds
Extremities:
   Inspect for needle marks or self-inflicted wounds

Baseline Vital Signs

BP: normal or increased, may also be absent or decreased in suicide attempt
HR: normal or increased, may also be absent or decreased in suicide attempt
RR: normal or increased, may also be absent or decreased in suicide attempt
Skin: normal; may be pale, cool, and clammy in patients experiencing fear and anxiousness
Pupils: normal or may be dilated or constricted in
   suicide attempt

Figure 26-3a   Assessment summary: behavioral emergency.

(Continued on the next page.)

EMERGENCY CARE PROTOCOL

BEHAVIORAL EMERGENCY

1. Ensure your own safety and be prepared to retreat if patient is violent.
2. Assess patient for possible self-inflicted injury.
3. Establish and maintain in-line spinal stabilization if spinal injury suspected.
4. Establish and maintain an open airway; insert a nasopharyngeal or oropharyngeal airway if patient is unresponsive and has no gag or cough reflex.
5. Suction secretions as necessary.
6. If breathing is inadequate, provide positive pressure ventilation with supplemental oxygen at a minimum rate of 12 ventilations/minute for an adult and 20 ventilations/minute for an infant or child.
7. If breathing is adequate, administer oxygen by nonrebreather mask at 15 lpm. If possible, deliver warm, humidified oxygen.
8. If no pulse is present, apply AED and follow AED protocol.
9. If patient is responding, keep him calm.
10. If patient becomes violent or threatens to injure himself, you, your partner, or others, restrain patient.
11. Perform an ongoing assessment every 5 minutes if patient is unstable or every 15 minutes if stable.

Figure 26-3b Emergency care protocol: behavioral emergency.

RESTRAINING A PATIENT

The patient who is out of control and not responding to interventions is a difficult problem for the EMT-B. *If no one is able to communicate with the patient and you believe that he may present a danger to himself, to you, or to others, you must notify the police.* Never leave such a patient alone; watch him constantly, and stay alert.

If you need to transport a violent patient against his will, you may need to use restraints. *Even if a violent patient comes with you voluntarily, be prepared to use restraints;* the situation may change suddenly.

Restraint should be avoided unless the patient is a danger to himself and/or others. *Restraints may require police authorization;* seek medical direction and follow local protocol. If you are not authorized by state law to use restraints, wait for someone with the proper authority.

Restraints used with a patient should be **humane restraints.** This means that they are padded so they will not injure a patient who struggles against them; use soft leather or cloth restraints, but never metal handcuffs. A violent physical struggle is usually brief, since most people cannot sustain the intensity of such a struggle; however, if you still feel the need for restraints, follow these guidelines (Figures 26-5a to d):

1. Gather enough people to overpower the patient rapidly *before* you attempt restraint. Effective teamwork is more important than the strength of any individual team member.
2. Plan your activities *before* you attempt restraint. Everyone involved should know what is going to happen.
3. Use only as much force as needed for restraint; never inflict pain or use unwarranted force in restraining a patient.
4. Estimate the range of motion of the patient's arms and legs, and stay beyond that range until you are ready to begin imposing restraint.
5. Once you have made the decision to restrain, *act quickly.* A key to effective restraint is taking the patient by surprise; delay or indecision could allow the patient to get the upper hand.
6. One rescuer should talk to the patient throughout the restraining process. However, you should never bargain with the patient or agree to remove the restraints if the patient promises to behave well.
7. Approach the patient with at least four rescuers at the same time; one person should be assigned to each of the patient's limbs.
8. Secure the patient's limbs with equipment approved by medical direction; as mentioned, restraints should be of soft leather or cloth. If available, use commercial wrist- and ankle-restraining straps.
9. Secure the patient to the stretcher with multiple straps—effective placement is around the patient's chest, waist, and thighs. Make sure none of the straps is unduly tight or impairs the patient's breathing.

EMERGENCY CARE ALGORITHM:
BEHAVIORAL EMERGENCY

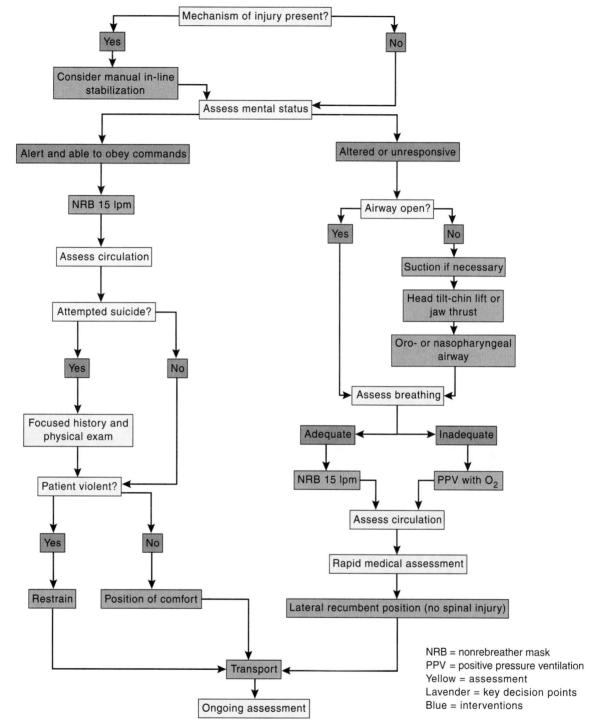

Figure 26-4 Emergency care algorithm: behavioral emergency.

RESTRAINING THE COMBATIVE PATIENT

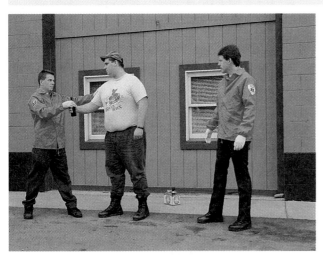

Figure 26-5a   If a possibility of danger exists, the patient should be interviewed with another EMT-B present. Identify yourselves and let the patient know what you expect.

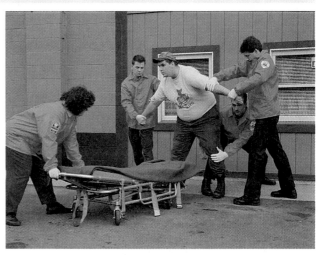

Figure 26-5b   Never try to restrain a patient until you have sufficient help and an appropriate plan. If necessary, create a safe zone and wait for police. Follow local protocol.

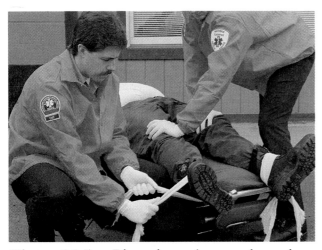

Figure 26-5c   Place the patient on the ambulance stretcher and apply ankle and wrist restraints.

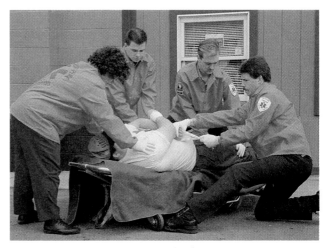

Figure 26-5d   One method is to pull arms tightly across the patient's chest and tie on opposite sides of the stretcher frame.

10. If the patient is spitting on rescuers, cover his face with a disposable surgical mask. If a mask is used, reassess airway and breathing frequently to ensure that the mask is not interfering with them or that the patient has not vomited.

11. Once you have applied restraints, do not remove them—not even during transport. Reassess the patient's circulation frequently to make sure the restraints are not binding.

Make sure you document on the prehospital care report why you felt it necessary to restrain the patient, and thoroughly document the technique you used for the restraint. Again, always avoid unnecessary force.

LEGAL CONSIDERATIONS

Every time you respond to a call as an emergency care provider, you have a chance of becoming involved with the legal system. That chance becomes greater when you are responding to patients with behavioral problems.

CONSENT

Simply stated, *consent* is permission to treat. Under most state laws, any adult of sound mind has the right to determine whether he will be treated or, more specifically, touched by another person in the course of treatment. In most states, that consent must also be informed. *Informed consent* means that the person who is to receive the treatment must understand what it involves. In practical terms, this means that, with every conscious, mentally competent adult, you must explain the treatment, its nature and its potential effects before starting it. Under laws in most states, forcing a person to have treatment against his will—that is, without consent—is grounds for a charge of assault and battery.

In most states, anyone aged 18 or over is considered an adult. In most states, people under the age of 18 are also considered "adult" (emancipated minors) if they are in the armed services or are married, pregnant, or a parent. If the patient is under the age of 18 and is not an emancipated minor, consent to treat should come from a parent, guardian, or blood relative. Consent should also come from a parent, guardian, or blood relative of a person who is considered to be mentally incompetent.

If you cannot find a responsible adult to consent to the treatment of a minor or of a mentally incompetent patient, or if an adult patient is unresponsive, you can still go ahead and treat. You will act in such cases on the principle of *implied consent*. This is the belief that the person who could grant consent would if he were present or able to do so.

These principles can be difficult to apply in the case of a patient suffering a behavioral emergency. Is he to be considered mentally competent? Is he able to give, or withhold, informed consent? Consult medical direction and/or carefully follow local protocols

REFUSAL OF CARE

Emotionally disturbed patients—especially those who are intoxicated or who have taken a drug overdose—commonly refuse treatment. If the disturbed person is alert and oriented, unless considered mentally incompetent, he still must legally provide consent before you can treat him. Under these situations, the patient, not concerned family members, must consent to the care. Depending on state and local law, a patient who is disoriented, in shock, mentally ill, or under the influence of drugs or alcohol may not be considered competent to refuse care.

Your best protection against legal problems when dealing with emotionally disturbed patients is to document carefully and thoroughly all aspects of the encounter. If a patient refuses care, complete a refusal of care form (or a similar form used in your jurisdiction), then have it signed and witnessed by a police officer.

If a patient threatens to hurt himself or others *and you can demonstrate reason to believe that the patient's threats are real,* you can transport that patient without his consent. Remember, however, that you

must be able to show that your belief that the patient poses a threat is reasonable. In such cases, make every effort to have law enforcement personnel participate in the transport of the patient. They can provide important corroboration for your actions.

USING REASONABLE FORCE

If it proves necessary to restrain a patient or to transport a patient without consent, make sure you use **reasonable force** when doing so. This is defined as the minimum amount of force required to keep the patient from injuring himself or others.

In most areas, police authorization is necessary to use reasonable force in restraining or transporting a patient without consent. Seek medical direction and follow local protocol. In most jurisdictions, an EMT-B can use reasonable force to defend against an attack by an emotionally disturbed patient without fearing legal consequences. The basic guideline in such circumstances is to avoid any act or use of physical force that may injure the patient during restraint.

The amount of force deemed *reasonable* depends upon the circumstances of the situation. As a general guide, you'll need to consider the following:

- *The size and strength of the patient*—What may seem a reasonable amount of force when used against a 275-pound weight lifter probably wouldn't be considered reasonable when used against a 150-pound person with limited mobility.
- *The type of behavior exhibited by the patient*—You would not be expected to use the same kind of force against a frightened, paranoid person as you would against a belligerent, aggressive person who is loudly and repeatedly threatening to kill you.
- *The mental state of the patient*—It would be considered reasonable to use more force on a patient who is agitated and threatening than on one who is quiet and subdued.
- *The method of restraint*—Soft restraints, commonly called humane restraints, and straps are generally considered reasonable; metal cuffs are not.

Caution: Always be aware that a patient who has become calm following a period of combativeness and aggression may suddenly revert to the earlier behavior. In such cases, you should use reasonable force to restrain the patient even though he has become calm.

POLICE AND MEDICAL DIRECTION

In any case where you might need to use reasonable force or transport without consent, the best way to protect yourself legally is to involve your chain of command. A good rule of thumb is this: Before you restrain any patient for any reason, *seek medical direction*. If medical direction advises restraint, you can use that later as justification for your actions, should they be questioned.

Remember that law enforcement personnel, too, should be involved when you need to restrain a patient or to transport without consent or if there is any threat of violence. Law enforcement personnel serve a two-fold purpose in cases like these: They can help protect you from injury, and they can serve as credible witnesses if a legal case should arise.

FALSE ACCUSATIONS

The best way to protect yourself against false accusations by a patient is to carefully and completely document everything that happens during the encounter—including detailed aspects of the patient's abnormal behavior. In most jurisdictions, anything

documented during the call is considered legally admissible evidence. Anything that is not documented is considered hearsay (not legally admissible).

Another source of protection is to have witnesses, preferably throughout the entire course of treatment, including transport. It is common for emotionally disturbed patients to accuse medical responders of sexual misconduct. To protect against these kinds of charges, consider employing these measures:

- Involving other medical responders who can testify that there was no misconduct
- Using medical responders that are the same gender as the patient
- Involving third-party witnesses
- Carefully documenting your physical assessment

Whenever possible, have witnesses sign a written report of the incident.

CASE STUDY FOLLOW-UP

SCENE SIZE-UP

You have been dispatched to Room 22 at King's Motel with a report of a woman bleeding. Because blood figures in the report, you don appropriate body substance isolation gear. You observe no immediate hazards at the scene and exit the ambulance. The motel manager meets you and leads you to the room, but indicates he has no idea of the problem. The door opens at your knock, and a woman, in some distress, says she's bleeding and asks for help. You enter the room cautiously and find in the bathroom the only occupant, a young woman, sitting on the bathroom floor bleeding from a wound on her left wrist. In her right hand she is holding a large hunting knife.

You say, "Miss, we're emergency medical technicians and we're here to help you. But first, could you please reach up and put the knife on top of the sink and slide back from it a little." The woman is sobbing heavily and doesn't move or give any sign that she's heard you. You say again, "Please, miss, we want to help you, but before we can you have to put the knife down. Just reach up and put it on the sink. Then move back, just a bit." This time, she hears you. She slowly raises her arm and places the knife on the edge of the sink. Then she half turns away and buries her face in her hands. You then move into the bathroom, picking up the knife and handing it to your partner, who secures it.

INITIAL ASSESSMENT

You introduce yourself and your partner to the patient and ask her name. She replies, "Maria Foster." You tell her once again that you have come to help

her. Your general impression is of a female in her early 20s who appears to be emotionally upset and is crying. She has an open wound to her left wrist. You ask, "Maria? May I call you Maria? Maria, may I please take a look at your wrist?" Maria nods yes, giving consent, and holds her wrist out toward you.

Bleeding from the wound has now stopped. The patient is alert and oriented. Her airway is open and her breathing is adequate. Her right radial pulse is present and her skin is slightly pale, cool, and moist. You explain, "Maria, you have lost some blood. I'd like to give you some oxygen. I think it would make you feel better and help you out a bit. Is that OK?" She nods her head again.

The injury to her wrist is not severe and blood loss has not been extensive. Maria's condition does not warrant a priority transport, so you proceed with the focused history and physical exam.

FOCUSED HISTORY AND PHYSICAL EXAM

You indicate to the motel manager that the situation is under control and ask him to wait outside the room. Then you ask Maria what happened.

She says, "No one cares. I got so tired of it. I just wanted it all over. All of it. I thought I'd come here where nobody knows me and slit my wrists and that would be it. Over. I had a couple of drinks and I was going to do it, I really was. I thought I could go through with it. I did one wrist and then I saw the blood and I chickened out. I called 911. Now I'm sorry I did. No, I'm not. Oh, I don't know. I'm so confused. I don't know . . ." She trails off into sobs.

You have listened carefully to Maria's story. You try to show your concern and acknowledge her feelings by saying, "I'm sorry that you're feeling so bad, Maria. I can understand how confused you feel. If it's OK, I'd like to ask you a few more questions and then see if I can help you with that wrist."

Maria nods her consent, so you go ahead with obtaining a SAMPLE history. You find that Maria has no other physical complaints. She has no known allergies, is on no medications, and has no significant past medical history. She last ate at about 4 o'clock yesterday afternoon and had about two glasses of rum over the 2 or 3 hours she was sitting in the room before cutting her wrist.

You ask if she inflicted any other wound to her body. She denies doing so. You inspect and palpate the area around the wrist wound. You note that a radial pulse is present. The skin below the wound is slightly pale and cool and dry to the touch. Maria is able to wiggle her fingers of her left hand and she can identify which of her fingers you are touching. You apply a dressing to the wound and bandage it. Your partner, meanwhile, obtains a set of baseline vital signs; they show a blood pressure of 148/84 mmHg, a heart rate of 94 per minute, and a respiration rate of 14 per minute.

You explain to Maria that you and your partner are going to put her on the stretcher and take her to Clarendon Hospital. You ask if there is anyone that you can have called to meet her at the hospital. Maria says nothing for a minute, then replies softly, "My mother." She gives you her mother's number and your partner calls it. Maria's mother agrees to come to the hospital. You move Maria into the ambulance and begin transport.

ONGOING ASSESSMENT

En route, you quickly repeat the initial assessment, reassess the wound to the wrist to ensure that it is not bleeding, and get another set of vital signs. You continue to talk to Maria and listen carefully to what she says to you. Upon arrival at the hospital, you transfer care of the patient to the emergency department staff. After completing the prehospital care report and preparing the ambulance to return to service, you go back to see how Maria is doing. Her mother is with her, and they both thank you for your help and showing that you care. Just then you receive a call for another run, so you wish Maria luck as you head back to the ambulance.

CHAPTER REVIEW

TERMS AND CONCEPTS

You may wish to review the following terms and concepts included in this chapter.

anxiety—a state of painful uneasiness about impending problems characterized by agitation and restlessness.
behavior—the way a person acts or performs.
behavioral emergency—a situation in which a person exhibits "abnormal" behavior.
bipolar disorder—a psychiatric condition, also known as manic-depressive disorder, characterized by wide swings between periods of depression and periods of elation and manic behavior.
depression—one of the most common psychiatric conditions, one characterized by deep feelings of sadness, worthlessness, and discouragement, feelings that often do not seem connected to the actual circumstances of the patient's life.

humane restraints—padded soft leather or cloth straps used to tie a patient down to keep them from hurting themselves or others.
paranoia—a highly exaggerated or unwarranted mistrust or suspiciousness.
phobia—an irrational fear of specific things, places, or situations.
reasonable force—the minimum amount of force required to keep a patient from injuring himself or others.
schizophrenia—the name given to a group of mental disorders characterized by debilitating distortions of speech and thought, bizarre delusions, hallucinations, social withdrawal, and lack of emotional expressiveness.
suicide—a willful act designed to end one's own life.

REVIEW QUESTIONS

1. List some of the clues that a behavioral problem may be due to physical rather than psychological causes.
2. Explain some of the causes that can lead to violence in the behavioral patient.
3. Explain basic steps to follow during the assessment of a potentially suicidal patient.
4. Explain basic steps to follow during assessment of a violent patient.
5. List some of the basic signs and symptoms of a behavioral emergency.
6. Explain the basic steps of emergency medical care in a behavioral emergency.
7. Explain what type of restraints should be used with the violent patient.
8. List factors that would be considered in determining if the force used with a patient was reasonable.
9. Explain the circumstances in which you can transport a patient without his consent.
10. Explain basic steps to protect yourself against false accusations by a patient.

CHAPTER 27

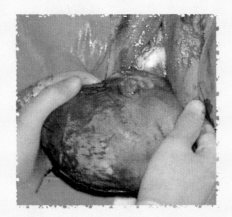

Obstetric and Gynecological Emergencies

INTRODUCTION

A pregnant woman is too often rushed to a hospital, usually because the EMT-B is afraid that the infant will be born before the mother can get there. In most cases there is no need for such haste. Childbirth is a normal, natural process. Only in a few situations involving complications do you need to see that the mother reaches the hospital quickly.

Care of patients with an emergency involving reproductive organs is not a common event. However, you must be prepared to deal with these emergencies in an absolutely professional, effective, and compassionate way. Be sure to review assessment and emergency medical care procedures for these kinds of emergencies as often as you can.

OBJECTIVES

Numbered objectives are from the United States Department of Transportation 1994 EMT-Basic National Standard Curriculum. Asterisked objectives, if any, pertain to material that is supplemental to the DOT curriculum.

COGNITIVE

4-9.1 Identify the following structures: uterus, vagina, fetus, placenta, umbilical cord, amniotic sac, perineum. (pp. 501, 503)

4-9.2 Identify and explain the use of the contents of an obstetrics kit. (p. 507)

4-9.3 Identify predelivery emergencies. (pp. 503–507)

4-9.4 State indications of an imminent delivery. (p. 507)

4-9.5 Differentiate the emergency medical care provided to a patient with predelivery emergencies from a normal delivery. (pp. 505–506, 509, 511–513)

4-9.6 State the steps in the predelivery preparation of the mother. (p. 509)

4-9.7 Establish the relationship between body substance isolation and childbirth. (p. 509)

4-9.8 State the steps to assist in the delivery. (pp. 509, 511–513)

4-9.9 Describe care of the infant as the head appears. (pp. 509, 511)

4-9.10 Describe how and when to cut the umbilical cord. (pp. 511, 512)

4-9.11 Discuss the steps in the delivery of the placenta. (p. 512)

4-9.12 List the steps in the emergency medical care of the mother post-delivery. (pp. 512–513)

4-9.13 Summarize neonatal resuscitation procedures. (pp. 519–520)

4-9.14 Describe the procedures for the following abnormal deliveries: breech birth, prolapsed cord, limb presentation. (pp. 513–514)

4-9.15 Differentiate the special considerations for multiple births. (p. 514)

4-9.16 Describe special considerations of meconium. (pp. 514–515)

4-9.17 Describe special considerations of a premature baby. (p. 515)

4-9.18 Discuss the emergency medical care of a patient with a gynecological emergency. (pp. 522, 524)

AFFECTIVE

4-9.19 Explain the rationale for understanding the implications of treating two patients (mother and baby). (pp. 507, 512)

PSYCHOMOTOR

4-9.20 Demonstrate the steps to assist in the normal cephalic delivery.

4-9.21 Demonstrate necessary care procedures of the fetus as the head appears.

4-9.22 Demonstrate infant neonatal procedures.

4-9.23 Demonstrate post-delivery care of the infant.

4-9.24 Demonstrate how and when to cut the umbilical cord.

4-9.25 Attend to the steps in the delivery of the placenta.

4-9.26 Demonstrate the post-delivery care of the mother.

4-9.27 Demonstrate the procedures for the following abnormal deliveries: vaginal bleeding, breech birth, prolapsed cord, limb presentation.

4-9.28 Demonstrate the steps in the emergency medical care of the mother with excessive bleeding.

4-9.29 Demonstrate completing a prehospital care report for patients with obstetrical/gynecological emergencies.

CASE STUDY

THE DISPATCH

EMS Unit 118—respond to Taggert's Laundromat on West Martin Street—a 30-year-old female in labor. Time out is 1926 hours.

ON ARRIVAL

Upon arrival, a man runs out of the Laundromat and tells you, "There is some woman in there about to have a baby. Boy is she screaming!" You and your partner proceed into the laundromat to find a female sitting on the floor in the corner, her anxious husband holding her hand. As you approach her, she says in a gasping breath, "I think the baby is coming."

How would you proceed?

During this chapter, you will learn how to recognize and provide emergency medical care for obstetric and gynecological emergencies. Later, we will return to the case study and put in context some of the information you learned.

CHILDBIRTH AND OBSTETRIC EMERGENCIES

ANATOMY OF PREGNANCY

You may want to review the material on the reproductive system in Chapter 4, "The Human Body." A general description of the major organs and structures involved in pregnancy (Figure 27-1) follows.

The **uterus** is the organ that contains the developing **fetus,** the unborn infant. Its special arrangement of smooth muscle and blood vessels allows for great expansion during pregnancy and forcible contractions during labor and delivery. The uterus also is capable of rapid contractions after delivery, which help to constrict blood vessels and prevent hemorrhage.

The neck of the uterus is called the **cervix.** The cervix contains a plug of mucus that seals the uterine opening, thereby preventing contamination from entering. The plug is discharged when the cervix starts to dilate, or open, and appears as pink-tinged mucus in the vaginal discharge. The expulsion of the plug signals the first stage of labor and is known as the **bloody show.**

The **placenta** is a disk-shaped inner lining of the uterus that begins to develop after the *ovum,* or egg, is fertilized and attaches itself to the uterine wall. Rich in blood vessels, the placenta is the sole organ through which the fetus receives oxygen and nourishment from the mother and discharges carbon dioxide and waste products. The exchange is made between the mother's and infant's blood streams within the placenta; however, the blood of the fetus and the blood of the mother do not mix.

After the infant is born, the placenta separates from the uterine wall and is delivered as the **afterbirth.** This usually weighs about a pound, or generally one-sixth of the infant's weight.

The **umbilical cord** is the unborn infant's lifeline, attaching the fetus to the placenta. It contains one vein and two arteries in a spiral arrangement that is covered by a protective substance called *Wharton's jelly.* The vessels in the umbilical cord are unique: the vein carries oxygenated blood and nutrients to the fetus, and the arteries carry deoxygenated blood and waste products back to the placenta. The structure of the cord—and the blood traveling through it—keep it from kinking. When the infant is born, the umbilical cord resembles a sturdy rope about 22 inches long and one inch in diameter.

The **amniotic sac,** or *bag of waters,* is filled with the amniotic fluid in which the infant floats, insulating and protecting it throughout the pregnancy. The amount of amniotic fluid varies from 500 to 1000 milliliters. At the onset of labor, the sac usually tears. This "rupturing of the bag of waters" is one of the first indications to the pregnant mother that her labor is starting. The amniotic fluid helps to lubricate the birth canal and remove any bacteria. During labor, part of the amniotic sac is forced ahead of the infant, serving as a resilient wedge to help dilate the cervix.

The lower part of the birth canal is called the **vagina.** About 8 to 12 centimeters in length, the vagina originates at the cervix of the uterus and extends through to an external opening of the body. During pregnancy, the vagina undergoes changes that prepare it for passage of the infant. The smooth muscle layer of the vagina allows it to stretch gently to accommodate the infant during delivery.

A full-term pregnancy lasts approximately 280 days from the first day of the last normal menstrual cycle. Each 3-month period of the approximately 9-month pregnancy is referred to as a *trimester.* Toward the end of a full-term pregnancy, in the third trimester, the fetus moves into a head-down position. When the head descends through the broad upper inlet of the mother's pelvis, the uterus moves downward and forward. Mothers can feel the difference and say that the infant has "dropped." This position is the one most common for the infant's passage through the cervix to the vagina.

ANATOMY OF PREGNANCY

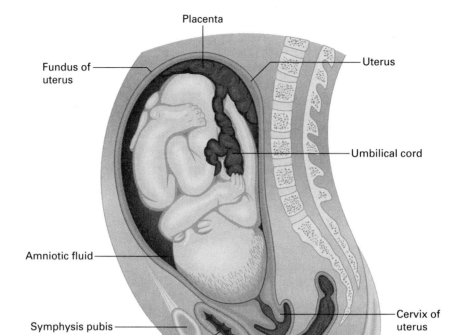

Figure 27-1 Anatomy of pregnancy.

STAGES OF LABOR

Labor is the term used to describe the process of birth. It consists of contractions of the uterine wall, which expel the fetus and the placenta out of the uterus and vagina. Normal labor can be divided into three stages—*dilation, expulsion,* and *placental* (Figure 27-2). The length of each stage varies in different women and under different circumstances.

FIRST STAGE: DILATION

During this first and longest stage, the cervix becomes fully dilated. This allows the infant's head to progress from the body of the uterus to the birth canal. Through uterine contractions, the cervix gradually dilates (stretches) and effaces (thins) until the opening is large enough to allow the infant to pass through.

The contractions usually begin as an aching sensation in the small of the back. Within a short time, the contractions become cramp-like pains in the lower abdomen. These recur at regular intervals, each one lasting about 30 to 60 seconds. At first, the contractions occur about 10 to 20 minutes apart and are not very severe. They may even stop completely for a while and then start again. Appearance of the plug of mucus (the bloody show) may occur before or during this stage of labor. Also before or during this stage, the amniotic sac may rupture, resulting in a brief flow of fluid from the vagina.

Stage one may continue for as long as 18 hours or more for a woman having her first child. Women who have had a child before may only experience 2 or 3 hours of early labor. The dilation stage ends when contractions are at regular 3- to 4-minute intervals, last at least 60 seconds each, and feel very intense.

SECOND STAGE: EXPULSION

During this stage, the infant moves through the vagina (the birth canal) and is born (Figures 27-3a to f). Contractions are closer together—2 to 3 minutes apart—and last longer—45 to 90 seconds each. As the infant moves downward, the mother experiences considerable pressure in her rectum, much like the feeling of a bowel movement. When the mother has this sensation, it is usually an indication that delivery is imminent.

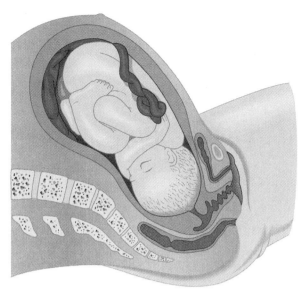

FIRST STAGE:
First uterine contraction to dilation of cervix

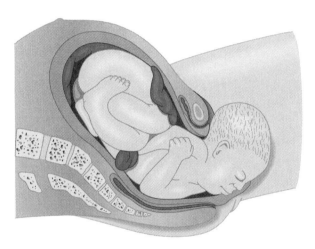

SECOND STAGE:
Birth of baby or expulsion

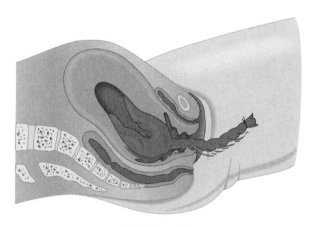

THIRD STAGE:
Delivery of placenta

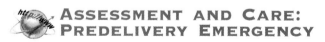

Figure 27-2   Stages of labor.

The tightening and bearing-down sensations will become stronger and more frequent. The mother will have an uncontrollable urge to push down, which she may do. There probably will be more bloody discharge from the vagina at this point. The **perineum,** the area of skin between the vagina and the anus, bulges significantly—a sign of impending birth.

Soon after, the infant's head appears at the opening of the birth canal. This is called **crowning.** At this point, the mother should be coached to push with each contraction. The shoulders and the rest of the infant's body follow.

THIRD STAGE: PLACENTAL

During this stage, the placenta separates from the uterine wall and is expelled from the uterus.

ASSESSMENT AND CARE: PREDELIVERY EMERGENCY

SCENE SIZE-UP

Information provided by the dispatcher may be the first indication that the patient is experiencing a potential **obstetric** emergency (an emergency having to do with pregnancy or childbirth). However, the stress and anxiety of the emergency may prevent the patient from relaying information accurately. Thus your scene size-up is very important in this situation. Remember that, as a general rule, any women of child-bearing age (about 12 to 50 years old) could potentially be experiencing an obstetric emergency. Use a high index of suspicion when assessing such a patient.

NORMAL DELIVERY

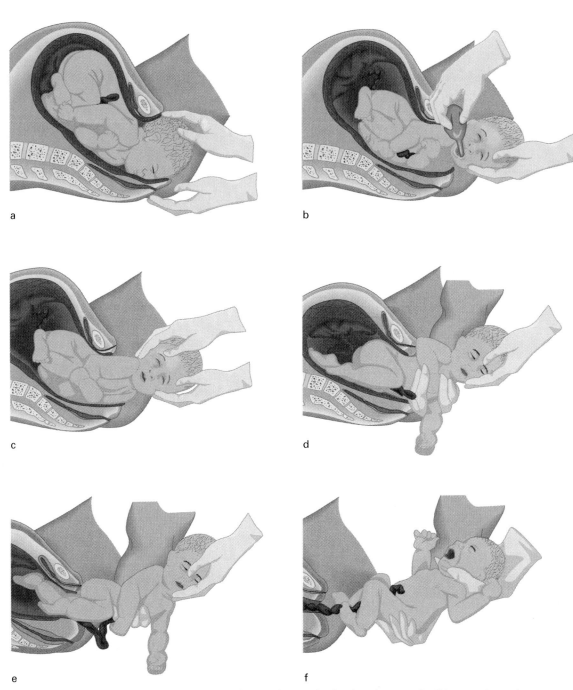

Figure 27-3 (a) The fetus moves down through the birth canal. (b) Suction the nose and mouth immediately upon delivery of the head. (c) Support the head to prevent an explosive delivery. (d) Deliver each shoulder. (e) Support the infant with both hands. (f) Keep the infant level with the vagina until the umbilical cord is cut.

INITIAL ASSESSMENT

After taking BSI precautions and making sure the scene is safe, perform an initial assessment, including the mental status, airway, breathing, and circulation of the patient. Use the same assessment and treatment techniques as for a patient who is not pregnant.

FOCUSED HISTORY AND PHYSICAL EXAM

Use SAMPLE questions including the OPQRST mnemonic to gather a history. Some patients may not realize that they are pregnant and experiencing an obstetric emergency. In this case, information collected in the history should provide the best evidence that the patient may be pregnant.

Include the following questions as appropriate:

- Are you experiencing any pain or discomfort?
  - What is the quality of the pain (dull, crampy, sharp, etc.)?
  - How intense is the pain?
  - Did the pain have a sudden or a gradual onset?
  - Does the pain radiate?
  - Can you point to the pain with one finger?
  - Is the pain constant? Does it come in regular or irregular intervals?
  - Are you nauseated? Have you thrown up?
  - Is the pain related to a menstrual cycle or sexual intercourse?
- When was your last menstrual period?
  - Date?
  - Was the volume and color of blood normal?
  - Have there been any episodes of bleeding between menstrual periods?
  - Have your periods been regular?
- Have you missed a menstrual period?
  - Is there any chance of pregnancy?
  - Is there any breast tenderness, an increase in urination, fatigue, nausea, or vomiting? (All are early indicators of pregnancy.)
- Have you had any unusual vaginal discharge?
  - What color was it?
  - Did it have an abnormal or foul odor?
  - How much was discharged?
- When (if patient knows she is pregnant) is your due date?
  - Have you had any prenatal care?
  - How many pregnancies have you had?
  - How many children do you have?
  - Did you have any complications with previous pregnancies?

If the obstetric patient is experiencing abdominal pain, perform a focused medical assessment that includes a thorough assessment of the abdominal region. Look for any abnormal distention or signs of injury. Palpation can help to determine the location of the pain as well as identify if there is any abdominal guarding, tenderness, or abnormal masses. You must consider conditions related to an acute abdomen in the patient with abdominal pain.

Also obtain a set of baseline vital signs.

Signs and Symptoms   Pregnancy is a normal process that is usually event-free. However, problems may occur, such as miscarriage (spontaneous abortion; early ending of the pregnancy before the baby is able to survive outside the uterus), seizures, vaginal bleeding not associated with the birth, or trauma. Characteristic signs and symptoms of each type of emergency are described on the following pages.

However, in general, a pregnant patient may be experiencing a predelivery emergency if she presents with one or more of the following:

- Abdominal pain, nausea, vomiting
- Vaginal bleeding, passage of tissue
- Weakness, dizziness
- Altered mental status
- Seizures
- Excessive swelling of the face and/or extremities
- Abdominal trauma
- Shock (hypoperfusion)

Note: Pregnancy may mask early signs and symptoms of shock (hypoperfusion). The initial indications may be very subtle or even absent. This is because a woman's blood volume is normally increased during pregnancy, which will mask a fall in blood pressure associated with shock. Also, the mother's body will shunt blood away from the fetus and redirect it back to the vital organs of the mother. So even though the mother seems well, the fetus could be in extreme distress. Any pregnant patient who is currently experiencing, or experienced prior to your arrival, some type of abnormality (pain, discomfort, or bleeding) needs to be seen by a physician.

EMERGENCY MEDICAL CARE

In general, provide the pregnant patient with the same emergency medical care you would provide to any patient with the same signs and symptoms.

However, for the pregnant patient who is close to full term (approaching the time of birth), take precautions against a condition known as **supine hypotensive syndrome.** This condition frequently results when the pregnant patient is supine and the combined weight of the enlarged uterus and fetus presses on the inferior vena cava, the great vein that collects blood from the lower body and delivers it to the heart.

The pressure may cause inadequate venous blood return to the heart and a drop in cardiac output (amount of blood pumped out of the left ventricle), which will result in hypotension (low blood pressure). If the mother experiences bleeding before delivery, the hypotension will be worsened. Watch for lower-than-expected blood pressure readings. Also be alert for syncope (fainting). To avoid supine hypotensive syndrome, the patient should be placed in a sitting position, if appropriate, or lying on her left side, which moves the uterus off the vena cava.

General guidelines for emergency medical care of a predelivery emergency include the following:

1. *Ensure adequate airway, breathing, and circulation.* Administer oxygen at 15 lpm by nonrebreather mask. (Note: In general, the pregnant patient and fetus consume a greater amount of oxygen than a nonpregnant patient. Therefore provide oxygen to any pregnant patient to help assure fetal oxygenation, or provide positive pressure ventilation with supplemental oxygen if breathing is inadequate.)

2. *Care for bleeding from the vagina.* If there is vaginal bleeding, place a sanitary napkin over the vaginal opening. Never pack the vagina in an attempt to control bleeding. Never touch the vaginal area. If the pad becomes soaked with blood, replace it. Save and transport with the patient any passed tissue or any evidence of blood loss (such as bloody sheets, towels, sanitary pads, or underwear).
3. *Treat for shock (hypoperfusion), if indicated.*
4. *Provide emergency medical care as you would for the nonpregnant patient based on any other signs and symptoms.*
5. *Transport the patient on her left side.* If she is on a backboard, tilt the board to the left.

ONGOING ASSESSMENT

Perform an ongoing assessment en route to the hospital. Repeat the initial assessment. Repeat vital signs. Check any interventions, being especially careful about oxygen mask fit and adequate flow of oxygen. Be attentive for and treat for any signs of developing shock (hypoperfusion). If the patient is stable, repeat the ongoing assessment every 15 minutes, if unstable every 5 minutes.

Note: If a pregnant patient dies in or as a result of an accident, CPR started immediately or within the first few minutes may save the life of the infant by continuing the oxygenation and circulation of the mother's blood. If you do begin CPR, it must be continued throughout transport and until the infant is surgically delivered at the hospital. The key to saving the infant is to prevent the mother's condition from deteriorating in the field. That is, protect the airway, support breathing and blood pressure, transport rapidly, and notify the receiving facility as soon as possible. Vigorous resuscitation of a mother to save a fetus is acceptable even if you believe that the mother is dead or is likely to die.

SPECIFIC PREDELIVERY EMERGENCIES

Miscarriage A **miscarriage,** or **spontaneous abortion,** may occur for any number of reasons and is defined as delivery of the fetus and placenta before the fetus is viable (can live on its own). Viability is usually considered to begin after the 20th week of pregnancy. The cause of a miscarriage often cannot be determined, and time should not be wasted trying to determine if a miscarriage has actually occurred.

The signs and symptoms of a possible miscarriage include:

- Cramp-like lower abdominal pain similar to labor
- Moderate-to-severe vaginal bleeding, which may be bright or dark red
- Passage of tissue or blood clots

In addition to the general guidelines for emergency medical care described above, be sure to ask when the patient's last menstrual period began. Provide emotional support to the mother and the members of her family throughout treatment and transport. Intense grief over loss of the pregnancy is normal and expected in both parents.

Seizures During Pregnancy Seizures during pregnancy can be a life-threatening emergency for the mother and the fetus. Provide emergency medical care the same as for any seizure patient. It is especially important to help protect the pregnant patient from injuring herself. Be sure to transport the patient on her left side. Since lights, noise, and movement can set off seizures in some conditions associated with pregnancy, transport the patient in as calm and quiet a manner as possible.

Vaginal Bleeding Vaginal bleeding may sometimes occur late in the pregnancy, with or without pain. If the bleeding is excessive, it can be a life-threatening emergency for the mother and fetus. For treatment, follow the general guidelines for emergency medical care described above. Be sure to place sanitary napkins externally over the vaginal opening and transport the patient as soon as possible. Be especially alert to the early signs and symptoms of shock (hypoperfusion).

Trauma to a Pregnant Woman A pregnant woman is subject to the same kind of trauma as any other person. Since the uterus and amniotic fluid are designed to protect the fetus, minor trauma to the abdomen usually does not cause injury to the infant. However, severe blunt trauma to the abdomen—especially late in the pregnancy—can damage the uterus and injure the fetus, as well as rupture the mother's, liver, spleen, or diaphragm.

Treat trauma to the pregnant patient the same as you would treat trauma to any other patient. Remember, however, that early signs of shock (hypoperfusion) may be minimal or absent in a pregnant patient, and if the patient starts to decompensate (fail to compensate for the condition and begin to deteriorate), she may do so more rapidly than a nonpregnant patient. Be sure to administer oxygen at 15 lpm by nonrebreather mask (if the patient's breathing is adequate) or positive pressure ventilation with supplemental oxygen (if the patient's breathing is inadequate) to any injured pregnant woman, and transport as soon as possible.

In addition to the general guidelines for emergency medical care described above, maintain a high index of suspicion for any trauma to the pregnant patient's abdomen, back, or pelvic region. Look closely for any abdominal injuries, especially in an unresponsive woman. Check for vaginal bleeding or possible rupturing of membranes and loss of amniotic fluid (however, do not touch the vaginal area). Transport as soon as possible, with the patient positioned on her left side. If you suspect neck or back injury, immobilize the patient using normal immobilization equipment and procedures. However, after immobilization, place pillows under the edge of the right side of the backboard to help tilt the patient to the left, thereby relieving pressure on the inferior vena cava during transport. Monitor and record vital signs continually.

SUMMARY: ASSESSMENT AND CARE—PREDELIVERY EMERGENCY

To review possible assessment findings and emergency care for a predelivery obstetric emergency, see Figures 27-4 and 27-5.

ASSESSMENT AND CARE: ACTIVE LABOR AND NORMAL DELIVERY

SCENE SIZE-UP, INITIAL ASSESSMENT, AND FOCUSED HISTORY AND PHYSICAL EXAM

For a woman in labor or having a normal delivery, the scene size-up, initial assessment, and focused history and physical exam are essentially the same as you would provide in a predelivery emergency, as just described. The difference now is that if you determine that the patient is in active labor (review the stages of labor described earlier in the chapter), your assessment and treatment goals now focus on assisting the mother with delivery and providing initial care to the **neonate** (the newborn infant).

As a general rule, it is best to transport a mother in labor so that the delivery can take place at a hospital. However, if delivery is expected within a few minutes, you will need to prepare to assist in the delivery at the scene. In order to determine if you should transport or commit to a delivery on scene, answer the following questions:

- Is this the patient's first delivery?
- How long has the patient been pregnant?
- Has there been any bleeding or discharge, (bloody show or amniotic fluid)?
- Are there any contractions or pain present?
- What is the frequency and duration of contractions?
- Is crowning occurring with contractions?
- Does the patient feel the need to push?
- Does the patient feel as if she is having a bowel movement with increasing pressure in the vaginal area?
- Is the abdomen (uterus) hard upon palpation?

Note: There are three cases in which you must assist in the delivery of the infant: if you have no suitable transportation; if the hospital or physician cannot be reached due to bad weather, a natural disaster, or some other kind of catastrophe; or if delivery is imminent. The answers to the questions above can help you determine if delivery is about to happen. Also see Signs and Symptoms, below, for indications that delivery is imminent.

Signs and Symptoms Delivery can probably be expected within a few minutes, if the following signs and symptoms are present:

- Crowning has occurred.
- Contractions are closer than 2 minutes apart, and they are intense and last from 30 to 90 seconds.
- The patient feels the infant's head moving down the birth canal (sensation of bowel movement).
- The patient has a strong urge to push.
- The patient's abdomen is very hard.

If birth is imminent with crowning, contact medical direction for a decision to commit to delivery on site. If delivery does not occur within 10 minutes, contact medical direction for permission to transport. If you determine that you must assist in the delivery of the infant, remember:

- Take all appropriate BSI precautions, including gloves, gown, and eye protection.
- Do not touch the patient's vaginal area, except during delivery and in the presence of your partner.
- Do not allow the patient to use the bathroom. She will feel as if she needs to move her bowels, but it is more likely that the infant's head is moving down the birth canal and pressing against the patient's rectum. If the patient does move her bowels or urinate, replace soiled linens with clean ones.
- Do not hold the mother's legs together. Do not do anything to attempt to delay delivery.
- Use a sterile obstetrics (OB) kit. Recommended equipment includes (Figure 27-6):
  - Surgical scissors or scalpel (for cutting the umbilical cord)
  - Cord clamps or cord ties
  - Umbilical tape or sterilized cord
  - Bulb syringe
  - Towels, five or more
  - Gauze sponges, 2 x 10
  - Sterile gloves
  - One infant blanket
  - Individually wrapped sanitary napkins, three or more
  - Large plastic bag, at least one
  - Germicidal wipes

If you are to assist the mother in delivery, stay calm and explain to her that you are trained to help. As much as possible, ensure the mother's comfort, modesty, and peace of mind. Try to limit distractions

ASSESSMENT SUMMARY

PREDELIVERY OBSTETRIC EMERGENCY

The following are findings that may be associated with a pre-delivery obstetric emergency.

SCENE SIZE-UP

Pay particular attention to your own safety. Look for:
- Mechanism of injury
- Blood in toilet or around patient
- Bleeding from the vagina
- Bloody tissue or blood clots

INITIAL ASSESSMENT

General Impression

Does patient appear to be pregnant?

Posture: lying still with knees to chest indicates severe abdominal pain, or supine

Any evidence of seizure activity?

Is umbilical cord or fetal body part other than the head present at vaginal opening?

Mental Status

Alert to unresponsive based on condition and potential blood loss

Airway

Potentially closed airway if mental status is altered

Breathing

Increased if associated with anxiety, pain, or blood loss

Circulation

Heart rate may be increased

Peripheral pulses may be weak or absent associated with blood loss

Skin may be cool, clammy, and pale

Status: *Priority patient if associated with shock, significant vaginal bleeding, or abnormal presenting part*

FOCUSED HISTORY AND PHYSICAL EXAM

SAMPLE History

Signs and symptoms:
  Abdominal pain, may be crampy

Vaginal bleeding, may be profuse or minimal, dark or bright red

Weakness, dizziness

Seizure activity

Peripheral edema

Signs and symptoms of shock

Fainting while lying supine (supine hypotensive syndrome)

History:
  What is the onset, provocation, quality, radiation, severity, and duration of the pain?

  When was your last menstrual period?

  Have you missed a menstrual period?

  Have you had any unusual vaginal discharge?

  When is your due date?

  Have you had previous problems with pregnancies?

  Have you been seeing a physician for this pregnancy?

  Do you get dizzy or faint while lying flat on your back? (supine hypotensive syndrome)

Physical Exam

Head, neck, and face:
  Edema to face and neck (may indicate preeclampsia)

Abdomen/genitalia:
  Large, palpable masses

  Is the abdomen/uterus rigid, soft, or tender?

  Any evidence of crowning or abnormal presenting part?

  Any passed tissue from the vagina?

  Vaginal bleeding, dark or bright red, may or may not be associated with pain

Extremities:
  Edema to hands and feet (may indicate preeclampsia)

Baseline Vital Signs

BP: may be normal, decreased in shock, or increased in preeclampsia

HR: may be normal or increased in shock

RR: may be normal or increased

Skin: may be normal or pale, cool, and clammy in shock

Pupils: may be dilated and sluggish

Figure 27-4a Assessment summary: predelivery obstetric emergency.

EMERGENCY CARE PROTOCOL

PREDELIVERY OBSTETRIC EMERGENCY

1. Establish and maintain an open airway; insert a nasopharyngeal or orpharyngeal airway if patient is unresponsive and has no gag or cough reflex.
2. Suction secretions as necessary.
3. If breathing is inadequate, provide positive pressure ventilation with supplemental oxygen at a minimum rate of 12 ventilations/minute for an adult and 20 ventilations/minute for an infant or child.
4. If breathing is adequate, administer oxygen by nonrebreather at 15 lpm.
5. If patient is pregnant, check for crowning or abnormal presenting part. If crowning is present, go to the protocol on "Active Labor and Delivery." If an abnormal presenting part is found, such as a prolapsed cord, hand, or foot, perform the following:
   a. Position patient in knee-chest position or elevate buttocks using pillows
   b. If umbilical cord is prolapsed, insert gloved hand into vagina and push presenting part of fetus away from cord.
   c. Cover presenting part with a sterile moist dressing.
   d. Rapidly transport patient and notify receiving facility of patient's condition.
6. If vaginal bleeding is present, place a sanitary napkin over vaginal opening. Do not insert anything into or pack the vagina.
7. Position patient on her left side to prevent or manage supine hypotensive syndrome. If patient is immobilized on a backboard, tilt right side of board to the left.
8. Transport.
9. Perform an ongoing assessment every 5 minutes if unstable, every 15 minutes if stable.

Figure 27-4b   Emergency care protocol: predelivery obstetric emergency.

and onlookers. Most importantly, be sure to recognize your own limitations. If you get into a situation you cannot handle, call medical direction for help and permission to transport.

EMERGENCY MEDICAL CARE

Be sure you are taking all appropriate BSI precautions. Wear protective gloves, gown, and eye protection. The amount of blood and body fluid exposure during delivery is usually significant. Handle blood and fluid-soaked dressings, pads, and linens carefully, and bag them in moisture-proof bags to prevent leakage. Seal and label the bags.

Emergency medical care of the patient in active labor for a normal delivery (Figures 27-7a to h) is as follows:

1. *Position the patient.* Have the patient lie on a firm surface with her knees drawn up and spread apart. Elevate the patient's buttocks several inches with a folded blanket, sheet, towels, or other clean objects. The patient's feet should be flat on the surface beneath her, which will help her brace herself. She should be several feet in from the edge of the surface to help provide extra support for the slippery infant as it is born. Support the mother's head, neck, and shoulders with pillows or folded blankets so she does not feel like she is slipping "downhill."

2. *Create a sterile field around the vaginal opening.* Use sheets from the OB kit, sterile towels, or paper barriers. Remove the patient's clothing or push it up above her waist. Place one sheet under the woman's hips, unfolding it toward her feet, and another sheet over her abdomen and legs. Place your OB kit or equipment close enough to reach, but away from the birth canal so it will not be contaminated by the vaginal discharge, blood, and amniotic fluid.

3. *Monitor the patient for vomiting.* Have your partner or a close family member stay at the patient's head. If she vomits, this person can be ready to turn her head to one side and clean out her mouth manually or with suction.

4. *Continually assess for crowning.*

5. *Place your gloved fingers on the bony part of the infant's skull when it crowns.* Exert very gentle pressure to prevent an explosive delivery. Avoid touching and exerting pressure on the infant's face and on any soft spot (fontanelle) on the head. With a sterile dressing, exert gentle pressure horizontally across the perineum to reduce the risk of traumatic tears.

6. *Rupture the amniotic sac if it is not already broken.* Use your fingers to rupture the sac, and

EMERGENCY CARE ALGORITHM:
PRE-DELIVERY OBSTETRIC EMERGENCY

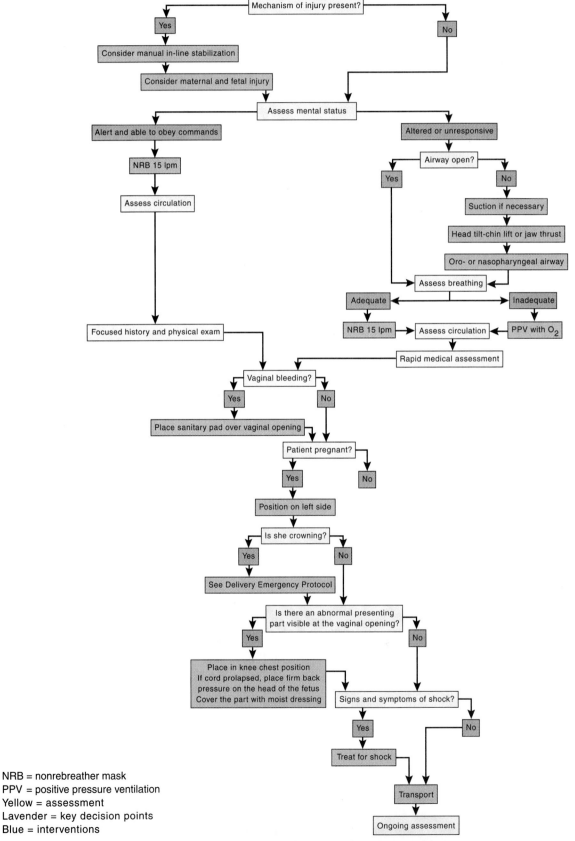

NRB = nonrebreather mask
PPV = positive pressure ventilation
Yellow = assessment
Lavender = key decision points
Blue = interventions

Figure 27-5   Emergency care algorithm: predelivery obstetric emergency.

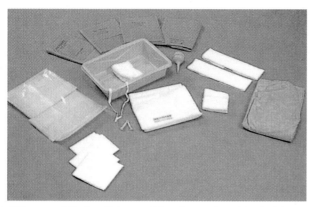

Figure 27-6   Disposable obstetrics (OB) kit.

then push it away from the infant's head and face as they appear.

7. *Determine the position of the umbilical cord.* As the infant's head is delivered, determine if the umbilical cord is around the infant's neck. If it is, use two fingers to slip the cord over the infant's shoulder. If you cannot move the cord, place two clamps 3 inches apart and cut between the clamps. Remove the cord from around the neck.

8. *Remove fluids from the infant's airway.* As soon as the head is delivered, support it with one hand and suction the mouth and nostrils two or three times each with a bulb syringe, or until clear of fluid and secretions. Suction the mouth first to avoid stimulating aspiration of any fluid still in the mouth or pharynx. Make sure you compress the bulb syringe *before* you bring it to the infant's face. Insert the tip of the compressed bulb 1.0 to 1.5 inches into the infant's mouth, slowly releasing the bulb to allow mucus and fluids to be drawn into the syringe. Avoid touching the back of the mouth. Remove the syringe, then discharge the contents onto a towel, and repeat. Use the same procedure to suction each nostril.

9. *As the torso and full body are expelled, support the newborn with both hands.* Never pull the infant from the vagina. The newborn will be slippery with a whitish, cheeselike substance *(vernix caseosa)* over its body. However, do not put your fingers in the infant's armpit; pressure there can damage nerve centers. Receive the newborn in a clean or sterile towel to help you hold it safely.

CHILDBIRTH

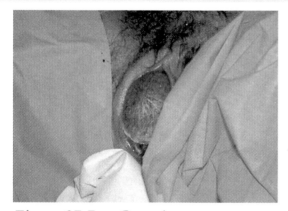

Figure 27-7a   Crowning.

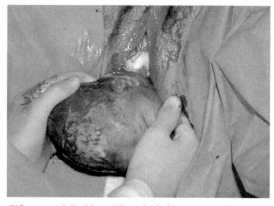

Figure 27-7b   Head delivers and turns.

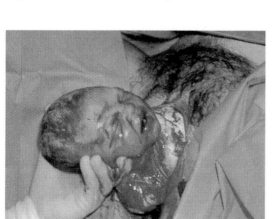

Figure 27-7c   Shoulders deliver.

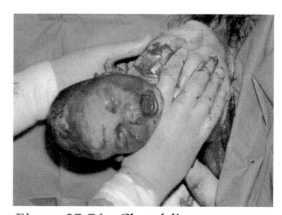

Figure 27-7d   Chest delivers.

(Continued on the next page.)

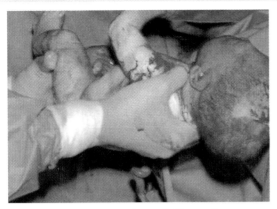

Figure 27-7e   Infant delivered.

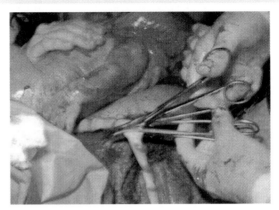

Figure 27-7f   Cutting of cord.

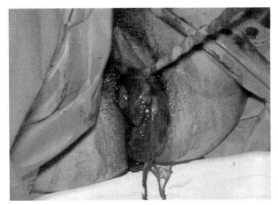

Figure 27-7g   Placenta begins delivery.

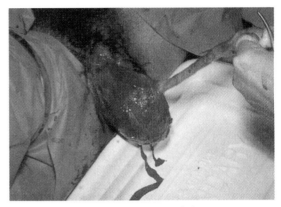

Figure 27-7h   Placenta delivers.

10. *Grasp the feet as they are born.* Do not pull on the umbilical cord as you lift or receive the infant.

11. *Clean the newborn's mouth and nose.* Wipe blood and mucus from the infant's mouth and nose with sterile gauze. Then suction the mouth and nose again. The infant will probably cry almost immediately.

12. *Dry, wrap, warm, and position the infant.* Dry the infant with towels. Place it in a warm blanket and on its back or side with the neck in a neutral position. Keep the infant level with the mother's vagina until the umbilical cord is cut.

13. *Assign your partner to monitor and complete initial care of the newborn.* You should complete emergency medical care of the mother.

14. *Clamp, tie, and cut the umbilical cord as pulsations cease (Figure 27-8).* Place two clamps or ties on the cord about three inches apart. The first clamp should be approximately four finger-widths (6 inches) from the infant. Use sterile surgical scissors or a scalpel to cut the cord between the two clamps. Periodically check the end of the cord for bleeding, and control any that may

occur by placing another clamp or tie proximal to the one you have already placed on the cord.

15. *Observe for delivery of the placenta.* While preparing the mother and infant for transport, continue to watch for delivery of the placenta. It usually is delivered within 10 minutes of the infant, and almost always within 20 minutes. When the placenta appears at the vagina, grasp it gently and rotate it. Never pull. Instead, slowly and gently guide the placenta and the attached membranes from the vagina. Do not delay transport while waiting for the delivery of the placenta.

16. *Wrap the delivered placenta.* When the placenta has completely delivered, wrap it in a towel and place it in a plastic bag for transport to the hospital. A physician will examine it to confirm that delivery was complete.

17. *Place one or two sanitary napkins over the vaginal opening.* Then lower the patient's legs and help her hold them together. Elevate her feet if necessary.

18. *Record the time of delivery and transport the mother, infant, and placenta to the hospital.* Keep mother and infant warm. Transport gently.

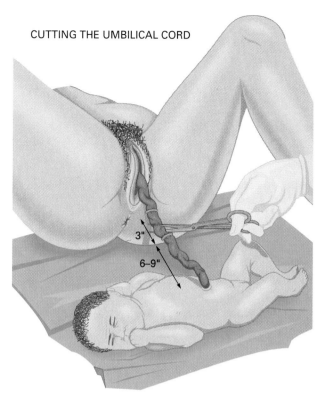

CUTTING THE UMBILICAL CORD

3"

6–9"

Figure 27-8   Cutting the umbilical cord.

Note that there will be vaginal bleeding after delivery. Up to 500 cc of blood loss is normal and well tolerated by the mother. However, if blood loss appears to be excessive, provide oxygen to the mother and massage the uterus as directed below. Massage helps to stimulate contractions, which decrease the uterine size and help to stop bleeding.

1. *Place the medial edge of one hand (fingers extended) horizontally across the abdomen, just above the symphysis pubis. This will help prevent the uterus from prolapsing with the massage.*
2. *Cup your other hand around the uterus. Use a kneading or circular motion to massage the area. It should feel like a hard grapefruit.*
3. *Also allow the infant to suckle on the mother's breast. This will release oxytocin, a naturally occurring hormone that will cause the uterus to contract.*
4. *If bleeding continues to appear to be excessive, check your massage technique, continue massage, and transport immediately.*

ONGOING ASSESSMENT

During the ongoing assessment, regardless of the estimated amount of blood loss after delivery, if the mother appears to be suffering shock (hypoperfusion), treat and transport immediately. You can initiate uterine massage during transport.

ASSESSMENT AND CARE: ACTIVE LABOR WITH ABNORMAL DELIVERY

SCENE SIZE-UP, INITIAL ASSESSMENT, AND FOCUSED HISTORY AND PHYSICAL EXAM

Just as you would perform a scene size-up, initial assessment, and focused history and physical exam on a patient having a normal delivery, so would you assess a patient who is experiencing a delivery emergency.

Signs and Symptoms   In general, you can recognize an abnormal delivery emergency by observing one or more of the following signs or symptoms:

• Any fetal presentation other than the normal crowning of the fetus head
• Abnormal color or smell of the amniotic fluid
• Labor before 38 weeks of pregnancy
• Recurrence of contractions after the first infant is born (indicating multiple births)

EMERGENCY MEDICAL CARE AND ONGOING ASSESSMENT

In general, emergency medical care of the mother and newborn is similar to that of a normal delivery. Exceptions are outlined below and include an emphasis on immediate transport, administration of high-flow oxygen, and continuous monitoring of vital signs during the ongoing assessment.

SPECIFIC ABNORMAL DELIVERY EMERGENCIES

Prolapsed Cord After the amniotic sac ruptures, the umbilical cord, rather than the head, may be the first part presenting at the vaginal opening. This is called a **prolapsed cord** (Figure 27-9). In this situation the umbilical cord may get compressed against the walls of the vagina by the pressure of the infant's head or buttocks. As a result the infant's supply of oxygenated blood can be cut off. This is a true emergency.

For a prolapsed cord, follow these guidelines:

1. Position the patient with her head down in a "knee-chest" position (kneeling and bent forward, face down, chest to knees), or raise her buttocks using pillows to allow gravity to reduce the pressure of the fetal head on the cord in the birth canal.
2. Insert a sterile, gloved hand into the vagina, and gently push the presenting part of the fetus, head or buttocks, back and away from the pulsating cord. (Note: This is the one time it is permissible to insert your hands into the mother's vagina.) Do *not* try to push the cord back into the vagina. *Follow local protocol and seek medical direction.*

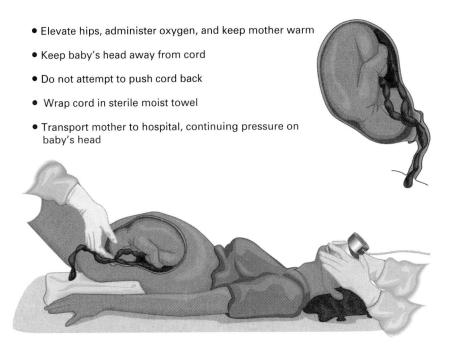

- Elevate hips, administer oxygen, and keep mother warm
- Keep baby's head away from cord
- Do not attempt to push cord back
- Wrap cord in sterile moist towel
- Transport mother to hospital, continuing pressure on baby's head

Figure 27-9   Prolapsed cord.

3. Cover the umbilical cord with a sterile towel moistened with a saline solution.
4. Transport the patient rapidly while maintaining pressure on the head or buttocks to keep pressure off the cord, and monitor pulsations in the cord. (Pulsations should be present.)

Breech Birth   A **breech birth** presentation is one in which the fetal buttocks or lower extremities are low in the uterus and are the first to be delivered (Figure 27-10). Delivery may be prolonged for these newborns, who are at great risk of delivery trauma. Transport immediately upon recognition of a breech presentation. Administer oxygen to the mother, and keep the mother in a supine head-down position with her pelvis elevated so gravity will discourage the movement of the fetus into the birth canal.

Limb Presentation   When one arm or one leg is the first to protrude from the birth canal, it is considered a **limb presentation.** The treatment necessary is the same as you would provide for a breech presentation. Transport immediately, because surgery is likely to be required. Administer oxygen to the mother, and keep the mother in a head-down position with her pelvis elevated so gravity will slow the progress of the fetus into the birth canal. *Never* pull on the infant by its arm or leg, and never attempt delivery in this situation. Have the mother pant if she has the urge to push with contractions.

Multiple Births   In a multiple birth the infants (twins, triplets, and so on) each may have its own placenta or the infants may share a placenta. Even if the mother is unaware that she is carrying more than one infant, you should be prepared for a multiple birth if one or more of the following is observed:

- The abdomen is still very large after one infant is delivered.
- Uterine contractions continue to be extremely strong after delivering the first infant.
- Uterine contractions begin again about 10 minutes after one infant has been delivered.
- The infant's size is small in proportion to the size of the mother's abdomen.

Follow the general guidelines for emergency medical care in a normal delivery, with the following exceptions: Be prepared to care for more than one infant. Call for assistance. Note that about one-third of the deliveries of the second infant will be breech, so assess carefully and take immediate action. If the second infant is not breech, handle the delivery as you would for a single infant. Expect and manage hemorrhage following the second birth. If the second infant has not delivered within 10 minutes of the first, transport the mother and the first infant to the hospital for delivery of the second infant.

Meconium   During a difficult labor the fetus may undergo significant distress. One result of this distress is the passing of a bowel movement in the amniotic fluid, causing the normally clear fluid to turn greenish or brownish yellow. This coloring is called **meconium staining.** If the infant aspirates into its lungs any of the meconium-stained fluid, infection and aspiration pneumonia can result. Meconium staining is more common in breech births.

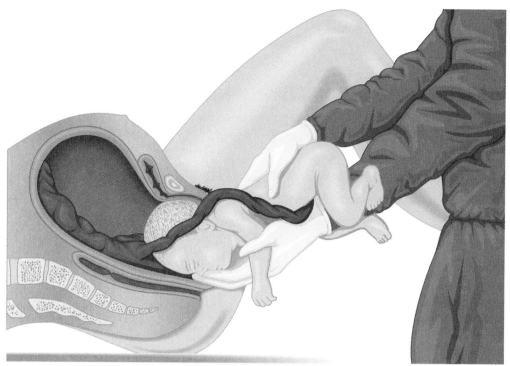

Figure 27-10   Breech delivery. Establish an airway during a prolonged delivery.

If you observe meconium staining of the amniotic fluid, suction the infant's mouth and nose as soon as the head emerges from the birth canal. *Do not stimulate the infant before you suction its mouth and nose.* The most critical aspect of treatment for meconium staining is to clear the mouth and nose before the infant takes its first breath. Transport the infant as soon as possible, maintaining the airway and supporting ventilation, if necessary, throughout transport.

Premature Birth An infant weighing less than $5\frac{1}{2}$ pounds, or an infant born before its 38th week of development is defined as a **premature infant** and requires special care. Because of their underdevelopment, premature babies are more susceptible to hypothermia and respiratory distress.

You can generally tell by appearance whether or not a infant is premature. A premature infant is thinner, smaller, and its skin will have a reddened and wrinkled appearance. There will be a single crease across the sole of the foot, there will be fuzzy scalp hair that is very fine, and the external ear cartilage will not be fully developed. A premature infant, because of its incomplete development, may require more vigorous resuscitation than a full-term infant.

Provide this additional care for a premature infant:

1. Be sure to dry the infant thoroughly and avoid heat loss. Keep the infant warm by using warmed blankets or a plastic bubble-bag swaddle, making sure that the head is covered.

2. Use gentle suction with a bulb syringe to keep the infant's nose and mouth clear of fluid.
3. Prevent bleeding from the umbilical cord. A premature infant cannot tolerate losing even the smallest amount of blood.
4. Administer supplemental oxygen by blowing oxygen across the infant's face, with the end of the oxygen tube approximately $\frac{1}{2}$ inch above the infant's mouth and nose. Never blow the oxygen directly into the face. Support ventilation if breathing is inadequate.
5. Premature babies are highly susceptible to infection. Prevent contamination and do not let anyone breathe into the infant's face.
6. Wrap the infant securely to keep it warm, and heat the vehicle during transport.

SUMMARY: ASSESSMENT AND CARE—ACTIVE LABOR AND DELIVERY

To review possible assessment findings and emergency care for an obstetric emergency associated with active labor and delivery, see Figures 27-11 and 27-12.

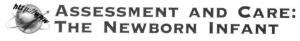 **ASSESSMENT AND CARE: THE NEWBORN INFANT**

Newborn infants can lose body heat quickly. Protecting them against heat loss preserves their energy and avoids the complex problem that hospitals face in try-

ASSESSMENT SUMMARY

OBSTETRIC EMERGENCY— ACTIVE LABOR AND DELIVERY

The following are findings that may be associated with an obstetric emergency occurring during active labor or delivery.

SCENE SIZE-UP

Pay particular attention to your own safety. Look for:
Mechanism of injury
Blood in toilet or around patient
Bleeding from vagina
Bloody tissue or blood clots
Fetus protruding from vagina
Mucus discharged, tinged with blood
Amniotic fluid
Meconium staining

INITIAL ASSESSMENT

General Impression

Does patient appear to be in full-term pregnancy?
Posture: lying still with knees to chest indicates severe abdominal pain, or supine
Any evidence of seizure activity?
Is umbilical cord or fetal body part other than the head present at vaginal opening?
Does patient appear to be having contractions that are intense, regular, frequent, and with a duration of about 60 seconds?

Mental Status

Alert

Airway

Open and usually not obstructed

Breathing

Increased due to pain

Circulation

Heart rate may be increased

Status: Priority patient if associated with shock, significant vaginal bleeding, or abnormal presenting part, or if greater than 10 minutes is spent attempting to perform delivery

FOCUSED HISTORY AND PHYSICAL EXAM

SAMPLE History

Signs and symptoms:
Abdominal pain due to contractions

True labor contractions:	Regular Occur at about 2-3 minute intervals Last about 30-90 seconds Are intense
False labor (Braxton-Hicks) contractions:	Irregular Interval time varies Duration varies Intensity varies May be relieved by walking

Vaginal discharge of amniotic fluid, clear with yellowish tint
Crowning
History:
Onset, provocation/palliation, quality, radiation, severity, and duration of pain
When was your last menstrual period?
Have you had any unusual vaginal discharge or bleeding?
When is your due date?
Have you had previous problems with pregnancies?
Have you been seeing a physician for this pregnancy?
Is this your first delivery?
Do you feel as if you are having a bowel movement?

Physical Exam

Abdomen/Genitalia:
Obvious protruded abdomen
Evidence of crowning or abnormal presenting part?
Any passed tissue from the vagina?
Vaginal bleeding, dark or bright red, may or may not be associated with pain
Amniotic fluid present
Meconium staining to amniotic fluid

Baseline Vital Signs

BP: may be normal or increased
HR: may be normal or increased
RR: may be normal or increased
Skin: normal
Pupils: normal size, equal, and reactive to light

Figure 27-11a *Assessment summary: obstetric emergency—active labor and delivery.*

✳ EMERGENCY CARE PROTOCOL

OBSTETRIC EMERGENCY—
ACTIVE LABOR AND DELIVERY

1. Place patient supine with knees drawn up and check for crowning.
2. If crowning is occurring, contractions are 2 minutes apart, intense, and lasting 30 to 90 seconds, and mother has urge to push, prepare to deliver.
3. Check for crowning or abnormal presenting part. If an abnormal presenting part is found, such as a prolapsed cord, hand, or foot, perform the following:
   a. Position patient in knee-chest position or elevate buttocks using pillows
   b. If umbilical cord is prolapsed, insert gloved hand into vagina and push presenting part of fetus away from cord.
   c. Cover presenting part with a sterile moist dressing.
   d. Rapidly transport patient and notify receiving facility of patient's condition.
   If the fetal head is crowning, proceed with delivery as described in steps 4 to 13.

4. Prepare OB kit and create sterile field around vaginal opening.
5. If amniotic sac is still intact, rupture it with your fingers and tear it away from infant's face.
6. As head and neck are delivered, inspect to determine if the umbilical cord is wrapped around the infant's neck. If it is, do the following:
   a. Slip cord over infant's head.
   b. If cord cannot be slipped over head, immediately clamp cord in two places and cut between clamps.
7. Suction mouth and nose as head is delivered.
8. Continue with delivery until entire body is expelled.
9. Keep infant level with mother. See "Emergency Care Protocol: Newborn Infant."
10. Place an umbilical clamp or tie about 6 inches from newborn's abdomen and a second one about 3 inches from the first. Cut the cord.
11. Deliver placenta. If greater than 10 minutes is spent waiting for placental delivery, transport.
12. Apply a sanitary napkin over vaginal opening.
13. Perform an ongoing assessment every 5 minutes if unstable, every 15 minutes if stable.

Figure 27-11b   Emergency care protocol: obstetric emergency—active labor and delivery.

ing to rewarm a cold infant. So immediately dry the infant. Be sure to dry the head well, and cover it. Then wrap the newborn in a blanket or a plastic bubble-bag swaddle. Repeat suctioning to make sure the infant's mouth and nostrils are clear.

ASSESSMENT

Perform a thorough assessment of the infant. You can use the Apgar scoring system to get a good overall indication of the baby's condition. The score should be determined at 60 seconds after birth, and then repeated in 4 minutes to obtain a 1 minute and a 5 minute score following birth. A change in the Apgar score may indicate improvement (higher score), worsening (lower score), or no change. To assess the newborn using the Apgar scoring system, you can use the letters in Apgar as a mnemonic to help you remember the parts of the assessment, as follows:

* *Appearance.*
  - If the skin of the newborn's entire body is blue (cyanotic) or pale, award 0 points.
  - If the newborn has blue hands and feet with pink skin at the core of the body (a condition called acrocyanosis), award 1 point.
  - If the skin of the extremities as well as the trunk is pink, award 2 points.
* *Pulse.* Heart rate is one of the most important signs of whether oxygen is reaching the newborn's tissues following birth. Count the heart rate for at least 30 seconds, preferably with a stethoscope. If you do not have a stethoscope, feel the pulse of the umbilical cord where it joins the abdomen or at the brachial artery.
  - If no pulse is present, award 0 points.
  - If the heart rate is under 100 (also a serious finding), award 1 point.
  - If the heart rate is over 100, award 2 points.
* *Grimace* (reflex irritability). Gently flick the soles of the newborn's feet, or observe the facial expressions during suctioning.
  - If the newborn displays no reflexive activity to your stimulation, award 0 points.
  - If the newborn displays only some facial grimace, award 1 point.
  - If your stimulation causes the newborn to grimace and cough, sneeze, or cry, award 2 points.
* *Activity.* This score refers to extremity reflexes/movement, or the degree of flexion of the arms and legs and the resistance to straightening them.

EMERGENCY CARE ALGORITHM:
OBSTETRIC EMERGENCY—ACTIVE LABOR AND DELIVERY

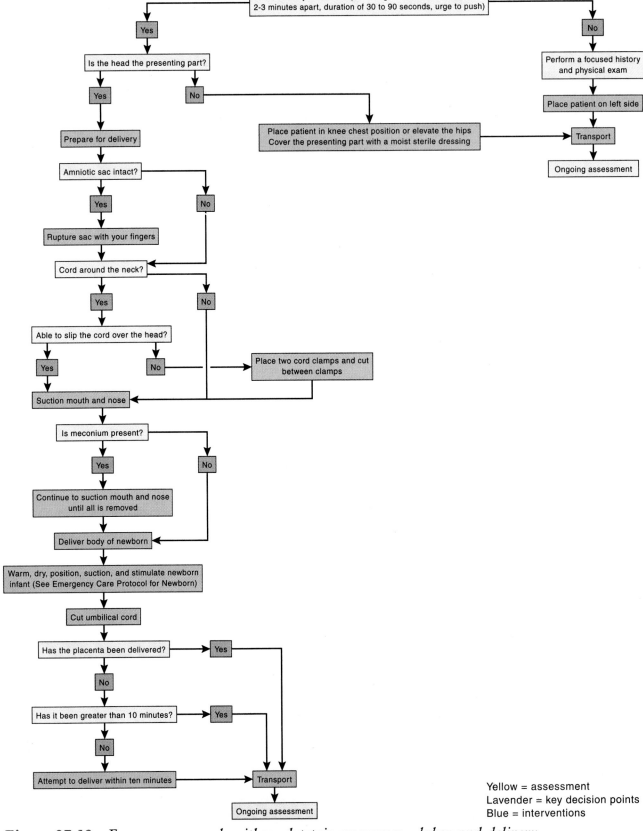

Figure 27-12   Emergency care algorithm: obstetric emergency—labor and delivery.

The normal newborn's elbows, knees, and hips are flexed, and you should encounter some degree of resistance when you try to extend them.

- If during your assessment, the newborn is limp and displays no extremity movement, award 0 points.
- If the newborn only displays some flexion without active movement, award 1 point.
- If the newborn is actively moving around, award 2 points.

• *Respiration.* Another important assessment sign is the newborn's breathing effort. The newborn should have regular respirations and a vigorous cry. Distress is indicated by irregular, shallow, gasping, or absent respirations.

- If the newborn displays no respiratory effort, award 0 points.
- If the newborn displays only a slow or irregular breathing effort with a weak cry, award 1 point.
- If the newborn displays good respirations and a strong cry, award 2 points.

At the conclusion of the assessment, you should have a numeric value that ranges from 0 to 10. Use the following guidelines to determine the significance of your finding:

• *7-10 points*—The newborn should be active and vigorous. Provide routine care.
• *4-6 points*—The newborn is moderately depressed. Provide stimulation and oxygen.
• *0-3 points*—The newborn is severely depressed. You will probably need to provide extensive care including oxygen with bag-valve-mask ventilations and CPR, as described on the next page.

Be sure to stimulate the newborn if it is still not breathing adequately. You can stimulate respirations by gently flicking the soles of the feet or by rubbing the back in a circular motion with three fingers (Fig-

ure 27-13). En route to the hospital, provide continual assessment for the newborn. Pay particular attention to body temperature, airway, breathing status, heart rate, color, and activity level. Contact medical direction to update them on the mother's and newborn's condition.

Signs and Symptoms Most newborns require no resuscitation beyond temperature maintenance, mild stimulation, and suctioning. Of those who do require additional resuscitation, most need oxygen or bag-valve-mask ventilations. A minority of the newborns will be so depressed that they also will need chest compressions or resuscitative medications.

Certain physical abnormalities, medical complications, or even distressed deliveries can lead to a severely depressed newborn in need of immediate and aggressive treatment. The signs of a severely depressed newborn are:

- Respiratory rate over 60 per minute
- Diminished breath sounds
- Heart rate over 180 per minute or under 100 per minute
- Obvious signs of trauma from the delivery process
- Poor or absent skeletal muscle tone
- Respiratory arrest, or severe distress
- Heavy meconium staining of amniotic fluid
- Weak pulses
- Cyanotic body (core and extremities)
- Poor peripheral perfusion
- Lack of or poor response to stimulation
- Apgar score under 4

EMERGENCY MEDICAL CARE

If one or more of the signs listed above are noted during your assessment following birth, you should gather the necessary equipment for neonatal resuscitation. It is important to remember that newborns

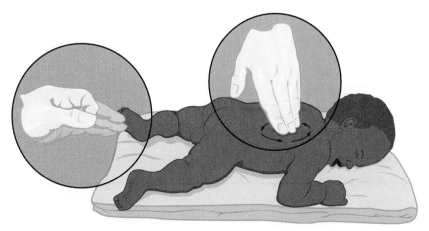

Figure 27-13   Stimulate the infant who is not breathing by flicking the soles of the feet or by rubbing the back.

cannot tolerate even brief periods of inadequate oxygenation without serious effects. *The establishment and maintenance of an adequate airway and breathing status is "cornerstone" treatment for any newborn infant.*

Keep in mind that most newborns do not require aggressive treatment. Approximately 80 percent require no resuscitation beyond keeping them warm and suctioning the airway. If their responses are slightly depressed, most will respond to oxygen blown by the face or to bag-valve-mask ventilations with supplemental oxygen. A small number may require chest compressions, and an even smaller number may require the medications or intubation that an advanced life support team can provide. The relative frequency of need for resuscitative measures is often shown as an inverted pyramid with the simple care most newborns require at the top (Figure 27-14).

Based on the signs and symptoms, you should provide the following treatment:

1. If the infant has bluish discoloration (cyanosis) of the skin, but has spontaneous breathing and an adequate heart rate (greater than 100 per minute), you should provide free-flow oxygen. Hold the tube $\frac{1}{2}$ inch from the nose and mouth and direct the oxygen flow across the mouth and nose (sometimes called the "blow-by" method—Figure 27-15). Remember to make sure the infant is kept warm.
2. Provide ventilations by bag-valve-mask with supplemental oxygen at the rate of 40-60 per minute (Figure 27-16a) if the newborn displays any of the following:

- The infant's breathing is shallow, slow, gasping, or absent following brief stimulation.
- The infant's heart rate is less than 100 beats per minute.
- The infant's core body remains cyanotic (blue) despite provision of blow-by oxygen.

Be sure to maintain a tight face mask seal, and provide the ventilations with just enough force to raise the infant's chest. Reassess after 30 seconds of ventilation. If the breathing and/or heart rate has not improved, continue ventilations and reassess every 30 seconds. If ventilation is required for more than 2 minutes and the infant's stomach becomes distended and impedes ventilation, it may be necessary to insert a gastric tube to relieve the distention. In some jurisdictions, this may be a procedure that EMT-Bs are trained to do (see Chapter 44, "Advanced Airway Management"); in other jurisdictions, this must be done only by ALS personnel.

3. If, despite adequate ventilations, the infant's heart rate drops to less than 60 beats per minute, or the heartbeat is between 60 and 80 beats per minute and is not rapidly increasing, continue ventilations and begin chest compressions.

Circle the torso with the fingers and place both thumbs on the lower third of the infant's sternum. If the infant is very small, you may need to overlap the thumbs. If the infant is very large, compress the sternum with the ring and middle fingers one finger's depth below the nipple line. Compress the chest $\frac{1}{2}$ to $\frac{3}{4}$ inch at 120 compressions per minute (Figure 27-16b).

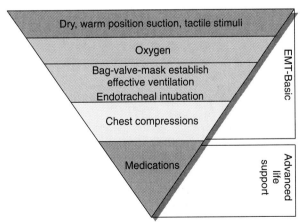

Figure 27-14 *The inverted pyramid for neonatal resuscitation shows that the majority of newborns will respond to simple routines of care; only a few will require aggressive resuscitation.*

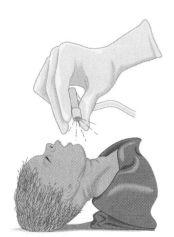

Figure 27-15 *Administration of oxygen to a newborn by placing the tube so that the oxygen blows by the infant's face.*

NEONATAL RESUSCITATION

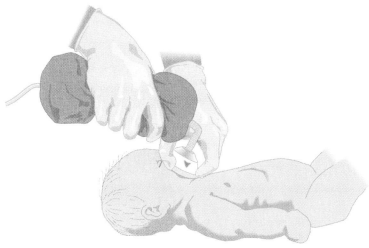

Figure 27-16a *To provide positive pressure ventilation, use a bag-valve mask. Maintain a good mask seal. Ventilate with just enough force to raise the infant's chest. Ventilate at a rate of 60 per minute for 30 seconds. Then reassess.*

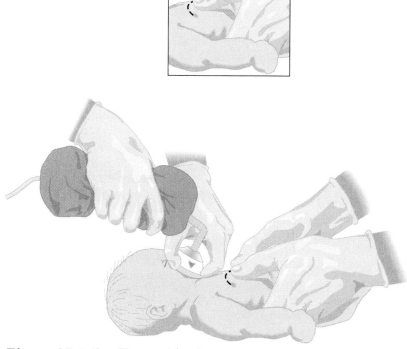

Figure 27-16b *To provide chest compressions, circle the torso with the fingers and place both thumbs on the lower third of the infant's sternum. If the infant is very small, you may need to overlap the thumbs. If the infant is very large, compress the sternum with the ring and middle fingers placed one finger's depth below the nipple line. Compress the chest $\frac{1}{2}$ to $\frac{3}{4}$ inch at the rate of 120 per minute.*

SUMMARY: CARE OF THE NEWBORN INFANT

To review emergency care for the newborn infant, see Figures 27-17 and 27-18.

GYNECOLOGICAL EMERGENCIES

ASSESSMENT AND CARE: GYNECOLOGICAL EMERGENCY

Your approach to the patient suffering a **gynecological** emergency (an emergency having to do with the female reproductive system) should progress as it would for any other patient.

SCENE SIZE-UP AND INITIAL ASSESSMENT

Complete a scene size-up, noting any mechanism of injury that may have caused abdominal or pelvic trauma. If this is the scene of a crime, such as sexual assault, do not approach the patient until the police assure you that the scene is secure.

After taking all appropriate BSI precautions, perform an initial assessment, evaluating mental status and assuring an open airway and adequate breathing and circulation. Consider having a female EMT-B assess the female sexual-assault victim when available.

FOCUSED HISTORY AND PHYSICAL EXAM

Get a SAMPLE history, using the OPQRST mnemonic and taking care to maintain a nonjudgmental attitude. In cases of sexual assault, your priority is to treat any injuries to the patient. Discreetly question the patient about any potential injuries, whether to the genitalia or other injuries.

As you perform a rapid trauma assessment, do your best to protect the patient's privacy by providing a cover such as a blanket or sheet. Note: *Do not examine the genitalia of a sexual assault victim unless there is profuse or life-threatening bleeding.* Try to estimate the volume of blood lost based on your findings of soiled clothes, patient history, and potential for developing signs and symptoms of shock (hypoperfusion). Obtain a set of baseline vital signs.

To help preserve evidence, discourage the sexual assault victim from taking a bath, douching, urinating, washing her hands, or cleaning wounds. Handle the patient's clothing as little as possible. Bag all items of clothing and other items separately. *Follow local protocol for crime scene protection.*

EMERGENCY CARE PROTOCOL

NEWBORN INFANT

1. If meconium is present, aggressively suction airway until clear.
2. Dry newborn with towels.
3. Wrap newborn in warm towels or blankets. Be sure to cover head and prevent hypothermia.
4. Position newborn on back, or in lateral recumbent position if large amount of secretions.
5. Stimulate newborn by rubbing its back or flicking soles of feet if breathing or activity is inadequate.
6. Perform an APGAR score 1 minute after birth.
7. If breathing is inadequate, perform positive pressure ventilation (PPV) with supplemental oxygen for 30 seconds to 1 minute. Then reassess. Continue PPV as necessary.
8. Assess pulse.
   - *If heart rate is greater than 100/minute,* assess color (see step 9).
   - *If heart rate is less than 100/minute but greater than 60/minute,* begin PPV with oxygen for 30 seconds to 1 minute. Then reassess heart rate.

If heart rate remains less than 100/minute, continue PPV with oxygen until rate exceeds 100/minute.
   - *If heart rate drops to less than 80/minute but greater than 60/minute,* perform aggressive ventilation. If heart rate does not increase above 80/minute, begin chest compressions at a rate of 120/minute.
   - *If at any time heart rate drops below 60/minute,* begin chest compressions and continue PPV.
9. Assess color. If body is cyanotic but breathing is adequate and heart rate is greater than 100/minute, administer blow-by oxygen until color improves. If heart rate is less than 100/minute, return to step 8.
10. Continue to reassess airway, suctioning secretions, and reassess breathing, heart rate, and skin color. Ensure infant is dry, wrapped, and warm.
11. Perform another APGAR score 5 minutes after birth
12. Transport.

Figure 27-17 Emergency care protocol: newborn infant.

EMERGENCY CARE ALGORITHM: NEWBORN CARE AND RESUSCITATION

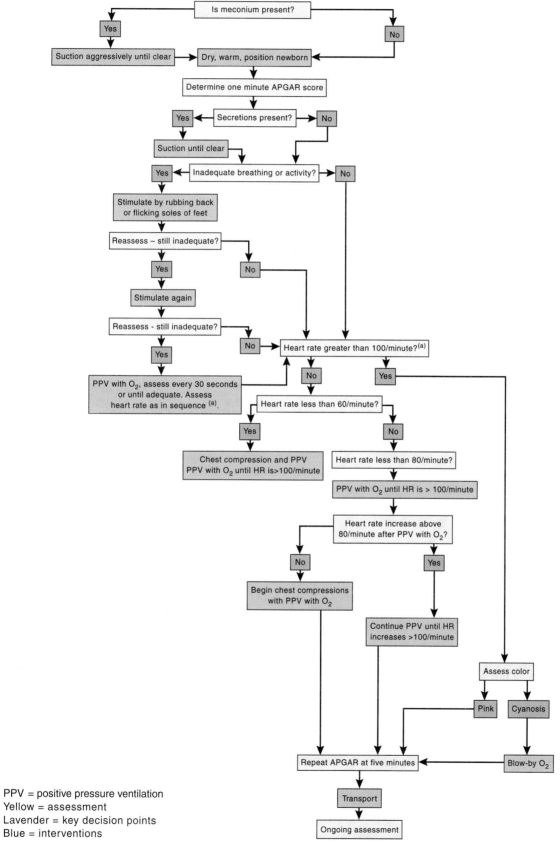

PPV = positive pressure ventilation
Yellow = assessment
Lavender = key decision points
Blue = interventions

Figure 27-18   Emergency care algorithm: newborn care and resuscitation.

Signs and Symptoms Injuries to the internal female genitalia are not common, because they are small and well protected, except during pregnancy when the uterus is enlarged. Injuries to the external female genitalia may result from straddle injuries or sexual assault, but they too are relatively uncommon.

Because the genital area is richly supplied with blood vessels and nerves, injuries can cause severe pain and considerable bleeding. The most common gynecological findings in the field are abdominal pain, vaginal bleeding, and soft tissue injuries. If blood loss is significant, the patient also may display the characteristic signs and symptoms of shock (hypoperfusion).

EMERGENCY MEDICAL CARE

Most injuries to the external female genitalia are soft tissue injuries and should be managed as such. Remember to take all appropriate BSI precautions, and follow these guidelines:

1. *Ensure an adequate airway, breathing, and circulation.* Administer high-flow oxygen and treat for shock (hypoperfusion), if indicated.
2. *Care for bleeding from the vagina.* If there is vaginal bleeding, place a sanitary napkin over the vaginal opening. *Never pack the vagina in an attempt to control bleeding.* If the pad becomes soaked with blood, replace it.
3. *Provide emergency medical care as you would for any patient based on any other signs and symptoms.*
4. *Transport.*

DETAILED PHYSICAL EXAM AND ONGOING ASSESSMENT

If time and the patient's condition permits, perform a detailed physical exam en route to the hospital to ensure that no injuries have been overlooked. Perform an ongoing assessment every 15 minutes if the patient is stable, every 5 minutes if the patient is unstable. Repeat the initial assessment and the focused history and physical exam. Repeat vital signs. Check any interventions, being especially careful about oxygen mask fit and adequate flow of oxygen. Be attentive for and treat for any signs of developing shock (hypoperfusion).

Patients who have been injured in a sexual assault also require emotional care and reassurance. Follow local protocol regarding the requirements for reporting sexual assaults.

ENRICHMENT

The enrichment section contains information that is valuable as background for the EMT-B but that goes substantially beyond the U.S. Department of Transportation (DOT) EMT-Basic curriculum.

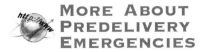

MORE ABOUT PREDELIVERY EMERGENCIES

PLACENTA PREVIA

When the fetus changes position or when the cervix begins to dilate, an abnormally low placenta—especially one that covers the uterine outlet—can either tear or separate from the uterus, resulting in hemorrhaging that is painless because the placenta has no nerve endings. This is a condition known as *placenta previa* (Figure 27-19). History and assessment findings consistent with placenta previa include:

- History of having borne more than two children
- History of early vaginal bleeding or spotting
- History of a previous cesarean section
- History of recent sexual intercourse
- Bright red vaginal bleeding during the third trimester
- A soft uterus without tenderness upon palpation
- Present fetal heart tones and movement

For treatment follow the general guidelines for emergency medical care of a predelivery emergency. Administer oxygen at 15 lpm by nonrebreather mask and provide immediate transport.

ABRUPTIO PLACENTA

In the condition known as *abruptio placenta* (Figure 27-20), the placenta separates from the uterine wall prematurely during the last trimester. Bleeding may be confined to the area behind the placenta, usually causing severe abdominal pain but little or no external vaginal bleeding. Pain is caused because sensory fibers in the uterus detect the placenta pulling away (abruption). Other history and assessment findings suggestive of abruptio placenta include:

PLACENTA PREVIA

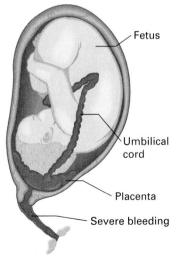

Figure 27-19 Placenta previa.

ABRUPTIO PLACENTA

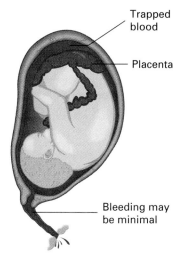

Trapped blood

Placenta

Bleeding may be minimal

Figure 27-20   Abruptio placenta.

- History of hypertension
- History of having borne more than two children
- History of previous abruption, or placenta previa
- History of recent strenuous exercise
- Abdominal trauma
- Sharp abdominal pain, usually severe in nature
- Possible dark red vaginal bleeding
- Observable blood loss typically out of proportion for the degree of shock (hypoperfusion)
- Possible uterine contractions
- Abdomen and uterus that are very tender to palpation; the abdomen may feel rigid and the uterus may feel very firm
- Fetal heart tones absent

For treatment follow the general guidelines for emergency medical care of a predelivery emergency. Administer oxygen at 15 lpm by nonrebreather mask and provide immediate transport.

TOXEMIA

A common condition affecting about one in twenty pregnant women is *toxemia,* or "poisoning" of the blood during pregnancy. Toxemia occurs most frequently in the last trimester and is most likely to affect women in their 20s who are pregnant for the first time. Women with a history of diabetes, heart disease, kidney problems, or high blood pressure are at the greatest risk, as are those whose mothers or sisters have had toxemia during pregnancy.

Toxemia is characterized by high blood pressure and swelling in the extremities. History and assessment findings also include:

- History of hypertension, diabetes, kidney (renal) disease, liver (hepatic) disease, or heart disease

- No previous pregnancies
- History of poor nutrition
- Sudden weight gain (2 pounds a week or more)
- Altered mental status
- Abdominal pain
- Blurred vision or spots before the eyes
- Excessive swelling of the face, fingers, legs, or feet
- Decreased urine output
- Severe, persistent headache
- Persistent vomiting
- Elevated blood pressure, usually greater than 140/90 mmHg (or a systolic increase of over 30 mmHg and/or a diastolic increase of over 15 mmHg of prepregnancy pressure)

The first stage of toxemia (*preeclampsia*) is characterized by high blood pressure, swelling, headaches, and visual disturbances. In the second stage of toxemia (*eclampsia*) life-threatening seizures occur. During a seizure, the placenta can separate from the uterine wall (abruption), causing death of the fetus and severe maternal hemorrhage. Death of the mother can also result from cerebral hemorrhage, respiratory arrest, kidney failure, or circulatory collapse. For treatment, follow the general guidelines for emergency medical care of a predelivery emergency. Be sure to administer oxygen at 15 lpm by nonrebreather mask, and keep suction close at hand. If a seizure begins, you may need to provide positive pressure ventilation during the seizure to prevent oxygen deprivation. Since lights, noise, and movement can set off seizures in patients with toxemia, transport the patient in as calm and quiet a manner as possible.

RUPTURED UTERUS

As the uterus enlarges during pregnancy, the uterine wall becomes extremely thin, especially around the cervix. This can lead to a spontaneous or traumatic rupture of the uterine wall, thereby releasing the fetus into the abdominal cavity (Figure 27-21). Mortality to the mother from a ruptured uterus is usually 5 to 20 percent; infant mortality is over 50 percent. A ruptured uterus requires immediate surgery.

The following history and assessment findings should alert you to this emergency:

- History of previous uterine rupture
- History or findings of abdominal trauma
- History of a large fetus
- History of having borne more than two children
- History of prolonged and difficult labor (which may force a large infant out through the uterine wall)
- History of prior Caesarean section or uterine surgery
- A tearing or shearing sensation in the abdomen
- Constant and severe abdominal pain
- Nausea

RUPTURED UTERUS

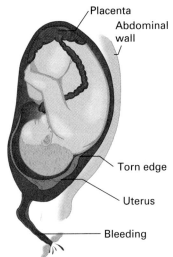

Figure 27-21   Ruptured uterus.

- Signs and symptoms of shock (hypoperfusion)
- Vaginal bleeding (typically minor bleeding, but could be heavy)
- Cessation of noticeable uterine contractions
- Ability to palpate the infant in the abdominal cavity

For treatment follow the general guidelines for emergency medical care of a predelivery emergency. Administer oxygen at 15 lpm by nonrebreather mask and provide immediate transport.

ECTOPIC PREGNANCY

In a normal pregnancy the ovum, or egg, is implanted in the uterus. In an ectopic pregnancy, the egg is implanted outside the uterus in one of the following locations: in a fallopian tube, on the abdominal peritoneal covering, on the outside wall of the uterus, on an ovary, or on the cervix. The placenta eventually invades surrounding tissue and, unable to accommodate the growing embryo, ultimately ruptures. Ectopic pregnancy is the leading cause of maternal death in the first trimester, and occurs in one of every two hundred pregnancies.

The following history and assessment findings should alert you to an ectopic pregnancy:

- History of previous ectopic pregnancies
- History of *pelvic inflammatory disease (PID)*
- History of missed menstrual cycles
- History of tubal surgery, including elective tubal ligation
- Sudden, sharp, or "knife-like" abdominal pain, localized on one side
- Vaginal spotting (light bleeding)
- Lower abdominal pain, possibly radiating to one or both shoulders
- Tender, bloated abdomen
- A palpable mass in the abdomen (either the embryo or a blood clot)
- Weakness or dizziness when sitting or standing
- Decreased blood pressure
- Increased pulse rate
- Signs of shock (hypoperfusion)
- Bluish discoloration around the navel, if the rupture occurred hours earlier
- Urge to defecate

For treatment follow the general guidelines for emergency medical care of a predelivery emergency. Be sure to treat the patient for shock (hypoperfusion), administer oxygen at 15 lpm by nonrebreather mask, constantly reassess vital signs, and provide immediate transport.

CASE STUDY FOLLOW-UP

SCENE SIZE-UP

You have been dispatched to the scene of a 30-year-old female experiencing active labor. She and her husband tell you that she was having contractions earlier that day, but they were short and slightly irregular, so she figured she would have time to get her laundry done before going to the hospital. Meantime, your partner has enlisted the help of some bystanders to bring in the stretcher and additional equipment from the ambulance.

INITIAL ASSESSMENT

Your general impression is that the patient, Ruth Baker, is experiencing uterine contractions and is in active labor. From the appearance of her slacks, it looks as if her water has already broken. You start to ask her questions, but every time she tries to answer you, her husband, Randy, cuts her off and finishes answering. Seeing this, your partner takes him aside and begins to question him about events prior to the emergency. This allows you to direct your attention to the patient.

You determine that she is alert and oriented with a patent airway and adequate breathing. Her pulse strong and regular, and her skin is warm and slightly sweaty. There is no evidence of bleeding so far. At this time you apply oxygen to the patient at 15 lpm by nonrebreather mask.

FOCUSED HISTORY AND PHYSICAL EXAM

During your focused history, you learn that this is Mrs. Baker's third child and the other pregnancies progressed without any complications. You also ask her about her due date, and she tells you "Not for two more weeks." The police have arrived and, at your request, they disperse the crowd so that you can continue the assessment with some privacy. Currently, contractions are occurring every 2 minutes, with a 50-second duration.

The patient cries out, "I think the baby is coming." You rapidly perform a visual inspection of the perineum and identify crowning, with the head bulging out further with each contraction. You also notice that the amniotic fluid appears to be clear.

At this point you advise the patient that delivery will take place here, and you ask her not to bear down until you have positioned her properly. Your partner notifies dispatch to send another unit for back-up.

You move Mrs. Baker to a supine position on the floor with her hips raised off the ground with some folded sheets. You then position Mr. Baker behind his wife so that he can support her during the delivery. Once she is positioned, and your equipment is ready, you encourage her to start pushing with the next contraction.

You continually support the infant during delivery, and verbally support Mrs. Baker to help her relax as best she can. As soon as the infant's head is born, you are very thorough in your suctioning of the newborn's mouth and nose. After full delivery of the infant, you clamp and cut the cord as appropriate while your partner begins to dry the infant. You dry the baby and wrap it in towels your partner has warmed in one of the laundromat dryers.

Your initial Apgar score of the newborn boy is 7, and after brief stimulation, the respiratory rate increases to 46 per minute with an adequate depth. The infant is starting to cry and is becoming more vigorous in muscular activity. Since there is some

cyanosis to the core and extremities, you provide blow-by oxygen.

ONGOING ASSESSMENT

You place both the mother and the child in the back of your ambulance. The father sits up front. Your partner has turned up the heat to be sure your two patients are warm enough. You ask Joe Garwood, an EMT-B from the back-up unit, to accompany you to the hospital to care for the mother while you focus your attention on the newborn. En route, the mother continues to have some minor vaginal bleeding and then delivers the placenta, which Joe places in a container for the emergency department staff. He then goes on to perform a uterine massage and bleeding soon stops.

The mother, although tired from the birthing process, is in good spirits and has no unusual complaint or distress. Her mental status is normal, vitals are stable, and she spends the rest of the trip thinking about the possible names for a boy that she and her husband have been discussing.

You repeat the Apgar score a second time and the newborn scores a 10. The baby has "pinked up" so that his color is now normal at the core and the extremities. His respirations are adequate at a rate of 48 per minute, and the heart rate is 146 and regular. The infant is actively moving around and has a good strong cry. You notify the hospital of the condition of the mother and newborn and arrive 10 minutes later.

After transferring care to the emergency department staff, you complete your prehospital care report and head back to the ambulance to get it ready for the next call. On your way out of the hospital, you stop to congratulate the new father and learn from him that the newborn will be named Jacob Allen Baker.

CHAPTER REVIEW

TERMS AND CONCEPTS

You may wish to review the following terms and concepts included in this chapter.

afterbirth—the placenta and other tissues that are expelled immediately after the birth of a child.

amniotic sac—a thin transparent membrane that forms the sac which holds the fetus suspended in amniotic fluid. Also called bag of waters.

bloody show—the mucus and blood that are expelled from the vagina as labor begins.

breech birth—a common abnormality of delivery in

which the fetal buttocks or lower extremities are low in the uterus and are the first to be delivered.

cervix—the neck of the uterus.

crowning—the stage in delivery when the fetal head presents at the vagina.

fetus—the child in the uterus from the third month of pregnancy to birth; prior to that time it is called an embryo.

gynecological—having to do with the female reproductive system.

labor—the physiological process by which the fetus is

expelled from the uterus into the vagina and then to the outside of the body. Also called childbirth.

limb presentation—when an arm or leg is the first fetal part to protrude from the vaginal opening.

meconium staining—a greenish or brownish yellow staining of the amniotic fluid, caused by a fetal bowel movement resulting from distress.

miscarriage—see spontaneous abortion.

neonate—a newborn infant up to 30 days of age.

obstetric—having to do with pregnancy or child-birth.

perineum—the area of skin between a female's vagina and anus.

placenta—the fetal organ through which the fetus exchanges nourishment and waste products during pregnancy.

premature infant—an infant weighing less than 5 pounds, or an infant born before its 38th week of gestation.

prolapsed cord—when the umbilical cord, rather than the head of the fetus, is the first part to protrude from the vagina.

spontaneous abortion—without apparent cause, the termination of a pregnancy before the fetus reaches the stage of viability, generally before the 20th week of pregnancy. Also called miscarriage.

supine hypotensive syndrome—inadequate return of venous blood to the heart, reduced cardiac output, and lowered blood pressure resulting from pressure on the inferior vena cava, caused by the weight of the uterus and fetus when the patient in late pregnancy is in a supine position.

umbilical cord—an extension of the placenta through which the fetus receives nourishment while in the uterus.

uterus—an organ of the female reproductive system for containing and nourishing the embryo and fetus from the time the fertilized egg is implanted to the time of birth.

vagina—the passageway through which the fetus is delivered. The lower part of the birth canal.

REVIEW QUESTIONS

1. List the signs and symptoms that would indicate a predelivery emergency, and describe the general guidelines for emergency medical care.
2. Describe signs that would indicate an imminent delivery.
3. Describe how to properly position a mother in active labor and how to create a sterile field around the vaginal opening.
4. Describe the emergency medical care for a patient in active labor for a normal delivery.
5. Describe how you would recognize an abnormal delivery.
6. Describe the specific steps you would take to provide emergency medical care for (a) a pro-lapsed cord, (b) a breech birth or limb presentation, (c) a multiple birth, (d) meconium staining, and (e) a premature birth.
7. Describe the initial care that is required for the majority (80 percent) of newborns that do not require aggressive resuscitation.
8. Describe the indications and procedures for neonatal resuscitation.
9. List the most commons signs and symptoms of a gynecological emergency.
10. Describe the general guidelines for emergency medical care of a gynecological emergency, including special consideration of the sexual assault victim.

CHAPTER 28

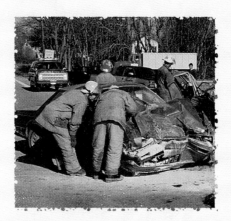

Mechanisms of Injury: Kinetics of Trauma

 ## INTRODUCTION

Since the early 1970s, trauma (injury) has been recognized as the leading cause of death for those between the ages of 14 and 40 and is the third leading cause of death for all age groups, after cardiovascular disease and cancer. Trauma makes up a significant percent of the calls to which prehospital personnel respond.

With any trauma patient, determining the possible extent of injury is critical to making good priority decisions regarding on-scene assessment and care vs. rapid transport with assessment and care continuing en route. To make these judgments, the EMT-Basic must not only recognize obvious injuries but also must maintain a high index of suspicion for hidden injuries. An understanding of mechanisms of injury is the chief component of this crucial assessment skill.

OBJECTIVES

Numbered objectives are from the United States Department of Transportation 1994 EMT-Basic National Standard Curriculum. Asterisked objectives, if any, pertain to material that is supplemental to the DOT curriculum.

COGNITIVE

3-1.4 Discuss common mechanisms of injury/nature of illness. (pp. 533–544)
* Explain how the following affect the force of impact: mass and velocity, acceleration and deceleration, energy changing form and direction. (pp. 530–532)

* Describe the three main impacts that occur in a vehicle collision. (pp. 532–533)
* Discuss the following mechanisms of injury and their effects on the human body: motor vehicle collisions, vehicle-pedestrian collisions, motorcycle collisions, falls, penetrating injuries, and blast injuries. (pp. 533–544)
* Discuss the steps of patient assessment, including the priority decision, as they relate to and are guided by the mechanism of injury. (pp. 544–546)

Objective 3-1.4 and additional objectives from DOT Lesson 3-1 are addressed in Chapter 8, "Scene Size-up."

CASE STUDY

THE DISPATCH

EMS Unit 632—proceed to 49 Elm Street—police are on the scene of a minor motor vehicle collision with a driver complaining of pain in his knees. Time out is 1307 hours.

ON ARRIVAL

The police officer greets you and explains that he was taking a report of a minor rear-end collision when the driver of the car that was struck from behind began

to complain of knee pain. As you approach the vehicle you notice that the driver is responsive and there are no cracks in the windshield of his car. Apparently the patient was waiting to make a left turn and another vehicle struck him from behind.

How would you assess and care for this patient?

During this chapter, you will learn special considerations in sizing up the mechanism of injury. Later, we will return to the case and apply what you have learned.

Mechanism of injury refers to how a person was injured. The mechanism may be a motor vehicle collision, a fall, a gunshot, or other. The science of analyzing mechanisms of injury, sometimes called the **kinetics of trauma,** helps you to predict the kind and extent of injuries as a basis for your priority decisions regarding continuing assessment, care, and transport (Figure 28-1).

THE KINETICS OF TRAUMA

Trauma is nearly always the result of two or more bodies colliding with each other. (Except for blast injuries caused by pressure waves, it is difficult to think of an injury that does not involve a collision of bodies—a passenger's head with a windshield, a knife

with someone's chest, and so on.) *Kinetics,* according to the dictionary, is "the branch of mechanics dealing with the motions of material bodies." So understanding kinetics is helpful in understanding mechanisms of injury and trauma.

How severely a person is injured depends on the force with which he collides with something—or something collides with him. This force depends partly on the energy contained in the moving body or bodies. The energy contained in a moving body is called **kinetic energy.**

MASS AND VELOCITY

The amount of kinetic energy a moving body contains depends on two factors: the body's *mass* (weight) and the body's *velocity* (speed). Kinetic energy in a moving body is calculated this way: the mass

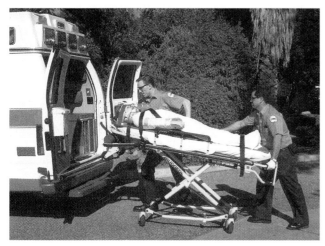

Figure 28-1   Is the patient a priority for transport? Analysis of the mechanism of injury may be a crucial element in the decision.

(weight in pounds), times the velocity (speed in feet per second) squared, divided by two. The formula can be written like this:

$$Kinetic\ energy = \frac{mass\ x\ velocity^2}{2}$$

This formula illustrates that as the mass of a moving object is doubled, its kinetic energy is also doubled. You would be injured twice as badly if you were hit by a 2-pound rock as if you were hit by a 1-pound rock thrown at the same speed.

However velocity is a much more significant factor than mass. Suppose you were hit by a rock thrown at a velocity of 1 foot per second, then hit by the same rock thrown again at 2 feet per second. The rock thrown at 2 feet per second would be not twice as harmful as at 1 foot per second, but four times as harmful—because the factor of velocity is squared.

Understanding the factor of velocity is important in evaluating mechanism of injury in vehicle collisions. During your scene size-up, as you try to get an idea of how seriously vehicle passengers may have been injured, it is important to get the best estimate you can of the speed the vehicle or vehicles were going at the time of collision, knowing that a high velocity collision will almost certainly have caused greater injury. (Also remember that the kinetic energy of two moving bodies that collide will be combined: Two vehicles that collide head on while each is moving at 30 mph will impact with the same force as one vehicle moving at 60 mph colliding with a tree.)

Understanding velocity also helps in understanding gunshot wounds and knife wounds. The great damage bullets do results not from their mass (a bullet doesn't weigh very much) but from their velocity. A bullet wound is potentially more traumatic than a knife wound (depending also on which organs and structures are struck). Even if the bullet is smaller and lighter than the knife blade, a bullet exploding from the barrel of a gun impacts the body at a relatively higher velocity than a knife blade propelled by a human hand.

ACCELERATION AND DECELERATION

The *law of inertia,* which is one of the *laws of motion* described by Sir Isaac Newton, states: *A body at rest will remain at rest, and a body in motion will remain in motion, unless acted upon by an outside force.* A person hit by a car and someone thrown several yards by an explosion are examples of bodies at rest that were put into motion by an outside force. Conversely, the person who has fallen onto a concrete pavement and the car that hits a guard rail are examples of bodies in motion that were stopped by an outside force.

The rate at which a body in motion increases its speed is known as *acceleration.* The rate at which a body in motion decreases its speed is known as *deceleration.* While mass and velocity are major factors in determining the force of impact, acceleration and deceleration also play key roles.

A faster change of speed (acceleration or deceleration) results in more force exerted. For example, two cars of the same weight moving at the same rate of speed have the same kinetic energy. If one car is braked to a gradual stop and the other is stopped suddenly by striking a telephone pole, however, the one with the faster rate of deceleration—the one that fetched up against the pole—exerts more force.

As another example, two people of the same size and weight riding in different cars at the same rate of speed have the same amount of kinetic energy. Suppose that one starts moving faster gradually by normal pressure on the gas pedal, and the other starts moving faster suddenly by being struck from behind by an out-of-control tractor trailer. The one with the faster rate of acceleration—the one struck from behind—will have his body jerked out from under his head and neck with sufficient force to cause a severe whiplash injury, while the one that accelerates gradually is not injured at all.

ENERGY CHANGES FORM AND DIRECTION

Energy travels in a straight line unless it meets and is deflected by some kind of interference. If kinetic energy, transmitted to a human body, continues to travel in a straight line without interruption, injury may not occur. However, energy traveling through the human body is frequently interrupted. The interruption may be due to a curve in the bone, an organ that is caught between two hard surfaces, or tissue that is pulled against a fixed point. Energy is then forced to change form because it can no longer travel in a straight line.

The result is either blunt or penetrating injury, which we will discuss later in the chapter.

IMPACTS

In the typical vehicular collision, there are actually three impacts, each of which is an opportunity for energy to be absorbed by the vehicle and the patient. First the vehicle is suddenly stopped and gets bent out of shape (Figure 28-2a). This is called the *vehicle collision*. Next the patient comes to a quick stop on some part or parts of the inside of the vehicle, such as the steering wheel, causing injury to the chest (Figure 28-2b). This is called the *body collision*. Finally,

there is the *organ collision* in which the patient's internal organs, which are all suspended in their places by tissue, come to a quick stop, sometimes striking an inside surface of the body (for example the inner chest wall or the inner skull) (Figure 28-2c).

Occasionally, there may be more impacts, such as the case of a motorcycle rider who hits a car and is thrown. The cyclist hits the handlebars of the motorcycle, then the hood of the car, and finally the ground. With the impact of the cyclist against the handlebars, car, and ground, the internal organs also strike the inner body. So there are six potential impacts—three body collisions and three organ collisions—each of which produces energy and potential injury.

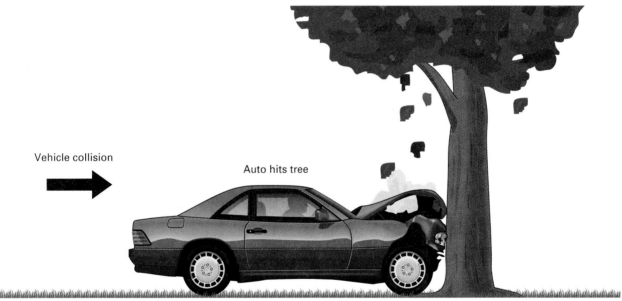

Figure 28-2a   Vehicle collision. The vehicle strikes an object.

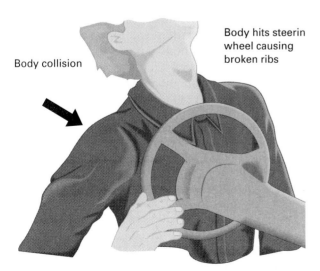

Figure 28-2b   Body collision. The occupant continues forward and strikes the inside of the automobile.

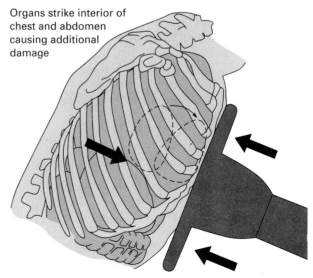

Figure 28-2c   Organ collision. The organs continue to move forward and strike the inside of the skull, chest, or abdomen.

By comparing the number of impacts, it is easy to understand why a person in or on a moving vehicle who gets thrown has a much greater chance for injury than one who is restrained or remains within the vehicle.

Your understanding of the kinetics of trauma also makes it clear why the faster a vehicle is traveling, the greater the kinetic energy—and the higher the rate of acceleration or deceleration, the greater the force. The greater these factors and the greater the number of impacts, the greater the potential for injury.

MECHANISMS OF INJURY

With a thorough understanding of mechanisms of injury, you will be able to arrive on the scene of a vehicle collision and determine, simply from looking at the damaged body of the vehicle, what types of traumatic injuries the patient is likely to have experienced. Or, you will be able to arrive at the scene of a fall and, judging by the patient's position, quickly estimate the types of injuries you will be called upon to treat. (As you read about the injuries that may be caused by various mechanisms of injury in the remainder of this chapter, keep in mind that later chapters in this Trauma module will deal with these kinds of injuries in more detail.)

Common mechanisms of injury include vehicular collisions, falls, penetrating gunshots or stabbings, and explosions. The fall is actually the most common mechanism of injury, accounting for more than half of all trauma incidents. Yet, while the fall is the most common mechanism of injury, it is not the most lethal. Over one-third of all deaths due to trauma occur from vehicle collisions.

VEHICLE COLLISIONS

As discussed earlier, velocity is a key factor in mechanism of injury. The greater the speed at collision, the greater the chance of life-threatening injury. If a ve-

hicle collided at high speed, your index of suspicion should include the possibility of the most severe injuries. Immediate assessment, aggressive treatment, and rapid transport are essential to saving occupants involved in these kinds of accidents.

You should also have a high index of suspicion in the following situations:

• *Death of another occupant of the vehicle*—A force severe enough to kill one passenger will almost certainly cause severe injuries, if not death, to all other passengers in the same compartment. So, even if another passenger does not appear to be badly injured, maintain a high level of suspicion that this passenger has potentially fatal injuries, which may be internal or otherwise hard to detect.

• *An unresponsive patient or patient with an altered mental status*—One of the earliest signs of brain injury is altered mental status or unresponsiveness. Upon your arrival at the collision, maintain a high index of suspicion if anyone reports that one of the passengers appeared "dazed" or has been "staring into space." A brief period of unresponsiveness or disorientation followed by a return of alertness may be a sign of brain injury. So if this has been reported to you about a patient whom you then examine and find to be alert, you should still consider him as a patient with an altered mental status.

Motor vehicle collisions can be classified as frontal, rear-end, lateral, and rotational and rollovers (Figure 28-3). Each type has a predictable pattern of injury.

FRONTAL IMPACT

In the frontal impact (Figure 28-4) the driver will continue to move forward at the same speed the vehicle is traveling (Figure 28-5). Then he will proceed to go either up and over the steering wheel, causing injuries to the head, neck, chest, and abdomen and

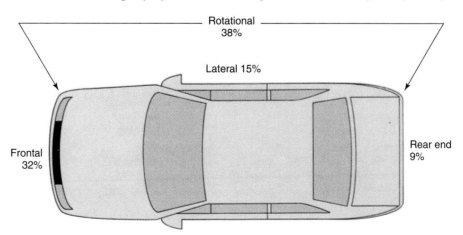

Figure 28-3 *Types of impacts in motor vehicle trauma and their incidence of frequency in urban areas (by percentage).*

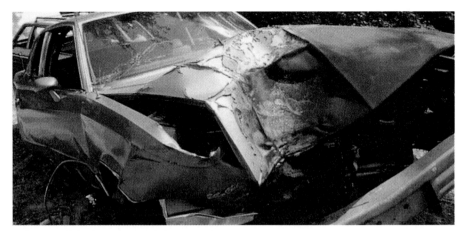

Figure 28-4   Frontal impact.

possible ejection through the windshield (Figure 28-6a), or he will go down and under the steering wheel, causing injuries to the knees, femurs, hips, acetabulum, and spine (Figure 28-6b).

If the unrestrained occupants of a vehicle involved in a collision travel in an up-and-over direction, they may be ejected from the vehicle. Partial ejection is also possible, for example the head protruding through the windshield. Severe soft tissue injuries, including avulsions and crushing injuries, often result. The chance of sustaining a fatal injury is increased by 300 percent when the occupant is ejected. The chance of cervical spine injury is increased by 1,300 percent.

Look for injuries to the abdomen, chest, face, head, and neck (Figure 28-7) when there is a frontal impact with the patient following an up-and-over pathway or with either full or partial ejection.

Abdomen   A damaged steering wheel or dashboard should cause you to suspect abdominal injury. As the abdomen strikes the steering wheel or dashboard, the liver, spleen, and hollow organs of the abdomen are compressed between the front and back abdominal walls and spine. The hollow organs are more easily displaced, leaving the solid liver and spleen to bear the brunt of the compression.

Chest   As the chest hits the steering wheel or dashboard, bones and soft tissues are both affected. The ribs and sternum may break, and the cartilage connecting the ribs to the sternum may separate. A torn intercostal artery can bleed 50 ccs per minute into the chest cavity with no blood seen externally.

The heart and lungs are the major organs affected. The heart suffers the effect of two forces:

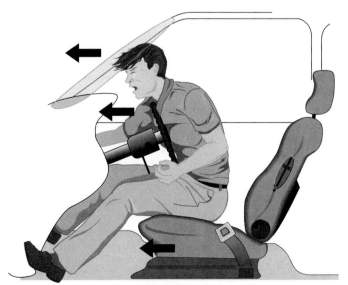

Figure 28-5   In a frontal collision, the occupant continues to move forward at the same speed the vehicle was moving.

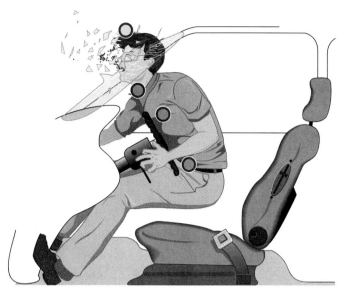

Figure 28-6a   The up-and-over pathway causes impact to the head, neck, chest, and abdomen.

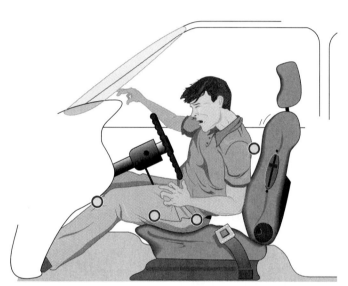

Figure 28-6b   The down-and-under pathway causes impact to the knees, femurs, hips, acetabulum, and spine.

compression and shear. The compression force occurs when the heart is caught between the sternum and the spine, which can result in a bruise to the heart muscle. The heart is suspended by the aorta, which is attached at the arch by a ligament. The shear force tends to pull the aorta at the ligament, which may tear or transect the aorta.

The lungs can also be affected. Air, trapped in the lungs by sudden closure of the epiglottis, is compressed between the ribs and spine. This kind of compression injury is called a "paper bag injury" because it is like blowing up a paper bag, then popping it between your hands. Air compressed inside the

limited areas of a lung can bruise or rupture the lung (Figure 28-8).

Face, Head, and Neck These parts of the body are next to impact the dashboard, windshield, or window. As you approach the vehicle, always check for the typical "spider web" windshield cracking, which is usually caused by a head striking the glass. Depending on the impact point and amount of glass, the face may have extensive soft-tissue damage. Head injuries also usually result when an occupant is ejected from the vehicle, and skull fracture may occur. Depending on the force involved, penetrating

DASHBOARD INJURIES

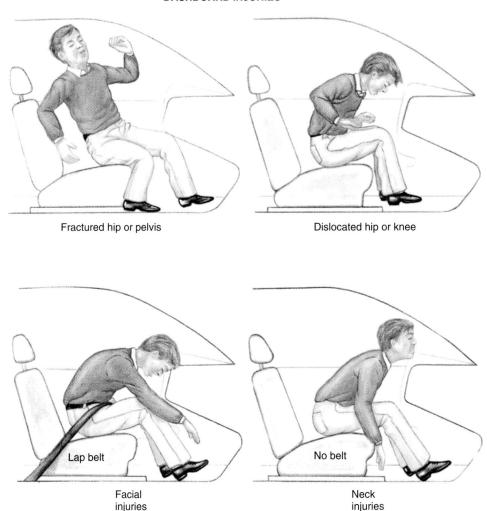

Fractured hip or pelvis

Dislocated hip or knee

Facial injuries

Neck injuries

Lap belt

No belt

Figure 28-7   Examples of mechanisms of injury associated with frontal impact.

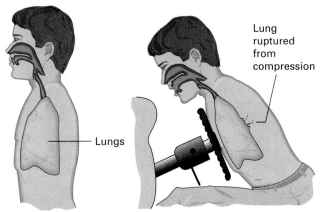

Figure 28-8   The "paper bag" syndrome results from compression of the chest against the steering column.

Lungs

Lung ruptured from compression

bone shards or a depressed skull fracture may result, lacerating the brain tissue.

Even in the absence of bone injury, the force of the impact may damage the brain. First, the floor of the skull is very rough, with many sharp projections. When the brain moves across these projections, it can become lacerated or bruised. Second, the brain may rebound against the opposite side of the skull from the original point of impact. The brain can be bruised on the side of the impact and/or on the opposite side as the brain hits the wall of the skull.

Because force travels in a straight line, energy not dissipated by the face or head will continue down the neck, with the potential for causing cervical spine injury. If the occupant is thrown forward at such an angle that the neck is either caught by the steering wheel or the dashboard, the trachea is in direct danger of being injured.

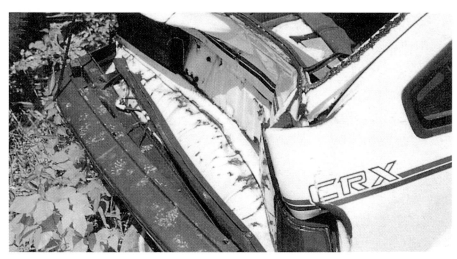

Figure 28-9   Rear impact.

REAR-END IMPACT

In a rear-end impact (Figure 28-9), the patient's head and neck are immediately whipped back. The body is propelled forward by the seat, while the head and neck, following the law of inertia, tend to remain at rest. Additionally, because the weight of the body exceeds that of the head, the body keeps moving while the head slows (Figure 28-10a).

If there is a head rest that has been properly positioned and seat belts are worn, injury is minimized. However if the vehicle does not have head rests or they are improperly positioned, the neck is hyperextended and the anterior ligaments are often stretched or torn. This is often referred to as a "whiplash" injury. An improperly positioned head rest that is pushed all the way down to restrain just the neck and not the head can actually contribute to the severity of the injury by creating a fulcrum to bend the neck over.

The injuries to be expected include the initial neck injury followed by either the frontal up and over or down and under injuries once the vehicle comes to a complete stop and the occupant jolts forward (Figure 28-10b).

LATERAL IMPACT

When a vehicle is struck laterally, or directly on the side, it can be crushed inward, impinging upon the occupants (Figure 28-11). Injuries may occur to the head, neck, chest, abdomen, and pelvis. You need to ask yourself who took the brunt of that collision and be very careful to examine carefully the side of the patient's body that bore the brunt of the lateral impact (Figure 28-12).

Head and Neck   As the energy of the impact is absorbed, the body is pushed laterally, out from under the head. This causes the head to move in the oppo-

site direction. The structures in the lateral areas of the neck are not as strong as in the anterior/posterior portion of the neck, thus resulting in more frequent muscle tears and ligament injuries. The vertebrae also

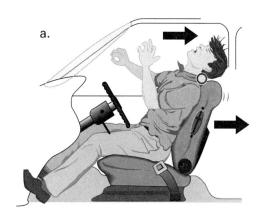

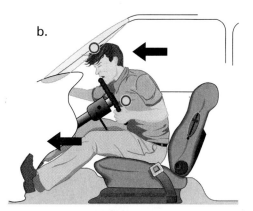

Figure 28-10   In a rear impact with an unrestrained occupant, initial movement is backward causing potential neck injury. The occupant then moves forward causing impact to the head and chest.

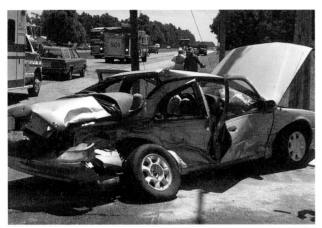

Figure 28-11 Lateral impact. (Robert J. Bennett)

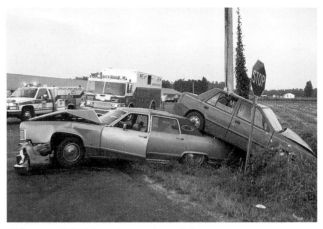

Figure 28-13 Rotational impact. (Robert J. Bennett)

are not designed for extreme lateral movement, and vertebral fractures are common. If there is more than one person in the passenger compartment, head injuries are frequently caused when heads collide.

Chest and Abdomen Injuries occur when the door strikes the side of the chest and abdomen. If the impact is on the shoulder, the energy traveling in a

straight line may dissipate at the curve in the clavicle, resulting in a fracture. If the arm is caught between the door and chest, or if the door hits the chest, fractured ribs and flail segments are possible. If the fractures occur low in the rib cage, the liver or spleen may be affected.

Pelvis The impact of the vehicle door to the chest wall also causes a lateral impact to the pelvis. Fractures of the pelvis and upper femur usually complete this pattern.

ROTATIONAL OR ROLLOVER CRASH

Injuries from rotational crashes (Figure 28-13) are not as easy to predict as those from other crashes. The vehicle spins around the point of impact causing the occupants who are not restrained to strike the mirror, posts, and doors, resulting in many injuries. Both head-on and lateral injury patterns occur.

During a rollover, the vehicle hits the ground multiple times and in various places (Figure 28-14).

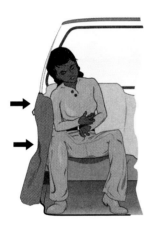

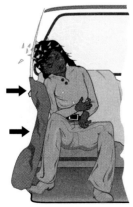

Figure 28-12 Lateral impact causes impact to the head, shoulder, lateral chest, lateral abdomen, lateral pelvis, and femur.

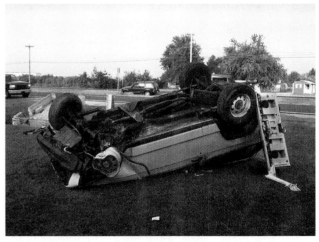

Figure 28-14 Rollover impact. (Robert J. Bennett)

The occupant changes direction every time the vehicle does (Figure 28-15). Vehicles with a high center of gravity, such as sports utility vehicles and vans, are more prone to rollovers. Every protruding object in the vehicle, including the rear-view mirror, the headrest, and the door handles, becomes a potentially lethal object.

While a specific pattern of injury is impossible to predict in a rollover, there are a few common characteristics. First, multiple systems injury is common. Second, ejection is common if the occupant was not restrained. Finally, crushing injuries to ejected occupants are common. Following the laws of motion, if you go straight through the windshield into the ditch, so does your vehicle, right into the ditch on top of you. Sometimes patients are thrown into other lanes of traffic too fast for oncoming vehicles to avoid.

VEHICLE-PEDESTRIAN COLLISION

When a vehicle hits a pedestrian, the extent of injury depends on how fast the vehicle was going, what part of the pedestrian's body was hit, how far the pedestrian was thrown, the surface the pedestrian landed on, and the body part that first struck the ground. There are likely to be very different patterns of injury in children than adults. This is because adults are larger and have a different weight distribution. Also, children and adults react to an impending collision very differently.

A child who is about to be hit by a vehicle—whether the child is walking or riding a bicycle—generally turns toward the oncoming vehicle, so injuries from the impact are generally to the front of the body. A very common pattern in a child struck by an auto is the combination of injuries to the femur, chest, abdomen, and head. Because a child is small and has a low center of gravity, a child struck by a ve-

hicle is usually thrown in front of the vehicle, and is often subsequently run over by the same vehicle that hit him. A child struck by the bumper may be thrown onto the hood and then, when the vehicle stops, be thrown off the car.

An adult, on the other hand, usually turns away from an oncoming vehicle, so the most common impact is to the side of the body. The bumper generally strikes the lower leg, typically causing fractures of the tibia and fibula. As the legs are propelled forward from the force of the vehicle, the adult generally falls backward and lands on the hood of the vehicle, resulting in injuries to the back, chest, shoulders, arms, and abdomen. If the adult continues across the hood and collides with the windshield, suspect serious head and neck injuries. Finally, the force of the moving vehicle throws the adult off the hood and to the ground.

RESTRAINTS: A CAUSE OF HIDDEN INJURIES

Hidden injuries may occur from the use of restraints in motor vehicles, including seat belts and air bags. Lap belts, when worn properly, distribute force across the iliac crests of the pelvis. The lap belt prevents the occupant from being ejected but, without a shoulder strap, it does not prevent the chest from striking the steering wheel or the head and neck from striking the dashboard or steering wheel. Compression fractures of the lumbar spine occur as the torso is forcibly flexed forward. If the seat belt is worn too low, it can dislocate the hips. Worn too high, it can cause abdominal compression and spinal fracture. A shoulder strap worn without a lap belt can result in severe neck injury.

Lap and shoulder belts that are properly positioned may reduce the force of the impact on any one point and, consequently, reduce the severity of the injuries. Properly applied lap belts and shoulder straps

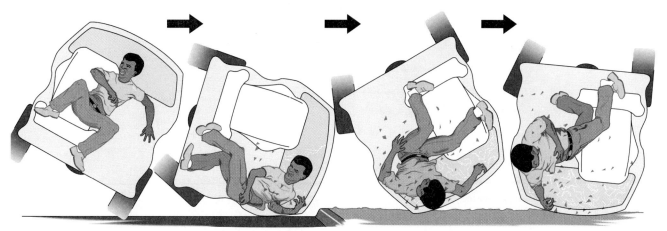

Figure 28-15   In a rollover of an unrestrained occupant, impact to the body is difficult to predict and commonly results in multiple system injury.

do not, however, prevent the head and neck from moving laterally or forward and back.

Air bags are triggered to inflate from the steering wheel or glove compartment when a collision occurs. They cushion the forward motion of the occupant, absorbing the energy from the collision and slowing the deceleration rate of the occupant. The bag deflates immediately after the impact. Thus, air bags work best in the first impact of a head-on collision. They do not work well in multiple collision events nor in rear-end, lateral, or rollover collisions. Air bags are most effective when used with seat belts. In fact, the air bag may not be effective without a seat belt.

Because the air bag deflates immediately after the impact, the driver may still hit the steering wheel. In any collision involving an air bag, the manufacturers of air bags recommend that rescuers lift the deployed air bag and check for deformation of the steering wheel. Any visible deformity of the steering wheel indicates potentially serious internal injury.

Airbags themselves may be the cause of eye, face, and neck injuries related to the explosive force of deployment. Deaths of children have been related to injury from airbags.

CONSIDERATIONS FOR INFANTS AND CHILDREN

The properly secured car seat restrains a child at three or four points: one or two points at mid-pelvis, and a point at each shoulder. During a collision, the part or parts of the body that are not restrained continue forward at the same speed the vehicle was traveling prior to the impact. As the child's head snaps forward, the neck is stretched against the resistance of the shoulder restraints. The result can be a spinal cord injury without injury to the vertebrae.

Even if the seat is facing backward, the same kind of injury can happen if the car seat is rotated into a reclining position. To prevent head snapping, the proper position for the car seat is to face backwards in the upright position, which will also prevent suffocation by a deployed air bag. To completely avoid injury from air bag deployment, children should always be restrained in the back seat of the vehicle and not in the front passenger seat.

MOTORCYCLE COLLISIONS

Motorcycle collisions account for a significant number of motor vehicle collisions that occur on and off our nation's highways (Figure 28-16). The incidence of morbidity (illness or injury) and mortality (death) is greatly affected by whether the rider is wearing a helmet. There are three main types of impact in motorcycle collisions: head-on, angular, and ejection. Ejection is most often associated with the head-on impact.

Head-on Impact   When this kind of impact occurs, the motorcycle tends to tip forward, due to the location of its center of gravity. This causes the rider to travel into the handlebars at the same speed the bike was traveling. Depending on what part of the rider's anatomy strikes the handlebars, a variety of injuries may occur.

Angular Impact   In angular motorcycle impacts, the rider strikes an object, usually a protruding object, at an angle. The object impacts whatever body part it comes into contact with, usually breaking or collapsing in on the rider. Examples include the edges of signs, outside mirrors on motor vehicles, or fence posts. The result can be severe avulsion injuries or even traumatic amputations.

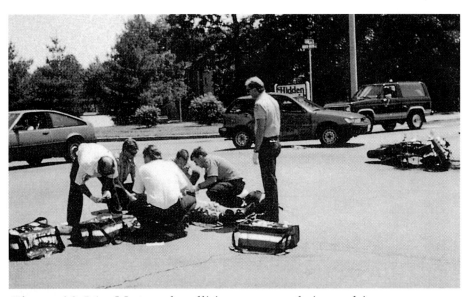

Figure 28-16 Motorcycle collisions can result in multi-system trauma due to multiple impacts to the rider.

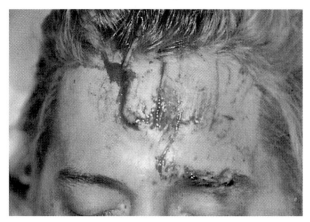

Figure 28-17   Soft-tissue injury to the fore-head.

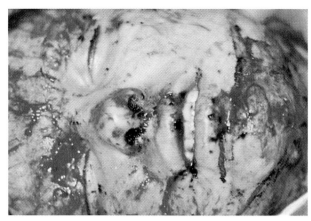

Figure 28-18   Soft-tissue injury to the face.

Ejection   After any motorcycle collision, ejection occurs if the rider clears the handlebars. Ejection continues until a body part impacts with the object of the collision, the ground, or both. Boots, leather clothing, and a helmet are used to help protect against soft tissue damage, commonly called "road rash," and against head and facial injuries (Figures 28-17 and 28-18). If the rider is not wearing a helmet, the incidence of severe head injury and death increases 300 percent, the same as that for auto ejections.

"Laying the Bike Down"   This is an evasive action on the part of the rider, designed to prevent ejection and separation of the driver from the bike in an impending collision. The bike is turned sideways and "laid down" with the driver's inside leg dragging on the pavement or ground. The driver tends to lose speed faster than the bike, thus moving the bike out from under the driver.

Abrasions can range from superficial ones, involving only the epidermis, to full-thickness abrasions, which extend through the subcutaneous tissue and, in severe cases to the covering over the bone. Abrasions can also be complicated by particles embedded in the tissue such as dirt, grass, or asphalt.

Burns are most often sustained when the inside leg does not clear the bike. The leg becomes caught between the exhaust pipe and the ground. The longer the contact with the hot pipe, the worse the burn.

All-Terrain Vehicles   ATVs are also very problematic since they are easily tipped over (Figure 28-19). The three-wheel versions have been pulled off the market. Even the four-wheel ATVs are quite unstable

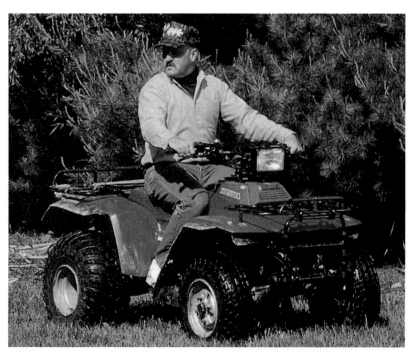

Figure 28-19   All terrain vehicles (ATVs) can cause multiple injuries due to the combination of speed and instability.

and can easily cause collisions similar to motorcycle collisions.

FALLS

Falls are the most common mechanism of injury. The severity of trauma depends on the distance, surface, and body part that impacted first. Associated factors are objects that interrupt the fall prior to landing.

In general, the greater the distance of the fall the more severe the injury, because increased height increases the velocity at impact. Some experts feel that the surface is more of a determining factor of injury than the height. A fall of 15 feet onto an unyielding surface is considered severe for an adult, and a fall of more than 10 feet can cause severe injuries in a child. Internal organ damage is frequent, and you should have a high index of suspicion regardless of how the patient looks at first.

The pattern of trauma injuries also depends on the body part that impacts first. As we pointed out earlier, *energy travels in a straight line until it is forced to curve.* At that point, energy changes form to dissipate, and injury occurs.

FEET-FIRST FALLS

A feet-first landing causes energy to travel up the skeletal system. Fractures of the heels and fractures or dislocations of the ankles are common (Figure 28-20). If the knees are flexed at the time of impact, the majority of energy will be dissipated at the knees and will preserve the rest of the skeletal system. If the person lands flat-footed with knees locked, however, energy will be transmitted up through the femurs to the hips and pelvis, possibly causing fractures.

If energy remains, the spine will absorb the force at every curve of the lumbar, mid-thoracic, and cervical spine. Experts tell us that the patient who fell three times his height or more will probably have a spinal injury resulting from the transmission of energy up through the legs and hips and into the spine.

In falls of more than 20 feet, the internal organs are likely to be injured from deceleration forces: the liver, spleen, kidney, and heart may be affected.

Extending the arms to break the fall as the body is thrown forward is natural. The first point of energy dissipation is at the wrist. A fracture of the wrist bones known as a Colles', or "silver fork," fracture is common. The elbow and shoulder are the next points of potential injury. If the body is thrown backward, the most common injuries are to the head, back, and pelvis.

HEAD-FIRST FALLS

In head-first falls, the pattern of injury begins with the arms and extends up to the shoulders. The head may be forcibly hyperextended, hyperflexed, or com-

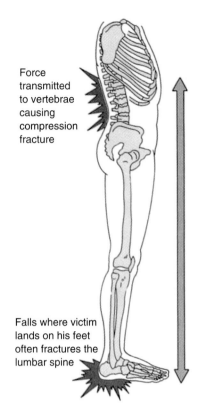

Force transmitted to vertebrae causing compression fracture

Falls where victim lands on his feet often fractures the lumbar spine

Figure 28-20   In falls the energy of impact is transmitted up the skeletal system.

pressed, all of which can cause extensive damage to the cervical spine. As the body continues its downward motion, the torso and legs are thrown either forward or backward. Chest, lower spine, and pelvic injuries are also common.

PENETRATING INJURIES

Penetrating injuries are caused by any object that can penetrate the surface of the body—such as bullets, darts, nails, and knives. The amount of damage that results depends on the amount of kinetic energy transferred to the tissue and the area of the body it penetrates. Of these two factors, the amount of kinetic energy transferred to the tissue is the greatest indicator of potential damage. For example, if the object is a knife, the low kinetic energy limits the damage to just the immediate site of impact and the underlying structures. On the other hand, the higher kinetic energy of a bullet results in tissue damage extending relatively far from the site of impact. If the kinetic energy produced by the bullet is totally absorbed by the body tissues, the bullet will not exit. If kinetic energy remains with the bullet, however, an exit wound will occur.

Penetrating injuries are classified as low-, medium-, and high-velocity (Figure 28-21).

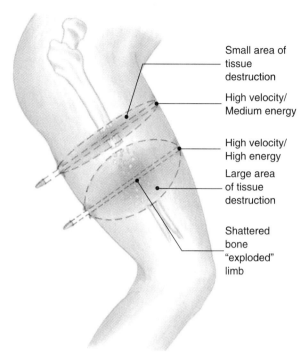

Small area of tissue destruction

High velocity/ Medium energy

High velocity/ High energy

Large area of tissue destruction

Shattered bone "exploded" limb

Figure 28-21   The severity of injury caused by penetrating trauma is related to the velocity of the penetrating object.

LOW-VELOCITY INJURIES

A knife or other object impaled in the body exerts damage to the immediate area of impact and its underlying structures. As the person tries to defend against an attack, wounds may occur. These are generally slash marks on the hands and arms that occur when the patient puts up one or both hands or arms to ward off the attacker or in an attempt to grab the knife.

The length of the object used in the stabbing also provides valuable clues. For example, a person stabbed from behind in the left upper chest with a short (3-inch) paring knife, may suffer a pneumothorax (air in the chest cavity). If stabbed with an 8-inch knife, the injuries may include lacerated pulmonary veins, lacerated aorta, even laceration to the heart itself. For this reason, if you know the type of knife and its length you should report it to the hospital staff.

MEDIUM- AND HIGH-VELOCITY INJURIES

Medium- and high-velocity projectiles are generally pellets or bullets. Most shotguns or handguns fire at medium velocity. High velocity weapons include high-power, high-speed rifles such as an M-16 or a 30-30 Winchester.

The damage caused by medium- and high-velocity projectiles depends on two factors: trajectory and dis-

sipation of energy. **Trajectory** is the path or motion of a projectile during its travel. Normally a bullet, once fired, follows a curved trajectory or path. However, the faster the bullet, the flatter the curve of the trajectory and the straighter the path of the bullet.

Dissipation of energy is the way energy is transferred to the human body from the force acting upon it. In the case of medium- and high-velocity projectile injuries, dissipation of energy is affected by drag, profile, and cavitation.

- **Drag**—The factors that slow a bullet down, such as wind resistance, constitute drag.
- **Profile**—The impact point of the bullet is its profile. The greater the size of the impact point, the more energy is transferred.
- **Cavitation**—Sometimes called pathway expansion, cavitation is the cavity in the body tissues formed by a pressure wave resulting from the kinetic energy of the bullet. Cavitation greatly extends the tissue damage beyond the initial bullet pathway. That is, the hole that is created in the tissues is larger than the diameter of the bullet. (Cavitation occurs with medium- and high-velocity projectiles but not generally with low-velocity projectiles.) Blown-out tissue caused by cavitation and carried along with the bullet explains why the exit wound is always larger than the entry wound. Remember to always assess for an exit wound.

Shotgun wounds differ significantly from rifle or handgun wounds, because shotguns have multiple pellets that spray in a pattern. The multiple pellets increase the impact surface area, thus increasing the amount of energy transferred to the tissues. Close-range shotgun wounds can cause devastating tissue damage, while long-range wounds may cause no more than relatively minor surface wounds (Figure 28-22).

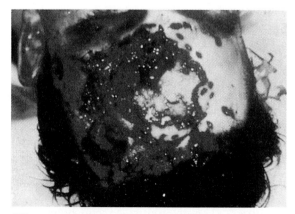

Figure 28-22   Wound resulting from close-range shotgun blast. Note the tattooing of the skin from the gunpowder.

GUNSHOT WOUNDS

Of fatal wounds that occur due to firearms, 49 percent occur to the torso, 42 percent to the head, and only 9 percent below the waist. Wounds also occur to the extremities.

Head The interior of the skull is a fixed space with little-to-no room for expansion. When the energy from a projectile enters the skull and starts to dissipate, brain tissue is naturally severely compressed.

Gunshot wounds to the face generally result in major soft-tissue injuries that immediately threaten the airway. It is very difficult to get a good seal when ventilating the patient who is lacking facial contours. Bleeding is extensive, and the airway is difficult to manage.

Chest Lung tissue is relatively tolerant of the cavitation caused by projectiles. The numerous air-filled alveoli form a spongy mass that is easily movable. Pneumothorax is a common result of injury to the chest and/or lung, with air or a combination of air and blood escaping into the chest cavity. Associated rib fractures may also occur.

The heart is not as tolerant of projectiles as are the lungs, but the outer covering of the pulmonary vessels, aorta, and heart are tough and elastic. These tissues may be able to seal themselves off from low-velocity projectile wounds, but medium- and high-velocity projectiles are likely to cause significant wounds to the heart and the great vessels that enter and exit the heart.

The lower boundary between the chest cavity and the abdomen is formed by the diaphragm. If a projectile strikes the lower part of the chest or upper abdomen during exhalation, the projectile is more likely to enter below the relaxed diaphragm and cause an abdominal wound. If the projectile strikes the same area during inhalation, the projectile is more likely to enter above the contracted diaphragm and cause a wound to the chest cavity. Suspect both thoracic and abdominal injury if the entrance wound is between the nipple line and the waist.

Abdomen The abdomen is often secondarily injured when the chest is injured. The abdominal cavity is large, and contains structures that are fluid-filled (such as the bladder), air-filled (such as the stomach), solid (such as the spleen), and bony structures (such as the pelvic bones). The air-filled and fluid-filled structures are more tolerant of cavitation than are the solid organs. The majority of abdominal wounds are not rapidly fatal, even though as many as 80 percent of those involving medium-velocity injuries require surgical repair.

Extremities The extremities contain bone, muscle, blood vessels, and nerves. Bone injury due to a projectile results in bony fragments becoming secondary missiles, lacerating surrounding vessels, muscles, and nerves. Muscle expands, resulting in capillary tears and swelling. Vessels can be severed, ripped, buckled, and/or obstructed. As a result, circulation and motor and sensory function to the extremity may be severely or totally compromised.

BLAST INJURIES

Blast injuries can occur as a result of explosions from, for example, natural gas, gasoline, fireworks, and grain elevators. Regardless of the cause, every explosion has three phases: primary, secondary, and tertiary (Figure 28-23). Each causes specific patterns of injury.

- *Primary phase injuries* are due to the pressure wave of the blast. These injuries primarily affect the gas-containing organs, such as the lungs, stomach, intestines, inner ears, and sinuses. Severe damage and death may occur from this phase without any external sign of injury.
- *Secondary phase injuries* are due to flying debris propelled by the force of the blast. Contrary to the injuries in the primary phase, the injuries of this phase are obvious. Most common are lacerations, impaled objects, fractures, and burns.
- *Tertiary phase injuries* occur when the patient is thrown away from the source of the blast. Injuries are much the same as would be expected from ejection from a vehicle. The pattern is dependent on the distance thrown and the point of impact.

Injuries sustained during the secondary and tertiary phases are the most obvious and are more easily accessed and treated. Injuries of the primary phase are most often ignored or unsuspected and, therefore, go untreated. Unfortunately, injuries of the primary phase are just as severe, if not more severe, than those obtained during the other phases. In general, the index of suspicion on all blast injury patients must remain high, regardless of the initial presentation.

THE GOLDEN HOUR

The "golden hour" has been established as a standard parameter for emergency care because studies have shown that a severely injured patient has the best chance for survival if surgical intervention takes place within one hour from time of injury. Some EMS services talk about the "platinum 10 minutes." This means that 10 minutes out of the golden hour is the maximum time the EMS team should devote to on-scene activities.

If a patient is not severely injured (or is without life-threatening medical problems), more time can and should be devoted to completing normal on-scene assessment and emergency care before transport is undertaken.

The key, of course, is the determination as to whether the patient is or is not (possibly) severely injured. It is to the patient's potential benefit to err on

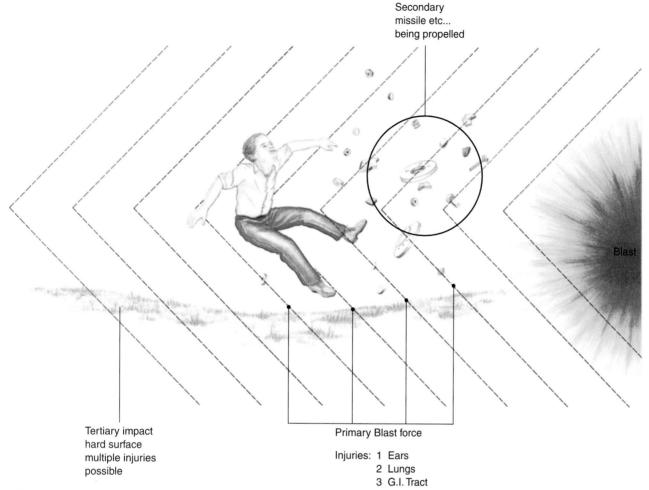

Figure 28-23   Blast injuries can cause injury with the initial blast, when the patient is struck by debris, or by the patient being thrown from the site of the blast.

the side of overestimating, rather than underestimating, the extent or severity of injuries. The harm that can be done by delaying transport when it is needed outweighs the good that can be done by completing on-scene assessment and care at a more deliberate pace. That is why EMT-Bs are taught to maintain a "high index of suspicion"—a presumption that a pa-

tient has severe injuries if there is any indication at all that this is possible, which is often based on findings at the scene as to the mechanism of injury and the amount of force that may have been delivered.

As you have learned in this chapter, a patient involved in trauma may have hidden, internal injuries. These may be far more serious than any of

TABLE 28-1

Significant Mechanisms of Injury

• Ejection from automobile • Death or altered mental status of a person in the same passenger compartment • Extrication time >20 minutes • Falls >20 feet • Rollover	
• High-speed auto crash	Initial speed >40 mph Major auto deformity >20 inches Intrusion into passenger compartment >12 inches
• Auto-pedestrian/auto-bicycle injury with significant (>5 mph) impact • Pedestrian thrown or run over • Motorcycle crash >20 mph or with separation of rider from bike	

the external injuries that you can observe. In fact, in some cases, there can be internal injuries with *no* external injuries that you can detect.

This is why, in instances of trauma, you must evaluate and rely on the mechanism of injury in your pri- ority *decision. Treatment and transport decisions must be based on the injuries the mechanism of injury tells you are POSSIBLE, even when the signs and symptoms that you can gather do not support this assumption.* (See Table 28-1 on the prior page.)

CASE STUDY FOLLOW-UP

SCENE SIZE-UP

Your initial call was for a minor collision with one patient complaining of knee pain. The police officer greeted you and explained that he was taking a report from the driver of a car that was struck from behind when he began to complain of the pain. He estimates the collision occurred at around 30 mph. He tells you that the other driver has been driven to the hospital by a friend.

The scene size-up reveals no obvious hazards; both vehicles have been moved off the road into a parking lot. You see only slight denting to the rear of your patient's vehicle. There is only one patient, and since his car wasn't damaged enough to interfere with the operation of the doors, gaining access to the patient is easy and will not require a rescue unit. You put on your disposable gloves and approach the vehicle.

INITIAL ASSESSMENT

You introduce yourself to the patient and ask him his name, and he says, "Call me Mike." You explain that, as a safety measure, your partner will get into the back seat and reach from behind to hold Mike's head still. There are no dents or damage to the steering wheel and no cracks in the windshield.

Your general impression is of a 40-year-old male in no obvious severe distress. Mike's chief complaint is pain in the knees, and he tells you privately that he did not have his seat belt on and went down and under the dashboard during the impact. He is alert and oriented. The airway, breathing, and circulation status are all fine. Because the mechanism of injury is not significant—and your general impression that Mike is not badly injured—you determine that he is a low priority for immediate transport and that you will proceed to conduct the focused history and physical exam at the scene.

You maintain a high index of suspicion, however, and will be ready to change your priority decision if you find out that the mechanism of injury was more severe than seems true at this point or if there is any deterioration in Mike's condition.

FOCUSED HISTORY AND PHYSICAL EXAM

You proceed with a rapid trauma exam and find no signs of injury. The knees, which Mike says continue to hurt, show no evidence of bruising, swelling, or deformity. A quick check of all four extremities reveals no loss of pulses or sensory or motor function. You obtain a set of baseline vitals, which are all within normal ranges. Rapid extrication technique is not warranted in this case, so you work with your partner and a police first responder to apply a cervical spine immobilization collar and a KED immobilization vest, then transfer and immobilize Mike to a long spine board.

Once he is secured, you reassess Mike's pulses and motor and sensory function in all four extremities. In the ambulance, you proceed to ask Mike the OPQRST and SAMPLE history questions and find out he now also has an ache in his lumbar spine, is allergic to sulfa drugs, takes medication for allergies to environmental substances, has a history of asthma which has not been bothering him recently, and last ate and drank at breakfast 2 hours ago. Mike states he was just waiting for the oncoming traffic to clear so he could make a left turn when suddenly the other car struck him from behind.

DETAILED PHYSICAL EXAM

Now there is time to conduct a detailed physical exam to make sure that no injuries have been overlooked. You make no additional findings.

ONGOING ASSESSMENT

Because Mike is stable, you conduct an ongoing assessment every 15 minutes on the way to the hospital. You repeat the initial assessment and vital signs. You check to be sure that he is securely immobilized with no loss of function to the extremities. To help him feel a little more comfortable, you apply a cold pack to his knees. You arrive at the hospital, transfer Mike to the care of the emergency department staff, and prepare your ambulance for the next call.

CHAPTER REVIEW

TERMS AND CONCEPTS

You may wish to review the following terms and concepts included in this chapter.

cavitation—a cavity formed by a pressure wave resulting from the kinetic energy of a bullet traveling through body tissue; also called pathway expansion.

dissipation of energy—the way energy is transferred to the human body by the forces acting upon it.

drag—the factors that slow a projectile.

kinetic energy—the energy contained by an object in motion. Kinetic energy equals mass (weight in pounds), times the velocity (feet per second) squared, divided by two.

kinetics of trauma—the science of analyzing mechanism of injury.

mechanism of injury—the factors and forces that cause traumatic injury.

profile—refers to the size and shape of a bullet's point of impact; the greater the point of impact the greater the injury.

trajectory—the path of a projectile during its travel; a trajectory may be flat or curved.

REVIEW QUESTIONS

1. Based on the formulas for kinetic energy and force, explain how the following are likely to affect the severity of an injury: (a) mass and velocity; (b) acceleration and deceleration.
2. Name and describe, in sequence, the three impacts that take place in a vehicular collision.
3. Name and describe four types of motorcycle collision.
4. Describe the path of energy and possible patterns of injury for each of the following kinds of falls:

(a) feet first; (b) landing on outstretched hands; (c) head first.
5. Define cavitation and tell which of the following kinds of weapons would be likely to produce it: knife, handgun, M-16 rifle.
6. Explain the cause of each of the following phases of blast injury: primary, secondary, and tertiary.
7. Name mechanisms of injury that should cause the EMT-B to have a high index of suspicion of significant injury.

CHAPTER 29

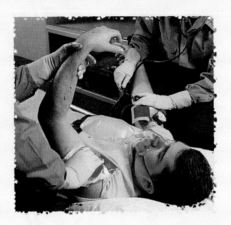

Bleeding and Shock

INTRODUCTION

B leeding can be a significant, life-threatening emergency. As an EMT-B you must be able to recognize obvious or external bleeding problems, as well as not-so-obvious internal bleeding problems. If either type of bleeding is left untreated, it has the potential to lead to rapid patient deterioration, shock (hypoperfusion), and death.

Control of severe external bleeding is performed during the initial assessment. Only airway and breathing have a higher priority. Internal bleeding and shock (hypoperfusion) are treated immediately following the initial assessment. Note that an important element of the emergency care of bleeding and shock (hypoperfusion) is to transport the patient to a medical facility as rapidly as possible.

OBJECTIVES

Numbered objectives are from the United States Department of Transportation 1994 EMT-Basic National Standard Curriculum. Asterisked objectives, if any, pertain to material that is supplemental to the DOT curriculum.

COGNITIVE

5-1. List the structure and function of the circulatory system. (p. 550)

5-1.2 Differentiate between arterial, venous, and capillary bleeding. (pp. 550, 552)

5-1.3 State methods of emergency medical care of external bleeding. (pp. 552–557)

5-1.4 Establish the relationship between body substance isolation and bleeding. (pp. 550, 552, 558, 559)

5-1.5 Establish the relationship between airway management and the trauma patient. (pp. 548, 552, 558, 559)

5-1.6 Establish the relationship between mechanism of injury and internal bleeding. (pp. 557–558)

5-1.7 List the signs of internal bleeding. (p. 558)

5-1.8 List the steps in emergency medical care of the patient with signs and symptoms of internal bleeding. (p. 558)

5-1.9 List signs and symptoms of shock (hypoperfusion). (pp. 559–560)

5-1.10 State the steps in the emergency medical care of the patient with signs and symptoms of shock (hypoperfusion). (pp. 560–562)

AFFECTIVE

5-1.11 Explain the sense of urgency to transport patients that are bleeding and show signs of shock (hypoperfusion). (pp. 548, 561)

PSYCHOMOTOR

5-1.12 Demonstrate direct pressure as a method of emergency medical care of external bleeding.

5-1.13 Demonstrate the use of diffuse pressure as a method of emergency medical care of external bleeding.

5-1.14 Demonstrate the use of pressure points and tourniquets as a method of emergency medical care for external bleeding.

5-1.15 Demonstrate the care of the patient exhibiting signs and symptoms of internal bleeding.

5-1.16 Demonstrate the care of the patient exhibiting signs and symptoms of shock (hypoperfusion).

5-1.17 Demonstrate completing a prehospital care report for the patient with bleeding and/or shock (hypoperfusion).

CASE STUDY

THE DISPATCH

EMS Unit 101—respond to Riverside High School at 1434 River Street for a reported stabbing—time out 1645 hours.

You ask the dispatcher if the police have been alerted. He doesn't know but will check. You and your partner decide that if police are not on the scene you will stage at the minimart down the street until the scene is secure.

The dispatcher comes back and advises you that the police are at the scene and have one person in custody. She says your patient is a male with a stab wound to the left upper abdomen with profuse bleeding.

ON ARRIVAL

You and your partner have put on your gloves, masks, eye protection, and gowns. As you pull into the high school parking lot, you notice a crowd of teenagers and adults gathered around a young male lying on the ground. You notify dispatch that you are "on arrival." Time is 1651.

A police officer approaches your unit. Your partner asks if the scene is secure. The officer states it is, and tells you they have one teenager in custody. You note that there is only one patient.

As you exit the vehicle and approach the patient, you see the young male, who appears to be a teenager, lying supine on the ground with a large penetrating wound to the left upper quadrant of the abdomen. The wound is bleeding profusely. There is no impaled object. No weapon is visible near the patient.

How would you proceed with this patient?

During this chapter, you will learn about bleeding and shock. Later, we will return to the case study and put in context some of the information you learned.

THE CIRCULATORY SYSTEM

The Heart, Blood Vessels, and Blood

To understand bleeding and shock, you should know the basic components of the circulatory system and how they work. Review the anatomy and physiology of the circulatory system in Chapter 4, "The Human Body," and in Chapter 15, "Cardiac Emergencies."

To review briefly, the circulatory system is responsible for providing the body with blood and a continuous supply of nutrients. It has three major components: the heart, blood vessels, and the blood.

- *The heart* is divided into two parts. The left side receives oxygen-rich blood from the lungs and pumps it to the body. The right side receives oxygen-depleted blood from the body and pumps it to the lungs.
- *Blood vessels* include the arteries, capillaries, and veins. The arteries function to carry oxygen-rich blood away from the heart to the body. The capillaries are a functional network of tiny blood vessels, which allow for oxygen and carbon dioxide to be exchanged with the body's cells. Veins carry oxygen-depleted blood from the body back to the heart.
- *Blood* contains red blood cells, white blood cells, plasma, and platelets. An average person weighing 150 pounds will have about 10–12 pints of total blood volume.

When the left side of the heart contracts, it sends a wave or pulsation of blood through the arteries. A pulse can be felt, or palpated, at any point where an artery passes over a bone near the skin surface. Pulse points include the central pulses—carotid and femoral—and peripheral pulses—radial, brachial, tibial, and dorsalis pedis.

Blood pressure is defined as the pressure exerted against the arterial walls during circulation, which can be measured with a sphygmomanometer (blood pressure cuff) and stethoscope, and reported as systolic and diastolic pressures. (See Chapter 5, "Baseline Vital Signs and History Taking.")

Perfusion

Perfusion is the delivery of oxygen and other nutrients to the cells of all organ systems and the effective elimination of carbon dioxide and other waste products, which results from the constant adequate circulation of blood through the capillaries.

Shock, or *hypoperfusion*, is the insufficient supply of oxygen and other nutrients to some of the body's cells and ineffective elimination of carbon dioxide and other waste products, which results from inadequate circulation of blood. It causes a state of profound depression of the vital processes of the body.

All parts of the body require some level of perfusion. However, some organ systems are especially sensitive to perfusion changes. The heart, for example, requires constant perfusion or it will not function properly. The brain and spinal cord can withstand a lack of perfusion for only 4 to 6 minutes before irreversible damage begins. The kidneys may be damaged if there is a lack of perfusion for more than 45 minutes. Skeletal muscle can withstand lack of perfusion for 2 hours before permanent damage occurs.

EXTERNAL BLEEDING

Body substance isolation precautions must be taken routinely to avoid exposure of skin and mucous membranes to blood and other body fluids. Wear personal protective equipment, including gloves and eyewear, and wash your hands before and after each run. BSI precautions are your best defense against transmission of infectious disease. (For more details, see Chapter 2, "The Well-being of the EMT-Basic.")

Severity

Your estimate of the severity of blood loss must be based on the patient's signs and symptoms (Figure 29-1). The sudden loss of 1 liter (1000 cc) of blood volume in the adult patient, $\frac{1}{2}$ liter (500 cc) of blood in children, and 100–200 cc in infants is considered serious. (For example, a 1-year-old baby has a total blood volume of only approximately 800 cc. A loss of 150 cc is considered significant, representing approximately 20 percent of the total volume.) If the patient exhibits signs and symptoms of shock (hypoperfusion), the bleeding is to be considered serious.

The natural response of the body to bleeding is blood vessel constriction and clotting. However, a serious injury can prevent that defense mechanism from working, resulting in uncontrolled bleeding. *Remember: Uncontrolled bleeding or significant blood loss can lead to shock (hypoperfusion) and quite possibly to death.*

Types of Bleeding

There are three types of bleeding—arterial, venous, and capillary. Each type can be life-threatening. Each has its own characteristics (Figure 29-2):

- *Arterial bleeding*—Bright red, spurting blood from a wound usually indicates a severed or damaged artery. The blood is bright red because it is rich in oxygen. Spurting generally coincides with the pulse or contraction of the heart. Arterial

THE FOUR STAGES OF HEMORRHAGE

CLASS 1	CLASS 2	CLASS 3	CLASS 4
Up to 15% blood loss	Up to 30% blood loss	Up to 40% blood loss	More than 40% blood loss

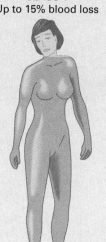 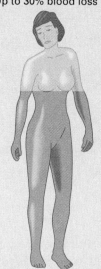 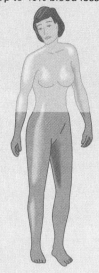 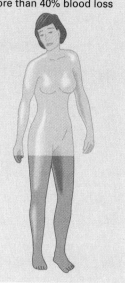

HOW THE BODY RESPONDS

The body compensates for blood loss by constricting blood vessels (vasoconstriction) in an effort to maintain blood pressure and delivery of oxygen to all organs of the body.

EFFECT ON PATIENT

• Patient remains alert.
• Blood pressure stays within normal limits.
• Pulse stays within normal limits or increases slightly; pulse quality remains strong.
• Respiratory rate and depth, skin color and temperature all remain normal.

*The average adult has 5 liters (1 liter = approximately 1 quart) of circulating blood; 15% is 750 ml (or about 3 cups). With internal bleeding 750 ml will occupy enough space in a limb to cause sweeling and pain. With bleeding into the body cavities, however, the blood will spread throughout the cavity, causing little, if any initial discomfort.

• Vasoconstriction continues to maintain adequate blood pressure, but with some difficulty now.
• Blood flow is shunted to vital organs, with decreased flow to intestines, kidneys, and skin.

EFFECT ON PATIENT

• Patient may become confused and restless.
• Skin turns pale, cool, and dry because of shunting of blood to vital organs.
• Diastolic pressure may rise or fall. It's more likely to rise (because of vasoconstriction) or stay the same in otherwise healthy patients with no underlying cardiovascular problems.
• Pulse pressure (difference between systolic and diastolic pressures) narrows.
• Sympathetic responses also cause rapid heart rate (over 100 beats per minute). Pulse quality weakens.
• Respiratory rate increases because of sympathetic stimulation.
• Delayed capillary refill.

• Compensatory mechanisms become overtaxed. Vasoconstriction, for example, can no longer sustain blood pressure, which now begins to fall.
• Cardiac output and tissue perfusion continue to decrease, becoming potentially life-threatening. (Even at this stage, however, the patient can still recover with prompt treatment.

EFFECT ON PATIENT

• Patient becomes more confused, restless, and anxious.
• Classic signs of shock appear—rapid heart rate, decreased blood pressure, rapid respiration and cool, clammy extremities.

• Compensatory vasaoconstriction now becomes a complicating factor in itself, further impairing tissue perfusion and cellular oxygenation.

EFFECT ON PATIENT

• Patient becomes lethargic, drowsy, or stuporous.
• Signs of shock become more pronounced. Blood pressure continues to fall.
• Lack of blood flow to the brain and other vital organs ultimately leads to organ failure and death.

Figure 29-1   The patient's signs and symptoms may indicate the severity of blood loss.

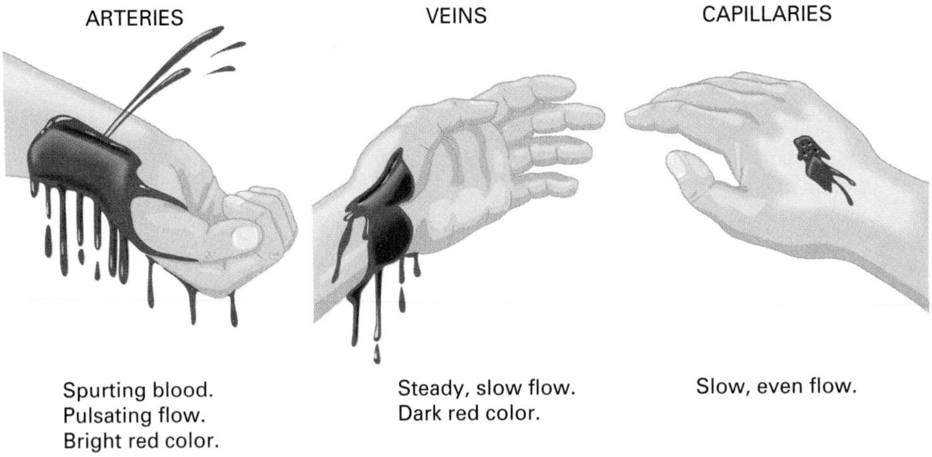

ARTERIES VEINS CAPILLARIES

Spurting blood.
Pulsating flow.
Bright red color.

Steady, slow flow.
Dark red color.

Slow, even flow.

Figure 29-2 Types of bleeding.

bleeding can be more difficult to control than any other type of bleeding because of the higher pressure in the arteries. As the patient's blood pressure decreases, the spurting may also decrease (a late sign of shock, or hypoperfusion).

- *Venous bleeding*—Dark red blood that flows steadily from a wound usually indicates a severed or damaged vein. When blood is dark red in color, it is depleted of oxygen. A steady flow usually indicates venous bleeding, because veins are under less pressure than arteries. Venous bleeding may be profuse, but it is usually easier to control than arterial bleeding because of its lower pressure.
- *Capillary bleeding*—Dark red, slowly oozing blood usually indicates damaged capillaries. In most cases capillary bleeding is easily controlled. This type of bleeding often clots spontaneously. However, if a large body surface is involved, bleeding may be profuse and the threat of infection great.

ASSESSMENT AND CARE: EXTERNAL BLEEDING

SCENE SIZE-UP AND INITIAL ASSESSMENT

Based on dispatch information, begin preparing for the call while still en route by putting on all the necessary personal protective equipment. If you are responding to a known scene of violence or to an accident, make certain that the appropriate support agencies have been notified (police have secured the scene, for example, or special extrication teams have been notified).

Upon arrival, make sure the scene is safe before you enter, and be sure to take notice of any potential mechanism of injury. Also note the number of patients at the scene. If more than one patient has profuse bleeding, more resources may be required to effectively treat them.

In most cases, get a general impression of the patient and the patient's mental status as you approach. When you reach the patient, assure the ABCs—airway, breathing, and circulation—and perform basic life support procedures as necessary. Serious bleeding, which is life-threatening, takes precedence over all other emergency medical care except that of the airway or breathing. In some cases, airway and breathing may be maintained at the same time as bleeding is brought under control.

EMERGENCY MEDICAL CARE

Severe external bleeding should be controlled during the initial assessment. Steps are listed below. A detailed discussion of each step is provided in the next segment.

1. *Maintain body substance isolation* by wearing all appropriate personal protective equipment.
2. *Apply direct pressure* to the site of the bleeding.
3. *Elevate the injured extremity.*
4. If direct pressure and elevation alone do not stop the bleeding, *use pressure points* to help stop bleeding in the upper and lower extremities.
5. *Immobilize injured extremities* to help control bleeding.
6. *As a last resort* to control bleeding of an amputated extremity, when all other methods of bleeding control have failed, *use a tourniquet.*
7. *Provide care for signs and symptoms of shock,* as detailed later in this chapter.

REMAINDER OF THE ASSESSMENT

After you have cared for life-threatening bleeding, continue to be alert for renewed bleeding as you progress through the focused history and physical exam, detailed physical exam, and ongoing assessment.

METHODS OF CONTROLLING EXTERNAL BLEEDING

DIRECT PRESSURE

The first method for controlling bleeding is direct pressure (Figures 29-3a to c). This is usually accomplished by placing a sterile gauze pad or dressing over the injury site and applying fingertip pressure directly to the point of bleeding. Large gaping wounds may require packing with sterile gauze and the application of direct hand pressure, if fingertip pressure fails (Figure 29-3d). If, during the initial assessment, you find a major bleed, apply pressure to the site with your gloved hand until dressings can be applied.

If bleeding persists, remove dressings and apply direct pressure to the point of bleeding. If diffuse bleeding is discovered, apply additional pressure.

ELEVATION

Elevation of an injured extremity should be used in conjunction with direct pressure to control bleeding. Elevate the arm or leg above the level of the heart to slow the flow of blood and aid in clotting.

If the extremity is painful, swollen, or deformed—indicating a possible bone or joint injury—elevate the extremity only after splinting.

PRESSURE POINTS

An artery that lies close to the surface of the skin over a bony prominence creates a pulse point. These sites are also called **pressure points** (Figure 29-4a). By compressing an artery at a pressure point (Figure 29-4b), arterial blood flow can be reduced in that extremity.

BLEEDING CONTROL BY DIRECT PRESSURE

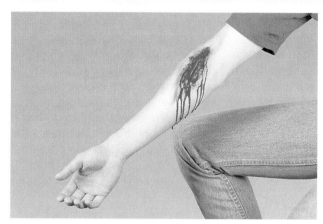

Figure 29-3a   Bleeding from a wound to the forearm.

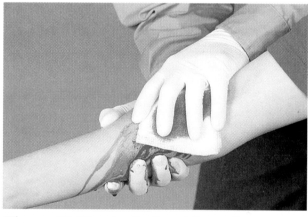

Figure 29-3b   Apply gloved fingertip pressure over a dressing directly on the point of bleeding.

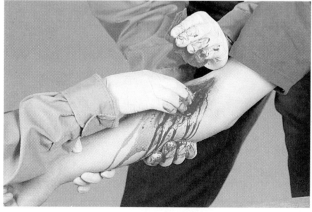

Figure 29-3c   If the bleeding does not stop, remove the dressing and apply direct pressure with gloved fingertips to the point of bleeding.

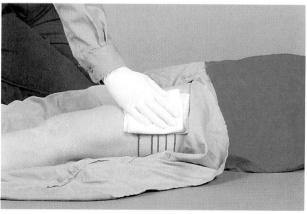

Figure 29-3d   Pack large gaping wounds with sterile gauze and apply direct pressure.

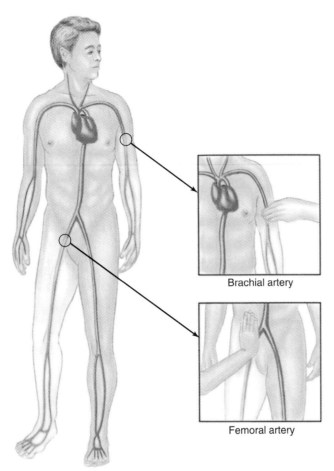

Brachial artery

Femoral artery

Figure 29-4a   Pressure points.

- For bleeding in the upper extremity, use the brachial pressure point (Figure 29-5a). It is located on the medial aspect of the arm, midway between the shoulder and the elbow. Use the flat surfaces of your fingers to compress the artery against the bone.
- For bleeding in a lower extremity, use the femoral pressure point, which is located in the crease between the abdomen and the groin (Figure 29-5b). It usually requires greater pressure than that applied to the brachial artery because there is more muscle mass to compress. After locating the femoral artery, use the heel of one hand to compress it.

Because a number of arteries supply each extremity, it may be necessary to apply pressure to a pressure point as well as direct pressure to the injury site to control major bleeding. Always reassess bleeding immediately after using a pressure point to assure that life-threatening bleeding has been controlled.

SPLINTS

Bleeding can be life-threatening in an open wound to an extremity with a possible bone or joint injury (one that presents as painful, swollen, or deformed). If left unsplinted, movement of broken bone ends or bone fragments can continue to damage surrounding tissues and blood vessels. Splinting the extremity may allow prompt control of bleeding associated with a possible bone injury. See Chapter 32, "Musculoskeletal Injuries," for more information on splints and splinting.

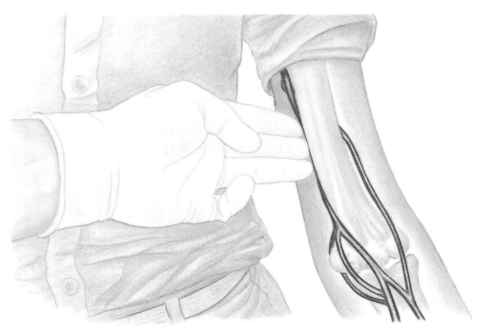

Figure 29-4b   Using pressure points can stop profuse bleeding in an arm or leg.

BLEEDING CONTROL WITH PRESSURE POINTS

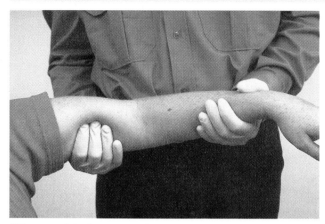

Figure 29-5a Apply pressure to the brachial artery pressure point to control bleeding from the arm.

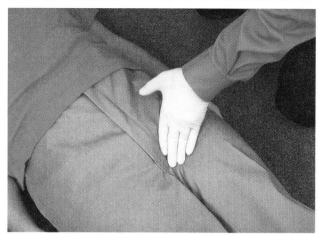

Figure 29-5b Apply pressure to the femoral artery pressure point to control bleeding from the leg.

PRESSURE SPLINTS

In addition to stabilizing bones, the inflated air splint (Figure 29-6a) exerts pressure that provides an extra measure of bleeding control. The pneumatic antishock garment (PASG—Figure 29-6b) can be used in a similar manner. If the injury is to the right leg, inflate only the right leg of the garment; if to the left leg, inflate the left leg. If there is injury to the pelvis, inflate the entire garment. (See, later in this chapter, information on use of the PASG to control shock. Follow local protocols and apply the PASG only with approval from medical direction.)

TOURNIQUETS

Tourniquets are used *only as a last resort* to control bleeding of an amputated extremity when all other methods have failed. Because it can cause all blood flow to an extremity to cease, a tourniquet should not be used for any injury other than an amputation. It can cause permanent damage to nerves, muscles, and blood vessels and may result in the loss of the affected extremity.

To apply a tourniquet, follow these directions (Figure 29-7):

1. Use a bandage four inches wide and four to six layers thick.

BLEEDING CONTROL WITH PRESSURE SPLINTS

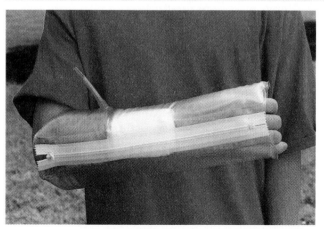

Figure 29-6a Air splints can be used to apply pressure and control bleeding from an extremity.

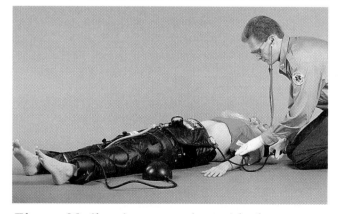

Figure 29-6b A pneumatic antishock garment (PASG) can be used to control severe bleeding in the lower extremities, with approval from medical direction.

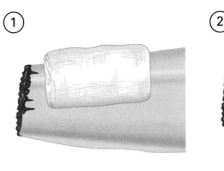
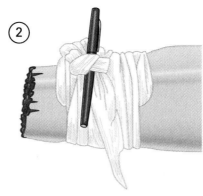
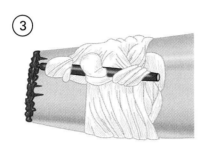

Figure 29-7 Application of tourniquet: (1) Apply pad. (2) Wrap a wide bandage around the extremity twice and tie it off. Then tie a stick-type object to the top. (3) Twist the stick-type object until bleeding stops. Secure it and document the time it was applied.

2. Wrap it around the extremity twice at a point proximal to the bleeding but as distal on the extremity and as close to the injury as possible.
3. Tie a knot in the bandage material, and place a stick-type object on top of it. Tie the ends of the bandage in a square knot over the stick-type object.
4. Twist the stick-type object until the bleeding stops.
5. After the bleeding has stopped, secure the stick-type object in place.
6. Notify other emergency personnel who will care for the patient that a tourniquet has been applied.
7. Document the use of the tourniquet and the time it was applied in the prehospital care report.

In some cases, a continuously inflated blood pressure cuff may be used as a tourniquet until bleeding stops. However, if this technique is used, the cuff needs to be monitored to maintain pressure.

When using any type of tourniquet, take the following precautions.

- Always use a wide bandage, never wire, a belt, or any other material that may cut the skin or underlying soft tissue.
- Once applied, secure the tourniquet tightly. Do not loosen or remove it unless you are directed to do so by medical direction. (A lethal effect known as tourniquet shock may result as toxins that have built up behind the tourniquet are suddenly released into the bloodstream.)
- Never apply a tourniquet directly over any joint, but as close to the injury as possible.
- Always make sure the tourniquet is in open view.

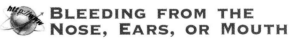

BLEEDING FROM THE NOSE, EARS, OR MOUTH

The EMT-B may encounter patients who are bleeding from the nose, ears, or mouth (Figure 29-8). These special areas may be cause for concern, because they can indicate a serious condition. Possible causes of bleeding from the nose, ears, or mouth include:

- Skull injury
- Facial trauma
- Digital trauma (nose picking)
- Sinusitis and other upper respiratory tract infections
- Hypertension (high blood pressure)
- Clotting disorders
- Esophageal disease

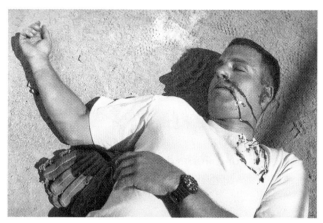

Figure 29-8   Bleeding from the nose, ears, or mouth could be a sign of serious illness or injury.

Any time you observe bleeding from a patient's ears or nose, suspect a possible skull fracture. If the patient has experienced a head injury, you should not attempt to stop the flow of blood, which could create pressure inside the skull causing even more damage. Instead, place a loose dressing around the area to collect the drainage and limit exposure to sources of infection.

Epistaxis, or nosebleed, is bleeding from the nose, which may result from injury, disease, or the environment. Usually this type of bleeding is more of an annoyance than a threat to life. However, in cases of extreme blood loss, shock (hypoperfusion) can develop.

To provide emergency medical care for nosebleed, place the patient in a sitting position and have him lean forward. Apply direct pressure by pinching the fleshy portion of the nostrils together (Figures 29-9a and b). Keep the patient as calm and as still as possible.

INTERNAL BLEEDING

Internal bleeding may result from a variety of causes, including blunt trauma, abnormal clotting within the body, rupture of a blood vessel or vascular structure, and as a result of certain fractures (especially pelvic fractures). Because it is not visible and seldom obvious, internal bleeding can result in severe blood loss with rapid progression of shock (hypoperfusion) and death—all in a matter of minutes.

SEVERITY

The severity of internal bleeding depends on the patient's overall condition, age, other medical condition, and source of the internal bleeding. The two most common sources of internal bleeding are injured or damaged internal organs and fractured extremities, especially fractures of the femur, hip, or pelvis. Always suspect internal bleeding if there are penetrating wounds to the skull, chest, or abdomen.

Suspicion and estimates of the severity of internal bleeding should be based on the mechanism of injury and signs and symptoms. *Always suspect internal bleeding in cases of unexplained shock (hypoperfusion).*

ASSESSMENT AND CARE: INTERNAL BLEEDING

SCENE SIZE-UP AND INITIAL ASSESSMENT

During your scene size-up, look for and evaluate potential mechanisms of injury. Your suspicion of internal bleeding may be based on the mechanism of injury you identify. Ask yourself questions such as *Did the patient fall? Is there a weapon or other item that might have caused trauma?* If, for example, the emergency involves a fall, motorcycle or automobile collision, pedestrian

CONTROLLING A NOSEBLEED

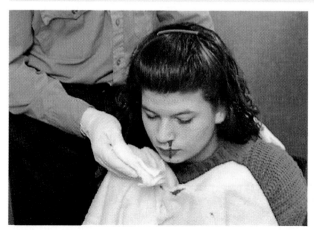

Figure 29-9a   Have the patient sit and lean forward.

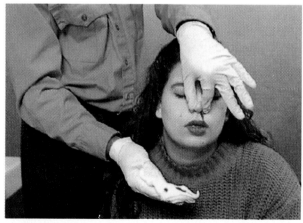

Figure 29-9b   Pinch the fleshy part of the nostrils together.

impacts, or blast, suspect blunt trauma and internal bleeding. Remember, too, that penetrating injuries can result in both external and internal bleeding.

When you are certain the scene is safe, approach the patient. Evaluate mental status and assure an open airway, adequate breathing, and adequate circulation. Provide basic life support as needed. Care for serious external bleeding.

FOCUSED HISTORY AND PHYSICAL EXAM

If the potential mechanism of injury and your general impression of the patient suggests internal bleeding, proceed to a thorough focused history and physical exam. If there is evidence of contusions, abrasions, deformity, impact marks, or swelling, treat the patient for internal bleeding. This is a priority patient; therefore, prepare for immediate transport.

Signs and Symptoms   Internal bleeding is not visible and may not be easily detectable. In some patients, by the time obvious signs and symptoms are present, it may be too late to provide effective emergency medical care. So be on guard for subtle changes in the patient's condition. Signs and symptoms of internal bleeding include:

- Pain, tenderness, swelling, or discoloration of suspected site of injury
- Bleeding from the mouth, rectum, vagina, or other orifice
- Vomiting bright red blood or blood the color of dark coffee grounds
- Dark, tarry stools, or stools with bright red blood
- Tender, rigid, and/or distended abdomen

Late signs and symptoms of internal bleeding, which indicate shock (hypoperfusion), are as follows:

- Anxiety, restlessness, combativeness, or altered mental status
- Weakness, faintness, or dizziness
- Thirst
- Shallow, rapid breathing
- Rapid, weak pulse
- Pale, cool, clammy skin
- Capillary refill greater than 2 seconds (most reliable in infants and children under 6)
- Dropping blood pressure
- Dilated pupils that are sluggish in responding to light
- Nausea and vomiting

EMERGENCY MEDICAL CARE

The goal of all emergency medical care for internal bleeding is to recognize its presence quickly, maintain the body's perfusion, and provide rapid transport to an appropriate medical facility.

1. *Take body substance isolation precautions* by wearing all appropriate personal protective equipment.
2. *Maintain an open airway and adequate breathing.* Provide positive pressure ventilation as necessary.
3. *Administer high-flow oxygen,* if you have not already done so in the initial assessment.
4. *Control external bleeding.* Splint any painful, swollen, or deformed extremity.
5. *Provide immediate transport* to critical patients with signs and symptoms of shock (hypoperfusion).
6. *Provide care for signs and symptoms of shock,* as detailed later in this chapter.

DETAILED PHYSICAL EXAM AND ONGOING ASSESSMENT

Continue to be alert for renewed bleeding as you progress through the detailed physical exam. Continually reevaluate the critical patient, performing an ongoing assessment every 5 minutes during transport.

SHOCK (HYPOPERFUSION)

Shock is known as **hypoperfusion** or *hypoperfusion syndrome.* It is the direct result of inadequate perfusion of tissue. When the cells of the body do not receive the oxygen and other nutrients they need, they begin to fail and die. If this condition persists, cell failure, organ failure, and death will follow (Figure 29-10). It is therefore imperative to the survival of the patient that shock (hypoperfusion) is recognized and treated promptly. Most forms of shock are not adequately treated in the field. Immediate transport is necessary.

Certain major organs of the body require an adequate blood flow in order to function properly. When bleeding continues unchecked, there is a reduction in circulating blood volume. In response, blood may be shunted or redirected from less important organs to more important organs. Since these important organs are located in the head and trunk, peripheral perfusion (to the extremities) and perfusion of the skin, for example, are drastically reduced.

Shock (hypoperfusion) should be suspected in any patient who has suffered or may have suffered trauma (Figure 29-11).

ASSESSMENT AND CARE: SHOCK (HYPOPERFUSION)

As in any case with potential for exposure to blood or body fluids, wear the appropriate personal protective equipment. If possible, put it on while en route to

CONTINUOUS CYCLE OF SHOCK

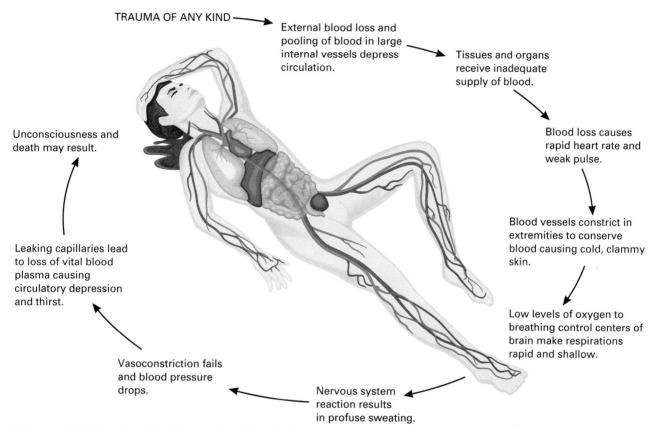

Figure 29-10   Continuous cycle of shock (hypoperfusion).

the scene to decrease the amount of time it takes to get to the patient.

SCENE SIZE-UP AND INITIAL ASSESSMENT

During scene size-up, be sure to take note of any potential mechanism of injury that may have caused external or internal bleeding. Penetrating injuries may prompt you to seek law enforcement resources and to reevaluate scene safety. When it is safe to approach the patient, assess the mental status to establish a baseline and perform the ABCs. Pay particular attention to airway maintenance and, if needed, provide positive pressure ventilation and high-flow oxygen.

FOCUSED HISTORY AND PHYSICAL EXAM

Monitor for signs and symptoms of shock (hypoperfusion) throughout the focused history and physical exam. Restlessness, anxiety, and an altered mental status may be the first signs of shock. If the patient ex-

hibits these signs, assess (or reassess) the patient for internal or external bleeding.

Monitor for peripheral perfusion and skin color, temperature, and condition, too. Peripheral blood flow will be decreased as internal bleeding progresses. This may cause weak, thready, or absent pulses in the distal extremities, and also cause the skin to become pale, cool, and clammy.

Signs and Symptoms When bleeding continues unchecked, the patient's vital signs will be affected. Establish a baseline as soon as possible. The signs and symptoms of shock are as follows (Figure 29-12):

- Mental status:
  - Restlessness
  - Anxiety
  - Altered mental status
- Peripheral perfusion and perfusion of the skin:
  - Pale, cool, clammy skin
  - Weak, thready, or absent peripheral pulses
  - Delayed capillary refill greater than 2 seconds in normal ambient air temperature (more reliable in infants and children under 6)

SHOCK

Watch for shock in all trauma patients. They can lose fluids not only externally through hemorrhage, or burns, but also internally through crush injuries and organ punctures.

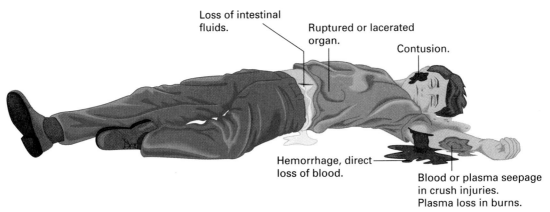

Loss of intestinal fluids.

Ruptured or lacerated organ.

Contusion.

Hemorrhage, direct loss of blood.

Blood or plasma seepage in crush injuries. Plasma loss in burns.

Figure 29-11   Shock as a result of trauma.

SIGNS AND SYMPTOMS OF SHOCK

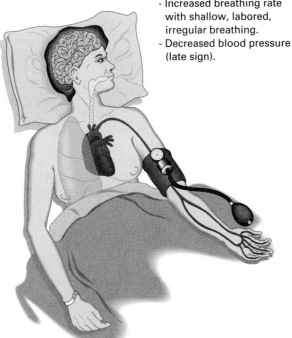

Mental status:

- Restlessness.
- Anxiety.
- Altered mental status.

Vital signs:

- Increased pulse rate (early sign) with weak and thready pulse.
- Increased breathing rate with shallow, labored, irregular breathing.
- Decreased blood pressure (late sign).

Peripheral perfusion:

- Pale, cool, clammy skin.
- Weak, thready, or absent peripheral pulses.
- Delayed capillary refill greater than two seconds in normal ambient air temperature (in infants and children only).

Other signs and symptoms:

- Dilated pupils.
- Marked thirst.
- Nausea and vomiting.
- Pallor.

Figure 29-12   Signs and symptoms of shock.

- Vital signs:
  - Increased pulse rate (early sign), with weak and thready pulse
  - Increased breathing rate that may be deep or shallow, labored, and irregular
  - Decreased blood pressure (late sign)
- Other signs and symptoms:
  - Dilated pupils (sluggish reaction)
  - Marked thirst
  - Nausea and vomiting
  - Pallor with cyanosis to the lips

Note: Infants and children can compensate, or maintain their blood pressure, until their blood volume is depleted by almost one-third. Then their condition will suddenly and radically deteriorate. If a child's blood pressure is dropping, it is an ominous sign.

EMERGENCY MEDICAL CARE

The treatment of shock (hypoperfusion) needs to occur early in the initial assessment and continue until transfer of care to the receiving medical facility is complete. The main priority in the care of this patient is to maintain perfusion to the vital organs and interrupt any progression or worsening of shock.

Emergency medical care of shock (hypoperfusion) is as follows (Figures 29-13a to d):

1. *Maintain body substance isolation precautions* by wearing the appropriate personal protective equipment during patient care.
2. *Maintain an open airway.* If breathing is adequate, *administer oxygen* via nonrebreather mask at 15 lpm. If breathing is inadequate, begin positive pressure ventilation with supplemental oxygen.

EMERGENCY CARE FOR SHOCK (HYPOPERFUSION)

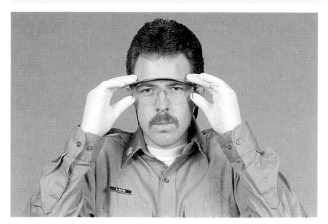

Figure 29-13a Take all necessary body substance isolation precautions.

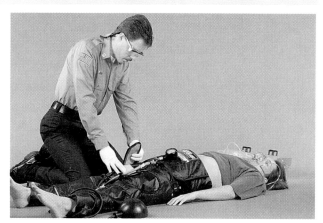

Figure 29-13b Administer oxygen by nonrebreather mask or positive pressure ventilation as needed. Apply the pneumatic antishock garment (PASG) if approved by medical direction.

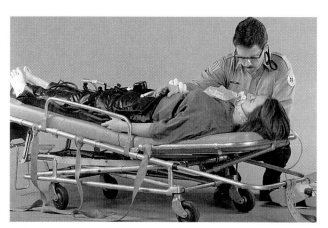

Figure 29-13c Elevate the lower extremities, if there are no serious injuries to the chest or abdomen and if no injury to the head, neck, or spine is suspected.

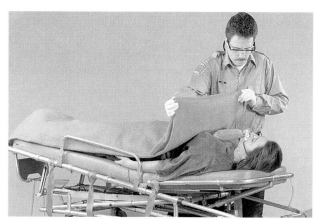

Figure 29-13d Cover the patient to prevent loss of body heat.

3. *Control any external bleeding* using the techniques described earlier in this chapter.
4. *If signs and symptoms of shock (hypoperfusion) are present, the lower abdomen is tender with a suspected pelvic injury (lower abdominal tenderness, pelvic instability), and there is no evidence of chest injury, apply and inflate the PASG (Figure 29-14), in accordance with local protocols and if approved by medical direction.* (For application of the PASG, see Figures 29-15a to i.)
5. *Elevate the lower extremities approximately 8 to 12 inches.* If the patient is on a long backboard, the foot of the board may be elevated, keeping the patient's body in line. (This positioning is controversial and may contribute to breathing diffi-

culty and other complications. Follow your local protocol.) *If the patient has injuries to the pelvis, lower extremities, head, chest, abdomen, neck, or spine, or if the shock may be due to cardiac compromise, keep the patient supine; do not elevate the feet.*
6. *Splint suspected bone or joint injuries.*
7. *Use a blanket to cover any patient suspected of suffering shock* (hypoperfusion) to prevent loss of body heat. Since the patient may have a decreased blood flow to nonvital organs, the body's heat regulation may be impaired.
8. *Transport the patient immediately.*

Note: Because of the ability of infants and children to compensate for shock by maintaining blood

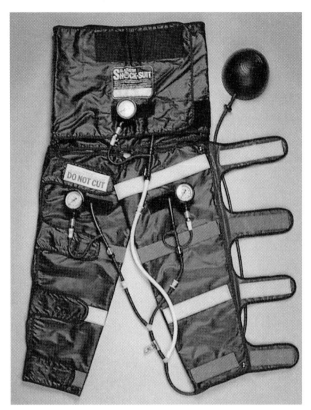

Figure 29-14   One type of pneumatic anti-shock garment (PASG)

pressure, followed by a sudden deterioration into severe and possibly irreversible shock, it is crucial in infants and children not to wait for signs of shock to appear but to treat the infant or child based on mechanism of injury or any suspicion of trauma. Remember also that a child's total blood volume is far less than that of an adult. Even a small loss of blood that would not be considered life-threatening for an adult should be considered critical in an infant or child. Immediate transport is crucial.

REMAINDER OF THE ASSESSMENT

Continue to assess the patient for changes in mental status and vital signs throughout the focused history and physical exam, detailed physical exam, and ongoing assessment. These may be conducted en route if early transport is initiated because of suspected shock.

SUMMARY: ASSESSMENT AND CARE

To review possible assessment findings and emergency care for bleeding and shock, see Figures 29-16 and 29-17.

ENRICHMENT

The enrichment section contains information that is valuable as background for the EMT-B but that goes substantially beyond the U.S. Department of Transportation (DOT) EMT-Basic curriculum.

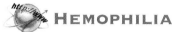 HEMOPHILIA

There are many different types of blood disorders. One you are likely to encounter from time to time is a clotting disorder called *hemophilia*. This disorder is a congenital disease (one the patient was born with) that prevents activation of the normal clotting mechanisms found in the blood. This means that even the smallest wound or cut in a patient with hemophilia can cause uncontrolled bleeding, usually into a joint space.

Bleeding in this patient is always considered to be significant. Provide emergency care for bleeding as for any patient. However, for the patient to obtain the special medication necessary to assist clot formation, transport to a medical facility immediately.

MORE ABOUT SHOCK

CAUSES OF SHOCK

There are four general causes of shock (hypoperfusion): fluid loss, pump failure, vasodilation (increased size of blood vessels), and hypoxia (inadequate oxygen).

- *Fluid loss*—Fluid can be lost from the circulatory system from injury that causes bleeding, burns that cause plasma loss, and dehydration. When the brain detects a fluid loss, it releases hormones that cause the heart to beat faster and blood vessels to decrease in size (vasoconstriction).
- *Pump failure*—If the heart is damaged (for example in a heart attack or trauma) and cannot pump enough blood to the body, it may lead to shock.
- *Vasodilation*—In some cases (as a result of spinal-cord damage, for example), the blood vessels will increase in size (dilate). When this happens, the heart is unable to keep perfusion and blood pressure at normal levels. There is not enough blood volume to fill the dilated vessels.
- *Hypoxia (inadequate oxygen)*—A severe chest injury, airway obstruction, or any other cause of respiratory difficulty may prevent an adequate amount of oxygen from entering the bloodstream. Without oxygen, perfusion is inadequate and the body's cells will begin to die.

TYPES OF SHOCK

Common types of shock include hypovolemic, vasogenic, anaphylactic, cardiogenic, and septic. Though there are different types, you do not need to be able to determine which type your patient might be suf-

APPLYING THE PASG

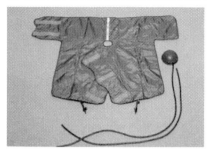

Figure 29-15a   Unfold PASG on a firm surface and open stop-cock valves.

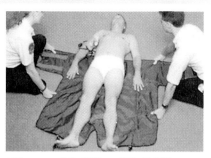

Figure 29-15b   Unfolding PASG on a long spine board or lifting apparatus is preferred. Then place or log roll the patient onto PASG so that it will be just below the patient's last rib.

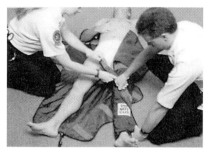

Figure 29-15c   Wrap the left leg of PASG around the patient's left leg and secure with Velcro strips.

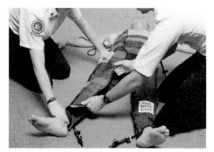

Figure 29-15d   Wrap the right leg of PASG around the patient's right leg and secure with Velcro strips.

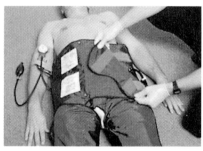

Figure 29-15e   Wrap the abdominal portion of PASG around the patient's abdomen and secure with Velcro strips.

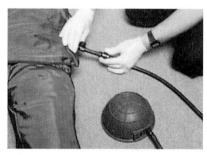

Figure 29-15f   Check tubes leading to pump and PASG and make sure stop-cock valves are open.

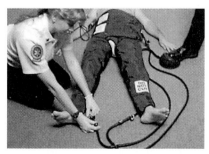

Figure 29-15g   Inflate with foot pump until systolic blood pressure stabilizes at 100 mmHg or until "pop-off" valve releases.

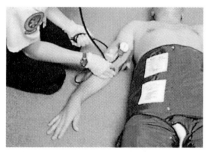

Figure 29-15h   Check the patient's blood pressure.

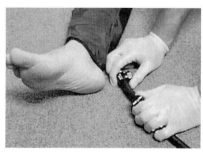

Figure 29-15i   Close stop-cock valve.

ASSESSMENT SUMMARY

BLEEDING AND SHOCK

The following are findings that may be associated with bleeding and shock.

SCENE SIZE-UP

Pay particular attention to your own safety. Look for:
Mechanism of injury
Splatters or pools of blood at scene
Blood-soaked clothing
Penetrating trauma
Blunt trauma

INITIAL ASSESSMENT

General Impression

Obvious massive external hemorrhage
Extremely pale color
Appears weak and ill

Mental Status

Alert to unresponsive, based on amount of blood loss
and shock
As blood loss continues, mental status decreases

Airway

May be closed if mental status is altered
May be bleeding in airway due to trauma

Breathing

Initially fast and normal to deeper volume
May become shallow and fast or slow as blood loss
and shock progress
May be absent or inadequate if bleeding in chest or
associated with chest injury
May be fast and shallow if abdominal injury is present

Circulation

Pulses possibly difficult to find due to extreme blood
loss
Increased heart rate that becomes extremely elevated,
then suddenly decreases with continued blood loss
Pulses becoming extremely weak or absent as blood
loss and shock continue
Skin becoming increasingly pale, cool, and clammy as
blood loss and shock progress

Status: Priority Patient

FOCUSED HISTORY AND PHYSICAL EXAM

Physical Exam

Head, Neck, and Face:
External bleeding
Blood from ear, nose, or mouth
Pupils dilated and sluggish to respond to light
Cyanosis
Pale oral mucosa
Chest:
Penetrating or blunt trauma to chest
Decreased breath sounds if bleeding into chest
cavity
Abdomen:
Rigid, distended abdomen
Discoloration around umbilicus or in the flank area
Penetrating or blunt trauma
Pain on palpation
Pelvis:
Unstable on palpation
Pain
Extremities:
Obvious external bleeding
Deformity or discoloration around femur(s)
Poor or absent peripheral pulses
Pale, cool, clammy skin
Cyanosis

Baseline Vital Signs

BP: decreasing or absent
HR: increased
RR: increased
Skin: pale, cool, clammy, cyanosis
Pupils: dilated and sluggish to respond

SAMPLE History

Signs and symptoms of blood loss and shock:
Anxiousness and anxiety
Decreasing mental status
Pale, cool, clammy skin
Decreasing blood pressure
Narrow pulse pressure
Tachycardia
Tachypnea
Poor or absent peripheral pulses
Dilated and sluggish pupils
Capillary refill greater than 2 seconds (infants and
children)

Figure 29-16a   Assessment summary: bleeding and shock.

EMERGENCY CARE PROTOCOL

BLEEDING AND SHOCK

1. Control any major life-threatening bleeding.
2. Establish manual in-line immobilization if spinal injury is suspected.
3. Establish and maintain open airway; insert naso-pharyngeal or oropharyngeal airway if patient is unresponsive and has no gag or cough reflex.
4. Suction secretions as necessary.
5. If breathing is inadequate, provide positive pressure ventilation with supplemental oxygen at a minimum rate of 12 ventilations/minute for an adult and 20 ventilations/minute for an infant or child.
6. If breathing is adequate, administer oxygen by nonrebreather mask at 15 lpm.
7. Control bleeding:
   Direct pressure (use fingertip pressure)
   Elevation
   Cold application
   Splint suspected fractures
8. If bleeding is not controlled, use appropriate pressure point until bleeding has stopped.
9. Apply sterile dressings and bandages.
10. Apply tourniquet only as last resort to control bleeding.
11. Maintain body temperature.
12. If abdominal tenderness and pelvic pain associated with signs and symptoms of shock, consider PASG.
13. Place patient supine. Legs may be elevated 8 to 12 inches. However, if injury to the pelvis, lower extremity, head, chest, abdomen, neck, or spine is suspected, do not elevate the legs.
14. If spinal injury suspected, immobilize patient to backboard.
15. Transport.
16. Perform ongoing assessment every 5 minutes.

Figure 29-16b   Emergency care protocol: bleeding and shock.

fering from. Most signs and symptoms of shock are common to all types; so, emergency medical treatment is the same.

- *Hypovolemic shock*—the result of a decrease in the volume of blood available for perfusion of the body's organs. The loss of blood in the circulatory system is caused either by external or internal bleeding. It may also result from a profound fluid loss from injury or illness, such as plasma loss due to burns or dehydration due to diarrhea, vomiting, or excessive urination.
- *Vasogenic shock*—usually the result of a spinal or head injury, which causes the nervous system to lose control over the vascular (vasogenic) system. Blood vessels dilate, causing blood to pool in the periphery (outer areas of the body away from the vital organs) and blood pressure to decrease.
- *Anaphylactic shock*—a result of the body's abnormal reaction to a foreign protein from a source such as a bee sting, food, or certain medications. The body reacts to the foreign substance by releasing chemicals that cause blood vessels to dilate and leak and the bronchioles to constrict. This reaction may have a rapid and severe onset. Without immediate emergency medical care, the patient may die. (See Chapter 20, "Allergic Reaction.")

- *Cardiogenic shock*—a result of inadequate pumping of the heart. Conditions that cause this include coronary artery disease, myocardial infarction (heart attack), heart valve disease, pulmonary embolism (blood clot), tension pneumothorax (air leak from the lung into the chest), or cardiac tamponade (fluid leaking in the sac surrounding the heart). Once cardiogenic shock begins, it is very difficult to reverse and must be treated very rapidly.
- *Septic shock*—a result of the toxins produced by a severe infection (usually bacterial in nature). The toxins cause a reaction that dilates the blood vessels and allows blood to pool in the extremities and fluid to leak from the blood vessels into the surrounding tissue.

STAGES OF SHOCK

Shock is progressive and advances in three distinct stages (Figure 29-18).

- *Compensatory shock*—In this first stage, the body is able to use its normal defense mechanisms to maintain perfusion and function. In most cases the patient does not exhibit any signs or symptoms. As the body detects a drop in blood pressure, it signals the heart to increase its rate and the blood vessels to constrict in an attempt to maintain the blood

EMERGENCY CARE ALGORITHM: BLEEDING AND SHOCK

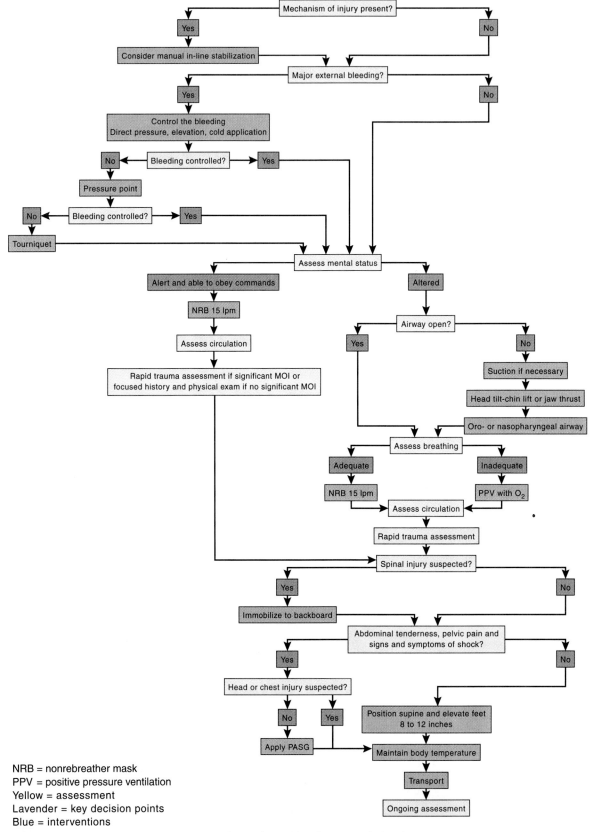

NRB = nonrebreather mask
PPV = positive pressure ventilation
Yellow = assessment
Lavender = key decision points
Blue = interventions

Figure 29-17 *Emergency care algorithm: bleeding and shock.*

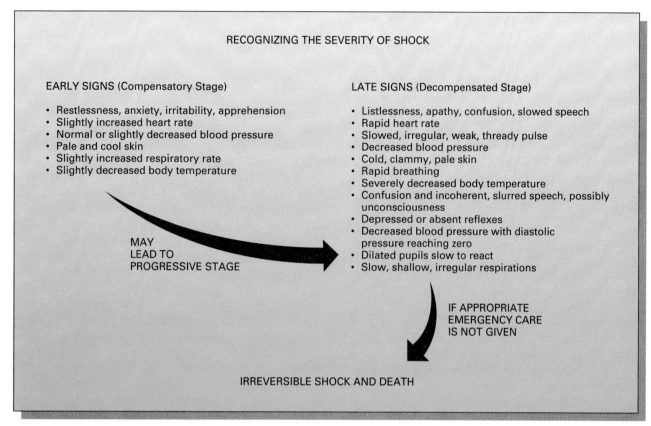

Figure 29-18   Recognizing the severity of shock.

pressure. If the blood loss is stopped, the body may replenish the lost volume within 24 hours.

- *Progressive (decompensated) shock*—The normal compensatory mechanisms of the body will work only for so long. If bleeding goes on uncontrolled, then the body works to maintain adequate perfusion to the vital organs. Blood will be shunted away from the less vital organs and redirected to the most vital organs—the brain, heart, and lungs. The

body will not be able to correct itself from this stage without outside intervention.

- *Irreversible shock*—This is the third and final stage, which cannot be reversed. Multi-system organ damage may produce signs and symptoms several days after the initial injury or illness as the body organs begin to die. Even with treatment, if shock has reached the irreversible stage, death will result.

CASE STUDY FOLLOW-UP

SCENE SIZE-UP

You and your partner have responded to a reported stabbing at Riverside High School. You arrive on the scene to find it has been secured. So you approach the patient, an unresponsive male lying supine on the ground with a large penetrating wound to the left upper quadrant of the abdomen. The wound is bleeding profusely. There is no impaled object, and no weapon visible.

INITIAL ASSESSMENT

Your general impression of the teenage patient is that he is critical and will require rapid transport to the hospital. You immediately tell your partner to get the stretcher. You begin to assess the patient's mental status and note that he is unresponsive to verbal stimuli but will grimace to painful stimuli. His airway is patent with rapid and shallow breathing at a rate of 34 per minute. You instruct one of the first responders to begin bag-value-mask ventilations with supplemental oxygen at 20/minute.

You cannot feel a radial pulse but can feel a carotid pulse which is weak and rapid with a rate of 120. Dark red blood is flowing profusely from the abdominal wound. You decide to quickly pack the wound with sterile dressings and tape the dressings in place.

Your partner and a first responder return with the stretcher and a pair of firefighter first responders who have just arrived on the scene. Since there are no other signs of external trauma, you decide not to use spinal precautions.

FOCUSED HISTORY AND PHYSICAL EXAM

Once the patient is on the stretcher and in the ambulance, you conduct a rapid trauma assessment that does not reveal signs or symptoms not already known, other than that the abdomen is rigid to palpation. The patient remains unresponsive.

Your partner obtains a set of vital signs. You notify the hospital via radio of your patient's condition and expected arrival in 7 minutes.

Your partner informs you that blood pressure is 72/40, pulse is 134, breathing is being assisted at a rate of 20, skin is pale, cool, and clammy. Although the external bleeding was profuse, you know that, because the wound site is the abdomen, the patient is most likely bleeding internally as well and suffering

from shock (hypoperfusion). You elevate the patient's feet approximately 8 to 12 inches, as you begin a rapid trauma assessment to find any additional wounds.

ONGOING ASSESSMENT

Transport time is short. There is time for only one ongoing assessment, which reveals no changes in the patient's condition. You arrive at the hospital and quickly unload the patient. You give a quick report to the waiting trauma team as you transfer care to them. You then begin the task of documenting the call on your prehospital care report. Your partner and the firefighters begin to clean and decontaminate the ambulance and equipment used during the call.

On the evening news, you learn that the patient died while in surgery. The next day you get a chance to talk to the Emergency Department physician who explains that the patient had a severely lacerated spleen and an abdomen filled with blood. You ask if you could have done anything different, or better, or faster. The doctor tells you there was nothing anyone could have done for this patient in the prehospital setting that you did not do, and she commends you for your work in attempting to control bleeding, assisting ventilations, and—especially—in transporting the patient without delay. The only satisfaction to be gained from this sad case is the knowledge that you were able to give the young patient the best possible chance.

CHAPTER REVIEW

TERMS AND CONCEPTS

You may wish to review the following terms and concepts included in this chapter.

epistaxis—bleeding from the nose resulting from injury, disease, or environment; a nosebleed.
pressure point—the point where an artery lies close

to the surface over a bony prominence. By compressing an artery at a pressure point, arterial blood flow can be reduced in an extremity.
shock (hypoperfusion)—the insufficient supply of oxygen and other nutrients to some of the body's cells that results from inadequate circulation of blood.

REVIEW QUESTIONS

1. Describe arterial, venous, and capillary bleeding.
2. List five ways to control external bleeding.
3. Explain (a) when and (b) how to use a tourniquet to control bleeding.
4. Name the two most common sources of internal bleeding.
5. List the signs and symptoms of internal bleeding, including late signs.
6. Describe emergency medical care of internal bleeding.
7. List the signs and symptoms of shock (hypoperfusion).
8. Describe emergency medical care of shock (hypoperfusion).

CHAPTER 30

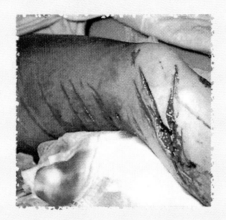

Soft Tissue Injuries

INTRODUCTION

Injuries to the soft tissues—the skin, muscles, nerves, blood vessels, and organs—are often dramatic but rarely life-threatening. However, they are serious if they lead to airway or breathing compromise, uncontrolled bleeding, or shock.

In general, emergency medical care emphasizes the control of bleeding, prevention of further injury, and reduction of the risk of infection. Unless life-threatening, care is usually accomplished after the initial assessment and prior to lifting and moving. Failure to recognize and provide care for soft tissue injuries may lead to severe, uncontrolled bleeding, possible additional injury including shock (hypoperfusion), or further contamination of the wound leading to an increased risk of infection.

OBJECTIVES

Numbered objectives are from the United States Department of Transportation 1994 EMT-Basic National Standard Curriculum. Asterisked objectives, if any, pertain to material that is supplemental to the DOT curriculum.

COGNITIVE

5-2.1   State the major functions of the skin. (p. 571)

5-2.2   List the layers of the skin. (p. 571)

5-2.3   Establish the relationship between body substance isolation (BSI) and soft tissue injuries. (pp. 572, 576)

5-2.4   List the types of closed soft tissue injuries. (pp. 571–572)

5-2.5   Describe the emergency medical care of the patient with a closed soft tissue injury. (pp. 572–573)

5-2.6   State the types of open soft tissue injuries. (pp. 573–576)

5-2.7   Describe the emergency medical care of the patient with an open soft tissue injury. (pp. 576, 578)

5-2.8   Discuss the emergency medical care considerations for a patient with a penetrating chest injury. (p. 578)

5-2.9   State the emergency medical care considerations for a patient with an open wound to the abdomen. (pp. 578–579)

5-2.10   Differentiate the care of an open wound to the chest from an open wound to the abdomen. (pp. 578–579)

5-2.21   List the functions of dressing and bandaging. (p. 581)

5-2.22   Describe the purpose of a bandage. (p. 581)

5-2.23   Describe the steps in applying a pressure dressing. (p. 582)

5-2.24   Establish the relationship between airway management and the patient with chest injury, burns, blunt, and penetrating injuries. (pp. 572, 578)

5-2.25   Describe the effects of improperly applied dressings, splints, and tourniquets. (p. 584)

5-2.26   Describe the emergency medical care of a patient with an impaled object. (pp. 579–580)

5-2.27   Describe the emergency medical care of a patient with an amputation. (pp. 580–581)

PSYCHOMOTOR

5-2.29   Demonstrate the steps in the emergency medical care of closed soft tissue injuries.

5-2.30   Demonstrate the steps in the emergency medical care of open soft tissue injuries.

5-2.31   Demonstrate the steps in the emergency medical care of a patient with an open chest wound.

5-2.32   Demonstrate the steps in the emergency medical care of a patient with open abdominal wounds.

5-2.33   Demonstrate the steps in the emergency medical care of a patient with an impaled object.

5-2.34   Demonstrate the steps in the emergency medical care of a patient with an amputation.

5-2.35   Demonstrate the steps in the emergency medical care of an amputated part.

5-2.40   Demonstrate completing a prehospital care report for patients with soft tissue injuries.

Additional objectives from DOT Lesson 5-2 are addressed in Chapter 31, "Burn Emergencies." Some of the objectives from DOT Lesson 5-2 are also addressed in Chapter 36, "Chest, Abdomen, and Genitalia Injuries."

C A S E   S T U D Y

THE DISPATCH

EMS Unit 14—respond to May's Coffee Shop at 154 Bayside Village for a man who was bitten by a dog while jogging—time out is 0740 hours.

ON ARRIVAL

While still en route, you get gloves, mask, and eye protection ready for both you and your partner—just in case. When your partner pulls up to the diner's parking lot, you spot the police unit. You ask one of the police officers where the dog is. She tells you the scene is safe and "the owner got the dog into the garage across the street. It's locked up for now."

The police officer affirms that there is only one patient. You and your partner exit the unit and move toward him. The jogger is sitting on the curb holding a towel to his left leg. As you approach him, you note that the bleeding has soaked through the towel.

"I'm Harvey Young," he calls out. "A dog bit me." How would you assess and care for this patient?

During this chapter, you will learn how to recognize and provide emergency care for soft tissue injuries. Later, we will return to the case study and put in context some of the information you learned.

THE SKIN

Review the description and function of the skin provided in Chapter 4, "The Human Body." You may recall that the skin is one of the most durable and largest organs of the body. It is composed of three layers—*the epidermis,* the *dermis,* and a *subcutaneous layer.* It protects the body from the environment, bacteria, and other organisms, and it helps to regulate the body's temperature. The skin also serves as a receptor organ that senses heat, cold, touch, pressure, and pain, and it aids in the elimination of water and various salts.

The term *wound* usually refers to an injury to the skin and underlying tissues. Wounds to the skin are categorized as *closed, open, single,* or *multiple.* These types of injuries are discussed in detail on the following pages.

CLOSED SOFT TISSUE INJURIES

A wound that is beneath unbroken skin is called a **closed injury.** There are three specific types of closed injuries: contusions, hematomas, and crush injuries.

CONTUSIONS

A **contusion,** or bruise, is an injury to the cells and blood vessels contained within the dermis (Figure 30-1). This type of injury will cause localized swelling and pain at the injury site. The patient may also have some discoloration at the injury site caused by blood leaking from damaged vessels and accumulating in the surrounding tissues.

HEMATOMAS

A **hematoma is** similar to a contusion, except that it usually involves damage to a larger blood vessel and a larger amount of tissue (Figure 30-2). It is characterized by a large lump with bluish discoloration caused by blood collecting beneath the skin. This blood may also separate tissues and pool in the pockets they form. A hematoma the size of the patient's fist can be equal to 10 percent blood loss, causing minimal signs and symptoms of shock (hypoperfusion).

CRUSH INJURIES

A **crush injury** is one in which force great enough to cause injury has been applied to the body. Severe blunt trauma or crushing force can cause serious damage to the underlying soft tissues with associated internal bleeding, resulting in shock (hypoperfusion).

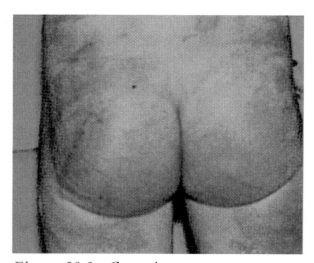

Figure 30-1   Contusions.

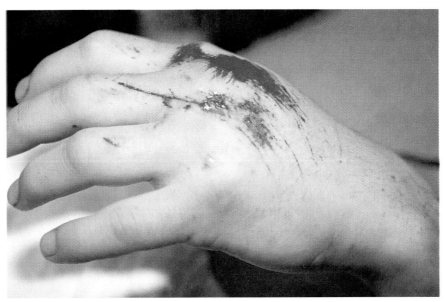

Figure 30-2   Hematoma.

Internal organs may actually rupture if a severe crush injury is sustained. Crush injuries can fall into either category, open or closed injuries. See Open Soft Tissue Injuries later in this chapter for more details.

ASSESSMENT AND CARE: CLOSED SOFT TISSUE INJURIES

SCENE SIZE-UP AND INITIAL ASSESSMENT

During your scene size-up, include a scan for the mechanism of injury. Be sure you have taken all body substance isolation (BSI) precautions before you approach the patient, including protective gloves.

When the scene is safe, approach the patient and conduct an initial assessment. If the mechanism of injury and your general impression of the patient suggest a possible spinal injury, establish in-line stabilization of the cervical spine. After assessing mental status and assuring adequate airway and breathing, check for and treat obvious signs of severe bleeding and shock. Administer oxygen by nonrebreather mask at 15 lpm, if indicated, or positive pressure ventilation with supplemental oxygen if breathing is inadequate.

FOCUSED HISTORY AND PHYSICAL EXAM

To begin the focused history and physical exam, reconsider the mechanism of injury to estimate the potential number and sites of impact to the patient. Perform a rapid trauma assessment, including a check for DCAP-BTLS. Assess baseline vital signs and take a SAMPLE history.

For patients without a significant mechanism of injury, the physical exam should be a focused trauma

assessment based on the components of the rapid trauma assessment for the specific injury site.

Signs and Symptoms Signs and symptoms of closed soft tissue injury include:

- Swelling, pain, and discoloration at the injury site
- Signs and symptoms of internal bleeding and shock (hypoperfusion) with severe injuries

EMERGENCY MEDICAL CARE

In general, small contusions do not require treatment. They usually heal by themselves. Larger contusions, hematomas, and crush injuries, however, can be an indication of serious underlying internal injuries and blood loss and can lead to compromised blood flow and nerve injury.

Steps to provide emergency medical care to closed soft tissue injuries are as follows:

1. *Take BSI precautions.* Since blood or body fluids may be present, be sure to wear protective gloves and other appropriate personal protective equipment. Remember to wash your hands thoroughly after the call, even if gloves were worn.
2. *Assure an open airway and adequate breathing.* Provide oxygen by nonrebreather mask at 15 lpm or positive pressure ventilation with supplemental oxygen as needed.
3. *Treat for shock (hypoperfusion), if necessary.* If you suspect significant blood loss, provide emergency care based on the mechanism of injury and the patient's signs and symptoms.
4. *Splint painful, swollen, deformed extremities.* Prevent a closed injury associated with possible bone

fracture from becoming an open injury, and relieve the patient's pain by immobilizing the injured extremity. The injured extremity should also be elevated, if possible.

DETAILED PHYSICAL EXAM AND ONGOING ASSESSMENT

If you performed a rapid trauma assessment, consider conducting a detailed physical exam. For the ongoing assessment, repeat the initial assessment and rapid or focused assessment, reassess and monitor vital signs, and recheck all interventions.

OPEN SOFT TISSUE INJURIES

When the skin breaks, the wound is called an **open injury.** In open injuries the patient is at risk for contamination with dirt and bacteria, which may lead to infection. Also, the open injury may be the first indicator of a deeper, more serious injury, such as a fracture or ruptured organ.

There are six general types of open injuries: abrasions, lacerations, avulsions, penetrations/punctures, amputations, and crush injuries (Figure 30-3).

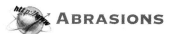 ## ABRASIONS

An **abrasion** generally is caused by scraping, rubbing, or shearing away of the epidermis, the outermost layer of the skin (Figure 30-4). Even though an abrasion is considered a superficial injury, it often is extremely painful because of the presence of exposed nerve endings. In most cases, blood will ooze from the wound (capillary bleeding), which can be controlled easily with direct pressure.

While small abrasions may not be life-threatening, abrasions to large areas of body surface may be cause for concern. For example, as a result of a motorcycle accident, a patient may slide across the pavement, causing head-to-toe abrasions ("road rash"). Bleeding in such a case may not be a serious threat; however, contamination, infection, and the potential for underlying injuries will be significant.

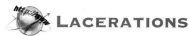 ## LACERATIONS

A break in the skin of varying depth, a **laceration** may be *linear* (regular) or *stellate* (irregular) (Figures 30-5 and 30-6a to b). Lacerations may bleed more than other types of open soft tissue injuries, especially when an artery is involved. Linear lacerations are usu-

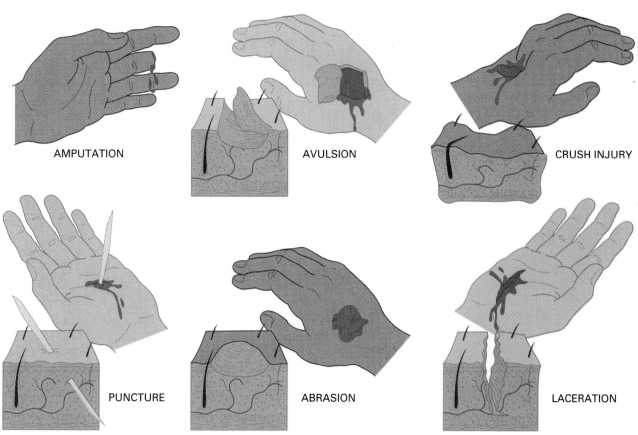

Figure 30-3 Classification of open injuries.

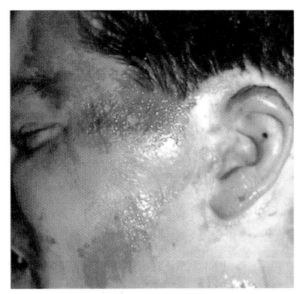

Figure 30-4   Abrasions.

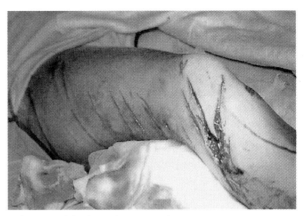

Figure 30-6a   Lacerations.

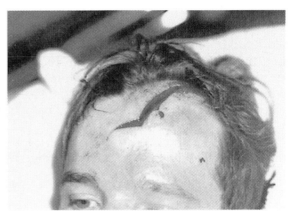

Figure 30-6b   Laceration.

ally caused by a knife, razor, or broken glass. They usually heal better than stellate injuries because the wound has smooth edges. Stellate lacerations are commonly caused by a blunt object. The edges of the wound will be jagged and healing may be prolonged.

AVULSIONS

An **avulsion** is a loose flap of skin and underlying soft tissue that has been torn loose or pulled completely off (Figures 30-7a to b). Bleeding may be severe due to blood vessel injury, although some blood vessels may tamponade (compress) themselves by retracting into the soft tissue. Healing will be prolonged and scarring may be extensive.

Avulsions are most commonly a result of accidents with industrial or home machinery and motor vehicles. They commonly involve the fingers, toes, hands, feet, forearms, legs, ears, and nose. A small amount of blood loss does not negate the possibility of a serious injury. The severity of an avulsion is di-

rectly related to the effectiveness of circulation and perfusion distal to the injury.

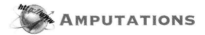

AMPUTATIONS

An **amputation** involves a disruption in the continuity of an extremity or other body part (Figures 30-8a to c). Amputations are the result of ripping or tearing forces often associated with industrial or motor vehicle accidents. Bleeding from amputations may be massive. However, in most cases due to the elasticity of the blood vessels, very little bleeding occurs. An incomplete amputation typically bleeds more than a complete amputation. Always consider shock (hypoperfusion) in cases of amputation.

PENETRATIONS/PUNCTURES

A **penetration/puncture** injury generally is the result of a sharp, pointed object being pushed or driven into the soft tissues (Figure 30-9). The entry wound may appear very small and cause little bleeding. However, such injuries may be deep, damaging, and cause severe internal bleeding. The overall severity of the injury depends on the location, the size of the penetrating object, the depth of penetration, and the

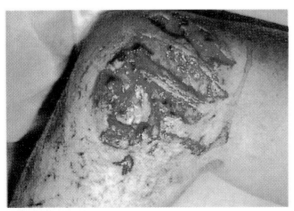

Figure 30-5   Lacerations and deep abrasions.

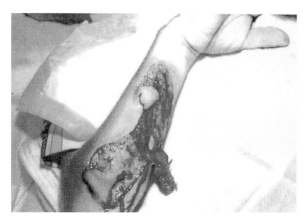

Figure 30-7a   Forearm avulsion.

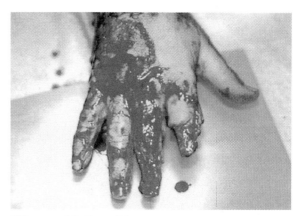

Figure 30-8a   Finger amputation.

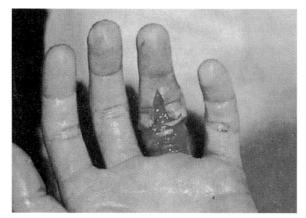

Figure 30-7b   Ring avulsion.

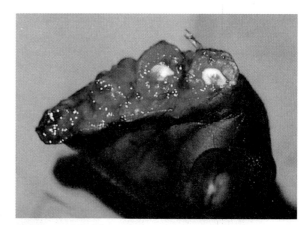

Figure 30-8b   Finger amputations.

forces involved in creating the injury. It can be difficult to determine the extent of injury based on the external wound. Therefore, treat these injuries with great caution.

Gunshots may cause both an entrance and an exit wound (Figures 30-10a to f). In general, the entrance wound is smaller than the exit wound and, if the patient was shot at close range, the entrance wound will be surrounded by powder burns. The exit wound is usually larger and will bleed more profusely. Remember to assess for the possibility of multiple gunshot wounds, especially in areas covered with hair.

Stab wounds may be easily detected or may be small and hidden by clothing or body parts, such as an extremity. Expose the patient and carefully inspect all areas of the body so that a potentially life-threatening injury is not missed. Always assess the patient for underlying internal injuries and shock (hypoperfusion).

CRUSH INJURIES

Usually the result of blunt trauma or crushing forces, crush injuries may not appear to be serious (Figure 30-11). The only external sign may be an injury site

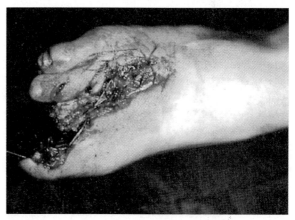

Figure 30-8c   Toe amputation.

that is painful, swollen, deformed. External bleeding may be minimal or absent. In fact, always suspect that there may be internal injury and severe internal bleeding in the presence of crush injuries.

Patients with crush injuries may appear to be unaffected at first. However, they can deteriorate rapidly into shock (hypoperfusion). This typically occurs when the object causing the crush injury is lifted

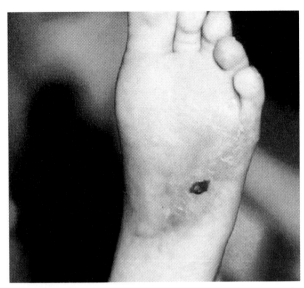

Figure 30-9   Penetration/puncture wound to the foot.

from the patient. The object will initially tamponade, or restrict, any bleeding while it is against the body. Then, when released, the blood vessels or internal organs will begin to bleed freely and profusely.

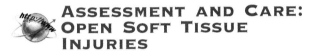

ASSESSMENT AND CARE: OPEN SOFT TISSUE INJURIES

If you are responding to a known scene of violence or to an accident, check with dispatch to make certain that the appropriate support agencies have been notified (police have secured the scene, for example, or special extrication teams have been notified). Since there is an increased likelihood of exposure to blood or body fluid when you treat a patient with open injuries, be sure to wear the appropriate personal protective equipment, including gloves and eye protection. In cases of potential splattering, a protective mask and gown should be worn.

SCENE SIZE-UP AND INITIAL ASSESSMENT

Make sure the scene is safe before you enter, and take notice of potential mechanisms of injury. Be prepared to stabilize the cervical spine if the mechanism of injury or signs and symptoms suggest it may be necessary.

In most cases, get a general impression of the patient and the patient's mental status as you approach. When you reach the patient, assure an open airway. If severe injuries are suspected or apparent and breathing is adequate, provide oxygen by nonrebreather mask at 15 lpm. If breathing is inadequate, initiate positive pressure ventilation with supplemental oxygen. Bring any severe bleeding under control.

FOCUSED HISTORY AND PHYSICAL EXAM

Begin the focused history and physical exam with a rapid trauma assessment. Assess baseline vital signs, and take a SAMPLE history. For patients without a significant mechanism of injury, perform a focused trauma assessment, using components of the rapid assessment for the specific injury site.

Signs and Symptoms   The signs and symptoms of open soft tissue injuries include:

- A break in the skin and external bleeding
- Localized swelling, pain, and discoloration at the injury site
- Possible signs and symptoms of internal bleeding and shock (hypoperfusion)

EMERGENCY MEDICAL CARE

Unless bleeding is severe, most emergency care for open soft tissue injuries is performed after the initial assessment.

1. *Take BSI precautions.*
2. *Assure an open airway and adequate breathing.* Provide oxygen by nonrebreather mask at 15 lpm or positive pressure ventilation with supplemental oxygen as needed.
3. *Expose the wound.* In order to completely assess the wound, expose the entire injury site. Cut away clothing and, if necessary, clear the area of blood and debris with sterile gauze, dressings, or the cleanest material available. Remember to thoroughly assess and evaluate the patient for additional wounds or injuries.
4. *Control the bleeding.* Use a pressure point if bleeding is not controlled with direct pressure and elevation. Use a tourniquet only as a last resort when all other methods to control bleeding have failed.
5. *Prevent further contamination.* Keep the wound as clean as possible. If there are loose particles of foreign material around the wound, wipe them away with a sterile gauze or similar clean material. Always wipe away from the wound never toward it. Never pick out embedded particles or debris.
6. *Dress and bandage the wound.* If not already done, apply a dry sterile dressing. Secure it with a bandage. Check distal pulses both before and after applying the bandage to be sure it is not too tight.
7. *Keep the patient calm and quiet.* Remember that an early sign of shock (hypoperfusion) is restlessness. In addition, the more excited a patient becomes, the higher the heart rate and blood pressure, which may lead to increased bleeding.
8. *Treat for shock (hypoperfusion).* If signs and symptoms are present, provide the appropriate care.
9. *Transport.*

GUNSHOT WOUNDS

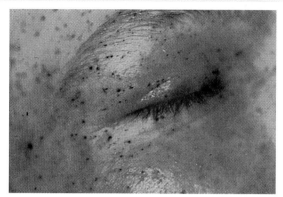

Figure 30-10a   Powder burns from gunshot.

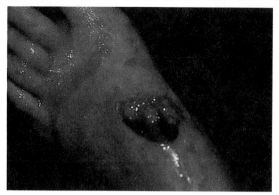

Figure 30-10b   Gunshot wound to the foot.

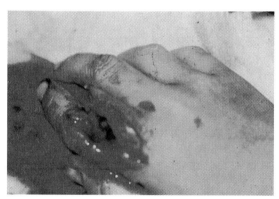

Figure 30-10c   Gunshot wound to the finger.

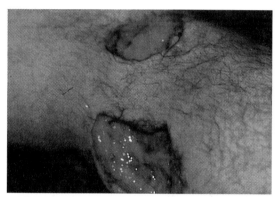

Figure 30-10d   Gunshot entrance and exit wounds to lower leg.

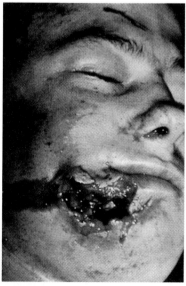

Figure 30-10e   Gunshot wound to chin.

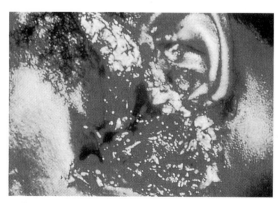

Figure 30-10f   Gunshot wound to side of head.

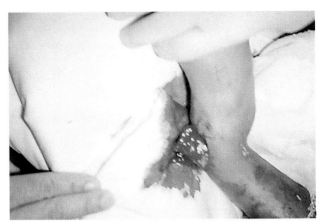

Figure 30-11 Crush injury, open wound.

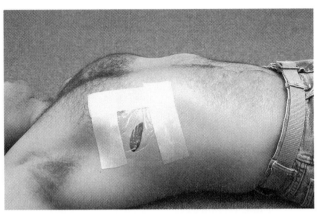

Figure 30-12 Open chest injury with occlusive dressing taped on three sides. (Shout Picture Library)

DETAILED PHYSICAL EXAM AND ONGOING ASSESSMENT

If a rapid trauma assessment was performed, consider performing a detailed physical exam en route. Perform an ongoing assessment by repeating the initial assessment, rapid or focused assessment, monitoring vital signs, and rechecking interventions.

SPECIAL CONSIDERATIONS

All of the above emergency care steps apply to the specific injuries discussed in additional detail below: chest injuries, abdominal injuries, impaled objects, amputations, and large open neck injuries. *In all of these cases, ensure an open airway; administer oxygen by nonrebreather mask at 15 lpm or, if breathing is inadequate, provide positive pressure ventilation with supplemental oxygen.*

Chest Injuries   A chest injury may prevent adequate respiration. In cases of penetrating chest wounds:

1. *Use an occlusive dressing to prevent air from entering the chest cavity through the wound* (a condition known as an *open pneumothorax*). An **occlusive dressing** (one that can form an air-tight seal), such as Vaseline gauze, household plastic wrap, or the plastic bag from a dressing or oxygen mask should be secured with tape on three sides (Figure 30-12). For an open chest wound, leave one side untaped in order to allow air to escape as the patient exhales. This will prevent a condition called *tension pneumothorax*, a severe build-up of air in the chest cavity that compresses the lungs and heart toward the uninjured side.

2. *If there is no suspected spinal injury, the patient may assume a position of comfort or any position that allows for easiest chest expansion.* (However, with any significant mechanism of injury to the chest, including gunshots, spinal injury should be assumed. Spinal immobilization must be established and maintained.)

Abdominal Injuries   Abdominal wounds sometimes result in an **evisceration** (internal abdominal organs protrude through the wound). Follow these guidelines when dealing with such an injury:

1. *Do not touch the abdominal organs or try to replace the exposed organs.* You may cause further damage and increase contamination of the organs and abdominal cavity.

2. *Cover the exposed organs.* Use a sterile dressing moistened with sterile water or saline. The dressing should be large enough to cover all of the protruding organs. Sterile gauze is preferred. Avoid all absorbent materials, such as toilet tissue or paper towels, which may cling to the organs. Then loosely cover the moistened dressing with an occlusive dressing (Figure 30-13). Maintain temperature with layers of a more bulky dressing, such as a particle-free bath blanket or towel. The

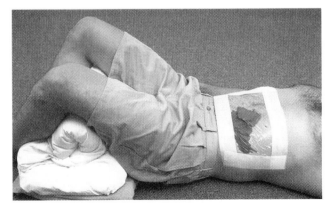

Figure 30-13 Cover the abdominal organs with moist sterile dressing and an occlusive covering.

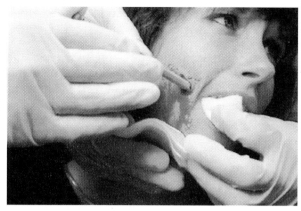

Figure 30-14   Impaled object in the cheek may be removed. Dress outside of wound and inside between cheek and teeth.

dressings may be held loosely in place with a bandage or clean sheet. Do not apply the abdominal portion of the PASG if it is used in your system.

3. *Flex the patient's hips and knees, if they are uninjured and if spinal injury is not suspected.* This will help to decrease the tension of the abdominal muscles. Placing pillows or other materials under the patient's knees also may be helpful. (However, suspect spinal injury with a significant mechanism of injury to the abdomen.)

Impaled Objects An **impaled object** (an object still embedded in a wound) should never be removed in the field, unless it is through the cheek or the neck and obstructing air flow through the trachea (Figure 30-14).

Emergency medical care for a patient with an impaled object includes the following (Figures 30-15a to c):

1. *Manually secure the object.* Prevent any motion, which can cause further damage and bleeding.

STABILIZING AN IMPALED OBJECT

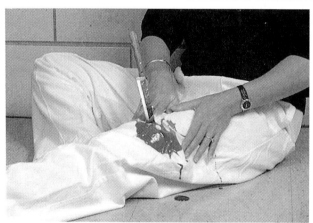

Figure 30-15a   An impaled kitchen knife.

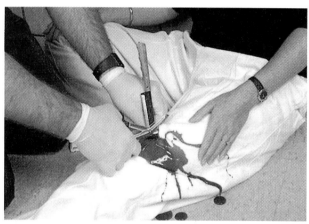

Figure 30-15b   Cut away clothing.

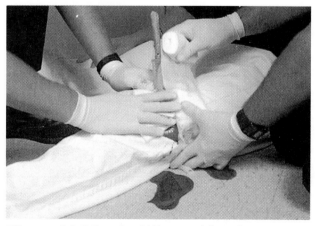

Figure 30-15c   Stabilize and bandage the object in place.

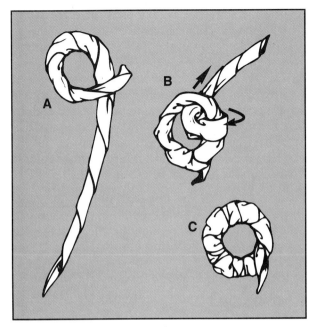

Figure 30-16 An impaled object can be encircled and immobilized with a ring pad, which can be improvised from a cravat, handkerchief, stocking, or small towel. Bandage in place.

2. *Expose the wound area.* Remove clothing from around the wound, but remember that care must be taken to cause no further motion of the object.
3. *Control bleeding.* Apply direct pressure to the wound edges. Avoid putting undue pressure on the impaled object.
4. *Use a bulky dressing to help stabilize the object.* Surround the entire impaled object with dressings. Pack them around the object, and tape it securely in place to avoid motion during transport. A ring or doughnut pad may be used to stabilize the object (Figure 30-16). If in the ab-

domen, do not inflate the abdominal portion of the PASG if it is used in your system.

Amputations In amputation injuries, you must care for the amputated part, as well as for the patient and the injury site. Your handling of the amputated part can have significant impact on the success of surgical reattachment.

First provide emergency medical care to the patient. Do not spend time looking for the amputated body part. If possible, other EMS or support personnel should be enlisted to search for any missing body parts. Once the body part is located, follow these guidelines (Figure 30-17):

1. *Wrap the part in a dry sterile gauze dressing.* (Check with local medical direction, which may dictate the use of moist dressings instead.) Never immerse the part in water or sterile saline, since this may damage it.
2. *Wrap or bag the amputated part in plastic.* Place it a plastic bag or plastic wrap in accordance with local protocol. Label the bag with the patient's name, date, and time the part was wrapped and bagged.
3. *Keep the amputated part cool.* Place the wrapped and bagged part in a cooler or other suitable container with an ice pack or ice on the bottom to keep the part cool. Do not place the part directly on the ice pack or ice unless well insulated to avoid any possibility of freezing the part. The container should also be marked with the patient's name, date, and body part.
4. *Transport the part with the patient, if at all possible.* In some cases, however, this may not be possible, especially when the part has not been located. In this instance, arrange for immediate transport of the body part, once it is found, to the same facility to which the patient has been transported.

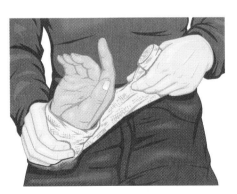
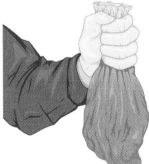
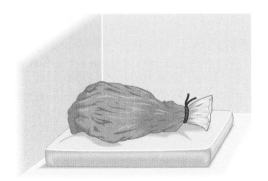

(1) Wrap completely in sterile dressings.

(2) Place in plastic bag and seal shut.

(3) Place sealed bag in a cooler or other suitable container to keep it cool.

Figure 30-17 Emergency care for amputated part. Follow local protocol.

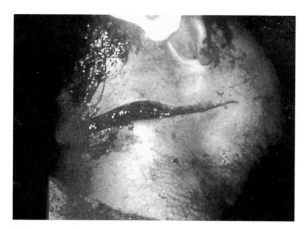

Figure 30-18   Open wound to the neck.

Note: If an amputation is incomplete and the body part is still partially attached, do not complete the amputation. Care for the wound as previously described, but also make sure that the partially amputated part is not twisted or constricted. Immobilize the injured area to prevent further injury.

Large Open Neck Injuries   In addition to severe bleeding from a wound involving the major blood vessels of the neck, there is the danger of air being sucked into a neck vein and carried to the heart, which can be lethal. Bleeding control and prevention of an **air embolism** (air bubble) are the major goals (Figure 30-18). Assess any neck wound for major blood vessel involvement. Arterial bleeding will be profuse with bright red blood spurting from the wound and is a grave sign. Venous bleeding will be dark red and flowing very steadily from the wound.

In general, follow these guidelines for care of a large open neck wound:

1. *Place a gloved hand over the wound to control bleeding.*
2. *Apply an occlusive dressing,* which should extend beyond all wound edges to avoid air or part of the dressing being sucked into the wound. Tape the dressing on all four sides.
3. *Cover the occlusive dressing with a regular dressing.*
4. *Apply only enough pressure to control the bleeding.* Compress the carotid artery only if it is severed and it is necessary to control bleeding.
5. *Once bleeding is controlled, apply a pressure dressing,* taking care not to restrict air flow or compress the major blood vessels in the neck. Such a dressing should not be applied circumferentially around the neck. (Direct pressure is preferred.)
6. *If there is a suspected spinal injury, provide appropriate immobilization.* Spinal injury should al-

ways be suspected with any significant injury or mechanism of injury to the neck.

DRESSINGS AND BANDAGES

DRESSINGS

A **dressing** covers an open wound to aid in the control of bleeding and to prevent further damage or contamination. The dressing should be **sterile,** or free of any organisms (bacteria, virus, or spore) that may cause infection. Commercially wrapped and packaged dressings are available in various types and sizes.

Common types of dressings include (Figures 30-19a to d):

- *Gauze pad*—Available in various sizes (2″ × 2″, 4″ × 4″, 5″ × 9″, and so on), a gauze pad is made of layered gauze.
- *Self-adhering dressing*—This type of dressing adheres to itself when overlapped. It is available in various sizes and may also be used as a roller bandage.
- *Universal or multi-trauma dressing*—This is a bulky dressing, usually 10″ × 36″, and is used on large areas such as abdominal wounds. (Also called ABD pads.)
- *Occlusive dressing*—This dressing creates an airtight seal for open abdominal, chest, and large neck injuries. A petroleum-type occlusive dressing is impregnated with petroleum to prevent adhering to the open wound. An improvised occlusive dressing may be made from sterile plastic wrap, plastic bags, or a similar material.

Note: Plastic is preferred over aluminum foil as an occlusive dressing, because foil has been found to cause further damage to exposed internal organs.

BANDAGES

Once a dressing is applied, a **bandage** is used to secure a dressing in place (Figures 30-20a to g). In most cases it is not necessary for a bandage to be sterile, but it should be clean and free of debris. Bandages that may be used as dressings are also available in various types and sizes. Common types of bandages include:

- *Self-adhering bandage*—This type of bandage adheres to itself when overlapped. It may be used as a dressing or as a roller bandage (Figures 30-21a to c).
- *Gauze rolls*—Available in various sizes, this bandage is rolled meshed gauze.
- *Triangular bandage*—This bandage is usually a forty-inch square piece of cloth (Figure 30-22). When folded to form a two- or three-inch-wide cravat, it may be used as a bandage to secure dressings.

DRESSINGS

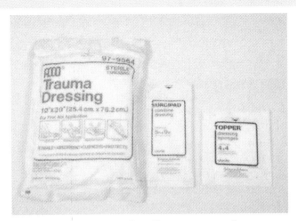

Figure 30-19a Sterile gauze pads.

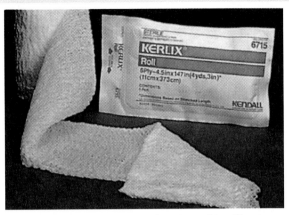

Figure 30-19b Nonelastic, self-adhering dressing and roller bandages.

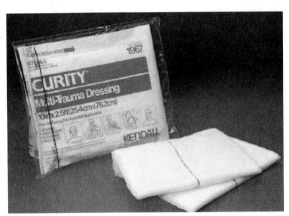

Figure 30-19c Multi-trauma dressings.

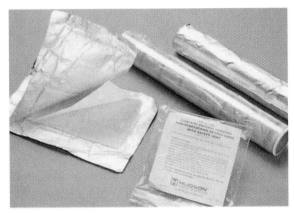

Figure 30-19d Occlusive and petroleum gauze dressings.

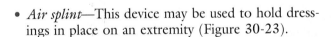

- *Air splint*—This device may be used to hold dressings in place on an extremity (Figure 30-23).

PRESSURE DRESSINGS

A pressure dressing can be used to maintain control of bleeding. Apply a pressure dressing in the following way:

1. *Cover the wound with several sterile gauze dressings or a sterile bulky dressing.*
2. *Apply hand pressure* over the wound until the bleeding is controlled.
3. *Bandage* firmly to create enough pressure to maintain control of the bleeding. Check distal pulses to be sure the bandage is not too tight. An air splint or blood pressure cuff can also be used to hold a pressure dressing in place. If a blood pressure cuff is used, be sure that distal pulses are still present after inflation.
4. If blood soaks through the original dressing and bandage, do not remove them as this will aggra-

vate the bleeding. Instead, *apply additional dressings and bandage over the original ones.*

GENERAL PRINCIPLES OF DRESSING AND BANDAGING

There are no hard-and-fast rules for dressing and bandaging wounds. Often, adaptability and creativity are far more important ingredients. In dressing and bandaging, use the materials you have on hand and the methods you can best adapt, as long as the following conditions generally are met:

- *Dressing materials should be as clean as possible.* Sterile materials are always preferable. When you open dressing packages or handle any materials you will use as dressings, do so carefully in order to keep those materials as free of dirt and debris as possible.
- *Do not bandage a dressing in place until bleeding has stopped.* The exception is a pressure dressing, which is designed to help stop hemorrhaging.

BANDAGING

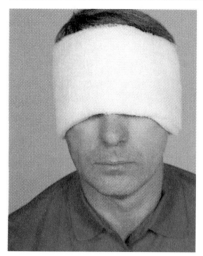

Figure 30-20a *Head and/or eye bandage.*

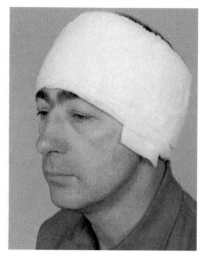

Figure 30-20b *Head and/or ear bandage.*

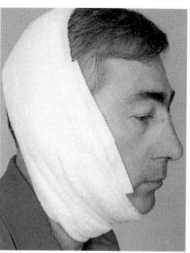

Figure 30-20c *Cheek bandage (be sure the mouth will open).*

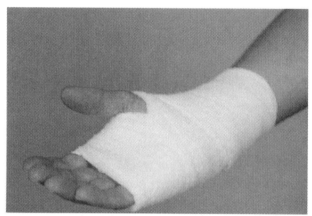

Figure 30-20d *Hand bandage.*

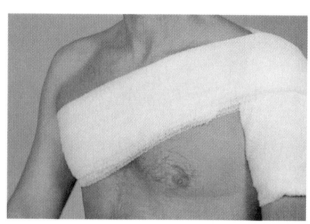

Figure 30-20e *Shoulder bandage.*

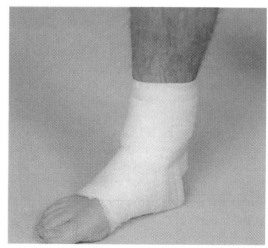

Figure 30-20f *Foot and/or ankle bandage.*

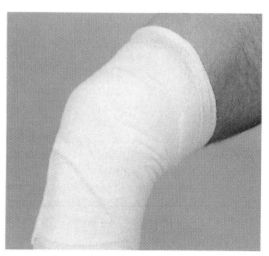

Figure 30-20g *Knee bandage.*

THE SELF-ADHERING ROLLER BANDAGE

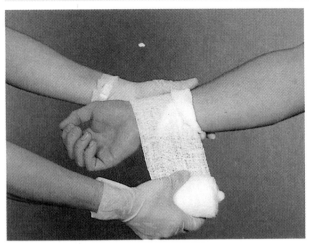

Figure 30-21a Secure the self-adhering roller bandage with several overlying wraps.

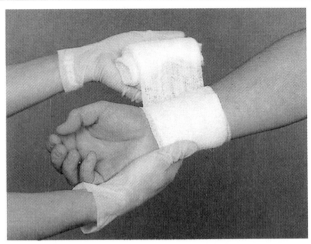

Figure 30-21b Overlap the bandage, keeping it snug.

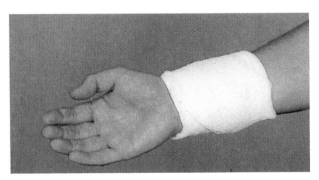

Figure 30-21c When the bandage covers an area larger than the wound, secure with tape or tie it in place.

- *A dressing should adequately cover the entire wound.* All edges of a dressing should be covered by the bandage. Tape bandages in place or secure with a square knot. Make sure there are no loose ends of cloth, gauze, or tape that could get caught when the patient is transported.
- *If possible, remove all jewelry* from the injured body part. Jewelry may cause further damage if swelling occurs.
- *Do not bandage a wound too loosely.* Bandages should not slip or shift and should not allow the dressing beneath to slip or shift.
- *Bandage wounds snugly, but not too tightly.* Be careful not to interfere with circulation. If the injured part involves the hands or feet, leave the tips of the toes or fingers exposed to allow for distal circulation assessments. For circumferential bandages, check distal pulses, motor, and sensory function before and after bandage application.

- *If you are bandaging a small wound on an extremity, cover a larger area with the bandage.* This will help avoid creating a pressure point, and it will distribute pressure more uniformly.
- *Always place the body part to be bandaged in the position in which it is to remain.* Avoid bandaging across a joint, and do not try bending a joint after the bandage has been applied.
- *Apply a tourniquet only as a last resort.* Since a tourniquet cuts off all circulation, it will cause severe damage to the distal extremity. Once in place, a tourniquet must not be removed in the field.

SUMMARY: ASSESSMENT AND CARE

To review possible assessment findings and emergency care for soft tissue injuries, see Figures 30-24 and 30-25.

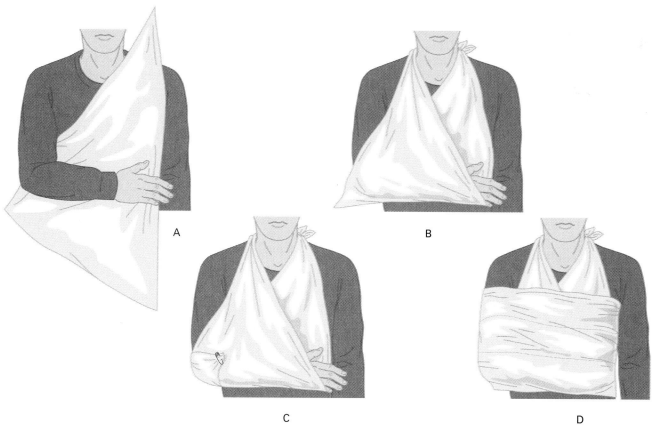

Figure 30-22   Triangular bandage as arm sling.

ENRICHMENT

The enrichment section contains information that is valuable as background for the EMT-B but that goes substantially beyond the U.S. Department of Transportation (DOT) EMT-Basic curriculum.

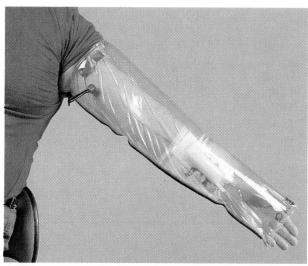

Figure 30-23   Example of inflatable air splint.

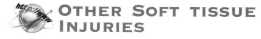

OTHER SOFT TISSUE INJURIES

BITES

Dog bites are a common type of animal bite. The soft tissue injuries caused by dog bites are usually to the hands, arms, and legs, although some occur on the head and face (Figure 30-26). The most common complications include infection, *cellulitis* (inflammation of skin cells), *tetanus* (lock jaw), and *septicemia* (blood infection). *Rabies* is also a concern, although rare. Human bites may cause *hepatitis* (inflammation of the liver).

Generally, bite wounds are a combination of penetration/puncture injuries and crush injuries, which may also involve internal organs and bones. Severity of a bite injury is related to the force of the animal's jaws. The most dangerous bite occurs from injuries over vascular areas. Human bites are probably the most difficult to manage in the long term because of the high rate of infection. (The human mouth carries a greater amount of bacteria.) The most frequent human bite locations are the ears, nose, and fingers.

Emergency care for bites is essentially the same as for other soft tissue injuries. However minor the wound may appear, the bite should be evaluated at a medical facility. In addition, always assure scene safety first. If possible, arrange for someone to contain or

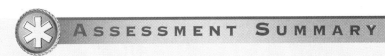

ASSESSMENT SUMMARY

SOFT TISSUE INJURY

The following are findings that may be associated with soft tissue injury.

SCENE SIZE-UP

Pay particular attention to your own safety. Look for:
　　Mechanism of injury
　　Splatters or pools of blood at scene
　　Blood-soaked clothing
　　Penetrating trauma
　　Blunt trauma

INITIAL ASSESSMENT

General Impression

Obvious massive external hemorrhage
Extremely pale color
Open or closed injuries to body

Mental Status

Alert to unresponsive, based on amount of blood loss
　　and shock
As blood loss continues, mental status decreases

Airway

May be closed if mental status is altered
May be bleeding in airway due to trauma

Breathing

Initially fast and normal to deeper tidal volume
May become shallow and fast or slow as blood loss
　　and shock progress
May be absent or inadequate if bleeding in chest or
　　associated with chest injury
May be fast and shallow if abdominal injury is present

Circulation

Pulses possibly difficult to find if extreme blood loss
Increased heart rate that becomes extremely ele-
　　vated, then suddenly decreases with continued
　　blood loss
Pulses becoming extremely weak or absent as blood
　　loss and shock continue
Skin becoming increasingly pale, cool, and clammy as
　　blood loss and shock progress

Status: Priority Patient if uncontrolled bleeding or shock is suspected

FOCUSED HISTORY AND PHYSICAL EXAM

Physical Exam

Head, neck, and face:
　　Look for large laceration to neck that may cause
　　　air emboli
Chest:
　　Open wound to chest
Abdomen:
　　Rigid, distended abdomen
　　Discoloration around umbilicus or in flank area
　　Penetrating or blunt trauma
　　Pain on palpation
　　Abdominal evisceration
Extremities:
　　Obvious external bleeding
　　Swelling, pain, and discoloration at injury site
　　Flaps or complete avulsions
　　Amputations

Baseline Vital Signs

BP: normal; may decrease or become absent in shock
HR: normal or increased in shock
RR: normal or increased in shock
Skin: normal or pale, cool, clammy, cyanotic in shock
Pupils: normal or dilated and sluggish to respond in
　　shock

SAMPLE History

Signs and symptoms of closed soft tissue injury:
　　Swelling
　　Pain
　　Discoloration
　　Shock if associated with internal injury
Signs and symptoms of open soft tissue injury:
　　Abrasions
　　Lacerations
　　Punctures
　　Avulsions
　　Amputations
　　Obvious external bleeding
　　Shock if associated with significant bleeding

Figure 30-24a　Assessment summary: soft tissue injury.

EMERGENCY CARE PROTOCOL

SOFT TISSUE INJURY

1. Establish manual in-line stabilization if spinal injury is suspected.
2. Control any major life-threatening bleeding.
3. Establish and maintain open airway, insert nasopharyngeal or oropharyngeal airway if patient is unresponsive and has no gag or cough reflex.
4. Suction secretions as necessary.
5. If breathing is inadequate, provide positive pressure ventilation with supplemental oxygen at a minimum rate of 12 ventilations/minute for an adult and 20 ventilations/minute for an infant or child.
6. If breathing is adequate, administer oxygen by nonrebreather mask at 15 lpm.
7. If open chest injury, apply non-porous dressing taped on three sides.
8. Control bleeding:
   Direct pressure (use fingertip pressure)
   Elevation
   Cold application
   Splint suspected fractures
9. If bleeding is not controlled, use appropriate pressure point until bleeding has stopped.
10. Apply sterile dressings and bandages.
11. Apply tourniquet only as last resort to control bleeding.
12. Maintain body temperature.
13. If abdominal tenderness and pelvic pain associated with signs and symptoms of shock, consider PASG.
14. Place patient supine. Legs may be elevated 8 to 12 inches.
15. If spinal injury suspected, immobilize patient to backboard.
16. Manage specific soft tissue injuries as follows:

Abdominal evisceration
Apply moist sterile dressing over wound and cover with a nonporous dressing taped on four sides. Position patient supine and flex knees.

Large laceration to neck
Apply direct pressure to stop bleeding. Apply a nonporous dressing taped on all four sides.

Open chest wound
Apply a nonporous dressing taped on three sides.

Impaled object
Apply dressings to wound and stabilize in place. Remove object only if impaled in cheek or obstructing ventilation in neck.

Avulsion
Do not complete avulsion. Rinse wound to clean off debris if necessary. Apply dressing and bandages to keep avulsed tissue in place. Splint extremity to limit movement.

Amputation (Partial)
Do not complete partial amputation. Realign extremity to as normal a position as possible. Apply sterile dressings. Splint to immobilize and limit movement. Be prepared to control bleeding.

Amputation (Complete)
Apply direct pressure to stump to control bleeding. Apply sterile dressings and bandages. Wrap part in a dry, sterile gauze dressing. Wrap or bag amputated part in plastic and place on cold pack or ice. Do not freeze. Transport with patient if possible.

17. Transport.
18. Perform ongoing assessment every 5 minutes if unstable and every 15 minutes if unstable.

Figure 30-24b Emergency care protocol: soft tissue injury.

isolate the animal, so that it will not interfere while you provide care to the patient.

CLAMPING INJURIES

You may encounter a patient who has a *clamping injury,* or a body part that is caught or strangled by some piece of machinery (Figure 30-27). Most clamping injuries involve a finger or hand that is caught in an opening (the mouth of a bottle, for example) and cannot be removed. Time is a factor because the longer a part remains in the clamping object, the more damage there may be.

In general, if a body part is trapped in a clamping object and the patient is stable, apply a lubricant (K-Y Jelly®, for example) and slowly attempt to wiggle the part loose. If possible, elevate the body part above the level of the patient's head to decrease circulation pressure as you attempt to remove the part.

If a clamping injury causes severe bleeding or shock (hypoperfusion) and if the patient cannot be rapidly disentangled, then immediately transport the

EMERGENCY CARE ALGORITHM: OPEN SOFT TISSUE INJURY

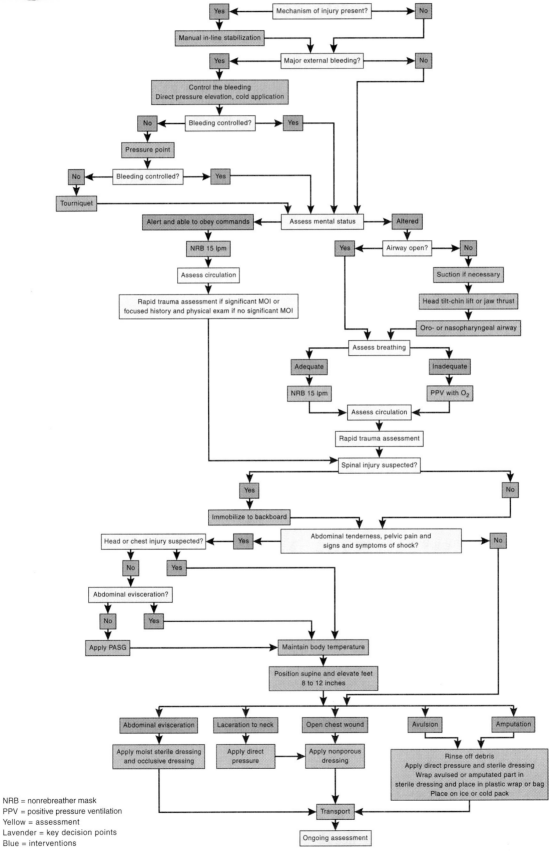

NRB = nonrebreather mask
PPV = positive pressure ventilation
Yellow = assessment
Lavender = key decision points
Blue = interventions

Figure 30-25 Emergency care algorithm: open soft tissue injury.

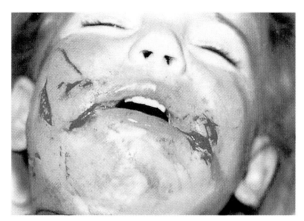

Figure 30-26   Dog bite.

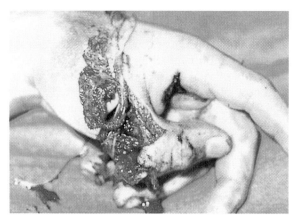

Figure 30-27   Clamping injury.

patient. Life-saving measures may then be initiated and the clamping object removed later by emergency department personnel. If the clamping object is too

large to transport, specialized personnel may be required to cut away parts of the machine or other clamping object and disentangle the patient.

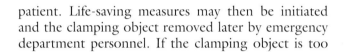

CASE STUDY FOLLOW-UP

SCENE SIZE-UP

You and your partner are at the scene of a reported dog bite. A male patient, who introduces himself as Harvey Young, is sitting on the curb, holding a towel on his left leg. Blood has soaked through. You find out that the dog is contained and isolated in a nearby garage and Harvey Young is the only patient.

INITIAL ASSESSMENT

Overall Mr. Young appears stable and is responsive, alert, and oriented. He is talking with you, so you know his airway is open. Breathing also appears to be adequate and normal and his color is good. You remove the towel and find two 3-inch lacerations on the calf of the lower leg. Bleeding is dark red and moderate in rate. The puncture is through all layers of the skin and appears to extend into the muscle.

You place a sterile gauze dressing over the wounds and apply direct pressure. You decide that while Mr. Young will require transport to the hospital, he is not in shock (hypoperfusion) and does not need priority transport.

FOCUSED HISTORY AND PHYSICAL EXAM

Mr. Young tells you he was jogging down the street when a dog "came out of nowhere." Usually dogs do not bother him, but this one came directly at him and bit his left lower leg. He did not fall or lose consciousness during the event. The dog's owner took control of the dog and gave the patient the towel for his leg.

Nothing else hurts him other than his leg. You do a rapid trauma assessment and see no other signs of external trauma. Your partner takes his vital signs, which appear normal: pulse 86, blood pressure 108/78, respirations 16, skin is pink, warm, and dry.

Mr. Young reports that he is not allergic to anything that he knows of, takes no medications on a daily basis, has no other medical problems or history, and last had a drink of water before jogging.

As you continue with direct pressure your partner has removed the patient's running shoe and sock. All responses appear to be normal: Mr. Young is able to feel sensation in his toes, is able to move his ankle and toes, and has a good pedal pulse with normal skin color.

Since bleeding has almost stopped, you apply a pressure bandage with a Kerlix® roll, which you secure with tape. You reassess distal pulse, motor function, and sensation, and find that they remain normal. Mr. Young asks if he really needs to go to the hospital. You explain that there is a risk of infection from the dog's saliva. Also, because the wound is deep it may need to be sutured. He agrees to go. You and your partner place him on the stretcher and load him into the ambulance.

Before you leave the scene you ask the police officer to get the dog owner's name and address and find out if the dog has had shots for rabies. She tells you that she already has the information, which she gives to you in written form. The dog has had rabies shots, and the owner is willing to cooperate in whatever way she can.

ONGOING ASSESSMENT

While you are en route to the hospital you reassess the distal pulses, motor function, and sensation. You take another set of vital signs and call the hospital to let them know of your patient's condition. Upon arrival, you give the triage nurse a brief report and he has you transfer Mr. Young to the minor surgical room. You then begin your documentation of the call as your partner readies the ambulance for the next patient.

Later in the week you find out from the triage nurse that Harvey Young's wound did need sutures, the dog checked out negative for rabies, and the patient was discharged after treatment.

CHAPTER REVIEW

TERMS AND CONCEPTS

You may wish to review the following terms and concepts included in this chapter.

abrasion—an open injury to the outermost layer of the skin (epidermis) caused by a scraping away, rubbing, or shearing away of the tissue.

air embolism—an air bubble that enters the bloodstream and obstructs a blood vessel.

amputation—an open injury caused by the ripping or tearing away of a limb, body part, or organ.

avulsion—an open injury characterized by a loose flap of skin and soft tissue that has been torn loose or pulled completely off.

bandage—any material used to secure a dressing in place.

closed injury—any injury in which the skin remains unbroken.

contusion—a closed injury to the cells and blood vessels contained within the dermis that is characterized by discoloration, swelling, and pain; a bruise.

crush injury—a closed or open injury to soft tissues and underlying organs that is the result of a crushing force applied to the body.

dressing—a sterile covering for an open wound that aids in the control of bleeding and prevention of further damage and contamination.

evisceration—a protrusion of organs from a wound.

hematoma—a closed injury to the soft tissues characterized by swelling and discoloration caused by a mass of blood beneath the epidermis.

impaled object—an object embedded in an injury to the body.

laceration—an open injury usually caused by forceful impact with a sharp object and characterized by a wound whose edges may be linear (smooth and regular) or stellate (jagged and irregular) in appearance.

occlusive dressing—a dressing that can form an airtight seal over a wound.

open injury—any injury in which the skin is broken as a result of trauma.

penetration/puncture—an open injury caused by a sharp, pointed object being pushed into the soft tissues.

sterile—free from living microorganisms such as bacteria, virus, or spores that may cause infection.

REVIEW QUESTIONS

1. Describe each of three types of closed soft tissue injuries.
2. Identify the general signs and symptoms of closed soft tissue injuries.
3. Outline the general emergency medical care for closed soft tissue injuries.
4. Describe each of six types of open soft tissue injuries.
5. Identify the general signs and symptoms of open soft tissue injuries.
6. Outline the general emergency medical care for open soft tissue injuries.
7. Describe the special considerations that must be taken when providing emergency medical care to patients with the following injuries: penetrating chest wounds, abdominal evisceration, impaled object, amputated part, and large open injury to the neck.
8. Describe the purpose of a dressing and name several available types.
9. Describe the purpose of a bandage and name several available types.
10. Describe the purpose of a pressure dressing and outline the steps for applying a pressure dressing.

CHAPTER 31

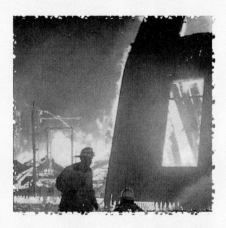

Burn Emergencies

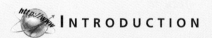 INTRODUCTION

Each year over two million people suffer burn injuries. Burn injuries are complicated because, contrary to what most people think, they are not just "skin deep." In addition to damaging the structure of the skin and compromising its functions, burn injuries impact most of the body's other systems in some way. For instance, burn injuries can impair the body's fluid and chemical balance and body temperature regulation, as well as its musculoskeletal, circulatory, and respiratory functions. Burn injuries may also affect a person's emotional well-being because of possible disfigurement and the need to cope with long healing processes.

In order to properly assess and provide emergency care for burn patients, EMT-Basics need to have a fundamental understanding of kinds of burns, how burn injuries are classified, and how they affect adult, child, and infant patients.

OBJECTIVES

Numbered objectives are from the United States Department of Transportation 1994 EMT-Basic National Standard Curriculum. Asterisked objectives, if any, pertain to material that is supplemental to the DOT curriculum.

COGNITIVE

5-2.1   State the major functions of the skin. (p. 593)

5-2.2   List the layers of the skin. (p. 593)

5-2.11   List the classifications of burns. (pp. 593–594)

5-2.12   Define superficial burn. (p. 594)

5-2.13   List the characteristics of a superficial burn. (pp. 594, 599)

5-2.14   Define partial thickness burn. (p. 594)

5-2.15   List the characteristics of a partial thickness burn. (pp. 594, 599)

5-2.16   Define full thickness burn. (p. 594)

5-2.17   List the characteristics of a full thickness burn. (pp. 594, 599)

5-2.18   Describe the emergency medical care of a patient with a superficial burn. (pp. 599–600)

5-2.19   Describe the emergency medical care of a patient with a partial thickness burn. (pp. 599–600)

5-2.20   Describe the emergency medical care of a patient with a full thickness burn. (pp. 599–600)

5-2.24   Establish the relationship between airway management and the patient with chest injury, burns, blunt and penetrating injuries. (pp. 593, 596, 598, 599, 601)

5-2.28   Describe the emergency care for a chemical burn. (pp. 600–601, 601–602)

5-2.29   Describe the emergency care for an electrical burn. (pp. 602–603)

PSYCHOMOTOR

5-2.36   Demonstrate the steps in the emergency medical care of a patient with superficial burns.

5-2.37   Demonstrate the steps in the emergency medical care of a patient with partial thickness burns.

5-2.38   Demonstrate the steps in the emergency medical care of a patient with full thickness burns.

5-2.39   Demonstrate the steps in the emergency medical care of a patient with a chemical burn.

Some of the above and additional objectives from DOT Lesson 5-2 are addressed in Chapter 30, "Soft Tissue Injuries."

CASE STUDY

THE DISPATCH

EMS Unit 101—respond with the fire department to 38 Blackstrap Road for a reported structure fire. Time out is 0235 hours. As you are getting into the ambulance you hear the fire department dispatcher alert the response companies that there is a man trapped on the second floor of the building. Reports are that the house is fully involved and a second alarm response has been requested. You look at your partner and you both know this could be a "bad" call if the patient has severe burn injuries.

Since you know that a fire like this may mean multiple patients, you request two more ambulances to respond to the fire scene for support. You and your partner don your body substance isolation clothing, just in case.

ON ARRIVAL

As you arrive on the scene, you notice that a firefighter is carrying a patient down a ladder from the second floor. Your partner gets the back of the ambulance ready by preparing the stretcher, turning on the heat, and arranging the burn supplies. You meet the firefighter at the bottom of the ladder and he tells you he found the patient, a male, on the second floor near a bedroom window.

How would you proceed to assess and care for this patient?

During this chapter you will learn about assessment and emergency care for a patient suffering from burn injuries. Later, we will return to the case and apply the procedures learned.

THE SKIN: STRUCTURE AND FUNCTION REVIEW

To understand how to classify burns, it is necessary first to understand the structure and function of the skin. (Review the information on the skin in Chapter 4, "The Human Body," and Chapter 30, "Soft Tissue Injuries," as well as reading the information in this chapter.)

The skin has a structure of three layers: the epidermis or outermost layer, the dermis or second layer, and the subcutaneous layer, the innermost layer which is composed of fatty connective tissue. The layers range in thickness from one cell to several layers of cells. The skin serves multiple functions. For instance, it:

- Provides a barrier against infection
- Provides protection from bacteria or other harmful agents found in the environment
- Insulates and protects underlying structures and body organs from injury
- Aids in the regulation of body temperature
- Provides for sensation transmission (hot, cold, pain, and touch)
- Aids in elimination of some of the body's wastes
- Contains fluids necessary to functioning of other organs and systems

It is important for you to be aware that all of the above functions can be impaired or destroyed by a burn injury.

AIRWAY, BREATHING, AND CIRCULATION

Most burn patients who die in the prehospital setting will die from an occluded airway, toxic inhalation, or other trauma, and not from the burn itself. Once the airway, breathing, and any life-threatening bleeding have been controlled, you will turn your attention to classifying the burn.

CLASSIFYING BURNS BY DEPTH

Burns are classified according to depth of the injury. Burn injuries involving the skin are classified as superficial, partial thickness, or full thickness burns (Figure 31-1). In most cases you can quickly classify the burn during the general impression and give a more detailed evaluation during the focused history and physical exam.

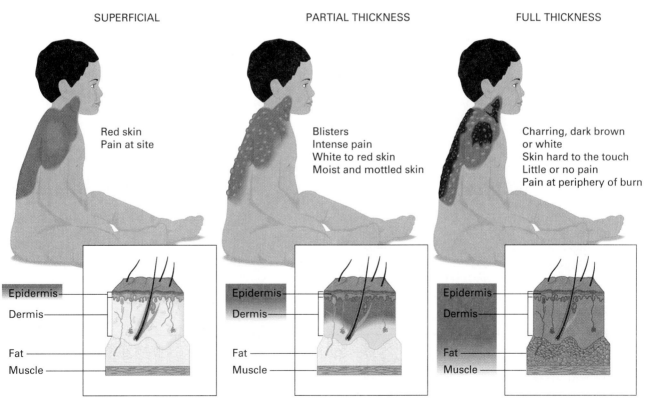

SUPERFICIAL

Red skin
Pain at site

Epidermis
Dermis
Fat
Muscle

PARTIAL THICKNESS

Blisters
Intense pain
White to red skin
Moist and mottled skin

Epidermis
Dermis
Fat
Muscle

FULL THICKNESS

Charring, dark brown
or white
Skin hard to the touch
Little or no pain
Pain at periphery of burn

Epidermis
Dermis
Fat
Muscle

Figure 31-1   Classification of burns by depth.

SUPERFICIAL BURNS

Also called a first-degree burn, a **superficial burn** is an injury that involves only the epidermis. Usually a superficial burn is caused by a flash (a sudden occurrence of heat or flame lasting only a few seconds), hot liquid, or the sun. The skin will appear pink to red and will be dry. In some cases there may be a slight swelling, but there will be no blisters.

Although superficial (not deep), these types of injuries may be very painful. Superficial burns, generally, will take several days to heal, not require much emergency medical care if only a small area is injured, and will cause the epidermis to peel but not cause any scarring. Examples of superficial burns include sunburn or a minor scald injury.

PARTIAL THICKNESS BURNS

Also called a second-degree burn, a **partial thickness burn** involves not only the epidermis but portions of the dermis as well. Partial thickness burns occur from contact with fire (flame or flash), hot liquids or objects, chemical substances, or the sun. The skin may appear white to cherry red, moist, and mottled. In addition, damage to the blood vessels causes plasma and tissue fluid to collect between the layers of skin and form blisters.

Partial thickness burns will cause intense pain resulting from nerve-ending damage. Examples of partial thickness burns include thermal flame burns or severe scaldings (Figure 31-2).

FULL THICKNESS BURNS

Also called a third-degree burn, a **full thickness burn** involves all of the layers of the skin and can extend beyond the subcutaneous layer into the muscle, bone, or organs below. This type of burn results from contact with extreme heat sources such as hot liquids or solids, flame, chemicals, or electricity. The skin will become dry, hard, tough, and leathery and may appear white and waxy to dark brown or black and charred. The tough and leathery dead soft tissue formed in the full thickness burn injury is called **eschar**.

Most full thickness burns will not be very painful because nerve endings will have been destroyed. However, in most such injuries there will be surrounding areas of partial thickness burns that may cause intense pain. Full thickness burns are often evident in patients who have been trapped in a confined space with flames or who have been exposed to a high heat source or chemical contact (Figure 31-3).

PARTIAL THICKNESS BURNS

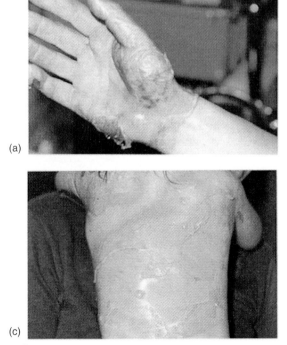
(a)

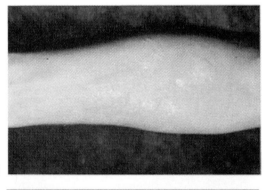
(b)

(c)

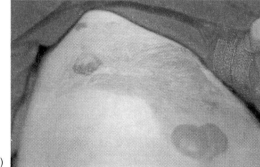
(d)

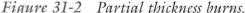
Figure 31-2   Partial thickness burns.

FULL THICKNESS BURNS

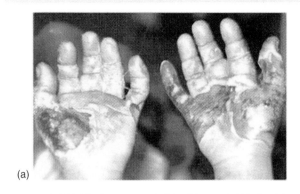

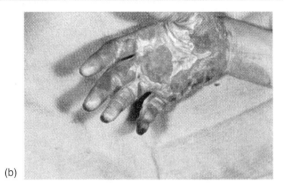

(a)

(b)

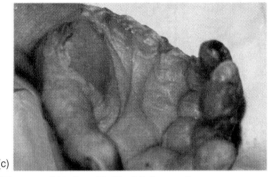

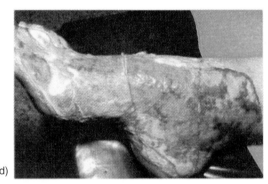

(c)

(d)

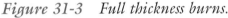

Figure 31-3   Full thickness burns.

DETERMINING THE SEVERITY OF BURN INJURIES

The EMT-B must classify the severity of the burn injury in order to provide the optimal emergency medical care, make the best patient transport decision, and give an accurate report to the receiving facility. In some areas, the estimate of burn injury severity may be crucial in deciding to which facility the patient will be transported—to a specialized burn center or to a regular hospital, for instance. In general, burns are classified as critical (Figure 31-4), moderate, or minor. See Table 31-1.

In addition to the depth of the injury (superficial, partial thickness, or full thickness) you will also consider other factors in determining the severity of a burn injury. For instance, you will often want to consider the source or agent of the burn. A small burn caused by an electrical source may give more cause for concern than a small thermal (heat) burn because of the electrical burn's potential for internal injury. Likewise, a chemical burn will vary in severity depending upon the type and strength of the chemical. Inhalation injuries or burns involving the airway are always considered critical.

The most important factors to consider in determining burn severity are percentage of body surface area involved, the location of the burn, the patient's age, and preexisting medical conditions.

BODY SURFACE AREA PERCENTAGE

The **rule of nines** is a standardized way to quickly determine the amount of skin surface, or the body surface area (BSA) percentage, of a burn (Figure 31-5). In an adult the head and neck together, each upper extremity, the chest, the abdomen, the upper back, the lower back, the anterior of each lower extremity, and the posterior of each lower extremity each represents a BSA of 9 percent. The genital region represents a 1 percent BSA. This rule will guide you in determining the burn severity, categorizing the patient for triage, and alerting the receiving facility as to the severity of the patient.

In infants and children there are different BSA percentages assigned to body regions because of their different proportional dimensions. The infant's or young child's head is much larger in relationship to the rest of the body than in adults. Therefore, for infants and young children the head and neck are counted as 18 percent, the chest and abdomen as 18 percent, the entire back as 18 percent, each upper extremity as 9 percent, and each lower extremity as 14 percent.

CRITICAL BURNS

Critical burns include:

- Full thickness burns involving hands, feet, face, or genitalia.

- Burns associated with respiratory injury.

- Full thickness burns covering more than 10% of body surface.

- Partial thickness burns covering more than 20% of body surface.

- Burns complicated by painful, swollen, deformed extremity (bone injury).

- Moderate burns in young children or elderly patients.

- Burns encompassing any body part, such as arm, leg, or chest.

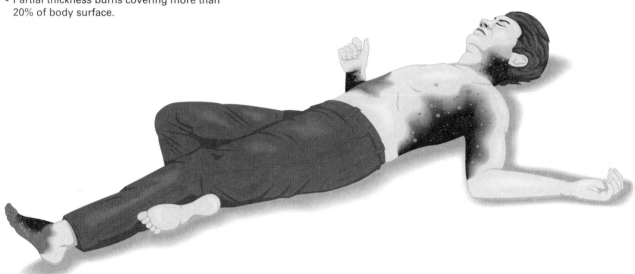

Figure 31-4 Critical burns.

An alternative way to determine the BSA estimate is to compare it to the *patient's* palm (of the hand) surface area, which equals approximately 1 percent of BSA. For example, if the burn area is equal to "7 palm surface areas," then the burn would be estimated at 7 percent BSA. You can use this method to estimate a burn area on any age patient.

In most cases you may find it useful to use the rule of nines in larger burn injuries and use the "palm" method for smaller burns. You can begin to estimate BSA during the initial assessment. Do not spend time trying to determine the exact percentage of BSA injured. The BSA percentage is an *estimate* only, and slight differences of percentages will not affect proper emergency medical care.

BURN INJURY LOCATION

Just as the depth of the burn injury and its body surface area are important so, too, is the location of the burn. Injuries to certain body areas are more critical than those to other areas. Burns of the face (Figure 31-6) are considered critical because of the potential for respiratory compromise or injuries to the eyes. Hands and feet are also given special consideration because of the potential for loss of function. Burn injuries to the genital or groin region are given special

consideration because of the potential for loss of genitourinary function and increased chances for infection.

Circumferential burns, which encircle a body area such as an arm, leg, or the chest—and especially ones that encircle joint areas—are critical because of the circulatory compromise and nerve damage that result from constriction or from swelling tissues. Burns that encircle the chest may impede respiratory function by limiting expansion of the chest.

AGE AND PREEXISTING MEDICAL CONDITIONS

Age of the patient is also used as a major factor in determining the severity of the burn injury. Children under 5 and adults over 55 have less tolerance for burn injuries. Children, in addition to BSA percentage differences, face other challenges of growth process impairment. Because of their relatively larger skin surface in relation to body mass, they have the potential for greater fluid loss in burn injuries than adults. Older adults have prolonged healing processes and may have underlying medical conditions that may affect their response to burn injuries.

Any preexisting illness or injury may increase the severity of a burn injury. A patient with an existing respiratory illness or condition may be adversely af-

TABLE 31-1

Determining Burn Severity Classification

	Adults	Children under 5
Critical Burns	• Any burn injury complicated by respiratory tract injuries or other accompanying major traumatic • Full or partial thickness burns involving the face, hands, feet, genitalia or respiratory tract • Any full thickness burn injury covering 10% or more BSA • Any partial thickness burn injury covering 20% or more BSA • Burn injuries complicated by a suspected fracture to an extremity • Any burn that encircles a body part, e.g., arm, leg, or chest • Any burn classified as moderate in an adult younger than 55 is considered critical in an adult older than 55	*As for adults plus . . .* • Any full or partial thickness burn greater than 20% BSA • Any burn, including a superficial burn, involving hands, feet, face, or genitalia • Any burn classified as moderate for an adult
Moderate Burns	• Full thickness burns with 2%–10% BSA, excluding the face, hands, feet, genitalia, or respiratory tract • Partial thickness burns with 20%–30% BSA involvement • Superficial burns greater than 50% BSA	• Any partial thickness burn of 10% to 20% BSA
Minor Burns	• Full thickness burns involving less than 2% BSA • Partial thickness burns less than 15% BSA • Superficial burns less than 50% BSA	• Any partial thickness burn less than 10% BSA

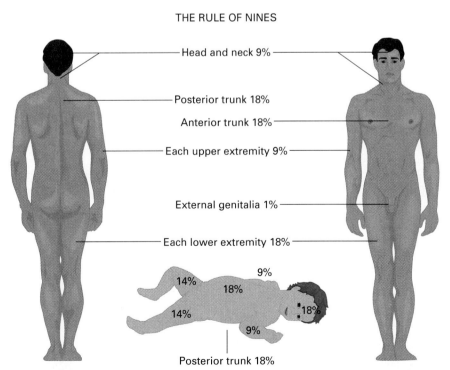

Figure 31-5   The "rule of nines" is a method for estimating how much body surface is burned.

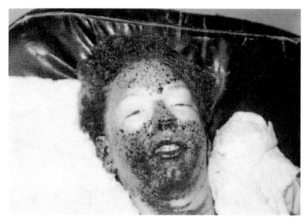

Figure 31-6 Burns to the face suggest respiratory tract involvement or injuries to the eyes.

fected if there is further respiratory compromise from a burn injury. A patient with an existing cardiovascular problem may have increased complications from a burn injury and resulting fluid loss. Diabetes will compromise the patient's ability to heal from the burns. You must always realize that what may seem like a minor burn in an otherwise healthy adult may be more severe in those patients with preexisting medical conditions. If the patient has experienced other injuries along with a burn injury, the life threat or potential for shock (hypoperfusion) may be increased, as well.

SPECIAL CONSIDERATIONS FOR INFANTS AND CHILDREN

As mentioned earlier, infants and children have a larger body surface in relation to mass than adults. For this reason, burn injuries can have increased effects on infants and children. Fluid and heat loss are greater in infants and children than in adults. A higher risk for shock (hypoperfusion), airway difficulties, and hypothermia are found with burn injuries to infants. Further differences in burn injury severity classification for children less than 5 years old are outlined in Table 31-1.

In addition to assessment and emergency medical care considerations, you must consider the possibility of child abuse when a child has a burn injury. (See information about assessing for and reporting child abuse in Chapter 38, "Infants and Children.")

ASSESSMENT AND CARE: BURN INJURIES

SCENE SIZE-UP

Your first priority is to determine whether the scene is safe to enter. Do not enter scenes for which you are not trained. If the patient is in an unsafe environment, such as a fire-engulfed building, and you do not have the proper equipment or training to enter, you must wait until properly equipped and trained personnel can safely remove the victim. Once the scene is safe to enter, you must take appropriate body substance isolation precautions and then begin assessing the mechanism of injury and number of patients.

INITIAL ASSESSMENT

Remember that removing the patient from the burn source does not completely stop the burning process. Burn injuries need to be "cooled down" within approximately the first 10 minutes of injury. Stop the burning process initially by using water or saline. As you continue working to stop the burning, attempt to remove any smoldering clothing and jewelry which will still be producing heat and may constrict swollen extremities. If any clothing still adheres to the patient, cut around the area. Do not attempt to remove the adhered portion, since this may cause further damage to the soft tissues. Do not keep the burn immersed, as this may cause hypothermia; cool for 60 to 120 seconds.

Once you have stopped the burning process, you can continue your initial assessment and evaluate the patient's airway, breathing, and mental status. Look for any indications that the airway may be injured or compromised, such as, sooty deposits in the mouth or nose, singed facial or nose hairs, signs of smoke inhalation, or any facial burns. A burn victim's first reaction when frightened or startled—such as when trapped in a confined space or startled by an explosion—is to deeply inhale. Air in these situations may be superheated and will have an adverse effect on the airway and respiratory function. Hence, you need to consider the likelihood of airway compromise and breathing difficulties. Provide oxygen by nonrebreather mask at 15 lpm or, if breathing is inadequate, provide positive pressure ventilation with supplemental oxygen.

To complete the initial assessment, assess the patient's circulation and determine whether the patient is a priority for transport. At this point you will need to make a rapid estimate of the severity of the burn, taking into account BSA percentage and any information you have gained about the burn source or agent and the age and medical condition of the patient that you have gained from bystanders or the patient himself. Remember not to spend too long estimating the exact BSA percentage of the burn; you can gather more information later in your assessment.

Most burns do not bleed and are not a cause of early shock. Therefore, if signs and symptoms of shock are present, look for other sources of blood loss or possible spinal injury. As in all traumatic emergencies, a burn injury patient is a priority for transport if he is unresponsive with no gag reflex or is responsive but not following commands, if he has airway compromise or difficulty breathing, if he shows signs of shock or uncontrolled bleeding, or if he presents with severe pain. *However, burn injury patients are also considered high priority for transport if their burn is classified as critical. This is why it is of utmost importance that you know how to estimate the severity of the patient's burn (review Table 31-1).*

Focused History and Physical Exam

After treating all life-threatening injuries, conduct the focused history and physical exam. You will reassess mechanism of injury and chief complaint. If the patient is alert and does not have a significant mechanism of injury, begin with a focused trauma assessment, but if the patient has an altered mental status and there is evidence of additional injuries, perform a rapid trauma assessment. Check for DCAP-BTLS and get a more accurate estimate of BSA percentage than the one you determined during the initial assessment. As you examine the patient, continue to remove his clothing and jewelry, but do not attempt to remove debris or any adhered clothing. Take and record the patient's baseline vital signs.

Obtain a SAMPLE history from the patient or from family and bystanders. However, if the patient's burn is considered critical or if he is a priority for transport for other reasons, you may not have time to obtain the answers to your questions at the scene. If possible, ask the following questions:

- How did the burn happen?
- What caused the burn?
- Was the patient exposed to an explosion or other significant mechanism of injury?
- Did the patient lose consciousness at any time?
- Was the patient confined in an enclosed space or found to inhale copious amounts of smoke?
- How long ago was the patient burned?
- What care was given by bystanders?
- If the burn involved chemicals, what chemical?
- If the burn was a scald, how did it happen? (If a scald or burn injury involves an infant, child, or elderly patient consider the possibility of abuse.)
- Does the patient have any history of significant heart disease, pulmonary problems, diabetes, or any other condition that might increase the burn severity or complicate treatment?

Signs and Symptoms In addition to estimating BSA and noting location of the burn injuries, watch for the following signs and symptoms of burn depth and possible inhalation injuries:

Superficial Burns
- Pink or red, dry skin
- Slight swelling
- Pain

Partial Thickness Burns
- White to cherry red skin
- Moist and mottled skin
- Blistering and intense pain

Full Thickness Burns
- Dry, hard, tough, and leathery skin that may appear white-waxy to dark brown or black and charred (eschar)
- Inability to feel pain because of damaged nerve endings

Inhalation Injuries
- Singed nasal hairs
- Facial burns
- Burned specks of carbon in the sputum
- A sooty or smoky smell on the breath
- Respiratory distress accompanied by restriction of chest wall movement, restlessness, chest tightness, stridor, wheezing, difficulty in swallowing, hoarseness, coughing, and cyanosis
- The presence of actual burns of the oral mucosa

Emergency Medical Care

There are many ways in which to care for burn injuries. You should check with your local medical director to determine the most appropriate emergency medical care for burn injuries in your region. The following steps in emergency medical care for burn injuries represent a general protocol in providing care. Particular attention is paid to preventing further contamination and injury.

1. *Remove the patient from the source of the burn and stop the burning process.* As mentioned earlier, you should not attempt to enter an unsafe environment and extricate the patient unless you have the proper training and equipment. Once the patient has been removed from the source of the burn, you can stop the burn process by using water or saline (Figure 31-7a), but do not keep it immersed. If the burn source is a semi-solid or liquid, e.g., tar, grease, or oil, cool the burn with water or saline to stop the burning process but do not attempt to remove the substance since this could cause further tissue damage. Dry chemicals should be brushed away before flushing with water. Remove any smoldering clothing and any jewelry. If any clothing remains adhered to the patient, cut around the area (Figure 31-7b). Do not attempt to remove the adhered portion.

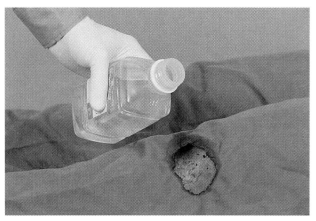

Figure 31-7a   Stop the burning process.

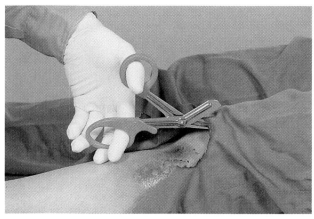

Figure 31-7b   Remove the smoldering clothing.

2. *Establish and maintain an airway and breathing.* Pay particular attention to evidence of inhalation injury to the patient's upper airway. Maintain an open airway and administer oxygen by nonrebreather mask at 15 lpm or, if breathing is inadequate, provide positive pressure ventilation with supplemental oxygen.
3. *Classify the severity of the burn and transport immediately if critical.* Take into account the factors mentioned earlier: BSA percentage, source or agent of the burn, location of the burn, age of patient, preexisting medical conditions. (Review Table 31-1.)
4. *Cover the burned area with a dry sterile dressing* (Figure 31-7c) or a sterile, particle-free disposable **burn sheet.** Continual use of a wet or moist dressing may cause hypothermia because of the loss of heat regulation in the burned area. However, some EMS systems use moist dressing on 10 percent BSA or less for partial thickness burn injuries. Check with local medical direction regarding the use of wet or moist dressings.
5. *Keep the patient warm and treat other injuries as needed.* Remember the burn injury will impair or destroy the skin's heat regulation function. Also remember that the burn may be accompanied by other injuries.
6. *Transport the patient to the appropriate facility,* depending upon the severity of the burn and local protocol for burn injuries.

SPECIAL CONSIDERATIONS FOR DRESSING BURNS

In dressing a burn, follow these guidelines:

- Avoid using any material that shreds or leaves particles since this may cause further contamination of the burn area.
- Never apply any type of ointments, lotions, or antiseptics to burn injuries. This may cause heat re-

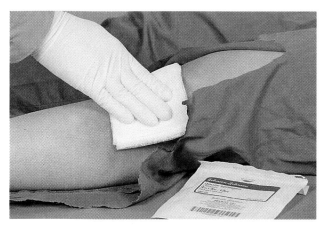

Figure 31-7c   Cover with dry sterile dressings.

tention and hospital personnel would most likely have to vigorously cleanse the area of any debris material.
- Never attempt to break or drain blisters. This may cause further contamination and potential for fluid loss.

Special areas of concern when applying burn dressings are the hands, the toes, and the eyes. In those areas, follow these guidelines.

For Burns of the Hands and Toes:

- Remove all rings and jewelry, which may constrict with swelling after the burn injury. Separate all digits with dry sterile dressing material to prevent adhering of burned areas (Figures 31-8a to c).

For Burns of the Eyes:

- Do not attempt to open eyelids if they are burned. Determine if the burn is thermal or chemical. If thermal, apply a dry, sterile dressing to BOTH eyes to prevent simultaneous movement of both eyes. Chemical burns should be flushed with water for at least 20 minutes while en route to the hospital.

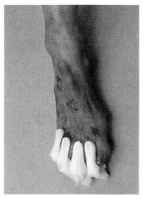

Figure 31-8a
Separate burned toes
with dry sterile gauze.

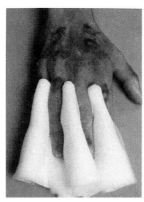

Figure 31-8b
Separate burned fin-
gers with dry sterile
gauze.

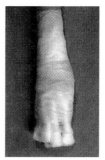

Figure 31-8c
Cover the burned
fingers or toes com-
pletely with dry ster-
ile dressings.

Flush the eye from the medial to the lateral side to avoid washing the chemical into the opposite eye (Figures 31-9 and 31-13). See more about chemical burns in the following section.

DETAILED PHYSICAL EXAM AND ONGOING ASSESSMENT

En route to the burn center or hospital, perform a detailed physical exam if warranted by suspicion of additional injuries and if time and the patient's condition permit. Perform the ongoing assessment. Monitor vital signs and check interventions every 5 minutes for unstable patients and every 15 minutes for stable patients. Continually evaluate the airway, especially if there are any burns to the face.

Note: *Swelling or closure of the airway may be rapid and emergency medical care will need to be quickly accomplished. Always consider advanced life support (ALS) response when dealing with airway complications in burn injuries.*

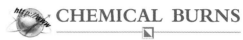

CHEMICAL BURNS

Chemical burns require immediate care, since the longer the chemical is in contact with the skin the greater the potential for injury (Figure 31-10). In many cases, emergency medical care may be started by people at the scene. Industrial sites may have special response teams or first responders and equipment available to provide initial emergency medical care. However, you should follow these rules when dealing with chemical burn injuries:

• *Protect yourself first.* As with other burn emergencies, never enter an unsafe scene. Chemical burns may involve a hazardous material incident which you may not be prepared to handle or that may cause you to become exposed. Wear gloves and eye protection at a minimum. In some cases of a large exposure you may have to wear an impervious (fluid-proof) gown or suit to prevent further contamination from the chemical(s).

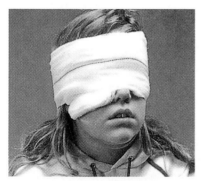

Figure 31-9 Apply sterile
gauze pads to both eyes.

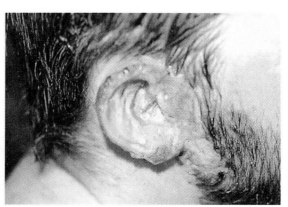

Figure 31-10 Chemical burn.

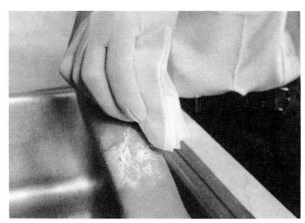

Figure 31-11   Lime powder should be brushed off the skin before flushing with water.

- *Dry chemicals, e.g., dry lime, should be brushed off before flushing with water* (Figure 31-11).
- *Most chemical burns can be flushed with copious amounts of water* (Figures 31-12 and 31-13). Always assure that the chemical is one that may be diluted with water. (Consult a hazardous materials guidebook.) There are some chemicals that may produce combustion when they come into contact with water. Minimize further wound contamination by making sure fluid runs away from the injury and not toward any uninjured areas. Remove all clothing and jewelry as in other burn injuries. *Continue to flush for at least 20 minutes while en route to the hospital.*

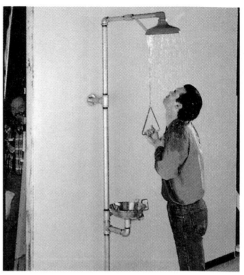

Figure 31-12   Flushing a chemical burn patient under an emergency wash/shower system at the worksite. (Courtesy of Lab Safety Supply)

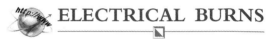 **ELECTRICAL BURNS**

Electrical burns, including those caused by electrical currents and lightning (Figures 31-14a to d), can cause severe damage not only to soft tissues but to the body as a whole.

Electrical energy will always seek to flow to ground, and as the energy enters the body it will seek the path of least resistance to exit the body. All tissues

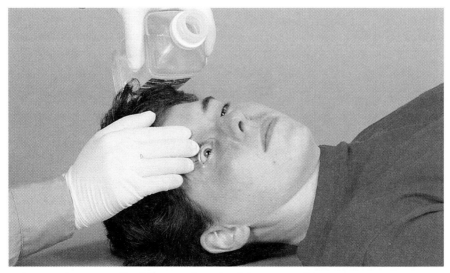

Figure 31-13   Flushing a chemical burn to the eye.

ELECTRICAL BURNS

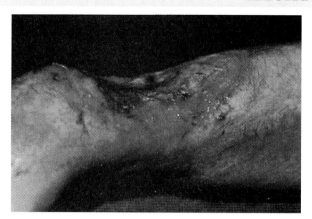

Figure 31-14a   Full thickness electrical burn.

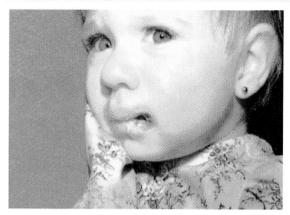

Figure 31-14b   Electrical burn caused by chewing on an electrical cord.

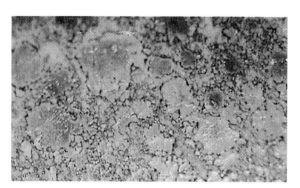

Figure 31-14c   Lightning burn.

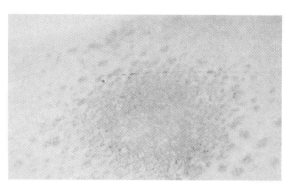

Figure 31-14d   Lightning burn.

between the entrance and exit of the current will potentially be injured due to the extreme heat created by the resistance of body structures to the electricity (Figure 31-15). Further, since the body, especially the heart, produces its own electrical energy from chemical reactions, electrical injuries can disturb or destroy these functions, causing irregular heartbeat or even cardiac arrest.

Scene safety is crucial in electrical burn injuries because of the extremely hazardous nature of the electrical source. Always assume the electrical source is still charged unless the power source has been completely shut down.

When caring for electrical burn injuries:

- *Never attempt to remove a patient from an electrical source unless trained and equipped to do so.*
- *Never touch a patient still in contact with the electrical source.*
- *Administer oxygen by nonrebreather mask* at 15 lpm or positive pressure ventilation with supplemental oxygen, if necessary.

- *Monitor the patient for cardiac arrest.* Be prepared to administer CPR and apply an automated external defibrillator (AED) as soon as possible.
- *Assess the patient for muscle tenderness* with or without twitching and any seizure activity.
- *Always assess for an entrance and exit burn injury.* All tissue in between is suspect for injury even if not readily visible. Emergency medical care for entrance and exit injuries are the same as for other thermal burns.
- *Transport the patient as soon as possible.* Most electrical burn injuries will have a slow onset and underlying tissue or organ damage may not be readily apparent. These patients should all be assumed to have critical injuries, even if burns appear insignificant.

SUMMARY: ASSESSMENT AND CARE

To review possible assessment findings and emergency care for burn emergencies, see Figures 31-16 and 31-17.

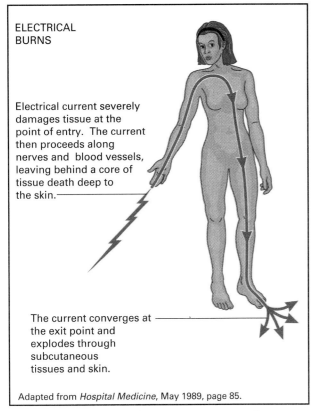

ELECTRICAL
BURNS

Electrical current severely
damages tissue at the
point of entry. The current
then proceeds along
nerves and blood vessels,
leaving behind a core of
tissue death deep to
the skin.

The current converges at
the exit point and
explodes through
subcutaneous
tissues and skin.

Adapted from *Hospital Medicine*, May 1989, page 85.

Figure 31-15 *Look for two separate burns when electricity is the cause of injury.*

ENRICHMENT

The enrichment section contains information that is valuable as background for the EMT-B but that goes substantially beyond the U.S. Department of Transportation (DOT) EMT-Basic curriculum.

As stated earlier in this chapter, burn injuries can not only impair or destroy the structure and functions of the skin, but they can also damage other body systems as well. This section will discuss some of the potential complications to body organ systems of the burn injury patient other than the skin. The organ systems discussed below are all essential for patient survival and successful recovery. Burn injuries that impair any of these functions can have a dramatic effect on the patient's outcome.

By providing the proper emergency medical care of the airway, preventing further contamination, and providing protection from further injury, you can decrease burn patient mortality considerably.

CIRCULATORY SYSTEM

Burn injuries can cause extreme fluid loss and increased stress on the heart. Burns increase the capillary permeability, or the ability of fluid to exit from the vessels. This decreases the fluid volume inside the vessels. Fluid also will leak from the damaged tissue cells to areas between the cells and cause edema, or swelling. In 24 hours after the injury, the edema may double in size from normal.

All of the above fluid loss can lead to shock (hypoperfusion). Major burns will need large amounts of fluid replacement during hospitalization. For example, a full or partial thickness burn area of 50 percent BSA in an average adult may need as much as 15 liters of fluid in the first 24 hours after a burn injury.

RESPIRATORY SYSTEM

Swelling in the face or throat may cause airway closure. Inhalation of superheated air may cause the lining of the larynx to swell (laryngeal edema) and may cause fluid to accumulate in the lungs. Smoke inhalation may cause respiratory arrest or compromise or poisoning from noxious fumes. If the chest is circumferentially burned, scarring may restrict chest expansion.

RENAL SYSTEM (KIDNEYS)

Decrease in blood flow caused by a burn (see Circulatory System, above) will, of course, cause decreased blood flow to the kidneys and a consequent decrease in urinary output. Also, the burn injury will cause many wastes to form in the blood because of cell destruction, such as myoglobin from muscle destruction. This is particularly true with electrical burns. Since the kidneys are responsible for filtering the contaminated blood, a blockage in the kidneys may also result. In the end this may cause all or part of the kidneys to stop functioning.

NERVOUS AND MUSCULOSKELETAL SYSTEMS

Burn injuries can destroy nerve endings in the burn area and cause loss of function to extremities or other body parts. An extremity burn may cause loss of function, long term muscle wasting, and joint dysfunction because of scarring. It should also be noted that patients who face loss of function, extreme pain, and scarring will also be prone to fear and anxiety. These patients may need both medical and psychological help to aid the healing process.

GASTROINTESTINAL SYSTEM

While a low priority for the EMT-B, this system plays an important role in the long term care and survival of severely burned patients. As blood flow is decreased, blood will be re-routed from this system to the rest of the body. Nausea or vomiting can further upset normal chemical balances, and long-term stress may cause ulcers. In order to promote healing and survival of burn patients, the gastrointestinal system must be kept functioning properly.

ASSESSMENT SUMMARY

BURN EMERGENCY

The following are findings that may be associated with a burn emergency.

SCENE SIZE-UP

Pay particular attention to your own safety. Look for:
- Burning structures or material
- Chemicals
- Electrical sources
- Confined spaces
- Burned clothing
- Obvious burns to patient's body
- Evidence of explosion
- Other blunt or penetrating trauma

INITIAL ASSESSMENT

General Impression

Stridor or crowing from upper airway
Obvious burns to body and clothing
Burns to neck and face
Singed hair, nasal hair, eyebrows, and other facial hair
Carbonaceous (black) sputum

Mental Status

Alert to unresponsive

Airway

Stridor (indicates upper airway burn)
Edema to oral mucosa and tongue
Burns around neck and face
Black inside mouth

Breathing

Normal to increased if airway or respiratory tract not involved
Increased or decreased, labored, and shallow if airway or respiratory tract burns

Circulation

Increase; may be decreased if severely hypoxic
Skin normal in unburned areas; may be cool, clammy and pale

Status: Priority patient if large body surface area burns, airway or respiratory tract is involved, critical burns are apparent, or burns involve hands, feet, face, or genitalia

FOCUSED HISTORY AND PHYSICAL EXAM

Physical Exam

Head, neck, and face:
- Burns
- Singed hair, eyebrows, facial and nasal hair
- Dark black (carbonaceous) sputum
- Swelling of tongue and oral mucosa
- Hoarseness
- Coughing (may cough up black sputum)
- Cyanosis
- Burns to the oral mucosa

Chest:
- Burns
- Wheezing
- Circumferential burns around thorax may impede ventilation
- Blunt or penetrating trauma if explosion or fall involved

Abdomen:
- Burns
- Blunt or penetrating trauma if explosion or fall involved

Extremities:
- Burns
- Circumferential burns may reduce distal circulation
- Swelling, pain, and discoloration if explosion or fall involved

Baseline Vital Signs

BP: normal, may decrease with severe burns after a few hours (if BP decreased at the scene, look for evidence of other trauma)
HR: normal or increased
RR: normal; increased and labored if respiratory tract burn involved
Skin: normal in unburned areas (if pale, cool, clammy immediately after burn may indicate shock from other trauma)
Pupils: normal

SAMPLE History

Signs and symptoms of superficial burns:
- Skin is pink or red, and dry
- Slight swelling
- Pain

Signs and symptoms of partial thickness burns:
- Skin is white to cherry red
- Moist and mottled
- Blisters
- Intense pain

Signs and symptoms of full thickness burns:
- Skin is dry, hard, tough, and leathery
- White-waxy, dark brown, or charred
- No pain in burned area
- Usually pain around the site of full thickness burn

Signs and symptoms of inhalation injury:
- Facial burns
- Singed nasal and facial hair, and eyebrows
- Black sputum
- Respiratory distress with labored breathing
- Coughing, hoarseness, cyanosis

Figure 31-16a Assessment summary: burn emergency.

EMERGENCY CARE PROTOCOL

BURN EMERGENCY

1. Remove patient from source of burn and stop burning process.
2. Establish manual in-line stabilization if spinal injury suspected.
3. Establish and maintain open airway; insert nasopharyngeal or oropharyngeal airway if patient is unresponsive and has no gag or cough reflex.
4. Suction secretions as necessary.
5. If breathing is inadequate, provide positive pressure ventilation with supplemental oxygen at a minimum rate of 12 ventilations/minute for an adult and 20 ventilations/minute for an infant or child.
6. If breathing is adequate, administer oxygen by nonrebreather mask at 15 lpm.
7. Estimate body surface area burn (% BSA) using rule of nines.
8. Determine depth of burn: superficial, partial thickness, and full thickness.
9. Apply sterile dressings and bandages or burn sheet.
10. If the burn is less than 10% BSA, dress wet. Dress all other burns dry.
11. Maintain body temperature.
12. Manage other associated injuries.
13. If spinal injury suspected, immobilize patient to backboard.
14. Manage specific burns as follows:

    Dry chemical burn
    Remove affected clothing, brush off dry chemical, then irrigate with large amounts of water for at least 20 minutes.

    Liquid chemical burn
    Remove affected clothing; irrigate with large amounts of water for at least 20 minutes.

    Burns to the hands and feet
    Remove all rings and jewelry; dress between digits.

    Chemical burns to the eyes
    Flush with large amounts of water for 20 minutes and continue to flush en route.

    Thermal burns to the eyes
    Do not attempt to open eyelids; apply dry sterile dressing to both eyes.

    Electrical burns
    Carefully monitor pulse and respiration; inspect for entrance and exit wound; assess for muscle tenderness; apply AED if patient is in cardiac arrest.

15. Transport.
16. Perform ongoing assessment every 5 minutes if unstable and every 15 minutes if stable.

Figure 31-16b   Emergency care protocol: burn emergency.

EMERGENCY CARE ALGORITHM:
BURN EMERGENCY

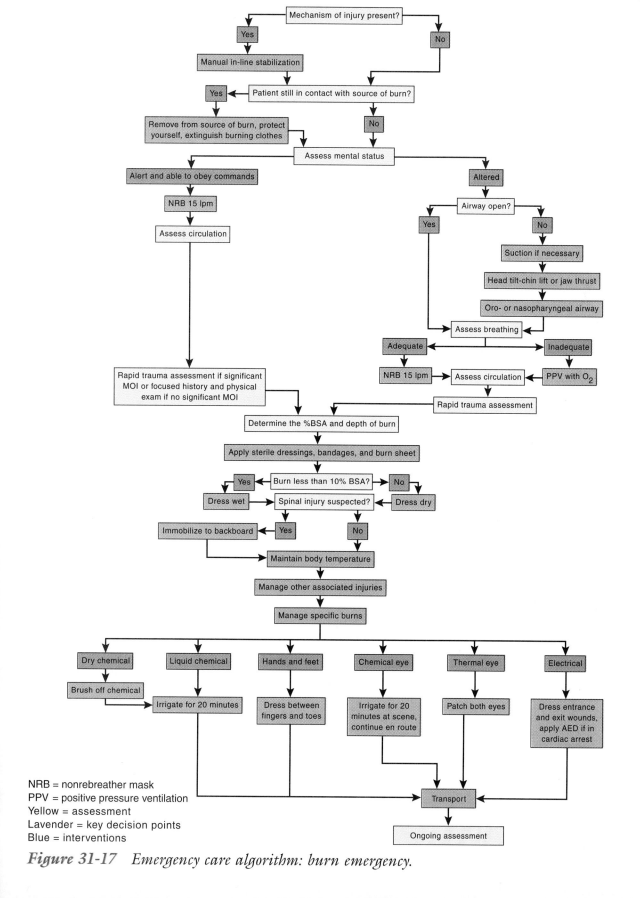

NRB = nonrebreather mask
PPV = positive pressure ventilation
Yellow = assessment
Lavender = key decision points
Blue = interventions

Figure 31-17 *Emergency care algorithm: burn emergency.*

CASE STUDY FOLLOW-UP

SCENE SIZE-UP

You and your partner have been dispatched to a reported structure fire. You have arrived on the scene of a fully involved structure fire with one patient trapped on the second floor. You have donned your gloves, mask, and eye protection. Since this is a "working" fire with one known patient already, you have called for additional units for assistance.

As you arrive, you spot a firefighter carrying the reported patient down the ladder. Your partner readies the back of the ambulance as you go to the patient.

INITIAL ASSESSMENT

You begin your assessment by noting that the patient, a male, has severe charring and other burns on the right half of his body and that he is unresponsive. His airway is open but breathing is shallow and rapid. His face is somewhat blackened. You immediately place him in the back of the ambulance on the stretcher. His pulse is weak and rapid and you consider him a high priority patient.

Your partner has inserted an airway adjunct and set up the bag-valve unit for positive pressure ventilation with supplemental oxygen. He begins ventilations while you stop the burning process. You begin to pour sterile saline over the patient's burned areas and at the same time begin to assess the severity of the burn. There are full thickness burns over the patient's right chest and abdomen both front and back, right arm, and leg. There is singed nasal hair and blackened areas around the face. You quickly estimate this to be about a full thickness burn over a 50 percent BSA and classify the patient as critical, in terms of burn severity.

You begin to remove clothing and jewelry, continuing to stop the burning process, then immediately begin transport to the local trauma center.

FOCUSED HISTORY AND PHYSICAL EXAM

The patient remains unresponsive as you begin to further assess and treat him. You have cooled the burn down and now cover the patient with a sterile burn sheet and place sterile dressings between his fingers and toes. You also cover the patient with several blankets to keep him warm. Your partner is continuing to ventilate the patient. You do a rapid trauma assessment, checking for any further injuries, but do not find any. You assess the patient's vital signs, and they are BP 98/68, pulse 124 rapid and weak, respirations assisted at 24 breaths per minute. Upon auscultation of the lungs you discover wheezing in all lung fields. You radio the hospital to advise them of the patient's status and estimated time of arrival. You are unable to obtain a SAMPLE history because the patient is unresponsive and his critical condition did not allow you time to question bystanders at the scene.

ONGOING ASSESSMENT

Since transport time is short, you conduct only one ongoing assessment. There is essentially no change in the patient's status and the positive pressure ventilations seem to be helping. At the hospital, you give a quick report to the hospital staff as you take the patient to the trauma room. The emergency department physician immediately prepares to intubate the patient as other personnel start fluid replacement.

You next begin the task of completing the prehospital care report as your partner readies the vehicle. The dispatcher advises you that you will be required back at the fire scene as quickly as possible.

CHAPTER REVIEW

TERMS AND CONCEPTS

You may wish to review the following terms and concepts included in this chapter.

burn sheet—commercially prepared sterile, particle-free, disposable sheet used to cover the entire body in severe burn injuries.

circumferential burn—burn that encircles a body area, e.g., arm, leg, or chest.

eschar—the hard, tough, leathery dead soft tissue formed as a result of a full thickness burn.

full thickness burn—burn that involves all of the layers of the skin and can extend beyond the subcu-

taneous layer into the muscle, bone, or organs below; also called a third-degree burn.

partial thickness burn—burn that involves the epidermis and portions of the dermis; also called a second-degree burn.

rule of nines—standardized format to quickly identify the amount of skin or body surface area (BSA) that has been burned.

superficial burn—burn that involves only the epidermis; also called a first-degree burn.

REVIEW QUESTIONS

1. Define and list the characteristics of superficial, partial thickness, and full thickness burns.
2. Define the rule of nines and describe how it is used on both adult and infant or child burn injury patients.
3. Using the rule of nines, name the percentage of body surface area (BSA) burned if (a) a 4-year-old child has superficial burn injuries to the front and back of both legs as well as the chest, abdomen and back; (b) an adult has partial thickness burn injuries to the front of one lower extremity and to the front and back of the other lower extremity.
4. Determine the burn severity classification for patients a and b in Question 3.
5. Describe the basic emergency care steps for burn injuries.
6. List the three things an EMT-B should not do when applying dry, sterile dressings to a burn injury patient.
7. List the emergency medical care guidelines for chemical burns.
8. List the emergency medical care guidelines for electrical burns.

CHAPTER 32

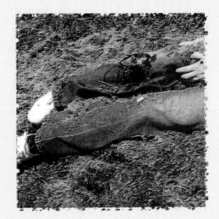

Musculoskeletal Injuries

INTRODUCTION

Injuries to muscles, joints, and bones are some of the most common emergencies you will encounter in the field. These injuries can range from the simple and non-life-threatening (such as a broken finger or sprained ankle) to the critical and life-threatening (such as a fracture of the femur or spine). Regardless of whether the injury is mild or severe, your ability to provide emergency care efficiently and quickly may prevent further painful and damaging injury and may even keep the patient from suffering permanent disability or death.

OBJECTIVES

Numbered objectives are from the United States Department of Transportation 1994 EMT-Basic National Standard Curriculum. Asterisked objectives, if any, pertain to material that is supplemental to the DOT curriculum.

COGNITIVE

5-3.1 Describe the function of the muscular system. (pp. 611–612)
5-3.2 Describe the function of the skeletal system. (p. 612)
5-3.3 List the major bones or bone groupings of the spinal column; the thorax; the upper extremities; the lower extremities. (pp. 611–612)
5-3.4 Differentiate between an open and a closed painful, swollen, deformed extremity. (p. 614)
5-3.5 State the reasons for splinting. (p. 615)
5-3.6 List the general rules of splinting. (pp. 617–620)
5-3.7 List the complications of splinting. (p. 622)

5-3.8 List the emergency medical care for a patient with a painful, swollen, deformed extremity. (pp. 615, 622–631)

AFFECTIVE

5-3.9 Explain the rationale for splinting at the scene versus load and go. (p. 615)
5-3.10 Explain the rationale for immobilization of the painful, swollen, deformed extremity. (p. 615)

PSYCHOMOTOR

5-3.11 Demonstrate the emergency medical care of a patient with a painful, swollen, deformed extremity.
5-3.12 Demonstrate completing a prehospital care report for patients with musculoskeletal injuries.

CASE STUDY

THE DISPATCH

Medic One—respond to the Peninsula High football field—you have a 17-year-old male patient complaining of leg pain. Time out is 1634 hours.

ON ARRIVAL

You are met by the football coach. He tells you his quarterback was tackled very hard. The patient cries out in pain, "My leg, my leg!"

How should you proceed to care for this patient?

During this chapter you will learn how to assess and treat a painful, swollen, or deformed extremity. Later we will return to the case and apply the knowledge and skills learned.

MUSCULOSKELETAL SYSTEM REVIEW

The two main parts of the musculoskeletal system, as is obvious from its name, are the muscles and the skeleton. The functions of the musculoskeletal system are:

• To give the body shape
• To protect the internal organs
• To provide for movement

The musculoskeletal system was presented in Chapter 4, "The Human Body," which you may wish to review now. Some major points about the musculoskeletal system are summarized below.

THE MUSCLES

There are three kinds of muscles: voluntary (skeletal), involuntary (smooth), and cardiac. Involuntary muscles are found in the walls of organs and help move food through the digestive system. Cardiac muscle is found only in the walls of the heart.

The kind of muscle that is pertinent to the topic of this chapter, musculoskeletal injuries, is *voluntary muscle*. Voluntary muscles are those that are under control of a person's will. They make possible all deliberate acts, such as walking, chewing, swallowing, smiling, frowning, talking, or moving the eyeballs. Often referred to as *skeletal muscles*, most voluntary muscles are generally attached at one or both ends to the skeleton.

The voluntary muscles form the major muscle mass of the body. Movements of the body are the result of work performed by the muscles. What enables muscle tissue to work is its ability to contract—to become shorter and thicker—when stimulated by a nerve impulse. In addition to enabling us to move, muscles help give our bodies their distinctive shapes.

Muscles can be injured in many ways. Overexerting a muscle may break fibers, and muscles subjected to trauma can be bruised, crushed, cut, torn, or otherwise injured, even if the skin is not broken. Muscles injured in any way tend to become swollen, tender, painful, or weak.

TENDONS AND LIGAMENTS

Tendons and ligaments (Figure 32-1) are, in a sense, the glue that holds the body together. Composed of specialized connective tissue, *tendons* connect muscle to bone while *ligaments* connect bone to bone. Ten-

dons and ligaments, as well as muscles, can be bruised, crushed, cut, or torn, and are included in the category of musculoskeletal injuries.

THE SKELETAL SYSTEM

The skeletal system (Figure 32-2) supports the body, allowing it to stand erect. Without its bones, the body would collapse. As the body's structural framework, the skeleton must be strong to provide support and protection, jointed to permit motion, and flexible to withstand stress. A major element in motion is the body's *joints*, or places where bones meet.

The skeletal system consists of six basic components: the skull, spinal column, thorax, pelvis, lower extremities, and upper extremities.

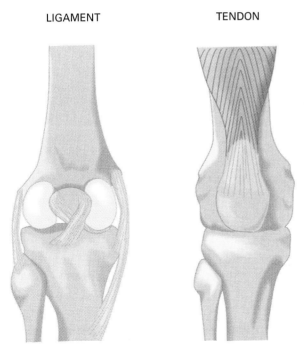

LIGAMENT   TENDON

Figure 32-1   Ligaments connect bone to bone. Tendons attach muscle to bone.

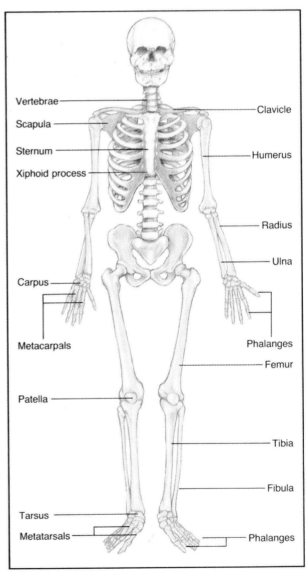

Figure 32-2   The skeletal system.

INJURIES TO BONES AND JOINTS

Several kinds of musculoskeletal injuries are possible. The first to come to mind is a *fracture* or, simply, a broken bone. A *strain* is an injury to a muscle or a muscle and tendon, possibly by being overextended or stretched. A *sprain* is an injury to a joint with possible damage to or tearing of ligaments. A *dislocation* is the displacement of a bone from its normal position in a joint.

All of these kinds of injuries may present with similar signs and symptoms: swelling, pain, or deformity. Sometimes there will be discoloration. Sometimes broken bones will break through the skin.

Musculoskeletal injuries are usually associated with external forces such as falls or vehicle collisions, though some may occur through disease (e.g., bone degeneration), particularly in elderly patients. The force applied to the body may cause injuries to the surrounding soft tissues (e.g., nerves and arteries), and even to body areas distant from the injury site. In assessing and treating injuries to the bones and joints, it is important to determine the mechanism of injury as well as the signs and symptoms of the injury itself.

MECHANISM OF INJURY

As you approach a patient with an injured extremity you can get a good idea of how much damage may have occurred by determining the mechanism of injury. The forces that may cause bone and joint injury include direct force, indirect force, and twisting force.

DIRECT FORCE

The injury from **direct force,** or a direct blow, occurs at the point of impact. For example, a man in an automobile accident who is not wearing a seat belt is thrust forward, the knees hitting the dashboard. As a result, the patella may be fractured.

INDIRECT FORCE

With **indirect force,** the force impacts on one end of a limb, causing injury some distance away from the point of impact. For instance, a woman is thrown from a horse and lands on two outstretched hands. One arm sustains a fractured wrist, while the clavicle (collarbone) at the end of the other arm is fractured.

TWISTING FORCE

In **twisting force,** one part of the extremity remains stationary while the rest twists. Take the case of the child running across a field who steps into a hole.

The child's foot is rammed snugly into the hole and stays stationary while her leg twists, fracturing the tibia and/or fibula. Bone and joint injuries from twisting force occur commonly in football or skiing accidents.

ASSESSMENT AND CARE: BONE OR JOINT INJURIES

SCENE SIZE-UP AND INITIAL ASSESSMENT

As you approach the patient with a possible bone or joint injury, take appropriate body substance isolation precautions and consider the mechanism of injury. During your scene size-up, ask questions of bystanders, family, and the patient. Is the cause of the injury a fall, ejection from a vehicle, high speed collision, or some other traumatic force? Try to imagine the forces the patient's body was subjected to and the direction in which those forces propelled the body.

During the initial assessment, your general impression of the patient's injury helps determine the priority of care and whether or not your patient has a life-threatening emergency. Though joint or bone injuries are rarely life threatening, you should check for obvious signs of severe hemorrhage and treat for shock. Any force significant enough to cause a major musculoskeletal injury can also cause internal injuries. When severe hemorrhage is not obvious, bleeding may be internal to the injury site. This is often the case during blunt trauma. Remember: if the mechanism of injury is severe, look for signs and symptoms of shock.

Pulselessness and cyanosis distal to an injured extremity is a serious condition. If this is apparent, transport the patient immediately after immobilizing the injury, immediately following your focused history and physical exam. Absent pulses sometimes indicate arterial compromise, which may cause impaired tissue perfusion, possible tissue death, and loss of the limb.

If the patient has a life-threatening condition that requires immediate transport but that is not directly related to or caused by the extremity injury, you will initiate transport and, if time and the patient's condition permit, immobilize the extremity injury en route. If the patient is immobilized to a spine board, this will provide temporary stability to the injured extremity.

FOCUSED HISTORY AND PHYSICAL EXAM

If the patient is unresponsive or the mechanism of injury is significant, begin the focused history and physical exam with a rapid trauma assessment. If the patient is responsive and the mechanism of injury is not significant, conduct a focused physical exam, inspecting and gently palpating the injured bone or joint. Be sure to assess the joints above and below any bone injury or the bones above and below any joint injury. As you examine the patient, be gentle and reassuring since musculoskeletal injuries are very frightening for the patient. Check for DCAP-BTLS at the injury site. In infants or children under 6 years of age who have suffered a bone or joint injury, check for a capillary refill time greater than 2 seconds.

Assess the baseline vitals and obtain a SAMPLE history from the patient. Don't forget to ask such basic questions as:

When did the injury occur?
What happened?
Where does it hurt?
What did you feel at the time of injury?

Most patients with significant musculoskeletal injury will complain of pain localized to the area of injury. The patient may also report feeling or hearing something snap.

Signs and Symptoms Bone and joint injuries can be one of two types (Figure 32-3):

- *Closed*—in which the overlying skin is intact
- *Open*—in which the skin over the fracture site has been broken; bone may or may not protrude through the wound

The signs and symptoms of bone and joint injury may include (Figure 32-4):

- Deformity or angulation—When compared to the normal extremity, there is a difference in the size or shape or the injured extremity is in an unnatural position
- Pain and tenderness
- Grating, or **crepitus,** the sound or feeling of broken fragments of bone grinding against each other
- Swelling
- Disfigurement—Either an indentation where tissues have separated or swelling indicating contracted tissue

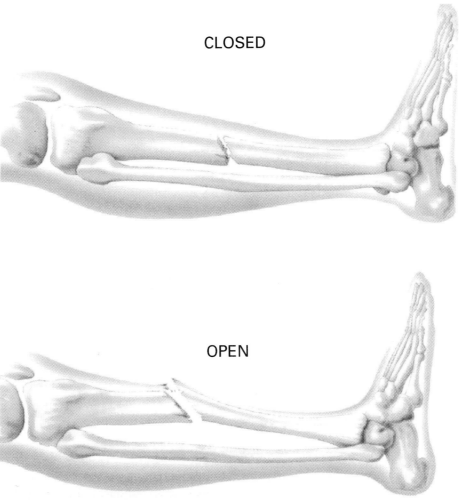

CLOSED

OPEN

Figure 32-3   Closed and open injuries.

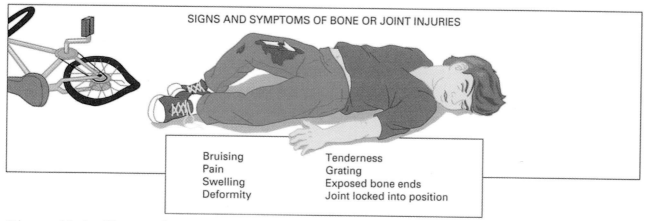

SIGNS AND SYMPTOMS OF BONE OR JOINT INJURIES

Bruising
Pain
Swelling
Deformity

Tenderness
Grating
Exposed bone ends
Joint locked into position

Figure 32-4   Signs and symptoms of bone or joint injuries.

- Severe weakness and loss of function
- Bruising (discoloration)
- Exposed bone ends
- Joint locked into position

Note that it is not necessary, and often not possible, to diagnose the nature of the injury in the prehospital setting. An extremity that is painful, swollen, or deformed may be the result of a fracture, sprain, strain, or dislocation. However, you should not waste time trying to figure out which kind of injury it is. Any painful, swollen, or deformed extremity should be given the emergency care that is outlined below.

EMERGENCY MEDICAL CARE

In some cases, the bone injury is the chief complaint. As stated previously, if the patient has a life-threatening condition caused by or directly related to the extremity injury, you will immobilize the injured extremity during your initial assessment. If the patient has a life-threatening condition not directly related to the extremity injury, you will initiate transport and immobilize the extremity en route if time and critical patient care permit.

Perform the following steps to immobilize a suspected fracture:

1. *Use proper body substance isolation techniques,* such as putting on disposable gloves, before you approach the patient.
2. *Administer oxygen if needed.*
3. *Maintain in-line spinal stabilization if spinal injury is suspected.*
4. *Splint bone and joint injuries.* Be sure to check the patient's distal pulses, motor function, and sensation both before and after splinting. Document your findings in the prehospital care report. Specifics on splinting are detailed in the next section.

5. *Apply cold packs to the painful, swollen, or deformed extremity* to reduce pain and swelling.
6. *Elevate the extremity* (if spinal injury is not suspected) and keep it elevated throughout transport.
7. *Transport.*

DETAILED PHYSICAL EXAM AND ONGOING ASSESSMENT

You may choose to conduct a detailed physical exam en route to the hospital for those patients who may have suffered multiple injuries to identify any other potential injuries that may require treatment. Next, perform the ongoing assessment, including a recheck of the patient's vital signs and interventions. Is the injured extremity properly immobilized? Make sure that the patient's distal pulses, motor function, and sensation have improved or have not deteriorated as a result of immobilization.

SUMMARY: ASSESSMENT AND CARE

To review possible assessment findings and emergency care for musculoskeletal injuries, see Figures 32-5 and 32-6.

BASICS OF SPLINTING

Any device used to immobilize a body part is a **splint.** A splint can be soft or rigid. It can be commercially manufactured or it can be improvised from virtually any object that can provide stability.

There are two basic reasons for splinting a bone or joint injury. First, splinting prevents movement of any bone fragments, bone ends, or dislocated joints, reducing the chance for further injury. Second,

ASSESSMENT SUMMARY

MUSCULOSKELETAL INJURY

The following are findings that may be associated with a musculoskeletal injury.

SCENE SIZE-UP

Pay particular attention to your own safety. Look for:
Mechanism of injury
    Ejection from a vehicle
    High speed collision
    Sports injury
    Fall
    Crushing force
    Gunshot wounds
    Evidence of other trauma

INITIAL ASSESSMENT

General Impression

Major bleeding associated with suspected fracture
Open fracture sites
Obvious deformity to extremities

Mental Status

Alert to unresponsive based on other injuries

Airway

Clear and open unless associated with facial fractures or other injuries

Breathing

Normal; increased if extreme pain or associated with shock or other injury

Circulation

Pulse is normal; may be increased in response to pain or shock
Skin is normal; may be cool, clammy, pale, and cyanotic in extremity if bone injury disrupts distal blood flow

Status: Priority patient if distal pulses are not present or if bone injury is associated with other life-threatening injuries such as severe blood loss, shock, or internal injuries

FOCUSED HISTORY AND PHYSICAL EXAM

Physical Exam

Pelvis:
    Pain
    Instability on compression
    Deformity
Extremities:
    Pain
    Deformity
    Tenderness on palpation
    Crepitus
    Loss of function distal to injury
    Open wounds
    Discoloration
    Exposed bone ends
    Abnormal inward or outward rotation of foot and leg (hip dislocation or femur fracture)

Baseline Vital Signs

BP: normal or may be decreased if there is other trauma and shock
HR: normal, or may be increased due to pain or other injuries, bleeding, or shock
RR: normal, or may be increased due to pain, other injuries, bleeding, or shock
Skin: normal, or may be pale, cool, clammy and cyanotic if the bone injury is interfering with distal circulation or associated with bleeding and shock
Pupils: normal or may be dilated and sluggish if associated with bleeding and shock

SAMPLE History

Signs and symptoms of an open fracture:
    Pain, deformity, swelling to long bone
    Open wound associated with suspected fracture site
    Exposed bone ends
Signs and symptoms of a closed fracture:
    Pain, deformity, swelling to long bone
Signs and symptoms of a dislocation:
    Pain, deformity, swelling to a joint
    Abnormal rotation of foot and leg (hip dislocation)

Figure 32-5a Assessment summary: musculoskeletal injury.

EMERGENCY CARE PROTOCOL

MUSCULOSKELETAL INJURY

1. Establish manual in-line stabilization if spinal injury is suspected.
2. Establish an open airway, and insert nasopharyngeal or oropharyngeal airway if patient is unresponsive and has no gag or cough reflex.
3. Suction secretions as necessary.
4. If breathing is inadequate, provide positive pressure ventilation with supplemental oxygen at a minimum rate of 12 ventilation/minute for an adult and 20 ventilation/minute for an infant or child.
5. If breathing is adequate, administer oxygen by nonrebreather mask at 15 lpm.
6. Control any major bleeding.
7. If priority patient, splint suspected fractures and dislocations en route to medical facility.
8. If spinal injury suspected, immobilize patient to a backboard.
9. Follow the general rules of splinting:
   a. Assess pulses, motor, and sensory function distal to injury before and after splinting.
   b. Immobilize joints above and below in long bone injury and bones above and below in joint injury.
   c. Dress and bandage all open wounds before splinting.
   d. If suspected fracture is grossly deformed or no distal circulation is present, apply gentle traction and attempt to realign. If excruciating pain or resistance is met, stop and splint in the position found.
   e. Splint suspected dislocations in position found unless distal pulses are absent. If no distal pulses, apply gentle traction and realign unless extreme pain or resistance is met. Splint in position found.
   f. Cold can be applied to deformity to reduce swelling and pain.
   g. Elevate extremity slightly to reduce swelling. Remove all jewelry on affected extremity.
   h. Reassess pulses, motor, and sensory function.
10. Suspected fractures or dislocations requiring special equipment or procedures:
    Hip Dislocation or Fracture
    Pad between legs and bind legs together or apply long board splints; place patient on backboard.
    Pelvis
    Apply PASG and inflate all three sections to splinting pressure, or pad between legs and bind legs together; place patient on a backboard.
    Femur
    Apply a traction splint; place on backboard.
    Shoulder
    Sling and swathe if in relatively normal position. Vacuum splint, wire ladder splints, or board splints if severely deformed.
    Clavicle
    Sling and swathe.
11. Transport.
12. Perform ongoing assessment every 5 minutes if unstable and every 15 minutes if stable.

Figure 32-5b   Emergency care protocol: musculoskeletal injury.

splints usually reduce pain and minimize the following common complications from bone and joint injuries:

- Damage to muscles, nerves, or blood vessels caused by movement of bone fragments or bone ends
- Conversion of a closed fracture to an open fracture (by breaking through the skin)
- Restriction of blood flow as a result of bone ends or dislocations compressing blood vessels
- Excessive bleeding from tissue damage caused by movement of bone ends
- Increased pain associated with movement of bone ends or dislocated bones
- Paralysis of the extremities resulting from a damaged spine

GENERAL RULES OF SPLINTING

Regardless of where you apply the splint, follow these general rules (Figures 32-7a to f):

- *Both before and after you apply the splint, assess the pulse, motor function, and sensation distal to the injury.* (Keep the mnemonic PMS for pulse, motor function, and sensation constantly in mind as you manage a suspected fracture.) You should evaluate these signs every 15 minutes after applying the splint to make sure the splint is not impairing circulation to the extremity.
- Immobilize the joints both above and below an injury to a long bone. (If the forearm is fractured, for

EMERGENCY CARE ALGORITHM: MUSCULOSKELETAL INJURY

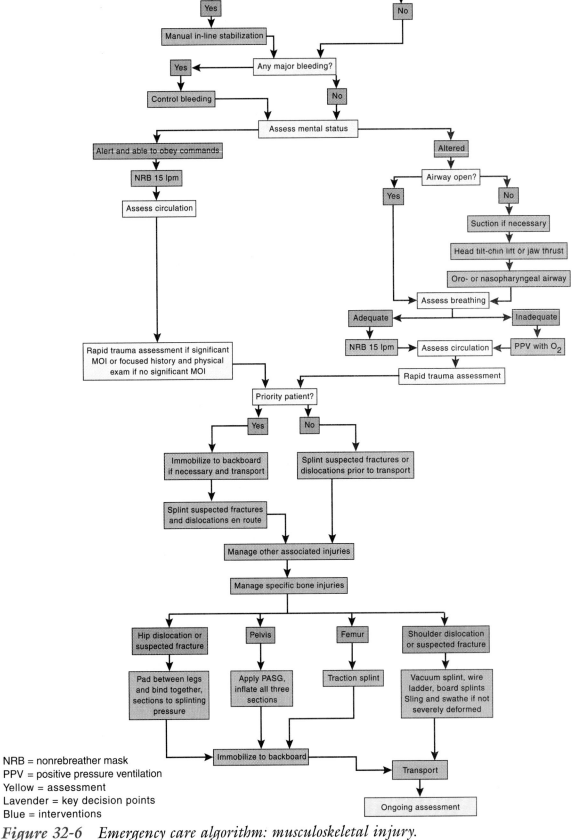

Figure 32-6 Emergency care algorithm: musculoskeletal injury.

GENERAL SPLINTING RULES

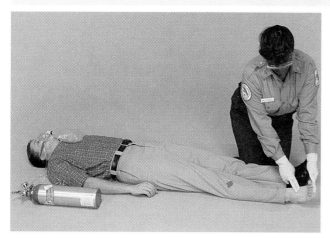

Figure 32-7a   *Assess the distal pulse and motor and sensory function.*

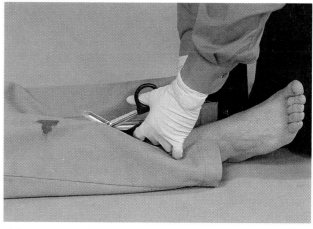

Figure 32-7b   *Cut away clothing to expose the injury site.*

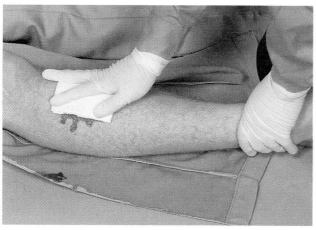

Figure 32-7c   *Place a sterile dressing over the open wound.*

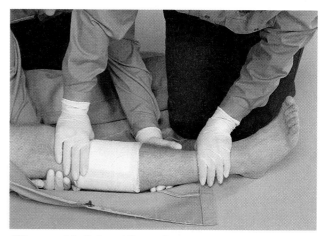

Figure 32-7d   *Align the extremity with gentle traction if there is severe deformity, absence of distal pulses, or cyanosis.*

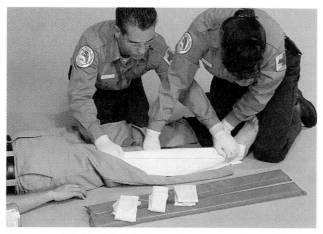

Figure 32-7e   *Pad the splint to prevent discomfort and unnecessary pressure. The correct size splint will immobilize the joint above and below the site of a bone injury.*

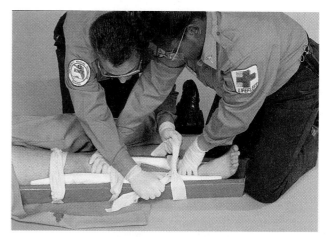

Figure 32-7f   *Maintain manual traction. Do not release until the splint has been applied. Assess distal pulse and motor and sensory function after the splint has been applied.*

example, immobilize both the wrist and the elbow.) Immobilize the bones above and below an injury to a joint. (If the elbow is injured, immobilize both the humerus of the upper arm and the radius and ulna of the forearm.)

- Remove or cut away all clothing around the injury site with a pair of bandage scissors so you won't accidentally move the fractured bone ends and complicate the injury. Remove all jewelry around the injury site, especially distally, because it may become entrapped by swelling. Bag the jewelry and either give it to a family member or see that it is transported with the patient.

- Cover all wounds, including open fractures, with sterile dressings before applying a splint, then gently bandage. Avoid excessive pressure on the wound.

- If there is a severe deformity or the distal extremity is cyanotic (bluish) or lacks pulses, align the injured limb with gentle manual traction (pulling) before splinting. As a general rule, make one attempt to align the extremity. *If pain, resistance, or crepitus increase, stop.* Generally, you should not try to align a wrist, elbow, knee, hip, or shoulder—major nerves and arteries close to these joints increase the chance of causing further damage. *Follow local protocol.*

- Never intentionally replace protruding bones or push them back below the skin. (Occasionally, during realignment, these will be drawn into the wound.)

- Pad each splint to prevent pressure and discomfort to the patient.

- Apply the splint before trying to move the patient. Do not release manual traction until after the splint has been applied.

- When in doubt, splint the injury.

- If the patient shows signs of shock, align the patient in the normal anatomical position, treat for shock, and transport immediately without taking the time to apply a splint.

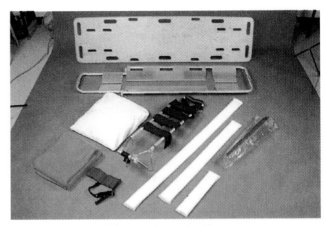

Figure 32-8   Examples of splints.

SPLINTING EQUIPMENT

Some splints are more suitable to certain types of injuries than others, but many are interchangeable (Figure 32-8). You will need to follow your local protocol in such cases. The general types of splints are rigid splints, traction splints, pressure splints, improvised splints, and the sling and swathe.

RIGID SPLINTS

Rigid splints are commercially manufactured splints made of wood, aluminum, wire, plastic, cardboard, or compressed wood fibers. Some are designed in specific shapes for arms and legs and are equipped with Velcro closures; others are pliable enough to be molded to fit any appendage. Some come with washable pads, but others must be padded before being applied.

TRACTION SPLINTS

Traction splints (Figure 32-9) provide a counter-pull, alleviating pain, reducing blood loss, and minimizing further injury. Traction splints are not intended to

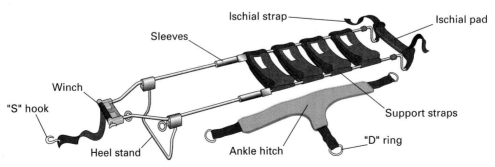

Figure 32-9   A bipolar traction splint.

reduce (correct) the fracture, but simply to immobilize the bone ends and prevent further injury. Several types of traction splints are available, and procedures vary according to the manufacturer. Specifics about traction splinting are detailed later in this chapter.

VACUUM SPLINTS

Vacuum splints (Figure 32-10a to c) are soft, pliable splints that are easily formed to deformed extremities. The air is then sucked out of the splint, causing it to become extremely rigid in its position of placement.

PRESSURE SPLINTS

The main type of pressure splint is an air splint. Air splints are soft and pliable before being inflated but rigid once they are applied and filled with air. Air splints cannot be sized, may impair circulation, may

interfere with the ability to assess pulses, and may lose or gain pressure with temperature and altitude changes. Seek medical direction and follow local protocol regarding their use.

The pneumatic antishock garment (PASG) is also sometimes used as a pressure splint to immobilize an injury to a lower extremity or the pelvis. (See Chapter 29, "Bleeding and Shock," for detailed information on PASG.) Follow local protocol, and never apply the PASG without approval from medical direction. The use of the PASG to splint a pelvic injury is illustrated under Splinting Specific Injuries later in this chapter.

IMPROVISED SPLINTS

You may be forced to improvise at the scene. Improvised splints can be made from a cardboard box, cane, ironing board, rolled-up magazine, umbrella,

APPLYING A VACUUM SPLINT

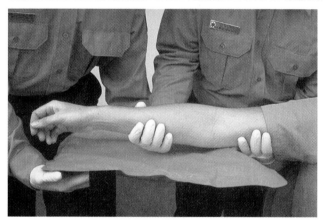

Figure 32-10a   Manually stabilize the suspected fracture and assess pulse, motor, and sensory function.

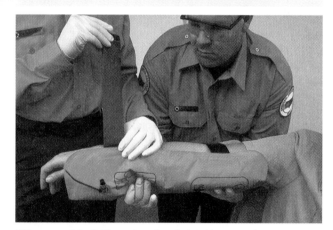

Figure 32-10b   Apply the splint and secure it to the extremity.

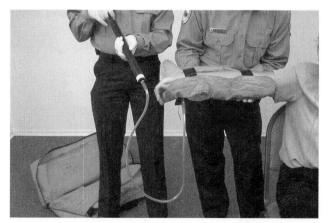

Figure 32-10c   Suction the air out of the splint until it is rigid. Reassess pulse, motor, and sensory function.

broom handle, catcher's shin guard, or any other similar object. An effective improvised splint must be:

- Light in weight, but firm and rigid
- Long enough to extend past the joints and prevent movement on either side of the fracture
- As wide as the thickest part of the fractured limb
- Padded well so the inner surfaces are not in contact with the skin

An ordinary bed pillow (Figure 32-11) or blanket roll can be an effective improvised splint when wrapped around the area and secured with several cravats.

SLING AND SWATHE

A sling and swathe is often used to provide stability to a painful and tender shoulder injury. A sling is a triangular bandage. The sling supports the patient's arm, while a swathe of cloth holds the patient's arm against the side of the chest. This minimizes the pain and further injury associated with arm and shoulder movement. (See instructions for applying a sling and swathe under Splinting Specific Injuries later in this chapter.)

HAZARDS OF IMPROPER SPLINTING

For all their obvious benefits to the patient with a bone or joint injury, splints can also cause complications if they are applied in the wrong manner. Improper splinting can:

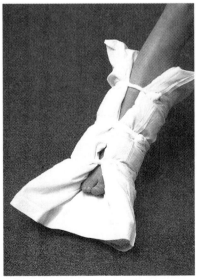

Figure 32-11 Pillow splint for injured foot or ankle.

- Compress the nerves, tissues, and blood vessels under the splint, aggravating the existing injury and causing new injury
- Delay the transport of a patient who has a life-threatening injury
- Reduce distal circulation, compromising the viability of the extremity
- Aggravate the bone or joint injury by allowing movement of the bone fragments or bone ends or by forcing bone ends beneath the skin surface
- Cause or aggravate damage to the tissues, nerves, blood vessels, or muscles due to excessive bone or joint movement

SPLINTING LONG BONE INJURIES

Special considerations must be taken into account when splinting long bones or joints. Remember that some long bone injuries may lead to serious internal bleeding. As you assess for DCAP-BTLS, look for the following signs and symptoms of long bone injury:

- Exposed bone ends
- Joints locked in position
- **Paresthesia,** a pricking or tingling feeling that indicates some loss of sensation
- Paralysis
- Pallor of the injury site

Assess the pulse, motor, and sensory function below the injury site. Assess the radial pulse for an upper extremity, the dorsal pedal or posterior tibial pulse for a lower extremity. Sensation is intact if the patient can tell you, without looking, which finger or toe you are touching and can feel painful stimuli. If the injury involves an upper extremity, motor function is intact if the patient can make a fist, undo the fist, spread the fingers, and make a hitchhiking sign with the thumb. If the injury involves a lower extremity, motor function is intact if the patient can tighten the kneecap and move the foot up and down as if pumping an automobile accelerator.

If the limb is severely deformed, cyanotic, or lacks distal pulses, align it with gentle traction. Provide steady, gentle pressure along with traction. If pain or crepitus increases, stop.

For specific guidelines on splinting a long bone injury see Figures 32-12a to f. In Figure 32-12e, you will see that the hand (or foot) must be immobilized in the position of function. The position of function for a hand is with the fingers curled as if holding a ball. You can put a roll of bandage in the patient's hand to support this position. The position of function for the foot is at a 90-degree angle to the leg with the foot bent at the normal angle to the leg, not pushed downward or upward toward the shin.

SPLINTING A LONG BONE

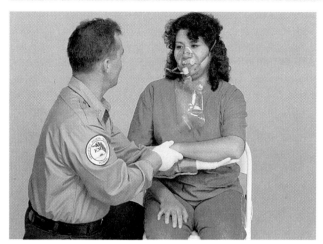

Figure 32-12a   Apply manual stabilization to the injured extremity.

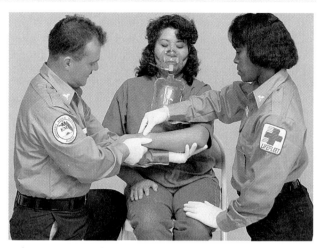

Figure 32-12b   Assess the distal pulse and motor and sensory function.

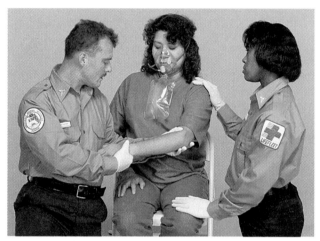

Figure 32-12c   If the deformity is severe, distal pulses are absent, or the distal extremity is cyanotic, align with gentle manual traction.

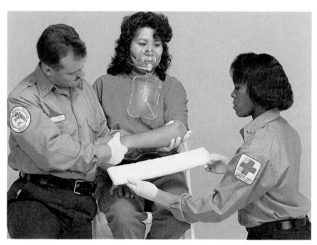

Figure 32-12d   Measure the splint for proper length.

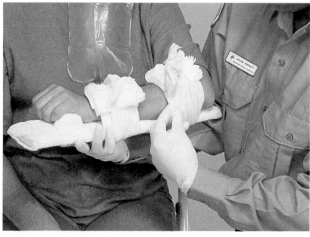

Figure 32-12e   Secure the entire injured extremity. The hand (or foot) must be immobilized in the position of function.

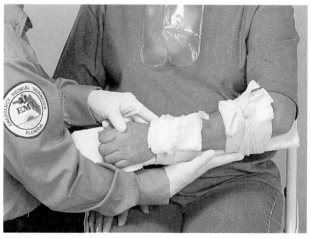

Figure 32-12f   Reassess the pulse and motor and sensory function.

SPLINTING JOINT INJURIES

A common joint injury is the displacement of a bone end from the joint, or dislocation. In a dislocation, the ligaments holding the bones in proper position are often stretched and sometimes are torn loose. Dislocations cause serious pain because the joint surfaces are rich in nerves.

The principal signs and symptoms of any type of joint injury are pain, swelling, deformity, and possible rigidity and loss of function. As with long bone injuries, assess the pulse, motor, and sensory function below the injury site. Look for paresthesia or paralysis, and if the distal extremity is cyanotic (bluish) or lacks pulses, align the joint with gentle traction. If pain or crepitus increases, stop. Remember not to spend time trying to differentiate a joint injury from a bone injury since it may be difficult to distinguish between the two; for both you will need to splint and transport.

For specific guidelines on splinting a joint injury see Figures 32-13a to c.

TRACTION SPLINTING

Fractures of the femur and some fractures below the knee can be successfully immobilized with a traction splint. A fractured femur is complicated because of the large muscle mass of the thigh that will contract and pull the fractured femur ends so that they override, or pass each other. This causes great pain and a lot of internal soft tissue injury and bleeding. Trac-

tion splinting serves to realign the fractured femur. This helps relieve pain and reduce the incidence of internal injuries that would occur if the patient were transported without immobilization. *Remember, though, that you don't have to be certain the femur has actually been fractured. If the thigh is painful, swollen, or deformed you should treat as if the femur is fractured.*

In general, you should *not* use a traction splint if:

- The injury is within one to two inches of the knee or ankle
- The knee itself has been injured
- The hip has been injured
- The pelvis has been injured
- There is partial amputation or avulsion with bone separation, and the distal limb is connected only by marginal tissue. (In such a case, using a traction splint would risk separation.)

See Figures 32-14a to l for instructions on applying a bipolar traction splint. See Figures 32-15a to f for instructions in applying a unipolar traction splint.

SPLINTING SPECIFIC INJURIES

Special techniques may be applied to the splinting of suspected bone and joint injuries to specific sites. Splinting techniques are illustrated in Figures 32-16 through 32-27 for the following: the shoulder, upper arm, elbow, forearm, wrist, hand, fingers, pelvis, hip, thigh, knee, lower leg, ankle, and foot.

SPLINTING A JOINT

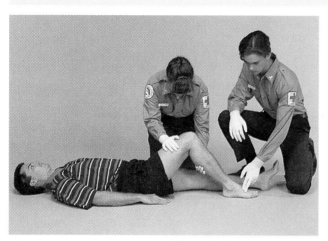

Figure 32-13a   Manually stabilize the joint in the position found. Then assess distal pulse and motor and sensory function.

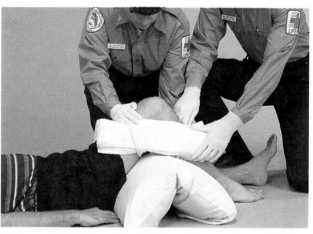

Figure 32-13b   Apply the splint to immobilize the bone above and below the joint.

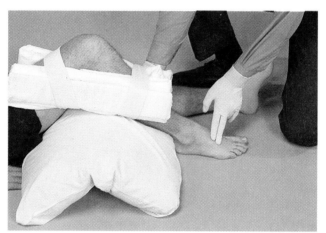

Figure 32-13c   Reassess distal pulses and motor and sensory function after splint is applied.

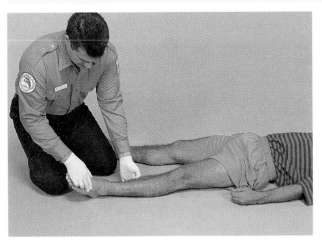

Figure 32-14a *Assess distal pulses and motor and sensory function.*

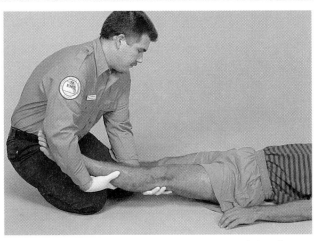

Figure 32-14b *Stabilize the injured leg by applying manual traction.*

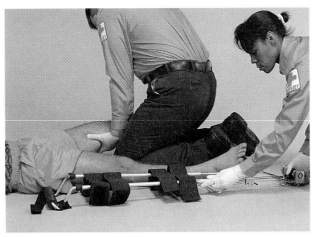

Figure 32-14c *Adjust the splint for proper length.*

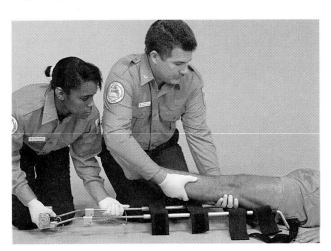

Figure 32-14d *Position the splint under the injured leg until the ischial pad rests against the bony prominence of the buttocks. Once the splint is in position, raise the heel stand.*

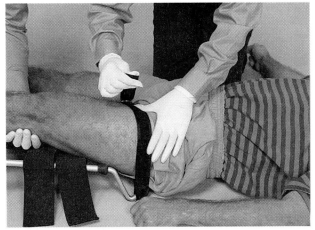

Figure 32-14e *Attach the ischial strap over the groin and thigh.*

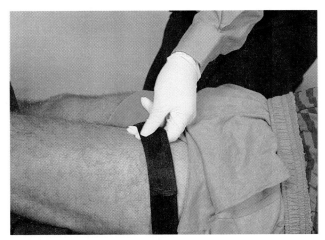

Figure 32-14f *Make sure the ischial strap is snug but not tight enough to reduce distal circulation.*

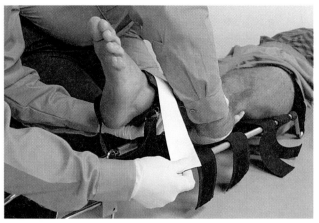

Figure 32-14g With the patient's foot in an upright position, secure the ankle hitch.

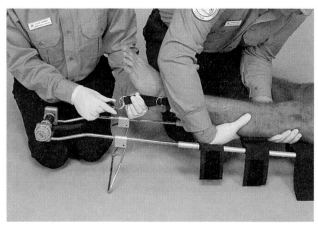

Figure 32-14h Attach the "S" hook to the "D" ring and apply mechanical traction. Full traction is achieved when the mechanical traction is equal to the manual traction and the pain and muscle spasms are reduced. In an unresponsive patient, adjust the traction until the injured leg is the same length as the uninjured leg.

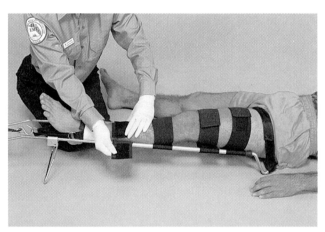

Figure 32-14i Fasten the leg support straps.

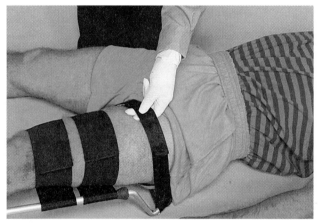

Figure 32-14j Reevaluate the ischial strap and ankle hitch to ensure that both are securely fastened.

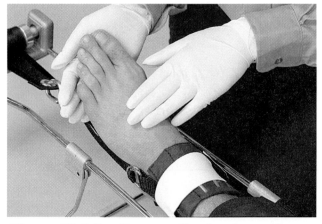

Figure 32-14k Reassess distal pulses and motor and sensory function.

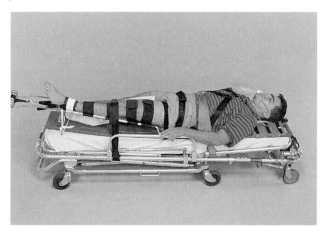

Figure 32-14l Place the patient on a long board and secure with straps. Pad between the splint and uninjured leg. Secure the splint to the backboard.

APPLYING A UNIPOLAR TRACTION SPLINT

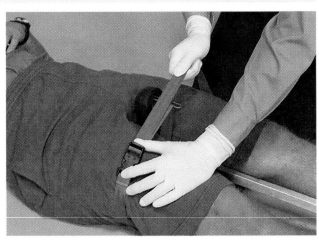

Figure 32-15a Place the splint along the medial aspect of the injured leg. Adjust it so that it extends about four inches beyond the heel.

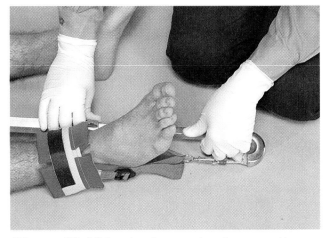

Figure 32-15b Secure the strap to the thigh.

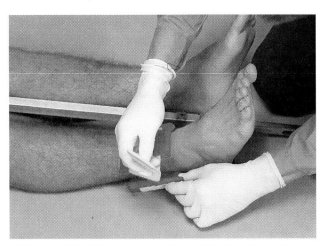

Figure 32-15c Apply the ankle hitch and attach it to the splint.

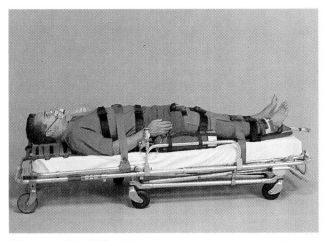

Figure 32-15d Apply traction by extending the splint. Adjust the splint to 10% of the patient's body weight.

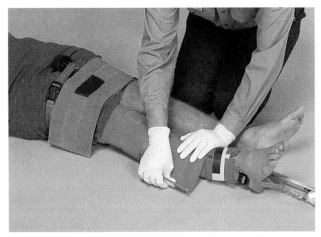

Figure 32-15e Apply the straps to secure leg to splint. Reassess distal pulses and motor and sensory function.

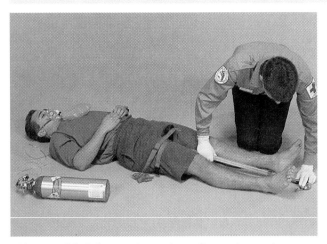

Figure 32-15f Place the patient onto a long backboard. Strap the ankles together and secure to the board.

SPLINTING SPECIFIC INJURIES

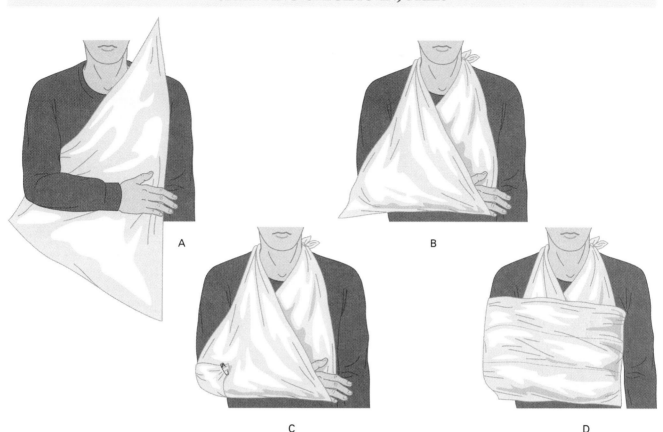

Figure 32-16 Application of sling and swathe. (A) Place one end of the base of an open triangular bandage across the shoulder of the uninjured side, the apex behind the elbow of the injured arm. Bend the arm at the elbow with the hand elevated 4 to 5 inches. (B) Bring the lower end of the bandage over the shoulder of the injured side. Tie it in a knot at the back of the neck. (C) Pin the apex to form a pocket at the elbow. (D) Immobilize the injured arm to the body with a swathe.

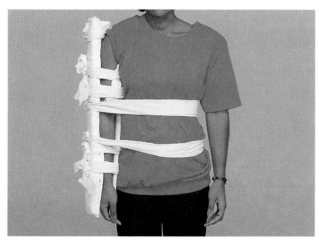

Figure 32-17a Fixed splint for humerus injury.

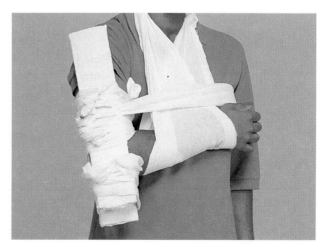

Figure 32-17b Fixation or rigid splint with a sling and swathe.

SPLINTING SPECIFIC INJURIES

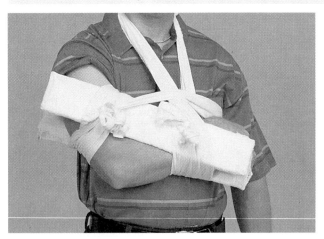

Figure 32-18a Immobilization of an elbow injury in a bent position.

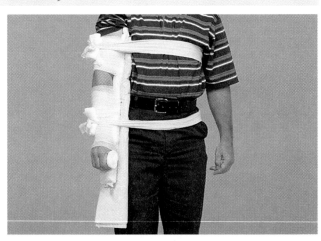

Figure 32-18b Immobilization of an elbow injury in a straight position.

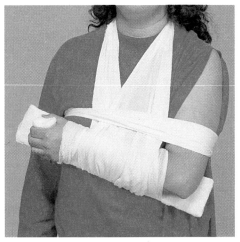

Figure 32-19a Immobilization of a bone injury to the forearm, wrist, or hand.

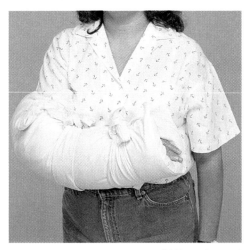

Figure 32-19b Immobilization of a bone injury to the forearm, wrist, or hand.

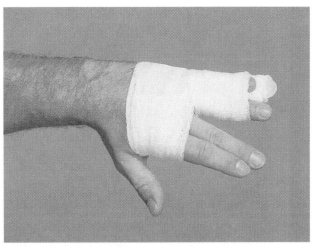

Figure 32-20 Bone injury to the finger splinted with a tongue depressor.

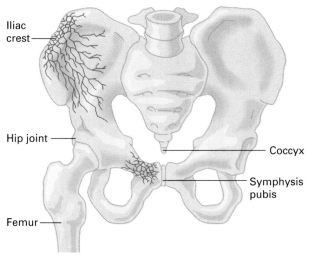

Figure 32-21 Common sites of injury to the pelvis.

SPLINTING SPECIFIC INJURIES

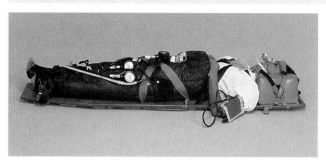

Figure 32-22   Use of the PASG is recommended to splint a suspected pelvic injury.

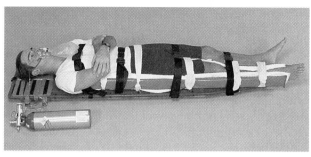

Figure 32-23   Rigid splint for hip injury.

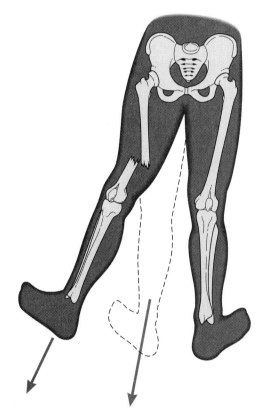

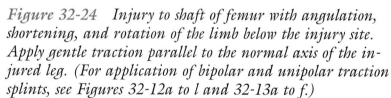

Figure 32-25   Immobilized knee injury in straight position.

Figure 32-24   Injury to shaft of femur with angulation, shortening, and rotation of the limb below the injury site. Apply gentle traction parallel to the normal axis of the injured leg. (For application of bipolar and unipolar traction splints, see Figures 32-12a to l and 32-13a to f.)

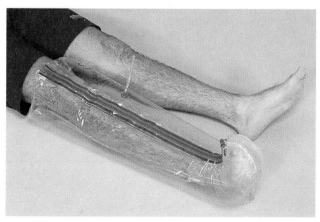

Figure 32-26   Immobilization of lower leg injury with air splint.

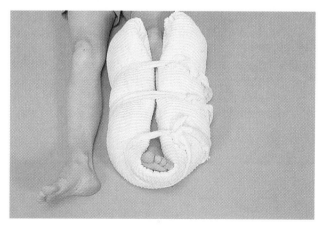

Figure 32-27   Immobilization of the ankle and foot with a blanket roll.

CASE STUDY FOLLOW-UP

SCENE SIZE-UP

You and your partner have just arrived at the high school football field. You have been dispatched to a 17-year-old male patient complaining of leg pain. The scene appears safe as you put on your disposable gloves and remove the stretcher from the ambulance. Your partner grabs the trauma kit. As you wheel the stretcher onto the field you are met by the football coach who tells you his quarterback, Tom Cvitanovic, was tackled. "He can't move his right leg. He got tackled pretty hard." The coach's remarks lead you to believe the mechanism of injury may mean a fracture due to direct force. You approach Tom and introduce yourself. Your partner asks, "What happened, and where is the pain?"

INITIAL ASSESSMENT

Tom complains of severe right leg pain and says his right arm hurts, too. Because he is talking clearly, you assume his airway is open. His breathing is adequate, his radial pulse is strong and 103 per minute. You do not believe he has a life-threatening condition. Tom then lets out a great groan, and says, "Oh, man, can't you do anything for the pain?!!" He seems frightened so you reassure him that he'll get care quickly. Your partner is at Tom's head maintaining manual in-line spinal stabilization. You decide to administer oxygen via a nonrebreather mask at 15 liters per minute.

FOCUSED HISTORY AND PHYSICAL EXAM

While your partner continues spinal stabilization, you perform a rapid trauma assessment; using the DCAP-BTLS mnemonic, you look and feel for signs of injury. Tom denies any neck pain. However, due to the mechanism of injury you apply a cervical spine immobilization collar as your partner continues to maintain manual stabilization.

You find that Tom's right arm is tender and swollen. Approximately 6 inches below Tom's right knee you see bone ends protruding through a fracture site. Pulse, motor, and sensory function are good below both injury sites.

You apply a cold pack to Tom's right arm and then take his baseline vitals. His blood pressure is 142/70 mmHg, respirations are 20 per minute, pulse is 120 per minute, skin warm and slightly sweaty. Skin color is normal. You obtain a SAMPLE history and learn that Tom denies any further pain or injury. He says he is allergic to aspirin and doesn't take any medication. He tells you that 3 years ago he broke the same leg and was hospitalized for almost a week. He had his last meal at noon. Then he describes how he was tackled by two, maybe three, other football players.

Following your local protocols, you decide to apply a vacuum splint to Tom's right arm. You cover the protruding bone ends below the knee with a trauma pad and note that there is very little bleeding. Following local protocols, and with your partner's assistance, you apply padded board splints to Tom's right leg. You recheck pulse, motor, and sensory function of Tom's injured arm and leg. There is no change. Once Tom is fully immobilized to a backboard, you load him into the ambulance for transport.

DETAILED PHYSICAL EXAM

Because Tom was tackled with such force, you conduct a detailed physical exam while en route to the hospital. You do not find any further injuries during the detailed physical exam.

ONGOING ASSESSMENT

You perform an ongoing assessment and find that Tom remains alert and oriented. His airway, breathing, and circulation remain adequate. You reassess vital signs, then recheck your medical interventions. The nonrebreather mask continues to deliver oxygen at 15 liters per minute. The vacuum splint is rigid, and the padded board splints are secure. You reassess pulses, motor function, and sensation to Tom's right arm and leg. You radio your report to the emergency department, continue your ongoing assessment, and reassure Tom that you are only 5 minutes away from the hospital.

A few weeks later, when you are reading the sports page, you spot a picture of Tom on the team bench with crutches propped up beside him. The season is nearly over, but Tom is only a junior and is expected to quarterback the team again next year.

CHAPTER REVIEW

TERMS AND CONCEPTS

You may wish to review the following terms and concepts included in this chapter.

crepitus—the sound or feel of broken fragments of bone grinding against each other.

direct force—a direct blow. Injuries from direct force occur at the point of impact.

indirect force—a force that causes injury some distance away from the point of impact.

paresthesia—a prickling or tingling feeling that indicates some loss of sensation.

splint—any device used to immobilize a body part.

twisting force—a force that twists a bone while one end is held stationary.

REVIEW QUESTIONS

1. List three functions of the musculoskeletal system.
2. Explain the difference between an open and a closed bone injury.
3. List the indications that would lead you to suspect a bone or joint injury.
4. Explain the reasons for splinting a bone or joint injury.
5. List the emergency medical care steps for treating a bone or joint injury.
6. Outline the general rules for splinting a bone or joint injury.
7. Describe the complications that can arise from improper splinting of a bone or joint.
8. List contraindications for (reasons for not using) a traction splint on a suspected femur fracture.

CHAPTER 33

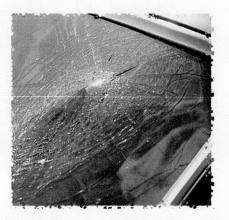

Injuries to the Head

INTRODUCTION

Injuries to the head pose some of the most serious situations you will face as an EMT-B. The patient is often confused or unresponsive, making assessment of his condition difficult. Drug and alcohol use will also cloud the assessment and make head injury diagnosis difficult. Head injuries to a patient can occur days or weeks before the onset of any signs or symptoms. In addition, many injuries to the head are life threatening. Such injuries are, in fact, a leading cause of death among this nation's young people. Many patients who survive head injuries suffer permanent disability. So it is clear that the cost of failing to recognize or properly treat such injuries can be very high.

Numbered objectives are from the United States Department of Transportation 1994 EMT-Basic National Standard Curriculum. Asterisked objectives, if any, pertain to material that is supplemental to the DOT curriculum.

COGNITIVE

5-4.1 State the components of the nervous system. (pp. 635–637)
5-4.2 List the functions of the central nervous system. (pp. 635–637)
5-4.3 Define the structure of the skeletal system as it relates to the nervous system. (pp. 635–636)
5-4.4 Relate mechanism of injury to potential

injuries of the head and spine. (pp. 637, 638, 642–643)
5-4.11 Establish the relationship between airway management and the patient with head and spine injuries. (pp. 638, 643, 644)

PSYCHOMOTOR

5-4.44 Demonstrate completing a prehospital care report for patients with head and spinal injuries.

The above and additional objectives from DOT Lesson 5–4 are also addressed in Chapter 34, "Injuries to the Spine."

CASE STUDY

THE DISPATCH

EMS Unit 504—proceed to 2516 Elmwood Street—unresponsive 18-year-old male. Time out is 1230 hours.

ON ARRIVAL

Family members are waiting outside as your unit approaches the house. An anxious woman begins to speak as soon as you open your door: "My son, we can't wake him up. We found him on his bed and we

can't wake him up! He just came home 20 minutes ago. He laughed and said he'd bumped his head playing basketball. But he seemed fine. I went to get him for lunch and we couldn't wake him up. He's in his room. Please hurry!"

How would you proceed to assess and care for this patient?

In this chapter, you will learn about assessment and care for a patient suffering from head injury. Later, we will return to the case study and apply the procedures learned.

Head injuries must be looked at with concern because the skull encases the structures of the central nervous system. The central nervous system, made up of the brain and the spinal cord, coordinates the functions of other body systems. Injury to it can have severe consequences.

ANATOMY OF THE SKULL AND BRAIN

The skull is the portion of the skeletal system that contains and protects the brain and the portion of the spinal cord that exits from the brain. At this point,

you may want to review the information about the skeletal and nervous systems that were presented in Chapter 4, "The Human Body."

THE SKULL

The brain, which occupies 80 to 90 percent of the space inside the skull, is surrounded by plates of large, flat bones that are fused together to form a helmet-like covering called the **cranial skull.** The remainder of the skull is made up of facial bones. Composed of 14 irregularly shaped bones, it is made up of the cheek, nose, and jaw bones (Figure 33-1). The **basilar skull,** or floor of the skull, is made up of many separate pieces of bone and is the weakest part

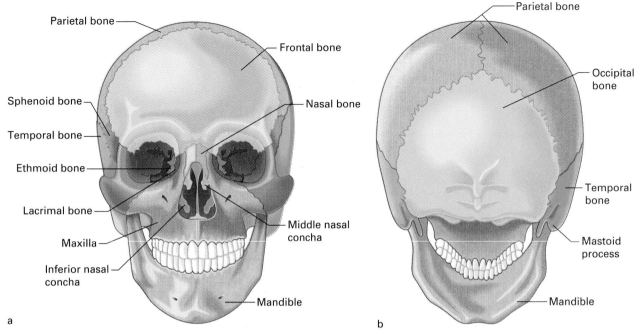

Figure 33-1   The skull.

of the skull. Some of its bones are thin and perforated extensively by the spinal cord, nerves, and blood vessels. The basilar skull has many bony ridges that can cause injury to the brain. Also, the skull tightly encloses the brain, severely limiting the swelling and bleeding that can occur around the brain.

THE BRAIN

Within the skull, the brain is cushioned in a dense, serous substance called **cerebrospinal fluid.** Produced by the brain, this fluid protects the brain and spinal cord against impact. The cerebrospinal fluid is clear and colorless, circulates throughout the skull and spinal column, and is reabsorbed by the circulatory system. The fluid not only cushions and protects but also performs a function similar to lymph fluid in combating infection and cleansing the brain and spinal cord. When both the skull and the membrane surrounding the brain are broken, cerebrospinal fluid leaks out, often through the nose and/or ears—a classic sign of basilar skull fracture.

THE MENINGES

Inside the skull, the surface of the brain is protected from injury by three **meninges,** or layers of tissue, that enclose the brain (Figure 33-2). The outermost is the **dura mater** ("hard mother"), composed of a double layer of tough, fibrous tissue. The next layer is the **arachnoid.** Beneath that, in contact with the brain, is the **pia mater** ("soft mother"). All three layers enclose not only the brain, but the brainstem and the spinal cord as well. The arachnoid membrane and

the pia mater are separated by a lattice of fibrous, spongy tissue filled with cerebrospinal fluid called the **subarachnoid space.**

Bleeding that occurs between the dura mater and the skull is called **epidural** and usually involves the brain's outermost arteries. Recognized and treated early, such bleeding may have no permanent consequences. **Subdural** bleeding, on the other hand, occurs beneath the dura and is usually venous. Bleeding that occurs between the arachnoid membrane and the surface of the brain is called **subarachnoid hemorrhage.** It can be fatal in minutes.

PARTS OF THE BRAIN

The brain is divided into three anatomical components:

- The **cerebrum**—The largest part of the brain, the cerebrum comprises three-fourths of the brain's volume. It is made up of four distinct lobes. It is responsible for most conscious and sensory functions, the emotions, and the personality. The cerebrum is not attached to the inside of the skull.
- The **cerebellum**—Sometimes called the "little brain," the cerebellum controls equilibrium and coordinates muscle activity. Tucked underneath the cerebrum, it controls muscle movement and coordination, predicts when to stop movement, and coordinates the reflexes that maintain posture and equilibrium.
- The **brainstem**—The brain's funnel-shaped inferior part, the brainstem, is the most primitive and best protected part of the brain. Tethered to the skull by numerous nerves and vessels, it controls

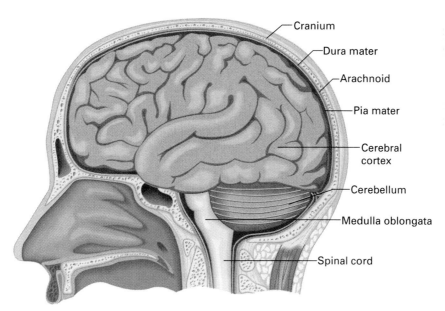

Figure 33-2   The meninges and brain.

most automatic functions of the body, including cardiac, respiratory, vasomotor (blood pressure), and other functions vital to life. The brainstem is made up of the pons, the midbrain, and the medulla, or medulla oblongata, which physically connects the brain to the spinal cord. All of the messages between the brain and the spinal cord pass through the medulla.

TYPES OF HEAD INJURY

Head injuries can involve the scalp, the skull, the brain itself, or combinations of these.

SCALP INJURIES

The scalp may be injured in the same way as any other soft tissue; it may be contused, lacerated, abraded, or avulsed. Because of the rich supply of blood vessels to the scalp, injuries of the scalp tend to bleed very heavily. In addition, the underlying fascia may be torn while the skin stays intact. Bleeding then occurs under the skin and may be confusing at first as you try to assess the patient. (The presence of blood under intact skin can mimic skull deformity.)

SKULL INJURIES

Because of the skull's spherical shape and its thickness, it is generally deformed only if the trauma is extreme. Skull deformities can be *open* (where there is a break in the continuity of the skin and bone) or *closed* (with the scalp intact).

The deformity itself does not cause disability or death; rather, it is the *underlying damage to the brain* that leads to serious consequences. The deformity

presents no danger if it is not accompanied by brain injury, hematoma, cerebrospinal fluid leakage, or subsequent infection.

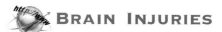 **BRAIN INJURIES**

As already explained, the brain itself is enclosed in the skull—a rigid, unyielding case. Injury can cause swelling of brain tissue or bleeding within the skull. Both conditions can cause increased pressure in the skull.

Brain injury may be direct (from penetrating trauma), indirect (from a blow to the skull), or secondary (for example, from a lack of oxygen, build-up of carbon dioxide, or change in blood pressure). The injury may be closed or open.

In cases of *closed head injury*, the scalp may be lacerated but the skull remains intact and there will be no opening to the brain. Brain damage within the intact skull can, nonetheless, be extensive. The amount of injury depends mainly on the mechanism of injury and the force involved. In general, brain tissue is susceptible to the same kinds of injury as any soft tissue, especially contusion and laceration.

An *open head injury* (Figure 33-3) involves a break in the skull, such as that caused by impact with a windshield or by an impaled object. It involves direct local damage to the involved tissue, but it can also result in brain damage due to infection, laceration of the brain tissue, or punctures of the brain by objects that invade the cranium after penetrating the skull.

Specific types of brain injuries include *concussion*, a temporary loss of the brain's ability to function; *contusion*, bruising or swelling of the brain; *hematoma*, pooling of blood within the brain; and *lacera-*

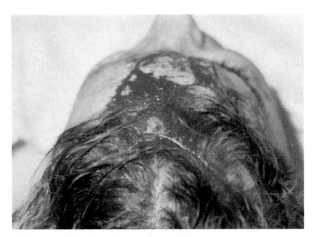

Figure 33-3 Open head injury.

tion, or tearing of the brain tissue. These types of injuries will be discussed at greater length in the Enrichment section at the end of this chapter.

ASSESSMENT AND CARE: HEAD INJURIES

You have studied many of the elements of assessment that apply to head injury—for example, the AVPU method of assessing mental status—in earlier chapters. We will review and develop these assessment elements on the following pages with particular emphasis on how they apply to a patient who has, or may be suspected to have, a head injury (Figure 33-4).

SCENE SIZE-UP

Because head injuries can be so serious, always be alert for signs of them during the scene size-up. Unresponsiveness or altered mental status, especially in trauma patients, should always suggest the possibility of head injury.

Other signs of head injury can be more obvious. These might include bleeding from the scalp or face or an apparent mechanism of injury, such as a fractured windshield at the scene of an automobile crash, a deformed helmet at a bicycling crash, or evidence of a fall (Figure 33-5).

Nontraumatic injuries to the brain can be caused by clots or hemorrhaging. Such injuries can cause altered mental status and present signs and symptoms similar to those in trauma cases. (See Chapter 18, "Altered Speech, Sensory, or Motor Function: Stroke Emergency.")

INITIAL ASSESSMENT

When performing the initial assessment, be alert for cervical spine injury. Forces applied to the head may have been strong enough to injure the cervical spine

as well. Manual in-line stabilization of the spine should be your first step (Figure 33-6).

If the patient is unresponsive or has an altered mental status, establish an airway using a jaw-thrust maneuver while holding in-line spinal stabilization. Maintain the patient's airway and provide oxygen by nonrebreather mask at 15 lpm if breathing is adequate, positive pressure ventilation with supplemental oxygen if breathing is inadequate. *Maintaining an adequate airway and providing oxygen are vital, because head injuries can become worse if there is an inadequate supply of oxygen to the brain.*

Mental Status A decreasing mental status is the most important sign in cases of suspected head injury. The mental status is initially assessed using the AVPU mnemonic (<u>A</u>lert, responds to <u>V</u>erbal stimulus, responds to <u>P</u>ainful stimulus, or <u>U</u>nresponsive). Keep in mind that the patient's mental status may change. For example, the patient may be alert but deteriorate slowly, or he may respond to verbal stimuli and deteriorate to responding to painful stimuli only.

A patient who responds to pain may do so in two ways. The patient may try to move away from or remove the pain. This is a *purposeful* response. Or the patient may respond by inappropriately moving parts of his body, reacting to the pain but not trying to stop it. This is a *nonpurposeful* response.

A nonpurposeful response to pain indicates a deeper state of unresponsiveness. Patients who respond nonpurposefully will usually do one of two things. They will posture by flexing their arms across their chest and extending their legs (**decorticate posturing** or flexion) which indicates an upper level brainstem injury, or they will extend both arms down at their sides, extend their legs, and sometimes arch their backs (**decerebrate posturing** or extension). Decerebrate posturing represents the lowest level of nonpurposeful pain response, indicating a lower level brainstem injury.

The lowest level on the AVPU scale is "unresponsive." A patient at this level exhibits no response at all to verbal or painful stimuli. This is an ominous sign in head injury.

Record your observations of mental status accurately, noting the types of stimuli administered and the patient's responses. You must determine a baseline for level of responsiveness and check repeatedly for signs of deterioration. For example, a patient who first responds to the loud calling of his name, but later only responds to a shoulder pinch with decorticate posturing, has a deteriorating level of responsiveness. Such deterioration of level of responsiveness in cases of head injury can be a sign of a serious problem.

A useful and more discriminating tool for determining a patient's level of responsiveness is the Glasgow

TRAUMA RESULTING IN INJURY TO BRAIN

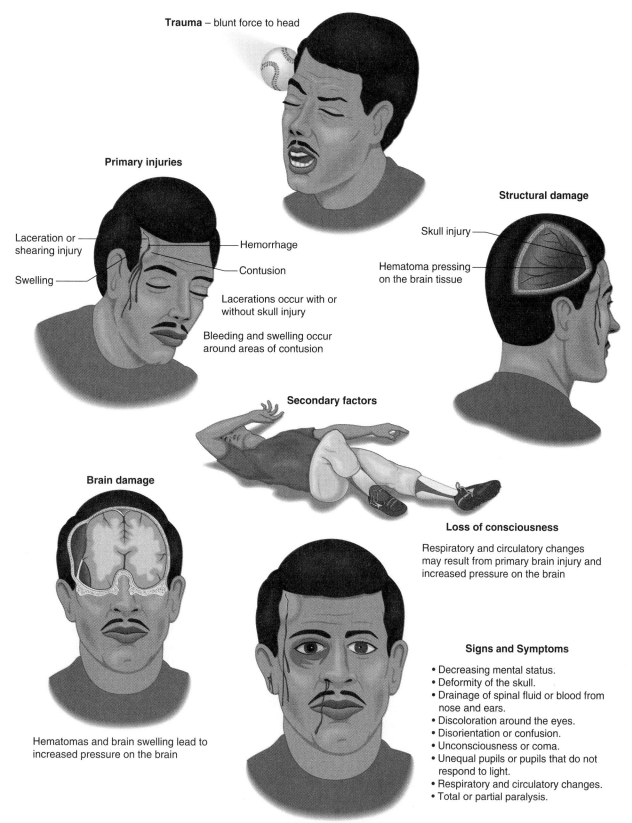

Trauma – blunt force to head

Primary injuries

Laceration or shearing injury

Swelling

Hemorrhage

Contusion

Lacerations occur with or without skull injury

Bleeding and swelling occur around areas of contusion

Structural damage

Skull injury

Hematoma pressing on the brain tissue

Secondary factors

Brain damage

Hematomas and brain swelling lead to increased pressure on the brain

Loss of consciousness

Respiratory and circulatory changes may result from primary brain injury and increased pressure on the brain

Signs and Symptoms

- Decreasing mental status.
- Deformity of the skull.
- Drainage of spinal fluid or blood from nose and ears.
- Discoloration around the eyes.
- Disorientation or confusion.
- Unconsciousness or coma.
- Unequal pupils or pupils that do not respond to light.
- Respiratory and circulatory changes.
- Total or partial paralysis.

Figure 33-4   Trauma to the head and resulting injury to the brain.

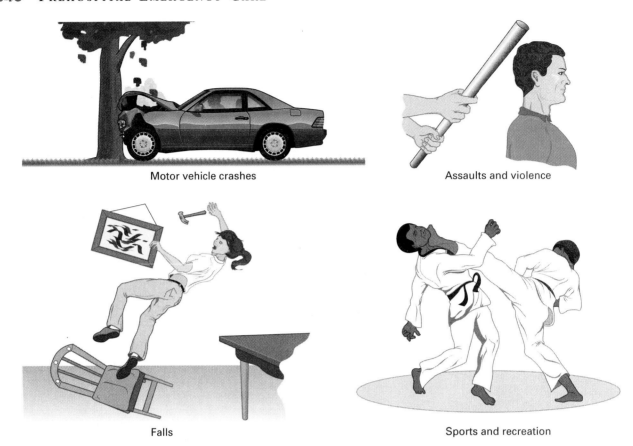

Motor vehicle crashes

Assaults and violence

Falls

Sports and recreation

Figure 33-5   Mechanisms of head injury.

Coma Scale (Figure 33-7). The scale is a measure of the patient's eye opening, verbal response, and motor response to different stimuli. In the prehospital setting, the numerical values on the scale are not as important as the types of response to specific stimuli.

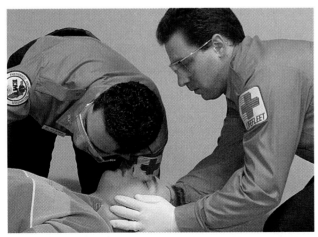

Figure 33-6   Establish and maintain spinal stabilization. Then open the airway and assess breathing.

Glasgow Coma Scale

Eye opening	Spontaneous	4	
	To Voice	3	
	To Pain	2	
	None	1	
Verbal response	Oriented	5	
	Confused	4	
	Inappropriate Words	3	
	Incomprehensible Sounds	2	
	None	1	
Motor response	Obeys Command	6	
	Localizes Pain	5	
	Withdraw (pain)	4	
	Flexion (pain)	3	
	Extension (pain)	2	
	None	1	
Glasgow coma score total			

Figure 33-7   Glasgow Coma Scale.

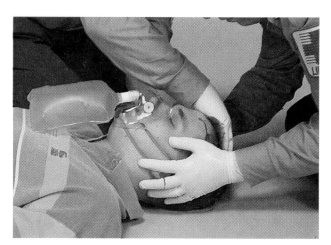

Figure 33-8   Inspect and carefully palpate the patient's head.

FOCUSED HISTORY AND PHYSICAL EXAM

When dealing with trauma patients who have head injuries, or suspected head injuries, you will next perform a rapid trauma assessment. After that, you will check vital signs and obtain a SAMPLE history. *Be aware, however, that such patients may become disoriented or unresponsive. If a patient is alert and oriented, you or your partner might wish to gather the SAMPLE history while the other performs the rapid trauma assessment.*

Remember that any patient who loses consciousness, even briefly, must be evaluated at the hospital. *A patient whose mental status worsens at any stage of the assessment or treatment process needs immediate transport and continuous monitoring during transport.*

Rapid Trauma Assessment   Perform a rapid trauma assessment, paying particular attention to the following parts of the exam in cases of suspected head injury:

- *The Head*—Use extreme care in checking the patient's head (Figure 33-8). Palpate for deformities, depressions, lacerations, or impaled objects around the head and face (Figure 33-9). Be careful not to jab or apply pressure to skull depressions or deformities.
- *The Eyes*
  1. Check the patient's pupils with a bright light. Are they equal in size? Do they react equally? If one or both are fixed and dilated, this may mean an increase in pressure in the brain (Figure 33-10).
  2. Check eye movements. Do the eyes track (follow movement normally)?
  3. Is there any discoloration? A purplish discoloration (bruising) of the soft tissues around one or both eyes—**raccoon sign**—may be an indication of intracranial injury. It is a late sign of skull fracture.
- *The Ears and Nose*
  1. Check both ears for leakage of blood or clear fluid; skull fracture or intracranial bleeding can cause both (see Figure 33-11).
  2. **Battle's sign,** a purplish discoloration (bruising) of the mastoid area behind the ear, is another late sign of skull fracture.
  3. Check the nose for leakage of blood or clear fluid, which can indicate skull fracture or intracranial injury.
- *Motor/Sensory Assessment*—To examine motor and sensory function, if the patient is alert, check his

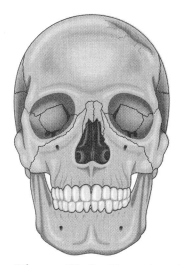
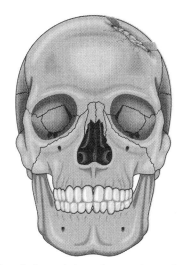
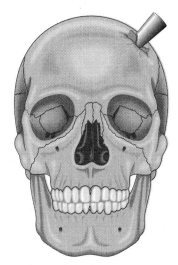

Figure 33-9   Examine the head for deformities, depressions, lacerations, or impaled objects.

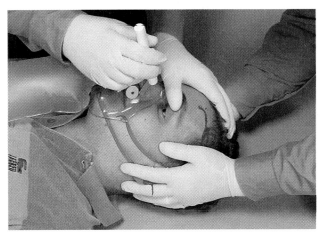

Figure 33-10   Assess pupils for size, equality, and reactivity.

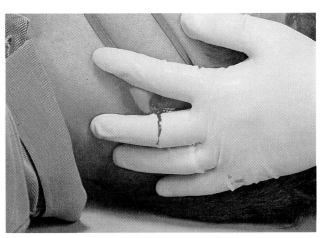

Figure 33-11   Blood and/or cerebrospinal fluid may leak from the ears or nose.

ability to move his fingers and toes. Have him squeeze your fingers with both hands simultaneously to test for equal grip strength. Ask the patient to tell which finger or toe you are touching without watching what you are doing. Pinch each extremity and ask if he can identify the pain. Ask if the patient feels any weakness on one side of the body compared to the other (Figure 33-12).

If the patient is only responsive to verbal or painful stimuli, motor and sensory function cannot be as accurately assessed, but watch for a response such as a grimace or withdrawal from a painful stimulus.

Baseline Vital Signs   Check and record vital signs every 5 minutes, staying alert to any changes. In cases of possible head injury, be alert to the following:

- *Blood Pressure*—If the systolic blood pressure is high or rising, suspect pressure inside the skull; if it is low or dropping, suspect blood loss that has led to shock. Low blood pressure in a head-injured patient almost always is due to bleeding elsewhere in the body (there is not enough space in the brain to permit enough bleeding to reduce blood pressure). It should be a signal to check the rest of the body for bleeding.
- *Pulse*—If the pulse is high or rising, suspect hemorrhage elsewhere in the body or early onset of hypoxia. If it is slow or dropping, suspect pressure inside the skull or severe hypoxia.
- *Respiration*—Assess the rate, depth, and pattern of respiration. The patient may display several different respiratory patterns if the brain is compressed from increased intracranial pressure resulting from swelling and/or bleeding inside the skull. The respirations may be extremely fast and shallow, completely irregular, or absent (apnea).

If definite signs of *severe* head injury exist, and if you have not already done so, begin positive pressure ventilation and consider hyperventilation at a rate of 20 ventilations per minute with supplemental oxygen. (Hyperventilation at a rate >20 may reduce cerebral blood flow and worsen the head injury.) A sign of severe head injury is **Cushing's reflex** in which the systolic blood pressure increases, the heart rate decreases, and the respiratory pattern changes.

If positive pressure ventilation is needed but significant signs and symptoms of severe head injury are *not* present, ventilate at a rate of 12/minute.

SAMPLE History   The SAMPLE history can provide vital information about the mechanism of injury. Remember that a head-injury patient may experience a deteriorating mental status. If he is unable to an-

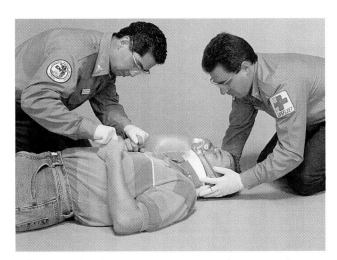

Figure 33-12   Assess motor and sensory function.

swer questions appropriately, try to obtain information from others at the scene. The following questions are particularly relevant in cases of head injury:

- When did the incident occur?
- What is the patient's chief complaint? Did he feel pain, tingling, numbness, or paralysis? Where? How have symptoms changed since the accident?
- How did the accident occur?
- *Did he lose consciousness at any time? This information is critically important in assessing a brain injury.* How long was the period of unresponsiveness? When did it occur in relation to the injury? Did the patient suddenly lose consciousness and then gradually reawaken, or did he pass out immediately, suddenly wake up, and then gradually lose consciousness again?
- Was the patient moved after the incident?
- Is there any history of a previous blow to the head? If so, when did it occur? Was the patient knocked unconscious? Sometimes a blow to the head days or weeks after an incident in which a patient was knocked unconscious can reinjure the brain.

Signs and Symptoms   Signs and symptoms of head injury include (Figure 33-13):

- Altered mental status—disorientation to unresponsiveness
- Decreasing mental status
- Irregular breathing pattern (severe)
- Increasing blood pressure and decreasing pulse (a late finding) (severe)
- Obvious signs of injury—contusions, lacerations, or hematomas to the scalp or deformity to the skull
- Blood or cerebrospinal fluid from ears or nose
- Discoloration (bruising) around the eyes in the absence of trauma to the eyes (raccoon sign)

- Discoloration (bruising) behind the ears, or mastoid process (Battle's sign)
- Absent motor or sensory function (severe or poor response)
- Nausea and/or vomiting; vomiting may be forceful or repeated
- Unequal pupil size with altered mental status (severe)
- Possible seizures
- Visible damage to the skull (visible through laceration in the scalp)
- Pain, tenderness, or swelling at the site of injury
- Nonpurposeful response to painful stimuli (severe)

EMERGENCY MEDICAL CARE

To treat a patient with head injury:

1. *Take body substance isolation precautions.*
2. *Take manual in-line spinal stabilization.*
   - Maintain neutral positioning of the head and neck manually, even after a cervical collar is applied, until the patient is completely immobilized to a backboard.
3. *Maintain a patent airway with adequate oxygenation.* Oxygen deficiency in the brain is the most frequent cause of death following head injury.
   - Use a jaw thrust to open the airway.
   - Remove any foreign bodies from the mouth, and suction blood and mucus.
   - Protect against aspiration by having suction available at all times and by being prepared to roll the secured patient to clear the airway.
   - Administer oxygen by nonrebreather mask at 15 lpm if breathing is adequate, or positive pressure ventilation with supplemental oxygen at 12/minute if breathing is inadequate and signs of head injury are present.

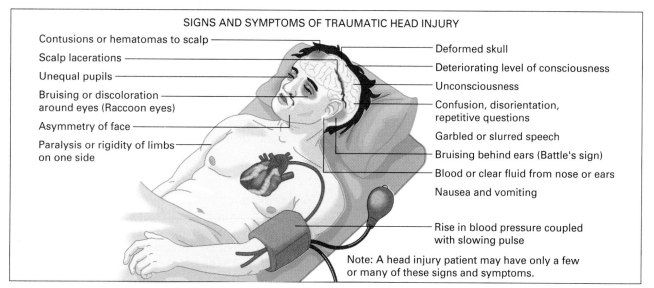

SIGNS AND SYMPTOMS OF TRAUMATIC HEAD INJURY

Contusions or hematomas to scalp
Scalp lacerations
Unequal pupils
Bruising or discoloration around eyes (Raccoon eyes)
Asymmetry of face
Paralysis or rigidity of limbs on one side

Deformed skull
Deteriorating level of consciousness
Unconsciousness
Confusion, disorientation, repetitive questions
Garbled or slurred speech
Bruising behind ears (Battle's sign)
Blood or clear fluid from nose or ears
Nausea and vomiting
Rise in blood pressure coupled with slowing pulse

Note: A head injury patient may have only a few or many of these signs and symptoms.

Figure 33-13   *Signs and symptoms of traumatic head injury.*

– Consider hyperventilation at a rate of 20 breaths per minute if signs of *severe* head injury are present—such as unequal pupils, increased systolic blood pressure, irregular or absent breathing (or Cushing's reflex: increased systolic blood pressure with decreased heart rate and changed breathing pattern), absent motor or sensory function, seizures, or nonpurposeful movement.

4. *Monitor the airway, breathing, pulse, and mental status for deterioration.* Any patient who deteriorates must be transported immediately.

5. *Control bleeding.* Face and scalp wounds may bleed heavily, but such bleeding is usually controlled easily.

 – Do not apply pressure to an open or depressed skull injury; doing so can drive pieces of fragmented bone into the brain tissue.

 – Dress and bandage open head wounds as indicated in the treatment of soft tissue injuries.

 – Do not attempt to stop the flow of blood or cerebrospinal fluid flowing from the ears or nose. Instead, cover loosely with a completely sterile gauze dressing to absorb, but not stop, the flow.

 – For other wounds, use gentle, continuous direct pressure with sterile gauze only as needed to control bleeding.

 – *Never try to remove a penetrating object.* Instead, immobilize the object in place and dress the wound.

6. *Be prepared for seizures.*

7. *Transport immediately.*

DETAILED PHYSICAL EXAM AND ONGOING ASSESSMENT

If time and the patient's condition permit, conduct a detailed physical examination during transport. This can be important in discovering any further injuries that may have been overlooked, especially if rapid transport has been initiated. Remember that the head-injured patient may not be able to identify other areas of pain.

Provide ongoing assessment during transport, paying close attention to the airway and mental status of the patient. Repeat the ongoing assessment every 5 minutes.

SUMMARY: ASSESSMENT AND CARE

To review possible assessment findings and emergency care for injuries to the head, see Figures 33-14 and 33-15.

ENRICHMENT

The enrichment section contains information that is valuable as background for the EMT-B but that goes substantially beyond the U.S. Department of Transportation (DOT) EMT-Basic curriculum.

MORE ABOUT BRAIN INJURIES

Concussion, contusion, subdural and epidural hematoma, and laceration—mentioned earlier in this chapter—are discussed more fully below. As you read about these types of brain injury, also consult Figure 33-16.

CONCUSSION

A **concussion** normally causes some disturbance in brain function ranging from momentary confusion to complete loss of responsiveness, and it usually causes headache. If the patient loses consciousness, it is usually brief (lasting only a few minutes) and does not recur.

Depending on where the force is absorbed in the brain, the signs of simple concussion might include the following:

* Momentary confusion
* Confusion that lasts for several minutes
* Inability to recall the incident and, sometimes, the period just before it (retrograde amnesia) and after it (antegrade amnesia)
* Repeated questioning about what happened
* Mild to moderate irritability or resistance to treatment
* Combativeness
* Irritability
* Inability to answer questions or obey commands appropriately
* Nausea and vomiting
* Restlessness

The key distinguishing factor in concussion is that its effects appear immediately or soon after impact, and then they disappear. An injury that causes symptoms that develop several minutes after an incident or symptoms that do not subside over time is not a concussion, but a more serious injury.

CONTUSION

A contusion, or bruising and swelling of the brain tissue, can accompany concussion. A contusion causes bleeding into the surrounding tissues and may or may not cause increased intracranial pressure, even in cases of open head injury. Contusion is usually caused by coup-contrecoup or acceleration/deceleration injury.

ASSESSMENT SUMMARY

HEAD INJURY

The following are findings that may be associated with a head injury.

SCENE SIZE-UP

Pay particular attention to your own safety. Look for:
Mechanism of injury
   Ejection from a vehicle
   High speed collision
   Sports injury
   Fall
   Crushing force
   Gun shot wounds
Evidence of other trauma
   Impact mark on windshield
   Deformed helmet
   Obvious scalp and skull injuries

INITIAL ASSESSMENT

General Impression

Altered mental status
Open fracture sites to skull
Obvious deformity to skull

Mental Status

Alert to unresponsive based on type and degree of head injury
Unresponsiveness or decreasing mental status associated with trauma to the head (a hallmark sign of head injury)
Decorticate or decerebrate (nonpurposeful) posturing to painful stimuli
Garbled or slurred speech

Airway

Assume airway is closed if patient has an altered mental status
May be occluded by bleeding associated with facial fractures
Be prepared to manage vomiting

Breathing

May be absent, inadequate, or normal
Abnormal breathing patterns may occur

Circulation

Pulse may be normal or decreased
Skin is normal

Status: Priority patient if patient never regains consciousness or has a decreasing mental status

FOCUSED HISTORY AND PHYSICAL EXAM

Physical Exam

Head:
   Open or closed wounds to the head or face
   Leakage of blood or cerebrospinal fluid from ears, nose, or mouth
   Discoloration around eyes (raccoon eyes) or behind ears (Battle's sign) (late signs)
   Unequal pupils or fixed and dilated pupil
Extremities:
   No response to pain or light touch
   Inability to move extremities

Baseline Vital Signs

BP: normal, may have a significantly increased systolic BP (Cushing's reflex)
HR: normal or bradycardia (Cushing's reflex); tachycardia may be associated with shock associated with bleeding from other injuries
RR: normal, irregular, decreased, or absent (Cushing's reflex)
Skin: normal or may be pale, cool, clammy if other injuries are present with bleeding and shock
Pupils: may be equal or unequal, reactive or unreactive; may be fixed and dilated

SAMPLE History

Signs and symptoms of an open or closed skull fracture:
   Pain, deformity, swelling
   Open wound associated with suspected fracture site
   Exposed bone ends
   Facial trauma
Penetrating injuries or impaled objects in the head
Cushing's reflex (triad): increased systolic blood pressure, decreased heart rate, abnormal respiratory pattern
Nausea and vomiting
Abnormal motor/sensory response
Patient loses responsiveness after impact to the head
Loss of responsiveness, followed by a lucid interval, then a gradual loss of responsiveness

Figure 33-14a   Assessment summary: head injury.

EMERGENCY CARE PROTOCOL

HEAD INJURY

1. Establish manual in-line stabilization.
2. Establish and maintain an open airway. Insert a nasopharyngeal or oropharyngeal airway if patient is unresponsive and has no gag or cough reflex.
3. Suction secretions as necessary.
4. If breathing is inadequate, provide positive pressure ventilation with supplemental oxygen at a minimum rate of 12 ventilations/minute for an adult and 20 ventilations/minute for an infant or child. Consider hyperventilation at 20 ventilations/minute if signs of severe head injury are present:*
5. If breathing is adequate, administer oxygen by nonrebreather mask at 15 lpm.
6. Control any major bleeding. Be careful not to apply excessive pressure to open skull fractures.
7. Immobilize patient to backboard.
8. Transport.
9. Perform an ongoing assessment every 5 minutes if unstable and every 15 minutes if stable. Be prepared for vomiting and seizures.

* The most current recommendation for hyperventilation in the severe head-injured patient is now at 20 ventilations/minute. Ventilation at a higher rate may reduce perfusion of the brain.

Figure 33-14b　Emergency care protocol: head injury.

In **coup-contrecoup injury,** there can be damage at the point of a blow to the head and/or damage on the side opposite the blow as the brain is propelled against the opposite side of the skull. In **acceleration/deceleration injury,** typical of a car crash, the head comes to a sudden stop but the brain continues to move back and forth inside the skull, resulting in bruising (possibly very severe) to the brain.

Signs and symptoms of contusion include the initial signs and symptoms of concussion plus one or more of the following:

- Decreasing mental status or unresponsiveness
- Paralysis
- Unequal pupils
- Vomiting
- Alteration of vital signs
- Profound personality changes

Contusion can lead to swelling of the brain tissue, which can result in permanent disability or death. You can improve the patient's chances of recovery by vigorous airway management, ventilation of the patient with high-concentration oxygen and immobilization of the cervical spine. Hyperventilation may also be considered.

SUBDURAL HEMATOMA

Bleeding into the skull occurs with a subdural hematoma when blood vessels on the surface of the brain are torn, causing bleeding between the brain and the dura mater, its protective covering. A subdural hematoma usually results from an impact that causes coup-contrecoup or acceleration/deceleration injury. The bleeding associated with subdural hematoma is usually venous, and skull fracture is not usually present.

Blood pooling causes pressure within the skull, and it displaces brain tissue as the blood accumulates. The bleeding, being venous, may clot quickly, and the displacement of brain tissue may be due to the clot. Subdural hematoma is the most common type of intracranial bleeding.

Signs and symptoms of subdural hematoma include the following:

- Deterioration in level of responsiveness
- Vomiting
- Dilation of one pupil
- Abnormal respirations or apnea
- Possible increasing systolic blood pressure
- Decreasing pulse rate

EPIDURAL HEMATOMA

Epidural hematoma accounts for only about 2 percent of all head injuries that require hospitalization. However, it is an extreme emergency that typically results from skull fracture. It most commonly occurs from low-velocity impact to the head or from deceleration injury.

In epidural hematoma, arterial bleeding pools between the skull and the protective covering of the brain. Bleeding is usually rapid, profuse, and severe. The bleeding expands rapidly in a small space, causing a dramatic rise in intracranial pressure.

Signs and symptoms of epidural hematoma include the following:

EMERGENCY CARE ALGORITHM: HEAD INJURY

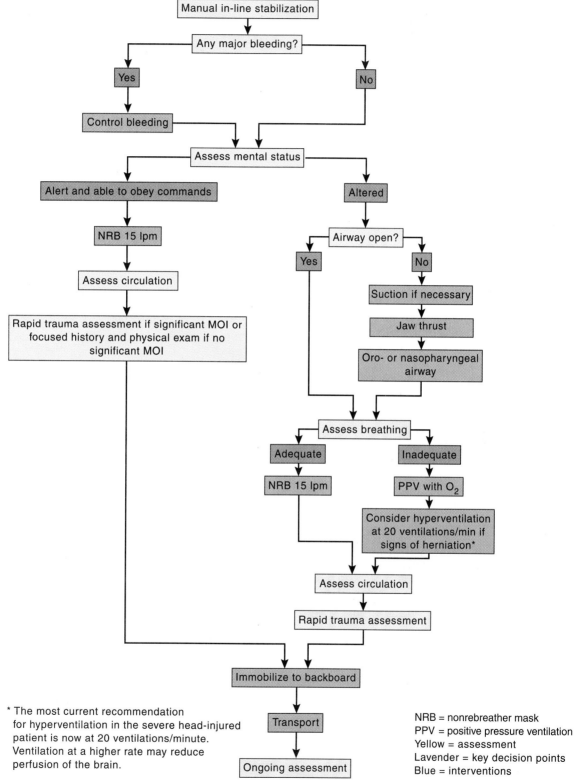

* The most current recommendation for hyperventilation in the severe head-injured patient is now at 20 ventilations/minute. Ventilation at a higher rate may reduce perfusion of the brain.

NRB = nonrebreather mask
PPV = positive pressure ventilation
Yellow = assessment
Lavender = key decision points
Blue = interventions

Figure 33-15   Emergency care algorithm: head injury.

BRAIN INJURIES

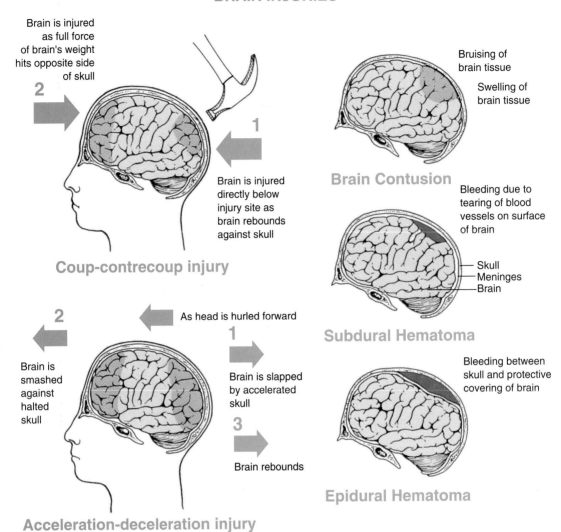

Brain is injured as full force of brain's weight hits opposite side of skull

2

1

Brain is injured directly below injury site as brain rebounds against skull

Coup-contrecoup injury

Bruising of brain tissue

Swelling of brain tissue

Brain Contusion

Bleeding due to tearing of blood vessels on surface of brain

— Skull
— Meninges
— Brain

Subdural Hematoma

2

As head is hurled forward

1

Brain is smashed against halted skull

Brain is slapped by accelerated skull

3

Brain rebounds

Bleeding between skull and protective covering of brain

Epidural Hematoma

Acceleration-deceleration injury

Figure 33-16   Types of brain injury.

- Loss of responsiveness followed by return of responsiveness (lucid interval) and then rapidly deteriorating responsiveness (a classic presentation, but rare)
- Decreasing mental status (a more common presentation than the classic lucid interval)
- Severe headache during periods of lucidity
- Pupil fixed and dilated on side of impact
- Seizures
- Increasing systolic blood pressure and decreasing heart rate

Late signs can include fixed, dilated pupils, absent reflexes, and decreasing vital signs. Immediate surgical repair is needed in cases of epidural hematoma. If it is treated early, the prognosis is generally good, since underlying brain damage is usually minimal.

LACERATION

Like contusion, a laceration of brain tissue can occur in either an open or closed head injury. Often it occurs when an object penetrates the skull and lacerates the brain. It is a permanent injury, almost always results in bleeding, and can cause massive disruption of the nervous system.

Remember that with isolated head trauma, a patient's blood pressure may go up and the pulse rate down (a late finding). If your patient has a subdural or epidural hematoma or laceration, but his blood pressure is dropping, you must consider that he is bleeding somewhere else in the body. If this is the case, continue to hyperventilate the patient and treat the underlying shock resulting from blood loss.

CASE STUDY FOLLOW-UP

SCENE SIZE-UP

You have been dispatched to an 18-year-old unresponsive male, Mike Ryan. As you arrive, his mother reports that he experienced a bump on the head that seemed minor. As you enter the young man's room, you find him supine on his bed. His breathing is deep and fast with snoring respirations.

INITIAL ASSESSMENT

You immediately establish in-line spinal stabilization and open Mike's airway using a jaw thrust. The snoring sounds disappear, but he continues to breathe rapidly and deeply. While holding his airway open, your partner pinches his shoulder muscle and holds it. His arms flex across his chest and his legs stiffen. Your partner inserts an oral airway. It is accepted without any gag reflex. You then provide positive pressure ventilation with supplemental oxygen at 20 breaths per minute because you suspect severe head injury.

FOCUSED HISTORY AND PHYSICAL EXAM

Your partner performs a rapid trauma assessment and takes vital signs. Mike's left pupil is dilated and unreactive to light. Vital signs are BP 190/72, pulse 62, and respirations are assisted at 20 per minute. Lungs are clear and there are no signs of injury to the rest of his body.

You obtain a SAMPLE history from the family. It reveals that Mike was knocked unconscious for about 3 minutes 2 weeks ago after a rollerblading accident. He said he was fine and never sought medical care. This morning he was playing basketball and, according to his brother Sean, was hit in the head with an elbow. After that, the two brothers walked home. Sean states he noticed that Mike was walking oddly and complained of being tired. Once home, Mike went up to his room to lie down.

When the exam and history findings are recorded, you and your partner prepare the patient for transport. You apply a cervical collar and move him onto a backboard. When immobilization is complete, Mike is taken to the ambulance.

ONGOING ASSESSMENT

En route to the hospital, you monitor Mike's airway, breathing, circulation, and level of responsiveness. You continue hyperventilation.

During transport, you note no change in Mike's condition. At the emergency department, he is transferred to the staff. You and your partner complete a prehospital care report and prepare the ambulance for another call.

A couple of months later, as you are passing the high school on the way to another call, you are happy to spot Mike and Sean walking toward the school. Mike seems to be fine.

CHAPTER REVIEW

TERMS AND CONCEPTS

You may wish to review the following terms and concepts included in this chapter.

acceleration/deceleration injury—a head injury typical of a car crash in which the head comes to a sudden stop, but the brain continues to move back and forth inside the skull, resulting in bruising to the brain.

arachnoid—middle layer of protective brain tissue (meninges).

basilar skull—floor of the skull.

Battle's sign—discoloration of the mastoid suggesting basilar skull deformation.

brainstem—the funnel-shaped inferior part of the brain that controls most automatic functions of the body. It is made up of the pons, the midbrain, and the medulla, which is the brain's connection to the spinal cord.

cerebellum—part of the brain controlling equilibrium and muscle coordination.

cerebrospinal fluid—serous substance that protects the brain.

cerebrum—largest part of the brain, responsible for most conscious and sensory functions, the emotions, and the personality.

concussion—temporary loss of brain function.

coup-contrecoup injury—a brain injury in which there may be damage at the point of a blow to the head and/or damage on the side opposite the blow as the brain is propelled against the opposite side of the skull.

cranial skull—helmet-like covering of the brain.

Cushing's reflex—a protective reflex by the body to try to maintain perfusion of the brain in a head-injured patient with an increase in intracranial pressure. The systolic blood pressure increases, heart rate decreases, and the respiratory pattern changes. This collective change in vital signs indicates a severe head injury.

decerebrate posturing—a posture in which the patient extends arms and legs and sometimes arches the back; a nonpurposful response to painful stimulus; a sign of deep unresponsiveness and serious brain injury.

decorticate posturing—a posture in which the patient flexes the arms across the chest and extends the legs; a nonpurposful response to painful stimulus; a sign of deep unresponsiveness and serious brain injury.

dura mater—outer layer of protective brain tissue (meninges).

epidural—between the dura mater and the skull.

meninges—layers of tissue protecting the brain. They include the dura mater, the arachnoid, and the pia mater.

pia mater—inner layer of protective brain tissue (meninges).

raccoon sign—discoloration of tissue around the eyes suggestive of basilar skull injury.

subarachnoid hemorrhage—bleeding that occurs between the arachnoid membrane and the surface of the brain.

subarachnoid space—a lattice of fibrous, spongy tissue filled with cerebrospinal fluid that separates the arachnoid membrane and the pia mater.

subdural—beneath the dura mater.

REVIEW QUESTIONS

1. Name the two parts of the central nervous system.
2. Define the meninges and name the three layers of the meninges.
3. Name the three anatomical components of the brain.
4. Describe an open and a closed head injury.
5. Name other types of injury that may be present and related to a head injury.
6. Name some of the major types of brain injury.
7. Explain why determining a baseline level of responsiveness is important in cases of head injury.
8. Explain why a SAMPLE history is important in cases of head injury.
9. List the signs and symptoms of head injury.
10. Outline the steps of emergency medical treatment in cases of head injury.

CHAPTER 34

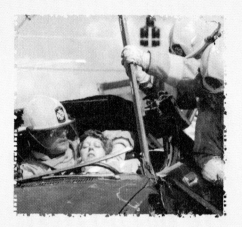

Injuries to the Spine

INTRODUCTION

Spine injuries are among the most formidable and traumatic you will manage as an EMT-Basic. Yet you may face the probability of such injuries on almost a daily basis. Automobile crashes, shallow-water diving accidents, motorcycle crashes, and falls are all common causes of spine injury. Likewise, accidents during skiing, sledding, football, and gymnastics can result in spine injury. It is your job as an EMT-B to recognize injuries that could damage the spinal column or spinal cord and provide appropriate emergency care. You must also be aware that improper movement and handling of patients in such situations can easily lead to permanent disability or even death.

OBJECTIVES

Numbered objectives are from the United States Department of Transportation 1994 EMT-Basic National Standard Curriculum. Asterisked objectives, if any, pertain to material that is supplemental to the DOT curriculum.

COGNITIVE

5-4.1 State the components of the nervous system. (pp. 653–654)

5-4.2 List the functions of the central nervous system. (pp. 653–654)

5-4.3 Define the structure of the skeletal system as it relates to the nervous system. (p. 654)

5-4.4 Relate mechanism of injury to potential injuries of the head and spine. (pp. 654–657, 660)

5-4.5 Describe the implications of not properly caring for potential spine injuries. (p. 651)

5-4.6 State the signs and symptoms of a potential spine injury. (pp. 660–661)

5-4.7 Describe the method of determining if a responsive patient may have a spine injury. (pp. 657–661)

5-4.8 Relate the airway emergency medical care techniques to the patient with a suspected spine injury. (pp. 657, 662, 663)

5-4.9 Describe how to stabilize the cervical spine. (pp. 661–662, 666)

5-4.10 Discuss indications for sizing and using a cervical spine immobilization device. (pp. 662, 666)

5-4.11 Establish the relationship between airway management and the patient with head and spine injuries. (pp. 657, 662, 663)

5-4.12 Describe a method for sizing a cervical spine immobilization device. (pp. 666, 668)

5-4.13 Describe how to log roll a patient with a suspected spine injury. (pp. 667, 672–673, 675–676)

5-4.14 Describe how to secure a patient to a long spine board. (pp. 666, 667–678, 670–679)

5-4.15 List instances when a short spine board should be used. (pp. 666, 674–676, 678–679)

5-4.16 Describe how to immobilize a patient using a short spine board. (pp. 674–676, 678–679)

5-4.17 Describe the indications for the use of rapid extrication. (pp. 679–680)

5-4.18 List steps in performing rapid extrication. (pp. 680–681)

5-4.19 State the circumstances when a helmet should be left on the patient. (pp. 682–683)

5-4.20 Discuss the circumstances when a helmet should be removed. (p. 682)

5-4.21 Identify different types of helmets. (p. 682)

5-4.22 Describe the unique characteristics of sports helmets. (p. 682)

5-4.23 Explain the preferred methods to remove a helmet. (pp. 682, 683–684)

5-4.24 Discuss alternative methods for removal of a helmet. (p. 685)

5-4.25 Describe how the patient's head is stabilized to remove the helmet. (pp. 682–685)

5-4.26 Differentiate how the head is stabilized with a helmet compared to without a helmet. (pp. 682–685)

AFFECTIVE

5-4.27 Explain the rationale for immobilization of the entire spine when a cervical spine injury is suspected. (p. 666)

5-4.28 Explain the rationale for utilizing immobilization methods apart from the straps on the cots. (pp. 666–681)

5-4.29 Explain the rationale for utilizing a short spine immobilization device when moving a patient from the sitting to the supine position. (pp. 673, 675–676, 678–681)

5-4.30 Explain the rationale for utilizing rapid extrication approaches only when they indeed will make the difference between life and death. (pp. 679–681)

5-4.31 Defend the reasons for leaving a helmet in place for transport of a patient. (p. 682)

5-4.32 Defend the reasons for removal of a helmet prior to transport of a patient. (p. 682)

PSYCHOMOTOR

5-4.33 Demonstrate opening the airway in a patient with suspected spinal cord injury.

5-4.34 Demonstrate evaluating a responsive patient with a suspected spinal cord injury.

5-4.35 Demonstrate stabilization of the cervical spine.

5-4.36 Demonstrate the four person log roll for a patient with a suspected spinal cord injury.

5-4.37 Demonstrate how to log roll a patient with a suspected spinal cord injury using two people.

5-4.38 Demonstrate securing a patient to a long spine board.

5-4.39 Demonstrate using the short board immobilization technique.

5-4.40 Demonstrate procedure for rapid extrication.

5-4.41 Demonstrate preferred methods for stabilization of a helmet.

5-4.42 Demonstrate helmet removal techniques.

5-4.43 Demonstrate alternative methods for stabilization of a helmet.

5-4.44 Demonstrate completing a prehospital care report for patients with head and spinal injuries.

Some of the above objectives from DOT Lesson 5-4 are also addressed in Chapter 33, "Injuries to the Head."

CASE STUDY

THE DISPATCH

EMS Unit 106—respond to Rita's Dance and Gym, 1403 Lisbon Road. You have a 12-year-old female patient who has fallen. Time out is 1552 hours.

ON ARRIVAL

Upon your arrival, an assistant at the gym tells you that a young girl fell during a gymnastics meet. She directs you into an open gymnasium. Across the floor, you see a crowd of people around a young girl lying on a mat. A woman is holding the girl still. The woman says, "She missed a maneuver off the top bar. She fell and hit the bottom bar with the middle of her back, then landed head first on the floor." The young girl is crying.

How would you proceed to assess and care for this patient?

During this chapter you will learn special considerations of assessment and emergency care for a patient suffering from a possible spine injury. Later we will return to the case and apply the procedures learned.

THE ANATOMY AND PHYSIOLOGY OF SPINE INJURY

To appreciate the potential severity of spine injuries, you should begin by understanding the relationship between the nervous system and the parts of the skeletal system most closely related to it, the skull and the spinal column. Before continuing, you may want to review the information about the skeletal and nervous systems that were presented in Chapter 4, "The Human Body," "Chapter 32, Musculoskeletal Injuries," and Chapter 33, "Injuries to the Head."

THE NERVOUS SYSTEM

Injuries to the spine have the potential for severity because within the spinal column is the spinal cord. This structure carries nerve impulses from most of the body to the brain and back to the body. A single spinal cord injury can affect several organs and bodily functions.

PARTS OF THE NERVOUS SYSTEM

The nervous system has two major functions: communication and control. It enables the individual to be aware of and to react to his environment. It also coordinates the responses of the body to changes in the environment and keeps body systems working together.

The nervous system consists of nerve centers and of nerves that branch off from the centers and lead to tissues and organs. Most nerve centers are in the brain and spinal cord.

The structural divisions of the nervous system (Figure 34-1) are these:

• The **central nervous system,** which consists of the brain and the spinal cord

• The **peripheral nervous system,** which consists of nerves located outside of the brain and spinal cord

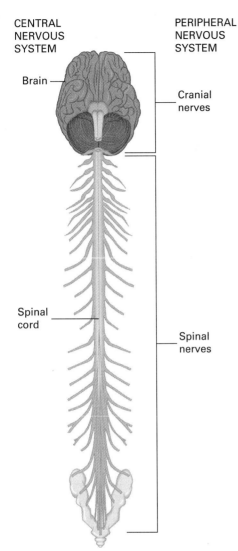

CENTRAL NERVOUS SYSTEM

PERIPHERAL NERVOUS SYSTEM

Brain

Cranial nerves

Spinal cord

Spinal nerves

Figure 34-1 Components of the central and peripheral nervous systems.

The functional divisions of the nervous system are these:

- The **voluntary nervous system,** which influences the activity of voluntary (skeletal) muscles and movements throughout the body
- The **autonomic nervous system,** which is automatic and influences the activities of involuntary muscles and glands; the autonomic system is partly independent of the rest of the nervous system

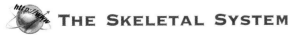

THE SKELETAL SYSTEM

The **skeletal system,** gives the body its framework, supports and protects vital organs, and permits motion. The bony framework of the body is held together by **ligaments,** tough, fibrous connective tissue. The skeleton is also flexible enough to absorb and protect against impacts and stress. The parts of the skeletal system that protect the most important parts of the nervous system are the skull and the spinal column.

THE SKULL

Resting at the top of the spinal column, the skull contains the brain. The skull has two parts; the cranium (or brain case) and the face.

THE SPINAL COLUMN

The **spinal column** is the principal support system of the body. Ribs originate from it to form the thoracic cavity, and the rest of the skeleton is directly or indirectly attached to the spine.

Amazingly mobile, the spinal column is made up of thirty-three irregularly shaped bones called **vertebrae.** Lying one on top of the other to form a strong, flexible column, the vertebrae are bound firmly together by strong ligaments. Between each two vertebrae is a fluid-filled pad of tough elastic cartilage called a **disc** that acts as a shock absorber. The spinal column (or vertebral column), which surrounds and protects the spinal cord, is divided into five parts (Figure 34-2):

- The **cervical spine**—The first seven vertebrae that form the neck. The cervical vertebrae are the most mobile and delicate; injury to the cervical spine is the most common cause of spinal cord injury.
- The **thoracic spine**—The twelve vertebrae directly below the cervical vertebrae that comprise the upper back
- The **lumbar spine**—The next five vertebrae that form the lower back
- The **sacral spine** (sacrum)—The next five vertebrae that are fused together and form the rigid posterior portion of the pelvis
- The **coccyx** (tailbone)—The four fused vertebrae that form the lower end of the spine

The **spinal cord,** composed of nervous tissue, exits the brain through an opening at the base of the skull. The cord is surrounded by a sheath of protective membranes (meninges) and a cushioning layer of cerebrospinal fluid. The cord narrows as it goes, filling 95 percent of the spinal column "canal" in the cervical vertebrae (neck), but only 60 percent in the lumbar area (lower back). All nerves to the trunk and extremities originate from the spinal cord. The spinal cord carries messages from the brain to the various parts of the body through nerve bundles.

COMMON MECHANISMS OF SPINE INJURY

The spine is quite strong and flexible, but it is particularly susceptible to injury from the following mechanisms (Figure 34-3):

Spinal curves   Vertebrae

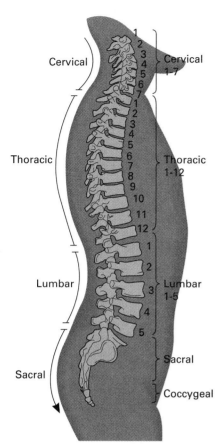

Cervical — Cervical 1-7

Thoracic — Thoracic 1-12

Lumbar — Lumbar 1-5

Sacral — Sacral

— Coccygeal

Figure 34-2   The spinal (vertebral) column.

- *Compression*—when the weight of the body is driven against the head. This is common in falls, diving accidents, motor vehicle crashes, or other accidents where a person impacts an object head first.
- *Flexion*—when there is severe forward movement of the head in which the chin meets the chest, or when the torso is excessively curled forward
- *Extension*—when there is severe backward movement of the head in which the neck is stretched, or when the torso is severely arched backward
- *Rotation*—when there is lateral movement of the head or spine beyond its normal rotation
- *Lateral Bending*—when the body is bent severely from the side
- *Distraction*—when the vertebrae and spinal cord are stretched and pulled apart. This is common in hangings.
- *Penetration*—when there is injury from gunshots, stabbings, or other types of penetrating trauma that involve the cranium or spinal column

You must suspect spine injury in any case that you believe involves one or more of these mecha-

nisms. Suspect spine injury even if the patient appears to be able to move normally. *Injured vertebrae that are still aligned, but unstable, can become unstable at any moment and damage or sever the spinal cord.*

 ## ASSESSMENT AND CARE: SPINE INJURY

SCENE SIZE-UP

Because suspicion of, and emergency care for, spine injury are most often based on mechanism of injury, the scene size-up is an extremely important phase of patient assessment.

Likely Mechanisms of Spinal Injury You should be especially alert to the possibility of spine injury when called to any of the following scenes, since all of them are likely to produce the mechanisms that may result in spinal injury:

- Motorcycle crashes
- Motor vehicle crashes
- Pedestrian-vehicle collisions
- Falls
- Blunt trauma
- Penetrating trauma to the head, neck, or torso
- Hangings
- Diving accidents or near-drownings
- Gunshot wounds to the head, neck, chest, abdomen, back, or pelvis
- Unresponsive trauma patient
- Electrical injuries

Gunshot wounds to the head, neck, chest, abdomen, back, or pelvis should always cause suspicion of injury to the vertebrae or spinal cord. Even if entrance and exit wounds are closely aligned and appear to indicate a clean, through wound, the bullet could have ricocheted and caused an injury to the vertebrae or spinal cord. Also, exploding fragments from other bones could have injured the spine. Therefore, with any gunshot wound to the body, immediately establish manual in-line spinal stabilization and take the necessary spinal precautions during your emergency care.

Also, suspect spine injury with any serious blunt injury to the head, neck, chest, abdomen, back, or pelvis—and even to the legs or arms. The energy of the impact can travel up the extremity to the spinal column.

Clues to Mechanism of Injury Upon arrival at the scene, scan it closely for evidence of a mechanism of injury that could cause damage to the vertebrae or spinal cord. Look up, down, and around the patient for signs that an injury has occurred. If an unresponsive patient is lying on the ground in a relatively open area near a tree, assume that the patient fell out of the tree until proven otherwise.

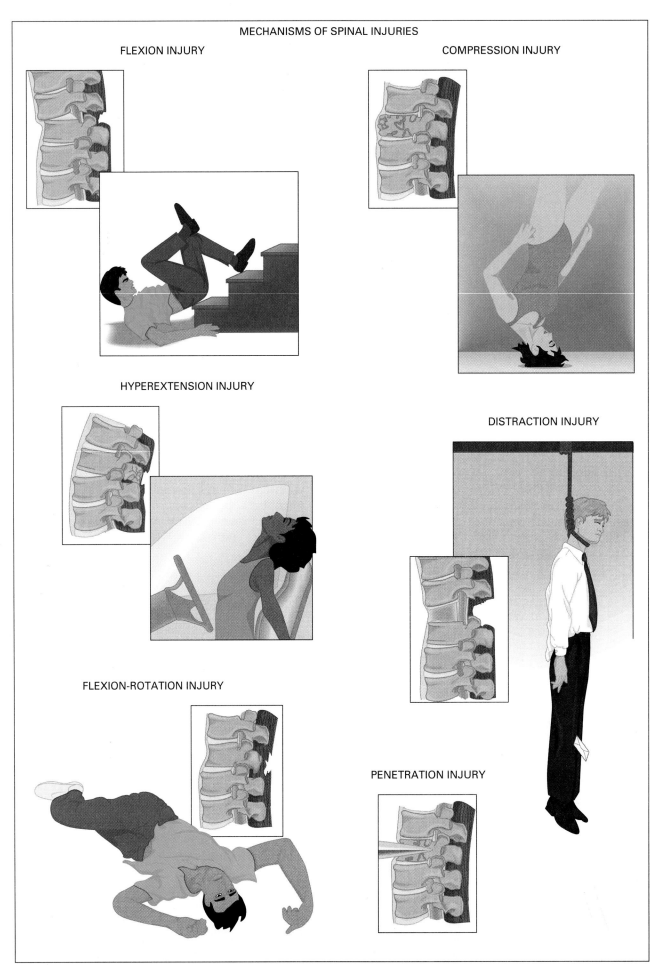

Figure 34-3   Mechanisms of spine injury.

Even though there may be no overt signs of trauma to the patient, a spine injury may nevertheless exist. In such a situation, opening the airway using a head-tilt, chin-lift maneuver (which requires extension of the head and neck) or failing to provide proper manual in-line spinal stabilization may produce catastrophic permanent injury or even be lethal to the patient. These dire results can be avoided if you perform a thorough assessment of the scene for mechanism of injury and maintain a high index of suspicion of spine injury.

You must deduce the mechanism of injury from the evidence at the scene and determine if such a mechanism could have injured the spine. For example, on arrival at the scene of an automobile collision, you may note minor damage to the front of the car. As you quickly scan the car, you note an impact mark on the front windshield on the driver's side apparently made by the driver's head. You also note that the patient is not wearing his lap or shoulder restraint.

This evidence should create a high index of suspicion that the patient was propelled forward in the crash and struck his head on the windshield. This would likely have caused the head and neck to bend (flex) forward during the forward movement and bend backward (hyperextend) during the rearward movement. Both motions are significant mechanisms of injury that might not be suspected if the damage to the vehicle were not observed.

You may arrive at a collision scene and find the patient walking around or sitting in the back of a police car. Remember that this does not rule out the possibility of spine injury. Many times, a patient with a stable spine injury does not exhibit signs and symptoms consistent with injury to the spine. Improper movement by either the patient or the EMT-B can easily cause the stable injury to become unstable, resulting in permanent neurologic damage or even death. You must maintain proper in-line spinal stabilization, even if the patient has moved prior to your arrival.

Always bear in mind that suspicion of injury to the spine based on the mechanism of injury sets the standard for subsequent emergency care for the patient. All assessment and care must be conducted with extreme caution to avoid excessive movement and manipulation of the body. *In-line spinal stabilization must be maintained throughout the entire patient contact.*

Initial Assessment

When performing the initial assessment, the general impression may not lead you to suspect a spine injury, since the signs and symptoms may not be very apparent. *Regardless of the lack of obvious trauma or patient complaints, however—based solely on a scene size-up that has suggested a mechanism of injury that could cause spine injury—you must adopt a high index of suspicion and must initiate immediate manual in-line spinal stabilization. Manual stabilization must not be released until the patient is securely strapped to a backboard with his head and neck immobilized.*

Whenever spine injury is suspected, you must open the airway using the jaw-thrust maneuver instead of the head-tilt, chin-lift maneuver. Do not turn the patient's head to the side to facilitate drainage of fluids from the airway. Instead, suction any secretions, blood, or vomitus from the patient's mouth.

Spinal cord damage from a cervical spine injury can block nerve impulses traveling from the brain to the diaphragm and intercostal muscles, which are necessary for adequate respiration. Inadequate or absent breathing may result. There may be very little or no movement of the chest and only slight movement of the abdominal muscles, or excessive abdominal muscle movement may be noted. Be prepared to provide positive pressure ventilation with supplemental oxygen.

The patient's pulse and skin color, temperature, and condition may appear normal in spite of injury to the vertebrae. However, an injury to the spinal cord can interrupt the transmission of impulses from the brain to the heart and the blood vessels that control blood pressure. You may find the radial pulse weak or absent due to a reduced blood pressure. The skin may be warm and dry below the site of spinal cord injury and cool, pale, and moist above the site of injury.

The mental status of a patient with spine injury may range from completely alert and oriented to unresponsive.

Based on the mechanism of injury, categorize the patient as either high or low priority for emergency care or transport. If the patient is unresponsive, is responsive but unable to obey your commands, or displays an abnormal respiratory pattern or obvious signs of spine injury such as numbness or paralysis, you must consider the patient a high priority for emergency care and prompt transportation.

Focused History and Physical Exam

Conduct the focused history and physical exam. Continue manual in-line spinal stabilization and reassess the patient's mental status. Conduct a rapid trauma assessment, followed by vital signs assessment and SAMPLE history.

Rapid Trauma Assessment Whether the patient is responsive or unresponsive, a rapid trauma assessment must be conducted when there is a mechanism of injury that causes suspicion of spine injury.

Instruct the patient to be still and not attempt to move. Do not attempt to unbutton or unzip clothing to expose the patient. Instead, reduce unnecessary movement by cutting clothing away. Inspect and palpate the head, neck, chest, abdomen, pelvis, extremities, and posterior body for DCAP-BTLS (deformities, contusions, abrasions, penetrations/punctures, burns, tenderness, lacerations, and swelling).

When spine injury is suspected, pay particular attention to the following during the rapid trauma assessment:

- *Injuries Associated with Spine Injury*—Watch for evidence of trauma to the head, posterior cervical region, anterior neck, chest, abdomen, back, and pelvis. Injuries to these areas also frequently cause spine injury.
- *Cervical Spine Immobilization Collar*—Following your assessment of the neck, apply the cervical spine immobilization collar (CSIC). The cervical collar is only an adjunct to full spinal immobilization; it does not provide complete immobilization by itself. Do not release manual in-line spinal stabilization until the patient is fully immobilized on a backboard. This will be done after the focused history and physical exam.
- *Assessing Pulses, Motor, and Sensory Function*—In the responsive patient, assess the pulses and motor and sensory function (Figures 34-4a to h) of each extremity. Check for the presence and strength of the radial pulses for the upper extremities, the pedal pulses for the lower extremities.

    Assess motor function by comparing the equality of strength. Have the patient grip your fingers with his hands simultaneously to assess equality of strength in the upper extremities. Have the patient gently push both his feet simultaneously against your hands to measure the equality of strength in the lower extremities.

    Check the sensory function by lightly touching the patient's fingers and toes on each extremity one at a time out of the patient's sight. As you do, ask:
    - Can you feel me touching your finger?
    - Can you tell me what hand and which finger I'm touching?
    - Can you feel me touching your toe?
    - Can you tell me which foot and what toe I'm touching?
    - Repeat the same sequence with painful stimuli by pinching or poking the extremity with a somewhat sharp object.

    If the patient is unresponsive, pinch the foot and hand to determine a sensory response. Compare the sensory function and strength in the upper and lower extremities. It is more common for spine injuries to cause paralysis to all four extremities (*quadriplegia*) or to the lower half of the body

only (*paraplegia*). Loss of function confined to the right or left side of the body (*hemiplegia*) is more typical of a brain injury or stroke.

- *Posterior Exam*—Carefully log roll the patient with in-line spinal stabilization to assess the posterior body. Palpate the area of the spine very gently. Evidence of deformity, tenderness, contusions, lacerations, punctures, or swelling to the spine or around the spine should heighten your suspicion that a spine injury truly exists. Muscle spasms along the spinal column are a protective reflex and a common indication that a spine injury has occurred.

Baseline Vital Signs Obtain and record a set of baseline vital signs. If the brain or spinal cord is damaged, baseline vital signs may reflect a condition referred to as **neurogenic shock,** which inhibits neural transmission to the arteries and arterioles. The blood pressure may be low and the heart rate slow. If the neurogenic shock is caused by spinal cord injury, it may be called **spinal shock.** With spinal shock, the skin is warm and dry and the patient will present with motor and/or sensory deficit. Closely reassess the patient for deterioration and report these findings to the emergency department. (See the Enrichment section later in this chapter for more on neurogenic and spinal shock.)

SAMPLE History Obtain a SAMPLE history from the responsive patient. Because of the seriousness of a spine injury, try to take this history as the rapid assessment is being conducted. Questions that might be asked in cases of suspected spine injury include the following:

- Does your neck or back hurt?
- Where does it hurt?
- Can you move your hands and feet?
- Do you have any pain or muscle spasms along your back or to the back of your neck?
- Do you have any numbness or tingling sensations in any of your arms or legs?
- Was the onset of pain associated with a fall or other injury?
- Did you move or did someone move you before our arrival?
- Were you up walking around before our arrival?

Also, assess for allergies, medications, past medical history, and the last intake of food or drink. Remember to ask about events prior to the onset of signs or symptoms, because they may provide evidence of or clarify the mechanism of injury.

If the patient is unresponsive, obtain the SAMPLE history from the bystanders at the scene. Try to determine the patient's mental status before your arrival, if the patient was moving any extremities, or if the patient was moved prior to your arrival.

ASSESSING MOTOR AND SENSORY FUNCTION

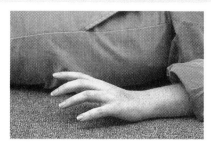

Figure 34-4a   Assess the patient's ability to move the hand.

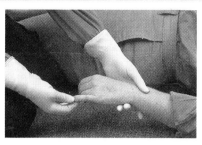

Figure 34-4b   Assess sensation in the fingers and hands.

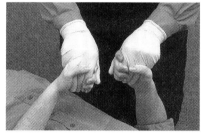

Figure 34-4c   Check for equal strength in the upper extremities.

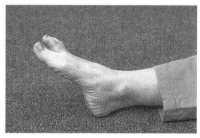

Figure 34-4d   Determine if the patient can move the feet.

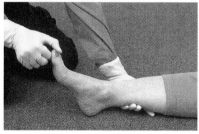

Figure 34-4e   Check for sensation by touching the toe and asking patient to identify which one you are touching.

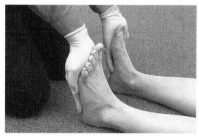

Figure 34-4f   Assess equality of strength in the lower extremities.

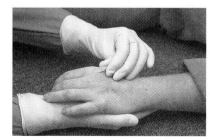

Figure 34-4g   If the patient is unresponsive or does not feel light touch, pinch the hand and watch and listen for a response.

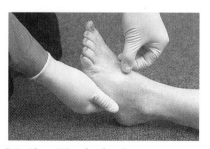

Figure 34-4h   Pinch the foot to assess sensation in the lower extremities if the unresponsive patient does not respond to light touch.

Signs and Symptoms Most often, you will take spinal precautions based solely on the mechanism of injury rather than on specific signs and symptoms of spine injury. It is imperative for you as an EMT-B to recognize that a patient's lack of pain in the spinal column or his ability to walk, to move his extremities, and to feel sensations do not rule out the possibility of spinal column (vertebrae) or spinal cord injury.

The following are signs and symptoms of spine injury (Figure 34-5):

- Tenderness in the area of injury, specifically along the spinal column.
- Pain associated with movement from spine injury may be localized. Ask the patient to pinpoint the location (by telling you where it is, not by trying to point to it). *Do not ask the patient to move to try to elicit a pain response. Do not move the patient to test for pain.*
- Pain independent of movement or palpation along the spinal column or in the lower legs. Such pain is generally intermittent instead of constant and may occur anywhere along the spinal column from the base of the head to the extreme lower back. If the lower spinal column is injured, the patient may complain of pain to the legs.

- Obvious deformity of the spine upon palpation. This is a rare assessment finding.
- Soft tissue injuries from trauma to the head and neck are associated with cervical spine injury. Soft tissue injuries to the shoulders, posterior thorax (back), or abdomen are associated with thoracic or lumbar spine injury. Lower extremity trauma is associated with lumbar and sacral spine injury.
- Numbness, weakness, tingling, or loss of sensation in the arms and/or legs.
- Loss of sensation or paralysis below the suspected level of injury or in the upper or upper and lower extremities. Paralysis of the extremities is a very reliable sign of spine injury.
- Loss of bowel or bladder control (incontinence).
- Priapism, a persistent erection of the penis resulting from injury to the spinal nerves to the genitals. It occurs soon after injury and is a classic sign of cervical spine injury.
- Impaired breathing, especially breathing that involves little or no chest movement and only slight abdominal movement, is an indication that the patient is breathing with the diaphragm alone. This diaphragmatic breathing is indicative of cervical spine injury. If injury to the nerve that controls the

SIGNS OF SYMPTOMS OF POSSIBLE SPINAL INJURY

- PAIN   Unprovoked pain in area of injury, along spine, in lower legs.

- TENDERNESS   Gentle touch of area may increase pain.

- DEFORMITY (rare)   There may be abnormal bend or bony prominence.

- SOFT TISSUE INJURY   Injury to the head, neck, or face may indicate cervical-spine injury. Injury to shoulders, back, and abdomen may indicate thoracic- or lumbar-spine injury. Injury to extremities may indicate lumbar- or sacral-spine injury.

- PARALYSIS   Inability to move or inability to feel sensation in some part of body may indicate spinal fracture with cord injury.

- PAINFUL MOVEMENT   Movement may increase pain. Never try to move the injured area.

- ALSO: Loss of bowel or bladder control, priapism, impaired breathing.

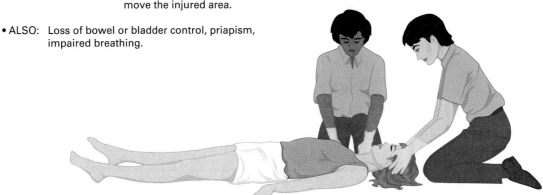

Figure 34-5   Signs and symptoms of possible spine injury.

diaphragm occurs, you may see either no breathing effort or an attempt to breathe using only the abdominal muscles.

Complications of Spine Injury Spine injury may produce catastrophic permanent damage. Three major complications of spine injury are these:

- *Inadequate Breathing Effort*—Paralysis of the respiratory muscles may occur with injury to the cervical spine. Rapid deterioration of the patient's condition and death may result without quick intervention by the EMT-B. The diaphragm may continue to function even if the chest wall muscles are paralyzed. The patient will display shallow, inadequate breathing with little movement of the chest or abdomen. Continuous positive pressure ventilation is necessary.
- *Paralysis*—Paralysis may occur below the site of spinal cord damage (Figure 34-6). If the damage is to the lower part of the spinal cord, paralysis is isolated to the lower half of the body (paraplegia). Damage to the spinal cord in the neck can produce complete paralysis of the entire body (quadriplegia). Paralysis to only one side of the body (hemiplegia) is more common in head injuries and stroke.
- *Inadequate Circulation*—Blood pressure and perfusion may be poor in the patient with spine injury. If the spinal cord nerve fibers traveling from the medulla in the brain to the blood vessels are damaged, the blood pressure control center (vasomotor center) can no longer maintain the muscle tone in the blood vessels. Below the point of spinal cord injury, the blood vessels dilate (increase in size) and

lower their resistance. Subsequently, blood begins to pool in the dilated vessels, the blood pressure drops, and the perfusion of other tissues of the body is reduced. Because of the blood vessel dilation, the skin is usually warm and dry, even though the tissue perfusion is poor. The heart rate typically remains normal or decreases slightly.

EMERGENCY MEDICAL CARE

In cases of suspected spine injury, it is **not** the role of the EMT-B to attempt to diagnose the condition or the site of the injury. The EMT-B must instead ensure that life-threatening conditions are cared for, that the possibility of further injury is reduced by careful handling of the patient, and that the patient is properly immobilized to a backboard and expeditiously transported to a medical facility.

When in doubt, immobilize the patient.

Remember that it is safer to err on the side of caution and completely immobilize a patient if spine injury is suspected. Immobilization devices can always be removed at the emergency department once the physician or x-rays prove no spine injury exists. Paralysis resulting from failure to immobilize a patient because he did not display signs and symptoms of spine injury cannot be so easily undone.

The general guidelines for emergency care of a suspected spine-injured patient are these:

1. *Take necessary body substance isolation precautions.*
2. *Establish manual in-line spinal stabilization immediately upon making contact with the patient*

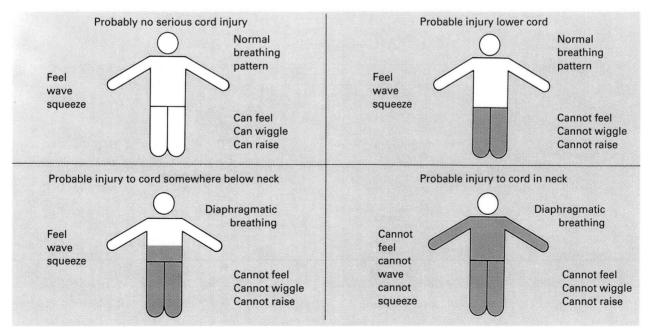

Figure 34-6 Signs and symptoms correlated to location of spinal-cord injury.

(Figures 34-7a to b). Ensure that the head is in a neutral, in-line position. That means bringing the head into a position in which the nose is in line with the navel (belly button) and the head is neither flexed forward nor extended backward. This manual stabilization must be maintained until the patient is completely secured and immobilized to the backboard.

If the patient complains of severe pain to the neck or cervical spine, or the head does not easily move, stabilize and maintain the head in the position found.

If a first responder is holding manual in-line spinal stabilization upon your arrival, instruct him not to let go. If he can continue with the stabilization, evaluate the position of the patient's head and make any necessary readjustments. If the first responder needs to be relieved, you should take over the in-line stabilization in a controlled manner. Replace the first responder's hands on the patient's head with yours one at a time so that stabilization is never lost or uncontrolled.

3. *When performing the initial assessment, open and maintain the airway with the jaw-thrust maneuver.* Insert an oropharyngeal or nasopharyngeal airway if necessary. Suction secretions without turning the patient's head. Provide positive pressure ventilation or oxygen via a nonrebreather device while manual in-line stabilization is maintained.

4. *Assess the pulse, motor function, and sensation in all extremities.* Record these and document any differences or changes in the neurologic status during your contact with the patient.

5. *Assess the cervical region and the neck* before applying the cervical spine immobilization collar. Gently palpate the cervical region for any deformities or tenderness.

6. *Apply a cervical spine immobilization collar.* Be sure that you are familiar with the type of cervical collar you are using. Refer to the manufacturer's instructions on proper sizing since each device is different. An improperly sized collar can cause more harm to the patient and further aggravate a potential spine injury. Information about sizing and applying the cervical spine immobilization collar is given on the next pages.

If the cervical spine immobilization collar does not fit properly, use a rolled towel or blanket instead. Loosely wrap the towel or blanket around the patient's neck to take the place of the cervical collar, taping the towel or blanket to the backboard. Maintain manual in-line stabilization.

7. *Immobilize the patient to a long backboard.* Steps for immobilization in a variety of different circumstances are illustrated and explained on the following pages.

8. *Once the patient is immobilized, reassess, record, and document the pulses and motor and sensory function in all extremities.*

9. *Transport to the hospital.*

DETAILED PHYSICAL EXAM

Perform the detailed exam en route to the hospital if time and the patient's condition permit. Remember that, because the patient will be completely immobilized to the backboard, your access to the head, neck, ears, and posterior body will be somewhat limited.

ESTABLISH MANUAL IN-LINE STABILIZATION

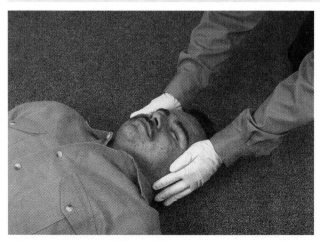

Figure 34-7a   Properly position your hands.

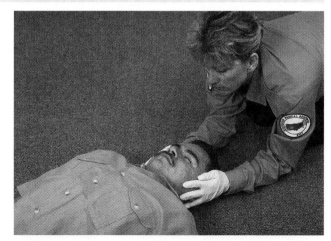

Figure 34-7b   Keep the head in a neutral position and the nose in-line with the patient's navel.

Inspect and palpate for further evidence of injury without unnecessarily moving the patient. Assess and record any change in motor and sensory function in the extremities.

ONGOING ASSESSMENT

Perform an ongoing assessment every 5 minutes en route to the hospital. Ensure that the airway is clear and that breathing is adequate. Reassess and record the baseline vital signs. Look for any changes in the pulse, skin condition, or blood pressure.

Because a spine injury is rarely an isolated injury, look for signs of shock (hypoperfusion): The skin becomes pale, cool and moist, the blood pressure falls, the heart rate increases, the patient's mental status decreases. Remember that a decreasing level of re-

sponsiveness is an early sign of head injury, while a rising systolic blood pressure and decreasing heart rate are late signs of head injury.

If the patient has any further complaints, repeat those necessary parts of the focused history and physical exam. Be aware of complaints of tingling, numbness, loss of sensation, or paralysis. Reevaluate any airway adjuncts, positive pressure ventilation devices, mask seal, oxygen therapy, splints, and immobilization devices. Record your findings in the prehospital care report and communicate them to the emergency department.

SUMMARY: ASSESSMENT AND CARE

To review possible assessment findings and emergency care for injuries to the spine, see Figures 34-8 and 34-9.

 ASSESSMENT SUMMARY

SPINE INJURY

The following are findings that may be associated with a spine injury.

SCENE SIZE-UP

Pay particular attention to your own safety. Look for:
Mechanism of injury
    Automobile crash
    Motorcycle crash
    Pedestrian-vehicle collision
    Fall
    Blunt trauma
    Penetrating trauma to the head, neck, and torso
    Hanging
    Diving accident or near-drowning
    Gunshot wound to head, neck, chest, abdomen, or
      pelvis
    Electrical injury

INITIAL ASSESSMENT

General Impression

Assume spinal injury based on mechanism of injury
Patient may be paralyzed and not moving

Mental Status

Alert to responsive, based on type and degree of injury

Airway

Assume airway is compromised if patient has an altered mental status

Breathing

May be absent, inadequate, or normal
Little or no movement of chest with slight or excessive abdominal muscle use may be present, depending on level of spinal cord injury

Circulation

Pulse and skin color vary, depending on injury
Pulse may be normal or decreased
Skin may be normal, or may be pale, cool, and clammy above site of injury and flushed, warm, and dry below site of injury

Status: Priority patient if evidence of a spinal injury or altered mental status exists

FOCUSED HISTORY AND PHYSICAL EXAM

Physical Exam

Head:
    Open or closed wounds to the head, neck, or face
Chest:
    Blunt or penetrating trauma to chest
Abdomen:
    Blunt or penetrating trauma to abdomen
Pelvis:
    Blunt or penetrating trauma to pelvic area
Extremities:
    No response to pain or light touch
    Inability to move extremities
    Numbness or tingling sensation in extremities

Figure 34-8a   Assessment summary: spine injury.

(continued on the next page)

ASSESSMENT SUMMARY

SPINE INJURY (CONTINUED)

Posterior body:
 Deformity to spinal column
 Evidence of trauma
 Swelling around spinal column
 Tenderness on palpation of spinal column
 Muscle spasms along spinal column
 Blunt or penetrating trauma to back

Baseline Vital Signs

BP: normal, or may be low
HR: normal, or bradycardia
RR: normal, irregular, decreased, or absent
Skin: normal, or may be pale, cool, clammy above site of injury and flushed, warm, dry below site of injury

Pupils: equal and reactive, may be sluggish to respond to light
Note: If the blood pressure is low, heart rate elevated, and skin is pale, cool, and clammy, suspect shock. Look for other trauma and treat for shock.

SAMPLE History

Tenderness in area of injury
Pain
Deformity to the spine
Soft tissue injuries to posterior body, neck, or cervical region
Numbness, tingling, weakness, or paralysis in arms and/or legs
Loss of bowel and bladder control
Priapism (persistent erection of penis)
Inadequate breathing or abnormal breathing patterns

EMERGENCY CARE PROTOCOL

SPINE INJURY

1. Establish manual in-line stabilization. Do not release it until patient is immobilized onto backboard.
2. Establish and maintain an open airway. Insert a nasopharyngeal or oropharyngeal airway if patient is unresponsive and has no gag or cough reflex.
3. Suction secretions as necessary.
4. If breathing is inadequate, provide positive pressure ventilation with supplemental oxygen at a minimum rate of 12 ventilations/minute for an adult and 20 ventilations/minute for an infant or child.
5. If breathing is adequate, administer oxygen by nonrebreather mask at 15 lpm.
6. Control any major bleeding.
7. Apply a cervical spinal immobilization collar.
8. Place patient on backboard, pad any voids, and apply a minimum of 3 straps, at chest, hips, and above knees. Once torso is secured, secure head in a head immobilization device.

- Standing patient: Immobilize using standing immobilization technique.
- Seated patient with critical injuries: Perform rapid extrication and immobilize to backboard as described in item 8.
- Seated patient with no critical injuries: Apply vest-type immobilization device. Extricate and immobilize to backboard as described in item 8.
- Supine or prone patient: Logroll patient onto backboard and immobilize as described in item 8.

9. If BP and HR are low and skin is flushed, suspect spinal shock. Treat for shock.
10. If BP is low, HR is elevated, and skin is pale, cool, and clammy, suspect hypovolemic shock. Look for other injuries and treat for shock.
11. Transport.
12. Perform an ongoing assessment every 5 minutes if unstable and every 15 minutes if stable. Be prepared for vomiting and seizures.

Figure 34-8b Emergency care protocol: spine injury.

EMERGENCY CARE ALGORITHM:
SPINE INJURY

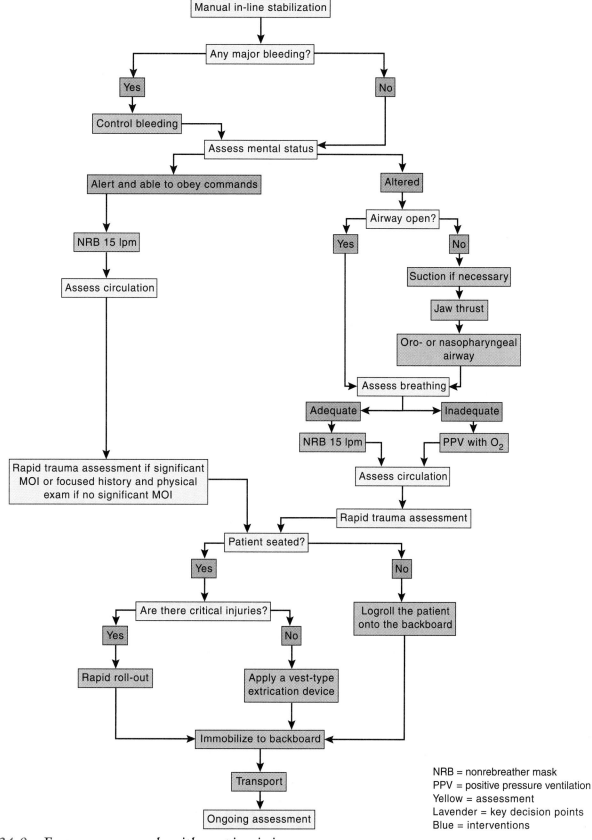

Figure 34-9 Emergency care algorithm: spine injury.

GUIDELINES FOR IMMOBILIZATION

As an EMT-B, you will encounter patients with spine injury or suspected spine injury in a variety of different circumstances. Some may be lying unresponsive on the ground. Others might be responsive, but seated in wrecked automobiles. Still others might be walking about. No matter what the circumstances, your task when you encounter a patient with suspected spine injury is to immobilize that patient safely and swiftly and transport him to a receiving facility. Mastering a variety of tools and techniques will help you carry out this task successfully.

TOOLS

The basic tools you will use in immobilizing patients are cervical spine immobilization collars, long backboards, and both rigid and vest-type short backboards.

CERVICAL SPINE IMMOBILIZATION COLLARS

A cervical spine immobilization collar should be used any time you suspect injury to the spine based on the mechanism of injury, the patient's history, or the signs and symptoms. There are several types of cervical collars (Figures 34-10a to c). *Never use a soft collar;* it permits too much movement.

The collar by itself does not immobilize the patient. The purpose of the collar is not to prevent the head from moving, but rather to prevent the head from moving in relation to the spine and to reduce the compression of the cervical spine during movement and transport of the patient. Even if you believe that the injury is only to the cervical (neck) area, the cervical collar is not enough. The entire spine must be stabilized and then immobilized. After a collar is applied, in-line manual stabilization must be maintained until the patient is fully secured to a backboard.

Sizing of the collar to the patient is based on the design of the device (Figures 34-11a to c). Be sure to use a collar of the proper size for the patient.

Using a collar that is too small will not restrain the patient's head adequately. Using a collar that is too large may cause extension of the patient's neck and aggravate the spine injury.

Cervical spine immobilization collars should be applied by two rescuers: One stabilizes the neck manually in the neutral position while the other applies the collar. Placement of the cervical collar should never obstruct the patient's airway. See Figures 34-12a to c and 34-13a to d for detailed descriptions of how to apply a cervical spine immobilization collar.

FULL BODY SPINAL IMMOBILIZATION DEVICES

Several different types of long board immobilization devices exist to provide stabilization and immobilization of the head, neck, torso, pelvis, and extremities (Figures 34-14a, b, d, and e). Generally, long backboards are used to immobilize patients who are found in a lying or standing position. They may also be used in conjunction with short backboards. For proper immobilization of a patient, padding, straps, and cravats are also used with the long board.

SHORT SPINAL IMMOBILIZATION DEVICES

The most common short spine device is the commercially made vest-type device with supplied straps for the head, chest, and legs (Figure 34-14f and g). A device now less commonly used than in the past is the rigid short spine board (Figure 34-14c). This device requires the addition of backboard straps, padding, tape, or cravats to secure the patient. Both vest-type and rigid devices provide stabilization and immobilization to the head, neck, and torso. They are most commonly used to immobilize noncritical sitting patients with suspected spine injuries.

Once again, it is very important to be completely familiar with the proper use of these devices to avoid further injury to the patient. For vest-type devices, follow all of the manufacturer's instructions regarding application and use of the device.

Both vest-type and rigid short boards should be used only to immobilize the patient while moving him from a sitting position, then immediately to a long board. Short devices cannot adequately immobilize a patient because they can't immobilize the surrounding joints of the head, torso, and legs.

OTHER IMMOBILIZATION EQUIPMENT

Whenever a patient is placed onto a backboard, he must be secured to the board with backboard straps and some type of head immobilizer. Techniques for using this equipment to immobilize a patient to a long backboard are discussed in the next section.

Straps or cravats should be placed to keep the patient from sliding up and down or laterally on the board. Place straps across the chest and under the armpits in a manner that does not interfere with the patient's breathing. Place straps across the pelvis and above the patient's knees.

Deceleration straps are another important adjunct to immobilization. These straps are fastened across the patient's shoulders. They help prevent the patient's torso from sliding up the backboard and compressing the cervical spine when the ambulance slows or stops during transport.

CERVICAL SPINE IMMOBILIZATION COLLARS

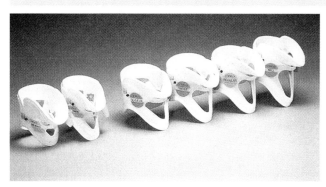

Figure 34-10a   Stifneck cervical spine immobilization collars. (Laerdal Medical Corporation).

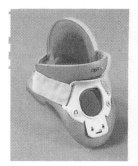

Figure 34-10c   Philadelphia Cervical Collar assembled and disassembled. (Philadelphia® Cervical Collar Co.).

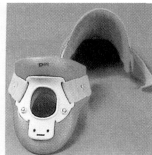

Figure 34-10b   The Stifneck® Select™ collar can be adjusted to fit all sizes. (Laerdal Medical Corporation/John Hill Photography).

IMMOBILIZATION TECHNIQUES

As previously noted, you will encounter patients with suspected spine injuries in a variety of circumstances. The guidelines that follow tell you how to use the tools we have just described to immobilize patients in the most common situations.

IMMOBILIZING A SUPINE OR PRONE PATIENT

When you encounter a supine or prone patient with a suspected spine injury, first ensure that all life-threatening situations have been managed, establish and maintain in-line manual spinal stabilization, and apply a cervical spine immobilization collar. Then you must immobilize the patient to a long backboard. A brief description of the four-rescuer log roll and immobilization procedures are provided in Figures 34-15a-h and 34-16a-e.

1. *Move the patient onto the spine board by log rolling the patient.* This move is ideally performed by at least four rescuers. One rescuer at the patient's head directs the movement and maintains in-line

stabilization of the patient. One to three other rescuers actually move the patient onto the backboard. As the patient is rolled onto his side, his posterior body should be carefully assessed if this has not been done during the initial assessment.

2. *Position the long spine board under the patient* by sliding the board under the patient during the log roll. Then place the patient on the board at the command of the rescuer who is maintaining in-line stabilization. Use a slide, proper lift, log roll, or scoop stretcher to position the patient on the backboard so that movement is as limited as possible. (The method used will depend on the situation, the scene, and available resources.)

3. *Place padding in the spaces between the patient and the board.* In an adult, pad under the head and torso, taking care to avoid extra movement. In an infant or child, pad under the shoulders (because the child's relatively larger head will otherwise cause the neck to flex forward) and anywhere along the length of the body as necessary to maintain a neutral position.

4. *Immobilize the patient's torso to the board with straps.* The strap across the chest should be tight

SIZING A CERVICAL SPINE IMMOBILIZATION COLLAR

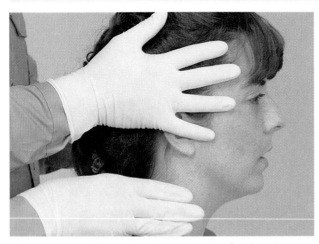

Figure 34-11a To size a cervical spine immobilization collar, first draw an imaginary line across the top of the shoulders and the bottom of the chin. Use your fingers to measure the distance from the shoulder to the chin.

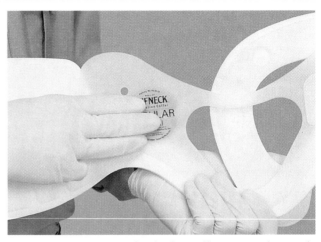

Figure 34-11b Check the collar you select. The distance between the sizing post (black fastener) and lower edge of the rigid plastic should match that of the number of stacked fingers previously measured against the patient's neck.

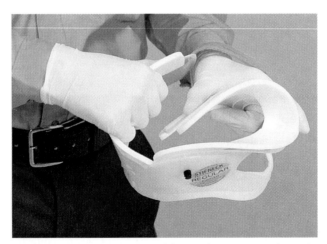

Figure 34-11c Assemble and preform the collar.

enough to prevent shifting of the torso but not so tight that it inhibits movement of the chest muscles and impairs breathing.

5. *Immobilize the patient's head to the board with a commercial head/cervical immobilization device or through the use of blanket rolls and tape.* Never place padding behind the neck itself. If the patient vomits, your strapping technique should be good enough to enable you to roll the patient onto his left side several times without any change in body position on the board.

6. *Secure the patient's legs to the board with straps.*

7. *Proceed with care as described earlier under Emergency Medical Care.*

If only two or three rescuers are available the log roll can be done using the techniques shown in Figures 34-17a to d and 34-18a to d.

APPLYING A CERVICAL SPINE IMMOBILIZATION COLLAR TO A SITTING PATIENT

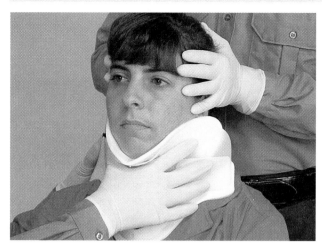

Figure 34-12a   After selecting the proper size, slide the cervical spine immobilization collar up the chest wall. The chin must cover the central fastener in the chin piece.

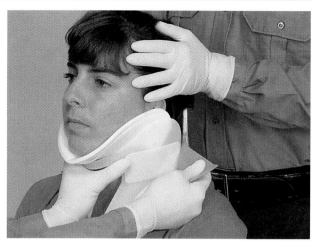

Figure 34-12b   Bring the collar around the neck and secure the Velcro. Recheck the position of the patient's head and collar for proper alignment. Make sure the patient's chin covers the central fastener of the chin piece.

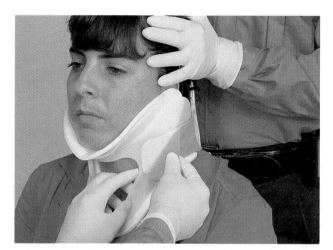

Figure 34-12c   If the chin is not covering the fastener of the chin piece, readjust the collar by tightening the Velcro until a proper sizing is obtained. If further tightening will cause hyperextension of the patient's head, then select the next smaller size.

APPLYING A CERVICAL SPINE IMMOBILIZATION COLLAR TO A SUPINE PATIENT

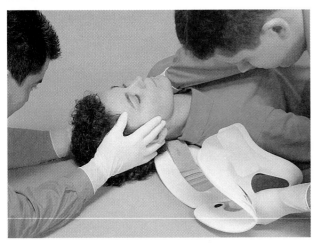

Figure 34-13a Slide the back portion of the cervical spine immobilization collar behind the patient's neck. Fold the loop Velcro inward on the foam padding.

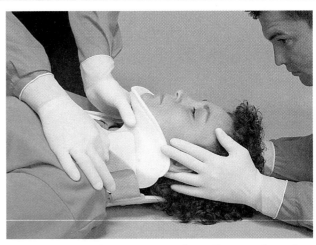

Figure 34-13b Position the collar so that the chin fits properly. Secure the collar by attaching the Velcro.

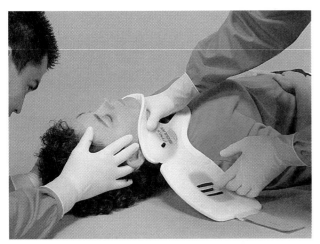

Figure 34-13c An alternative method of applying the collar to a supine patient is to start by positioning the chin piece and then sliding the back portion of the collar behind the patient's neck.

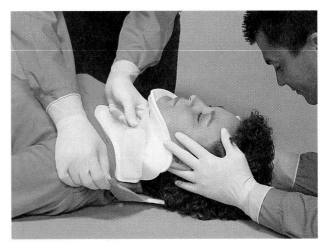

Figure 34-13d Hold the collar in place by grasping the trachea hole. Attach the loop Velcro so it mates with (and is parallel to) the hook Velcro.

IMMOBILIZING A STANDING PATIENT

It is not uncommon to find patients with suspected spine injuries standing or walking around at the scene of an accident. Never permit such patients to sit down or to walk to the cot and lie down on a backboard. In such cases, you should instead use a standing long board technique to assist the patient from a standing to a supine position while keeping his spine aligned. This technique is outlined below and also illustrated in Figures 34-19a to d.

1. *One EMT-B should immediately take normal manual in-line spinal stabilization measures while another EMT-B applies a cervical collar.*
2. *Position the long board behind the patient. Examine the back carefully.*
3. *Two EMT-Bs should stand on either side of the patient to support him. Each should place one arm under the patient's armpit and grasp the highest reachable handhold on the long board. The EMT-Bs' other hands should be holding the pa-*

EXAMPLES OF IMMOBILIZATION DEVICES

Always follow local protocol in purchasing and using immobilization devices

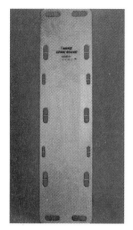

Figure 34-14a
Long board.

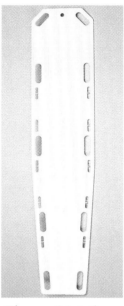

Figure 34-14b
Fiberglass back-
board.

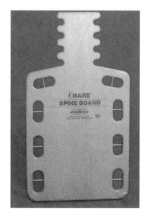

Figure 34-14c
Short board.

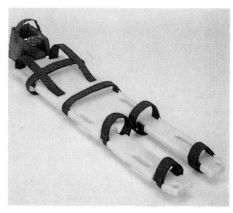

Figure 34-14d   Full body splint.

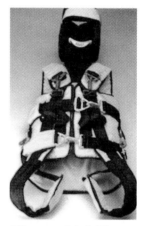

Figure 34-14f
Corset-type half-
back immobilizer.

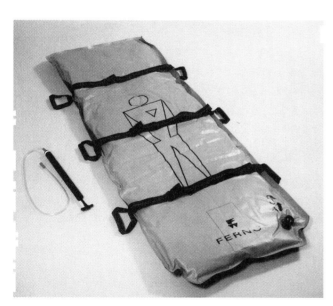

Figure 34-14e   Full body vacuum splint.
(Ferno Corporation)

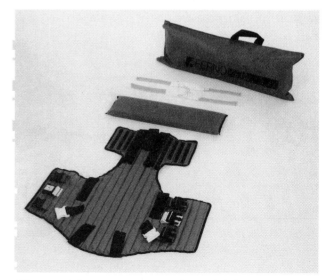

Figure 34-14g   K.E.D. (Kendrick Extrication
Device) (Ferno Corporation)

FOUR-RESCUER LOG ROLL AND LONG SPINE BOARD IMMOBILIZATION

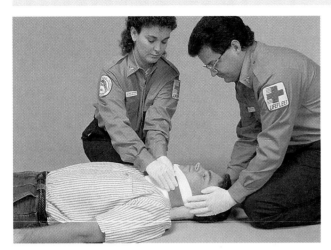

Figure 34-15a *Establish and maintain in-line stabilization. Apply a rigid cervical spine immobilization collar.*

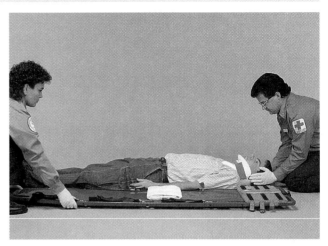

Figure 34-15b *Place a long spine board parallel to the patient. If possible, pad the voids under the head and torso.*

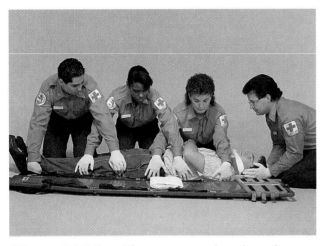

Figure 34-15c *Three rescuers kneel at the patient's side opposite the board, leaving space to roll the patient toward them.*

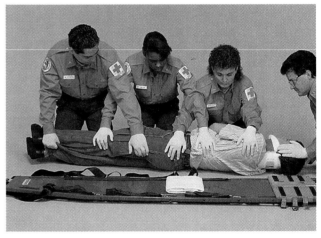

Figure 34-15d *The EMT-B at the head directs the others to roll the patient as a unit onto his side. Assess the patient's posterior side.*

tient's elbows to steady and support him. The third EMT-B maintains in-line manual stabilization.

4. *The EMT-Bs at the sides of the patient should each place a leg behind the board. They should then slowly tip the board backward and begin lowering it to the ground while the third EMT-B maintains stabilization.* Be sure to inform the patient what you are going to do before you begin to tip the board backward.

5. *Once the board is lying level on the ground, one EMT-B maintains manual stabilization while the others perform the necessary assessment and care. The patient is then immobilized on the backboard following the guidelines for prone and supine patients given earlier.*

6. *Proceed with care as described earlier under Emergency Medical Care.*

This technique can also be adapted for use by two EMT-Bs as illustrated in Figures 34-20a to d.

FOUR-RESCUER LOG ROLL AND LONG SPINE BOARD IMMOBILIZATION

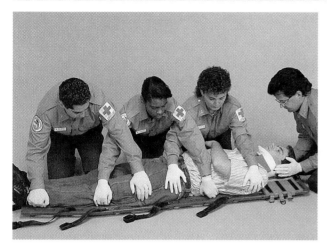

Figure 34-15e   The EMT-B at the waist reaches over, grasps the spine board, and pulls it into position against the patient. (This can also be done by a fifth rescuer.) The EMT-B at the head instructs the rescuers to roll the patient onto the spine board.

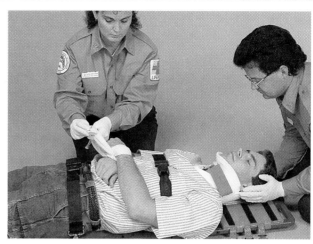

Figure 34-15f   Secure the patient to the board with straps. Loosely tie the wrists together.

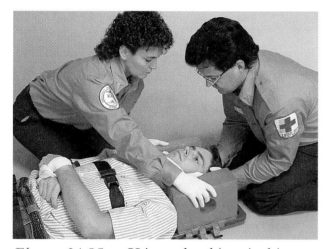

Figure 34-15g   Using a head/cervical immobilizer, secure the patient's head to the spine board.

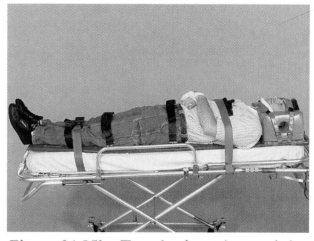

Figure 34-15h   Transfer the patient and the spine board as a unit. Secure the patient and the spine board to cot.

IMMOBILIZING A SEATED PATIENT

If the suspected spine-injured patient is found in a seated position, a short spinal immobilization device will be used. This will minimize movement and aggravation of potential spine injury while the patient is being transferred to a long board for complete immobilization.

The following are general steps to follow. The steps involved in using a vest-type device are illustrated in Figures 34-21a to h.

1. *Use manual in-line spinal stabilization and apply a cervical collar.* Assess pulses and motor and sensory function in all four extremities.
2. *Position the short spinal device behind the patient. Examine the back carefully.* Be careful not to have the EMT-B holding in-line spinal stabilization move excessively or move the patient as the device is positioned. You should slide the board behind the patient and as far into the seat as you can. The top of the board should be level with

IMMOBILIZING A PATIENT TO A LONG BOARD

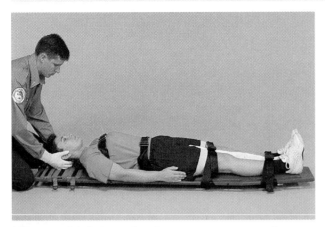

Figure 34-16a　Apply straps to secure the patient to the backboard. Place one strap at the level of the chest, one at the hip, one above the knee, and another below the knee. Pad between the legs.

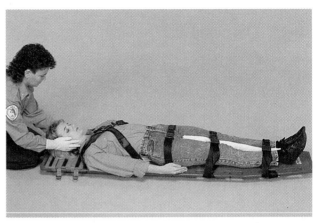

Figure 34-16b　An "X" strap method secures the torso to the backboard. Also apply one strap at the hip, one above the knee, and one below the knee.

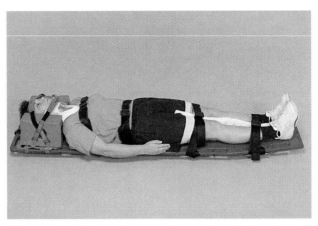

Figure 34-16c　Secure the patient's head to the backboard with a head immobilization device.

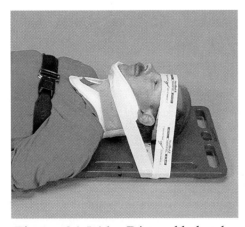

Figure 34-16d　Disposable head immobilization device.

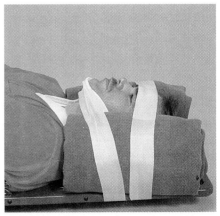

Figure 34-16e　Blanket rolls and tape can be used.

THREE-RESCUER LOG ROLL

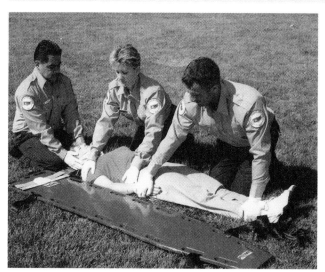

Figure 34-17a   Maintain in-line spinal sta-bilization while preparing for log roll.

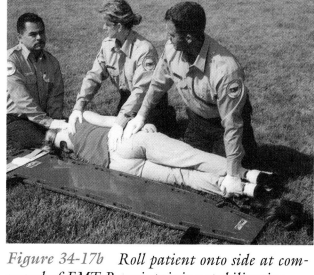

Figure 34-17b   Roll patient onto side at com-mand of EMT-B maintaining stabilization. Inspect the back.

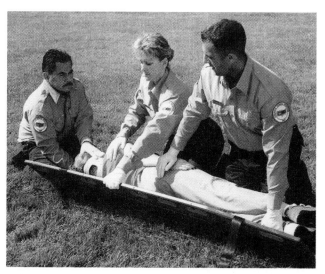

Figure 34-17c   Move spine board into place.

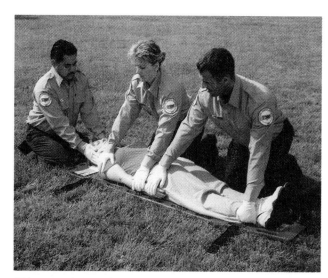

Figure 34-17d   Lower patient onto spine board at command of EMT-B maintaining in-line stabilization. Center patient on board.

the top of the patient's head, and the bottom of the board should not extend past the coccyx. The body flaps should fit snugly under the patient's arm pits.

3. *Secure the device to the patient's torso.* Make sure the straps are tight enough to prevent movement of the device laterally or vertically. If the device has straps that circle the legs, apply and tighten these after the chest straps are applied.

4. *Pad behind the patient's head to ensure neutral alignment of the head and neck with the remainder of the spine.* Excessive padding will cause the head and neck to flex forward, whereas lack of padding will allow the head and neck to be extended.

5. *Secure the patient's head to the device.* Maintain manual in-line spinal stabilization even though the head is secured to the device. Securing the head is the last step in the application of the de-vice.

TWO-RESCUER LOG ROLL

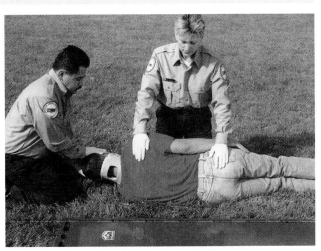

Figure 34-18a   Maintain an open airway and in-line spinal stabilization while applying a cervical spine immobilization collar.

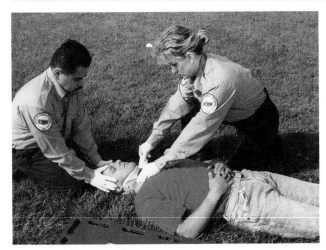

Figure 34-18b   Maintain in-line support while moving patient onto the side.

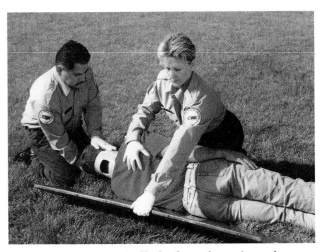

Figure 34-18c   Pull the board against the patient.

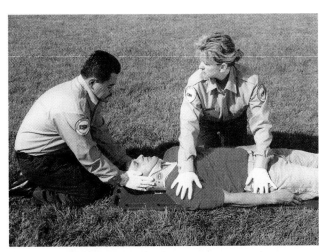

Figure 34-18d   Roll the patient gently onto the board and secure.

6. *Position a long backboard under or next to the patient's buttocks and rotate him until his back is in line with the backboard. Lower the patient onto the backboard while maintaining manual in-line spinal stabilization.* If it is not possible to get a long backboard next to the patient, lift the patient under his arms and legs and lower him onto the long board.

7. *Follow the guidelines for immobilizing a patient to a long backboard given above. Release manual in-line spinal stabilization only when the patient is completely secured to the backboard. Assess*

pulses and motor and sensory function and record your findings on the prehospital care report.

8. *Proceed with care as described earlier under Emergency Medical Care.*

There are several special considerations to be aware of when using a short spinal device:

- Do any assessment of the back, scapula, arms, or clavicles before you apply the board.
- Angle the board to fit between the arms of the rescuer who is stabilizing the patient's head without jarring the rescuer's arms.

IMMOBILIZING A STANDING PATIENT—THREE EMT-B'S

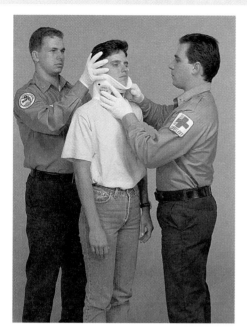

Figure 34-19a   Apply a cervical spine immobilization collar while in-line stabilization is being held.

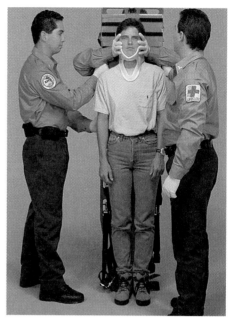

Figure 34-19b   Position the backboard behind the patient and align it properly. Check the position of the board from the front of the patient.

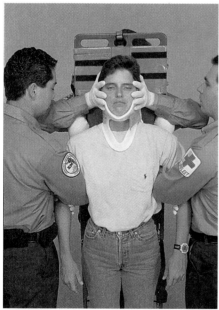

Figure 34-19c   The EMT-Bs at the sides of the patient place their hands under each arm and grasp the next highest handhold. Their other hands grasp the elbows of the patient to provide additional stabilization on the board.

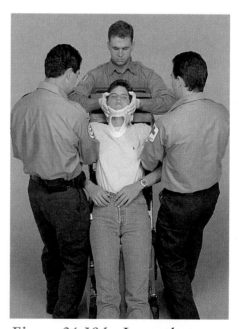

Figure 34-19d   Lower the patient to the ground. Continue holding in-line stabilization until the patient is completely immobilized to the backboard with a head/cervical immobilization device and straps.

IMMOBILIZING A STANDING PATIENT—TWO EMT-BS

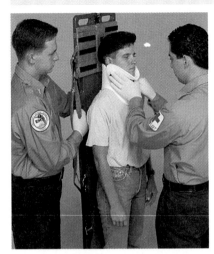

Figure 34-20a *Apply a cervical spine immobilization collar and position the long board behind the patient.*

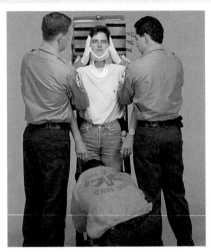

Figure 34-20b *The EMT-Bs on each side of the patient hold the long board in place and hold the patient's head in a neutral in-line position.*

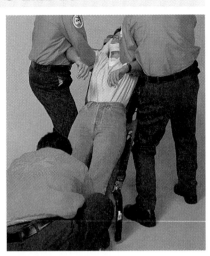

Figure 34-20c *Each EMT-B then places the leg closest to the board behind it and lowers the board to the ground.*

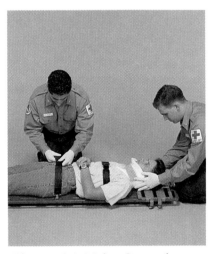

Figure 34-20d *Once the patient is horizontal on the ground, one EMT-B takes over in-line stabilization until the patient is completely immobilized.*

- As mentioned above, push the spine board as far down into the seat as possible. If you don't, the board may shift and the patient's cervical spine may compress. The top of the board must be level with the top of the patient's head; the base of the board must not extend past the coccyx.

- Never place a chin cup or chin strap on the patient. They will prevent the patient from opening his mouth if he needs to vomit.
- When applying the first strap to the torso, take care not to apply the strap too tightly, which could cause abdominal injury or impair breathing.

IMMOBILIZING A SEATED PATIENT WITH A FERNO K.E.D. EXTRICATION DEVICE

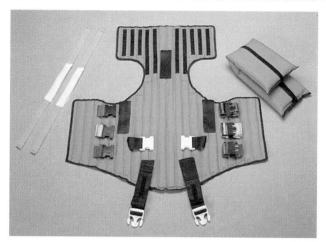

Figure 34-21a   The Ferno (K.E.D.) Extrication Device.

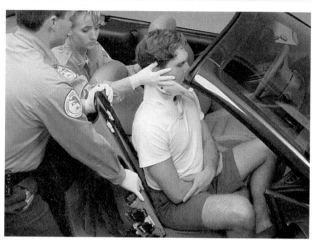

Figure 34-21b   After a cervical spine immobilization collar has been applied, slip the K.E.D. behind the patient and center it.

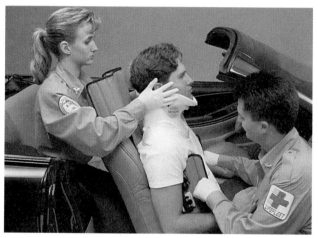

Figure 34-21c   Properly align the device. Then wrap the vest around the patient's torso.

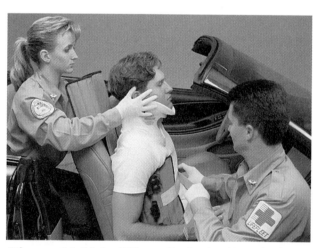

Figure 34-21d   When the device is tucked well up into the arm pits, secure the chest straps.

(continued on the next page)

- Always tighten the torso and leg straps before securing the patient's head to the device. This prevents accidental movement of the patient's cervical spine.
- Never allow buckles to be placed midsternum where they would interfere with proper hand placement if CPR becomes necessary.
- Never pad between the cervical collar and the board; doing so creates a pivot point that may cause hyperextension of the cervical spine when the head is secured.
- Assess pulses and motor and sensory function before and after applying the device.

RAPID EXTRICATION

There are times when you will have to move a patient with a suspected spine injury before immobilizing him to a long backboard or even to a short spinal device. There are three situations in which such movement is permissible. They are as follows:

- The scene is not safe (because of the threat of fire or explosion, chemical spills, or gunfire for example).
- The patient's condition is so unstable that you need to move and transport him immediately.
- The patient blocks your access to a second, more seriously injured patient.

IMMOBILIZING A SEATED PATIENT WITH A FERNO K.E.D. EXTRICATION DEVICE

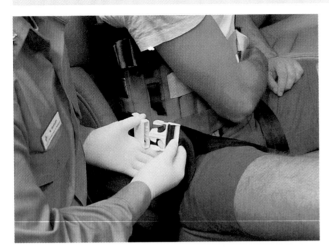

Figure 34-21e   Secure the leg straps.

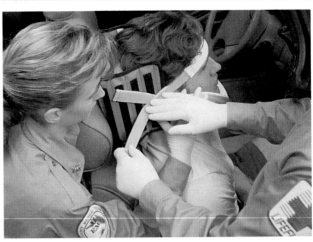

Figure 34-21f   Secure the patient's head with the Velcro head straps.

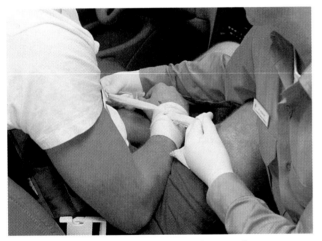

Figure 34-21g   Tie the hands together.

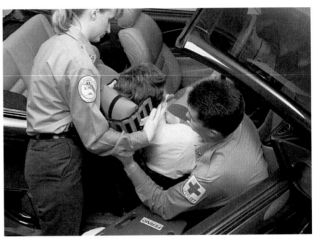

Figure 34-21h   Pivot patient onto the back-board while maintaining in-line stabilization.

In these circumstances—when the time saved by immediate extrication will make the difference between life and death—a **rapid extrication** will be performed. Rapid extrication eliminates the delay inherent in the use of spinal immobilization devices. Time is critical in the situations described above; therefore, the benefit of rapid transport outweighs the risk of movement during extrication.

Rapid extrication requires constant cervical spine stabilization and good communication among the EMT-Bs moving the patient. The patient's entanglement with seat belts, wreckage, or other objects can complicate rapid extrication procedures, so all rescuers need to be aware of the patient's position as well as any potential problems as the extrication is proceeding.

In rapid extrication, the patient is brought into alignment with manual in-line spinal stabilization and a cervical spine immobilization collar is applied. A long backboard is positioned next to him. The patient is quickly transferred to the long backboard while manual in-line spinal stabilization is maintained. The rapid extrication procedure is described in more detail in Figures 34-22a to f.

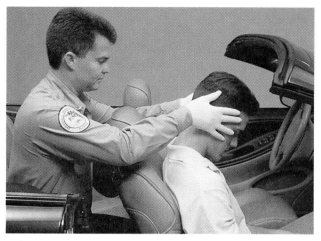

Figure 34-22a Bring the patient's head into a neutral in-line position. This is best achieved from behind or to the side of the patient.

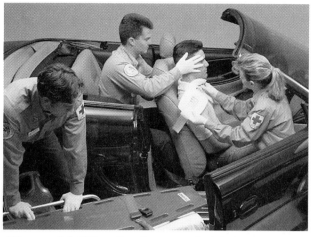

Figure 34-22b Perform an initial assessment and rapid trauma assessment. Then apply a cervical spine immobilization collar.

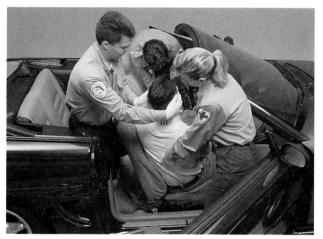

Figure 34-22c Support the patient's thorax. Rotate the patient until his back is facing the open car door. Bring the patient's legs and feet up onto the car seat.

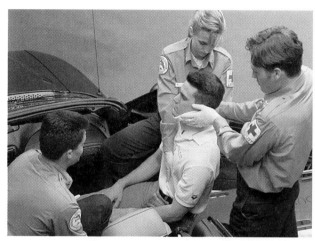

Figure 34-22d Bring the board in line with the patient and against the buttocks. Stabilize the cot under the board. Begin to lower the patient onto the board.

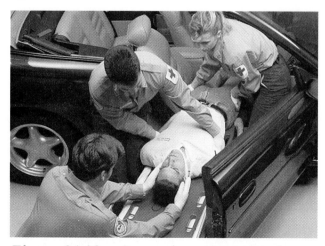

Figure 34-22e Lower the patient onto the board. Dependent on the structure of the car, it may be necessary to change positions to maintain in-line stabilization while lowering the patient onto the board.

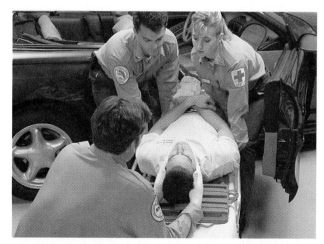

Figure 34-22f As one EMT-B maintains in-line stabilization, the other EMT-Bs support the patient as they slide him onto the backboard in 6-inch to 12-inch increments.

HELMET REMOVAL

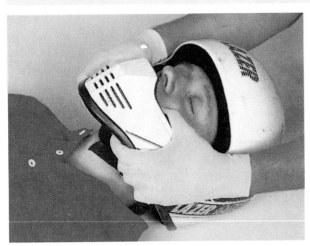

Figure 34-23a One rescuer applies stabilization by placing hands on each side of the helmet with fingers on the patient's mandible. This prevents slippage if the strap is loose.

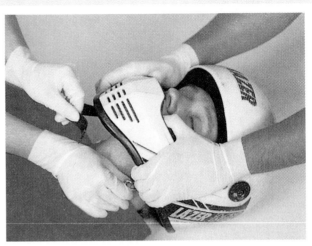

Figure 34-23b A second rescuer loosens the strap at the D-rings while stabilization is maintained.

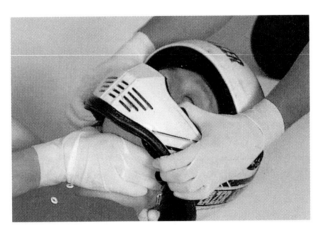

Figure 34-23c The second rescuer places one hand on the mandible at the angle, thumb on one side, long and index fingers on the other.

SPECIAL CONSIDERATIONS

Handling and immobilization of patients with suspected spine injuries can be complicated by a variety of factors. Two of the more common such situations you will encounter involve suspected spine injury in people wearing helmets and suspected spine injury in infants and children.

HELMETS

Activities such as bicycle riding, motorcycle riding, and playing football can easily lead to accidents involving mechanisms that can produce spine injury. People taking part in such activities often wear helmets, and you may arrive at an accident scene to en-counter a patient still wearing a helmet. Thorough assessment of a patient is difficult under any circumstances; the presence of a helmet makes the task still more difficult. But removal of a helmet (see Figures 34-23 and 34-24) should not be an automatic step. Such removal could risk aggravating the spine injury, if one exists. You should first assess the patient wearing the helmet in the following areas:

- Assess the patient's airway and breathing.
- Assess the fit of the helmet and the likelihood of movement of the patient's head within the helmet.
- Determine your ability to gain access to the patient's airway if intervention should be necessary to assist his breathing.

HELMET REMOVAL

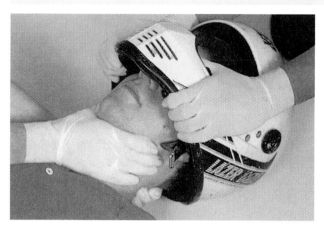

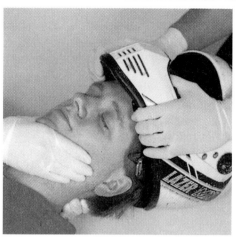

Figure 34-23d   With the other hand, the second rescuer holds the occipital region. This maneuver transfers the stabilization responsibility to the second rescuer. The rescuer at the top removes the helmet in two steps, allowing the second rescuer to readjust his hand position under the occipital region. Three factors should be kept in mind: (a) The helmet is egg-shaped and therefore must be expanded laterally to clear the ears. (b) If the helmet provides full facial coverage, glasses must be removed first. (c) If the helmet provides full facial coverage, the nose will impede removal. To clear the nose, the helmet must be tilted backward and raised over it.

Figure 34-23e   Throughout the removal process, the second rescuer maintains in-line stabilization from below in order to prevent head tilt.

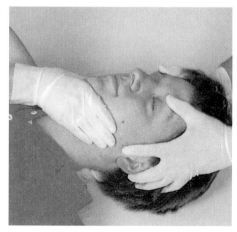

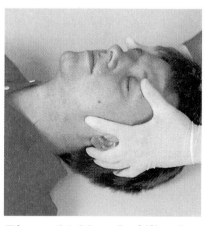

Figure 34-23f   After the helmet has been removed, the rescuer at the top replaces his hands on either side of the patient's head with palms over the ears, taking over stabilization.

Figure 34-23g   Stabilization is maintained from above until a cervical spine immobilization collar and complete immobilization to the backboard is achieved.

You should *leave the helmet in place* if your assessment reveals the following:

- The helmet fits well, and there is little or no movement of the patient's head inside the helmet.
- There are no impending airway or breathing problems.
- Removal of the helmet would cause further injury to the patient.
- You can properly immobilize the spine with the helmet in place.
- The helmet doesn't interfere with your ability to assess and reassess airway and breathing.

You should *remove the helmet* if your assessment reveals the following:

- The helmet interferes with your ability to assess or reassess airway and breathing.
- The helmet interferes with your ability to adequately manage the airway or breathing.
- The helmet does not fit well and allows excessive movement of the head inside the helmet. If this is a problem, you can carefully place padding between the helmet and the head to control the movement of the patient's head.
- The helmet interferes with proper spinal immobilization.
- The patient is in cardiac arrest.

HELMET REMOVAL

There are two basic types of helmets: sports helmets (such as those worn for football) and motorcycle helmets. Typically, sports helmets have an opening in the front and allow much easier access to the airway. Face masks on football helmets can be removed either by cutting the plastic clips that hold the mask to the helmet or by unsnapping the face mask retainers. Motorcycle helmets, on the other hand, generally cover the full face and have a shield that prevents access to the airway.

The techniques for the removal of motorcycle and sports helmets are illustrated in Figures 34-23a to g and 34-24a to d. The general steps for removal of a helmet are these:

1. Take the patient's eyeglasses off before you attempt to remove the helmet.
2. One rescuer should stabilize the helmet by placing hands on each side of the helmet with fingers on the mandible (lower jaw) to prevent movement.
3. A second rescuer should loosen the chin strap.
4. The second rescuer should place one hand anteriorly on the mandible at the angle of the jaw

and the other hand at the back of the head.
5. The rescuer holding the helmet should pull the sides of the helmet apart (to provide clearance for the ears), gently slip the helmet halfway off the patient's head, then stop.
6. The rescuer who is maintaining stabilization of the neck should reposition, sliding his hand under the patient's head to keep the head from falling back after the helmet is completely removed.
7. The first rescuer should remove the helmet completely.
8. The patient should then be immobilized as described earlier.

FOOTBALL INJURIES

When dealing with football injuries, the EMT-B has to take into consideration the equipment football players wear. In most cases, an injured player is wearing not only a helmet but also shoulder pads. Usually the shoulder pads and the helmet elevate the player's head, neck, and shoulders off the ground, almost in a neutral position. Because of this, you should leave the helmet on the player unless it is absolutely necessary to remove it. Removing the helmet while leaving the shoulder pads on will cause the head to drop and hyperextend the neck. Removal of the shoulder pads is difficult because the player is usually on his back and the attempt may cause unnecessary movement, risking aggravation of his injury.

As mentioned above, the face mask can be removed and airway control established and maintained with the helmet left on. If the head is loose in the helmet, you can pad the inside of the helmet to secure the player's head in the helmet. Log rolling a player with shoulder pads onto a long board may be difficult, so flat lifting might be the preferable technique.

INFANTS AND CHILDREN

When treating infants or children, use a rigid board appropriate for the child's size, following the guidelines outlined earlier for general immobilization. However, the following special considerations should apply when immobilizing infants or children:

- Pad from the shoulders to the heels of an infant or a child, if necessary, to maintain neutral in-line immobilization. Remember that the larger head of the infant or young child causes the head and neck to flex when supine. Use padding to eliminate flexion and maintain neutral alignment of the head, neck, and spine.

HELMET REMOVAL—ALTERNATIVE METHOD

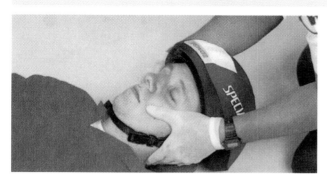

Figure 34-24a   Apply steady stabilization with the neck in neutral position.

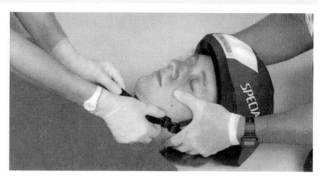

Figure 34-24b   Remove the chin strap.

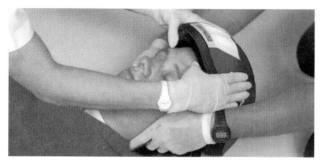

Figure 34-24c   Remove the helmet by pulling out laterally on each side.

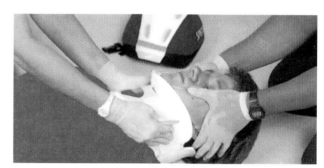

Figure 34-24d   Apply a suitable cervical spine immobilization collar and secure the patient to a long board.

• Make sure the cervical collar fits properly before applying it to an infant or child. If you don't have a collar that fits, immobilize the neck with a rolled towel, tape the towel to the backboard, and manually support the patient's head in a neutral in-line position. An improperly fitted collar will do more harm than good.

IMMOBILIZATION WITH A CAR SEAT

If you are at an automobile collision involving a child in a car seat, you can use that car seat to stabilize the child for transport, unless the child needs to be transferred to a backboard for care. Depending on the size of the child and the type of car seat he is in, you may need to pad around the child to prevent unnecessary movement.

Then follow these steps:

1. Apply manual in-line cervical stabilization.
2. Assess the infant or child to ensure that there are no life-threatening injuries or other reasons for removal from the car seat.
3. Carefully place towel rolls on both sides of the child's head between the head and the car seat to support the head. Secure with tape across the child's forehead to each side of the seat.
4. Determine that the child is secure in the seat and that there is not a lot of room between the child and the seat. If there is too much room, fill the spaces on each side of the child with padding and then resecure the straps around the child. Use tape if necessary.
5. Transport the child in a regular seated position with the car seat securely belted to the ambulance seat.

ENRICHMENT

The enrichment section contains information that is valuable as background for the EMT-B but that goes substantially beyond the U.S. Department of Transportation (DOT) EMT-Basic curriculum.

NEUROGENIC SHOCK (SPINAL SHOCK)

Neurogenic shock results from injury either to the brain or to the spinal cord, resulting in an interruption of nerve impulses to the arteries. When the arteries lose the nervous impulses from the brain and spinal cord, they relax and vasodilate (enlarge). This enlargement causes a relative hypovolemia within the circulatory system. That is, there is more space than there is blood to fill the arteries. Because of this, the patient becomes hypotensive (has lowered blood pressure).

Spinal shock results specifically from injury to the spinal cord, usually high in the cervical spine. In addition to the interruption of nerve impulses to the arteries, there is also an interruption of impulses to the peripheral nervous system, causing paralysis and loss of sensation. Sympathetic nerve impulses to the adrenal glands are lost, which prevents the release of epinephrine and norepinephrine. This causes vessel dilation (red skin) and sweat gland malfunction (dry skin). With the blood pooling in the body and the lack of circulating hormones (epinephrine and norepinephrine), the patient's physical signs are different from those of hypovolemic shock. The skin will be warm and dry and may appear slightly pink or red in color. The patient's pulse is typically 60 to 100 beats per minute, unlike the rapid rates usually found in hypovolemia.

Treatment for neurogenic shock or spinal shock is much the same as for any other shock (see Chapter 29). Cervical spinal control must be applied and the patient must be kept warm and completely immobilized to the backboard.

CASE STUDY FOLLOW-UP

SCENE SIZE-UP

You are dispatched to a gymnastics meet for a 12-year-old girl who has fallen during the competition. As you arrive on the scene, you are directed into the gymnasium by an assistant. The lights are bright and the music is loud. You and your partner make your way around various pieces of gymnastics equipment to the far side of the gym, where a small group of girls, some in tears, are crowded around a young girl supine on the mat. Immediately above her are a set of uneven parallel bars at approximate heights of 10 and 6 feet. A woman, who identifies herself as the coach, is kneeling next to the girl and holding her head and body still. The coach says, "She missed a maneuver off the top bar. She fell and hit the bottom bar with the middle of her back, then landed head first on the floor."

INITIAL ASSESSMENT

Recognizing the mechanism of injury, your partner immediately brings the patient's head and neck into a neutral position and establishes manual in-line spinal stabilization. You and your partner introduce yourselves and instruct the patient not to move. The young girl cries out, "My legs are numb and tingly! Am I going to be paralyzed?" You ask, "Can you tell me your name?" She says, "Carrie." "Well, Carrie," you say, "we're going to take good care of you and get you to the hospital where the doctors can figure out what's wrong and treat it."

Carrie's airway is patent and her breathing is rapid but adequate at a rate of approximately 28 per minute. Her radial pulse is strong and estimated at a rapid 125 per minute. Her skin is slightly cool to touch, slightly pale, and dry. You note, however, that the gymnasium temperature is relatively cool.

FOCUSED HISTORY AND PHYSICAL EXAM

You ask the coach if she actually saw the accident. You also ask if the patient attempted to get up or if she moved or was moved after the fall. The coach explains that she was standing next to Carrie when she fell. Because of how she landed, the coach immediately went to her side and instructed her to keep extremely still.

Because of the significant mechanism of injury, you proceed with a rapid trauma assessment. Very gently, you assess the head and find a contusion along the scalp line above the right eye. You ask, "Carrie, does your neck or back hurt?" She cries, "I don't know. I just feel my legs are numb and tingly." As you carefully palpate her neck, Carrie complains of tenderness to the cervical region at about the level of the sixth vertebrae. You apply a cervical collar. The chest, abdomen, and pelvis have no signs of injury.

You place the patient on oxygen via a nonrebreather mask at 15 liters per minute.

Following your inspection and palpation of her arms and determining that radial pulses are present bilaterally, you ask, "Can you move your hands just very slightly for me?" The patient complies and waves her hands slightly. You encourage her, "That's very good, Carrie." Keeping your hand out of her sight, you touch the little finger of her left hand and ask, "Can you tell me which hand and finger I'm touching?" Carrie replies, "My left hand, the pinkie." You touch her right hand and she again replies correctly. You then apply pinches to both hands and she identifies them correctly. Finally, you have her grip your fingers simultaneously and find the strength to be equal and strong in both upper extremities. Both radial pulses are strong.

You then inspect and carefully palpate the lower extremities for any signs of injury. The pedal pulses are present bilaterally. You instruct her to wave her foot very gently. She is able to move both feet. You touch the big toe on the right foot and ask, "Can you tell me which foot and toe I am touching?" She cries, "No!" Stabilizing the leg to avoid unsuspected and exaggerated movement, you pinch the top of the left foot. Carrie states, "I can feel that on my left foot." You repeat the same on the right foot and get a response to the pinch.

You enlist the help of the coach, who is familiar with log rolling, and instruct her to position herself at Carrie's feet. You position the backboard next to the patient. At the direction of your partner holding in-line stabilization at Carrie's head, you log roll her up and quickly assess her back, finding no deformities but some tenderness in the lumbar region. The backboard is positioned under her and she is rolled back onto it. A void behind the lumbar region is padded and straps are applied to the torso and legs and secured. A head/cervical immobilization device is applied and secured. Your partner releases manual in-line spinal stabilization and moves to the side to take the baseline vital signs. The blood pressure is 104/76, the heart rate is 118 per minute, the skin is slightly cool to touch, slightly pale, and dry. You obtain a SAMPLE history from the patient.

Carrie's parents have been notified by the gym staff. You and your partner meanwhile transfer Carrie to the ambulance and begin transport.

DETAILED PHYSICAL EXAM

En route, you conduct a detailed physical exam, which does not reveal any other signs of injury or changes from the focused history and physical exam.

ONGOING ASSESSMENT

During the ongoing assessment, you reevaluate the spinal immobilization. All straps are secure and all pads properly positioned. Carrie complains of some discomfort to her back but says it is from the hard backboard. You reassess her pulses and motor and sensory function in all the extremities and find no change. You reassess and record the baseline vital signs.

Upon arrival at the emergency department, you help the hospital staff gently transfer the backboard to the emergency department bed. You provide an oral report regarding your findings. You briefly reassure Carrie then proceed to the EMS room to complete your prehospital care report as your partner restocks the ambulance. You finally notify dispatch that you are prepared for another call.

Later that day, on another call to the same hospital, you find time to check on Carrie's condition. The emergency medicine physician states that she suffered a spinal contusion and will completely recover. He praises the coach's work in keeping Carrie still until EMS arrived. He thanks you and your partner for the very detailed information provided both orally and in the prehospital care report regarding the scene characteristics and mechanism of injury. He also states, "Very nice immobilization job."

CHAPTER REVIEW

TERMS AND CONCEPTS

You may wish to review the following terms and concepts included in this chapter.

autonomic nervous system—part of the nervous system that influences involuntary muscles and glands.

central nervous system—the portion of the nervous system consisting of the brain and the spinal cord.

cervical spine—the first seven vertebrae; the neck.

coccyx—the four fused vertebrae that form the lower end of the spine; the tailbone.

disc—fluid-filled pad of cartilage between two vertebrae.

ligaments—bands of fibrous tissue that connect bones about a joint and support organs.

lumbar spine—the five vertebrae that form the lower back.

neurogenic shock—type of shock common in cases of damage to the brain or spinal cord that results in vasodilation and relative hypovolemia. See also *spinal shock.*

peripheral nervous system—structures of the nervous system outside the brain and spinal cord.

rapid extrication—a technique using manual stabilization rather than application of an immobilization device for the purpose of speeding extrication when the time saved will make the difference between life and death.

sacral spine—the five fused vertebrae that form the rigid back of the pelvis; the sacrum.

skeletal system—the bony framework of the body.

spinal column—the 33 vertebrae that enclose and protect the spinal cord.

spinal cord—a column of nervous tissue that exits from the brain and extends the length of the spinal column. All nerves to the trunk and extremities originate from the spinal cord.

spinal shock—shock caused by injury to the spinal cord, causing vasodilation and relative hypovolemia (neurogenic shock) as well as paralysis and loss of sensation below the level of the spinal cord injury. Signs include normal to low heart rate and warm, dry, pink skin.

thoracic spine—the twelve vertebrae directly below the cervical vertebrae that comprise the upper back.

vertebrae—bones of the spinal column.

voluntary nervous system—part of the nervous system that influences voluntary muscles and movements of the body.

REVIEW QUESTIONS

1. Describe the relationship between the spinal column and the spinal cord.
2. Name the most common mechanisms of spine injury.
3. List the signs and symptoms of potential spine injury.
4. Explain the types of stabilization and immobilization that must be applied in cases of suspected spine injury.
5. Describe how the airway is managed in a suspected spine-injured patient.
6. Explain the purpose and use of the cervical spine immobilization collar.
7. Explain how to assess motor and sensory function in a patient with suspected spine injury.
8. Explain the use of long and short spinal immobilization devices for seated patients with suspected spine injuries.
9. Under what circumstances is rapid extrication appropriate?
10. Under what circumstances should you leave a helmet in place in a patient with suspected spine injury?

CHAPTER 35

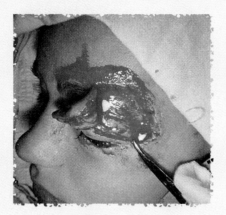

Eye, Face, and Neck Injuries

INTRODUCTION

If you have ever experienced a serious eye, face, or neck injury, you can appreciate a patient's fear and panic associated with one of these emergencies. Aside from the pain, injuries to the eye cause emotional duress as the patient thinks about the possible loss of vision, and the patient who suffers a facial injury may fear permanent scarring or disfigurement.

As an EMT-Basic, you must remain aware that injuries to the eyes, face, or neck have a high probability of causing airway compromise, severe bleeding, and shock. Additionally, injury to the face and neck is likely to be associated with spinal injury. While caring for the sometimes dramatic or horrific injuries themselves, you must always maintain a high index of suspicion for spinal injury and give first priority to care for life-threatening compromise of the airway and circulation.

OBJECTIVES

Numbered objectives are from the United States Department of Transportation 1994 EMT-Basic National Standard Curriculum. Asterisked objectives, if any, pertain to material that is supplemental to the DOT curriculum.

COGNITIVE

* List the major anatomical structures of the eye, face, and neck. (p. 691)
* Describe the relationship between eye, face, and neck injuries and the personal protection and safety of the EMT-B. (p. 693)
* List the overall assessment procedures for eye, face, and neck injuries. (p. 693)
* Describe the general assessment procedures for eye injuries, including use of the penlight. (p. 694)
* List the basic rules for emergency medical care for eye injuries. (p. 694)
* List specific common eye injuries and describe their appropriate emergency medical care. (pp. 694–698)
* Describe emergency medical care for eye-injured patients wearing contact lenses. (pp. 699, 701)
* Describe the general assessment and care guidelines for face injuries. (pp. 701–703)
* List the signs and symptoms and describe the emergency medical care for injuries to the midface, upper jaw, and lower jaw. (pp. 703–704)
* Describe the emergency medical care for an object impaled in the cheek. (p. 704)
* Describe the emergency medical care for injuries to the nose and ear. (pp. 704–705)
* List special signs or symptoms of injury to the neck. (p. 705)
* Describe the emergency medical care for injuries to the neck. (pp. 705–707)

AFFECTIVE

* Recognize and respect the feelings of a patient suffering eye, face, or neck injury. (pp. 689, 693, 698)

PSYCHOMOTOR

* Demonstrate the steps in the emergency medical care of common eye injuries.
* Demonstrate the steps in the removal of soft and hard contact lenses from eye-injured patients.
* Demonstrate the steps in the emergency medical care of various types of face, jaw, and neck injuries, including care for avulsed teeth and for severed blood vessels to the neck.

CASE STUDY

THE DISPATCH

EMS Unit 201—respond to 400 Mill Street—you have a 22-year-old male patient complaining of blindness and severe eye pain. Time out is 1345 hours.

ON ARRIVAL

As you pull into the patient's driveway, a neighbor greets you: "He's in the house!" Crossing the patient's driveway, you see battery jumper cables linking two cars together. Beneath the hood of one of the cars, you see powdery white battery acid sprayed across the engine. Once inside the patient's home, you hear someone screaming, "My eyes! My eyes! I can't see!"

How would you proceed to assess and care for this patient?

During this chapter, you will learn special considerations of assessment and emergency care for a patient suffering eye, face, and neck injuries. Later, we will return to the case and apply the procedures learned.

ANATOMY OF THE EYE, FACE, AND NECK

THE EYE

The globe of the eye, or eyeball (Figure 35-1), is a sphere approximately 1 inch in diameter. It is covered with a tough outer coat called the **sclera** (the exposed portion of the sclera is "the white of the eye"). The clear front portion of the eye, the **cornea,** covers the dark center, the **pupil,** and the colored portion, the **iris.** The cornea is the window through which light enters the eye. It is extremely sensitive and susceptible to injury. A superficial scratch or the smallest foreign object can cause extreme pain with redness and a flow of tears.

The pupil is the opening that expands or contracts to allow more or less light into the eye through the **lens,** just behind the pupil. The lens focuses light on the **retina,** or back of the eye. The inner surface of the eyelids and the exposed portion of the sclera are lined with a paper-thin covering called the **conjunctiva.** The conjunctiva does not cover the cornea.

The interior of the eye contains the **anterior chamber** (front chamber) which is filled with a watery fluid called the **aqueous humor.** Behind the lens is the large **vitreous body,** which is filled with a clear jelly called the **vitreous humor.** The bony structures of the skull that surround the eyes are called the **orbits,** or sockets.

All of the structures of the eyes, the muscles that hold the eyes in position, and the orbits of the eyes are susceptible to trauma ranging from minor abrasion and irritation to impaled objects that invade the interior of the eye to extrusions in which an eye is pulled out of its socket.

THE FACE

The bones of the face were introduced in Chapter 4, "The Human Body." The face has fourteen bones. Thirteen—including the orbits of the eyes, the nasal bones, the zygomatic bones (cheekbones), and the maxillae (fused upper jaw bones)—are immovable. One, the mandible (lower jaw), moves on hinge joints.

The face is extremely vascular (contains many blood vessels), and facial injuries, even otherwise minor ones, may bleed profusely. Blood and pieces of broken bone, teeth, and other tissues may cause airway compromise when the face is injured.

Remember that the facial bones are part of the skull and help to protect the brain. Compromise of the facial structures (Figure 35-2) can also cause a closed or an open brain injury with possible leakage of cerebrospinal fluid from the nose or ears. Also remember that a mechanism of injury that causes trauma to the face is likely, as well, to have caused injury to the spine.

THE NECK

The major blood vessels and structures of the neck were introduced in Chapter 4, "The Human Body." The neck contains the major (carotid) arteries and (jugular) veins that carry blood to and from the head. It also contains major structures of the airway, including the trachea and the larynx. Injuries to the neck (Figure 35-3) can cause life-threatening bleeding and airway compromise that can be very difficult to control. Damage to structures of the airway are, of course, serious life threats. The posterior neck contains the cervical spine, and any injury to the neck should automatically be assumed to have caused spinal injury.

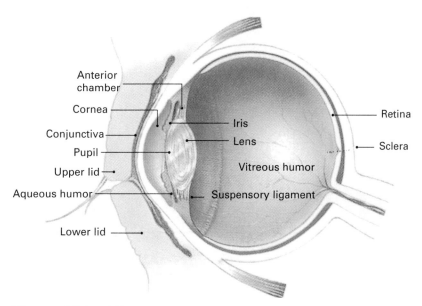

Figure 35-1   The eye.

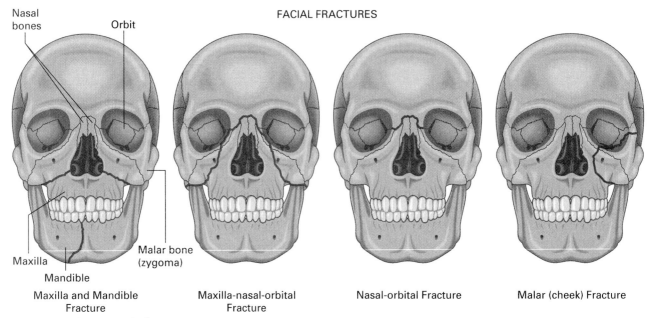

FACIAL FRACTURES

Nasal bones

Orbit

Maxilla

Mandible

Malar bone (zygoma)

Maxilla and Mandible Fracture

Maxilla-nasal-orbital Fracture

Nasal-orbital Fracture

Malar (cheek) Fracture

Figure 35-2   Facial fractures.

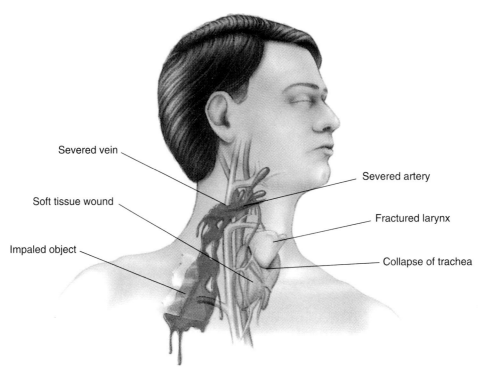

COMMON NECK AND THROAT INJURIES

Severed vein

Soft tissue wound

Impaled object

Severed artery

Fractured larynx

Collapse of trachea

Figure 35-3   Common neck and throat injuries.

EYE, FACE, AND NECK INJURIES

The eyes, face, and neck may be subject to a wide variety of injuries. However, these injuries may present you with some challenges in common:

- *Eye, face, and neck injuries can hemorrhage profusely and require that you take body substance isolation precautions.* You will need to wear disposable gloves and possibly protective eyewear, mask, and gown.
- *Many injuries to the eyes, face, and neck are the result of assault.* In addition, injuries to the neck may be caused by accidental or intentional hanging.
- *You may need to treat emotional trauma as well as physical trauma.* The responsive patient who has suffered an eye injury fears blindness. A face injury arouses fear of permanent facial disfigurement or scarring. A neck injury may cause fear of immediate lethal bleeding or choking. These patients, and their friends and family at the scene, can be emotionally distraught or panicked. You will need to display a calm and reassuring manner to gain the patient's confidence so you can begin care and treatment of the physical trauma.

ASSESSMENT AND CARE: EYE, FACE, AND NECK INJURIES

The assessment procedures and considerations described here will apply, overall, to the specific eye, face, and neck injuries described in the rest of this chapter.

SCENE SIZE-UP

Because mechanism of injury will guide your treatment, you will want to think about the forces behind the injury as soon as you get the dispatcher's call. During the scene size-up it may be difficult to gather information from the patient, because he is likely to be in a state of extreme pain and emotionally distraught. Try to determine the mechanism of injury or nature of the problem from bystanders, friends, or family. Make sure to protect your own safety and call for police back-up if the mechanism of injury involves an assault.

INITIAL ASSESSMENT

While conducting your initial assessment, keep in mind that severe trauma to the face and throat can cause altered mental status, airway compromise, and spinal injury. Establish manual in-line stabilization of the head and neck on first contact with the patient. Open the airway with a jaw-thrust maneuver and suc-

tion vomitus and other substances as needed. Consider advanced life support back-up, if available, since advanced airway procedures may be required. Provide oxygen at 15 lpm by nonrebreather mask if breathing is adequate; provide positive pressure ventilation with supplemental oxygen if breathing is inadequate. Control severe bleeding.

In making a priority decision, consider any patient with chemical burns to the eye, an impaled object in the eye, an extruded eyeball, or severe injuries to the face or throat to be a high priority for immediate transport with assessment and care continuing en route.

FOCUSED HISTORY AND PHYSICAL EXAM

For any patient who is unresponsive or with a significant mechanism of injury, begin the focused history and physical exam by conducting a rapid trauma assessment. Conduct a focused trauma assessment of the injury site if the patient is responsive or the mechanism of injury is not significant. Inspect and gently palpate for any sign of injury to the eye sockets or bones of the cheek, nose, or jaw. Check for DCAP-BTLS (deformities, contusions, abrasions, punctures/penetrations, burns, tenderness, lacerations, swelling) and check for crepitation in facial injuries. If the patient has suffered an eye injury, you will want to use a small pen light to examine the eyes. Never push directly on the eyes.

Record baseline vitals and, in patients with severe bleeding, be prepared to treat for shock. Obtain a SAMPLE history and use the OPQRST mnemonic to assess the pain. Particularly in the case of eye injuries where time could mean the difference between sight and loss of vision, make sure to ask the patient or bystanders questions regarding the events leading up to the injury.

Signs and symptoms of eye, face, and neck injuries, as well as emergency care steps, are detailed throughout this chapter within the sections on the particular injuries you will encounter.

DETAILED PHYSICAL EXAM AND ONGOING ASSESSMENT

If the patient is unresponsive or the mechanism of injury was significant—and if time and the patient's condition permit—conduct a detailed physical exam to identify any additional injuries. Conduct an ongoing assessment—repeating the initial assessment and vital signs, repeating the rapid or focused trauma assessment, and checking interventions. Monitor especially for deterioration of mental status, airway, or breathing. Conduct the ongoing assessment every 5 minutes if the patient is unstable or every 15 minutes if the patient is stable.

INJURIES TO THE EYE

While usually not life-threatening, an injury to the eye can take away the precious gift of sight. Time is a critical consideration in your treatment, particularly in cases such as chemical burns, impaled objects in the eye, or extruded eyeballs.

ASSESSMENT AND CARE GUIDELINES

When you conduct the focused history and physical exam on a patient with an eye injury, assess the eyes separately and together with a small penlight (Figure 35-4a) to evaluate:

- *The orbits* (eye sockets) for bruising, swelling, laceration, and tenderness
- *The lids* for bruising, swelling, and laceration
- *The conjunctivae* for redness, pus, and foreign bodies
- *The globe* for redness, abnormal coloring, and laceration
- *The pupils* for size, shape, equality, and reactivity to light

Additionally, ask the patient to follow your finger (Figure 35-4b) as you move it left and right, up and down, to evaluate:

- *Eye movements in all directions* for abnormal gaze, paralysis of gaze, or pain on movement

Suspect significant damage if the patient has loss of vision that does not improve when he blinks, loses part of the field of vision, has severe pain in the eye, has double vision, or is unusually sensitive to light.

Regardless of the injury, remember the following basic rules when giving emergency medical care for eye injuries:

- If the eye is swollen shut, avoid any unnecessary manipulation in examining the eye.
- Do not try to force the eyelid open unless you have to wash out chemicals.
- Consult medical direction or local protocol before irrigating. Some jurisdictions do not permit irrigating an injured eye, except in the case of a chemical burn.
- Do not put salve or medicine in an injured eye.
- Do not remove blood or blood clots from the eye. Sponge blood from the face to help keep the patient comfortable, but leave the eye alone.
- Have the patient lie down and keep quiet. Never let a patient with an eye injury walk without help, especially up or down stairs.
- Limit use of the uninjured eye. It is usually best to cover it along with the injured eye. Eyes move together, and if the patient is using the uninjured eye, chances are the injured eye is moving, too.
- Give the patient nothing by mouth in case general anesthesia is required at the hospital.
- Every patient with an eye injury must be transported for evaluation by a physician.

Foreign Object in the Eye   Foreign objects—such as particles of dirt, sand, cinders, coal dust, or fine pieces of metal—can be blown or driven into the eye

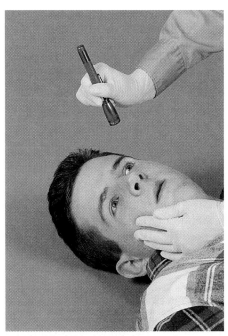

Figure 35-4a   Inspect the eyes for any abnormality.

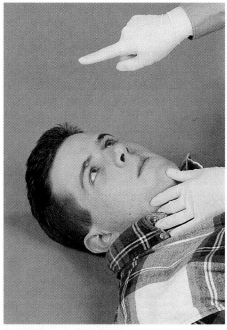

Figure 35-4b   Assess the patient's ability to move the eyes in any direction.

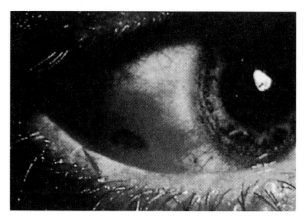

Figure 35-5   Foreign object lodged in the eye.

and lodged there (Figure 35-5). A flow of tears washes out many of these substances before any harm is done. A patient with a foreign object in the eye will complain of feeling the object, and the globe will appear red. During the SAMPLE history, determine if the patient or others made any attempt to remove the object, possibly causing abrasions to the cornea.

Generally, it is safer to transport the patient for further medical evaluation than to attempt to remove foreign particles from the eye in the field. You should attempt removal only of objects in the conjunctiva, not of those on the cornea or lodged in the globe.

If you need to remove a foreign particle from the conjunctiva, use the following techniques if permitted by medical direction or local protocol: If possible, flush the eye with clean water, holding the eyelids apart (Figure 35-6). *Remember that some EMS systems do not recommend flushing the eye except in cases of chemical burns.*

If you cannot flush the eye, the removal technique depends on where the object is located. To re-

move an object from the white of the eye, pull down the lower lid while the patient looks up or pull up the upper lid while the patient looks down. Then remove the object with a piece of sterile gauze or a swab (Figure 35-7).

If the object is under the upper lid, draw the upper lid down over the lower lid. As the upper lid returns to its normal position, the undersurfaces will be drawn over the lower lashes, removing the object. If the object remains, grasp the lashes of the upper lid and turn the lid upward over a cotton swab or similar object. Carefully remove the object with the corner of a piece of sterile gauze or a swab (Figures 35-8a to d). If the object is under the lower lid, pull down the lid and remove the object with sterile gauze or a swab.

If a foreign object becomes lodged in the eyeball, do not attempt to disturb it. Place a bandage over

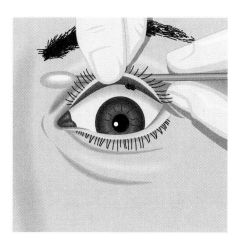

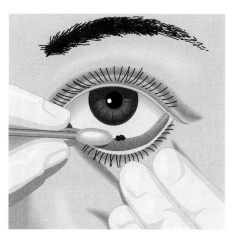

Figure 35-7   To remove particles from the white of the eye, pull down the lower lid while the patient looks up or pull up the upper lid while the patient looks down.

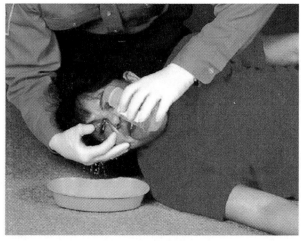

Figure 35-6   Flushing foreign particle from the eye.

REMOVAL OF FOREIGN OBJECT—UPPER EYELID

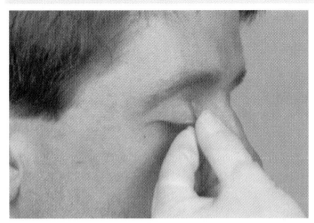

Figure 35-8a   Grasp eyelash between thumb and forefinger while patient is told to look downward.

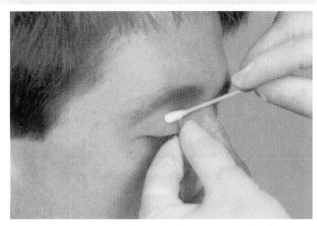

Figure 35-8b   Place applicator swab along center of upper eyelid.

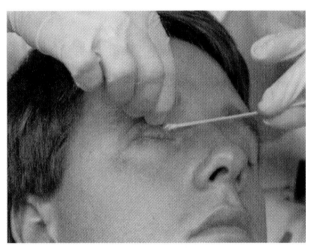

Figure 35-8c   Pull eyelid forward and upward over applicator swab.

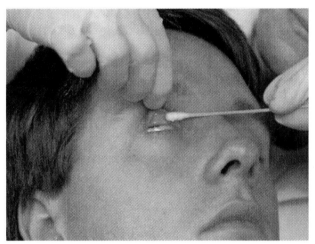

Figure 35-8d   Undersurface of eyelid is exposed and foreign object can be gently removed with a sterile, moistened applicator swab.

both eyes and transport the patient as soon as possible.

Injury to the Orbits   Trauma to the face may result in the fracture of one or several of the bones that form the orbits of the eyes (Figure 35-9). If fracture of the orbits is suspected, establish and maintain spinal immobilization. Injuries serious enough to cause orbital fractures may also cause cervical spine trauma. As you inspect and palpate for signs of injury to the orbits, remember to check for DCAP-BTLS.

The signs and symptoms of orbital fracture include the following: double vision; a marked decrease in vision; loss of sensation above the eyebrow, over the cheek, or in the upper lip; nasal discharge; tenderness to palpation; bony "step-off" (defect in

smooth contour of bone); or paralysis of upward gaze in the involved eye (the patient's eye will not be able to follow your finger upward).

Orbital fractures may require hospitalization and possible surgery. If the signs and symptoms lead you to suspect possible fracture, take the following emergency care steps: If the eyeball has not been injured, place cold packs over the injured eye to reduce swelling and transport the patient in a sitting position. If you suspect injury to the eyeball, avoid using cold packs and transport the patient in a supine position.

Lid Injury   Lid injuries include bruising (black eyes), burns, and lacerations (Figure 35-10). Because the eyelid is richly supplied with blood vessels, lacer-

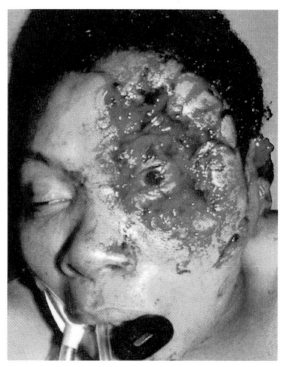

Figure 35-9   Eye orbit injury.

ations can cause profuse bleeding. Anything that lacerates the lid can also cause damage to the eyeball, so assess the injury carefully. Remember to carefully inspect the area around the lid injury for DCAP-BTLS.

To treat a lid injury: Control bleeding with light pressure from a dressing; use no pressure at all if the eyeball itself may be injured. Cover the lid with sterile gauze soaked in saline to keep the wound from drying. Preserve any avulsed skin and transport it with the patient for possible grafting. If eyeball injury is not suspected, cover the injured lid with cold compresses to reduce swelling. Cover the uninjured eye with a bandage to decrease movement, and transport.

Injury to the Globe   Injuries to the globe of the eye include bruising, lacerations, foreign objects, and abrasions. Overnight use of contact lenses (even extended-wear lenses) can cause corneal abrasions, inflammation of the conjunctiva, and corneal ulcers. Deep lacerations can cut the cornea, causing the contents of the eyeball to spill out.

Some injuries to the globe—such as lacerations or embedded objects—are immediately apparent. Other signs and symptoms of injury to the globe may include a pear- or irregular-shaped eyeball and blood in the anterior chamber of the eye. Note that a high-speed activity such as grinding can lead to penetration of the globe with minimal external signs. Globe injuries should be treated with great caution.

Injuries to the globe are best treated at the hospital. In the field: Apply patches lightly to both eyes. Do not use a patch or any kind of pressure if you suspect a ruptured eyeball, since pressure can force the eye contents to leak out. Apply an eye shield to the injured eye. Keep the patient supine, and transport.

Chemical Burn to the Eye   A chemical burn to the eye (Figure 35-11) represents a dire emergency. Permanent damage can occur within seconds, and the first 10 minutes following injury often determine the final outcome. *Remember that burning and tissue damage will continue to occur as long as any substance is left in the eye, even if that substance is diluted.* If, during your scene size-up and initial assessment, you determine the mechanism of injury is a chemical to the eye, *you must begin treatment immediately!*

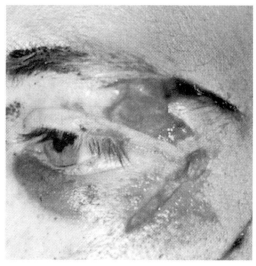

Figure 35-10   Eyelid injury.

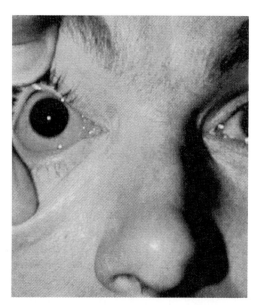

Figure 35-11   Chemical burns of the eye.

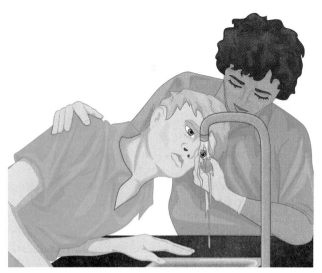

Figure 35-12   Irrigate the chemical burn to the eye with large amounts of water.

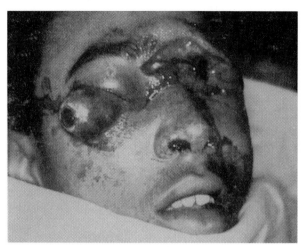

Figure 35-13   Extruded eyeball.

The signs and symptoms of chemical burns to the eye include: irritated, swollen eyelids; redness of the eye or red streaks across the surface of the eye; blurred or diminished vision; excruciating pain in the eyes; or irritated, burned skin around the eyes.

In all chemical burns of the eye, immediately upon contact with the patient begin irrigation with water or saline (Figure 35-12). It need not be sterile, but it should be clean. Hold the eyelids open so all chemicals can be washed out from behind the lids. Continuously irrigate the eye for at least 20 minutes—or if the injury involves alkali, for at least an hour—or until arrival at the hospital. Use running water or continually pour the water or saline from the inside corner, across the eyeball to the outside edge, taking care not to contaminate the uninjured eye. You may have to force the lids open, since the patient may be unable to do so because of pain. If available at the site, have the patient irrigate the eye(s) with an eye wash system. *Do not use any irrigants other than saline or water. Never irrigate the eye with any chemical antidote, including diluted vinegar, sodium bicarbonate, or alcohol.*

Contact lenses must be removed or flushed out; left in, they will trap chemicals between the contact lens and the cornea; see the section on contact lens removal later. Remove any solid particles from the surface of the eye with a moistened cotton swab. Place the patient on his side on the stretcher, with a basin or towels under his head, and continue irrigation throughout transport.

Following irrigation, avoid contaminating your own eyes by washing your hands thoroughly and using a nail brush to clean under your fingernails.

Impaled Object in the Eye or Extruded Eyeball
Impaled or embedded objects in the eye should not be removed. Field care consists of stabilizing the object to prevent accidental movement or removal until the patient receives further medical attention.

During a serious injury, the eyeball may be forced or extruded out of the socket (Figure 35-13). Never attempt to replace the eye in the socket. An impaled object in the eye or an extruded eyeball is a true emergency.

Although an impaled object in the eye or extruded eyeball should be treated with great urgency, you should not manipulate the eye during treatment. Treatment for both is the same (Figures 35-14a to d): Place the patient supine and immobilize the head. Encircle the eye and the impaled object or extruded eyeball with a gauze dressing or other suitable material, such as soft, sterile cloth. Do not apply pressure. You can cut a hole in a single bulky dressing to accommodate an impaled object. Place a metal shield, crushed paper cup, or cone over the impaled object or extruded eyeball. Do not use a Styrofoam cup, since it can crumble. The impaled object or eyeball should not touch the top or sides of the cup.

Hold the cup and dressing in place with a self-adhering bandage or roller bandage that covers both eyes. Do not wrap the bandage over the cup, which can push the cup down onto the impaled object or extruded eyeball. Make sure you bandage both eyes to prevent eye movement. If the patient is unresponsive, close the uninjured eye before bandaging to prevent drying, which can cause additional eye injury.

Give the patient nothing by mouth. Never leave the patient alone, as he might panic with both eyes covered. Transport immediately.

SUMMARY: EMERGENCY CARE— EYE INJURIES

To review possible emergency care for eye injuries, see Figure 35-15.

EMERGENCY CARE—IMPALED OBJECT IN THE EYE

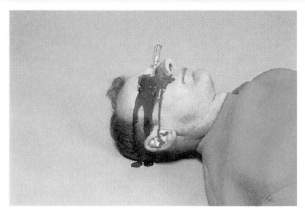

Figure 35-14a Impaled object in the eye.

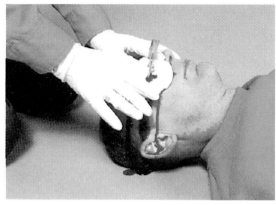

Figure 35-14b Place padding around the object.

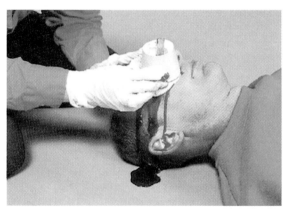

Figure 35-14c Stabilize the impaled object with a cup.

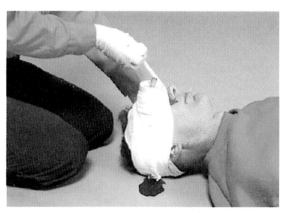

Figure 35-14d Bandage the cup in place.

REMOVING CONTACT LENSES

Eye injuries are often further complicated by the presence of contact lenses. To detect lenses, shine a penlight into the eye. A soft lens will show up as a shadow on the outer portion of the eye, while a hard lens will show up as a shadow over the iris. Some patients wear a contact lens in only one eye, so do not dismiss the possibility of contact lenses after examining only one eye. Some patients, especially the elderly, wear both contact lenses and eyeglasses, so you also can't dismiss the possibility of contact lenses just because the patient is wearing eyeglasses.

When determining whether to remove contact lenses, seek medical direction and follow local protocol. Generally, you should remove contact lenses if:

* There has been a chemical burn to the eye.
* The patient is unresponsive, is wearing hard contact lenses, and transport time will be lengthy or delayed.

Generally, you should not remove contact lenses if:

* The eyeball is injured (other than a chemical burn).
* Transport time is short enough to allow emergency department personnel to remove the lens.

Removing Soft Contact Lenses Even though they are designed for extended wear, soft contact lenses can cause damage if left in for a long time. Over time, they can also gradually dehydrate and shrink, adhering to the cornea and making removal difficult.

Soft lenses are slightly larger than a dime and cover all of the cornea and some of the sclera. One way to remove them is to place several drops of saline on the lens, then gently lift the lens off the eye by pinching the lens between your thumb and index finger.

You can also remove soft lenses with the following method (Figure 35-16):

1. With your middle fingertip on the lower lid, pull the lid down.

EMERGENCY CARE PROTOCOL

EYE INJURY

1. Consider manual in-line stabilization based on mechanism of injury. Do not release it until patient is immobilized onto backboard.
2. Establish and maintain an open airway. Insert a nasopharyngeal or oropharyngeal airway if patient is unresponsive and has no gag or cough reflex.
3. Suction secretions as necessary.
4. If breathing is inadequate, provide positive pressure ventilation with supplemental oxygen at a minimum rate of 12 ventilations/minute for an adult and 20 ventilations/minute for an infant or child.
5. If breathing is adequate, administer oxygen by nonrebreather mask at 15 lpm.
6. Control any major bleeding.
7. Place patient in a supine position.
8. Treat the specific eye injury as follows:
   Foreign Object in Eye
   If possible, transport patient for further evaluation and removal of object by emergency department staff.
   Only attempt removal of objects in the conjunctiva. Do not attempt removal of objects on or lodged in the cornea.
   To remove a foreign object from the conjunctiva:
   Flush with water.
   If not successful and under the upper lid, draw upper lid down over lower lid.
   If object remains, lift lid with cotton swab or similar object and remove with corner of sterile gauze or swab.

Orbital Injury
If eyeball has not been injured, place ice packs over injured eye.
If eyeball is injured, do not use cold packs. (Refer to management of globe injury.)

Lid Injury
Control bleeding with light pressure; do not use pressure if eyeball is injured.
Cover lid with sterile gauze soaked in saline.
Preserve avulsed skin and transport with patient.
If eyeball injury is not suspected, cover lid with cold compress.
Patch both eyes.

Injury to the Globe
Apply patches to both eyes.
Do not apply any type of pressure.
Apply an eye shield to injured eye.
Keep patient supine.

Chemical Burn to Eye
Begin irrigation with water or saline immediately and for at least 20 minutes at the scene.
Do not contaminate uninjured eye.
Force lids open if necessary to flush.
Remove contact lenses.
Remove solid particles from eye surface with moistened cotton swab.
Continue to irrigate en route to medical facility.

9. Immobilize patient to backboard if you suspect spine injury.
10. Transport.
11. Perform an ongoing assessment every 5 minutes if unstable and every 15 minutes if stable.

Figure 35-15   Emergency care protocol: eye injury.

2. Place your index fingertip on the lower edge of the lens, then slide the lens down to the sclera, or white of the eye.
3. Compress the lens gently between your thumb and index finger, allowing air to get underneath it, and remove it from the eye.
4. If the lens has dehydrated on the eye, run sterile saline across the eye surface, slide the lens off the cornea, and pinch it up to remove it.
5. Store the removed soft contact lens in water or a saline solution.

Removing Hard Contact Lenses Even though soft contact lenses are more popular, hard contact lenses are still in use. About the size of a shirt but-

ton, they fit over the cornea. To remove (Figure 35-17):

1. Separate the eyelids.
2. Position the visible lens over the cornea by manipulating the eyelids.
3. Place your thumbs gently on the top and bottom eyelids, and open the eyelids wide.
4. Gently press the eyelids down and forward to the edges of the lens.
5. Press the lower eyelid slightly harder and move it under the bottom edge of the lens.
6. Moving the eyelids toward each other, slide the lens out between them.

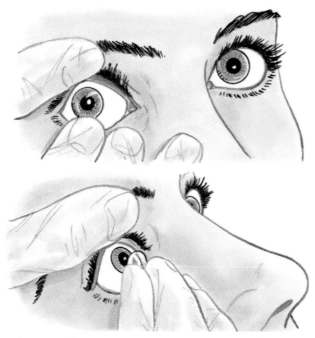

Figure 35-16   Removing soft contact lenses.

You can also use a suction cup moistened with saline to remove hard contact lenses (Figure 35-18).

 ## INJURIES TO THE FACE

The specialized structures of the face, prone to injury because of their location, can be permanently and irreversibly damaged (Figures 35-19a and b and 35-20a to d). Injuries to the face are quite common. Approximately 75 percent of all those involved in motor vehicle accidents sustain at least minor facial trauma. While some injuries to the face are minor, many such injuries are life-threatening because they compromise the upper airway. In addition, many injuries of the face stem from impacts strong enough to cause cervical spine damage or skull fracture.

ASSESSMENT AND CARE GUIDELINES

There are some special assessment considerations you should heed for injuries to the face, mouth, or jaw. During your scene size-up, it is especially important to consider the mechanism of facial injury. For example, during a head-on collision, did the patient's head strike the windshield? If so, what was the estimated speed of travel? In patients with trauma to the face, mouth, or jaw, you should suspect possible spinal cord injuries. Patients who sustain significant trauma to the face may also have fractures of the jaw and damage to or loss of teeth.

In any case of severe facial trauma, suspect cervical spine injury. Establish manual in-line stabilization of the spine on first contact with the patient and maintain it until the patient can be completely immo-

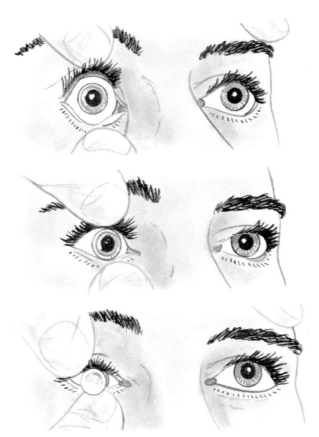

Figure 35-17   Removing hard corneal contact lenses.

bilized to a long backboard. An added benefit of cervical spine stabilization and immobilization is the stabilization of facial bones. During your initial assessment immediately manage airway, breathing, and circulation problems. Severe trauma to the face may also cause an altered mental status from possible head injury or hypoxia from airway compromise.

In patients with a significant mechanism of injury, conduct a rapid trauma assessment. Inspect and pal-

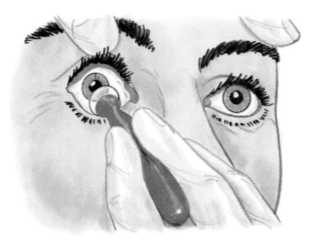

Figure 35-18   Using a moistened suction cup to remove hard contact lens.

INJURIES TO THE FACE

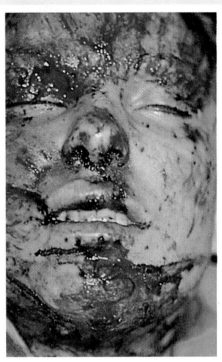

Figure 35-19a

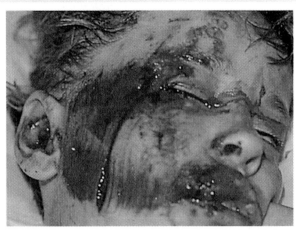

Figure 35-19b

pate for DCAP-BTLS and crepitation of the face. When the mandible (lower jaw) is fractured, it is generally broken in at least two places and will be unstable. Bruising and swelling may be obvious. Fracture of the maxilla (upper jaw) is often accompanied by a black eye. The face may appear elongated, and the patient's bite will no longer be even. Again, swelling may be noticeable.

Remember that, in the field, you do not need to diagnose whether a fracture has actually occurred. If the patient has any of the DCAP-BTLS signs or symptoms to the face, mouth, or jaw—in particular pain, swelling, deformity, crepitation, discoloration, or instability—provide emergency care as follows:

1. Establish and maintain in-line spinal stabilization.
2. In establishing and maintaining a patent airway, do not use airway adjuncts, which can force debris further down the throat and aggravate existing injuries. Instead, do the following:
   - Inspect the mouth for small fragments of teeth or broken dentures, bits of bone, pieces of flesh, or foreign objects (such as pieces of broken glass). Pick them from the mouth or remove them with finger sweeps as thoroughly as possible.
   - If dentures are in the mouth and are secure and unbroken, leave them in place; they can

help support the structures of the mouth. If dentures are broken or loose, remove them. Transport any dentures or pieces of dentures with the patient so the surgeon can use them to establish proper alignment when wiring the jaw.
   - In facial injury, the tongue may lose its support structure and may fall back, occluding the airway. Open the airway using a jaw-thrust maneuver and, if necessary, grasp the tongue to pull it forward.
   - Suction any blood, vomitus, secretions, or small debris from the mouth and throat throughout treatment and transport.
   - *Request advanced life support back-up, if needed and available, to provide advanced airway management.*
3. Provide oxygen by nonrebreather mask at 15 lpm or, if breathing is inadequate, begin positive pressure ventilation with supplemental oxygen.
4. Control severe bleeding. Several major arteries run through the face, and they can bleed profusely and rapidly enough to cause death. Use direct pressure and pressure dressings. Apply pressure gently if you suspect that bones under the wound may be fractured or shattered.
5. If nerves, tendons, or blood vessels have been exposed, cover them with a moist, sterile dressing.
6. If a tooth has been lost, try to find it. The tooth may be reimplanted. To treat for an avulsed tooth:

INJURIES TO THE MOUTH, JAW, CHEEK, AND CHIN

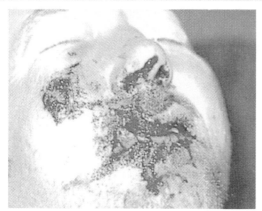

Figure 35-20a   Injuries to the mouth, jaw, cheek, and chin.

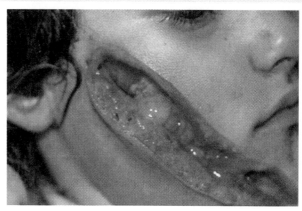

Figure 35-20b   Injuries to the jaw, cheek, and chin.

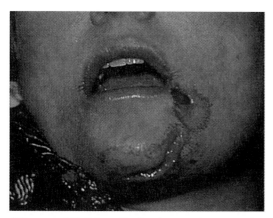

Figure 35-20c   Injuries to the mouth, cheek, and chin.

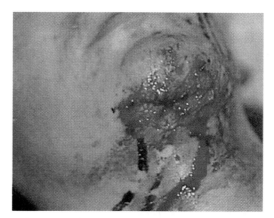

Figure 35-20d   Injuries to the chin.

- Rinse the tooth with saline to gently remove any debris; never scrub the tooth. Transport the tooth in a cup of saline or wrapped in gauze soaked in sterile saline. *Seek medical direction and follow local protocol.* Never wrap the tooth in dry gauze, and guard against the tooth drying out.
- Never handle the tooth by the root; there may still be ligament fibers attached that could enable successful reimplantation.
- If you cannot find teeth that have been knocked out, assume that the patient has swallowed or aspirated them.
- Control bleeding from the tooth socket with a gauze pad.
7. Treat for shock and transport.

Injury to the Mid-Face, Upper Jaw, or Lower Jaw
Mid face and jaw injuries (Figure 35-21) may be simple, such as undisplaced nasal fractures, or extensive, involving severe lacerations, bony fractures, and nerve damage. Such injuries can result from a blunt instrument, a blow from the fist, an automobile accident, or a gunshot.

Signs and symptoms of fracture or other severe trauma to the mid-face, upper jaw, and lower jaw include:

- Numbness or pain
- Distortion of facial features
- Crepitation
- Irregularities in the facial bones that can be felt before swelling occurs
- Severe bruising and swelling; black eyes
- Distance between the eyes too wide or eyes unlevel
- Bleeding from the nose and mouth
- Double vision (when the orbit is fractured)
- Limited jaw motion
- Movement of the maxilla
- Teeth not meeting normally
- Hematoma (collection of blood) under the tongue
- Limited jaw motion

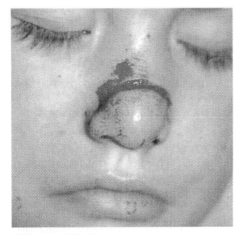

Figure 35-21 Soft tissue and bone injury to the mandible.

- Mouth open or patient unable to open the mouth
- Saliva mixed with blood flowing from the mouth
- Drooling (pain prevents the patient from swallowing)
- Painful or difficult speech
- Missing, loosened, or uneven teeth (even if teeth are not missing, the patient may complain that teeth do not "fit together right")
- Pain around the ears

As emphasized earlier, as an EMT-B you do not need to diagnose whether a facial fracture has actually occurred. If there is a significant mechanism of injury and any of the signs and symptoms listed above, treat as if a fracture has occurred. Your first priorities are establishing and maintaining a patent airway, supporting breathing as necessary, and controlling life-threatening bleeding. Remember to request advanced life support back-up if needed and available, because patients with severe facial trauma may require advanced airway procedures. Also assess for spine injury, skull and/or brain injury, eye injury, and facial burns, which are commonly associated with facial injury.

Object Impaled in the Cheek If the patient has a foreign object impaled in the cheek, stabilize it with bulky dressings and transport the patient. If the object has penetrated all the way through the cheek and is loose—so that it may fall into the mouth, obstructing the airway—you need to remove it.

To remove an impaled object from the cheek:

1. Pull or push the object out of the cheek in the same direction in which it entered the cheek.
2. Pack dressing material between the patient's teeth and the wound. Leave some of the dressing outside the mouth and tape it there to prevent the patient from swallowing the dressing. Monitor closely to make sure the dressing doesn't become loose and compromise the airway.
3. Dress and bandage the outside of the wound to control bleeding.
4. Consider requesting ALS back-up if advanced airway procedures may be needed.
5. Suction the mouth and throat frequently throughout transport.

Injury to the Nose Soft tissue injuries to the nose should be assessed and cared for as you would other soft tissue injuries (Figures 35-22a and b). Take special care to maintain an open airway, and position the patient so that blood does not drain into the throat. Nosebleeds are a relatively common reason for emergency calls. For information on the emergency medical care of nosebleeds, see Chapter 29, "Bleeding and Shock." Never pack the injured nose; clear or bloody fluids can indicate a skull fracture, and packing the nose can create dangerous pressure.

INJURIES TO THE NOSE

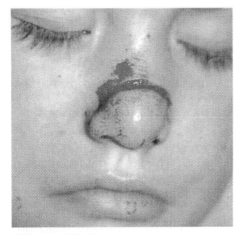

Figure 35-22a

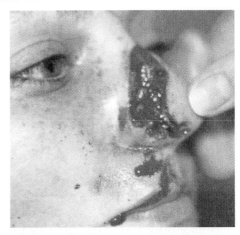

Figure 35-22b

Foreign objects in the nose usually occur among small children. To treat, reassure and calm the child and parent, then transport the patient. Do not try to remove the object.

Nasal fractures are the most common type of facial fracture because of the delicate structure of the nose. The most common signs and symptoms are swelling and deformity. To treat, apply cold compresses to reduce swelling, then transport.

Injury to the Ear   Cuts and lacerations of the ear are common (Figures 35-23a and b). Occasionally, a section of the ear may be severed. Assess and treat as for other soft tissue injuries. Save any avulsed parts; wrap avulsed parts in saline-soaked gauze, and transport with the patient. When dressing an injured ear, place part of the dressing between the ear and the side of the head. As a general rule, don't probe into the ear. Never pack the ear to stop bleeding from the ear canal. Clear or bloody fluid draining from the ear can indicate a skull fracture. Place a loose, clean dressing across the opening of the ear to absorb blood and fluids, but do not exert pressure to stop the bleeding.

Foreign objects in the external ear are a common problem among children. Do not attempt to remove the object. Instead, reassure the patient and parent and transport the patient to the hospital.

SUMMARY: EMERGENCY CARE— FACIAL INJURIES

To review possible emergency care for facial injuries, see Figure 35-24.

INJURIES TO THE NECK

The neck can be injured by any blunt or penetrating trauma (Figures 35-25a and b). Common causes include hanging (accidental or intentional), impact with a steering wheel, knife wounds, gunshot wounds, or running or riding into a stretched wire or clothesline. In cases of accidental or intentional hanging, call law enforcement. If the neck is lacerated, bleeding from a major artery or vein can occur. Air bubbles may enter a lacerated vein. Other common consequences of neck injuries are a fractured larynx and a collapsed trachea. And finally, do not overlook the possibility of a cervical spine injury.

Besides obvious lacerations or other wounds, signs and symptoms of an injured neck include:

- Obvious swelling or bruising
- Difficulty speaking
- Loss of the voice
- Airway obstruction that is not obviously due to other sources (such obstruction may be caused by swelling of the throat)
- Crepitation heard during speaking or breathing as air escapes from an injured larynx
- Displacement of the trachea to one side (also a sign of possible chest injury)

Maintaining an airway is extremely important in neck injuries, because—in addition to swelling or presence of crushing of airway structures or debris such as bone fragments—blood will clot when it is exposed to air and can threaten the airway. Also maintain a high index of suspicion for possible cervical spine injury.

To treat a neck injury, use proper BSI precautions, establish and maintain in-line spinal stabilization, establish a patent airway, provide high flow oxygen or positive pressure ventilation with supplemental oxygen as necessary, control severe bleeding, treat for shock, and transport. Consider requesting ALS backup if advanced airway management is needed.

If one of the major blood vessels of the neck is severed, follow the guidelines for care that were outlined in Chapter 30, "Soft Tissue Injuries," and are

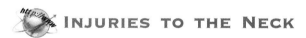

INJURIES TO THE EAR

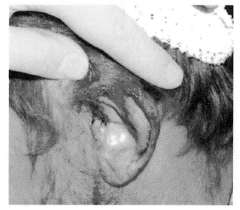

Figure 35-23a

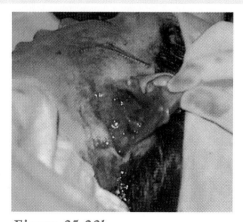

Figure 35-23b

FACIAL INJURY

1. Establish manual in-line stabilization. Do not release it until patient is immobilized onto backboard.
2. Establish and maintain an open airway. Avoid using a nasopharyngeal airway if there is midface or nasal trauma; avoid using an oropharyngeal airway if there is trauma to the oral cavity.
3. Suction blood and secretions as necessary. Remove any broken teeth or loose bone fragments from the mouth.
4. If dentures are in the mouth and secure, leave them in place. If the dentures are loose, remove them.
5. If breathing is inadequate, provide positive pressure ventilation with supplemental oxygen at a minimum rate of 12 ventilations/minute for an adult and 20 ventilations/minute for an infant or child.
6. If breathing is adequate, administer oxygen by nonrebreather mask at 15 lpm.
7. Control any major bleeding.
8. Apply a moist sterile dressing to any exposed nerves, tendons, or blood vessels.
9. Treat specific injuries as follows:
   Avulsed Tooth
   Rinse with saline; do not scrub or handle tooth by the root.
   Place in cup with sterile saline or wrap in gauze soaked in sterile saline.
   Do not wrap in dry gauze.
   Control the bleeding from the tooth socket with a gauze pad. Make sure that the pad does not work loose and become an airway obstruction.

Foreign Object in the Cheek
If object did not penetrate completely through the cheek or is not loose, use bulky dressings to stabilize object in place.
If object penetrated through to other side of cheek and is loose, do the following:
Push or pull object out of cheek in same direction it entered.
Pack with dressings between teeth and wound; make sure dressings do not work loose and become an airway obstruction.
Dress and bandage outside of wound.
Suction blood as necessary.
Injury to Nose
Manage as a soft tissue injury.
Position patient to allow blood to drain.
Do not pack the nose.
Transport if foreign body is in nose.
Apply cold compresses if nose fracture is suspected.
Injury to Ear
Manage as a soft tissue injury.
Save avulsed parts; wrap in saline-soaked gauze and transport with patient.
Place part of dressing between ear and side of head.
Do not probe into ear.
Do not pack the ear.
Place a loose dressing over ear to absorb blood and fluid; do not apply pressure.
Do not attempt to remove foreign objects in ear.
10. Immobilize patient to backboard if you suspect spine injury.
11. Transport.
12. Perform an ongoing assessment every 5 minutes if unstable and every 15 minutes if stable.

Figure 35-24   Emergency care protocol: facial injury.

INJURIES TO THE NECK

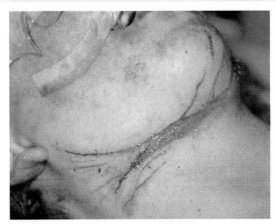

Figure 35-25a

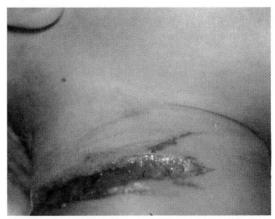

Figure 35-25b

summarized in Figures 35-26a to d. When treating bleeding wounds to the neck, never probe open wounds or use circumferential bandages, which can interfere with blood flow to the brain on the uninjured side of the neck and can also impair respiration.

SUMMARY: EMERGENCY CARE— NECK INJURIES

To review possible emergency care for neck injuries, see Figure 35-27.

EMERGENCY CARE—SEVERED BLOOD VESSEL OF THE NECK

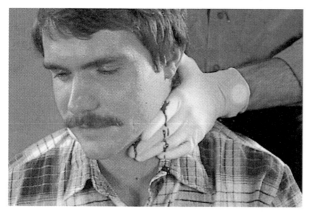

Figure 35-26a   Place a gloved hand over the wound to control bleeding. Apply pressure to the carotid artery only if necessary to control bleeding. Never apply pressure to both sides of the neck at the same time.

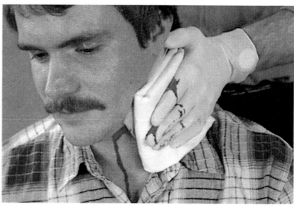

Figure 35-26b   Apply an occlusive dressing, which should extend beyond all edges of the wound to avoid being sucked into the wound. Cover the occlusive dressing with a regular dressing. Apply only enough pressure to control the bleeding.

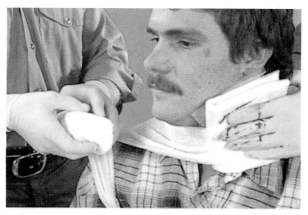

Figure 35-26c   Once bleeding is controlled, apply a pressure dressing. A figure-eight wrap of bandage over the dressing, across one shoulder, across the back, under the opposite armpit, and anchored at the shoulder.

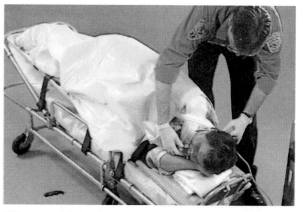

Figure 35-26d   If spinal injury is not suspected, position the patient on his left side, head tilted downward. (If spinal injury is suspected and patient is immobilized to a spine board, board and patient can be turned and tilted as a unit.) Continue administration of oxygen. Care for shock, and transport.

EMERGENCY CARE PROTOCOL

NECK INJURY

1. Establish manual in-line stabilization. Do not release it until patient is immobilized onto backboard.
2. Control any major bleeding from the neck by applying direct pressure.
3. Establish and maintain an open airway. Avoid using a nasopharyngeal airway if there is midface or nasal trauma; avoid using an oropharyngeal airway if there is trauma to the oral cavity.
4. Suction secretions as necessary.
5. If breathing is inadequate, provide positive pressure ventilation with supplemental oxygen at a minimum rate of 12 ventilations/minute for an adult and 20 ventilations/minute for an infant or child.
6. If breathing is adequate, administer oxygen by nonrebreather mask at 15 lpm.
7. Apply a nonporous dressing taped on four sides.
8. Immobilize patient to backboard if you suspect spine injury.
9. Transport.
10. Perform an ongoing assessment every 5 minutes if unstable and every 15 minutes if stable.

Figure 35-27   Emergency care protocol: neck injury.

CASE STUDY FOLLOW-UP

SCENE SIZE-UP

You and your partner have been dispatched to a 22-year-old male patient complaining of blindness and severe eye pain. As you approach the patient's driveway, you see no safety hazards. Walking past two vehicles with jumper cables, you begin to think the mechanism of injury might be an exploding car battery. The sight of white battery acid sprayed across the car hood and a brief talk with a neighbor confirm your suspicion. The neighbor tells you the patient was smoking a cigarette over the car battery when there was a big explosion.

Once inside the patient's house you find him running around the living room with a wet towel wrapped around his face. You try to calm him. He tells you his name is Hector Fernandez. He says he can't see, and it hurts "really bad!"

INITIAL ASSESSMENT

Since he is talking to you and answers questions appropriately, you determine that Hector's airway, breathing, and mental status are adequate. He denies breathing difficulty but tells you both eyes are extremely painful. Your general impression is that Hector seems alert and oriented, but he needs eye care immediately or he'll be in danger of losing his sight.

Quickly you walk the patient into the kitchen. You ask if he is wearing contact lenses. He says "no." You direct the patient to lean over the sink. Next you turn on the faucet and direct Hector to lean under it. You have him turn his head from side to side so that the water runs from the medial to the lateral side of each eye in turn.

FOCUSED HISTORY AND PHYSICAL EXAM

You are unable to conduct an exam of Hector's eyes while he is irrigating them at the kitchen sink, but your partner is able to take Hector's baseline vitals. He reports Hector's pulse at 120, his blood pressure 140/80. His skin is warm and dry. His respirations are regular at 24 per minute. Meanwhile, you are able to gather a SAMPLE history from Hector who replies to your questions while continuing to keep his eyes under the running water. He describes the pain to his eyes as "about 7 or 8" on a scale of 1 to 10. He reports no known allergies and is not taking any medications or seeing a doctor for any medical problems. His last oral intake was lunch about an hour ago. Events leading to the present problem were, as described by the neighbor, an explosion of battery acid while he was working on his car.

While you are busy treating Hector's eyes, your partner conducts a rapid trauma assessment to see if there were further injuries from the battery explosion. He feels for DCAP-BTLS and does not find any further trauma.

After 20 minutes of irrigation, Hector's pain decreases. He says, "I can see, now—some." You place Hector on his side on the stretcher with a basin under his head. You continue irrigation with your ambulance's bottled water and transport.

ONGOING ASSESSMENT

You perform an ongoing assessment. Hector's vital signs are stable, and you reassess his eyesight to find that it continues to improve. Once at the hospital, you transfer Hector to the care of emergency department personnel, provide an oral report, complete your prehospital care report, and prepare the ambulance for return to service.

CHAPTER REVIEW

TERMS AND CONCEPTS

You may wish to review the following terms and concepts included in this chapter.

anterior chamber—the front chamber of the eye containing the aqueous humor.
aqueous humor—the watery fluid that fills the anterior chamber of the eye.
conjunctiva—the thin covering of the inner eyelids and exposed portion of the sclera of the eye.
cornea—the clear front portion of the eye that covers the pupil and the iris.
iris—the colored portion of the eye that surrounds the pupil.
lens—the portion of the eye behind the pupil that focuses light on the retina.

orbits—the bony structures that surround the eyes; the eye sockets.
pupil—the dark center of the eye; the opening that expands or contracts to allow more or less light into the eye.
retina—the back of the eye.
sclera—the outer coating of the eye; the exposed portion is "the white of the eye."
vitreous body—the large chamber of the eye, containing the vitreous humor.
vitreous humor—the clear jelly that fills the large chamber of the eye.

REVIEW QUESTIONS

1. Describe the emergency care that may need to be undertaken during initial assessment of eye, face, or neck injuries.
2. Explain why, during initial assessment, you should consider requesting advanced life support back-up for injuries to the eyes, face, or neck.
3. Describe how to conduct the physical exam of a patient with an eye injury.
4. List the basic rules of emergency care for eye injuries.
5. Describe the emergency care steps for a patient with a foreign object (a) located on the white of the eye; (b) located under the upper eyelid; and (c) lodged in the eyeball.
6. Describe the emergency care steps for a patient with a chemical burn to the eye.
7. List the reasons for removing, and the reasons for not removing, contact lenses from a patient with an eye injury.
8. List the general emergency medical care guidelines for injuries to the face, mouth, and jaw.
9. Describe the care for a foreign object in the nose or ear.
10. In addition to obvious lacerations or wounds, list the signs and symptoms of neck injury.

CHAPTER 36

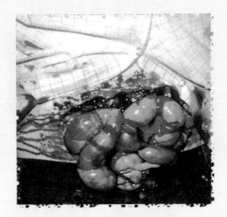

Chest, Abdomen, and Genitalia Injuries

INTRODUCTION

Most injuries to the chest or abdomen are not characterized by large, gaping wounds. Unlike some injuries to the extremities, they rarely involve bones protruding through the skin. Injuries to the chest and abdomen, in fact, are often not very dramatic in appearance and can be easily overlooked in the physical assessment. The patient may actually be complaining of much more pain from injuries to bones and joints or from surface lacerations and abrasions. Initially, the patient may not even realize that he has a serious injury to the chest or abdomen.

It is important to understand, however, that the chest and abdomen contain vital organs and that injuries to the chest and abdomen are often lethal. Chest injuries can cause a disturbance in respiration, oxygen exchange, and circulation. Abdominal injuries may produce severe internal bleeding and shock (hypoperfusion). Rely on the mechanism of injury, a high index of suspicion, and careful physical examination to determine and then care for life-threatening injuries to the chest and abdomen.

OBJECTIVES

Numbered objectives are from the United States Department of Transportation 1994 EMT-Basic National Standard Curriculum. Asterisked objectives, if any, pertain to material that is supplemental to the DOT curriculum.

COGNITIVE

5-2.8 Discuss the emergency medical care considerations for a patient with a penetrating chest injury. (pp. 717–719)

5-2.9 State the emergency medical care considerations for a patient with an open wound to the abdomen. (pp. 726–727)

5-2.10 Differentiate the care of an open wound to the chest from an open wound to the abdomen. (pp. 717–719, 726–727)

* Review the anatomy of the chest cavity as it pertains to chest injuries. (pp. 712–714)
* Identify signs and symptoms of possible life-threatening chest injuries. (pp. 716–717)

* Describe emergency medical care for life-threatening chest injuries. (pp. 718–719)
* Review the anatomy of the abdomen. (pp. 722, 724)
* Recognize the common signs and symptoms of abdominal injuries. (pp. 725–726)
* Describe the emergency medical care for a suspected abdominal injury. (pp. 726–727)
* Describe the emergency medical care for genitalia injuries. (pp. 727, 729)

PSYCHOMOTOR

5-2.31 Demonstrate the steps in the emergency medical care of a patient with an open chest wound.

5-2.32 Demonstrate the steps in the emergency medical care of a patient with open abdominal wounds.

The numbered objectives are also addressed in Chapter 30, "Soft Tissue Injuries."

CASE STUDY

THE DISPATCH

EMS Unit 106—respond to the corner of Market Street and Breaden Avenue—you have a man down with an unknown problem—be advised that this was called in by a person driving by. Time out is 2206 hours.

ON ARRIVAL

As you and your partner are turning the corner onto Market Street, you note what appears to be a man lying in a prone position on the sidewalk. You pull up to the scene and turn on the driver-side scene lights. You look for any other people or activity. It is a cold

night and the patient is dressed in a heavy overcoat. You can hear him moaning as you step out of the ambulance. As you approach the patient, you indicate "Sir, we are emergency medical technicians, and we are here to help you. Can you tell me if you are hurt or ill?" The patient responds with a moan.

How would you proceed to assess and care for this patient?

During this chapter, you will learn about assessment and emergency medical care for patients suffering from chest, abdomen, and genitalia injuries. Later, we will return to the case study and put in context some of the information you learned.

THE CHEST

ANATOMY OF THE CHEST

Before reading this section on chest injuries, it may be helpful for you to review Chapter 4 "The Human Body," for descriptions of the structures and organs of the chest, as well as the anatomy and physiology of the circulatory and respiratory systems.

To recap briefly, the chest cavity is also known as the *thoracic cavity* (Figure 36-1). It is a cavity surrounded by the ribs, which form a bony cage around the organs of the respiratory and circulatory systems. The thoracic cavity is bordered inferiorly by the *diaphragm*, which separates it from the abdominal cavity. A hollow area, the *mediastinum,* is located in the middle of the thoracic cavity between the right and left lungs. The mediastinum houses the trachea (conduit to the lungs), the *venae cavae* (the two great veins that collect blood from the upper and lower body and return it to the heart), the *aorta* (the great artery carrying blood from the heart to the body), the *esophagus* (the tubelike structure that connects the pharynx with the stomach), and the *heart.*

With this collection of vital organs, it is easy to see why injury to the chest can be life threatening.

 CHEST INJURIES

There are two general categories of chest injuries: open and closed. Closed injuries to the chest are the result of blunt trauma applied to the chest cavity,

CHEST CAVITY

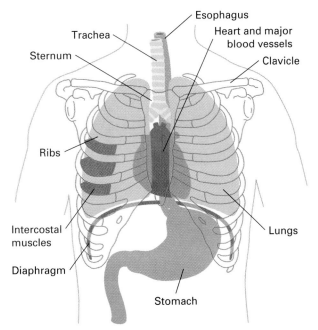

Figure 36-1 The chest cavity.

which can cause extensive damage to the ribs and internal organs. Blunt trauma is often associated with falls, automobile crashes, and blows to the chest.

An open chest injury is the result of a penetrating chest wound caused by a knife, gunshot, or a wide variety of other objects such as ice picks, screwdrivers, letter openers, broken glass, nails, and car keys. A knife or similar object damages the tissues and organs along the path of penetration. A bullet, however, can make a tiny entrance wound to the chest in one area, ricochet around, and cause extensive internal damage throughout the chest cavity, and may create a second, or exit wound, that is typically larger than the entrance wound if the bullet leaves the body. A bullet, because of its velocity, also causes cavitation—a hollowing-out of tissues along the path of the bullet that is much greater in diameter than the bullet itself.

The heart is a special type of contractile muscle. It can be injured by both penetrating and blunt trauma: a knife or bullet, a fractured rib that slices into the heart or lung, or even the simple transmission of kinetic energy from a blow to the chest or impact with a steering wheel. Injury to the heart can lead to ineffective pumping or to severe blood loss.

The major vessels in the chest carry large amounts of blood, some at very high pressures, and if injured can result in immediate death.

The organs and structures responsible for breathing are also contained in the chest. Inhalation occurs when the muscles between the ribs, the *intercostal muscles,* pull the ribs upward to increase the size of the rib cage. Also, the diaphragm contracts and moves slightly downward and flares the bottom portion of the ribs outward. This expands the space in the thoracic cavity, thus generating negative pressure, or a vacuum, which causes the lungs to inflate and "pull in" air from the atmosphere. (Any gas will flow from a higher pressure to a lower pressure area. When the thoracic cavity expands and the lungs inflate, the pressure inside the lungs is lower than in the atmosphere and, as a consequence, atmospheric air flows into the airway and lungs. The reverse happens during exhalation when the intercostal muscles and diaphragm relax, the thoracic cavity gets smaller, and the pressure in the lungs becomes higher than in the atmosphere, so that air flows out of the lungs.)

It is easy to see that the ability of the lungs to inflate will be seriously impeded when there is an open chest wound—when the chest wall is penetrated and air flows into the thoracic cavity around the lungs. (Air in the chest cavity is called a **pneumothorax** (Figure 36-16), from *pneumo,* meaning "air," and *thorax,* meaning "chest.") Pneumothorax can also be caused even when there is no open wound to the chest: For example, a fractured rib can penetrate a lung, causing air to flow from the lung into the surrounding chest cavity, collapsing the lung.

An open chest wound can pull air into the thoracic cavity, sometimes with a noticeable sucking sound. This is referred to as a **sucking chest wound.** There are two problems in managing an open or sucking chest wound. One is preventing additional air from being sucked into the chest cavity, and the other is avoiding trapping the air that is already in the chest cavity. Air trapped in the chest cavity can expand and build up enough pressure not only to collapse the lung on the injured side but also eventually to collapse the lung on the uninjured side and to compress the large vessels and the heart. This is a truly life-threatening condition called a **tension pneumothorax** (Figure 36-16).

Cover a sucking chest wound with your gloved hand on first identifying it, then tape it on three sides. This will prevent both pulling in additional air and trapping air that is already in the cavity. (A tension pneumothorax that is caused by air leaking into the chest cavity from a damaged lung with *no* opening through the outer chest wall cannot be managed by EMT-Bs in the prehospital setting. Rapid transport is especially critical in this situation.)

Another life-threatening chest injury is a (usually) closed injury that occurs when two or more adjacent ribs are broken in two or more places. This creates a segment that is completely unattached to the rest of the rib cage, an injury known as a **flail segment** (Figure 36-2). Because it is unattached, a flail segment will "flail around" on its own, actually moving in the opposite direction to the rest of the rib cage during respiration. When the rib cage moves outward on inhalation, the flail segment will move inward. When the rib cage moves inward on exhalation, the flail segment will move outward. This contrary movement of the flail segment is called **paradoxical movement**

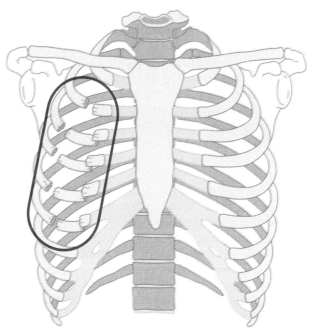

Figure 36-2   Flail segment occurs when blunt trauma causes fracture of two or more ribs, each in two or more places.

(Figure 36-3). Paradoxical movement may not always be seen because of shallow breathing in response to the rib injury. A large unstable flail segment is life-threatening because it interferes with proper expansion of the chest cavity, causing intrathoracic pressure changes and severe respiratory distress or inadequate respiration and rapid patient deterioration.

Later in this chapter we will discuss how to identify a flail segment early (it is often more easily felt than seen and therefore can be overlooked during initial assessment, a dangerous problem since it is a life-

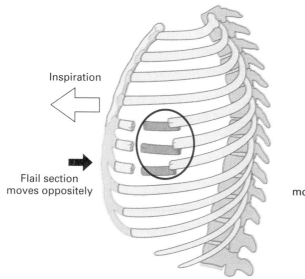

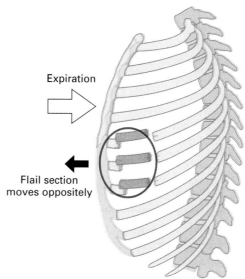

Inspiration

Flail section moves oppositely

Expiration

Flail section moves oppositely

Figure 36-3   Paradoxical movement.

threatening injury). We will also discuss how to stabilize a flail segment with your hand, then splint it.

Remember that a patient who has suffered a chest injury may appear relatively well at first, but can deteriorate suddenly and rapidly. The patient may not complain about a chest injury. In fact, the patient's chief complaint related to the chest may only be shortness of breath. It is your responsibility to suspect a potential chest injury based on mechanism of injury and a high index of suspicion, to adequately assess the patient, and to provide the necessary emergency medical care.

An open (sucking) chest wound and paradoxical movement (flail segment) are the two immediately life-threatening chest injuries that require management in the prehospital setting. Because they are life-threatening, they must be managed immediately upon identification. Other injuries to the internal organs and structures of the chest cannot be directly treated in the field. Early recognition and rapid transport will be critical.

ASSESSMENT AND CARE: CHEST INJURIES

SCENE SIZE-UP

Conducting a scene size-up to ensure your safety and that of your partner is especially important when the chest injury was a result of violence with a knife or gun. When you arrive on the scene, a threat to your safety may still exist. *Do not enter the scene of a shooting or stabbing until the police secure it and tell you it is safe to enter.* Also remember to take all BSI precautions. Since bleeding is often found with both blunt and penetrating injuries, it is necessary to be wearing gloves and eye protection before entering the scene.

While the scene is being cleared of safety hazards, concentrate on the mechanism of injury. Ask bystanders to tell you what happened. Scan the scene. Blunt trauma commonly occurs in sports accidents, falls, blows to the chest during fights, and most commonly automobile crashes. Penetrating trauma most often is associated with violence.

As you consider the mechanism of injury, it is important to look for and note the following:

- *Was the patient involved in a sports accident?* Did the patient take a direct blow to the chest? A direct blow to the anterior chest by a football helmet, a line-drive baseball, a hockey puck, an elbow during a rebound in basketball, or other similar mechanisms can produce serious injury.
- *Did the patient fall?* How far did the patient fall? How did he land? What did he hit on the way down? In what position was he found? What caused him to fall? What did he land on?

- *Was there a fight?* Was the patient punched or kicked in the chest? Were any weapons involved in the fight, such as a knife, gun, club, rocks, bottles? Is there a bloody object found at the scene that could have penetrated the chest? Did the patient feel a sting or hear a pop and suddenly become short of breath?
- *Is there any evidence that a shooting took place?* Were gunshots heard? Are there spent shell casings on the ground? Did dispatch indicate that this was a shooting?
- *Was the patient involved in an auto collision?* How fast was the car traveling? Where is the impact to the vehicle (and therefore to the patient)? Is the steering wheel bent, broken, or damaged? Is there damage to the dashboard on the passenger side? Is there an impact mark to the windshield indicating the patient was violently thrown forward? Was the patient wearing a seat belt? Were both the shoulder and lap belts worn properly? Did the airbag deploy? Is there any protruding metal or object in the vehicle that may have penetrated the chest?
- *Was the patient crushed between two objects?* Was the patient possibly run over by a heavy object?
- *Was an explosion involved?* Blast injuries can cause blunt injury from the blast wave and penetrating injury from flying debris that become penetrating objects.

INITIAL ASSESSMENT

As soon as you have determined that the scene is safe, proceed with the initial assessment. If there is a significant mechanism of injury and a high index of suspicion for blunt trauma to the chest, establish and maintain in-line spinal stabilization. (A blow to the chest can be forceful enough to cause spine injury.) Form a general impression of the patient: Is the patient severely cyanotic? Does he appear to be in extreme respiratory distress? Is he breathing shallowly and rapidly? Is he holding his arms tightly against his chest to splint the movement? Does he appear to be in extreme pain? Are there any open wounds to the chest? Is the chest moving unevenly when he breathes?

Clothing can disguise a life-threatening sucking wound or flail segment. If the mechanism of injury indicates possible chest injury or the patient shows any signs of respiratory distress, *quickly expose the chest and examine it.* If you note an open wound to the anterior, lateral, or posterior chest, *immediately* seal it with a gloved hand. If there is paradoxical movement, *immediately* place a gloved hand over the flail segment to splint it in an inward position.

Continue with the initial assessment and determine the patient's mental status. An altered mental status or unresponsiveness may be an indication of severe hypoxia (oxygen deficiency) resulting from a significant chest injury. Visually inspect the airway in the patient with an altered mental status. Look for blood or other potential obstructions. Also, listen and feel for air movement. Because spinal injury should be suspected if the chest injury is due to blunt trauma, perform the jaw-thrust maneuver to open the airway if necessary.

Note the patient's speech pattern. Does the patient speak a few words and then gasp for a breath? This would indicate severe respiratory distress. Many chest injuries produce ineffective ventilation. In some cases where the chest wall is injured and the ribs fractured, the pain is so severe that the patient purposely will breathe with extremely shallow, fast breaths in an attempt to reduce the pain. This can easily lead to hypoxia from inadequate breathing.

Carefully assess the breathing status. If breathing is adequate, administer oxygen with a nonrebreather mask at 15 lpm. If breathing is inadequate, positive pressure ventilation with supplemental oxygen should be initiated immediately (Figure 36-4).

If a tension pneumothorax exists, it will be increasingly difficult to ventilate the patient. (Expanding pressure in the chest cavity makes it increasingly difficult to inflate the lungs.) The pulses may be weak and fast if the injury is associated with bleeding in the chest or compression of the heart. Cyanosis would be an indicator of poor oxygenation and ventilation. Pale skin may indicate blood loss or poor pumping function of the heart. The skin may be moist and cool to the touch.

All of these are indications of chest injury. The patient with a chest injury is considered a high priority because of the possibility of rapid deterioration, ineffective ventilation, and poor oxygenation. Immediate transport, with assessment and care continuing en route, must be considered.

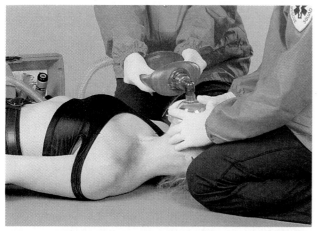

Figure 36-4   Provide positive pressure ventilation with supplemental oxygen if breathing is inadequate.

Note: If you suspect that the patient has been shot or stabbed, the patient complains of breathing difficulty, or the breathing rate or depth appears to be abnormal, it is vital that the patient is log rolled to assess the posterior body for another potentially life-threatening open (entrance or exit) wound.

FOCUSED HISTORY AND PHYSICAL EXAM

To perform the focused history and physical exam, begin with a rapid trauma assessment. It is very likely that other injuries exist, especially if the mechanism of injury suggests blunt trauma. Inspect and palpate for deformities, contusions, abrasions, punctures/penetrations, burns, tenderness, lacerations, and swelling (DCAP-BTLS).

Assess the breathing status. Cyanosis to the face, inside the mouth, or under the tongue indicates poor oxygenation. Be sure that the patient is on high-flow oxygen or is being ventilated adequately. If the cyanosis is severe or progressively gets worse, reevaluate the breathing status and consider positive pressure ventilation.

Assess the neck for subcutaneous emphysema, jugular vein distention, and tracheal deviation. Air tends to flow upward; therefore, with chest injury *subcutaneous emphysema* (air trapped under the skin giving it a bubbly inflated appearance) is usually present in the upper chest and neck. *Jugular vein distention* is an indication of possible cardiac injury or tension pneumothorax. Also, in a tension pneumothorax, the trachea will move toward the side of the uninjured lung (*trachael deviation*). The build-up of pressure in a tension pneumothorax will also cause the heart and large vessels to be compressed, causing a decreased blood flow to the heart and ineffective pumping which produce signs and symptoms of shock (hypoperfusion). Jugular vein distention and tracheal deviation are very late signs of a tension pneumothorax. Signs and symptoms of respiratory distress are better indicators.

If a spinal injury is suspected, apply a cervical spine immobilization collar. Most immobilization collars have a large opening on the anterior side allowing for reassessment of the jugular veins and trachea. Do not release manual in-line stabilization until the patient is completely immobilized to a backboard.

If you have not already done so, expose the chest by cutting the clothing. Inspect the chest carefully and thoroughly for any open wounds. If a penetrating injury is suspected, log roll the patient and inspect the back for open wounds. Also, lift the arm and inspect the axillary (armpit) area. An open wound to the back or side of the chest is just as lethal as one to the anterior chest. If an open wound is found there, immediately seal it by placing a gloved hand over the wound. If paradoxical movement is noted, immediately stabilize the segment with your hand by applying inward pressure to the flail area.

Look for retractions of the muscles, contusions, lacerations, or any other signs that blunt force may have been applied to the chest. Inspect the chest if the patient was a driver involved in an automobile crash. A bent or damaged steering wheel and positive markings on the patient's chest are indications of possible severe chest injury, especially if the driver was not wearing a seat belt. Air leaking from the respiratory tract or an injured lung may produce subcutaneous emphysema.

Palpate the chest, checking for symmetry (equal movement of both sides), paradoxical movement, swelling, and deformities. Fractures of the ribs may produce *crepitation* (a grating sound or sensation) and are usually accompanied by excruciating pain upon palpation. You will likely find that the patient with an injury to the chest wall or injury to the ribs will place his arm over the injured area to guard and splint it during breathing (Figure 36-5).

Auscultate the breath sounds bilaterally. Determine if the breath sounds are clear and equal, decreased or absent on one side, or decreased or absent on both sides. Decreased or absent breath sounds may indicate a collapsed lung or air or blood in the thoracic cavity. The patient in severe pain from a chest wall injury may have decreased or absent breath sounds bilaterally, which may indicate that both lungs are collapsed. A tension pneumothorax usually produces absent breath sounds on the injured side and decreased breath sounds on the side of the uninjured lung. Closely reevaluate the breathing status and determine if positive pressure ventilation should be initiated.

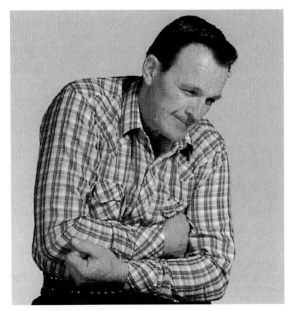

Figure 36-5 Typical "guarded" position of a patient with a rib injury.

Inspect the abdomen for excessive muscle movement during breathing. This may be an indication of severe respiratory distress associated with a chest injury.

Assess the baseline vital signs. The blood pressure may be low due to either bleeding or compression of the heart. The breathing rate can be significantly increased. Pain associated with chest injury may cause the patient's breathing to be very fast and shallow. The pulse is usually rapid and may be weak. The skin may appear cyanotic or pale, cool, and moist. *An increasing heart rate and decreasing blood pressure associated with increasing respiratory distress is an ominous sign of severe chest injury. Immediate transport should be considered.*

Obtain a SAMPLE history from the responsive patient. If the patient is unresponsive or is unable to answer your questions, attempt to gather information from others at the scene.

Signs and Symptoms Whether the injury is open or closed, certain signs and symptoms will occur in major chest trauma, many of them simultaneously (Figure 36-6). The major indications of chest trauma are:

- Cyanosis to the fingernails or fingertips, lips, or face
- Dyspnea (shortness of breath) or difficulty in breathing
- Breathing rate that is faster or slower than normal and usually shallow
- Contusions, lacerations, punctures, swelling, or other obvious signs of trauma to the chest
- Coughing up frothy blood
- Signs of shock (hypoperfusion)
- Decreasing blood pressure with a pulse that is becoming faster and weaker.
- Tracheal deviation
- Paradoxical movement of a segment of the chest wall
- Open wound that may or may not produce a sucking sound
- Distended jugular veins
- Absent or decreased breath sounds upon auscultation
- Pain at the injury site, especially pain that increases with inhalation and exhalation
- Failure of the chest to expand normally during inhalation

Not all of these signs need to be present in order to suspect serious chest injury. Sometimes only subtle signs of pain or symptoms of slight breathing difficulty are present. Consideration of the mechanism of injury and signs of trauma to the chest cavity should heighten your suspicion that a serious chest injury has occurred. Also, remember that an altered mental status, alcohol intoxication, or head injury can decrease

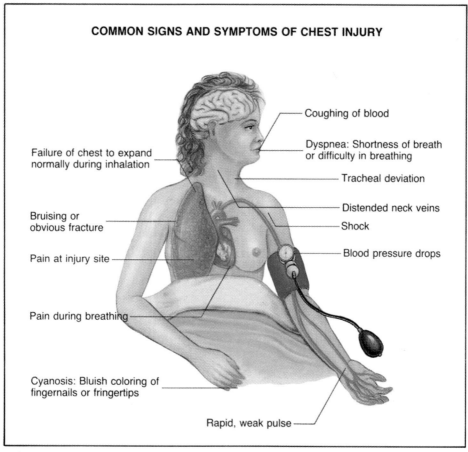

Figure 36-6 Common signs and symptoms of chest injury.

the patient's ability to complain of symptoms that might indicate chest injury.

GENERAL EMERGENCY MEDICAL CARE—CHEST INJURY

Chest injuries can be life-threatening. Therefore, prompt recognition and emergency medical care is essential to the patient's survival. An open chest wound, a flail segment that produces paradoxical movement, and inadequate breathing are all conditions that must be managed immediately upon identification.

1. *Maintain an open airway.* If the patient's condition continues to deteriorate, it may be necessary to insert a nasopharyngeal or oropharyngeal airway. Suction any secretions, blood, or vomitus. Remember that signs of inadequate breathing may occur from an occluded airway and not necessarily from a worsening chest injury. Continuously reassess the airway.

2. *Continue oxygen therapy.* Because most chest injuries produce disturbances in oxygen and carbon dioxide exchange in the lungs, the cells may

not be receiving an adequate amount of oxygen. This leads to cellular hypoxia (oxygen deficiency). It is essential that high flow oxygen (at 15 lpm) is continuously administered to all patients with suspected chest injury.

3. *Reevaluate breathing status.* Chest injuries can cause sudden and rapid deterioration. You should carefully and continuously reassess the breathing status and circulation. If at any time signs of inadequate breathing appear, immediately begin positive pressure ventilation with supplemental oxygen.

4. *Stabilize an impaled object in place.* If an impaled object is found, do not remove it. Stabilize the object with bulky gauze and bandages to prevent excessive movement.

5. *Completely immobilize the patient if spinal injury is suspected.* A cervical spinal immobilization collar must be applied and the patient must be immobilized to a backboard with straps and a head immobilization device.

6. *Treat the patient for shock (hypoperfusion) if signs and symptoms are present.* Many chest injuries involve blood loss or cardiac compromise from compression of the heart.

EMERGENCY MEDICAL CARE—OPEN CHEST WOUND

The open chest wound is an immediately life-threatening emergency that can lead to rapid deterioration and death if not managed properly. Emergency medical care includes the general care we have just detailed, plus the following:

1. *Immediately seal the open wound with your gloved hand.* Do not delay in order to find a dressing.
2. *Apply an occlusive dressing to seal the wound* (not a regular porous dressing, which would allow air to enter easily). Plastic wrap from an oxygen mask, the wrap covering an intravenous fluid bag, or Vaseline gauze may be used. The occlusive dressing should be a few inches wider than the wound. Place it over the entire wound and tape it on three sides (Figure 36-7). During inhalation, the dressing is sucked up against the wound, preventing air from entering. The side that is not taped allows for air that has built up in the thoracic cavity to escape during exhalation (Figure 36-8). An alternative method is to tape the dressing on four sides and occasionally lift a corner during expiration to relieve any pressure.
3. *Position the patient.* The patient may be positioned on the injured side so the uninjured lung can inflate more fully. This should be done only if no suspected spinal injury exists.
4. *Continuously assess the patient's respiratory status.* If the patient's condition begins to deteriorate and you notice more severe signs and symptoms of respiratory distress along with signs of shock (hypoperfusion), a tension pneumothorax may be developing. The occlusive dressing, even if taped on only three sides, may have become obstructed by trauma or clotted blood, preventing air from exiting the open wound in the chest, or air may be entering the thoracic cavity from a hole in the lung. The following are signs and symptoms that indicate a complication associated with the sealed wound and a developing tension pneumothorax. *The first three are the most important to recognize.*

   – Difficulty breathing, with increased respiratory distress and dyspnea (shortness of breath)
   – Tachypnea (breathing rate faster than normal)
   – Severely decreased or absent breath sounds on the injured side
   – Cyanosis
   – Tachycardia (heart rate faster than normal)
   – Decreasing blood pressure with a narrowing pulse pressure
   – Jugular vein distention (late sign)
   – Tracheal deviation (late sign)
   – Unequal movement of the chest wall (the injured side remains hyperinflated and will not move equally with the uninjured side)
   – Extreme anxiety and apprehension
   – Increased resistance to positive pressure ventilation

If these signs and symptoms develop after the occlusive dressing has been applied, you must lift a corner of the dressing for a few seconds to allow the air to escape during expiration. A rush of air may be heard or felt, and immediate relief of the signs and

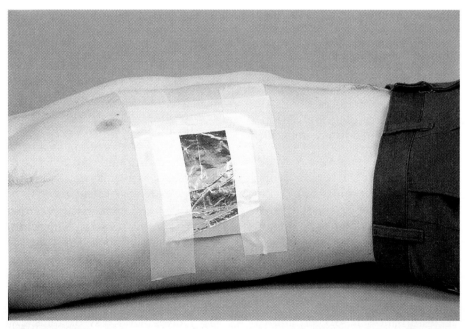

Figure 36-7   For an open chest wound, position an occlusive dressing directly on the chest wall. Tape it on three sides.

On inspiration, dressing seals
wound, preventing air entry

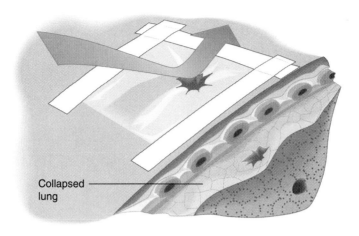

Collapsed —————————
lung

Expiration allows trapped air to escape
through untaped section of dressing

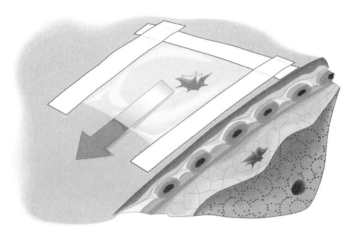

*Figure 36-8 By taping the occlusive dressing on
three sides, you create a flutter valve that helps to prevent tension pneumothorax.*

symptoms of severe compromise should occur. Reseal
the wound with the occlusive dressing. It may be
necessary to repeat this procedure several times.

EMERGENCY MEDICAL CARE— FLAIL SEGMENT

Paradoxical movement of a flail segment should be
initially splinted in an inward position by placing your
hand over the unstable flail segment (Figure 36-9a).
If the patient is breathing inadequately, initiate positive pressure ventilation during the initial assessment.
Paradoxical movement can also be stabilized by placing bulky dressings, a pillow, or towels over the unstable segment (Figure 36-9b), or by securing the patient's arm to his body (Figure 36-9c). Additional
care is as detailed on page 717.

DETAILED PHYSICAL EXAM AND ONGOING ASSESSMENT

En route to the hospital, if time and the patient's
condition permit, perform a detailed physical exam to
assess for any problems that may have been overlooked during the rapid trauma assessment. If the patient's condition is critical, performing a detailed
physical exam is less important than frequently performing an ongoing assessment.

During the ongoing assessment evaluate the effectiveness of your treatment and assess for further
deterioration of the patient's condition. Signs and
symptoms of increasing breathing difficulty, decreasing mental status, decreasing breath sounds, worsening cyanosis, and shock (hypoperfusion) should
prompt you to reevaluate your treatment and to

STABLIZING A FLAIL SEGMENT

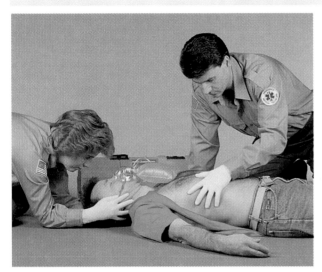

Figure 36-9a   Initially stabilize the flail segment with your gloved hand.

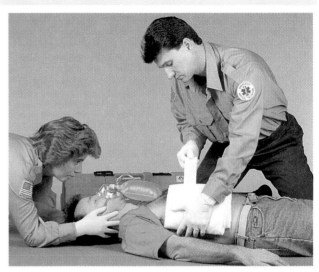

Figure 36-9b   Stabilize the flail segment by applying a bulky dressing or clean towel to the chest.

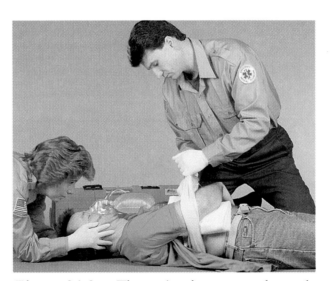

Figure 36-9c   The patient's arm can be used to help splint the flail segment.

perform a detailed physical exam or to repeat the rapid trauma assessment, looking for signs of injury that might have been missed initially. It may be necessary to reconsider the need to provide positive pressure ventilation if it has not already been initiated. Look for signs of a developing tension pneumothorax. If an occlusive dressing is in place, lift it to relieve any pressure that has potentially built up.

Reassess and record the baseline vital signs. A decreasing blood pressure, increasing heart rate, in-creasing respiratory rate, and cyanotic, cool, moist skin may indicate a worsening chest injury or shock (hypoperfusion) from blood loss.

SUMMARY: ASSESSMENT AND CARE—CHEST INJURIES

To review possible assessment findings and emergency care for chest injuries, see Figures 36-10 and 36-11.

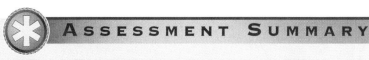

CHEST INJURY

The following are findings that may be associated with a chest injury.

SCENE SIZE-UP

Pay particular attention to your own safety. Look for:
Mechanism of injury
    Automobile crash, bent steering wheel
    Sports accident, especially blow to chest as from football helmet, baseball
    Fall
    Gunshot wound
    Fight, especially with blow to chest
    Crush injury
    Explosion

INITIAL ASSESSMENT

General Impression

Severe cyanosis
Extreme respiratory distress
Patient splinting chest with arm
Obvious open wound to chest
Uneven chest wall movement
Speech pattern: gasping for breath between words

Mental Status

Alert to unresponsive, based on type and degree of injury
Unresponsiveness or decreasing mental status associated with hypoxia and hypoperfusion

Airway

Assume airway is closed if patient has an altered mental status

Breathing

May be absent, inadequate, or normal
May be very shallow if ribs are fractured
May be labored

Circulation

Pulse and skin color vary depending on injury
Pulse may be normal
Pulse is increased if hypoxia, blood loss, or tension pneumothorax
Skin may be normal if minor chest injury
Cyanosis if perfusion disturbance or hypoxia

Status: Priority patient if any chest injury

FOCUSED HISTORY AND PHYSICAL EXAM

Physical Exam

Head:
    Cyanotic tongue, oral mucous membranes, and face

    Assess neck for subcutaneous emphysema
    Jugular venous distention and tracheal deviation are late signs of tension pneumothorax
Chest:
    Evidence of blunt trauma to chest: contusions, lacerations
    Penetrating trauma to chest: knife, gunshot wounds (look for exit wound)
    Retractions of suprasternal notch, supraclavicular spaces, lateral neck
    Palpate for symmetry, deformities, crepitation, pain
    Paradoxical movement indicates flail segment
    Breath sounds may be diminished or absent on one side or both
Abdomen:
    Excessive movement during breathing indicates severe respiratory distress
Extremities:
    Weak peripheral pulses may indicate a tension pneumothorax or poor perfusion
    Pulse that weakens with inspiration may indicate a tension pneumothorax
Posterior Body:
    Inspect for entrance and exit wounds
    Evidence or blunt trauma

Baseline Vital Signs

BP: normal; may be low if severe hypoxia, blood loss, tension pneumothorax, or cardiac tamponade
HR: normal, or tachycardia due to severe hypoxia, blood loss, tension pneumothorax, or cardiac tamponade
RR: normal, irregular, decreased, absent, or labored
Skin: normal; may be pale, cool, clammy if severe hypoxia, blood loss, tension pneumothorax, or cardiac tamponade
Pupils: equal and reactive, may be sluggish to respond to light

SAMPLE History

Dyspnea
Coughing up frothy blood
Pain at site of injury
Cyanosis
Obvious trauma to chest
Shock
Decreasing blood pressure with increasing pulse that becomes weaker
Tracheal deviation and distended neck veins
Paradoxical movement of chest
Absent or decreased chest sounds
Failure of chest to rise with inhalation

Figure 36-10a   Assessment summary: chest injury.

✳ EMERGENCY CARE PROTOCOL

CHEST INJURY

1. Establish manual in-line stabilization. Do not release it until patient is immobilized onto backboard.
2. If obvious open wounds to chest are found during the general impression, place gloved hand over them until they can be covered with a nonporous dressing taped on three sides.
3. Establish and maintain an open airway. Insert a nasopharyngeal or oropharyngeal airway if patient is unresponsive and has no gag or cough reflex.
4. Suction secretions as necessary.
5. If breathing is inadequate, provide positive pressure ventilation with supplemental oxygen at a minimum rate of 12 ventilations/minute for an adult and 20 ventilations/minute for an infant or child.
6. If breathing is adequate, administer oxygen by nonrebreather mask at 15 lpm.
7. Control any major bleeding.
8. Treat the specific condition or wound:

Impaled Object
Stabilize impaled object in place.
Open Chest Wound
Place gloved hand over wound immediately.
Apply an occlusive, or nonporous, dressing taped on three sides.
Fail Segment (Paradoxical Chest Wall Movement)
If inadequate breathing, begin positive pressure ventilation, which will splint segment internally.
Place gloved hand over segment, then stabilize with blanket, pillow, bulky dressing, or patient's own arm.

9. Treat for shock.
10. Immobilize to backboard if you suspect spine injury.
11. Transport.
12. Perform an ongoing assessment every 5 minutes if unstable an every 15 minutes if stable.
13. If open chest wound is occluded with a dressing and patient suddenly begins to deteriorate, lift dressing off wound during exhalation to relieve trapped air, then reapply dressing.

Figure 36-10   continued

THE ABDOMEN
◼

ANATOMY OF THE ABDOMINAL CAVITY

It may be helpful for you to review Chapter 4, "The Human Body," for a description of the abdominal cavity and the organs therein. A brief description follows.

The abdominal cavity contains the major organs of the digestive, urinary and endocrine systems. The abdomen is separated from the chest cavity superiorly by the diaphragm. The inferior border is the heavy, bony pelvic ring. Tough, thick, flat muscles form the bulk of the anterior border along with the lower portion of the rib cage. Posteriorly, the spinal column and strong muscles provide protection.

The abdominal cavity is lined by a two-layer sheathlike membrane called the *peritoneum*. The innermost lining—the *visceral peritoneum*—adheres to and supports the organs. The *parietal peritoneum* is the outer lining that adheres to the walls of the abdominal cavity. Between the two layers is a small amount of fluid that serves as a lubricant to reduce friction when the surfaces rub over each other. The potential space between the visceral and parietal peritonia is called the *peritoneal cavity*. Some organs in the posterior abdominal cavity lie partially or completely outside of the peritoneum. They are said to be *retroperitoneal*.

The abdomen contains vascular structures (blood vessels) as well as solid and hollow organs:

- *Hollow organs* include the stomach, gallbladder, urinary bladder, small intestine, and large intestine. They contain few blood vessels. If ruptured or lacerated they do not bleed very much, but they spill their contents into the abdominal cavity, causing irritation and inflammation of the peritoneal lining known as *peritonitis*. The leaking contents might include gastric juices from the stomach, highly acidic and partially digested food from the upper small intestine, bacteria from the large intestine, or urine from the bladder.
- *Solid organs* include the liver, spleen, pancreas, and kidney, which usually contain a very rich blood supply. A solid organ may bleed into the capsule that surrounds it for some time before the capsule ruptures and allows the blood to spill into the abdominal cavity. The major complication associated with the laceration or tearing of a solid organ is major bleeding and severe shock (hypoperfusion).

EMERGENCY CARE ALGORITHM: CHEST INJURY

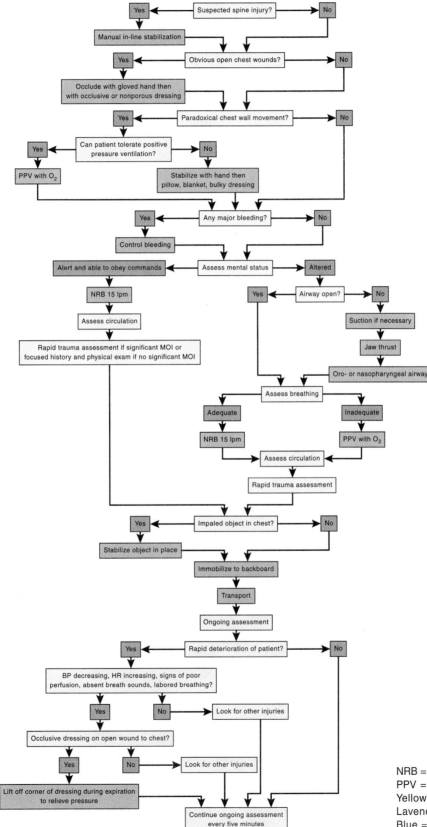

Figure 36-11 *Emergency care algorithm: chest injury.*

NRB = nonrebreather mask
PPV = positive pressure ventilation
Yellow = assessment
Lavender = key decision points
Blue = interventions

- *Vascular structures* include the abdominal aorta and inferior vena cava. They are primarily stationary, very large, and carry large amounts of blood. If lacerated, ruptured, or torn, the vessels will bleed massively and rapidly lead to severe shock (hypoperfusion) and death.

ABDOMINAL INJURIES

Abdominal injuries are caused by either blunt trauma or penetrating trauma. The mechanisms of injury are very similar to those of chest injury. Blunt trauma to the abdomen is especially lethal because of the large number of organs that can be affected.

Like chest injuries, injuries to the abdomen are classified as either open or closed. Open injuries result from penetrating trauma from bullets, knives, ice picks, sharp metal, broken glass, screwdrivers, and any other sharp object that you can think of.

Bullets, once they enter the body, can involve almost any organ or structure. If the patient is shot in the abdomen, the bullet could have entered the chest, fractured the pelvis, or lodged in the spinal column. The entrance wound may be to the anterior abdomen and the exit wound to the posterior thorax. Also, the patient may have been shot in the chest, with the bullet traveling through the diaphragm and into the abdomen. With any gunshot wound, be highly suspicious that many other organs, bones, and vessels have also been injured. Always search for an exit wound. If you focus on just the entrance wound, you could easily miss the potentially life-threatening exit wound.

Open wounds to the abdomen are much more dramatic and easier to find upon assessment than closed wounds. For example, a severe form of an open wound to the abdomen is an evisceration, in which organs are protruding through the skin. However, closed abdominal wounds could be much more dangerous. Blunt trauma applied to the abdomen can crush, tear, or rupture a large number of organs causing severe internal bleeding. You must look at the mechanism of injury and physical assessment findings, as well as maintain a very high index of suspicion that a closed abdominal injury exists.

ASSESSMENT AND CARE: ABDOMINAL INJURIES

Assessment of the patient with a suspected abdominal injury is very similar to that for a patient with a suspected chest injury. Consider the mechanism of injury, patient complaints, signs, and symptoms.

SCENE SIZE-UP

The scene size-up can provide you with clues as to whether the trauma was caused by blunt or penetrating forces. Once you have ensured your own safety,

scan the scene and develop suspicions of what may have caused injury. Look for evidence of knives, guns, sharp metal, and other objects that may have penetrated the body. Ask the police or bystanders at the scene if a gun was involved or if gunshots were heard. If the penetrating object is located, estimate the length and width (stabbing) or caliber (gunshot). This may be important information for the physician. However, do not spend valuable time looking for a weapon and trying to identify its characteristics.

Remember, do not expect abdominal (or chest) wounds to jump out at you if the patient is clothed. Suspicion of a penetrating wound should prompt you to expose and inspect the entire body for open wounds.

Blunt trauma is associated with motor-vehicle crashes, falls, pedestrian-vehicle collisions, motorcycle collisions, assaults, heavy objects thrown at or falling on the patient, and crushing injuries from machinery or other heavy equipment. The motor vehicle collision is by far the most common cause of blunt trauma to the abdomen. Attempt to determine the following when a motor vehicle collision is involved:

- Type of vehicle
- Approximate speed the vehicle was traveling (fast, slow, stationary)
- Type of collision and point(s) of impact
- Whether the patient was the driver, passenger, or a pedestrian
- Where the patient is found and his position
- Whether or not the patient was thrown from the vehicle
- Impact marks to the windshield, steering wheel, and dashboard
- Whether or not a seat belt was used. If so, try to determine if both the shoulder and lap belts were properly positioned.

Many times abdominal injuries produce only subtle signs and symptoms. Therefore, you must base your suspicions on the mechanism of injury. Also remember that alcohol intoxication, head injury, and the influence of other drugs and substances may reduce the patient's response to pain.

INITIAL ASSESSMENT

As you approach the patient, begin to form a general impression as the first step of the initial assessment. Typically, you will find the patient with an abdominal injury lying extremely still with knees flexed up toward the chest (Figure 36-12). This is done to decrease the tension on the abdominal muscles and reduce the abdominal pain. The patient may be moaning and complaining of severe pain. If spinal injury is suspected, establish in-line spinal stabilization.

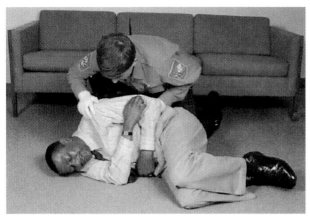

Figure 36-12   Patients with abdominal injuries often lie with legs drawn up in the fetal position.

Ensure an open airway and adequate breathing. Inspect the airway for evidence of bloody vomitus that may be associated with the injury and suction if necessary. Deliver oxygen by a nonrebreather mask at 15 lpm if breathing is adequate. If performing positive pressure ventilation, be sure supplemental oxygen is connected to the ventilation device. Assess circulation. The radial pulse may be weak or absent due to associated bleeding. The heart rate is typically increased beyond the normal limit. The skin may appear to be pale, moist, and cool. These are all signs of shock, which indicates a severe abdominal injury and blood loss, and criteria to establish the patient as a priority for immediate transport.

FOCUSED HISTORY AND PHYSICAL EXAM

During your focused history and physical exam, consider the patient's complaints and the mechanism of injury. Whether the injury is due to blunt or penetrating trauma, it is essential that the entire body is exposed and a rapid trauma assessment performed to identify other potential injuries. Since abdominal injuries can produce very severe pain, the patient may not complain of any other injuries. If you allow yourself to develop tunnel vision and not inspect other areas of the body, you can easily miss life-threatening injuries. First inspect the head, neck, and chest. If the patient has been shot in the abdomen, it is necessary for you to examine the chest for a possible exit wound or another gunshot wound.

Apply a cervical spinal immobilization collar if a spinal injury is suspected. Do not release manual inline spinal stabilization until the patient is completely immobilized to a backboard.

Inspect the abdomen. Look for contusions, lacerations, abrasions, and punctures. Determine if the abdomen appears to be distended. (If it is, several liters of blood may have been lost into the abdominal cavity.

It takes about a liter of blood to expand the abdominal girth by one inch.) Inspect around the umbilicus (navel) and the flank areas for discoloration and bruising, which also indicate that bleeding is occurring inside the abdomen. Look for bruising over the lower abdomen that could be caused by an improperly worn lap belt if the patient was involved in a motor-vehicle collision.

Inspect and provide emergency medical care for any abdominal evisceration (a large open wound with organs or tissue protruding). Then palpate the abdomen, starting from the point farthest away from the pain. Note any tenderness or masses. If the patient has a decreased mental status, watch the face for a grimace as you palpate. The abdomen may be rigid from contraction of the abdominal muscles. The patient may be voluntarily contracting the muscles as to guard against pain during your assessment, or the muscles may be involuntarily contracted by a reflex.

Assess the extremities for injury. Check and compare the strength of the pulses of both the upper and lower extremities. Abdominal aortic injury may cause the pulses of the lower extremities to be weaker than the upper extremities or even absent. If no pedal (foot) pulses are found, check for popliteal (back of the knee) or femoral (thigh) pulses. These should be equal to or stronger than the radial pulse, even in shock (hypoperfusion). Keep in mind that blood loss and shock will reduce the pulse strength in the most distal pulses. Also assess motor and sensory function.

Log roll the patient and inspect the entire back and lumbar region for any signs of trauma. If the patient is suspected of having a spinal injury, log roll the patient onto a backboard at this time.

Assess baseline vital signs, especially for indications of blood loss and shock. A low blood pressure, tachycardia (rapid heart beat), pale, cool, and moist skin would be good indicators that the patient is in shock. The breathing rate is typically fast and shallow in abdominal injuries due to the increase in pain associated with deep breathing.

From the responsive patient, obtain a SAMPLE history. The abdominal pain can be evaluated using the OPQRST mnemonic to help you. If the patient is unresponsive, ascertain as much information as possible from bystanders at the scene. The signs and symptoms and events prior to the injury are extremely important points of information to gather.

Signs and Symptoms   Patients with abdominal injury may exhibit the following signs and symptoms:

- Contusions, abrasions, lacerations, punctures, or other signs of blunt or penetrating trauma
- Pain that may initially be mild, then worsening
- Tenderness on palpation to areas other than the site of injury
- Rigid abdominal muscles

- Patient lies with his legs drawn up to the chest in an attempt to reduce the pain
- Distended abdomen
- Discoloration around the umbilicus or to the flank (late finding)
- Rapid shallow breathing
- Signs of shock
- Nausea and vomiting (the vomitus may contain blood)
- Abdominal cramping possibly present
- Pain may radiate to either shoulder
- Weakness

A mechanism of injury involving either blunt or penetrating trauma, early signs and symptoms of shock (hypoperfusion), shallow rapid respirations, and abdominal pain and rigidity are all very significant and early signs of a serious abdominal injury. Any patient who complains of abdominal pain should be taken seriously and assessed carefully.

GENERAL EMERGENCY MEDICAL CARE— ABDOMINAL INJURY

Emergency medical care is basically the same for both open and closed abdominal injuries: aggressive management of the airway, breathing, and circulation. Since you are limited in the emergency medical care you can provide for abdominal injury, early recognition and prompt transport is a key element.

1. *Maintain an open airway.* Reassess the airway continuously. The patient may suddenly vomit, which can easily occlude the airway. Suction any vomitus, blood, or other secretions from the mouth. If the condition continues to deteriorate, it may be necessary to perform a jaw-thrust maneuver and to insert an oropharyngeal or nasopharyngeal airway.
2. *Continue oxygen therapy.* Administer oxygen by a nonrebreather mask at 15 lpm.
3. *Reassess the breathing status.* If the breathing becomes inadequate, begin positive pressure ventilation. Be sure that supplemental oxygen is connected to the ventilation device.
4. *Treat for shock (hypoperfusion).*
5. *Control any external bleeding.* Apply a dry sterile dressing to open wounds to the abdomen. In case of an evisceration, see the guidelines in the next segment for preparing a dressing.
6. *Position the patient.* Place the patient in a supine position with legs flexed at the knees (legs brought up toward the chest) if no injury to the lower extremities, hips, pelvis, or spine is suspected. Remember not to give anything by mouth, even if the patient complains of thirst. Do not allow the patient to eat or drink any amount of food or liquid. If spinal injury is suspected, immobilize the patient to a backboard.

7. *Stabilize an impaled object.* Do not remove it. Dress the wound around the impaled object to control the bleeding. Stabilize the object with bulky dressings and bandages to prevent movement.
8. *Apply the pneumatic antishock garment (PASG),* if indicated and allowed by local protocol. The PASG may be applied if the abdominal injury is closed, pain is noted to the pelvis, and signs and symptoms of shock are present Follow local protocol.
9. *Transport as quickly as possible.*

EMERGENCY MEDICAL CARE— ABDOMINAL EVISCERATION

A large open wound to the abdomen may allow organs to protrude. Do not touch or attempt to replace the protruding organs. In caring for an evisceration, follow the general guidelines above for abdominal injury, except dress the evisceration in the following way (Figures 36-13a to c):

1. *Expose the wound.* Cut away clothing if necessary. Do not touch or attempt to replace any of the organs.
2. *Position the patient* on his back and flex the legs up toward the chest if spinal injury is not suspected.
3. *Prepare a clean, sterile dressing* by soaking it with saline or sterile water. Apply the dressing over the protruding organs. Do not use absorbent cotton or any other material that might cling to the organs when wet, such as paper towels or toilet tissue.
4. *Cover the moist dressing with an occlusive dressing* to retain moisture and warmth. Plastic wrap will do. Avoid the use of aluminum foil if possible, since it may lacerate the protruding organs. Secure the dressing in place with tape, cravats, or a bandage.
5. *Administer high-flow oxygen. Be prepared to treat for shock.*

En route to the hospital, if time and the patient's condition permit, perform a detailed physical exam to assess for any problems that may have been overlooked. If the patient's condition is critical, performing a detailed physical exam is less important than performing frequent ongoing assessment.

During the ongoing assessment, monitor the patient for further deterioration. Also, the ongoing assessment may indicate if your emergency medical care has been effective. Reassess and record baseline vital signs, paying particular attention to signs of shock (hypoperfusion). Monitor for an increasing heart rate, decreasing blood pressure, decreasing level of consciousness, and pale, cool, moist skin. If you note

DRESSING AN ABDOMINAL EVISCERATION

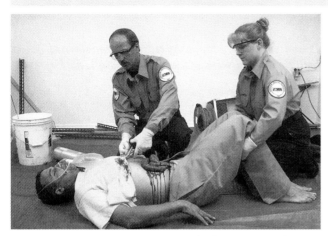

Figure 36-13a   Cut away clothing from the wound and support the knees in a flexed position.

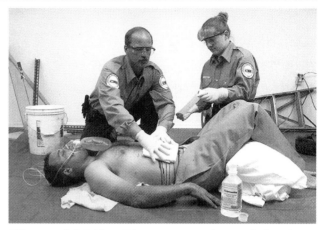

Figure 36-13b   Place a premoistened dressing over the wound (follow local protocol) and gently tape it in place. Do not attempt to replace intestines within the abdomen.

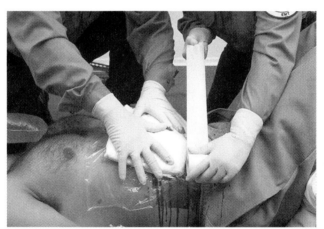

Figure 36-13c   Apply an occlusive covering (follow local protocol). Tape it loosely to keep the dressing moist.

deterioration, reevaluate the priority status of the patient and expedite transport.

SUMMARY: ASSESSMENT AND CARE—ABDOMINAL INJURIES

To review possible assessment findings and emergency care for abdominal injuries, see Figures 36-14 and 36-15.

THE GENITALIA

While injuries to the genitalia are rarely life threatening, they are typically extremely painful and could be quite embarrassing for the patient.

• *Injuries to the male genitalia* include lacerations, abrasions, avulsions, penetrations, and contusions. They usually produce excruciating pain and cause great concern to the patient. The penis is very vascular and can bleed excessively. An injury to the penis or scrotum should be treated as a soft-tissue injury, which can be controlled with direct pressure. Cold compresses also may be applied to the scrotum to reduce the pain and swelling associated with injury. If the penis has been avulsed or amputated, apply direct pressure to control the bleeding. If the amputated or avulsed part is located, wrap it in a sterile dressing moistened with sterile saline, place it in a plastic bag, and keep it cool by placing the bag on a cold pack or ice that has been wrapped in a towel. Provide oxygen at 15 lpm by nonrebreather mask, carefully assess for

ASSESSMENT SUMMARY

ABDOMINAL INJURY

The following are findings that may be associated with an abdominal injury.

SCENE SIZE-UP

Pay particular attention to your own safety. Look for:
Mechanism of injury
  Automobile crash, bent steering wheel
  Sports accident, especially blow to abdomen
  Gunshot wound
  Fight, especially with hard, direct blow to abdomen
  Crush injury
  Explosion

INITIAL ASSESSMENT

General Impression

Patient lying very still with knees flexed up toward chest
Obvious open wound to abdomen
Severe abdominal pain

Mental Status

Alert to unresponsive, based on type and degree of injury
Unresponsiveness or decreasing mental status associated with hypoperfusion

Airway

Assume airway is closed if patient has altered mental status

Breathing

Normal
May be fast and shallow due to pain associated with breathing
Labored breathing may be present if diaphragm is injured

Circulation

Pulse and skin color vary depending on injury
Pulse is increased in shock state and in association with severe pain
Skin will be pale, cool, and clammy in shock state

Priority Status: Priority patient if abdominal injury associated with severe pain or signs and symptoms of shock

FOCUSED HISTORY AND PHYSICAL EXAM

Physical Exam

Head:
  Pale oral mucous membranes in shock state
  Pupils may be sluggish to respond in shock state
Chest:
  Decreased breath sounds bilaterally if breathing is shallow due to pain
Abdomen:
  Contusions, lacerations, punctures, abrasions, or other evidence of trauma
  Inspect for distention
  Discoloration around umbilicus and in flank areas (late sign of intra-abdominal bleeding)
  Inspect for abdominal evisceration
  Palpate for rigidity and guarding
  Pain on palpation
  Palpate for masses
Extremities:
  Weak peripheral pulses indicate poor perfusion
  Difference in strength of pulses in upper and lower extremities may indicate aortic injury
Posterior Body:
  Evidence of blunt or penetrating trauma

Baseline Vital Signs

BP: may be low due to blood loss
HR: tachycardia due to severe pain and blood loss
RR: normal; may be increased due to pain, or labored if diaphragm injured
Skin: pale, cool, clammy if blood loss and shock
Pupils: may be sluggish to respond to light due to poor perfusion

Figure 36-14a Assessment summary: abdominal injury.

EMERGENCY CARE PROTOCOL

ABDOMINAL INJURY

1. Establish manual in-line stabilization. Do not release it until patient is immobilized onto backboard.
2. Establish and maintain an open airway. Insert a nasopharyngeal or oropharyngeal airway if patient is unresponsive and has no gag or cough reflex.
3. Suction secretions as necessary.
4. If breathing is inadequate, provide positive pressure ventilation with supplemental oxygen at a minimum rate of 12 ventilations/minute for an adult and 20 ventilations/minute for an infant or child.
5. If breathing is adequate, administer oxygen by nonrebreather mask at 15 lpm.
6. Control any major bleeding.

7. Treat the specific condition or wound:
   Impaled Object
   Stabilize impaled object in place.
   Abdominal Evisceration
   Place a moist, sterile dressing over entire wound, overlapping by 2 inches.
   Apply an occlusive dressing taped on all four sides.
   Flex knees up toward chest.
   Open Wound to Abdomen
   Apply a dressing over the wound.
8. Treat for shock.
9. Immobilize to backboard if you suspect spine injury.
10. Transport.
11. Perform an ongoing assessment every 5 minutes if unstable an every 15 minutes if stable.

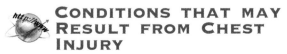

Figure 36-14b   Emergency care protocol: abdominal injury.

signs and symptoms of shock, and transport the patient with any amputated parts.

• *Injuries to the female genitalia* can occur due to straddle injuries, sexual assault, blunt trauma, abortion attempts, lacerations following childbirth, and from foreign bodies inserted into the vagina. Because a large number of nerves are located in this area, injuries usually produce excruciating pain and cause great concern to the patient. The female genital area is very vascular and can bleed profusely. Control any bleeding with direct pressure, using moistened compresses such as a sterile sanitary napkin. Never pack or place dressings inside the vagina. Carefully assess for signs and symptoms of shock, provide oxygen at 15 lpm by nonrebreather mask, and transport.

ENRICHMENT

The enrichment section contains information that is valuable as background for the EMT-B but that goes substantially beyond the U.S. Department of Transportation (DOT) EMT-Basic curriculum.

CONDITIONS THAT MAY RESULT FROM CHEST INJURY

Though several conditions may result from an injury to the chest (Figures 36-16 and 36-17), emergency medical care is basically the same for each: aggressive management of the airway, breathing, and circulation. Some of these conditions were introduced and briefly discussed earlier in this chapter but are presented in more detail on the following pages.

FLAIL SEGMENT

A flail segment occurs when two or more consecutive ribs have been fractured in two or more places producing a freely moving section of chest wall. During normal inhalation, the pressure in the chest is less than the pressure outside of the chest. With a flail segment, the patient cannot generate the normal negative pressure within the chest. This reduces the volume that can be breathed in, leading to hypoxia (oxygen deficiency) and poor oxygenation. During exhalation, the flail segment is forced outward as the remainder of the chest is moving back into a normal position. This creates a motion, or paradoxical movement, that is opposite the normal chest wall movement during inhalation and exhalation. Even though the flail segment requires immediate recognition and management, the underlying contusion to the lung is a more serious injury resulting from the blunt force applied to the chest.

Stabilization of the segment reduces the paradoxical movement and improves ventilation. As previously discussed, stabilization is achieved by splinting the flail segment. Because lung contusion and lung collapse are associated with a flail segment, positive pressure ventilation with supplemental oxygen is the ideal treatment. It expands the alveoli that are col-

EMERGENCY CARE ALGORITHM:
ABDOMINAL INJURY

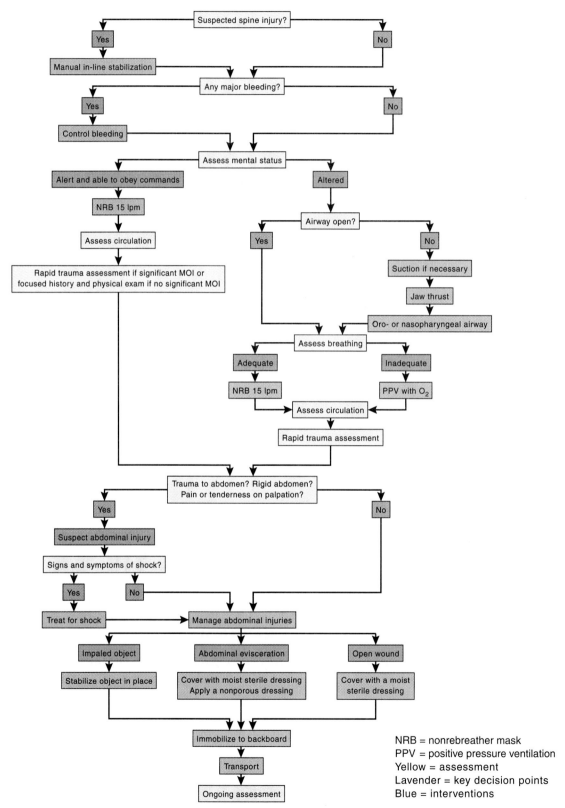

Figure 36-15 Emergency care algorithm: abdominal injury.

HEMOTHORAX

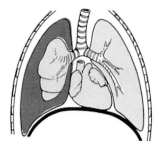

Blood leaks into the chest cavity from lacerated vessels or the lung itself and the lung compresses.

PNEUMOTHORAX

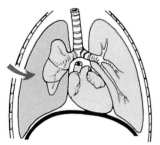

Air enters the chest cavity through a sucking wound or leaks from a lacerated lung. The lung cannot expand.

SPONTANEOUS PNEUMOTHORAX

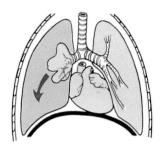

Air leaks into the chest from a weak area in the (nontrauma) lung surface and the lung collapses.

TENSION PNEUMOTHORAX

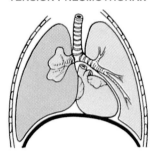

Air continuously leaks out the lung. It collapses, pressure rises, and the collapsed lung is forced against the heart and other lung.

MEDIASTINAL SHIFT

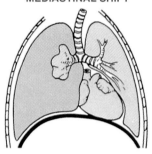

Usually caused by severe tension pneumothorax.

HEMOPNEUMOTHORAX

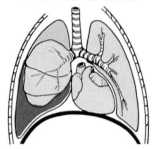

Air and blood leak into the chest cavity from an injured lung putting pressure on heart and uninjured lung.

Figure 36-16   Complications of chest injury.   *(continued on the next page)*

lapsed, greatly reducing the amount of hypoxia (oxygen deficiency) by forcing ventilation and increasing oxygenation.

PULMONARY CONTUSION

Pulmonary (lung) contusions are often a serious consequence of a flail segment. They can lead to death. Bleeding occurs in and around the alveoli and into the interstitial space that separates the alveoli and capillaries. This greatly reduces the exchange of oxygen and carbon dioxide, leading to severe hypoxia (oxygen deficiency).

A patient who has suffered a direct blow or any other blunt trauma to the chest should be suspected of having a pulmonary contusion. Such injuries are often seen in association with a flail chest.

The amount of respiratory distress depends on the amount of damaged lung tissue. Other signs and symptoms include dyspnea (shortness of breath), cyanosis, and signs of blunt trauma to the chest. As mentioned earlier, positive pressure ventilation with supplemental oxygen are required emergency care for this condition.

PNEUMOTHORAX

A pneumothorax is the accumulation of air in the thoracic cavity, causing collapse of a portion of the lung. It is usually due to either blunt or penetrating trauma. Blunt trauma may cause a fractured rib to penetrate the lung, leaving a hole that leaks air. Also, the lung may rupture if, upon impact and chest compression, the patient's epiglottis is closed over the trachea. This causes a "paper-bag effect" similar to an inflated paper bag that is sealed and ruptures when it is compressed between the hands. The resultant hole in the visceral pleura of the lung allows air to enter the thoracic cavity. Penetrating trauma is another way the lung can be punctured.

The accumulation of air in the thoracic cavity causes the lung on the injured side to collapse, either partially or fully. This results in a decrease in gas available within the alveoli, which causes a reduction of oxygen delivered to the cells of the body. Signs and symptoms of a pneumothorax include chest pain that worsens with deep inspiration, dyspnea (shortness of breath), tachypnea (faster than normal rate of breathing), and decreased or absent breath sounds on the affected side.

LACERATED AORTA

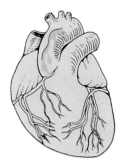

Lacerations of the great or major blood vessels.

TRAUMATIC ASPHYXIA

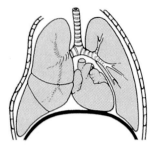

Severe chest compression puts pressure on heart and forces blood back into veins of the neck. It may cause severe lung damage.

PERICARDIAL TAMPONADE

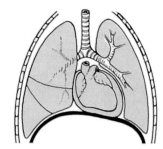

Blood or other fluid in the pericardial sac outside the heart exerts pressure on the heart.

TRAUMATIC EMPHYSEMA

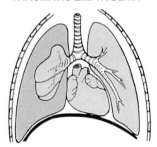

A sudden compression injury occurs when the glottis is closed. The air sacs (alveoli) in the lungs rupture and leak air.

LUNG CONTUSION

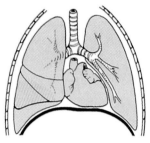

Usually caused by high velocity blunt trauma with bruising and bleeding from the lung.

RUPTURED DIAPHRAGM

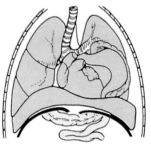

Usually caused by blunt trauma to one side or multiple trauma, often involving the pelvis.

Figure 36-16   Complications of chest injury. (continued)

A patient may suffer a pneumothorax in the absence of blunt or penetrating trauma to the chest. This condition is called a *spontaneous pneumothorax*, because it occurs without an external cause. It usually is the result of a congenitally weak area on the surface of the lung, which ruptures and allows air to enter the thoracic cavity. Spontaneous pneumothorax is common among smokers and emphysema patients. A sudden onset of dyspnea (shortness of breath), respiratory distress, sharp chest pain, and absent breath sounds on one side are typical signs and symptoms.

OPEN PNEUMOTHORAX

An open pneumothorax is a result of an open wound to the chest created by a penetrating object. Air may be heard escaping or entering through the chest wound, creating a bubbling or sucking sound. For this reason, an open pneumothorax is often referred to as a "sucking chest wound," as discussed earlier in this chapter. The signs and symptoms of an open pneumothorax are the same as for a closed pneumothorax, with the exception of the presence of an open wound the chest. You must immediately occlude an open wound to the chest. Initially seal it with your gloved hand and then with an occlusive dressing.

TENSION PNEUMOTHORAX

A tension pneumothorax is an immediately life-threatening condition resulting from a pneumothorax that continues to trap air in the thoracic cavity with no relief or escape. With each breath, a massive volume of air accumulates in the thoracic cavity on the injured side. This completely collapses the injured lung and begins to compress and shift the mediastinum over to the uninjured side. The uninjured lung, heart, and large veins are compressed, leading to poor cardiac output, ineffective ventilation, inadequate oxygenation, and severe hypoxia. Death can occur rapidly.

Rapid deterioration, severe respiratory distress, signs of shock (hypoperfusion), and absent breath sounds on one side of the chest should alert you to a possible tension pneumothorax. Other signs and symptoms include cyanosis, unequal movement of the chest, distended neck veins, diminished breath sounds

TRAUMATIC CARDIAC INJURIES

Trauma to the chest can induce three types of cardiac injury.
Determining the nature of the injury is difficult and emergency
care in the field is frequently limited to support of vital functions.

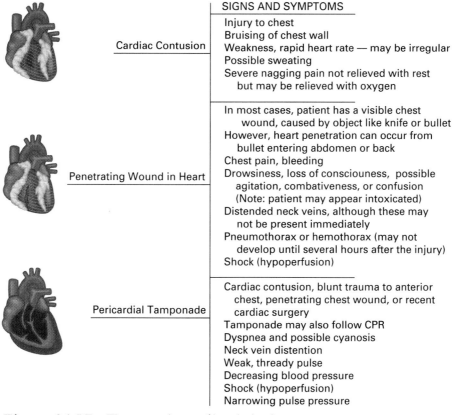

	SIGNS AND SYMPTOMS
Cardiac Contusion	Injury to chest Bruising of chest wall Weakness, rapid heart rate — may be irregular Possible sweating Severe nagging pain not relieved with rest but may be relieved with oxygen

Penetrating Wound in Heart	In most cases, patient has a visible chest
	   wound, caused by object like knife or bullet
	However, heart penetration can occur from
	   bullet entering abdomen or back
	Chest pain, bleeding
	Drowsiness, loss of consciousness, possible
	   agitation, combativeness, or confusion
	   (Note: patient may appear intoxicated)
	Distended neck veins, although these may
	   not be present immediately
	Pneumothorax or hemothorax (may not
	   develop until several hours after the injury)
	Shock (hypoperfusion)

Pericardial Tamponade	Cardiac contusion, blunt trauma to anterior
	   chest, penetrating chest wound, or recent
	   cardiac surgery
	Tamponade may also follow CPR
	Dyspnea and possible cyanosis
	Neck vein distention
	Weak, thready pulse
	Decreasing blood pressure
	Shock (hypoperfusion)
	Narrowing pulse pressure

Figure 36-17   Traumatic cardiac injuries.

on the side opposite to the injury, and deviation of the trachea to the uninjured side. Remember that this condition may develop following the application of an occlusive dressing to an open chest wound. Alleviate the pressure by lifting the dressing and allowing air to escape during expiration, even if it is taped on only three sides. If you suspect a tension pneumothorax, rapid transport is critical.

HEMOTHORAX

With a hemothorax, the thoracic cavity is filled with blood rather than air (*hemo* means "blood"). As the blood continues to collect, the lung is compressed. A hemopneumothorax, which is the collection of both blood and air (*hemo*, "blood"; *pneumo*, "air"), also may occur.

A hemothorax may be the result of blunt or penetrating trauma to the chest and may be associated with open or closed injuries. The bleeding usually originates from lacerated blood vessels in the chest wall or chest cavity caused by penetrating objects or fractured ribs. The patient can lose a significant

amount of blood in the chest, which results in severe shock. Early signs and symptoms of hemothorax are usually the same as for shock. Signs and symptoms of respiratory distress develop late. In addition, bleeding in and around the lung will commonly produce a pink or red frothy sputum when the patient coughs. Care is the same as for pneumothorax and shock.

TRAUMATIC ASPHYXIA

Traumatic asphyxia is brought about when severe and sudden compression of the thorax causes a rapid increase in the pressure in the chest. The heart and lungs are usually severely compressed by the sternum and ribs, causing a backflow of blood out of the right ventricle and into the veins of the head, shoulders, and upper chest. The patient often looks as if he has been strangled.

The signs and symptoms of traumatic asphyxia include bluish or purple discoloration of the face, head, neck, and shoulders; jugular vein distention; bloodshot eyes that are protruding from the socket; cyanotic and swollen tongue and lips; bleeding of the

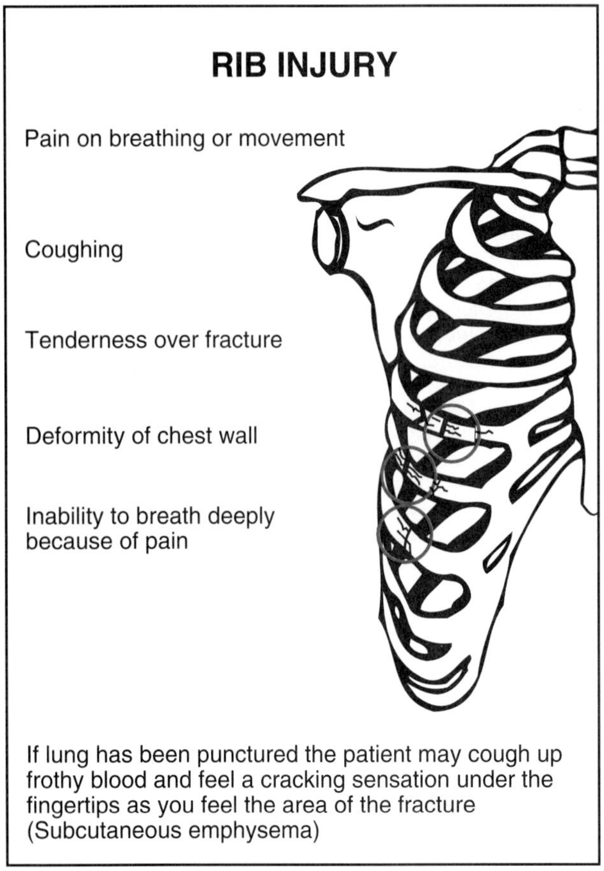

RIB INJURY

Pain on breathing or movement

Coughing

Tenderness over fracture

Deformity of chest wall

Inability to breath deeply because of pain

If lung has been punctured the patient may cough up frothy blood and feel a cracking sensation under the fingertips as you feel the area of the fracture (Subcutaneous emphysema)

Figure 36-18 Rib injury.

conjunctiva (area found under the lower eyelid). Provide emergency care for any wounds to the chest and for shock.

CARDIAC CONTUSION

Cardiac contusion is a common cardiac injury following severe blunt trauma to the chest. It occurs as the heart is violently compressed between the sternum and the spinal column. An actual bruise may occur to the heart wall. Also, the heart wall could be ruptured or a disturbance in its electrical conduction system may occur. The right ventricle, directly beneath the sternum, is the most likely area of the heart to be injured.

Signs and symptoms of cardiac contusion are chest pain or chest discomfort; signs of blunt trauma to the chest, including bruises, swelling, crepitation (grating sensation), and deformity; tachycardia (faster than normal heart rate) is very common; an irregular pulse may be noted. Prompt transport is required.

PERICARDIAL TAMPONADE

Blunt or penetrating trauma may cause bleeding into the tough fibrous sac that surrounds the heart—the pericardial sac. Since this sac cannot expand with the filling blood, the result is compression of the heart, which causes cardiac output to drop significantly and blood to back up in the venous system. This condition is known as pericardial tamponade. It is a life-threatening condition that requires prompt recognition and transport.

The most common cause of a pericardial tamponade is a penetrating wound to the heart from a knife or similar object. Bullets may also cause it, but more often a bullet wound directly to the heart causes immediate death.

The signs and symptoms of pericardial tamponade are very similar to those of tension pneumothorax, except that breath sounds remain normal in pericardial tamponade because only the heart is involved and not the lungs. Signs and symptoms will progressively worsen as the pericardial sac fills with more blood. They include jugular vein distention; signs of shock (hypoperfusion); tachycardia, with a heart rate that is extremely high in severe cases; decreased blood pressure; narrow pulse pressure (less than 30 mmHg); and weak pulses, with radial pulses disappearing or diminishing during inhalation.

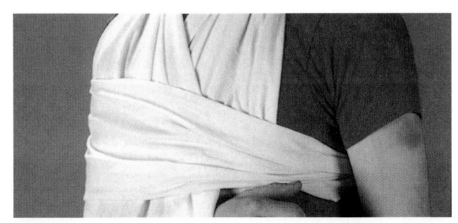

Figure 36-19 Apply a sling and swathe to stabilize the area of rib injury.

RIB INJURY

While a fractured rib is not life-threatening, it can cause life-threatening damage to other structures and organs. The most commonly fractured ribs are the third through the eighth. The most common site of fracture is on the lateral aspect of the chest. The intercostal artery or vein may be lacerated as a result of the fracture and cause bleeding into the chest cavity.

Rib fractures in children are less common because of a more resilient cartilage that does not break easily. The mechanism of injury should heighten your suspicion that chest injury may have occurred.

The most common signs and symptoms of rib injury include (Figure 36-18) pain, often excruciating, with movement and breathing; crepitation (grating sensation); tenderness upon palpation; deformity of the chest wall; inability to breathe deeply; coughing; and tachypnea (rapid breathing) that may be shallow.

If a simple rib fracture is suspected, the patient usually presents in the guarded position holding his arm over the injured site. You can use the arm to splint the injury by placing it over the injury site and applying a sling and swathe to hold it in place (Figure 36-19). The patient could also be given a pillow to hold it firmly over the injury in order to manually splint it. Do not completely wrap the chest or apply the swathe snugly. This would impede normal ventilation.

CASE STUDY FOLLOW-UP

SCENE SIZE-UP

You have been dispatched to a street corner for a man down. As you drive up to the scene, no bystanders appear to be present. It is dark outside, so you turn on the scene lights and very carefully assess for hazards. None are observed so you and your partner exit the ambulance. However, you still have your guard up. As you approach the patient, you note that he is lying in a prone position on the sidewalk. He is dressed in a heavy overcoat, and he is moaning. No visible blood is noted. You and your partner tell the patient you are emergency medical technicians and are there to help. The patient responds with a moan.

INITIAL ASSESSMENT

Because you are unaware of the mechanism of injury or nature of the illness, your partner establishes in-line spinal stabilization. You log roll the patient as a unit with spinal precautions being maintained. You ask, "Sir, are you hurt or ill?" The patient only responds with a moan. There still does not appear to be any visible injury or bleeding anywhere to the body. The airway is open and clear of any secretions or vomitus. The breathing is rapid and shallow at a rate of approximately 40 per minute. You prepare the bag-valve-mask device and instruct your partner to begin ventilating with supplemental oxygen. He kneels at the head of the patient, holding in-line stabilization with his upper legs. The radial pulse is weak and very rapid. The skin is cool, moist, and pale. You identify this patient as a high priority.

FOCUSED HISTORY AND PHYSICAL EXAM

In-line spinal stabilization is maintained by your partner as he continues to ventilate the patient with a bag-valve-mask device. The patient is still responding to verbal commands only with moans. There is no evidence of trauma to the head. The pupils are equal and reactive, but sluggish to respond. The jugular veins are flat and the trachea is mid-line. You quickly expose the chest and find what appears to be a small caliber gun shot wound to the right anterior aspect of the chest at about the third intercostal on the mid-clavicular line. A bubbly crackle is heard when the patient inhales spontaneously. You immediately place your gloved hand over the wound. You then apply the plastic wrap from the oxygen tubing over the wound and tape it on three sides.

The patient is log rolled and you closely inspect the back for an exit wound and find none. You also assess the axillary region for any other wounds to the chest. Auscultation of the lungs reveals significantly decreased breath to the right and good breath sounds on the left. There is no evidence of any wounds or trauma to the abdomen or pelvis. Palpation of the abdomen does not elicit a moan or other pain response. The extremities are quickly inspected. Pedal pulses are absent and the radial pulses are extremely weak and fast. A pinch to the extremities causes the patient to moan.

The carotid pulse is 138 per minute. The spontaneous respiratory rate is 35 and shallow. The blood pressure is 80/60 mmHg. The skin is cyanotic, pale, cool, and moist. A SAMPLE history is unobtainable.

You apply a cervical spine immobilization collar and immobilize the patient to a backboard with straps and a head immobilization device. You place the patient in the back of the ambulance and transport rapidly.

DETAILED PHYSICAL EXAM

The patient's condition is critical and unstable. Most of your time en route is devoted to an ongoing assessment, but you are able to quickly conduct a detailed physical exam to check for any injuries you might have missed in the darkness at the scene. You find no injuries other than the gunshot entrance wound.

ONGOING ASSESSMENT

En route to the hospital, the mental status remains unchanged. A nasopharyngeal airway is inserted and ventilation reassessed. Positive pressure ventilation is continued with supplemental oxygen. The pulse rate has decreased slightly to 130 per minute. The cyanosis has subsided slightly. The skin remains pale, cool, and moist. You record the vital signs.

Suddenly you notice that it is becoming extremely difficulty to ventilate the patient. The heart rate has increased to 148 per minute and the skin is becoming severely cyanotic. You immediately lift the corner of the occlusive dressing off the wound and note the sound of air escaping. Almost immediately the patient's condition improves and you replace the dressing. You contact the hospital and give a report.

Upon arrival at the hospital, you give an oral report to the physician who is waiting for you at the door. The patient is transferred to the hospital bed in the trauma room. While your partner cleans the ambulance and gathers the necessary supplies, you complete the prehospital care report. You check on the patient prior to leaving and are told by the physician that he is now in surgery. His prognosis is unknown. You clear the hospital and mark back in service.

CHAPTER REVIEW

TERMS AND CONCEPTS

You may wish to review the following terms and concepts included in this chapter.

flail segment—two or more consecutive ribs that are fractured in two or more places.
paradoxical movement—a segment of the chest wall moves inward during inhalation and outward during exhalation; see also flail segment.

pneumothorax—air in the chest cavity, outside the lungs.
sucking chest wound—an open wound to the chest that permits air to enter into the thoracic cavity.
tension pneumothorax—a condition in which the build-up of air and pressure in the thoracic cavity of the injured lung is so severe that it begins to shift to the uninjured side, resulting in compression of the heart, large vessels, and the uninjured lung.

REVIEW QUESTIONS

1. Identify and describe the two general categories of injuries to the chest.
2. List the signs and symptoms associated with major chest trauma.
3. Describe the general guidelines for emergency medical care of trauma to the chest.
4. Describe additional emergency medical care required for (a) an impaled object to the chest, (b) an open wound to the chest, and (c) a flail segment (paradoxical movement).
5. List the signs and symptoms associated with trauma to the abdomen.
6. Describe the general guidelines for emergency medical care of both open and closed abdominal injuries.
7. Describe emergency medical care for an abdominal evisceration.
8. Describe the general emergency care for injuries to the male or female genitalia.

CHAPTER 37

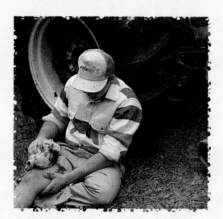

Agricultural and Industrial Emergencies

INTRODUCTION

There is some form of agricultural activity in every state in the United States. Agriculture-related accidents usually involve heavy machinery and specialized equipment, which can present unique challenges to EMT-Basics and other emergency care personnel.

Injuries that occur on a farm also occur in urban areas, since farm-type machinery is used for many applications. The equipment in many industries is similar: The pizza dough roller works on the same principles as the printing press or the agricultural combine, for example. Workers who do snow removal, construction work, and factory work also use similar machinery—and are prone to similar accidents.

OBJECTIVES

Numbered objectives are from the United States Department of Transportation 1994 EMT-Basic National Standard Curriculum. Asterisked objectives, if any, pertain to material that is supplemental to the DOT curriculum.

COGNITIVE

* Describe the general guidelines for emergency care of agricultural injuries and related industrial injuries. (p. 740)

* Identify the mechanisms of injury responsible for the majority of agricultural accidents. (p. 741)
* List the general guidelines for stabilizing and shutting down, agricultural equipment and other machinery. (pp. 741–742)
* List the common accidents/mechanisms of injury associated with various types of agricultural machinery, storage devices, and livestock. (pp. 740–746)
* List the general guidelines for industrial rescue. (p. 746)

CASE STUDY

THE DISPATCH

EMS Unit 1—proceed to the old Fenwick place—unknown medical emergency called in by a family member—time out 1300 hours.

ON ARRIVAL

Upon arrival the only thing you notice as unusual is the pickup parked in front of the house. Its engine is running. When you knock on the door, Ms. Fenwick—the granddaughter—races out past you.

"Let's go!" she commands. "Old Dad's out in the new field. Fainted or something. Old Ma is with him." She throws some blankets and a jug of water into the pickup and pulls out before you can ask a question.

You and your partner return to your vehicle and follow her. She leads you to a newly plowed field. As she slows down, you look in the near distance to see old Mr. Fenwick slumped on the ground not far from his tractor.

How would you proceed?

During this chapter, you will learn about types of accidents that commonly happen in agricultural and industrial settings. Later, we will return to the case study and put in context some of the information you learned.

RESPONSE TO AGRICULTURAL AND INDUSTRIAL EMERGENCIES

Farm accidents and industrial accidents often involve unique mechanisms of injury. The outcome of an accident involving agricultural or industrial machinery is likely to be severe trauma. This may involve a combination of open and closed musculoskeletal and soft tissue injuries—both penetrating and blunt force trauma—with crush injuries, avulsions, and amputations being common (Figures 37-1a to f).

The assessment guidelines that follow apply to trauma; however, be aware that farm accidents can also involve other problems such as near-drownings or poisonings, which will be discussed later.

ASSESSMENT AND CARE: AGRICULTURAL AND INDUSTRIAL EMERGENCIES

SCENE SIZE-UP

Before you begin any rescue at an agricultural or industrial accident, perform a scene size-up. Make sure you will not be exposed to gases, fumes, chemicals, unstable equipment, or livestock. If necessary, wait for fire personnel or specialized hazardous materials teams to control the scene. If there has been a tractor accident, call for the fire department to handle fire

INJURIES SUSTAINED FROM FARM MACHINERY

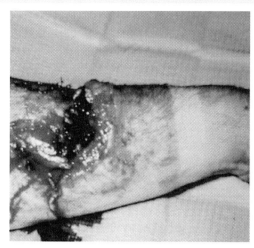

Figure 37-1a   Arm injured in a PTO (power takeoff) shaft.

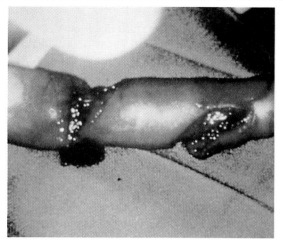

Figure 37-1b   Arm injured in an auger.

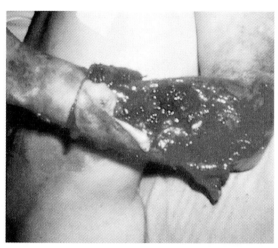

Figure 37-1c   Arm injured in an auger.

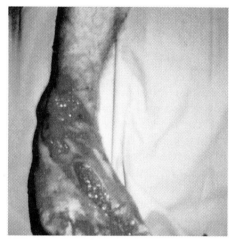

Figure 37-1d   Foot injured in an auger.

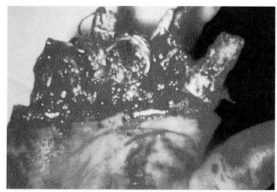

Figure 37-1e   Hand injured in snapping rolls.

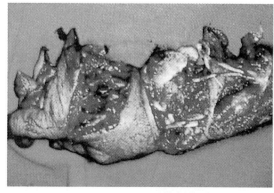

Figure 37-1f   Hand and arm injured in a hay baler.

that may ignite from spilled fuel and hot hydraulic fluid. The EMS team will extricate and treat the patient.

Note that a scene is not safe until machinery is stabilized and shut down and other hazards such as leaking fuel have been controlled. If rescue must be conducted in an agricultural storage area, *do not attempt rescue alone,* and all rescuers must wear the appropriate personal protective equipment, including a self-contained breathing apparatus (SCBA) and lifeline.

INITIAL ASSESSMENT

When the scene is safe, perform an initial assessment. Bear in mind that the tremendous kinetic energy involved in agricultural machinery can cause extensive injuries. Always assume spinal injury, and establish manual in-line stabilization on first contact with the patient. Assess the patient's mental status. Manage any life-threatening problems with the airway, breathing, and circulation. Make a priority decision for further care and transport.

FOCUSED HISTORY AND PHYSICAL EXAM

After you have identified and cared for life-threatening injuries, perform a focused history and physical exam. If the mechanism of injury is significant or the patient has an altered mental status, perform a rapid trauma assessment, checking for DCAP-BTLS. Bear in mind that chest injuries—including pneumothorax and sucking chest wounds—and abdominal injuries are common with accidents involving farm and industrial machinery, as are bone and joint injuries to the extremities. Record baseline vital signs and gather the SAMPLE history from the patient or bystanders. Obtain as much information as possible about events leading to the injury. If there were no witnesses to the accident, this information may have to be surmised from the mechanism of injury as determined from your scene size-up.

EMERGENCY MEDICAL CARE

In general, provide emergency care to a patient injured in a farm accident in the same way you would treat any patient with similar injuries:

1. *Establish a patent airway.* While maintaining manual in-line stabilization, use a jaw-thrust maneuver to open the airway. Suction the airway and insert an airway adjunct if appropriate. Consider calling for ALS back-up, especially if there has been trauma to the face or neck that will require advanced airway procedures.
2. *Administer oxygen by nonrebreather mask at 15 lpm if breathing is adequate; if breathing is inad-*
equate, initiate positive pressure ventilation with supplemental oxygen.
3. *Control severe bleeding.* (If pressure from the farm or industrial equipment is tamponading bleeding by the pressure it places on the injury, consider leaving the equipment in place and transporting it with the patient.) Be prepared to initiate CPR and consider AED as soon as available if the patient becomes pulseless.
4. *If the patient was exposed to chemicals or manure, remove all exposed clothing and flush the patient with copious amounts of water before transport.* Check for burns from spilled engine coolants, transmission fluid, hydraulic fluid, and battery acid.
5. *Preserve all avulsed body parts,* however mangled their appearance, and transport them with the patient.
6. *Stabilize all injuries.* Splint and immobilize bone or joint injuries. (If the patient is a high priority for transport, splinting may need to be done en route.)
7. *Immobilize the patient to a long backboard.*
8. *Treat for shock and transport.*

DETAILED PHYSICAL EXAM AND ONGOING ASSESSMENT

If time and the patient's condition permit, perform a detailed physical exam en route. Perform an ongoing assessment, repeating the initial assessment and rapid trauma exam, monitoring vital signs, and checking interventions. Be prepared to adjust care if the patient's condition begins to deteriorate.

CHARACTERISTICS OF AGRICULTURAL ACCIDENTS

Farmers work long hours, often seven days a week. During that time they are exposed to heat, cold, and unstable weather conditions, as well as excessive noise and vibration. They often use old equipment because of the tremendous expense of replacement, and many accidents occur during maintenance and repair of these complicated machines (Figures 37-2a to d).

These factors and a number of others contribute to making agricultural accidents most often the cause of serious injury:

- Many farmers do not use personal protective equipment.
- When a worker becomes entangled in equipment, lengthy extrication is often required, which aggravates and increases the severity of injuries.

FARM EQUIPMENT

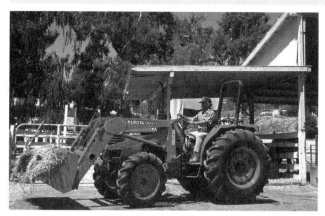

Figure 37-2a   Tractor: front loader. (Kubota Tractor Corporation)

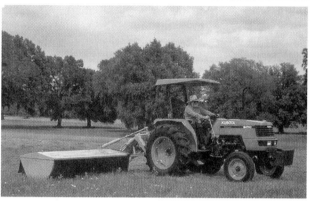

Figure 37-2b   Tractor with high residue shredder. (Kubota Tractor Corporation)

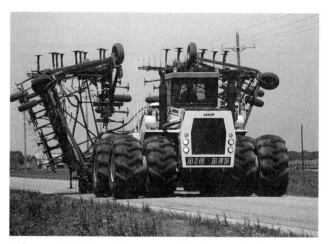

Figure 37-2c   Tractor with 72-inch planter. (Grant Heilman/Grant Heilman Photography, Inc.)

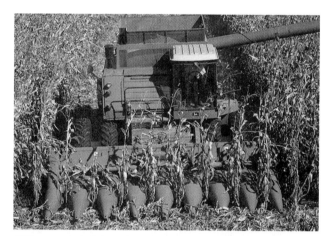

Figure 37-2d   Combine with 8-row head. (Arthur C. Smith III/Grant Heilman Photography, Inc.)

- Since many farmers work alone in remote areas, they may not be missed for hours. Many die from injuries that would not have been fatal if they had been discovered in time.
- There usually is no phone on the scene. In addition, rural areas often have no 911 service and no central dispatch.
- Long transport times contribute to the severity of injuries. Farms in rural areas can be long distances from hospitals.

MECHANISMS OF INJURY

The mechanisms of injury commonly involved in agricultural equipment accidents include:

- *Pinch points*—two objects meet to cause a pinching or pulling action
- *Wrap points*—an aggressive component of machinery moves in a circular motion
- *Shear points*—two objects move close enough together to cause a cutting action

- *Crush points*—two large objects come together to cause a crushing action
  Stored energy—hazards remain after the machinery is shut down

Agricultural accidents most often occur when the patient was in the process of maintaining or repairing a piece of equipment. Most trauma involves the hands and arms. Common types of injuries are abrasions, lacerations, contusions, punctures, sprains, strains, and fractures, eye injuries, concussion, avulsions, amputations, burns, and bites from farm animals.

STABILIZING AND SHUTTING DOWN AGRICULTURAL EQUIPMENT

GENERAL GUIDELINES

Before a patient can be extricated from agricultural equipment, the machine needs to be stabilized and shut down. To stabilize agricultural equipment, block or chock the wheels, set the parking brake, or tie it to another vehicle. Once stabilized, shut it down using the following procedure:

1. Enter the cab or climb onto the operator's platform. Locate the ignition switch or the key and throttle. *If you have any concern that you have not located the correct controls, do not touch them. Wait for help.*
2. Slow the engine down with the throttle, and then switch off the key. If the engine runs on diesel fuel, you may need to use a fuel or air shut-off lever instead of a key.
3. If you cannot shut down the engine from the cab or operator's platform, try the shut-off valve at the bottom of the fuel tank.
4. If that does not work, try using vise-grip pliers to clamp the fuel line shut. (The fuel line is a single metal or rubber pipe about one-half inch in diameter.)
5. If the patient is in a life-threatening situation and all other attempts to shut down the engine have failed, then discharge a twenty-pound CO_2 fire extinguisher into the air intake. (Warning: This technique can cause extensive damage to the engine.)

TRACTORS

Before you attempt to rescue a patient from a tractor accident, stabilize the tractor and shut down the engine. Tractor engines can be fueled by gasoline, diesel, or propane. Fuel leaks, fires, and explosions are common. Note also that many fatal farm injuries result from a tractor turning over backward or rolling to the side.

To stabilize a tractor, even when it is upright, lock up the rear wheels with two one-ton cable hoists (come-alongs) and three chains:

1. Wrap one chain around the rear tire and through the high slot in the rim.
2. Wrap the second chain around the same tire and through the low slot in the rim.
3. Attach the third chain to the front of the tractor and stretch it to the hoist.
4. Attach the other hoist to the two rear chains. If the tractor does not have slots in the rims, stretch the hoist and chains across the rear tire to a strong point on the rear of the tractor. Make sure you do not lift the secure tire off the ground during hoisting.

To extricate the patient, try the simplest method first. For example, you might be able to remove soil from beneath the patient with a shovel to create enough space to free the patient. If the steering wheel is trapping the patient's arm to the ground, cut

the steering wheel. In some cases, you might have to lift the tractor from the patient.

To lift a tractor:

1. Build a cross-crib capable of supporting the tractor. The crib should be as wide as possible, and the crib box should not be taller than it is wide. The crib should come to within about two inches of the axle or platform where you plan to lift.
2. Place the cribbing and lifting devices on a firm, solid surface. If the tractor is on soft ground or blacktop, use quarter-inch tread plates or similar equipment.
3. Place a steel plate on the cribbing to provide structural strength to the lifting system.
4. Place one or two high-pressure airbags on the steel plate, and then inflate them to lift the tractor. You may also place airbags on either side of the rear wheel, inflate them simultaneously to place pressure against the tire, and then rest the tractor on the cribbing until another airbag is placed under the tire.
5. If you do not have airbags, use power spreaders or hydraulic rams, hand-powered hydraulic jacks, or manual jacks, anchoring them against the steel plate.
6. Use cranes, wreckers, or boom trucks to lift extremely large tractors.

Any time you lift or remove an overturned tractor from an operator, continuously monitor the center of gravity. Watch for unstable conditions, such as changes of the angle between the lifting surface of the tool and the tractor or sinking of the tractor on the opposite side. Always lock the wheels in position before lifting the tractor.

To perform the lift as safely as possible, one rescuer should give lifting instructions while the others carry out the lift. If you use more than one lifting device, use extra care in coordinating the lift to keep the load from shifting. Constantly monitor the patient to make sure that the portion being lifted is moving properly and that another part is not putting more pressure on the patient.

POWER TAKEOFF SHAFTS

The power takeoff (PTO) shaft is a specially designed shaft that connects the tractor's engine to other agricultural implements, such as mowers, corn pickers, forage harvesters, and augers.

PTO-related accidents occur when clothing gets caught in the spinning shaft and pulls the worker in. Arms and legs may be amputated. The worker's body also may be wrapped around the shaft. Because of the energy involved, injuries to the patient can be very traumatic and may require rapid treatment and transport. Aggressively control bleeding with universal or multi-trauma dressings at the site of an avulsion or amputation. If advanced care is available (air transport, ground paramedics), call for it as soon as possible.

To free the patient, in some cases, find the end of the wrap where the clothing is only a layer thick. Use rescue knives to cut at that point. If you cannot free the patient by cutting the clothing, you will need to remove the PTO shaft.

1. Place a fire pry bar at least 42 inches long into the implement side of the PTO shaft. (Some PTOs will free-wheel in either direction when the power is shut off.)
2. Uncouple the shaft. Slide it apart. If necessary, transport it with the patient to the hospital.
3. If you cannot uncouple the shaft, cut it with a power saw, portable band saw, gasoline circular saw, or hack saw. Lock the PTO shaft in place with a fire pry bar through the universal joint on both ends before you begin to cut.

COMBINES

The combine is a complex machine made of many parts joined by welding, screws, nuts, bolts, and rivets. It is assembled with multiple augers, shafts, belts, pulleys, roller chains, and sprockets. However, instead of becoming overwhelmed by the complexity of it, look at the single part in which the patient is entrapped.

A common source of injury is the auger, which is used to move the threshed, separated, and cleaned grain from the cleaning shoe to the wagon for transport. The auger is the rotating part of a screw conveyor. It can pull in victims with extreme force, often causing complete amputations of extremities. Other sources of injury are the heads, which have oscillating cutting bars; reels, with hardened steel tines that can impale the patient; and snapping rollers, which cause severe crushing injuries.

To extricate a patient, identify the mechanism of injury and then follow these guidelines:

1. Never use the self-reversing feature on a combine to remove a trapped patient.
2. Always remember that stored energy can cause significant injury as you release parts of agricultural equipment. Use pry bars or other tools to prevent motion.
3. Spread snapping rollers on older equipment with power rescue tools, hand rescue tools, wooden wedges, and airbags. The rollers on newer equipment cannot be spread with conventional rescue tools.
4. Always lock the hydraulic system. A pipe or bar near the hydraulic cylinder will lock the header.

5. Just behind the combine header is a coupling device that attaches the head to the drive mechanism. It may be a shaft with a pin in it or a set of flat gears wrapped with a roller chain. Remove this device.
6. If you have to use an oxyacetylene torch to cut parts of the combine, reduce the risk of fire. Before cutting, wash down the combine and the surrounding soil with water. Then flush the inside of the combine header, feeder house, and main combine.
7. If the patient is trapped in the auger, disconnect the auger drive. Use a large pipe wrench on the shaft to prevent stored energy from reversing the auger.
8. Entanglement in an auger is usually too severe to handle in the field. If an auger has caused an avulsion, *do not try to disentangle the patient.* Instead, cut the auger free and transport it with the patient. Avoid excessive vibration or movement during cutting, and try to cut at a spot weld.

CORN PICKERS

A corn picker removes the kernels from the cob as it is picked. It may be mounted on a tractor, pulled behind a tractor, or it may be self-propelled. Corn pickers use a system of rollers, chains, belts, and blades to remove the ears from stalks and to remove the leafy cover of the corn.

Most injuries from corn pickers involve entrapment of the hands and arms and range from limited trauma to complete amputation. Some injuries can be fatal. When dealing with corn pickers, follow these steps:

1. Spread the snapping rolls with a portable power kit (two wooden wedges combined with two small hydraulic wedges). Insert one wedge at the top of the rolls, and the other below. Equip the bottom wedge with a rope so you can pull it through from above. You can also use high-pressure airbags or power hydraulic tools with the wooden wedges.
2. Once the rolls have been released, take great care to avoid an uncontrolled release of the springs. Release the tension by adjusting the nuts of bolts. Then remove the bolts that fasten the bearing housing to the side of the husking bed housing.
3. To remove the husking bed, take the machine apart with wrenches or cut the bolt heads with an air chisel.

HAY BALERS

Balers are designed to bale hay, straw, corn stalks, and other forage into uniform shapes. Either oscillating forks or a short auger move forage into the bale chamber. On round balers, a series of flat belts rotate around the perimeter of the bale chamber to form the bale one thin layer at a time. The pick-up assembly is a series of hardened metal tines that rotate on a shaft and rake the cut forage into a header.

A worker can be picked up and pulled into the header assembly. He can be entrapped up to the shoulders, and tines can cause penetrating wounds in the abdomen and chest. Avulsions of varying degrees can be caused by the cross auger.

To rescue a patient entrapped in a hay baler, follow the guidelines below. If the tailgate is open when you arrive, lock the tailgate from falling before you attempt the rescue. Some balers have a mechanical locking device or a hydraulic valve used as a safety lock. Then:

1. Disassemble the tines, which are held by one or two small bolts.
2. If the patient is entrapped in the cross auger, first try to loosen the drive belts driving the auger. Use a pipe wrench to hold onto the input shaft as you cut the chain or belt to prevent motion. Release stored energy slowly by hand.
3. If you cannot loosen the drive belts, raise the auger with power rescue tools, an airbag, power hydraulic tools, or a bottle jack and cribbing.
4. Never use oxyacetylene torches on a hay baler. Balers are filled with fine dust that can ignite with a single spark.
5. If the patient is entrapped in a set of smooth rollers, remove the mounting bolts on both ends of the housing to remove the bearings.

AGRICULTURAL STORAGE DEVICES

Suffocation and inhalation of toxic gases can occur in accidents involving grain tanks, silos, and manure storage areas and structures.

GRAIN TANKS

Usually loaded by augers, grain bins come in a variety of sizes. Workers who enter one to get grain flowing can be buried with grain in seconds. Because most bins unload from the center, most patients are found in the middle of the bin.

The temperature of stored grains is low, even in summer. A patient's resulting hypothermia may prolong survival. For that reason, always assume a patient is alive, even if the patient has been trapped for a long period of time.

Note: Never enter the structure without the help of other rescuers, without being tied to a safety lifeline, and without wearing a disposable mechanical filter respirator rated for dust particles. Call for extrication teams and fire personnel immediately.

To rescue a patient from a grain tank:

1. Turn off electric power to the structure as soon as possible. Keep fans working until the actual extrication begins, since they may deliver more air to the patient but could hamper rescue operations.
2. Make sure the fire department has a charged fire line available as the side of the bin is breached.
3. Cut an 18-inch triangle in the side wall. Make it as high as you can but still below the surface of the grain. Do not open the triangle until you have cut another hole on the opposite wall. Then open the holes at the same time to allow grain to flow out of the bin evenly. This will help prevent structural failure. Cut additional holes as needed. Holes *must* be cut in the middle of the bin sheets, avoiding bolts, seams, and stiffeners. Do not use augers, openings in doors, or doors to unload the grain bin.
4. As soon as the patient is exposed, secure him with a lifeline. If you do not, the patient will flow with the grain.
5. Use whatever is available to shore the grain away from the trapped patient, such as plywood, metal sheets, spine boards, or a 55-gallon drum.
6. Your top priority for patient care is airway management. The airway may be filled with grain, so aggressive suctioning and clearing may be necessary. Suction and clear the patient's airway in the bin while the extrication team prepares the patient for removal.
7. Immobilize the spine before you try to remove the patient from the grain bin.
8. Remove as much grain from around the patient as possible before extrication. Pulling against the force of the grain can cause further injury.

SILOS

Silos are used to store chopped grain or hay as feed for livestock. They may be constructed of clay blocks, concrete blocks, steel sheets, poured concrete, or steel glass-lined sheets.

When crops are stored in silos, gases are formed by natural chemical fermentation. Fermenting crops can release high levels of carbon monoxide, methane, and oxides of nitrogen ("silo gas"). Red-brown to yellow-green in color, silo gas smells like household bleach and will kill within minutes in high concentrations.

Because it is heavier than air, silo gas flows down the side chute and out the open silo door. People working around the base of the silo or in the feed room or adjacent barn can be exposed to dangerous levels of silo gas.

The severity of injury to the patient depends on the length of exposure. Low concentrations of silo gas can irritate the nose, throat, airways, and lungs. Common reactions to mild exposure include eye irritation, cough, labored breathing, fatigue, nausea, vomiting, cyanosis, and dizziness or sleepiness.

The presence of silo gas may be recognized by the following signs:

- Bleach-like odor
- Yellowish or reddish vapor hovering over the product
- Stains of red, yellow, or brown on the product or other surfaces touched by the gas
- Dead birds or insects near the silo
- Nearby livestock with signs of illness

When rescuing a patient exposed to silo gas, follow these guidelines:

1. Put on a self-contained breathing apparatus (SCBA) before you enter the silo. All rescuers working around or in the silo should be wearing one, even if there are no immediate signs of the gas.
2. If the patient is breathing, immediately administer oxygen by way of a self-contained breathing apparatus (SCBA) and a connecting tube. (If the patient is no longer near the silo, oxygen can be administered in the usual way by nonrebreather mask.)
3. If rescue will be delayed, run the silo blower to purge the air in the silo.
4. All patients exposed to silo gas must be transported to a hospital for further care. Complications such as severe pulmonary edema can develop up to 12 hours after the incident.

MANURE STORAGE

Large livestock facilities handle manure by flushing down the confinement buildings with water. The liquid is then sent to an open pond for storage. In some cases, liquid manure is stored in a structure similar to a silo. There are two potential injuries from liquid manure: drowning and inhaling toxic fumes. (The liquid manure releases ammonia, carbon monoxide, carbon dioxide, methane, and hydrogen sulfide.)

Agitation of a manure pit can cause the sudden release of hydrogen sulfide. Signs and symptoms of hydrogen sulfide intoxication may include cough, irritation of mucous membranes, nausea, and pulmonary edema. High concentrations can cause respiratory paralysis and sudden collapse.

In rescuing a patient exposed to manure:

1. Put on a self-contained breathing apparatus (SCBA) and a lifeline before you begin rescue. All rescue personnel who enter a livestock confinement house should be wearing SCBAs and lifelines.
2. Treat the patient who has suffered immersion in liquid manure as you would a near-drowning in water. If the patient is breathing at all, immediately administer a self-contained breathing apparatus (SCBA). Use a connecting tube to deliver supplemental oxygen.
3. Remove the patient's clothing and flush the patient's body with water. Green soap should be used to clean everyone who had contact with the manure.
4. Transport the patient to the hospital. Be sure that materials contaminated with manure are not put in the ambulance or helicopter, since fumes can overcome the crew.

AGRICULTURAL CHEMICALS

Thousands of pesticides are currently used in agriculture to control insects, plant growth, fungi, rodents, birds, and bacteria. Pesticide poisoning may be overlooked because signs and symptoms are similar to those of heat exhaustion, food poisoning, asthma, congestive heart failure, smoke inhalation, influenza, or other illnesses. Common symptoms include excessive tearing, drooling, abdominal cramps, bowel movement, cough, wheezing, bizarre behavior, and seizures.

When farm workers do not wear personal protective equipment such as eyewear or fail to wash properly, pesticides can enter the body through the eyes and skin, as well as through inhalation and swallowing. If you suspect exposure or poisoning, follow these guidelines:

1. Put on protective clothing before entering the scene. If appropriate, call a specialized hazardous materials team for decontamination.
2. If you know that a patient has been exposed to a particular pesticide, check the label for instructions and precautions. If possible, take the label to the hospital with you.
3. Remove all the patient's clothing and flush the patient with water. Follow appropriate decontamination procedures.

INJURIES FROM LIVESTOCK

Many agricultural injuries are caused by livestock or by tasks involving livestock production. Common types of trauma include soft-tissue injuries, concussions, sprains and fractures, and spinal, chest, and abdominal injuries. Common mechanisms of injury include falling on slippery floors and getting bitten, thrown, knocked down, stepped on, kicked, or punctured by an animal.

Treat a patient for a livestock injury as you would any patient with a similar injury. However, remember never to enter a livestock building or open lot until all animals are secure. Also, if animal feces are on the wound, flush the injury site before dressing and bandaging.

INDUSTRIAL RESCUE

While some industrial injuries may seem complex, you can prepare for emergency care by observing what goes on around you. The equipment in many industries is similar—the pizza dough roller works on the same principles as the printing press or the agricultural combine, for example.

For the greatest effectiveness, learn the basic components of machinery and the working principles of each component, including pulleys, belts, rotating shafts, bearings, and augers. Apply that understanding to specific pieces of machinery in emergency situations.

In any industrial rescue, follow these guidelines:

- If you are not familiar with the company's operations, check with staff to determine potential hazards at the scene. Make sure all hazards are controlled before you approach the patient.
- Never assume any machine is locked and secured. Verify with company officials that all valves, switches, and levers that allow a machine to operate have been padlocked to the off position.
- If the patient is in a confined space, or if he has been injured by an airborne or spilled agent, wait for specialized personnel or hazardous materials teams to arrive and decontaminate the scene and the patient.

CASE STUDY FOLLOW-UP

SCENE SIZE-UP

You have been dispatched to the farm of a 70-year-old male, Mr. Charles Fenwick, who is experiencing an unknown medical emergency. You follow his granddaughter to the scene of the emergency at the edge of a newly plowed field. Mr. Fenwick is sitting on the ground, leaning on his wife's shoulder.

As you approach the patient, your partner goes to the tractor, which is several yards away. He surveys the scene for hazards and checks to be sure the tractor engine is turned off.

It is not yet clear whether the patient is suffering from a medical problem or trauma.

INITIAL ASSESSMENT

Once you decide the scene is safe, you kneel beside the patient and ask: "Are you okay?" "Not as okay as I'd like," he responds. Mental status and airway seem adequate. "Did you fall from the tractor?" you ask. "No, no," he coughs and motions with his hands. "I got down. Dizzy." Mrs. Fenwick tells you her husband told her he felt dizzy and nauseated. You conclude that his problem is medical.

You notice that the patient has labored breathing. His skin is pale, cool, and dry. You administer oxygen via nonrebreather mask at 15 lpm.

FOCUSED HISTORY AND PHYSICAL EXAM

You ask Mr. Fenwick if he has any pain. He shakes his head no. His wife tells you that he didn't eat his lunch. When his granddaughter also tells you that he was working by the silo, you begin to suspect inhalation of noxious gases.

"Did you smell anything unusual while you worked there?" you ask the patient. Mr. Fenwick nods his head. "Smells like bleach over there, I noticed," says the granddaughter. "Anyone else working around there today?" you ask. Mr. Fenwick says no. You alert his wife and granddaughter to keep everyone away from the silo until it can be checked out.

As you perform a rapid medical assessment, Mrs. Fenwick tells you the patient had a "small heart attack" two years ago. He is not taking medication of any kind and has no current illnesses or allergies. His last oral intake was at breakfast nearly 8 hours ago.

While your partner prepares Mr. Fenwick for transport, you obtain a baseline set of vitals, including respiratory rate, heart rate, and blood pressure—which are all above normal.

You are not sure whether Mr. Fenwick's problem has resulted from inhaling silo gas, from his heart problem, or simply from hunger because he skipped lunch. However, the oxygen you are administering and transport to the hospital are appropriate for any of these possibilities.

DETAILED PHYSICAL EXAM

You decide that during the 35 minutes it will take you to get to the hospital, you will perform a detailed physical exam to be sure you have not overlooked any signs of trauma and to see if you can discover any additional information related to the patient's problem. You complete the exam but make no additional pertinent findings.

ONGOING ASSESSMENT

En route to the hospital, you perform an ongoing assessment every 15 minutes. You repeat the initial assessment and the rapid medical assessment, monitor vitals, and check to be sure that the nonrebreather mask is placed correctly and oxygen is flowing adequately. Throughout the trip the patient remains responsive. Breathing appears to be adequate. There are no significant changes in his condition.

You also contact dispatch to request a hazmat expert to check out the silo at the Fenwick farm.

After you deliver the patient to the emergency department personnel, you complete a prehospital care report and prepare the ambulance for your next call.

Two weeks later you meet Mr. Fenwick in town. He appears well. He tells you that "Sure enough, it was silo gas." He adds happily that he won't have the problem any more, because his granddaughter and her husband have decided to take over the farm. They are working to improve the silo's ventilation system.

CHAPTER REVIEW

REVIEW QUESTIONS

1. Briefly describe sizing up the scene of an agricultural accident. Describe what you can do to ensure scene safety.
2. List the specialized personnel that may be necessary to control the scene of an agricultural accident.
3. List mechanisms of injury associated with agricultural machinery.
4. List the general guidelines for stabilizing and shutting down agricultural equipment.
5. Describe accidents/mechanisms of injury associated with tractors, power takeoff shafts (PTOs), combines, corn pickers, and hay balers.
6. Describe accidents/mechanisms of injury associated with storage areas and storage devices.
7. Describe accidents/mechanisms of injury associated with farm animals.
8. List the general guidelines that should be applied to rescue in an industrial setting.

CHAPTER 38

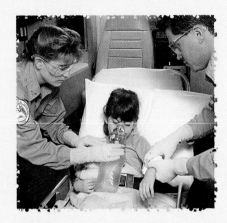

Infants and Children

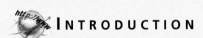 INTRODUCTION

Nearly 45,000 children die in the United States each year. Approximately one in four children will sustain an injury during their childhood that will require medical attention. Trauma is the leading cause of fatal injuries in children under the age of 14, particularly motor vehicle crashes, drownings, burns, poisonings, and falls. Of medical problems, respiratory problems are the most serious.

If asked, experienced EMS providers would probably concur that dealing with infants and children is one of the most (if not the most) stressful situations they encounter during their EMS career. This is mainly due to the relative infrequency of dealing with pediatric patients, the particularities of assessment and treatment, and having to deal with the emotions of the pediatric patient, the distressed parents, and probably the feelings they have themselves. Despite this, you must be able to prevent the emotions you experience from interfering with the task at hand: assessing and treating the young patient.

While your assessment approach to the ill or injured child is somewhat different from your approach to an adult, the basic treatment goals are the same.

OBJECTIVES

Numbered objectives are from the United States Department of Transportation 1994 EMT-Basic National Standard Curriculum. Asterisked objectives, if any, pertain to material that is supplemental to the DOT curriculum.

COGNITIVE

6-1.1 Identify the developmental considerations for the following age groups (pp. 750–752):
– infants
– toddlers
– pre-school
– school age
– adolescent

6-1.2 Describe the differences in anatomy and physiology of the infant, child, and adult patient. (pp. 752–754)

6-1.3 Differentiate the response of the ill or injured infant or child from that of an adult. (pp. 751–752)

6-1.4 Indicate various causes of respiratory emergencies. (pp. 754–755)

6-1.5 Differentiate between respiratory distress and respiratory failure. (pp. 754–755)

6-1.6 List the steps in the management of foreign body airway obstruction. (pp. 762–764)

6-1.7 Summarize emergency medical care strategies for respiratory distress and respiratory failure. (pp. 759–767)

6-1.8 Identify the signs and symptoms of shock (hypoperfusion) in the infant and child patient. (pp. 771–772)

6-1.9 Describe the method of determining end organ perfusion in the infant and child patient. (p. 757)

6-1.10 State the usual causes of cardiac arrest in infants and children versus adults. (p. 754)

6-1.11 List the common causes of seizures in the infant and child patient. (p. 768)

6-1.12 Describe the management of seizures in the infant and child patient. (p. 768)

6-1.13 Differentiate between the injury patterns in adults, infants, and children. (p. 776)

6-1.14 Discuss the field management of the infant and child trauma patient. (pp. 776–778)

6-1.15 Summarize the indicators of possible child abuse and neglect. (p. 778)

6-1.16 Describe the medical legal responsibilities in suspected child abuse. (p. 780)

6-1.17 Recognize the need for EMT-Basic debriefing following a difficult infant or child transport. (pp. 775, 780)

AFFECTIVE

6-1.18 Explain the rationale for having knowledge and skills appropriate for dealing with the infant and child patient. (pp. 750–751)

6-1.19 Attend to the feelings of the family when dealing with an ill or injured infant or child. (p. 750)

6-1.20 Understand the provider's own response (emotional) to caring for infants or children. (pp. 775, 780)

PSYCHOMOTOR

6-1.21 Demonstrate the techniques of foreign body airway obstruction removal in the infant.

6-1.22 Demonstrate the techniques of foreign body airway obstruction removal in the child.

6-1.23 Demonstrate the assessment of the infant and child.

6-1.24 Demonstrate bag-valve-mask artificial ventilations for the infant.

6-1.25 Demonstrate bag-valve-mask artificial ventilations for the child.

6-1.26 Demonstrate oxygen delivery for the infant and child.

CASE STUDY

THE DISPATCH

EMS Unit 101—respond to 24313 South Avenue for an 11-month-old infant—unknown medical emergency. Time out is 1651 hours.

ON ARRIVAL

As you turn onto the busy street, you see a man frantically waving at you and pointing to the residence. You position your ambulance in front of the house, out of traffic flow. The man, who you assume to be the infant's father, is almost in tears as he says to you "Oh god—please hurry, something is wrong with Jason. I don't think he's breathing." Almost simultaneously, the mother bursts out of the front door running toward you, carrying an infant in her arms. She runs to you, crying, and thrusts the infant into your arms. Every fiber in your body tightens as you realize the infant is blue, limp, and not breathing.

How would you proceed to assess and care for this patient?

During this chapter you will learn about special assessment and emergency care considerations when dealing with infants and children. Later, we will return to the case and apply the procedures learned.

DEALING WITH CAREGIVERS

When a child is critically ill or injured, you may have more than one person to care for. The parent or other caregiver may also need attention. Some caregivers are calm, cooperative, and even helpful (especially if they are experienced). Others may be perceived by the EMT-B as a hindrance. It is not uncommon for a caregiver to be upset, to cry, to blame himself, or to get mad at someone—even you. You need to listen carefully to these feelings and remain nonjudgmental. While taking the history and inquiring about the circumstances of the event, let caregivers verbalize their emotions. Conclude with something brief and supportive like, "Thanks for telling me this. We'll do the very best we can for Susie." Furthermore, remember that calm, supportive interaction with the child's family is in the child's best interest: Calm caregivers = calm child; agitated caregivers = agitated child.

What emotionally distressed caregivers most need to see from you is that you are competent, calm, and confident. Do not allow yourself to display doubt or indecision, as this will certainly reduce their confidence in you.

In addition to the guilt, anger, concern, and apprehension that caregivers may be feeling, be aware that caregivers may not understand emergency medical procedures. Keep the caregiver informed as to what you are doing and on the condition of the child. Usually it is best to keep your language jargon-free, but use your judgment. Some caregivers, especially if they are professionals or highly educated, may feel more reassured if you use technical terminology. Also, do not lie to the caregiver. If the child is very seriously injured, do not say "Everything will be OK." This type of false reassurance is not only unethical, it will certainly make matters worse when the true condition of the child is revealed.

You will probably need to question the caregivers and other witnesses to get a history of the incident. Remember to ask them how their child normally acts and whether a particular characteristic you may discover during assessment is normal for this child. While caregivers typically don't have medical training, they are experts on what is normal for their child; listen to what they say. If possible, enlist their help in treating their child—allowing them to hold the child, when appropriate, or assist in administering oxygen. This approach allows the caregivers to feel that they are participants in their child's care, and not just bystanders.

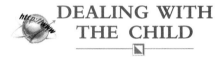 ## DEALING WITH THE CHILD

DEVELOPMENTAL CHARACTERISTICS

What you can expect from a pediatric patient depends to some degree on age. Many growth and development considerations come into play. Children can be classified in the following age groups:

Neonate refers to the first 4 weeks of life.
Infant refers to a child up to 12 months.
Toddler refers to a child 1 year to 3 years of age.
Preschooler refers to a child between the ages of 3 and 6.
School age usually refers to a child between 6 and 12 years of age.
Adolescent refers to a person between 12 and 18 years of age.

The reason for becoming familiar with this classification is simple. Each age group has different emotional and physical characteristics that may complicate your assessment and treatment. Some characteristics are common within each age group. Knowing these characteristics will enable you to develop a strategy for assessment.

Be aware, however, of one finding that is difficult to assess in most of these age groups: pain. Young children often lack the body awareness and vocabulary to describe the exact location and nature of the pain they are experiencing. Pain, especially when accompanied by bleeding, is usually so frightening that they cannot separate the emotional component from the physical. Ask the caregivers, if possible, how the child usually responds to pain in order to get some idea of how typical the reactions are. It is important to realize that all patients feel pain, even the neonate and young infant. Therefore, you must be considerate when providing emergency care to all age groups when pain is or may be involved.

NEONATES (0-4 WEEKS)

Newborn babies are totally dependent upon others for their survival. While neonates are a sub-group of infants, it is important to recognize the first 4 weeks of life as a very different time as far as growth and development are concerned. Birth defects (or congenital anomalies) and unintentional injuries are common causes of emergencies in this age group. However, neonates typically do not present any special assessment challenges.

INFANTS (0-1 YEAR)

Up to 6 months, babies will usually let you undress them, lay them on a warm, flat surface, and touch them with warm hands and equipment (stethoscope, splints, and so on). Infants can recognize their caregiver's face and voice and are emotionally tied to that person. Older infants will be distressed and almost always cry if separated from their caregiver. Complete your scene size-up and initial assessment as thoroughly as possible while you view the infant from across the room. Then, if possible, allow a familiar person to hold the baby while you complete your examination. Your assessment should start with the feet or the trunk and end with the head. Initial stimulation around the highly sensory area of the face will frighten infants and small children.

TODDLERS (1-3 YEARS)

Toddlers may be more challenging to assess than infants and neonates. They have numerous "do not like . . ." considerations which will challenge your skills:

- They do not like to be touched, so limit your touch to necessary assessment and management needs.
- They do not like to be separated from their caregiver. If possible, the caregiver should be present and in view of the toddler at all times.
- They do not like having their clothing removed. You should therefore remove (as necessary), examine, and replace. (It's a good idea to enlist the help of the caregivers in this).
- They do not like having an oxygen mask over their face. To them it is frightening and noisy, and they will resist it. (Alternative methods of oxygen administration are offered later in this chapter).

- They do not like needles, they fear pain, and may actually believe that the injury or illness they have is some form of punishment. It is not uncommon to have an injured, crying child apologize for being hurt.

Remain calm, speak soothingly, and try to distract the child with a favorite toy or somehow engage his interest. Decide which parts of the physical assessment are essential and get through them as best as you can. Also, try using a toe-to-head or trunk-to-head approach when performing your physical exam for the stable toddler. Since this group is often reliant on security objects such as a stuffed toy or blanket, try to allow the toddler to take this object with him.

PRESCHOOLERS (3-6 YEARS)

This age group has concrete thinking and interprets literally what they hear. At the same time, they have vivid imaginations and are able to dramatize events. They still believe that an illness or injury is their own fault and will view it as punishment. They are modest, resisting your attempt to unclothe them for assessment. While their vocabulary is larger, they may still confuse common words. You should explain medical procedures slowly and in simple terms they can understand: "Now I'm going to press on your tummy to see if everything's okay. Tell me if it hurts." or "Now I'm going to shine my light in your eyes." Allow the child to see your equipment in full view before you use it, if possible, and let the child touch the stethoscope or other equipment. Put it first on the child's leg or the caregiver's hand so that the preschooler can see it is not threatening. If you use a stethoscope with a rubber ring on the diaphragm, it will not be as cold.

Have a caregiver present if possible. Have the caregiver hold the child in his lap if the child is not critically ill or injured. Otherwise, the child will almost certainly squirm, thrash, and even try to run away. If necessary, set a few ground rules: "It's okay to cry. I know this hurts. But biting and kicking are not okay."

Children these ages are aware of death and are afraid of pain, blood, and permanent injuries. They also fear loss of body integrity. Be tactful and direct in dealing with physical fears. Cover bleeding injuries as soon as possible. Explain the obvious: "Your arm is hurt, but it can be fixed. We'll take you to the hospital where they can help fix you." Be sensitive to a child who is toilet trained and becomes overwhelmed by a bowel or bladder accident brought on by the illness or injury. Let the child hold his security object.

SCHOOL AGE (6-12 YEARS)

Usually children from this age on are more cooperative, even curious. They are able to rationalize. This age group can be the easiest to manage because most school-age children have an understanding of what EMS is about. They understand that you are there to help them. They also have a simple understanding of their body. It is easy to engage their interest in the procedures or your equipment. They will be fascinated by the contents of each cabinet in the ambulance. However, keep in mind that an illness or injury may cause children to emotionally regress. A 6-year-old may throw a temper tantrum like a 2-year-old after an injury. On the other hand, the child may act exceptionally mature. Maturity levels are highly individualized at this age.

Honesty is very important with school-age children. Treat them with respect and try to make them partners in their care. Information is reassuring to them and may need to be repeated until they understand, so explain each procedure in detail using appropriate language. Concerns about death and disability emerge at this age.

Children this age and even younger know that they need to take care of what they are wearing and sometimes get very anxious if you cut their clothes. Modesty and body image also are issues at this age. Explain gently but firmly, "I need to cut this sleeve off so that I can look at your arm." Be aware that pain, the sight of blood, permanent injuries, and disfigurement are still real fears for them. Take advantage of their increased vocabulary skills by explaining their physical injuries.

ADOLESCENTS (12–18 YEARS)

Adolescents use concrete thinking and are developing their abstract thinking skills. Children in this age group also generally believe that nothing bad can happen to them, or in other words, that they are invincible. Hence, they may take risks that lead to trauma. However, if injured or ill, they will still fear the possibility of disability and disfigurement.

Some experts suggest using a relaxed, rather than a professional, approach when performing a history and physical exam—especially if the situation involves conflict with an authority figure like a teacher, police officer, or caregiver. Asking the same questions to the adolescent when he is alone with you may generate very different answers than when he is with an authority figure. Smile, speak softly, and speak slowly. If the adolescent trusts you, he will be more likely to give you truthful information.

Most adolescents, either patients or their peers, will be reluctant to disclose information about their sexual history, drug use, personal habits, and illegal activities; ask for only the information that you need, and explain why you need it. Sometimes the presence of a peer, caregiver, or close friend is both physically and emotionally reassuring. Acknowledge the patient's friends, and allow them to help by notifying caregivers, holding equipment, and so on. You may need to explain to the patient that it is all right to react to pain, since you need to know what hurts.

Adolescents are preoccupied by their bodies and extremely concerned about modesty. An injury intensifies this preoccupation. They may ask about their greatest fears—for example, whether a facial cut will leave a scar or whether a broken leg signals the end of their basketball career. Be honest—up to a point. If available, have a same-sex provider conduct examinations of the genital area. Such exams are rarely necessary in the prehospital setting, generally required only when there is severe bleeding from the genital area. When it is necessary, if at all possible save this exam for last.

Occasionally you may encounter an adolescent who appears to be overreacting to the illness or injury. This age group is capable of hysterical reaction and may become involved in "mass hysteria." Be tolerant of this reaction and try not to get caught up in it or become angry.

ANATOMICAL DIFFERENCES

As mentioned earlier, most emergencies involving children are managed in the same way as those involving adults experiencing the same emergency. However, there are certain modifications you may need to make based on the anatomical and physiological development of children. When you are treating a child, be aware of some of the following special conditions and situations. Also be aware that the most significant of these differences typically concern the airway (Figure 38-1):

- *Infants have proportionally larger tongues than adults as compared to the size of the mouth.* You need to carefully assess the airway in a child with an altered mental status because it is easy for his airway to become occluded by his tongue.
- *The diameter of a newborn's trachea is only about 4 to 5 mm or about one-third the diameter of a dime,* compared to the 20 mm diameter of the adult trachea. This means that injury to the trachea (caused by inhaling steam or toxic fumes, for example) can cause life-threatening airway swelling not only faster but with less exposure to the fumes/gas/steam than in an adult.
- *Children's heads are proportionally larger than adults'.* This predisposes them to head injuries when involved in falls, auto accidents, and other types of trauma. The large occiput (back) of the child's head causes the neck to flex forward if the child is supine on a flat surface. To prevent this during immobilization, the EMT-B should place a small amount of padding under the shoulders to maintain neutral alignment of the airway and cervical spine (Figure 38-2). Until a child's body

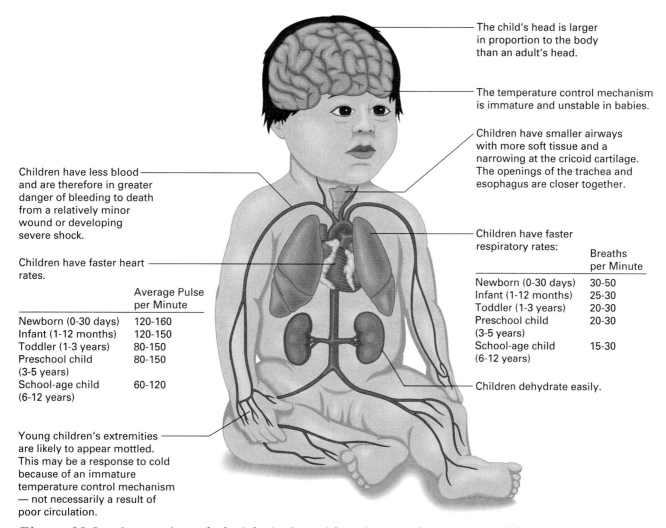

The child's head is larger in proportion to the body than an adult's head.

The temperature control mechanism is immature and unstable in babies.

Children have smaller airways with more soft tissue and a narrowing at the cricoid cartilage. The openings of the trachea and esophagus are closer together.

Children have less blood and are therefore in greater danger of bleeding to death from a relatively minor wound or developing severe shock.

Children have faster heart rates.

	Average Pulse per Minute
Newborn (0-30 days)	120-160
Infant (1-12 months)	120-150
Toddler (1-3 years)	80-150
Preschool child (3-5 years)	80-150
School-age child (6-12 years)	60-120

Children have faster respiratory rates:

	Breaths per Minute
Newborn (0-30 days)	30-50
Infant (1-12 months)	25-30
Toddler (1-3 years)	20-30
Preschool child (3-5 years)	20-30
School-age child (6-12 years)	15-30

Children dehydrate easily.

Young children's extremities are likely to appear mottled. This may be a response to cold because of an immature temperature control mechanism — not necessarily a result of poor circulation.

Figure 38-1   Anatomic and physiological considerations in the infant and child.

proportionately catches up with the head at approximately 8 or 9 years of age, padding is necessary.

- *Infants younger than 9 months typically cannot fully support their own heads.* Always support a baby's head when you pick him up.
- *A child's skin surface is large compared to his body mass,* making children more susceptible to hypothermia in cold environments. This means that you should take great care in protecting the young patient from extremes in the environment.

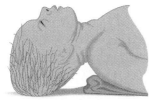

Figure 38-2   Pad behind the shoulders to maintain airway alignment.

- *Infants have a "soft-spot" on their head* from incomplete closure of the skeletal plates that make up the skull. Typically, the soft-spot (the **anterior fontanelle**) closes between 12 and 18 months of age. Be careful when handling an infant not to press on or poke into the fontanelle.
- *The child's ribs are much more pliable than the adult's.* This means that the rib cage cannot protect the internal organs as effectively. While this flexibility decreases the likelihood of rib fractures, it increases the likelihood of internal organ damage with blunt trauma to the chest.
- *The child's abdominal musculature is less well developed than the adult's,* increasing the likelihood of internal organ damage with blunt trauma to the abdomen.
- *Infants and children have a faster metabolic rate.* This means the cells in their body use oxygen from the blood stream faster than in adults, and periods of apnea (absence of breathing), hypoventilation (depressed breathing), or poor oxygenation can be more dangerous. Central nervous system damage

can occur more quickly, with more serious injuries affecting respiratory function, resulting in poor ventilation and/or oxygenation.

- *Infants and children have a smaller circulating blood volume than adult*s because of their smaller size. This means you must stop any bleeding as quickly as possible, since what would be a comparatively small blood loss in an adult would constitute a major hemorrhage for a child.

AIRWAY AND BREATHING PROBLEMS IN INFANTS AND CHILDREN

If *anything* should be emphasized when dealing with the assessment and treatment of infants or children, it is the assessment, establishment, and maintenance of the airway and respiratory function. The primary goal in treating any infant or child patient is the anticipation and recognition of respiratory problems, and to support any function that is compromised or lost. This is because, *failure to properly assess, establish, and maintain the airway, ventilatory, or oxygenation status will defeat any other or subsequent treatment, without exception!* Make no mistakes regarding this aspect of prehospital care.

The respiratory system, as a reminder, is responsible for providing the body with fresh oxygen for the blood as well as removing carbon dioxide and other wastes. Unfortunately, failure of this system is relatively common in pediatric patients. Further, failure of respiratory function can lead rapidly to cardiac arrest. In fact, *while cardiovascular disease is the leading medical cause of cardiac arrest in the adult, the leading medical cause of cardiac arrest in the infant or child patient is failure of the respiratory system.*

Compensatory mechanisms, which attempt to maintain normal physiological functioning, will often run at maximum in infants and children until total exhaustion occurs, leading to rapid respiratory deterioration and cardiac arrest. Therefore, even when the initial assessment of the respiratory status appears normal, you should maintain a high index of suspicion regarding the patency of the airway and adequacy of respiratory function. Even if it seems obvious that the patient is suffering from some other form of life threat (e.g., severe hemorrhage, head injury), do not drop your guard concerning proper airway management and oxygenation.

Determining the origin of the respiratory dysfunction may not be possible in the prehospital setting, but such a determination is not necessary in order to initiate appropriate treatment. You should focus your attention on the presenting signs and symptoms of respiratory dysfunction (the indications that there is respiratory dysfunction, without regard

to what may have caused it) and provide emergency care.

It will, however, be important for you to recognize the difference between upper airway obstruction (from a foreign body) and obstruction caused by a respiratory condition. The methods for removing a foreign body from a pediatric patient's airway could be deadly if applied to a patient with a condition such as epiglottitis (see Pediatric Respiratory Emergencies in the Enrichment section at the end of this chapter). Any attempt to put an object, such as your fingers or suction equipment, into the throat of a child with epiglottitis can cause fatal swelling or spasm

EARLY RESPIRATORY DISTRESS

If the infant or child is displaying the signs in the following list, but is still maintaining an adequate respiratory depth and rate, the patient is said to be in **early respiratory distress,** otherwise known as **"compensated respiratory distress."** *The patient in early respiratory distress is still in serious trouble. The patient can progress from early (compensated) respiratory distress to decompensated respiratory failure and respiratory arrest in minutes.* Signs of early respiratory distress include (Figure 38-3):

- An increase in respiratory rate above the normal rate for the child's age
- Nasal flaring

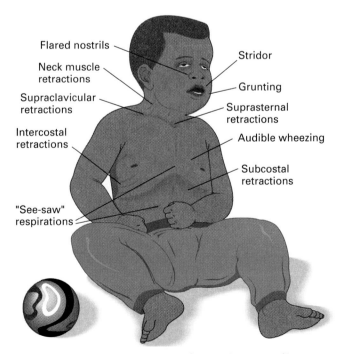

SIGNS OF EARLY RESPIRATORY DISTRESS

Flared nostrils

Neck muscle retractions

Supraclavicular retractions

Intercostal retractions

"See-saw" respirations

Stridor

Grunting

Suprasternal retractions

Audible wheezing

Subcostal retractions

Figure 38-3   Signs of early respiratory distress.

- Intercostal retractions on inspiration (retractions of the tissues and muscle between the ribs)
- Supraclavicular and subcostal retractions on inspiration (retractions of the tissues above the clavicles and beneath the margin of the ribs)
- Neck muscle retractions
- Audible breathing noises such as stridor, wheezing, or grunting
- "See-saw" respirations (extreme inspiratory effort draws the chest in and forces the abdomen out)

If these signs are present, provide oxygen (by methods to be described later in this chapter) and prompt transport to the hospital.

DECOMPENSATED RESPIRATORY FAILURE

The EMT-B may also encounter an infant or child in the advanced stage called **decompensated respiratory failure,** which is characterized by the signs of early respiratory distress (compensated respiratory failure) that were listed above, plus any of the following:

- Respiratory rate over 60 per minute
- Cyanosis (blue color)
- Decreased muscle tone
- Severe use of accessory muscles to aid in respirations
- Poor peripheral perfusion
- Altered mental status (in relation to the patient's developmental stage)
- Grunting (may also be present in early respiratory distress)
- Head bobbing

If these signs are present, provide positive pressure ventilation with supplemental oxygen and prompt transport to the hospital.

RESPIRATORY ARREST

Finally, **respiratory arrest** occurs when the compensatory mechanisms designed to maintain oxygenation of the blood have failed. Indications of respiratory arrest include:

- Respiratory rate less than 10 per minute (or absent breathing)
- Irregular respirations
- Limp muscle tone
- Unresponsiveness
- Slower than normal or absent heart rate
- Weak or absent peripheral pulses
- Hypotension (low blood pressure) in patients over 3 years of age

Remember, cardiopulmonary arrest in children is usually preceded by the *progressive* failure of the respiratory system. If any of the conditions listed here are present, the patient should be treated aggressively with oxygenation and positive pressure ventilation, and transported immediately to the hospital.

AIRWAY OBSTRUCTION

The patient may also present with some type of airway obstruction, since children often place things in their mouths. Keep a high index of suspicion for an obstructed airway in infants and children, because by the time you arrive they may be in a stage of compensated or decompensated respiratory failure—possibly even respiratory arrest.

As a general rule, the presentation and treatment goals of a choking infant or child mirror those of an adult. The difference, however, is how you attempt to relieve a complete obstruction.

In a *partial airway obstruction,* some air is still getting past the obstruction. Indications of a partial airway obstruction include:

- Patient may still be alert, pink, with peripheral perfusion
- Skin may be normal or slightly pale with peripheral perfusion present
- Stridor may be present (an inspiratory, high-pitched sound indicative of blockage at the level of the vocal cords)
- Retractions of intercostal, supraclavicular, and subcostal tissues
- Possible crowing or other noisy respirations
- Patient may be crying
- Forceful cough may still be present

If the patient is displaying the above signs and is still maintaining an adequate respiratory volume, general treatment principles include allowing the patient to assume a position of comfort (except do not lay the patient down). Enlist the help of the parents or caregivers while you administer oxygen. Encourage the patient to cough if a tangible obstruction is present. Limit your exam so as not to further agitate the patient, and transport.

Indications of a *complete airway obstruction* include:

- No crying, or talking
- Ineffective or absent cough
- Altered mental status, including possible loss of responsiveness
- Cyanosis probable

If the patient is displaying the above signs and is not maintaining an adequate respiratory volume, general treatment procedures should be based on foreign body airway obstruction procedures for an infant or child. These will be discussed later under Emergency Medical Care—Foreign Body Airway Obstruction.

ASSESSMENT AND CARE: RESPIRATORY EMERGENCIES

SCENE SIZE-UP

The scene size-up can provide many clues to the nature of the emergency, the initial status of the infant or child, and obstacles that may hamper extrication to the ambulance. Sometimes the EMT-B may believe that, because the call involves a child, there will be no threat to EMS providers (as compared to a bar fight, auto accident, or unknown medical emergency). Never get a false sense of security that the scene will be safe. The child may be a victim of violence that is ongoing or can erupt again; adults at the scene may be prone to hysterical or violent responses because of the stress of the emergency; or the child may have fallen victim to a poison or hazardous substance that can also affect EMS workers and others at the scene.

INITIAL ASSESSMENT

Remember that infants and young children may not have the mental capabilities to recognize or understand why someone unknown to them (the EMT-B) is coming toward them intently. You may scare them to a point where they become agitated, cry, and/or resist your assessment efforts.

Therefore, your initial assessment should begin "at the doorway." You should gather as much information about the young patient as possible as you observe him from across the room, while he is interacting with his caregiver and environment and has possibly not yet noticed or reacted to your presence.

This visual assessment of the patient's general condition is done in only a few moments as you scan the environment. Naturally, if you see signs of impending respiratory arrest or other life-threatening conditions, you will want to begin treatment immediately.

Form a general impression as to whether this is a "well" versus a "sick" child based on the overall appearance and activity (or lack of activity) of the infant/child in his surroundings. Does the patient:

- Display normal behavior for his age (as discussed earlier)?
- Move about spontaneously? (or) seem lethargic?
- Appear attentive and recognize the parents or caregivers?
- Maintain any eye contact (appropriate for the patient's age)?
- Seem easily consoled by the parents or caregiver? (or) seem inconsolable?
- Respond to parent or caregiver calling him? (or) respond inappropriately? (or) not respond at all?

A relatively "well" baby will be interactive with both the caregiver and the environment, will be ac-tively moving, have good color, and a good strong cry. Although noisy and mentally trying at times, a crying baby is (at least) a breathing baby. A "sick" baby upon initial visual assessment will be limp or flaccid, have a weak or absent cry, not interact with the environment or parents, possibly have poor skin color, and will not seem to notice your approach.

During your initial assessment, you should be acutely aware of alterations in the respiratory effort. Respirations can be counted by watching the chest rise or by placing your hand on the patient's abdomen. Adequate breathing can be assessed by watching for rise and fall of the chest at the child's clavicles. Because the clavicles are the highest point of the chest (and the last to fill with air), movement there signifies good expansion of the lung.

Because of the importance of the respiratory system in successful management of the infant or child, be alert for the following as clues to the infant or child's airway and respiratory status: rapid breathing, noisy breathing, and diminished breathing.

- *Rapid Breathing*—As a general rule, children breathe faster than adults. The key to recognizing rapid breathing is to be familiar with normal ranges of respirations (25 to 50 per minute in an infant; 15 to 30 per minute in a child) and to repeat assessment of respiratory rate frequently, each time counting the rate over a complete minute. In cases of rapid breathing (tachypnea) look for breathing through the mouth, flaring of the nostrils, retractions, and/or the use of accessory muscles. Also check for cyanosis around the mouth and changes in mental status. Possible causes of rapid breathing are:
  - Oxygen deficiency (hypoxia)
  - Head injury
  - Fever, which raises the metabolic rate, increasing the need for oxygen
  - Diabetes, when glucose levels get very high
  - Aspirin overdoses and other forms of poisoning
  - Stress or fear
- *Noisy Breathing*—Children *normally* breathe more loudly through the mouth than adults because of anatomical differences. Check with a caregiver if you hear an unusual sound to determine whether it is normal. When assessing breath sounds with a stethoscope, listen along both midaxillary lines (below the armpits). This is necessary since breath sounds typically transmit very easily from one side of the child's small chest to the other. Listening midaxillary will reduce the amount of sound you are hearing that is transmitted from the opposite side. The following is a checklist of sounds characteristically produced by certain problems:
  - *Coughing, gagging,* or *gasping* will be violent when the child breathes in a foreign body or bodily secretions, creating a partial blockage of

the airway. (If blockage is complete, however, there will be no cough or gasp.)

- *Crackles* (sometimes called rales), sounds that resemble the noise of rolling a few strands of hair near the ear, are commonly heard on listening to chest sounds when certain respiratory diseases have caused fluid to accumulate in the alveoli.
- *Wheezing* is caused by air moving at a high rate through narrowed bronchioles, is more "musical" than crackles, and may sometimes be a whistle. Wheezing sounds are caused by medical emergencies that cause narrowing of the lower airway (or bronchospasm) and can also be caused by aspiration of blood, vomitus, or foreign objects. Wheezing is usually heard on exhalation.
- *Stridor* (as discussed earlier) is a harsh, high-pitched sound that occurs typically during inspiration. It results from severe obstruction in the upper airway, as in the case of swelling to the larynx. Because stridor occurs only with upper airway problems, if it is absent, the cause of the emergency is more likely due to emergencies involving the lower portions of the airway.

- *Diminished Breathing*—When something (blood, fluid, or air) is preventing the lungs from inflating, there is a loss of breath sounds. The causes of diminished breathing can include obstruction, medical problems, or traumatic injuries like a pneumothorax (air in the chest cavity, collapsing one or both lungs). Consider providing positive pressure ventilation to the infant or child if breath sounds are not obvious.

Assess circulation by determining the quality of the pulse, skin, and capillary refill. If perfusion is inadequate, the patient will exhibit signs of shock (Figure 38-18) and should be treated for shock. If perfusion is adequate, all of the following assessment determinations will be normal (or acceptable):

- Capillary refill, for the patient under 6 years—Assess this as follows: Lightly grasp the pediatric patient's finger, and with the finger in a flexed (but relaxed) position, apply enough pressure to the middle of the nail bed to turn it white. Then, suddenly release the pressure and count in seconds how long it takes for the nail bed to return from white to its original pinkish color. If the color returns within 2 seconds, peripheral perfusion is adequate.
- Pulse rate and strength
- Strength of peripheral versus core pulses
- Warmth and color of the hands and feet
- Urinary output—a sign of the adequacy of kidney perfusion
- Mental status

Interventions during the initial assessment should be as follows: If the airway is not clear, open it by a head-tilt, chin-lift or a jaw-thrust maneuver and, if necessary, suction. Then assess the breathing status; if it is not adequate, provide positive pressure ventilation with supplemental oxygen immediately. If it is adequate, provide oxygen by a nonrebreather mask. (Review Chapter 14, "Respiratory Emergencies," for a full review of assessing the airway and respiratory status.) Then assess circulation and, if necessary, control bleeding and treat for shock.

From the information you have gathered thus far, you need to make a determination (based on your scene size-up and initial assessment, including your general impression of sickness or wellness) whether or not the patient should be a priority for immediate transport. *Any patient with signs and symptoms of early respiratory distress should be considered a priority patient.*

FOCUSED HISTORY AND PHYSICAL EXAM

You can begin your focused history and physical exam at the scene. For this part of the assessment, follow the guidelines in the earlier section under Dealing with the Child as well as the general procedures listed in Table 38-1, adapting them to the patient's age and situation.

While performing your focused history and physical exam for a medical emergency, gather the history first, then perform the physical exam and gather the baseline vital signs. (If it is for a trauma emergency, perform the physical exam and gather vital signs before obtaining the history.)

Complete the SAMPLE history, using the OPQRST mnemonic if pain is identified during your assessment. If the developmental age of the patient allows, the EMT-B should gather this history from the patient; if not, question the family or bystanders. While gathering the SAMPLE history, be sure to find out if any care or treatment has been rendered already, and, if so, whether it was effective. Also remember to ask if all shots and immunizations are up to date.

When performing the physical exam on an infant or young child, you should follow a toe-to-head or trunk-to-head approach. This means you will assess the extremities and core of the patient's body prior to the head. Although this is age- and situation-dependent, it will allow you to gather the most physical exam information while, at the same time, increasing the infant's or child's anxiety level as little as possible. If the patient is unresponsive, you can follow the traditional head-to-toe assessment format performed in the adult patient to identify any life threats as early as possible.

If this is a medical problem and the patient is responsive, you may perform a focused medical assess-

TABLE 38-1

Ten Tips for Examining Infants and Children

- *When examining an infant or child . . .*

1. If possible, have only one EMT-B deal with the infant or child. This reduces the fear the patient may experience by being assessed by two unknown individuals.
2. Get down to the child's eye level. Towering above an infant or child will only increase his fear and anxiety. In fact, sit down next to the child whenever possible.
3. With children under school age start the assessment with your hands and save stethoscopes, blood pressure cuffs, and scissors until you have developed some trust with the child. Keep the most painful parts of the examination for the end.
4. Speak in a calm, quiet voice and maintain eye contact as much as possible. Even infants will respond to a calm voice, and an apparently unresponsive child may actually hear much of what you say.
5. Never become impatient or lose your temper. This will just ignite the patient's temper. Switch off with a partner or take a brief "time out" for yourself, if you need to.
6. Avoid questions that require yes or no answers. Given the choice, a child will almost always say "no" when asked if you can do something to him. Instead, ask questions in this format: "Would you like your mother to take off your shirt, or may I do it?"
7. Involve the caregivers (or a familiar person) as much as possible during care and transport.
8. Be honest. For instance, you might say, "It will hurt when I touch you here, but it will only last a moment. If you feel like crying, it's okay." Children can tolerate pain if they are prepared for it and are given adequate support.
9. Ask children for their help and assure them that they are doing a good job. Have toys, stickers, or other "rewards" to console and encourage a child.
10. Be gentle. Use all appropriate measures to reduce the amount of pain that a child must endure. If you must restrain a child, be sure that it is absolutely necessary. Use only the minimum degree of restraint to be safe and allow you to provide good care. As a general rule, "humane" (soft) restraints are much better than "mechanical" ones.

ment, concentrating on the areas related to the problem. If trauma is suspected or the patient is unresponsive or unable to communicate clearly, perform a complete rapid trauma assessment. Since injuries present the same in adults and children, you will be looking for the same indicators of injury. Use the DCAP-BTLS mnemonic (deformities, contusions, abrasions, penetrations/punctures, burns, tenderness, lacerations, swelling) while assessing each part of the body.

As you go on to assess the baseline vital signs in infants and children, you should be aware that vital signs play only a limited role in your determination of the patient's overall status. Instead, pay more attention to the general impression you developed of the child's appearance of "sickness" or "wellness." This is because, as mentioned earlier, infants and children have excellent compensatory mechanisms that delay deterioration. It is only after the exhaustion of these mechanisms that you may see indicative changes in the vital signs. By then, the changes may occur very quickly, and the child's condition typically deteriorates rapidly. Here, then, are some special considerations, for assessing the vitals:

- *Respirations*—Obtain the respiratory rate at regular intervals, based on techniques and normal ranges discussed earlier.
- *Pulse*—It is very difficult to feel a carotid pulse in infants and toddlers because their necks are short

and fat. To assess circulation, use the radial pulse in a child and the brachial pulse in an infant (Figure 38-4a). Still another alternative is the femoral pulse near the crease between the pelvis and thigh. It is located by identifying the midpoint of an imaginary line extending from the anterior superior iliac spine to the symphysis pubis, then moving your fingertip about two finger breadths inferior (Figure 38-4b).

Another means of assessing heart rate is by auscultation of the apical pulse (at the apex of the heart). To locate it, place your hand over the fourth or fifth intercostal space on the left midclavicular line. Place your stethoscope here and count each "lub-dub" as one beat. Remember, this method will provide you with a heart rate, but it is not a measure of perfusion.

To evaluate circulation status you will want to compare central or core pulses with peripheral pulses. The farther away from the heart the peripheral pulse can be detected, the better the perfusion status.

- *Skin*—Check capillary refill, as discussed earlier, in children under 6. Check skin color (e.g., pink, blue, flushed, yellow), relative temperature (the back of your hand on the patient's forehead or abdomen), and condition (dry or sweaty).
- *Pupils*—Check for size, equality, and reactivity of pupils by shining your penlight into the eyes, espe-

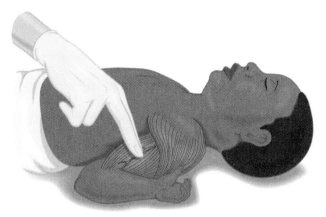

Figure 38-4a   Taking the brachial pulse.

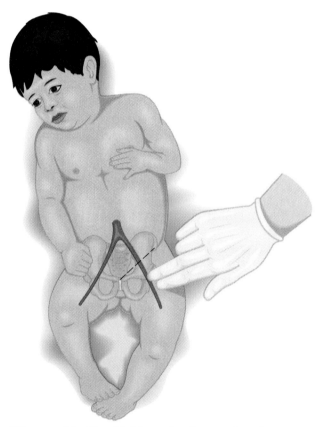

Figure 38-4b   Taking the femoral pulse.

cially if trauma is suspected or the patient is unresponsive.

• *Blood Pressure*—Do not attempt to take the blood pressure of a child under the age of 3. Instead, rely on other indicators of perfusion discussed earlier. In children over 3, be sure that you check the blood pressure with a correct-size cuff; it should cover about two-thirds of the upper arm. Do not take a blood pressure if the appropriate equipment is not available.

Signs and Symptoms   The signs of respiratory distress are significant findings when present, and require your immediate attention whether or not you know the exact cause of the respiratory distress. These have been discussed in detail earlier in this chapter, grouped as those that appear early, those that appear when compensation is failing, and those that appear with respiratory arrest (see Early Respiratory Distress, Decompensated Respiratory Failure, and Respiratory Arrest, earlier in this chapter).

EMERGENCY MEDICAL CARE—RESPIRATORY EMERGENCIES

When any of the signs of a respiratory emergency are present, provide care as described below. For more detail on all of these techniques, including adaptations for infants and children, review Chapter 7, "Airway Management, Ventilation, and Oxygen Therapy."

1. *Establish and maintain a patent airway.* Perform the head-tilt, chin-lift, but with caution. Since the infant's airway is much smaller and more flexible, excessive hyperextension of the head can result in the airway "kinking" (like a garden hose), actually resulting in airway occlusion. Extend the head only enough to ensure a patent airway; once that point is reached, stop there (Figure 38-5). Also, when performing a chin lift, little or no pressure should be applied to the soft tissue under the chin, which will occlude, rather than open, the airway. In pediatric patients with possible spine injury, you should perform a manual jaw-thrust technique to help establish the airway (Figure 38-6).

2. *Suction any secretions, vomitus, or blood.* Remember that the suctioning process temporarily prevents air from being breathed into the lungs. When suctioning an infant or child, be sure not to suction any longer than 5 to 10 seconds at a time, so as not to promote hypoxia. Use appropriately sized equipment (Figure 38-7). Be careful not to damage tissues while inserting and moving the suctioning device in the mouth. If the patient is responsive and has a gag reflex, be careful not to suction deeply enough to cause the patient to vomit.

3. *If you need to assist ventilations, maintain a patent airway with an oropharyngeal or nasopharyngeal airway.* Use an oropharyngeal airway (Figure 38-8) if there is no gag reflex. Use a nasopharyngeal airway (Figure 38-9) if the patient cannot tolerate an oral airway. Remember, however, that nasopharyngeal airways should be avoided in patients with possible head trauma.

4. *Initiate positive pressure ventilation.* If the infant or child is in decompensated respiratory failure

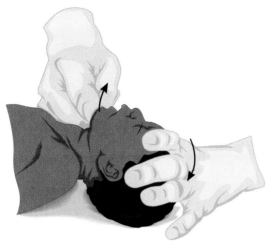

Figure 38-5 Head-tilt, chin-lift maneuver in the infant. Avoid overextension.

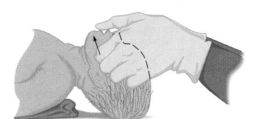

Figure 38-6 Jaw-thrust maneuver in the infant.

or respiratory arrest—that is, with inadequate breathing or not breathing—you should start positive pressure ventilation. Supplemental oxygen should be attached to the ventilation device as soon as practical.

When using a mouth-to-mask device, be sure to use a one-way valve to prevent disease transmission. If using a bag-valve-mask device, be sure to use an appropriate-sized bag. Infants and chil-

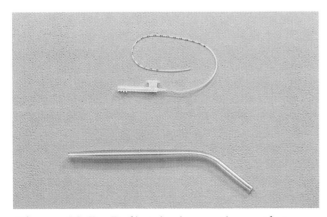

Figure 38-7 Pediatric size suction catheters. Top: soft suction catheter. Bottom: rigid or hard suction catheter.

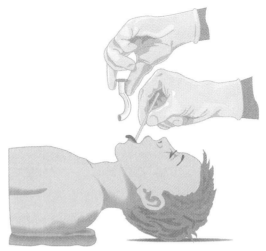

Figure 38-8 Inserting an oropharyngeal airway in an infant with the use of a tongue blade.

dren need a respiratory tidal volume of 10-15 ml/kg. Therefore, BVM devices ranging from 250-500 ml should be used for infants weighing less than 7 kg; 750-ml BVM devices are for children weighing 7 to 35 kg; and adult-sized devices may be used for children over 35 kg. Select an appropriate-size mask that fits over the bridge of the nose and into the cleft above the chin (Figure 38–10a). Ensure a good mask seal by using one or two hands to hold the mask to the face (Figures 38–10b and c). A two-handed seal is preferred to ensure delivery of an adequate tidal volume.

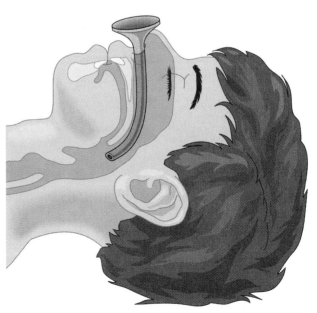

Figure 38-9 Proper placement of nasopharyngeal airway in a child.

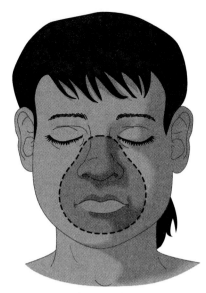

Figure 38-10a   The mask should fit on the bridge of the nose and the cleft above the chin.

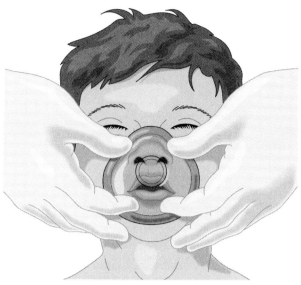

Figure 38-10b   Two-handed face mask seal.

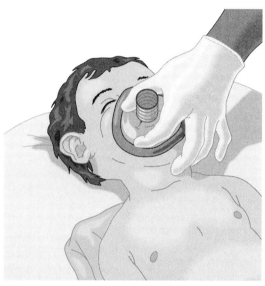

Figure 38-10c   One-handed face mask seal.

The infant or child patient should be ventilated at a minimum rate of 20 per minute. Be sure to breathe into the pocket mask or squeeze the BVM bag slowly and evenly to ensure adequate chest rise. If regurgitation is a problem, pressing on the cricoid cartilage (the ring of cartilage just below the larynx) will help alleviate it.

5. *Maintain oxygen therapy.* If the patient is breathing adequately but has other signs of early respiratory distress, administer oxygen at 15 lpm via a nonrebreather mask. If the patient will not tolerate the mask, try a "blow-by" method. Push the oxygen tubing through a hole created in the bottom of a disposable cup (not Styrofoam, which flakes), and hold it near the patient's mouth. This may be less frightening to younger patients, who may be curious and interested in the cup (Figure 38-11a). You may also hold the end of the oxygen tubing close to the patient's face to administer the oxygen (Figure 38-11b). In general, you can use the following guidelines for ventilation and oxygenation:

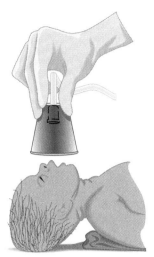

Figure 38-11a *"Blow-by" oxygen administration using oxygen tubing and a paper cup.*

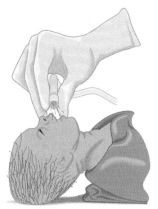

Figure 38-11b *"Blow-by" oxygen administration holding the tubing approximately 2 inches from the patient's face.*

Provide oxygen at 15 lpm via a nonrebreather mask to all infants and children who:

– Have indications of early respiratory distress but still have an adequate respiratory effort

Provide positive pressure ventilation (with supplemental oxygen) for all infants and children who:

– Have respiratory distress and altered mental status
– Have cyanosis present despite oxygen via a nonrebreather mask
– Display respiratory distress with poor muscle tone
– Are in respiratory failure or in respiratory arrest

6. *Position the patient.* Patients who are in mild respiratory distress will probably prefer to be sitting in the lap of the caregiver. If the patient is unresponsive, place him in a lateral recumbent position to help prevent aspiration, and have suction available.

It may be necessary to immobilize the infant or child to prevent possible aggravation of an existing spine injury. In addition, any pediatric patient with an altered mental status, and no caregiver who is able to give you a history that would rule out trauma, should be immobilized as well. The key in immobilizing the infant or child patient is to remember to place a folded towel (or similar item), beneath the shoulder blades to keep the head from flexing forward. For more about immobilizing an infant or child, see the Enrichment section at the end of the Chapter.

7. *Transport.* Any pediatric patient with a respiratory complaint, or with evidence of respiratory distress, needs to be transported to a medical facility for further evaluation.

EMERGENCY MEDICAL CARE— FOREIGN BODY AIRWAY OBSTRUCTION

If you notice a high resistance to airflow after initiating positive pressure ventilation on a patient with respiratory failure or respiratory arrest, attempt once to reposition the airway and reventilate. If, after repositioning, the airway is still not patent, and there are no indications that the child is suffering from an illness, assume the infant or child has an airway obstructed by a foreign body—especially if the child was observed to be eating or playing with small objects and then suddenly began to choke or stopped breathing.

Perform the next steps immediately, but only if you are sure that the obstruction is not caused by a respiratory disease. Remember that putting anything in the mouth of a pediatric patient with respiratory disease can cause fatal swelling or spasms of the airway:

If the patient is an infant less than 1 year of age:

1. Position the patient prone on your forearm in a head-down position, supporting the infant's head with your hand and supporting your arm on your thigh (Figure 38-12).
2. Deliver 5 sharp back-blows between the shoulder blades.
3. Transfer the patient to a supine, head-down position on your other forearm, and deliver 5 chest thrusts using 2 fingertips positioned one fingerwidth beneath the nipple line (Figure 38-13).
4. Assess (by looking) in the oral cavity for the foreign body. Should it become dislodged and visible, pluck or sweep (Figure 38-14) the foreign body out with a finger. If it is not visible, do not perform a "blind" finger sweep.
5. Attempt to ventilate. If ventilation is unsuccessful, repeat steps 1-4 twice and then transport immedi-

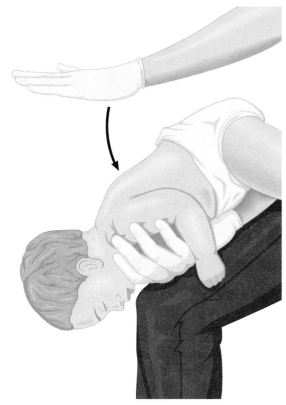

Figure 38-12   Position the infant to deliver back blows.

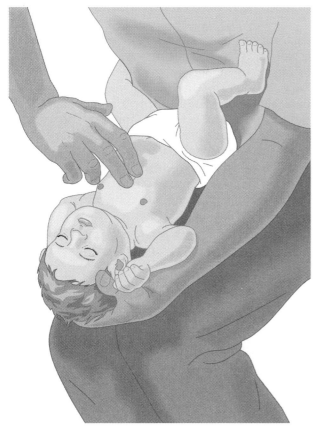

Figure 38-13   Position the infant to deliver chest thrusts.

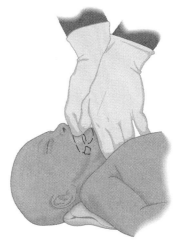

Figure 38-14   Use the finger sweep only when the foreign body is visible.

ately, continuing to repeat the steps en route until the obstruction is dislodged or until arrival at the medical facility. Consider ALS back-up.

If the patient is older than 1 year of age and is choking but still responsive, perform the Heimlich maneuver (abdominal thrusts) as follows:

1. Assure the patient that you are there to help.
2. Position yourself behind the child, and reach your arms around his abdomen (Figure 38-15).
3. Locate the navel and place the thumb side of one clenched fist midway between the navel and the xiphoid process (cartilage extending downward from the sternum).
4. Wrap the other hand over the clenched hand.
5. Deliver abdominal thrusts inward and upward, at a 45-degree angle toward the head
6. Continue to deliver the abdominal thrusts until the object is dislodged or the patient becomes unresponsive. If the patient becomes unresponsive, place the child in a supine position and continue to provide abdominal thrusts as described below for an unresponsive child. Immediately transport, continuing abdominal thrusts en route.

If the patient is older than 1 year and is unresponsive, perform abdominal thrusts as follows:

1. Straddle the supine patient's hips or thighs, facing his head (Figure 38-16).
2. Place the finger of one hand in the patient's navel, place the heel of the other hand directly in front of it, midline, your fingers pointing toward the head. By using this technique for hand placement, you will be above the navel, and well below the diaphragm (which is the proper area to deliver the abdominal thrusts).

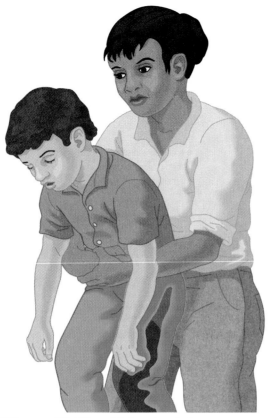

Figure 38-15   Abdominal thrusts on a choking but responsive child.

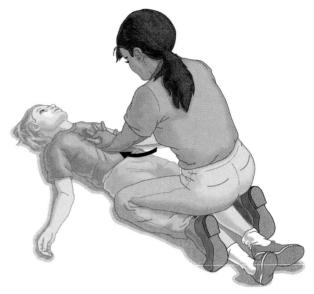

Figure 38-16   Abdominal thrusts on a child who is unresponsive.

3. Deliver 5 abdominal thrusts, at about a 45-degree angle to the patient's body.
4. Return to the side of the patient's head (quickly), look inside the mouth and retrieve any foreign body you can see. (Never perform a "blind" finger sweep except on an adult).
5. Attempt to ventilate the patient. If unsuccessful, repeat steps 1-4 twice until the object is dislodged and the airway is clear. If the airway remains obstructed, immediately transport and continue to perform steps 1-4 en route to the medical facility.

After you have successfully dislodged the foreign object, in each of the above instances you will manually open the patient's airway. If breathing is adequate, apply oxygen at 15 lpm with a nonrebreather mask. If breathing is not adequate perform positive pressure ventilation with supplemental oxygen. Diligently monitor the pulse.

DETAILED PHYSICAL EXAM AND ONGOING ASSESSMENT

If time and the patient's condition permit, perform a detailed physical exam for an unresponsive or trauma patient to check for any injuries or problems that may have been overlooked earlier.

The ongoing assessment must be performed on all patients to continuously monitor for changes in the patient's mental status, airway, breathing, and circulation status (be sure to watch any patient with respiratory distress for the development of respiratory failure; remember that compensatory mechanisms fail rapidly, and without warning). Also assess and record the vital signs and check interventions. Repeat the ongoing assessment at least every 5 minutes or as frequently as possible for the pediatric patient with respiratory distress. Communicate your findings and treatment to the receiving medical facility.

SUMMARY: ASSESSMENT AND CARE—RESPIRATORY EMERGENCIES

To review possible assessment findings and emergency care for respiratory emergencies in the infant or child, see Figures 38-17 and 38-18.

ASSESSMENT SUMMARY

RESPIRATORY EMERGENCIES IN THE INFANT OR CHILD

The following are findings that may be associated with a respiratory emergency in the infant or child.

SCENE SIZE-UP

Ensure your own safety. Look for:

Mechanism of injury; toxic inhalation or hazardous materials; patient in a confined space; evidence of poisoning; metered dose inhalers or nebulizers

INITIAL ASSESSMENT

General Impression

Is the child "sick" or "well"? Displaying normal behavior for his age? Moving spontaneously or lethargic or flaccid? Maintaining eye contact?

If older than 2 months does he recognize his parents? Respond when the parent calls his name?

Is he sitting up, leaning forward, neck jutting out, drooling?

Mental status (depending on age of patient)

Alert to unresponsive; decreasing mental status; increased anxiety; disorientation; restlessness

Seizure activity; weak or absent cry

Does not react with environment

Does not seem to notice your presence

Cannot be consoled by parent

Airway

Occluded by tongue, secretions, blood, or vomitus

Signs of laryngeal edema (stridor, crowing)

Swollen tongue; drooling

Harsh cough that sounds like a "seal bark"

Breathing

Tachypnea (>50 respirations /minute in an infant and >30 respirations/minute in child)

Inadequate ventilation

Wheezing; crackles

Mouth breathing; accessory muscle use; nasal flaring

Coughing, gagging, or gasping

Circulation

Weak pulses; tachycardia; bradycardia

Red, warm, and dry skin

Pale, cool, clammy skin; cyanosis

Capillary refill that is delayed >2 seconds

Status: *Priority patient if showing signs and symptoms of respiratory failure or respiratory distress*

FOCUSED HISTORY AND PHYSICAL EXAM

Physical Exam

Head, neck, and face
  Edema to face, hands, neck, and lips
  Hives; itching
  Warm, tingling feeling
  Difficulty in swallowing; coughed up mucus
  Itchy and watery eyes; runny or stuffy nose
  Runny or stuffy nose
  Coughed-up mucus
  Headache
  Stiff neck
  Bulging anterior fontanelle (infants <1 year) may indicate head injury
  Neck jutted out and drooling
  Evidence of trauma to the head, neck, or face

Chest
  Retractions; accessor muscle use
  Wheezing in all lung lobes; crackles
  Evidence of trauma to the chest

Abdomen
  Nausea/vomiting
  Abdominal cramping
  Diarrhea; loss of bowel control
  Excessive abdominal muscle use
  Evidence of trauma to abdomen

Extremities
  Warm, tingling feeling in hands and feet
  Itching, especially hands and feet
  Edema to hands and feet
  Cool, pale, cyanotic hands and feet
  Red, warm, dry skin
  Weak or absent peripheral pulses
  Poor skin turgor

SAMPLE History

Signs/symptoms of early respiratory distress:
  Tachypnea
  Nasal flaring
  Retractions
  Stridor, wheezing, or grunting
  "See-saw" respirations

Signs/symptoms of decompensated respiratory failure:
  Tachypnea >60/minute
  Cyanosis
  Deceased muscle tone
  Poor peripheral perfusion

(continued on the next page)

Figure 38-17a   Assessment summary: respiratory emergency in the infant or child.

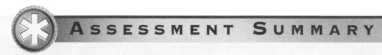

RESPIRATORY EMERGENCY IN THE INFANT OR CHILD (CONTINUED)

Altered mental status
Grunting
Head bobbing
Signs of respiratory arrest:
Respiratory rate less than 10/minute
Irregular respirations
Flaccid (limp) muscles
Unresponsiveness
Bradycardia
Weak or absent peripheral pulses
Hypotension

Baseline vital signs

BP: Take BP in children >3 years of age; BP may be decreased with severe respiratory failure.
HR: tachycardia with weak peripheral pulses that progresses to bradycardia
RR: tachypnea; may have wheezing and labored breathing; bradypnea is sign of impending respiratory failure and respiratory arrest
Skin: usually pale, cool, clammy and cyanotic; may be red, warm, dry; hives, itching if allergic reaction
Pupils: normal to dilated; sluggish to respond to light

EMERGENCY CARE PROTOCOL

RESPIRATORY EMERGENCY IN THE INFANT OR CHILD

1. Establish and maintain open airway extending head only enough to allow open airway and avoid hyperextension.
2. If complete foreign body airway obstruction suspected, perform the following:

   Infant (<1 year of age)
   a. Position head down.
   b. Deliver 5 back-blows.
   c. Deliver 5 chest thrusts.
   d. Assess inside mouth; finger sweep only if object is visualized.
   e. Attempt to ventilate.
   f. Perform two sets; begin immediate transport if airway not cleared.
   g. Continue until obstruction dislodged.

   Responsive child with complete airway obstruction
   a. Deliver 5–10 abdominal thrusts.
   b. Repeat twice until obstruction dislodged or child becomes unresponsive.
   c. Begin immediate transport; continue abdominal thrusts en route.

   Unresponsive child with complete airway obstruction
   a. Deliver 5–10 abdominal thrusts.
   b. Assess inside mouth; if child <8 years, finger sweep only if object is visualized; if child >8 years, perform blind finger sweep.
   c. Attempt to ventilate.
   d. Continue until obstruction dislodged or two sets performed.
   e. Begin immediate transport; continue abdominal thrusts en route.

3. If infant or child has incomplete obstruction, apply nonrebreather mask, allow patient to assume position of comfort, and encourage patient to cough forcefully; do not delay transport; continue en route. If obstruction becomes complete, perform foreign body airway maneuver.
4. Suction secretions no longer than 5 to 10 seconds each time.
5. Provide positive pressure ventilation with supplemental oxygen via reservoir at a minimum rate of 20 ventilations/ minute if:
   Respiratory failure
   Respiratory arrest
   Inadequate breathing
   Respiratory distress and altered mental status
   Cyanosis present despite oxygen delivery by nonrebreather mask
   Respiratory distress with poor muscle tone
6. If breathing is adequate, administer oxygen via nonrebreather mask at 15 lpm; consider blow-by oxygen in infants and very young children.
7. If signs and symptoms of allergic reaction and respiratory distress and/or hypotension, and with permission from medical direction, administer epinephrine by patient-prescribed auto-injector: **epinephrine pediatric dose: 0.15 mg**
8. If signs and symptoms of respiratory distress and wheezing and if patient has a prescribed metered-dose inhaler, and with permission from medical direction, administer the MDI.
9. Consider calling Advanced Life Support.
10. Expedite transport.
11. Perform an ongoing assessment every 5 minutes.

Figure 38-17b Emergency care protocol: respiratory emergency in the infant or child.

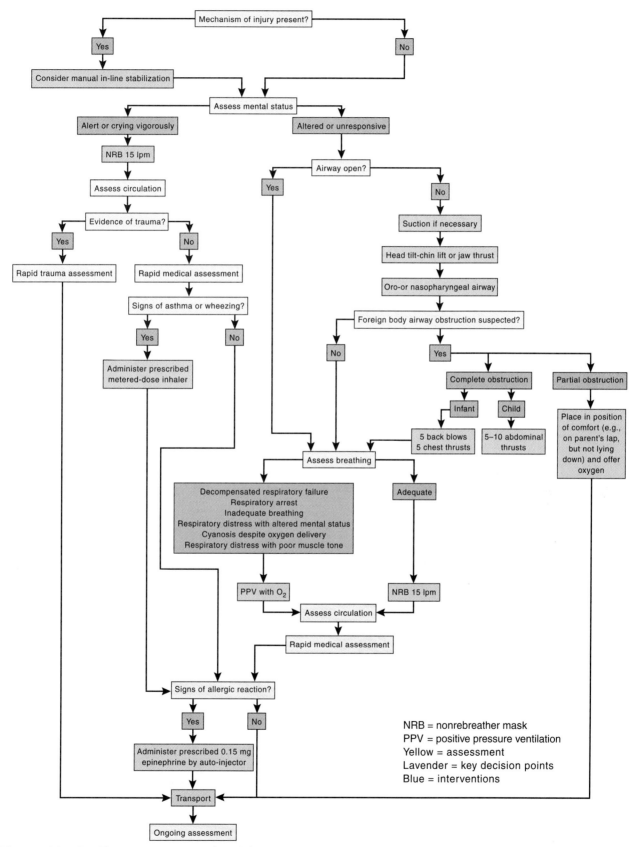

Figure 38-18   Emergency care algorithm respiratory emergency in the infant or child.

MEDICAL PROBLEMS COMMON TO INFANTS AND CHILDREN

The previous section dealt with respiratory emergencies in infants and children and, although it is a common medical problem, it was given its own section because the respiratory system is affected by—and usually is an early indicator of—other medical problems. Remember that regardless of the type of medical emergency, maintaining airway and adequate breathing are the primary goals. Remember also, the general principles and steps of assessment—scene size-up, initial assessment, focused history and physical exam, detailed physical exam (when appropriate), and ongoing assessment—will be the same no matter what medical emergency precipitates the call.

On the following pages, additional medical emergencies of which you should be aware are discussed with general principles of assessment and care as they would apply.

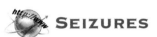 **SEIZURES**

Seizures in infants and children may be caused by any condition that would also produce seizures in adults: epilepsy, head injury, meningitis, oxygen deficiency, drug overdose, and low blood sugar (hypoglycemia). However, adults seldom have febrile seizures (seizures caused by fever), but children may. The risk of seizures is high among children up to age 2, and approximately 5 percent of children have febrile seizures. Although these childhood seizures may be frightening, they generally have no permanent adverse effects.

ASSESSMENT CONSIDERATIONS

During the seizure, the child's arms and legs become rigid, the back arches, the muscles may twitch or jerk in spasm, the eyes roll up and become fixed, the pupils dilate, and the breathing is often irregular or ineffective. The patient may lose bladder and bowel control and will be completely unresponsive. If the seizure lasts long enough, the skin will turn cyanotic from ineffective respirations. Also, the muscle spasms will prevent the child from swallowing. Hence, excessive saliva coming from the mouth is a common finding (saliva is also more copious during the seizure). If saliva is trapped in the throat, the child will make a gurgling sound with respirations.

While obtaining the SAMPLE history, ascertain whether the child has had prior seizures and, if so, find out whether this is the child's normal seizure pattern. You will also want to determine whether the child has taken his anti-seizure medications, if any have been prescribed.

EMERGENCY MEDICAL CARE

A single seizure is usually self-limiting, ends within minutes, is generalized in nature (all muscles involved), and does not recur. If the child has a single seizure, maintain an airway and be sure that he does not injure himself. Transport as soon as possible after the single seizure.

1. *Assure airway is open.*
2. *Position the patient on his side* if there is no possibility of cervical spine trauma, and make sure it will not be possible for him to strike any nearby objects and injure himself.
3. *Be prepared to suction.*
4. *Provide oxygen or ventilate as appropriate.* Provide oxygen at 15 lpm by nonrebreather mask or, if in respiratory arrest or severe respiratory distress, provide positive pressure ventilation with supplemental oxygen.
5. *Transport.* Although brief seizures are generally not harmful, there may be a more dangerous underlying condition.

If seizures last longer than 10 minutes or recur without a recovery period, this is a condition called *status epilepticus, which is a true medical emergency.* Provide positive pressure ventilation with supplemental oxygen during a prolonged seizure, if possible. After the seizure has ended, it may still be necessary to provide positive pressure ventilation. Provide rapid transport to the hospital, paying particular attention to maintaining the airway and protecting the patient from injury.

To review emergency care for seizures in the infant or child, see Figure 38-19.

ALTERED MENTAL STATUS

An altered mental status can be the reason for the emergency call (mother informs you the baby "just isn't acting right"), or a sign or result of the initial reason for the emergency call (a patient with a diabetic condition who, as a result, becomes unresponsive). In any instance, it is more important to assess and treat any life-threatening conditions associated with the altered mental status than to treat the altered mental status itself. Your pediatric patient could have an altered mental status for the same reason an adult patient would, such as hypoglycemia, poisoning, post-seizure, severe blood infection, or head injury from trauma.

EMERGENCY CARE PROTOCOL

SEIZURES IN THE INFANT OR CHILD

1. Establish and maintain open airway, extending head only enough to allow open airway and avoid hyperextension.
2. Protect infant or child from injuring himself; place him on his left side.
3. Suction secretions no longer than 5 to 10 seconds each time.
4. Provide positive pressure ventilation with supplemental oxygen via reservoir at a minimum rate of 20 ventilations/minute if breathing is inadequate.
5. If breathing is adequate, administer oxygen via nonrebreather mask at 15 lpm; consider blow-by oxygen in infants and very young children.

6. If seizure activity is due to fever (febrile seizure), remove clothing, cool infant or child by fanning, sponge with tepid water. Do not use ice or cold water.
7. Expedite transport in any of the following:
   a. Epileptic seizures lasting >10 minutes
   b. Two or more epileptic seizures without a period of consciousness between them
   c. Febrile seizures lasting >15 minutes
   d. Seizure due to any other cause (e.g., hypoxia, head injury)
8. Consider calling Advanced Life Support.
9. Expedite transport.
10. Perform an ongoing assessment every 5 minutes.

Figure 38-19   Emergency care protocol: seizures in the infant or child.

ASSESSMENT CONSIDERATIONS

The child's level of maturity will greatly influence the format of your assessment of mental status. If using AVPU or the Glasgow Coma Scale, you will need to modify them for a child. Ask the child simple questions. If the child appears to be lethargic, inconsolable, or agitated, ask the caregivers if this is a typical or an unusual response.

To assess the unresponsive infant or child, shout to elicit a response to verbal stimulus. Inflict a pinch to see if the child will respond to pain. *Never shake an infant or child for any reason.*

EMERGENCY MEDICAL CARE

Treatment of a pediatric patient with an altered mental status is aimed at managing life threats such as airway compromise. Treatment procedures include:

1. *Assure patency of the airway,* using manual and mechanical airway procedures as appropriate.
2. *Be prepared to suction the airway.*
3. *Administer oxygen* at 15 lpm or positive pressure ventilation with supplemental oxygen, as needed.
4. *Expedite transport.* A pediatric patient with an altered mental status is always a high priority.

To review emergency care for an altered mental status in the infant or child, see Figure 38-20.

EMERGENCY CARE PROTOCOL

ALTERED MENTAL STATUS IN THE INFANT OR CHILD

1. Establish and maintain open airway, extending head only enough to allow open airway and avoid hyperextension.
2. Suction secretions no longer than 5 to 10 seconds each time.
3. Provide positive pressure ventilation with supplemental oxygen at a minimum rate of 20 ventilations/ minute if breathing is inadequate.

4. If breathing is adequate, administer oxygen via nonrebreather mask at 15 lpm; consider blow-by oxygen in infants and very young children.
5. If signs and symptoms of hypoglycemia are present and child is a known diabetic on medication for the condition, consider oral glucose if child is able to swallow and medical direction approves.
6. Consider calling Advanced Life Support.
7. Expedite transport.
8. Perform an ongoing assessment every 5 minutes.

Figure 38-20   Emergency care protocol: altered mental status in the infant or child.

EMERGENCY CARE PROTOCOL

POISONING IN THE INFANT OR CHILD

1. Extend the head only enough to allow an open airway; avoid hyperextension.
2. Suction secretions no longer than 5 to 10 seconds each time.
3. Provide positive pressure ventilation with supplemental oxygen at a minimum rate of 20 ventilations/minute if breathing is inadequate.
4. If breathing is adequate, administer oxygen via nonrebreather mask at 15 lpm; consider blow-by oxygen in infants and very young children.
5. Treat the specific poisoning:

   Ingestion

   If patient is alert and able to swallow, and with permission from medical direction, consider activated charcoal at 12.5 to 25 grams in ingested poisons. Activated charcoal is contraindicated in the following:
   – Altered mental status
   – Ingestion of acids or alkalis
   – Patient is unable to swallow

   Inhalation

   Remove from toxic environment. Maximize oxygenation by nonrebreather mask at 15 lpm if breathing adequately or by positive pressure ventilation if breathing inadequately.

   Absorption

   Flush with water for 20 minutes at the scene. If eyes are involved, continue to flush en route.

   Injection

   Carefully monitor airway and breathing. If allergic reaction, and with order from medical direction, consider administration of epinephrine by auto-injector at 0.15 mg. Apply a constricting band proximal to site of bite or injection.
6. Consider calling Advanced Life Support.
7. Expedite transport.
8. Perform an ongoing assessment every 5 minutes.

Figure 38-21   Emergency care protocol: poisoning in the infant or child.

POISONINGS

Poisonings constitute a large number of emergency runs for pediatric patients. Due to children's inquisitive nature, they are always moving about and getting into things.

ASSESSMENT CONSIDERATIONS

For these patients a thorough focused history and physical exam is critically important. Since poisons can enter the body through numerous routes (ingestion, inhalation, absorption, injection), it is important for the EMT-B to gather as much information as possible regarding the type of overdose prior to transporting the patient to the hospital.

For specifics on assessment and management see Chapter 21, "Poisoning Emergencies."

EMERGENCY MEDICAL CARE

Emergency treatment of poisoned patients is geared toward the effects of the poisoning on the patient, rather than treating the specific type of poisoning. General emergency care for a pediatric patient suffering from a poisoning is as follows:

If the patient is alert:

1. *Contact medical direction or the local poison control center* regarding the use of activated charcoal if a poison was ingested.
2. *Provide oxygen* at 15 lpm by nonrebreather mask or positive pressure ventilation if necessary.
3. *Transport* any patient who was poisoned. Conduct an ongoing assessment en route, closely monitoring for a change in mental status or for airway or breathing compromise.

If the patient is initially unresponsive, or becomes unresponsive en route:

1. *Establish and maintain an open airway, and be prepared to suction.*
2. *Provide oxygen* at 15 lpm by nonrebreather mask; provide positive pressure ventilation with supplemental oxygen if the breathing is inadequate.
3. *Expedite transport.*
4. *Perform a rapid trauma assessment* to identify or rule out trauma as a cause of the altered mental status.

To review emergency care for poisoning in the infant or child, see Figure 38-21.

EMERGENCY CARE PROTOCOL

FEVER IN THE INFANT OR CHILD

1. Establish and maintain open airway, extending head only enough to allow open airway and avoid hyperextension.
2. Suction secretions no longer than 5 to 10 seconds each time.
3. Provide positive pressure ventilation with supplemental oxygen via reservoir at 20 ventilations/minute if breathing is inadequate.
4. If breathing is adequate, administer oxygen via nonrebreather mask at 15 lpm; consider blow-by oxygen in infants and very young children.

5. If seizure activity is due to fever (febrile seizure), remove clothing, cool infant or child by fanning, sponge with tepid water. Do not use ice or cold water.
6. Febrile seizures >15 minutes are a dire emergency and require expeditious transport and consideration for Advanced Life Support.
7. Consider calling Advanced Life Support.
8. Transport.
9. Perform an ongoing assessment every 5 minutes.

Figure 38-22 Emergency care protocol: fever in the infant or child.

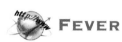 FEVER

Young children can develop fevers of up to 105 degrees Fahrenheit (40.6°C) quickly. Causes of high temperature include infection (including meningitis), and heat exposure (from being left in a hot car, for instance).

ASSESSMENT CONSIDERATIONS

The degree of temperature is not always of the greatest concern, but how quickly the temperature "spikes." If the temperature rises rapidly, a febrile seizure (a seizure caused by a high body temperature) may result. Not all high temperatures produce seizures.

In addition to seizures, another common result of fever is dehydration, the abnormal loss of fluids and electrolytes. Signs and symptoms include nausea, loss of appetite, vomiting, and possible fainting. A dehydrated child's pulse will be weak and rapid, the skin pale, the eyes sunken, and the mucous membranes will be dry and parched. When you pinch the skin, it will stay "tented." Dehydration in the infant may also result in a sunken fontanelle. The caregiver may indicate a decrease in frequency of urination by reporting fewer diaper changes than usual.

EMERGENCY MEDICAL CARE

Based on local protocol, lower the body temperature, administer oxygen at 15 lpm via a nonrebreather mask, and remove the child's clothes down to his diaper or underwear. Sponge the child's skin with a tepid towel to help drop the temperature. Do not use alcohol to sponge—the body will absorb it, and it

may cause hypothermia. Remove the child from the hot environment if the fever is related to the environment. Transport the patient and remain alert for seizures.

To review emergency care for fever in the infant or child, see Figure 38-22.

SHOCK (HYPOPERFUSION)

Severe shock (hypoperfusion) in children is unusual because their blood vessels constrict efficiently, which helps to maintain blood pressure. However, when blood pressure drops, it will usually drop rapidly and may precipitate cardiac arrest. Remember, however, that hypoperfusion and cardiac arrest is *rarely* due to cardiac compromise. In other words, failure of another body system (mainly respiratory) is what causes the cardiovascular system to fail, leading to hypoperfusion and/or cardiac arrest.

Newborns have been known to go into shock due to loss of body heat. They have immature thermoregulatory systems and cannot shiver or warm themselves through muscular activity. Additionally, their skin surface area is large in relation to their body weight which increases their rate of heat loss.

Shock can also be precipitated by certain medical problems that can cause the same response in adults. Common findings include diarrhea and dehydration, trauma, vomiting, blood loss, infection, and abdominal injuries. Less common causes of shock are allergic reactions, poisoning, or cardiac events.

The goal of treatment is to correct any abnormalities that may compound the hypoperfusion state (e.g., hypoxia, continued blood loss). Refer to Chapter 29, "Bleeding and Shock," for a complete discussion of assessment findings and treatment goals.

SIGNS OF SHOCK (HYPOPERFUSION) IN A CHILD

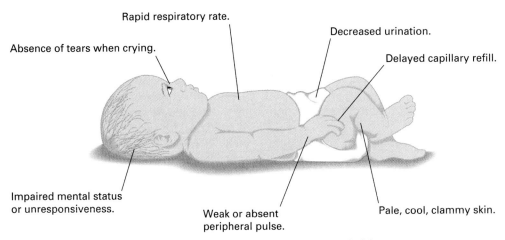

Figure 38-23 Signs of shock (hypoperfusion) in a child.

ASSESSMENT CONSIDERATIONS

Signs of shock include rapid respiratory rate, pale, cool, clammy skin, decreased mental status, prolonged capillary refill (under age 6), and weak or absent peripheral pulses (Figure 38-23). The important delineating factor between the adult and pediatric patient is that the onset of these signs in children may be sudden, occurring quickly as their compensatory mechanisms become exhausted and fail. This also means that *when pediatric patients deteriorate because of hypoperfusion, they deteriorate faster and more severely than adults.*

EMERGENCY MEDICAL CARE

1. *Assure an open airway and provide oxygen* at 15 lpm by nonrebreather mask.
2. *Provide positive pressure ventilation* with supplemental oxygen if breathing is inadequate.
3. *Control any bleeding if present.*
4. *Have the child lie supine; if possible raise the legs* to help venous return to the core.
5. *Keep the patient warm and as calm as possible.* If the patient is a newborn, preheat an isolette or your ambulance to at least 98°F (36.5°C) for full-term babies. If you do not have an isolette, wrap the baby in warm blankets (pre-warmed, if possible), then aluminum foil, to preserve body heat. Be sure that the baby's head (but not the baby's face) is covered.
6. *Transport* to the emergency department quickly.

To review emergency care for hypoperfusion in the infant or child, see Figure 38-24.

NEAR-DROWNING

Submersion can occur in *any* amount of water—from the ocean, to the bathtub, to a bucket. The main cause of death in infants or children who are submerged is not the aspiration of fluid (although it can occur in a small percentage of patients). Rather it is the hypoxia that occurs secondary to glottic closure reflex that occurs when the water comes in contact with the glottic opening. In other words, the majority of deaths are "dry drownings" where the person dies from suffocation, and fluid does not enter the lungs.

ASSESSMENT CONSIDERATIONS

When confronted with a near-drowning emergency, you need to be aware of the possibility of trauma and/or hypothermia. Infants and children are especially prone to hypothermia.

In any near-drowning emergency, you should also be on the alert for secondary drowning syndrome, a deterioration that takes place after normal breathing is restored—from minutes to hours after the event. For a more detailed discussion of near-drowning and other water emergencies, see Chapter 25, "Drowning, Near-Drowning, and Diving Emergencies."

EMERGENCY MEDICAL CARE

In the case of a cold water submersion, you should be particularly aggressive and persistent about resuscitating a pediatric patient. In response to the cold water, the mammalian dive reflex will slow down blood perfusion and metabolism. This means that the residual

EMERGENCY CARE PROTOCOL

HYPOPERFUSION IN THE INFANT OR CHILD

1. Establish and maintain open airway, extending head only enough to allow open airway and avoid hyperextension.
2. Suction secretions no longer than 5 to 10 seconds each time.
3. Provide positive pressure ventilation with supplemental oxygen at a minimum rate of 20 ventilations/minute if breathing is inadequate.
4. If breathing is adequate, administer oxygen via nonrebreather mask at 15 lpm; consider blow-by oxygen in infants and very young children.
5. If hypoperfusion is due to blood loss, control any external bleeding with direct pressure. If internal bleeding is suspected, transport immediately and expeditiously.
6. Keep the patient warm. If hypothermia is suspected, wrap patient in warm blankets and place ambulance heater on high. Cover infant or child's head. (Note: All patients in shock should be kept warm.)
7. Consider calling Advanced Life Support.
8. Expedite transport.
9. Perform an ongoing assessment every 5 minutes.

Figure 38-24   Emergency care protocol: hyperfusion in the infant or child.

oxygen in the blood will last longer for the brain to consume, and numerous cases of "saves" have been reported even after prolonged submersion in cold water (30 minutes or more). If you are unclear about the exact length of time under water, always give the patient the benefit of the doubt and initiate resuscitation.

1. *Remove the patient from the water.* Be sure that the person who rescues the patient is properly trained and equipped for water rescue.
2. *Assume that a spinal injury has occurred* and provide full immobilization while establishing an airway.
3. *Clear the airway, and provide positive pressure ventilation* with oxygen if breathing is inadequate or absent.
4. *Check circulation. Provide CPR as needed. Attach the AED in children older than 8 years.* If hypothermia is suspected, deliver only one set of three stacked shocks.
5. *Maintain the above treatment en route,* and monitor the airway closely for regurgitation.

To review emergency care for near-drowning in the infant or child, see Figure 38-25.

EMERGENCY CARE PROTOCOL

NEAR-DROWNING IN THE INFANT OR CHILD

1. Remove infant or child from water. If diving was involved in children or adolescents, consider in-line spinal stabilization and complete spinal immobilization.
2. Establish and maintain open airway, extending head only enough to allow open airway and avoid hyperextension.
3. Suction secretions no longer than 5 to 10 seconds each time.
4. Provide positive pressure ventilation with supplemental oxygen at a minimum rate of 20 ventilations/minute if breathing is inadequate.
5. Perform chest compression if no pulse is present. If child is older than 8 years, apply AED. Contact medical direction otherwise for orders. If hypothermia suspected, deliver only one set of three stacked shocks.
6. If breathing is adequate, administer oxygen via nonrebreather mask at 15 lpm; consider blow-by oxygen in infants and very young children.
7. If hypothermia is suspected, remove wet clothing, wrap patient in warm blankets and place ambulance heater on high. Cover infant or child's head.
8. Consider calling Advanced Life Support.
9. Expedite transport.
10. Perform an ongoing assessment every 5 minutes.

Figure 38-25   Emergency care protocol: near-drowning in the infant or child.

SUDDEN INFANT DEATH SYNDROME

Sudden infant death syndrome (SIDS), commonly known as crib death or cot death, is defined as the sudden and unexpected death of an infant or young child in which an autopsy fails to identify the cause of death. It is the leading cause of death among infants between 1 month and 1 year of age with a peak incidence around 4 months. SIDS is a post-mortem diagnosis, not one that can be made in the field. While the facts behind SIDS will be outlined here, *do not make a firm diagnosis to a family member.*

To date, no reliable ways to predict or prevent SIDS are known. It almost always occurs while the baby is sleeping. The typical SIDS case involves an apparently healthy infant, frequently born premature, and usually between the age of 4 weeks and 7 months, who suddenly dies during a sleep period in his crib. No illness need be present, though the baby may have had recent cold symptoms. There is usually no indication of struggle. Sometimes, though, the child has obviously changed position near the time of death.

There is much confusion about SIDS among both the general public and the medical profession. Not until recently has serious medical research on SIDS been conducted. However, its exact cause is still unknown.

ASSESSMENT CONSIDERATIONS

SIDS cannot be diagnosed in the field. When you arrive in response to the emergency call, you will find the patient in cardiac arrest and you will proceed with care as you would for any patient in this condition. Do not delay resuscitation (as described below) but, as practical, obtain a brief SAMPLE history of the infant and observe the surroundings, including:

- Physical appearance of the baby
- Position of the baby in the crib
- Physical appearance of the crib
- Presence of objects in the crib
- Unusual or dangerous items in the room (such as plastic bags)
- Appearance of the room/house
- Presence of medication, even if it is for adults
- Circumstances concerning discovery of the unresponsive child
- Time the baby was put to bed or fell asleep
- Problems at birth
- General health
- Any recent illnesses
- Date and result of last physical exam

Be very careful not to convey by the wording of your questions or your manner any suspicion that the parents may be responsible for the child's condition.

EMERGENCY MEDICAL CARE

When you find an infant in respiratory and cardiac arrest—a condition for which SIDS is one, but only one, possible cause—proceed as follows:

1. *Immediately try to resuscitate.* Attempt aggressive resuscitation of the baby. The exceptions are rigor mortis (when joints become rigid) and dependent lividity (discoloration created by gravity causing the blood to pool in the lowest body areas). If the patient displays rigor mortis or lividity, he should be left in the position found and local authorities should be called according to local protocol.
2. *Encourage the caregivers to talk and tell their story.*
3. *Do not provide false reassurances.*
4. *Transport the infant* to the hospital, making sure that you tell the caregivers where you are taking the child and provide clear directions about how to get there. Encourage them to have someone else drive them, and remind them to arrange for care of any siblings.
5. *Deliver the baby into the hands of the emergency department staff.* Be careful of what you say to your colleagues at the hospital. Casual comments such as "smothered" or "injured" may be overheard by the family and cause unnecessary emotional distress. Never say anything that the family may overhear which makes them feel they are to blame or are being blamed for the infant's death.

To review emergency care for sudden infant death syndrome in the infant or child, see Figure 38-26.

AIDING FAMILY MEMBERS IN SIDS EMERGENCIES

The reactions of family members to the SIDS incident will be varied. One of the most common immediate reactions of caregivers to SIDS is shock and disbelief. This may cause family members to become immobilized—incapable of making decisions. Or this may cause them to act as if they are cold and unfeeling. It is not that they do not care, just that they are having a hard time facing reality.

It may be difficult for you to deal with extreme reactions. Some caregivers may physically act out their emotions, resulting in hysteria, crying, or wailing. Caregivers may be confused and overwhelmed with guilty feelings, unfairly venting their anger and frustration on each other—or on you.

Do not dismiss the caregivers because they are not the patients in the traditional sense of the word. The tendency is to ignore the mother's bar-

EMERGENCY CARE PROTOCOL

SUDDEN INFANT DEATH SYNDROME

1. If rigor mortis and dependent lividity are present, do not attempt to resuscitate. Turn your attention to supporting the parents.
2. Attempt resuscitation if any chance of survival exists:
   a. Establish and maintain open airway, extending head only enough to allow open airway and avoid hyperextension.
   b. Suction secretions.
   c. Provide positive pressure ventilation with supplemental oxygen via reservoir at 20 ventilations/minute and chest compressions at a rate of at least 120/minute.
   d. Consider calling Advanced Life Support.
   e. Expedite transport.
   f. Perform an ongoing assessment every 5 minutes.
3. Care for the caregivers or parents.
   a. Encourage them to talk and tell their story.
   b. Do not provide false reassurances.
   c. Avoid any statements that might place blame on the caregiver or parents.
4. If resuscitation is not attempted, contact coroner or follow your local protocol regarding moving the infant or transport.

Figure 38-26   Emergency care protocol: sudden infant death syndrome.

rage of questions concerning her child, and to tell her politely to go away. While you are there to give medical care and not to become personally "involved," you must still understand that these caregivers and family members need your care also. Small, often nonverbal, gestures on your part are very important. By simply sitting with the caregivers, you are showing them that someone cares. Offer to be of assistance to them—to make phone calls or to get them coffee. A sympathetic ear may be all they need.

Don't neglect your own emotional turmoil. After a SIDS call, it is common for rescuers to experience anxiety, guilt, or anger. Ignoring your emotions will not cause them to go away. You should talk out your feelings with the Critical Incident Stress Debriefing (CISD) team, colleagues, friends, or your spouse.

TRAUMA IN INFANTS AND CHILDREN

Trauma is the leading cause of death in children from ages 1 to 14. Each year, thousands of children die from unintentional injury and more are permanently disabled. Fifty percent of deaths from trauma occur within the first hour after an injury. The primary killer of American children is the automobile; however, children may experience trauma while riding bicycles, all-terrain vehicles, and motorcycles, climbing trees, as pedestrians, during recreational activities, and even homicide and suicide.

Blunt trauma is the most common injury in children. Quite frequently, a child will be severely injured but display no early, obvious signs. (Review Chapter 28, "Mechanisms of Injury: Kinetics of Trauma.") At the scene, try to reconstruct the incident and understand the mechanism of injury.

When assessing mechanism of injury during the scene size-up, remember not only to look at the vehicle (or other object) that caused the trauma, but to look at the size of the patient in relation to what they came into contact with. The following are mechanisms of injury and the common patterns of injury to expect in infants and children:

- Unrestrained children in cars will probably suffer head and neck injuries because the child's head is proportionally larger than the adult's, and it is likely to come into contact with the interior of the car (e.g., the dashboard).
- Restrained passengers will probably suffer abdominal and/or lumbar injuries from the stress applied by the seat belt during the accident. This is especially true if the child was improperly restrained in the automobile.
- If the child was struck while riding a bike, he is likely to sustain head injuries, spinal injuries, and abdominal injuries because these areas of the body are typically near the same height as the bumper and hood of a car.
- If the young patient was struck by a car while walking, suspect head injuries, chest injuries, and lower extremity injuries. Again, a quick estimation of the pain site as well as the height of the bumper and hood on the car can help localize where the patient suffered trauma.
- If the patient was diving into water or fell from a height, suspect head and spinal injuries.
- If the mechanism of injury involved burns, be aware that the burns may be more severe to the in-

fant or child because his skin is not as thick or durable as an adult's. Also remember that the inhalation of smoke, toxic fumes, or super-heated air during a fire can cause airway swelling more rapidly and severely than in adults.

- Sports injuries typically involve injuries to the head and neck.
- Unfortunately, child abuse is another cause of trauma. A discussion of child abuse will follow later in the chapter.

TRAUMA AND THE INFANT'S OR CHILD'S ANATOMY

While a full discussion of trauma is presented in Chapters 28 through 37, the following will be a brief overview of injures as they relate to the infant or child patient. The EMT-B should remember that the treatment emphasis (regardless of injury) will always be airway, breathing, and circulatory management and consideration of spinal immobilization.

ASSESSMENT CONSIDERATIONS

Because of differences in infant and child anatomy, as compared to adult anatomy, there are some special considerations for the assessment of the infant or child trauma patient. Some of these considerations for injuries to the head, chest, abdomen, and extremities are discussed below.

Head Head injuries are common in children because of the relatively larger size of the child's head compared to the body. The weight of the head will carry it forward in advance of the body. Often in trauma the head is the first thing to strike an object. Common findings of head injury include:

- Nausea and vomiting
- Respiratory arrest (common to serious head injuries)
- Facial and scalp injuries (in infants and children, blood loss can be profound enough to cause hypoperfusion)

The most common cause of hypoxia in the unresponsive head injury patient is the tongue obstructing the airway. Therefore, an important consideration in the initial assessment is the airway.

Be aware that hypoperfusion is not typically one of the signs of closed head injury. If signs of hypoperfusion are present with a closed head injury, you should suspect that other injuries (e.g., internal injuries) are more likely causing the hypoperfusion.

Chest Remember that infants and children have ribs that are more pliable than adult ribs. This means that the young patient is less likely to suffer rib fractures, but is more likely to sustain internal damage (lung injury, heart wall injury) because the ribs do not protect these structures very well from forces applied to the chest. Even when you see minimal signs of external trauma, still suspect serious intrathoracic injuries.

Abdomen The abdominal muscles are not as developed in the child as in the adult and, therefore, they cannot offer as much protection from blunt trauma. If you have a patient who is deteriorating rapidly without external signs of injury, suspect hidden injuries of the abdomen. Consider any trauma to the abdomen as a serious injury, and transport the patient immediately.

Finally, be aware that younger patients are primarily "diaphragmatic breathers." Excessive gastric insufflation (air in the stomach) can distend the abdomen enough to interfere with normal diaphragm movement and also with lung inflation. This will impede normal ventilation or positive pressure ventilation. Do not generate high airway pressures while providing positive pressure ventilations to an infant or child, because this will cause air to enter the stomach. Slow delivery of ventilations over 1 to 1½ seconds with just enough volume to cause the chest to rise will decrease the incidence of gastric distention. Cricoid pressure will also reduce the incidence of gastric distention during ventilation. If gastric distention develops, it can be relieved by placing a gastric tube through the esophagus into the stomach—a procedure that may be performed by EMT-Bs in some jurisdictions, by ALS teams in others (see Chapter 45, "Advanced Airway Management").

Extremities The presentation of injuries to the extremities is the same for infants, children, and adults, and assessment and treatment of them is essentially the same. However, you should be sure to use the appropriately sized immobilization equipment rather than trying to "make-shift" an adult device to fit an infant or child.

EMERGENCY MEDICAL CARE— TRAUMA IN INFANTS AND CHILDREN

As with an adult, the priorities in treating an infant or child trauma patient center around airway management, breathing, and circulatory support as follows:

1. *Establish and maintain in-line spine stabilization and the airway,* using a jaw thrust.
2. *Suction as necessary.* Constantly reassess for hemorrhage into the mouth.
3. *Provide oxygen* at 15 lpm by nonrebreather mask if ventilations are adequate, or initiate positive pressure ventilation with supplemental oxygen if breathing is inadequate.

4. *Provide complete spinal immobilization* (a discussion of infant/child immobilization is given under Enrichment at the end of this chapter). Never use sandbags as a means to secure the head to a long spinal board. If it ever becomes necessary to roll the backboard with the patient secured (for vomiting), the heavy sandbags will put unnecessary pressure on the head.

5. *Transport* to a hospital. See Table 38-2 for criteria that may require transport to a trauma center.

Note that use of the PASG to control any major bleeding should be determined by local protocol. As a general rule, you should only use the PASG on pediatric patients if all of the following conditions are met:

• The garment fits the child (do not place an infant in one leg of a PASG trouser).
• The abdomen compartment is not inflated. (This could compromise respiration.)
• Proper indications for PASG use are present (i.e., trauma with signs of severe hypoperfusion and pelvic instability).

Infants and children under the age of 5 suffer more severe consequences from burns than do older children and adults. They are more at risk for hypothermia, fluid loss, and other effects, partly because of their greater skin surface in relation to body mass. In a trauma emergency that involves burns remember to cover the burn with dry sterile burn dressing and keep the patient warm. If the burns meet the criteria for burn center admission in your area, transport to that facility. Review the special segments on infants and children in Chapter 31, "Burn Emergencies."

To review emergency care for trauma in the infant or child, see Figure 38-27.

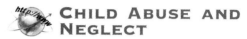

CHILD ABUSE AND NEGLECT

The estimated number of children who are abused and/or neglected in the United States is staggering. Estimates range between 500,000 and 4 million cases annually with thousands of abused children dying. In fact, child abuse has been the only major cause of infant and child death to increase in the last 30 years.

TABLE 38-2

Transporting the Traumatized Infant or Child

You should transport the traumatized child to a hospital specializing in trauma care or a Level 1 Pediatric Trauma Center when one or more of the following criteria has been met:
MECHANISM OF INJURY Pedestrian struck at speeds of 10 mph or greater, or thrown Unrestrained occupant at speeds of 20 mph or greater Restrained occupant at speeds of 40 mph or greater Hit by a vehicle at speeds of 20 mph or greater or at an unknown speed Ejected from the vehicle or thrown in the air greater than 5 feet Fell from a height of 10 feet or greater Prolonged extrication of 20 minutes or greater Motor vehicle crash when another occupant is killed Pulled from or dragged underneath a vehicle or run over by a vehicle's wheels When in doubt, assume the worst
GROSS LOCATION OF INJURY High suspicion of cervical spine injury Uncontrolled hemorrhage Obvious open injuries to extremities in which the bone is certain to be broken Severe maxillofacial injuries Unstable chest injuries and/or major pelvic injuries Penetrating or crush injury to the head, neck, chest, abdomen, or pelvis Neurologic injuries producing prolonged loss of consciousness, altered mental status, abnormal body posturing, seizures Major amputations Tracheal or laryngeal injuries Burns greater than 20% of body surface area or with suspected smoke inhalation
PHYSIOLOGICAL DISTRESS Any injury that produces hypoperfusion or respiratory distress Any child with a Pediatric Trauma Score of 8 or less (see Enrichment section) Any child with a Glasgow Coma Score of 12 or less Any child with a history of respiratory or cardiopulmonary arrest caused by the injury

EMERGENCY CARE PROTOCOL

TRAUMA IN THE INFANT OR CHILD

1. Establish and maintain in-line spine stabilization and open the airway, using jaw-thrust maneuver.
2. Suction secretions no longer than 5 to 10 seconds each time.
3. Provide positive pressure ventilation with supplemental oxygen at a minimum rate of 20 ventilations/minute if breathing is inadequate.
4. If breathing is adequate, administer oxygen via nonrebreather mask at 15 lpm; consider blow-by oxygen in infants and very young children.
5. Occlude any open wounds to the chest with a nonporous dressing taped on three sides.
6. Manage abdominal evisceration by applying a moist sterile dressing to exposed organs, covered by a nonporous dressing secured in place.
7. If spinal injury is suspected, completely immobilize patient to a long board.
8. Consider calling Advanced Life Support.
9. If a pelvic injury is suspected and the patient has abdominal pain, apply the PASG according to local protocol.
10. Expedite transport.
11. Splint fractures and dress wounds.
12. Perform an ongoing assessment every 5 minutes.

Figure 38-27 Emergency care protocol: trauma in the infant or child.

Physical abuse takes place when improper or excessive action is taken so as to injure or cause harm. **Neglect** is the provision of inadequate attention or respect to someone who has a claim to that attention. The adult (usually a caregiver) who abuses a child often behaves in an evasive manner, volunteering little information or giving contradictory information about what has happened to the child. The caregiver may show outright hostility toward the child or toward another caregiver in the household and rarely shows any guilt. The abused child will usually show fear when asked to describe how the injury occurred.

In many cases, a child will be victim of a combination of physical, emotional, and sexual abuse and neglect. General indicators of abuse and/or neglect include (Figures 38-28a to f).

- Multiple abrasions, lacerations, incisions, bruises, broken bones
- Multiple injuries or bruises in various stages of healing
- Injuries on both the front and back or on both sides of the child's body
- Unusual wounds (such as cigarette burns)
- A fearful child
- Injuries to the genitals
- Injuries, often lethal, to the brain or spinal cord that occur when the infant or child is violently shaken (known as "shaken baby syndrome")
- Situations in which the injuries do not match the mechanism of injury described by the caregivers or the patient
- Lack of adult supervision
- Untreated chronic illnesses (e.g., no medication for an asthmatic)
- Malnourishment and unsafe living environment
- Delay in reporting injuries

Bruises that are true accidents are often found on the lower arms, knees, shins, iliac crests, forehead, and under the chin. "Suspicious" bruises are found on the buttocks, genitalia, thighs, ears, side of face, trunk, and upper arms.

EMERGENCY MEDICAL CARE GUIDELINES FOR CHILD ABUSE

You should be familiar with several important guidelines when called to a possible child abuse situation. While the following care steps assume that a caregiver is the abuser, remember that a child may also be abused by a relative, sibling, or neighbor.

- *Gaining entry*—If the call came from outside the family, the caregivers may resist, and entry should be handled by the police. If you are asked to help the child, calm the caregivers and suggest by your actions that you are there to help and render emergency care to the child. Speak in a low, firm voice. If the scene is—or becomes—dangerous, request law enforcement to be dispatched.
- *Dealing with the child*—Speak softly and call the child by his first name. Do not ask the child to recreate the situation or answer questions while he is still in the crisis environment, with the possible abuser still present.
- *Examining the child*—If you have reason to suspect abuse, perform a head-to-toe (toe-to-head or trunk-to-head for an infant or toddler) rapid trauma assessment, searching for DCAP-BTLS and clues to internal injury. Look carefully for signs of head

CHILD ABUSE AND NEGLECT

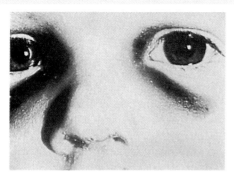

Figure 38-28a   Child physical abuse.

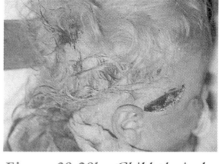

Figure 38-28b   Child physical abuse.

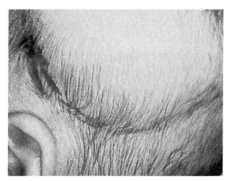

Figure 38-28c   Child neglect from lack of appropriate medical care.

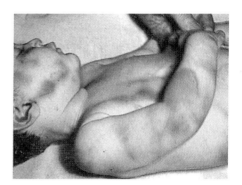

Figure 38-29d   Child abuse death from multiple injuries.

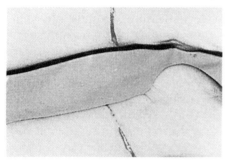

Figure 38-28e   Physical abuse—restraining by tying.

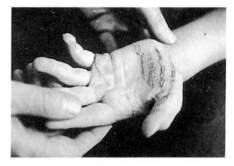

Figure 38-28f   Physical abuse—burns from hand held onto an electric stove.

trauma, closely examining the ears and nose for blood or cerebrospinal fluid and the eyes for pupillary changes. Conduct the examination in a matter-of-fact fashion, and keep your suspicions to yourself. Also note all that you have observed at the scene (e.g., condition of the home; any objects that might have been used to hurt the child, such as a belt or straps).

- *Dealing with the caregivers*—After administering emergency care, tell the caregivers that the child should be taken to the hospital for further care. In a separate room from the child, ask the caregivers to describe how the injury occurred. (This will permit the hospital staff, social service workers, or others later to compare the child's account with that of the caregivers.) *Do not question the caregivers about abuse, or act accusatory in any way. This is inappropriate and will only delay transport.* Simply gather information concerning the injuries as you would for any other problem.
- *Transporting the child*—Do not allow the child to be left alone with the suspected abuser. This may

EMERGENCY CARE PROTOCOL

ABUSE AND NEGLECT IN THE INFANT OR CHILD

1. Consider law enforcement to gain entry or if the scene becomes unstable or dangerous.
2. Establish and maintain open airway, extending head only enough to allow open airway and avoid hyperextension. If spinal injury is suspected, provide in-line spine stabilization and perform a jaw-thrust maneuver.
3. Suction secretions no longer than 5 to 10 seconds each time.
4. Provide positive pressure ventilation with supplemental oxygen at a minimum rate of 20 ventilations/minute if breathing is inadequate.
5. If breathing is adequate, administer oxygen via nonrebreather mask at 15 lpm; consider blow-by oxygen in infants and very young children.
6. Manage immediately life-threatening wounds.
7. If spinal injury is suspected, completely immobilize patient to a long board.
8. Consider calling Advanced Life Support if a priority patient.
9. Expedite transport.
10. Splint fractures and dress wounds.
11. Perform an ongoing assessment every 5 minutes.
12. Special considerations when dealing with child abuse and neglect:
    a. Speak softly and call the child by his first name.
    b. Do not ask the child to recreate the situation or answer questions while still in the abusive environment.
    c. Your main goal is to conduct an assessment and treat the injured infant or child. You are not there to investigate a crime; however, note and report objectively what was observed at the scene.
    d. Do not question the caregivers about the abuse, but ask what had happened.
    e. Do not let the child be left alone with the suspected or possible abuser.
    f. Provide accurate and objective documentation in the EMS report.

Figure 38-29   Emergency care protocol: abuse and neglect in the infant or child.

provide the opportunity for further abuse or intimidation.

• *Providing documentation*—When you reach the hospital, privately convey your suspicions and findings to the physician. Know your state's reporting laws for child abuse. Document everything, but be objective, not subjective. It is not your role to write "The patient was abused." Rather, by your accurate and detailed description of the injuries and history, the person reading the run report will be able to come up with this conclusion. Record all of your findings regarding the assessment, the conditions of the home, the behavior or the caregivers, and so on. Make drawings of injury patterns or locations of injuries. Maintain total confidentiality regarding the incident; do not share it with your family or friends.

It is critical that you be aware of the reporting laws in your own state and the reporting protocols for your EMS system. Aspects of the law to know are:

• Who must report the abuse
• What types of abuse and neglect must be reported
• To whom the reports are to be made
• What information a reporter must give
• What immunity the reporter is granted
• Criminal penalties for failing to report

Child-abuse cases are particularly painful for EMS providers. Be sure you talk out your feelings with someone you can trust (making sure not to divulge particulars of the case). Feelings of anger, revulsion, frustration, and helplessness are normal. In most instances, there is no "perfect" solution, whether the child remains in the home or is placed elsewhere. Yet, an EMT-B's skillful interviewing and reporting can make a positive difference, even in bad situations.

To review emergency care for abuse and neglect in the infant or child, see Figure 38-29.

INFANTS AND CHILDREN WITH SPECIAL NEEDS

Advances in medical technology have made it possible for many children who require advanced support (e.g., mechanical ventilation, supplemental tube feedings, intravenous medications) to live at home with skilled members of the family managing their needs. This has created a new and interesting challenge for the EMS provider.

Before a child is discharged home, the caregivers are taught to manage the needs of their child. Routine care and simple procedures are usually accomplished without any problems, but occasionally, something out of the ordinary happens and the caregiver accesses the EMS system. The most common problems you will encounter involve complications with tracheostomy tubes, failures of mechanical ventilators, problems with the venous access devices known as central lines, and feeding tubes in children who cannot be fed by mouth.

TRACHEOSTOMY TUBES

Tracheostomy tubes are placed through a surgical incision in the neck (called a stoma) directly into the trachea to provide a secure airway. Tracheostomy tubes are short plastic tubes with an external flange that are held in place with a tie of some sort (Figure 38-30).

In children with tracheostomy tubes, the body's natural ability to filter the air and to rid the airway of secretions are absent because the upper airway is bypassed. Accumulation of mucus can lead to obstruction of the airway. The airway can be easily cleared by suctioning the tube with a suction catheter that is half the diameter of the tube itself. Select the proper size catheter and measure against a new tracheostomy tube of the same size so that it will advance 0.5 cm beyond the tip. A small amount of sterile saline (1 ml) injected into the tube prior to suctioning will help to loosen mucus and make suctioning more productive. To avoid depriving the child of oxygen, suction for only 3 to 4 seconds at a time and hyperventilate the child (provide extra oxygen through a positive pressure ventilation device) between suctioning. The child will grimace and attempt to cough while you suction. This is normal. Repeat until the airway is clear.

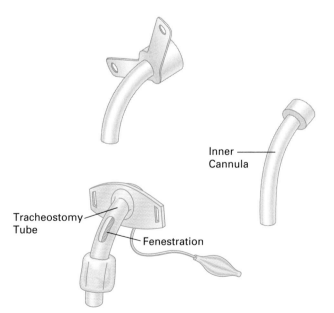

Figure 38-30 Tracheostomy tubes. Top: Plastic tube. Bottom: Metal tube with inner cannula.

Other common problems with tracheostomy tubes are bleeding, infection around the site, an air leak around the tube, or dislodgment of the tube. If a tube has become dislodged and the airway is compromised, bag-valve-mask or pocket-mask ventilations may not be effective. Two options exist in this situation: (1) Seal the mask around the mouth and nose, cover the stoma completely with your hand, and attempt to ventilate through the mouth and nose (usually there will still be a connection of the trachea to the mouth and nose, even though it has been bypassed by the stoma in the neck); or (2) Seal the mask over the stoma, cover the mouth and nose completely with your hand, and attempt to ventilate through the stoma. In any case, the child with a dislodged tracheostomy tube should be transported to the hospital.

If the problem is bleeding around the site of the stoma (excessive coughing can tear the soft mucous membranes and cause bleeding), be sure to continually suction out the blood so the patient does not aspirate it. General care steps for children with tracheostomy tubes are:

1. Maintain a patent airway.
2. Suction out any foreign material or fluid.
3. Provide supplemental oxygen. (Positive pressure ventilation can be provided by attaching the bag-valve-mask device directly to the standard fitting on the tracheostomy tube.)
4. Maintain a position of comfort for the patient.
5. Transport for evaluation at the hospital.

Often, the situation has become more than the caregiver could manage and this prompted the call for assistance, but once you are there the caregiver can function as an excellent resource and help you perform many necessary interventions.

HOME ARTIFICIAL VENTILATORS

Home ventilators automatically assist breathing in a patient who cannot breathe adequately on his own. Home ventilator malfunctions are usually due to mechanical failures, power outages, or a diminished oxygen supply. Ventilators have back-up batteries in the event of a power failure, but these usually have a short life. You may be notified in advance if a child comes home on a home ventilator so that you will be ready to assist the family in the event of a malfunction. The best course of action is to manually ventilate the child and help the caregiver to troubleshoot the problem with the ventilator. If the problem cannot be remedied:

1. Establish and maintain an open airway.
2. Provide positive pressure ventilation with supple-

mental oxygen at a rate of one every three seconds.
3. Transport to the hospital.

CENTRAL LINES

A central line is a long-term venous access device—a way of getting needed medications or other substances into the child's bloodstream by cannulating a vein. Common names for these devices include Hickman/Broviac, Groshong, Port-a-Cath, Infus-A-Port, and Mediport. Intravenous access is normally outside the area of practice for an EMT-B, so if you are called to take care of a child with an indwelling catheter (a permanently placed IV site), it may be necessary to transport quickly to get experienced help.

The call to EMS most commonly occurs when the site around the device has become infected or when the device is not flushing properly and has clotted off. Because these devices (unlike an everyday IV in a hand or arm) are placed very near to the heart in the body's central circulation, the risk of an overwhelming infection is very high. You may also be called to assist if the device has cracked or has otherwise ruptured. Often this occurs in the exposed portion of the catheter where the catheter can be clamped. If the device cracks beneath the skin, significant bleeding may result. Emergency management includes:

1. Correct and maintain any inadequacies to the child's airway, breathing, or circulation, as in any emergency call.
2. Apply pressure directly to the device to control the bleeding.
3. Transport to the hospital so that the device can be evaluated and repaired, if necessary.

GASTROSTOMY TUBES

Gastrostomy tubes are placed into the stomach through the abdominal wall in children who require long-term gastric feeding—patients who cannot be fed by mouth.

Another means of accomplishing gastric feeding is the surgical placement of a "feeding button." The feeding button is a small silicon device that protrudes slightly from the abdominal wall and accepts a feeding tube through its one-way valve. The feeding button is popular in children who require long-term feedings because it is cosmetically more pleasing than a tube and allows the child greater mobility.

Problems with gastrostomy tubes are usually not acute. You may be called to assist when a tube has dislodged or when the area around it has become infected. Emergency management includes:

1. Maintain an adequate airway and breathing status.
2. Be prepared to suction.

3. Be alert for changes in mental status. If the patient is also a diabetic, he will become hypoglycemic quickly if he cannot be fed.
4. Provide oxygen as necessary.
5. Transport the patient in a Fowler's position, or on his right side with the head elevated.

SHUNTS

Certain patients who have medical illnesses or anatomical defects are predisposed to an excessive accumulation of cerebrospinal fluid in the brain. Since the skull is a fixed size and cannot expand to accommodate the extra fluid, pressure builds within the skull which results in compression of the brain. To alleviate this, a device called a shunt is surgically placed, extending from the brain to the abdomen in order to drain this extra fluid. The EMT-B may also find a reservoir on the side of the skull.

When this shunt malfunctions, the CSF will accumulate in the brain and the patient may experience signs characteristic of head-injured patients. They may display changes in their mental status, seizures, loss of motor or sensory function, vomiting, and respiratory depression. The treatment is geared to supporting depressed or lost functions:

1. Manage the airway. Be alert for occlusion by the tongue if the mental status is decreased.
2. Initiate positive pressure ventilation if the breathing is inadequate. (Respiratory arrest is common.)
3. Position the patient on his left side and be prepared to suction.
4. Provide rapid transport to the hospital. This can be a truly life-threatening situation.

TAKING CARE OF YOURSELF

Taking care of a critically ill or injured child is perhaps one of the most challenging facets of an EMS career. The death of a child has a profound effect on each and every one of us. Almost half of the children in the United States who die from unintentional injuries are pronounced dead either at the scene or in the emergency department. EMT-Bs who are treating infants or children commonly experience stress and anxiety from:

- Lack of experience in treating children (from the relative infrequency of treating children)
- The fear of failure
- Identifying patients with their own children (e.g., "This could be my daughter . . .")

To help alleviate stress:

- Understand that much of what you learned about adults applies to children; typically it is not what you do but how you do it that varies when your patient is an infant or child.

- Learn skills and practice with equipment and examining children; the best defense against anxiety is preparation.
- Focus on the task at hand while treating infants and children. In other words, temporarily separate how you feel from what you must do.

As a professional EMT-B, you need to control your emotions so that you can render the best possible assistance to your patient and be supportive of other victims. But after the incident is over, you still need to deal with those feelings.

Most EMS systems have their own Critical Incident Stress Debriefing Team or have ready access to one. The CISD team is set up to defuse the stress that certain events can create. Use them. If not, find a trusted friend who will listen to you and allow you to talk about the way you feel. Stress-induced burnout is a leading reason why people do not remain in this field.

ENRICHMENT

The enrichment section contains information that is valuable as background for the EMT-B but that goes substantially beyond the U.S. Department of Transportation (DOT) EMT-Basic curriculum.

Since airway and respiratory problems are the most common findings in pediatric emergencies, in this segment we will discuss conditions that are often the cause of pediatric respiratory distress complaints. In addition, we will provide information on infectious diseases, pediatric trauma scoring, and infant car seat immobilization.

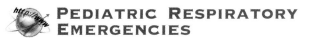

PEDIATRIC RESPIRATORY EMERGENCIES

CROUP

Croup is a common infection of the upper airway, usually caused by a virus but sometimes by bacteria. It has a slow onset of symptoms, is accompanied by a low grade fever, and it is most common in children between 1 and 3 years of age.

The infection causes swelling beneath the glottis and progressively narrows the airway (Figure 38-31). The child is typically hoarse, coughs with a harsh "seal bark," and produces stridor upon inhalation. High-pitched squeaking sounds may also be present. As the condition worsens, further obstructing the airway, you will see the classic signs of respiratory distress: nasal flaring, tugging at the throat, retraction of muscles around the rib cage, restlessness, a rising pulse rate, and cyanosis.

Severe attacks can be dangerous, and you should treat as follows:

1. Apply humidified oxygen by a mask held slightly away from the patient's face.
2. Keep the patient in a position of comfort, either propped up or in a caregiver's arms.
3. Transport the patient to the hospital with as little disturbance as possible.
4. Be aware that cool night air may reduce the swelling in the airway, bringing relief. You may need to explain the original signs to emergency department personnel if the patient appears much better after transport.

EPIGLOTTITIS

A condition that resembles croup, epiglottitis is caused by a bacterial infection that inflames and

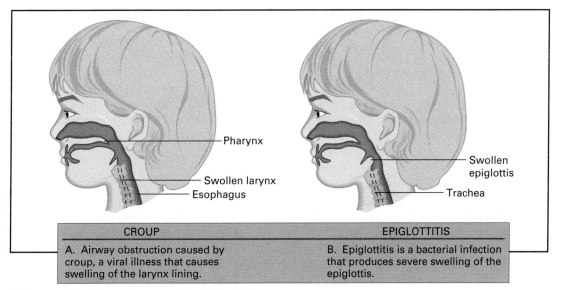

Figure 38-31 Croup and epiglottitis.

causes swelling of the epiglottis (Figure 38-31). The most common age group affected is 3 to 7 years. *Epiglottitis is life-threatening; if left untreated it has a 50 percent mortality rate. The onset is usually rapid and is accompanied by a high temperature.*

Signs and symptoms of epiglottitis are:

- Pain on swallowing
- High fever (102° to 104°F)
- Drooling (because it is painful to swallow)
- Mouth breathing
- Changes in voice quality and pain upon speaking
- The patient insists on sitting up and leaning forward (tripod position).
- The patient's chin and neck are thrust outward.
- The patient is usually not hoarse and may not struggle to breathe, although there may be a short "croak" during inhalation.
- As the attack worsens, the patient may appear strikingly still.

If you suspect epiglottitis, be calm and gentle and treat as follows:

1. Do not attempt to place anything in the child's mouth since this can increase swelling of the epiglottis and cause laryngospasm that can completely block the airway. Nothing in the mouth means no oropharyngeal airway, no suctioning equipment, and no fingers!
2. Allow the child to assume a position of comfort (usually sitting upright, leaning forward).
3. Provide oxygen at 15 lpm. Let the child hold the mask, or turn the oxygen on full and hold it a few inches away from the child's face. Be careful that it does not cause irritation or coughing. If the child's airway is completely obstructed, provide bag-valve-mask ventilations with supplemental oxygen, forcing oxygen past the swollen epiglottis and spasmed larynx.
4. Transport. Patients with epiglottitis may need endotracheal intubation or a surgical airway, and this should be done in a controlled setting such as an emergency department or operating room.

ASTHMA

Asthma is common in children, particularly those with allergies. Every asthmatic attack should be regarded as a serious medical emergency. The mortality rate from asthma increases annually in the United States. Acute asthmatic attacks occur when the bronchioles spasm and constrict and the bronchial membranes swell, reducing the airway size and producing large amounts of mucus. Signs of asthma attacks include wheezing, shortness of breath, cough, faster breathing than normal and increased heart rate. For a more detailed discussion of asthma signs, symptoms, and emergency medical care see Chapter 14, "Respiratory Emergencies."

Get the patient's SAMPLE history from the caregivers by asking:

- How long has the child been wheezing?
- How much fluid has he taken during this period?
- Has he had a recent cold or other infection, particularly one involving the respiratory tract?
- Has he had any medication for this attack? What is it? When? How much? (It is especially important to ask about metered dose inhalers.) Does he take steroids?
- Does he have any known allergies to drugs, foods, pollens, or other inhalants?
- Has he ever been hospitalized for an acute asthmatic attack? Was it an ICU admission (was the child in an intensive care unit)? How recently and how often? Has the patient ever required a mechanical ventilator during an attack?

During the physical exam of the patient, pay particular attention to:

- *Position*—Children with mild attacks of asthma often appear agitated and prefer to sit, but will lie still. Children with severe attacks seem exhausted and unable to move. Frequently they prefer to lean forward, bracing themselves on their elbows (tripod position). Children under the age of 2 often show no agitation and will lie on their backs, even when this increases their difficulty in breathing.
- *Mental status*—Sleepiness and changes in mental status are progressively more serious signs of hypoxia, acidosis, and retention of carbon dioxide.
- *Vital signs*—As an attack worsens, the pulse grows faster and weaker. Blood pressure may fall. Bradycardia (slower-than-normal heart rate) is an ominous sign of impending respiratory and potential cardiac arrest.
- *Skin color and condition*—Pinch the skin to look for evidence of dehydration ("tenting"). Check for cyanosis of the tongue and mucous membranes, suggesting hypoxia.
- *Respirations*—A mild to moderate attack of asthma is characterized by loud breathing sounds, loud wheezes, and occasional crackles. As the attack worsens, the breath sounds become less audible and are completely absent in a severe attack. Auscultate the entire chest, since localized wheezes suggest a foreign body obstruction, while asthma causes generalized wheezes.

Because of the emotional component of asthma (stress makes it worse), try to be as calm and reassuring as possible and follow these treatment steps.

1. Apply humidified oxygen at 15 lpm by nonrebreather mask. Assist ventilations if breathing is not adequate.
2. Allow the child to assume a position of comfort.
3. If the child has a prescribed inhaler, follow the same emergency care procedures for administra-

tion of the medication via MDI as for the adult. (Review Chapter 14, "Respiratory Emergencies," for information on prescribed inhalers.) Be sure to consult medical direction for permission to administer it.

4. Usually, you will need to transport the patient for further care.

Note: A severe attack that cannot be managed with medication is called status asthmaticus and is extremely serious. Consider ALS back-up, if available.

BRONCHIOLITIS

Bronchiolitis is easily confused with asthma but is caused when the bronchioles (small bronchi) in the lungs become inflamed by a viral infection. During exhalations, the child will wheeze loudly and have other signs similar to those of asthma. Usually, however, the child's age can help you distinguish between asthma and bronchiolitis. Children under 1 year almost never have asthma; children over 2 almost never have bronchiolitis.

Collect the same history and perform the same assessment as you would for asthma. Generally speaking, management of bronchiolitis is almost identical to that for other types of respiratory distress:

1. Apply humidified oxygen at 15 lpm by nonrebreather mask, and assist breathing as necessary.
2. Let the child assume a position of comfort or place him in a Fowler's position with his neck slightly extended if this position is more comfortable.
3. Monitor the pulse rate and mental status while you transport the child to the hospital.

CARDIAC ARREST

Although cardiac arrest is not a respiratory problem per se, it is a very real concern if the patient's respiratory status deteriorates. Almost all cardiac arrests in children result from airway obstruction and respiratory arrest; most of the remaining are caused by shock (hypoperfusion). It is extremely important to aggressively manage both respiratory problems and shock before they progress to cardiac arrest. Provide positive pressure ventilations if breathing is inadequate or signs of respiratory failure are present. Chest compressions may be necessary if the heart rate drops below 80 beats per minute in an infant and below 60 beat per minute in a child.

Signs of cardiac arrest in a child are:

- Unresponsiveness
- Gasping or no respiratory sounds
- No audible heart sounds
- Chest is not moving
- Pale or blue skin

- Absent pulse (assess the brachial pulse in the infant, the carotid pulse in the child over 8 years of age)

Your goal is to keep the brain viable. Standing orders that provide you with orderly direction of treatment, easy access to paramedic back-up, and continuous assessment are important. Unless too much time has elapsed between the arrest and initiation of artificial ventilation, the child may recover with minimal or no neurologic deficit—even following comparatively long periods of arrest.

Key components of management include the following steps:

1. Provide positive pressure ventilation with supplemental oxygen.
2. Perform CPR effectively with minimal interruption. (AED should not be applied to a child 8 years of age or less.) Also contact medical direction.
3. Call for ALS back-up.
4. Transport rapidly to the closest medical facility capable of handling a patient in cardiac arrest.

For a review of artificial ventilation and CPR techniques, see Appendix 1, "Basic Life Support."

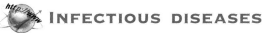 **INFECTIOUS DISEASES**

MENINGITIS

In meningitis, the lining of the brain and spinal cord (the meninges) are infected by either bacteria or viruses. These infections can be rapidly fatal, so they must be assessed promptly and treated in a timely and appropriate manner. Some pediatricians suggest that fever in a child younger than 3 months should be considered meningitis until proven otherwise.

Signs and symptoms of meningitis in children include recent ear or respiratory tract infection, high fever, lethargy, irritability, or vomiting. They generally do not have headaches or stiff necks but are lethargic and will not eat. The fontanelle may be bulging unless the child is dehydrated. Movement is painful.

If you suspect meningitis, you should complete the assessment rapidly and transport to the hospital. If the child is in shock (hypoperfusion), provide oxygen at 15 lpm by nonrebreather mask.

PEDIATRIC FIELD SCORING

Pediatric field scoring is a useful tool for rapidly determining the severity of injury in a child. One such scoring method is the Pediatric Trauma Score (PTS) (Table 38-3). Familiarity with and use of this tool will provide uniform methods for evaluating major body systems. It works by assigning a numeric score to each major body system. Unlike other field scoring

TABLE 38-3

The Pediatric Trauma Score

Start scoring at 0, and either add (denoted by the "+" sign), or subtract (denoted by the "−" sign) the number of points that correspond with your assessment finding.

Size/Weight
* +2 Heavier than 20 kilograms (44 pounds)
* +1 Between 10 and 20 kilograms (22 to 44 pounds)
* −1 Less than 10 kilograms (22 pounds)

Airway
* +2 No assistance needed aside from making sure that an unresponsive child's head does not flex forward on the chest
* +1 Constant observation required to maintain the patient's position or open airway. Also if supplemental oxygen is needed
* −1 Invasive techniques required, such as endotracheal intubation

Systolic Blood Pressure
Systolic pressures greater than 90 mmHg are adequate, and pressures of 50 mmHg or less are immediately life-threatening. Children with pressures between these two points may be in hypovolemic shock, but their blood vessels can constrict so efficiently that their blood pressure will not drop until they lose approximately one-fourth of the circulating blood volume. Monitor these in-between children closely.
* +2 Systolic blood pressure greater than 90 mmHg
* +1 90 to 50 mmHg
* −1 Less than 50 mmHg
If the proper-sized cuff is not available, or the patient is under 3 years of age, use this circulatory assessment instead:
* +2 Pulse palpable at the wrist
* +1 Pulse palpable at groin
* −1 No pulses palpable

Central Nervous System
Head injury occurs at the moment of impact. Any child who loses consciousness for any length of time as a result of injury may have sustained damage to the central nervous system either from a direct blow or from secondary injuries.
* +2 Fully alert, no loss of consciousness
* +1 Loss of consciousness in any degree for any length of time
* −1 Comatose and unresponsive

Wounds
These include abrasions, burns, lacerations, penetrating injuries, or missile injuries.
* +2 No wounds
* +1 Minor wounds, including abrasions and lacerations
* −1 Major open wounds, penetrating wounds, burns, tissue loss, or avulsions

Suspicion of Fractures
* +2 No fracture
* +1 Simple closed fracture, tibia-fibula
* −1 Open fracture(s), multiple fractures

Devised by J. J. Tepas, M.D., and validated by Diane Threadgill Alred, R.N.

systems, this one takes the differences in children's weights into consideration—for example, it recognizes that a toddler struck by a car will be injured more severely than a 10-year-old.

Practice with this scoring system is necessary for you to become proficient. Although using it may seem burdensome at first, it is actually very simple to use when you become familiar with it.

With a PTS of 0, the child will certainly die, even though the scores can go as low as −6. A PTS of +6 means that the child has a 30 percent chance of dying, and a PTS of +8 means a 1 percent chance of dying. If the PTS is +8 or lower, rapidly transport the child to a pediatric trauma center if one is available. All traumatized children should be transported to a hospital.

INFANT AND CHILD CAR SEATS IN TRAUMA

Because of child-restraint laws in many states, you will encounter an increasing number of children involved in motor vehicle crashes who are in child safety seats. These seats, if properly installed, are designed to hold a child in place during impact, particularly from head-on or rear-end collisions. Their effectiveness in broadside or rotating crashes is not yet clear. A survey by the National SafeKids Campaign disclosed that more than half of all children are either buckled incorrectly into child safety seats or don't use restraints at all. The most common mistakes caregivers make include choosing an inappropriate seat size for the child, improperly threading the safety belt through the seat, and failing to make the safety strap fit snugly enough.

You may transport small children in their own car seats under some circumstances. Often the child is reassured by being in his familiar seat. If the child is already seated in a car seat when you arrive on the scene of a motor vehicle crash, consider immobilizing the child in his own child safety seat as long as the plastic shell is not cracked and the metal tubes do not have jagged metal edges exposed and the patient is not in need of immediate resuscitation. If the child is not already in a safety seat, do not put him in a safety seat just for immobilization. Any child who requires resuscitation must be removed from the safety seat and immobilized on a spine board.

IMMOBILIZING AN INFANT OR CHILD IN A CAR SEAT

You can immobilize a child in the seat by stabilizing his head between two rolled towels and running one band of tape across his forehead and around the seat and a second band of tape across his upper lip and around the seat. This type of taping provides two solid points of contact on one bone and does not interfere with the integrity of the airway. Use folded blankets or towels to pad any spaces between the child and the seat to immobilize the child's trunk. Be sure that you can still adequately evaluate respiration. Do not use sandbags since they press downward on the shoulders, may impede breathing, and may destabilize clavicle injuries. If the caregiver is riding in the same ambulance, position the seat so that the child can see him without turning his head, if possible.

REMOVING THE INFANT OR CHILD FROM A CAR SEAT

It may be necessary for the EMT-B to remove an infant or child from a car seat in order to treat or assess the patient. If that is the case, follow these guidelines:

1. Establish cervical spine stabilization manually, while your partner cuts the restraining straps, and lifts the front guard of the car seat.
2. Apply a cervical spine immobilization collar (appropriately sized for the child—see item 8), or similar device, to offer mechanical support to continued manual in-line stabilization.
3. Position the entire car seat in the center of the backboard to which the patient will ultimately be secured. With a coordinated effort, tilt the car seat backwards until resting on the backboard. Take care not to let the patient slide out.
4. The EMT-B at the head calls for a coordinated movement of the patient, following the long axis of the body, moving the patient onto the backboard, supporting the head, neck, and trunk.
5. Remember that the back of the infant's or child's head is large and can cause the head and neck to flex forward. If necessary, place a small folded towel beneath the shoulders of the patient to prevent flexion of the head and neck.
6. While you maintain manual in-line spinal stabilization, have your partner place rolled-up towels on both sides of the patient to help pad spaces prior to securing the patient with straps.
7. Secure the patient to the board using straps or wide tape. Position the securing straps across the chest, hips, and legs.
8. Finish the immobilization by placing a cervical immobilization device (CID), or other such device (you can use rolled towels), on each side of the patient's head. Finally, secure the head to the backboard using tape across the forehead and cervical collar. (Avoid taping across the chin.)

Remember that almost any child under age 5 will resist being restrained. Sometimes laying a hand gently on the forehead will keep the patient from fighting against the straps. You may have to manually stabilize the cervical spine until arrival in the emergency department and hospital personnel take over. To minimize the emotional stress for the child, have a caregiver close enough to maintain eye contact with, talk to, and touch the child.

There are a number of pediatric immobilization devices on the market today. The "baby" size cervical collars are designed to fit a child at or about 24 months of age. Don't try to force a larger collar on a small child. If you do not have a cervical collar of the correct size, improvise one by rolling up a towel, taping it, laying it in a horseshoe shape over the neck, and taping down the ends. In addition you may find specialized child-size immobilizers. Each manufacturer produces a slightly different product and it is up to your system to decide which type to use.

FOUR-POINT IMMOBILIZATION OF AN INFANT OR CHILD

If some very simple rules of immobilization are followed, adult equipment, (such as a KED—Kendrick Extrication Device—or like product) can be modified to immobilize the child properly. When you must immobilize an infant or child to a stretcher, be aware that most straps attached to stretchers are designed to accommodate an adult. One way to accommodate children and infants is to use a four-point safety harness as shown in Figures 38–32a to e.

A PEDIATRIC IMMOBILIZATION SYSTEM

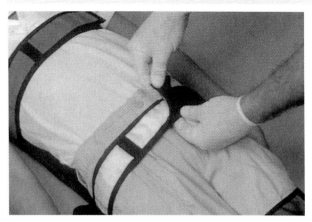

Figure 38-32a   *Adjust the color-coded straps to fit the child.*

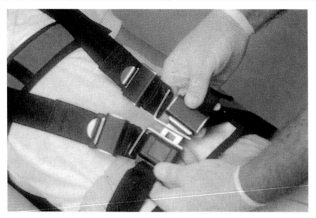

Figure 38-32b   *Attach the four-point safety harness.*

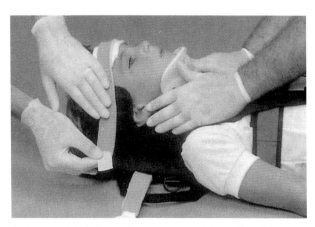

Figure 38-32c   *Fasten the adjustable head support system.*

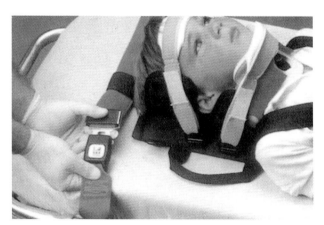

Figure 38-32d   *Fasten the loops at both ends to connect to cot straps.*

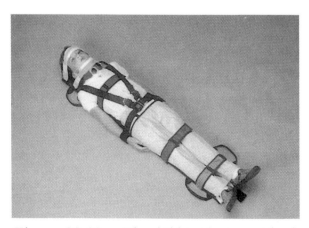

Figure 38-32e   *The child patient completely immobilized.*

CASE STUDY FOLLOW-UP

SCENE SIZE-UP

You have been dispatched to an 11-month-old infant with an unknown medical problem. Having parked your ambulance out of the flow of traffic, you have almost no time for further scene size-up as the parents come running out of the house and thrust an infant into your arms, exclaiming, "Oh, help! Help! Jason's not breathing!"

INITIAL ASSESSMENT

As soon as you see the infant, you identify cyanosis, flaccid muscles, and an absence of any response to the environment. It is obvious that this child is terribly ill, with ominous signs of respiratory arrest. As you immediately attempt to open the airway and assess for respirations, your EMT-B partner takes the parents and directs the mother to the passenger side of the ambulance, with the father to follow in a private vehicle to the hospital.

With little Jason in your arms, you rapidly proceed into the back of the ambulance. Your immediate opening of the airway did not result in spontaneous respirations. The mother cries from the front of the unit, "What's wrong with my baby!"

After confirming breathlessness, you attempt to provide positive pressure ventilation without success. You reposition Jason's airway and attempt ventilation again. Still no success. Your partner starts the unit moving to the hospital. Jason's color worsens.

FOCUSED HISTORY AND PHYSICAL EXAM

Since Jason is still suffering from a life threat, you have not proceeded to the formal focused history and physical exam. However, your partner quickly asks Jason's mother if he had shown any signs of illness. She shouts back to you, "He was absolutely fine." Because Jason's mother says he was not ill (which tends to indicate the problem is not related to a respiratory disease), and because repositioning the airway was unsuccessful, you now assume that Jason's airway is obstructed by a foreign body.

You lay Jason face down on your forearm and perform five back-blows. His condition does not improve, so you turn him over into a supine position on your other forearm and deliver five chest-thrusts.

After the next reassessment, Jason is still not breathing, and ventilations are still impossible. You repeat the sequence of five back blows and five chest thrusts. This time, when you look into Jason's mouth, you see what looks like a peanut in the back of the throat. You hook it out with your little finger.

Jason is still not breathing so you insert an oropharyngeal airway and provide positive pressure ventilations using a BVM with oxygen attached. This time, you are able to make Jason's chest rise with each ventilation, so you know that you have succeeded in unblocking his airway. You continue ventilations at 20 breaths per minute while assessing the pulse. The brachial pulse is currently 110/minute, and peripheral perfusion seems sluggish. Through her tears, the mother states that Jason was alone in the living room when he pulled himself up against a coffee table that had snacks in a bowl. When she returned into the living room, she says he was "just lying on the floor, gazing up, not moving—that's when I called."

ONGOING ASSESSMENT

You are still about 4 minutes away from the hospital when you notice that Jason's color has changed from blue to a normal pink. His muscle tone has returned, and he is moving around actively. You stop the ventilations and assess Jason's spontaneous respiratory effort. You find it to be at a rate of 30 per minute and with a normal depth. Jason starts crying as you now apply oxygen at 15 lpm via a nonrebreather mask. You've never been so happy to hear a crying baby before! Jason's mother starts crying all over again when she hears him—this time tears of joy. Peripheral perfusion has returned to normal by the time you arrive at the hospital.

You communicate your assessment and treatment to the receiving facility and complete the appropriate paperwork. Before leaving the hospital, you stop in Jason's room and find him to be alert and responsive to his surroundings. Both parents start crying again when they see you. The mother hugs you and your partner and the father slaps you hard on the back as they thank you for saving their son's life.

You and your partner give each other a couple of happy grins as you mark back in service, prepared for the next call.

CHAPTER REVIEW

TERMS AND CONCEPTS

You may wish to review the following terms and concepts included in this chapter.

adolescent—a person 12 to 18 years of age.

anterior fontanelle—the "soft-spot" on the top of an infant's head where the plates of the skull have not yet formed together.

compensated respiratory distress—see early respiratory distress.

decompensated respiratory failure—when the respiratory compensatory mechanisms have begun to fail and respiration becomes inadequate.

early respiratory distress—increased respiratory effort due to impaired respiratory function.

infant—a child up to 12 months.

neglect—the provision of insufficient attention or respect to someone who has a claim to that attention.

neonate—an infant in the first 4 weeks of life.

physical abuse—improper or excessive action taken so as to injure or cause harm.

preschooler—a child 3 to 6 years of age.

respiratory arrest—cessation of respiratory function.

school age—a child 6 to 12 years of age.

sudden infant death syndrome (SIDS)—the sudden and unexpected death of an infant or young child in which an autopsy fails to identify the cause of death. SIDS typically occurs while the infant is asleep.

toddler—a child 1 to 3 years of age.

REVIEW QUESTIONS

1. Describe differences in anatomy and physiology of the infant and child as compared to the adult patient.
2. Differentiate between early (compensated) respiratory distress and decompensated respiratory failure.
3. List the signs of an obstructed airway.
4. Describe the methods of determining end organ perfusion in the infant and child patient.
5. List the common causes of seizures in the infant and child patient and describe the management of seizures for the pediatric patient.
6. Describe the patterns of injury most likely to occur when pediatric patients are victims of trauma.
7. List the indicators of possible child abuse and neglect.
8. List five advanced support devices for children who receive home care; for each device, briefly state its general purpose, one or more problems that may prompt a call to EMS, and appropriate emergency care steps.
9. Discuss ways the EMT-B can deal with the emotional consequences of a difficult infant or child transport.

CHAPTER 39

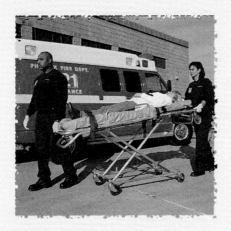

Moving Patients

INTRODUCTION

There may be occasions when you find it necessary to move a patient before providing complete assessment or medical care. Such emergency or urgent moves must be made in the safest way possible, causing the least possible chance of further injury to the patient. Once the patient is in a safe place and you have completed on-scene assessment and emergency care, you need to determine the best way to move the patient to and from the ambulance. Your choices will be based on the patient's injuries or medical condition, the patient's mental status, the environment, and the available resources (rescuers and equipment).

Generally, the best way to move a patient in any circumstance is the easiest way that will not cause injury or pain to your patient or to yourself. Let your equipment do the work whenever possible. If you must lift, if possible do it with a device designed for that purpose. As a rule, get as much help as you can to carry patients and equipment. Never risk falling or injuring yourself. Follow the rules of body mechanics.

OBJECTIVES

Numbered objectives are from the United States Department of Transportation 1994 EMT-Basic National Standard Curriculum. Asterisked objectives, if any, pertain to material that is supplemental to the DOT curriculum.

COGNITIVE

1-6.3   Describe the safe lifting of cots and stretchers. (p. 793)

1-6.10   Discuss the general considerations of moving patients. (pp. 792–798)

1-6.11   State three situations that may require the use of an emergency move. (p. 793)

1-6.12   Identify the following patient carrying devices: (pp. 798–806):
- Wheeled ambulance stretcher
- Portable ambulance stretcher
- Stair chair
- Scoop stretcher
- Long spine board
- Basket stretcher
- Flexible stretcher

PSYCHOMOTOR OBJECTIVES

1-6.14   Working with a partner, prepare each of the following devices for use, transfer a patient to the device, properly position the patient on the device, move the device to the ambulance, and load the patient into the ambulance:
- Wheeled ambulance stretcher
- Portable ambulance stretcher
- Stair chair
- Scoop stretcher
- Long spine board
- Basket stretcher
- Flexible stretcher

1-6.15   Working with a partner, the EMT-Basic will demonstrate techniques for the transfer of a patient from an ambulance stretcher to a hospital stretcher.

Additional objectives from DOT lesson 1-6 are addressed in Chapter 6, "Preparing to Lift and Move Patients."

CASE STUDY

THE DISPATCH

EMS Unit 101—proceed to 605 Lindsey Drive in Rockaway—a 72-year-old patient has a routine transfer to Dover General. Time out is 0910 hours.

ON ARRIVAL

You are a probationary EMT-B accompanied by a training officer and an experienced EMT-B. Your training officer tells you that she knows the patient, Amanda Sanchez, and that this is one of three prescheduled visits Mrs. Sanchez takes to the hospital dialysis center every week. She tells you the patient cannot walk without assistance and will need help getting down one flight of stairs. As your partner parks the ambulance, he remarks that there is still snow and probably ice on the walk to the house.

How would you proceed to package and transport this patient?

During this chapter, you will read about special considerations that can ensure your own well-being while moving patients safely. Later, we will return to the case study and apply the procedures learned.

LIFTING AND MOVING PATIENTS

There are three categories of patient moves: an emergency move, an urgent move, and a nonurgent move. In general, an **emergency move** should be performed when there is *immediate danger to the patient or to* the rescuer. An **urgent move** is performed when the patient is suffering *an immediate threat to life* and the patient must be moved quickly and transported for care. Finally, a **nonurgent move** is defined as one in which *no immediate threat to life* exists and the patient can be moved in a normal manner when ready for transport.

Reminder: Whenever you carry or move a patient, apply the basic principles of body mechanics to ensure your own safety. Maintain a straight, rigid back by contracting the abdominal and gluteal muscles. Bend at the hips, not at the waist. Keep your head in a neutral position, not flexed forward or extended back, and use your leg muscles, not your back, to lift, move, or drag the patient. (See Table 39-1 for a summary of body mechanics and Chapter 6, "Preparing to Lift and Move Patients," for detailed discussion.)

EMERGENCY MOVES

Top priority in emergency care is to maintain the patient's airway, breathing, and circulation. The rule of thumb is to control any life-threatening problems and stabilize the patient before moving him. However, when the scene of an accident is unstable, or threatening to your life and the patient's, your priority changes. You must move the patient first. Make an emergency move only when no other options are available. Follow local protocol. Always take appropriate precautions to be sure you do not become an additional victim of the emergency.

In general, an emergency move should be performed when there is immediate danger to the patient or to the rescuer. Consider an emergency move under the following conditions:

- *Immediate environmental danger to the patient or rescuer, such as*
  - *Fire or danger of fire.* Fire should always be considered a grave threat, not only to patients, but to rescuers.
  - *Exposure to explosives or other hazardous materials.* When a patient is directly exposed to substances that can cause grave injury or death, move the patient immediately.
  - *Inability to protect the patient from other hazards at the scene.* Move the patient to safety when, for example, you haven't the resources to protect him from uncontrolled traffic, physically unsta-

ble surroundings, extreme weather conditions, or hostile crowds.
- *Inability to gain access to other patients who need life-saving care.* In cases where more than one patient has been injured, you may need to move one in order to gain access to another. This may apply to moving a moderately injured person in order to gain access to one who has life-threatening injuries.
- *Inability to provide life-saving care because of the patient's location or position.* There will be times when you need to change a patient's position to control hemorrhage, for instance, or to perform CPR.

Remember: The greatest danger to the patient in any emergency move is the possibility of aggravating a spinal injury. Yet, it is impossible to move a patient quickly and still provide as much protection to the spine as would an interim immobilization device such as a spine board. In every such emergency, however, make every effort to provide as much protection to the spine as possible. And always make sure you pull the patient in the direction of the long axis of the body.

Three types of emergency moves are the armpit-forearm drag, the shirt drag, and the blanket drag.

THE ARMPIT-FOREARM DRAG

In general, if the patient is on the floor or ground, you can move him by inserting your hands under the patient's armpits from the back. Grasp the patient's left forearm with your right hand, the right forearm with your left hand, and drag. Make sure you pull the patient in the direction of the long axis of the body (Figure 39-1).

THE SHIRT DRAG

If the patient is wearing a shirt, you can use it to support the patient's head and pull (Figure 39-2). Note that the shirt drag cannot be used if the patient is wearing only a T-shirt.

TABLE 39-1

Summary of Proper Body Mechanics

- Use teamwork, equipment, and imagination to make sure you are always in the position of using proper body mechanics.
- Use the power-lift and power-grip techniques as a best defense against injury.
- Reduce the height or distance through which an object must be moved. Lift in stages if necessary.
- Lift an object as close to your body as possible to avoid back injury.
- Avoid using back muscles to lift.
- Use legs, hips, and gluteal muscles plus abdominal muscles for safe, powerful lifts.
- While you are carrying an object, keep shoulders, hips, and feet in alignment.
- Use the proper posture—ears, shoulders, and hips in vertical alignment—when standing and sitting.
- Improve personal physical fitness to build strength and manage stress.

Note: Body mechanics are discussed in detail in Chapter 6, "Preparing to Lift and Move Patients."

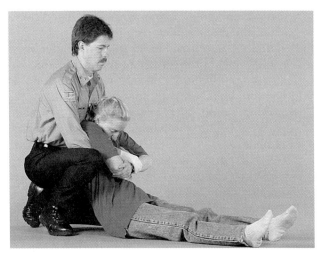

Figure 39-1   The armpit-forearm drag. Slide your hands under the patient's armpits and grasp the forearms. Drag along the long axis of the patient's body.

1. Fasten the patient's hands or wrists loosely together. If possible, link them to a belt or pants with a small Velcro strap or self-adherent bandage. This will serve to prevent the patient's arms from flopping or slipping out of the shirt.
2. Grasp the neck and shoulders of the shirt so that the patient's head rests on your fists.
3. Then using the shirt as a handle, pull the patient toward you. Be careful not to strangle the patient. The pulling power should engage the armpits, not the neck. Reposition your hands if you notice excessive pressure or strain from the shirt on the patient's neck.

THE BLANKET DRAG

The blanket drag is an effective way for a single rescuer to move a patient to safety (Figure 39-3). If you do not have a blanket, use a coat to drag the patient. Follow these steps.

1. Spread a blanket alongside the patient. Gather about half into lengthwise pleats.
2. Roll the patient away from you onto his side. Tuck the pleated part of the blanket as far beneath the patient as you can.
3. Roll the patient back onto the center of the blanket and onto his back.
4. Wrap the blanket securely around the patient.
5. Grab the part of the blanket that is beneath the patient's head, and drag the patient toward you.

URGENT MOVES

Many times a patient in a motor vehicle collision must be quickly removed from the vehicle for emergency care and immediate transport, and the application of a short spine board or vest to immobilize the spine would take too much time. The rapid extrication move is designed for this situation.

RAPID EXTRICATION

See Chapter 34, "Injuries to the Spine," for detailed discussion and illustrations of rapid extrication. A summary of the rapid extrication procedure follows.

1. One rescuer should bring the patient's head into a neutral in-line position and provide manual stabilization. This is best achieved from behind or to the side of the patient.
2. A second rescuer should apply a cervical-spine immobilization device as a third places a long

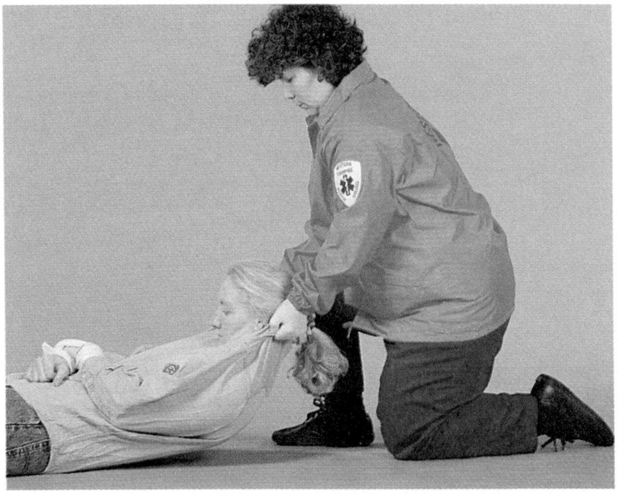

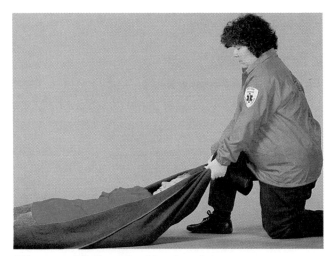

Figure 39-2   The shirt drag.

Figure 39-3   The blanket drag.

backboard near the door. The third rescuer should then move to the passenger seat.

3. The second rescuer should support the patient's thorax as the third frees the patient's legs from the pedals or from under the dashboard.

4. At the direction of the second rescuer, he and the third rescuer rotate the patient in several short, coordinated moves until the patient's back is in the open doorway and his feet are on the seat.

5. Since the first rescuer can no longer support the patient's head, another rescuer should support the head until the first rescuer exits the vehicle and takes over supporting the head from the door opening.

6. The end of the long backboard is placed on the seat next to the patient's buttocks. Assistants support the other end of the board as the first and second rescuers lower the patient onto it, the first maintaining in-line stabilization of the head and neck.

7. The second and third rescuers should then slide the patient into the proper position on the board in short, coordinated moves as the first continues manual stabilization.

Several variations of this technique are possible. The most critical factor is that this procedure must be accomplished rapidly, but without any compromise to the patient's spine. In addition, operating inside a vehicle places the rescuer's lower back in a vulnerable position. Whenever possible, you should support your weight with a free arm or by resting your chest against the seat backs.

NONURGENT MOVES

When there is no immediate threat to life, take the time to choose the best equipment and positioning for moving the patient safely. Generally, the best way to move a patient is the easiest way that will not cause injury or pain. That includes "walking" the patient, if he is able, while supporting him. Never walk a patient who becomes lightheaded or sweaty upon standing or who is having chest pain or respiratory problems, has an injured lower extremity, or has suspected spinal injury.

Whenever you move, lift, or carry a patient, remember to move him as a unit. Keep the patient's head and neck in a neutral position. If you suspect head, neck, or spinal injury, take all necessary spinal precautions. Be sure that all rescuers understand what is to be done before any move is attempted, and make one rescuer responsible for giving commands.

There are many ways to move patients. You are only limited by your imagination and the basic principles of body mechanics and patient safety and comfort. The direct ground lift, extremity lift, direct carry, and draw sheet methods are accepted nonur-

gent moves that provide the greatest safety to both you and the patient.

DIRECT GROUND LIFT

Note that the direct ground lift is not recommended for a heavier patient. When lifting a patient from the ground, it is usually safer and more mechanically efficient to use a long backboard. However, when this cannot be accomplished, follow these steps (Figures 39-4a to c):

1. Two or three rescuers should line up on the same side of the patient.

2. Each rescuer should kneel on one knee, preferably the same knee for all rescuers.

3. The second rescuer should place the patient's arms on the chest if possible.

4. The first rescuer should then cradle the patient's head by placing one arm under the patient's neck and shoulder. Then he should place his other arm under the patient's lower back.

5. The second rescuer should place one arm under the patient's knees and one arm above the buttocks.

6. If a third rescuer is available, he should place both arms under the waist. The other two rescuers then should slide their arms either up to the midback or down to the buttocks as appropriate.

7. On signal from the first rescuer, they should lift the patient to their knees and roll the patient in toward their chests.

8. On signal from the first rescuer, they should stand and move the patient to the stretcher or other patient-carrying device.

9. To lower the patient, the steps are reversed.

Remember that you should bend at the hips and not at the waist, your back should remain straight, and the lifting force should be generated from your legs and buttocks, not the back.

EXTREMITY LIFT

Use the extremity lift to move a patient from the ground to a patient carrying device (Figures 39-5a and b). Note that this lift should not be used on a patient with suspected spinal or extremity injuries.

1. The first rescuer should kneel at the patient's head. A second rescuer should kneel at the patient's side by the knees.

2. The first rescuer should place one hand under each of the patient's shoulders, while the second rescuer grasps the patient's wrists.

3. The first rescuer should slip his hands under the patient's arms and grasp the patient's wrists.

DIRECT GROUND LIFG

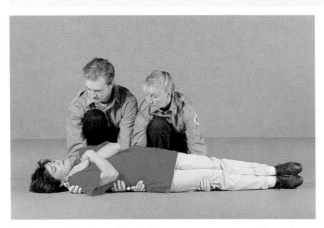

Figure 39-4a   Position your arms under the patient. Be sure to cradle the head. If a third rescuer is available, he should slide both arms under the waist while the first two rescuers move their arms up and down as appropriate.

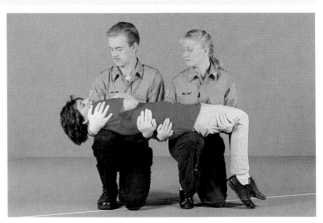

Figure 39-4b   Lift the patient to your knees and roll toward your chests.

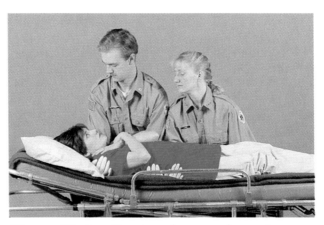

Figure 39-4c   On signal, move the patient to the carrying device.

4. The second rescuer can then slip his hands under the patient's knees.
5. Both rescuers should move up to a crouching position, keeping their backs straight and heads in neutral alignment.
6. On signal from the first rescuer, they should stand up simultaneously and move with the patient to a stretcher or other patient carrying device.

While lifting the patient, each rescuer must maintain a straight back and contract the abdominal muscles. The rescuer's head must remain in line with the back. (If the head were to be extended backward, the rescuer would be forced to use the lower back muscles. Flexing the head forward would also put undo force on the lumbar discs.) When lifting the patient, the rescuer should drive upward with leg and gluteal muscles.

DIRECT CARRY METHOD

The direct carry is one way of transferring a supine patient from a bed to a wheeled stretcher or from any patient carrying device to another (Figures 39-6a to c).

1. Position the wheeled stretcher perpendicular to the bed, with the head of the device at the foot of the bed.
2. Prepare the wheeled stretcher by unbuckling straps and removing other items. Both rescuers should stand between the bed and stretcher, facing the patient.
3. The first rescuer then slides an arm under the patient's neck and cups the patient's shoulder.
4. After the second rescuer slides a hand under the patient's hip and lifts slightly, the first rescuer should slide an arm under the patient's back.

EXTREMITY LIFT

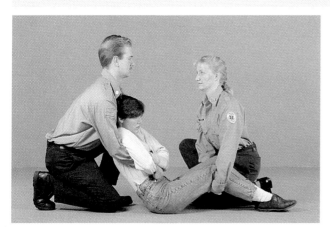

Figure 39-5a One rescuer should put one hand under each arm and grasp the wrists. The other should slip hands under the knees.

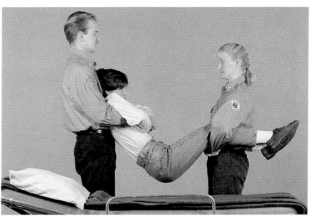

Figure 39-5b Both rescuers should move up to a crouching and then standing position.

DIRECT CARRY

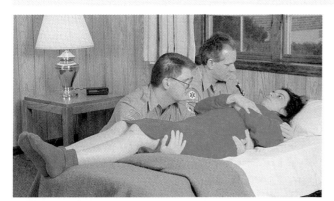

Figure 39-6a Position your arms under the patient and slide the patient to the edge of the bed.

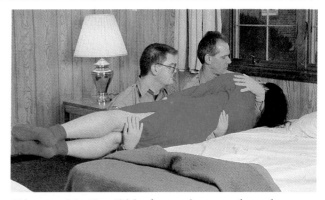

Figure 39-6b Lift the patient and curl toward your chests.

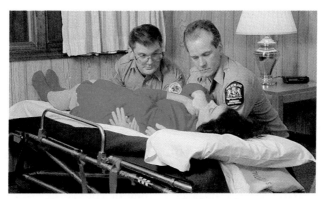

Figure 39-6c Rotate and place the patient gently on the carrying device.

DRAW SHEET METHOD

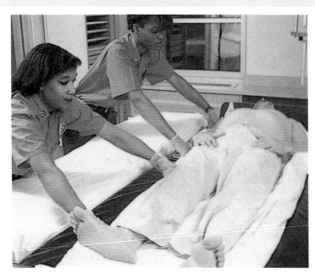

Figure 39-7a *Reach across the stretcher and grasp the sheet firmly.*

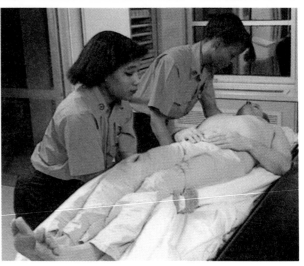

Figure 39-7b *Slide the patient gently onto the carrying device.*

The second rescuer then places his arms under the patient's hips and calves.

5. The rescuers slide the patient to the edge of the bed, lift and curl the patient to their chests, and then rotate and place the patient gently onto the wheeled stretcher.

DRAW SHEET METHOD

Another way of transferring a supine patient from a bed to a wheeled stretcher or from any patient carrying device to another is the draw sheet method (Figures 39-7a and b).

1. Loosen the bottom sheet of the bed.
2. Position the wheeled stretcher next to the bed. Prepare it by adjusting height, lowering rails, unbuckling straps, and so on.
3. Reach across the stretcher and grasp the sheet firmly at the patient's head, chest, hips, and knees. As you reach across the stretcher, use your hips to support yourself against the stretcher.
4. Slide the patient gently onto the wheeled stretcher. Be sure to contract your abdominal and gluteal muscles to splint the lower back.

PACKAGING FOR TRANSPORTATION

Packaging simply means readying the patient for transport. That is, once the patient is stabilized and all interventions have been checked, you must be able to select and prepare the appropriate carrying device, safely transfer and secure the patient to the carrying

device, and finally move the patient and carrying device to the ambulance for loading and unloading.

Some general considerations: Make sure the carrying device is locked in the open position before positioning the patient. Use an appropriate lifting, moving, or carrying technique to place the patient on the carrying device. Generally, place a sheet or blanket on the carrying device and, when the patient is positioned, cover him as appropriate with sheets or blankets to maintain body temperature. Then secure him with straps. Make certain all straps and ties are tucked in or positioned so that they will not cause you to trip and fall. When the patient is placed in the ambulance, be sure both the patient and the carrying device are secured properly before the ambulance moves.

Note: If you suspect head, neck, or spinal injury, take all necessary spinal precautions before, during, and after packaging.

EQUIPMENT

Both medical and trauma patients need to be moved, packaged, and transported in ways that will not make their conditions worse. To be able to make the best choices of equipment for your patients, learn the advantages and disadvantages of each type (Table 39-2). Practice often, and follow manufacturer instructions for inspection, cleaning, repair, and upkeep.

WHEELED STRETCHER

The wheeled stretcher (also called an ambulance gurney or cot) is the patient carrying device most commonly used by rescue personnel. It is also the safest and most comfortable means of transferring a patient.

TABLE 39-2

Patient Carrying Devices

Device	Advantages	Disadvantages
Wheeled Stretcher	Enables movement without carrying Accommodates variety of positions, heights, lengths Safe traversal of stairways and curbs Can be lifted or lowered from ends or sides Durable Mechanically simple Comfortable	Difficult to load and unload by two rescuers X-ray opacity
Portable Stretcher	Light weight Compact Excellent for use as auxiliary stretcher Can be used in spaces too confined or narrow for wheeled stretcher Some models have folding wheels and posts for easier movement Easily loaded and off-loaded Can be folded for storage	Must be carried Metal styles interfere with some X-rays
Stair Chair	Good for use on stairways, narrow corridors and doorways, small elevators Some models can be converted into portable stretchers	Must be carried Does not accommodate trauma patients Should not be used for patients with altered mental status Fairly complex Consumes considerable space
Backboard	Good spinal immobilizer Good lifting device Can float Light Compact Can serve as CPR surface Mechanically simple X-ray translucency Can be carried and loaded from ends or sides Integrates well with various other equipment	Must be carried Usually must be left with patient Unstable for moves up or down inclines Uncomfortable May develop splinters May weaken with time
Scoop Stretcher	Can be used in confined areas in which other stretchers will not fit Allows easy application of restraints Integrates well with various other equipment	Must be carried Requires padding of head and body prominences Should be prewarmed if air temperature is cold Not recommended for patients with suspected spinal injury Consumes considerable space
Basket Stretcher	Good for traversing rough terrain Can be fitted with flotation harness for water rescue Extremely durable Can be carried from sides or ends Integrates well with various other equipment	Must be carried Bulky High cost Usually must be left with patient Metal style interferes with some X-rays Needs special training for use in rope or ladder rescues
Flexible Stretcher	Especially useful for narrow and restricted hallways Can be carried from sides or ends	Must be carried

Most wheeled stretchers are designed to accommodate weights up to 400 pounds and can be adapted to almost any patient position. They also can serve as a means of securing and carrying equipment to the patient's location.

To roll a wheeled stretcher, the rescuer at the head pushes and the rescuer at the foot guides. One limitation of the device is that rolling is usually restricted to smooth terrain. However, four rescuers—one at each corner—can keep it stable and move it

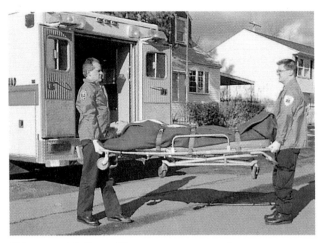

Figure 39-8a   Two-rescuer stretcher carry.

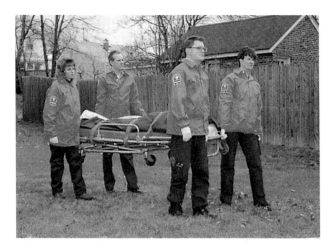

Figure 39-8b   Four-rescuer stretcher carry.

over rough ground. Two rescuers can carry a wheeled stretcher in narrow spaces. However, they would need to face each other from opposite ends, the stretcher could be easily unbalanced, and the lift and carry would require considerable strength (Figures 39-8a and b).

There are two basic types of wheeled stretchers in the United States: the lift-in cot and the roll-in cot (Figures 39-9a and b). Each weighs about 70 pounds and is constructed of aluminum alloy. The lift-in cot requires two attendants, one on each side, when loading and unloading from the ambulance (Figures 39-10a to f). The roll-in cot uses special wheels at the head to simplify the loading and unloading procedure (Figures 39-11a and b). The roll-in type significantly reduces the amount of twisting and lifting that is required of rescuers.

Trained emergency personnel should stay with a patient on a wheeled stretcher at all times. The patient should never be left unattended, even when secured. Before loading a wheeled stretcher into the ambulance, be sure there is enough lifting power. Load hanging stretchers before wheeled stretchers. Once in the ambulance, be sure the stretchers and patients are secure before the ambulance moves.

PORTABLE STRETCHER

The portable ambulance stretcher is standard equipment (Figures 39-12a and b). It is usually made of a continuous tubular metal frame, canvas or coated fabric bottom, and straps to secure the patient (Figure 39-12a). It is a conventional carrying device that is particularly useful when the patient must be removed from a space too confined or narrow for a wheeled stretcher. It is often used as an auxiliary to the wheeled stretcher when there is more than one patient to transport. It can be loaded easily into an ambulance and off-loaded easily once in the ambulance.

The portable ambulance stretcher generally is available in three styles: the basic model, the basic with folding wheels and posts, and the breakaway. The

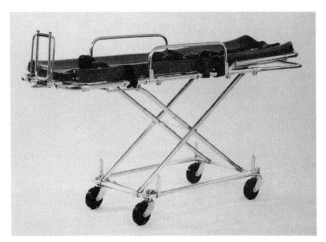

Figure 39-9a   Wheeled stretcher, lift-in type.
(Ferno Corporation)

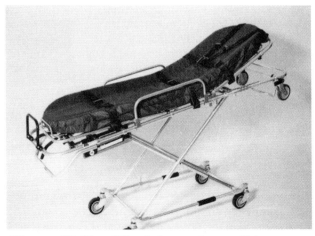

Figure 39-9b   Wheeled stretcher, roll-in type.
(Ferno Corporation)

LOADING THE LIFT-IN WHEELED STRETCHER

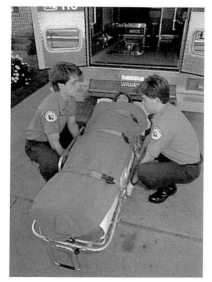

Figure 39-10a *Using the principles of body mechanics, prepare to lift.*

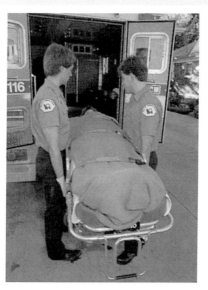

Figure 39-10b *Lift the stretcher to standing position.*

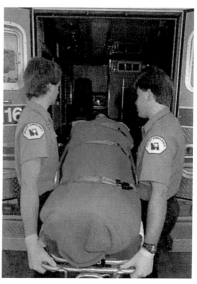

Figure 39-10c *Move the patient and stretcher into the ambulance.*

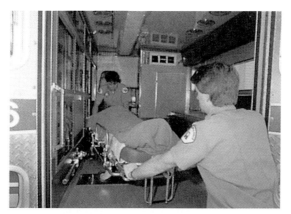

Figure 39-10d *Move front of stretcher into securing device.*

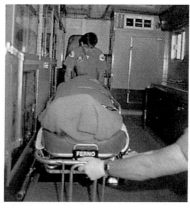

Figure 39-10e *Secure rear of stretcher in place.*

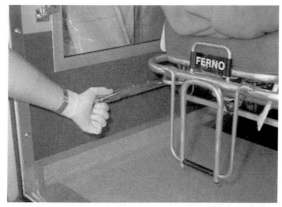

Figure 39-10f *Make certain both front and rear catches are engaged and securing stretcher.*

LOADING THE ROLL-IN WHEELED STRETCHER

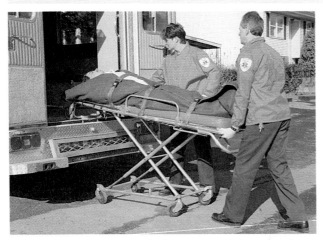

Figure 39-11a Roll the front of the stretcher into the ambulance until the safety mechanism engages.

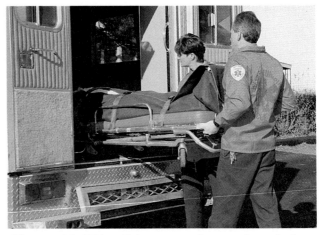

Figure 39-11b Disengage the carriage lock at the foot and roll the stretcher into the ambulance into locked position.

basic model is used as an auxiliary stretcher, which can be placed on the squad bench or suspended from hanging hardware inside the ambulance. It is very light and, though it has a load capacity of up to 350 pounds, it is not recommended for that much weight. Most models can be folded in half for storage.

One type of portable stretcher is the pole stretcher or canvas litter (Figures 39-12b), which has been used worldwide for centuries. It is lightweight and folds compactly. The vinyl-coated model is easy to clean. It is comfortable for the patient, especially when the head is padded, though it should not be used when spinal immobilization is necessary unless it is used with a long backboard. One drawback is that care must be taken when placing the patient on rocky ground for any length of time. Soft-tissue injury may result. When the canvas pole stretcher is to be used to transport a patient, care should be taken to see that the crosspieces are locked in place. When lifting a pa-

tient on a pole stretcher, it is preferable to have four or more rescuers.

STAIR CHAIR

A stair chair (Figure 39-13) is useful when a wheeled stretcher cannot traverse narrow corridors and doorways, small elevators, and stairways. Some models can be converted into portable stretchers. Do not use a stair chair when the patient has an altered mental status, suspected spinal injury, or injuries to the lower extremities.

To move a patient up or down stairs on a stair chair, explain to the patient everything you plan to do. Check to be sure all straps are secure. Then the rescuers should proceed with the following (Figures 39-14a and b).

1. One rescuer should stand behind the chair at the head, and another should stand at the foot facing the patient. A third rescuer, if available, should pre-

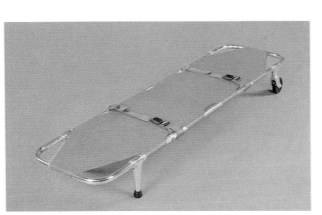

Figure 39-12a Portable ambulance stretcher with continuous tubular metal frame.

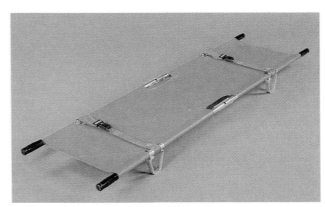

Figure 39-12b Pole stretcher, or canvas litter.

MOVING A PATIENT IN A STAIR CHAIR

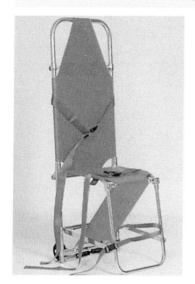

Figure 39-13   Stair chair.

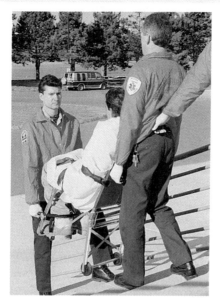

Figure 39-14a   Moving a properly secured patient in a stair chair up steps—spotter above.

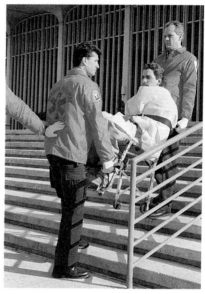

Figure 39-14b   Moving a properly secured patient in a stair chair down steps—spotter below.

pare to "spot" by standing behind the rescuer who will be moving backward (up or down the stairs).

2. As the chair is tilted back by the rescuer at the head, the rescuer at the foot should grasp the chair by its legs.

3. Both rescuers should lift and begin to carry simultaneously. If the chair has wheels, they should not be allowed to touch the steps.

4. As the rescuers descend (or ascend) with the patient, the spotter should count out the steps and identify upcoming conditions.

BACKBOARDS

Standard operating equipment in any emergency vehicle is the backboard (Figures 39-15a to c). It can protect the patient from rocky ground surfaces, and it acts as a spinal immobilizer. Straps and a head immobilizer device usually can be applied and secured without problems.

Many varieties of long and short backboards are manufactured. Traditionally, they are made of wood. The more popular models are plastic and lightweight, with molded handholds. Two common styles of backboard are the Farrington, which is rectangular with rounded corners, and the Ohio, which has mitered corners and tapering sides. The Ohio has the advantage of fitting into most basket stretchers and can be more easily maneuvered into car-door openings.

Short backboards usually are used to immobilize noncritical sitting patients before moving them. One

special type of short backboard is the vest-type or corset-type immobilizer such as the Ferno Kendrick Extrication Device (K.E.D.). Once a short backboard is applied, the patient should be placed on a long backboard. See Chapter 34, "Injuries to the Spine," for detailed descriptions, step-by-step instructions, and illustrations for applying backboards.

SCOOP STRETCHER

Designed for patients weighing up to 300 pounds, the scoop or orthopedic stretcher is made to be assembled and disassembled around the patient (Figure 39-16). An advantage is that it can be used in confined areas where other conventional stretchers will not fit. A disadvantage is that it is all metal, which picks up the temperature of the environment. Note also that the scoop stretcher is not recommended for patients with suspected spinal injury.

To use a scoop stretcher properly, you must have access to the patient from all sides. At least two rescuers are required—one to prepare and position the stretcher and one to move the patient. Follow these steps (Figures 39-17a to f):

1. Adjust the stretcher to the length of the patient.

2. Separate the stretcher halves, and place one on each side of the patient. Keeping the patient's spine in-line, gently roll the patient onto one side. Slide half of the stretcher under the patient.

3. If you have not been able to examine the patient's

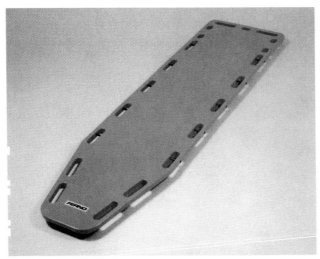

Figure 39-15a Traditional wooden long backboard. (Ferno Corporation)

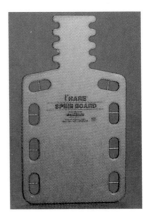

Figure 39-15b Short wooden backboard.

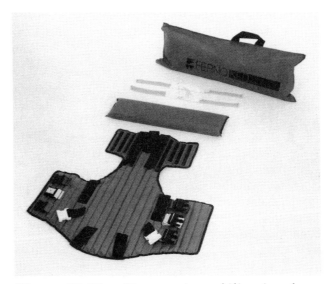

Figure 39-15c Vest-type immobilization device.

back before this time, do so now. Then return the patient to a supine position.

4. Assemble the head end of the scoop stretcher.
5. Roll the patient's body to the other side. Swing the remaining half of the stretcher into a closed (assembled) position. Latch the foot end of the stretcher.
6. Pad the patient's head and any bony prominence with a pillow or a folded sheet.
7. Secure the patient with at least three body straps.

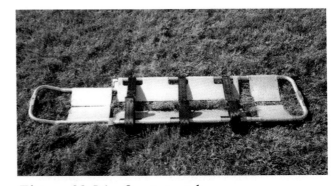

Figure 39-16 Scoop stretcher.

APPLYING THE SCOOP STRETCHER

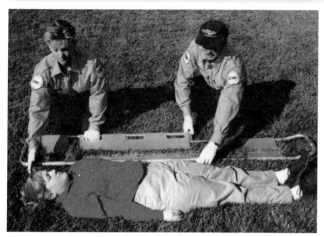

Figure 39-17a   *Adjust length of the scoop stretcher.*

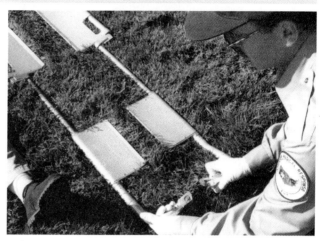

Figure 39-17b   *Separate the stretcher halves.*

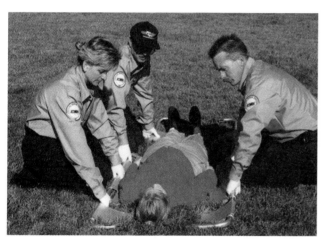

Figure 39-17c   *Gently slide half of the stretcher under the patient.*

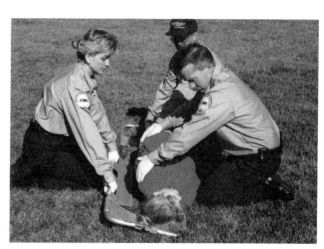

Figure 39-17d   *Swing the remaining half of the stretcher into a closed position.*

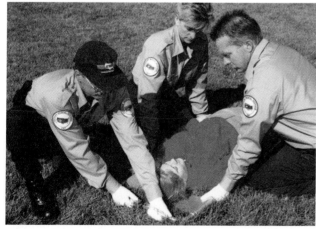

Figure 39-17e   *Close and lock the stretcher halves.*

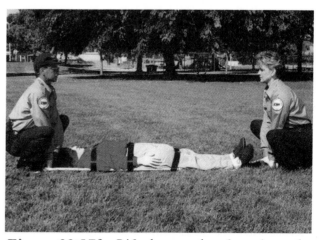

Figure 39-17f   *Lift the stretcher from its ends.*

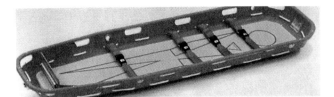

Figure 39-18a   Basket stretcher.

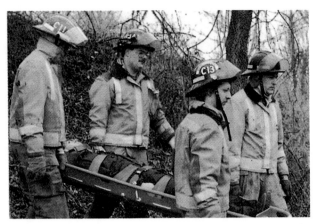

Figure 39-18b   Using a basket stretcher to move a patient over rough terrain.

BASKET STRETCHER

Most commonly called the *Stokes basket,* a basket stretcher is shaped like a long basket and comes in two basic styles (Figures 39-18a and b). One style has a welded metal frame fitted with a contoured chicken-wire web. The other style has a tubular aluminum frame riveted to a molded polyethylene shell. Either will accommodate a scoop stretcher or Ohio-type backboard. Basket stretchers will fit onto wheeled stretchers and can work with any vehicle large enough to accommodate them.

A basket stretcher has the advantage of enabling you to completely immobilize a patient who is already on a backboard and to move him over any kind of terrain. The lightweight polyethylene style slides easily and smoothly over snow and rough terrain while protecting the patient from branches and twigs. Note: Do *not* move a patient in a basket stretcher by rope or ladder unless you have been specifically trained to do so.

Place the mattress from a wheeled stretcher into a basket stretcher to increase patient comfort and insulate him from the cold. If you choose not to use a

mattress, be sure to pad the patient's head. If you anticipate especially rough transport, pad the edges of the patient's body with rolled blankets and strap him securely into place with nylon webbing.

FLEXIBLE STRETCHER

A flexible (or Reeves) stretcher is a special transfer device made of canvas or synthetic materials (Figure 39-19). It has six large lifting and carrying handles, three on each side. It is especially useful for narrow and restricted hallways such as those found in mobile homes. A patient on a backboard can be placed inside the flexible stretcher for moves down stairs or over rough terrain.

PATIENT POSITIONING

Generally, a patient is placed on a carrying device in a supine or sitting position, unless the patient's condition dictates otherwise.

- An unresponsive patient (with *no* suspected head, neck, or spinal injury) should placed in a left lateral recumbent position (coma or recovery position)—to face the rescuer once in the ambulance. This position will aid in draining fluids or vomitus from the mouth and help prevent aspiration into the lungs.
- A patient with chest pain or discomfort or with breathing difficulties should be placed in a position of comfort, usually sitting up, if hypotension is not present.
- A patient with suspected spinal injury should be immobilized on a long backboard. Once immobilized, the patient and backboard can be tilted as a

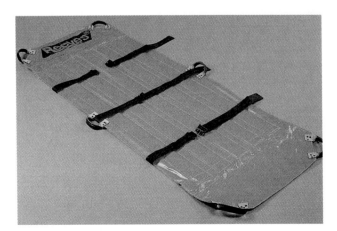

Figure 39-19   Flexible stretcher.

unit to place the patient on his left side for drainage from the mouth.

- A patient in shock (hypoperfusion) should be supine. His legs or the foot end of the backboard may be elevated 8 to 12 inches, depending on local protocol. This position is controversial because of its potential for impeding ventilation.
- An alert patient who is nauseated or vomiting should be transported in a sitting or a recovery position. That position should allow you to manage the patient's airway.
- A pregnant patient in her third trimester should be positioned on her left side.

Consider the following suggestions when moving and positioning patients with special needs:

- *Pregnant women.* In general, a pregnant woman will probably feel more comfortable on her left side. That position takes the weight of the baby off the large blood vessels and nerves in the abdomen, preventing supine hypotensive syndrome (dizziness, drop in blood pressure, and decreased cardiac output). If there is excess vaginal bleeding, place the woman in a supine position with feet elevated 10 to 12 inches. If you suspect a prolapsed umbilical cord, place the woman on her back and elevate her hips with a pillow. Follow local protocol. (See Chapter 27, "Obstetric and Gynecological Emergencies," for details on these conditions.)
- *Infants and toddlers.* An infant or toddler who is not critically injured can usually be carried easily in an infant car seat. When possible, use the child's own car seat to reduce fear of being in an unfamiliar environment. You can also use the car seat as an immobilizer. Simply pack the space around the child with rolled towels or folded sheets taped as padding. (See Chapter 38, "Infants and Children," for more information on immobilization of infants and toddlers.)
- *Elderly patients.* A possible limitation in an elderly patient is osteoporosis, a loss of mass that makes the bones extremely brittle and prone to fracture. In these cases, take extra care to avoid accidental injury. Also take time to make sure the patient understands what is happening and where you are taking him.
- *Handicapped patients.* Use common sense in handling patients who are handicapped. The nature of the handicap will let you know how to compensate. If, for example, the patient has fused joints or twisted limbs, position the patient to provide the greatest comfort. Take extra care in strapping. Whenever possible, use a rolled towel or other padding to support areas that might need it. Ask the patient to explain what positions are possible and comfortable for him.

ENRICHMENT

The enrichment section contains information that is valuable as background for the EMT-B but that goes substantially beyond the U.S. Department of Transportation (DOT) EMT-Basic curriculum.

PACKAGING PATIENTS FOR AIR TRANSPORT

When the distance to the appropriate hospital is great and/or the patient's condition is critical, the use of a helicopter or fixed-wing aircraft for patient transportation might be considered. (See Chapter 40, "Ambulance Operations," for more detail on helicopter transport.) In this situation, there are some special considerations in the packaging of the patient to assure the safety of the patient, rescuers, and helicopter crew. Follow local protocols for use of air ambulance service. Following are some basic guidelines for preparing a patient for air transport:

1. Be sure that a patient who has been contaminated by a hazardous material has been thoroughly decontaminated. Especially in the confined space of a helicopter, it is possible for the crew to be overcome by hazardous fumes and lose control of the craft.
2. If at all possible, have the patient's airway managed with an endotracheal tube prior to the arrival of the aircraft.
3. Leave the chest accessible if the patient is intubated so the aircraft crew can assess the patient's breath sounds prior to transport.
4. If the patient is to be transported by helicopter and is immobilized on a backboard, be sure the board is one that can be accommodated in the model of helicopter that will respond.
5. Be sure the patient is well secured to the backboard so as not to be jostled while moving to the aircraft or in flight.
6. Secure all equipment, blankets, sheets, and so on with tape so they cannot blow off the patient and into the rotor or engine of the aircraft. Secure all loose equipment at the scene.
7. Communicate to the patient what you are doing and prepare him to expect the noise and rotor wash of an incoming helicopter.
8. Cover the patient's eyes, ears, and exposed wounds to protect them from the noise and rotor wash.
9. Consider having an engine company wet the landing zone to prevent dust and debris from being blown onto the rescuers, crew, and patient.

10. All rescuers should remove any loose clothing or hats to avoid their being blown into the rotor or engine.
11. Do not approach the aircraft with the patient until instructed by the pilot or crew. Unless otherwise instructed, let the crew assist you in loading the aircraft.
12. When moving the patient to be loaded into a he-

licopter, lay an IV bag on the patient's chest instead of having it held up by a rescuer.
13. When loading a patient into a helicopter, minimize the number of people under the rotors at all times.

Refer to local protocols and air transportation companies for further guidelines.

CASE STUDY FOLLOW-UP

SCENE SIZE-UP

You have been dispatched to a 72-year-old female patient, Amanda Sanchez, to take her on a routine transfer to the hospital dialysis center. As your partners unload the stair chair and blankets from the ambulance, you shovel the short walk to the front of the house and apply salt. While you are upstairs, the ice will have a chance to melt.

The patient's daughter opens the door and sends you up a flight of narrow stairs to the bedroom. Mrs. Sanchez greets you there, and you notice that she is using a walker. Your partners take in the stair chair and prepare it for the patient.

PATIENT ASSESSMENT

The training officer suggests that you practice taking a SAMPLE history and vital signs.

LIFTING AND MOVING THE PATIENT

After taking a history and vital signs, you listen as your training officer explains the procedure to the patient. She explains that you and your partner will place Mrs. Sanchez on the hospital blanket in the stair chair, tuck her in so she'll be warm, and secure her for a safe trip down the stairs.

Mrs. Sanchez asks if she will need her winter overcoat. Your partner explains that a warm hat and scarf would be okay, but the overcoat may be too bulky for the move. He promises her the blankets and the ambulance will keep her warm. He also says she can take the coat with her in case she needs it later. You and your partners then package the patient and move her to the stairwell.

At the top of the stairs, your training officer explains exactly what will be done next, while you and your partner quickly check the straps. When she's finished, the training officer says, "Mrs. Sanchez, remember? You may feel as if you're falling for a second. But you won't fall. We'll be holding you. Is it okay that we begin now?"

Mrs. Sanchez agrees, and you get behind the chair at the head. Your partner, who is taller than you, stands at the foot facing the patient. The training officer gets in position to spot behind your partner, one hand on his back. As you tilt the chair back, your partner grasps it by its legs. Your training officer tells you how many steps there are ahead. Both of you lift simultaneously and start the descent. The trainer-spotter counts out.

You and your partner place the stair chair down at the bottom of the steps to rest for a minute. Mrs. Sanchez's daughter opens the front door, and the training officer checks to see that the walkway is clear of obstacles and ice. When you are all assured it is safe, you wheel the chair out to the ambulance and load the patient onto the ambulance cot.

ONGOING ASSESSMENT

Inside the ambulance, you make certain the patient is comfortable, loosening her scarf and the blankets. You perform an ongoing assessment en route and arrive at the hospital without any change in the patient's condition. You and your partners transfer Mrs. Sanchez to the hospital staff, complete the necessary paperwork, and then proceed to ready the ambulance for the next call.

CHAPTER REVIEW

TERMS AND CONCEPTS

You may wish to review the following terms and concepts included in this chapter.

emergency move—a move that should be performed when there is immediate danger to the patient or to the rescuer.

nonurgent move—a move made when no immediate threat to life exists.

urgent move—a move made because there is an immediate threat to life due to the patient's condition and the patient must be moved quickly for transport.

REVIEW QUESTIONS

1. Name the three categories of patient moves, and explain when each should be used.
2. Explain, briefly, how to perform (a) an armpit-forearm drag, (b) a shirt drag, and (c) a blanket drag.
3. Name the greatest danger to the patient in any emergency move and explain how to minimize that danger.
4. Explain, briefly, how to perform a rapid extrication from a vehicle.
5. Explain, briefly, how to perform (a) a direct ground lift, (b) an extremity lift, (c) a direct carry, and (d) the draw sheet method.
6. Name the most commonly used patient carrying device and explain one advantage and one disadvantage of its use.
7. Name types of patient-carrying devices you would consider using if the spaces you need to traverse are too narrow or too confined for a wheeled stretcher.
8. Name the patient carrying device you would consider using if the terrain is especially rough.
9. Name patient conditions for which the stair chair should not be used.
10. Name two positions in which a patient would usually be positioned on a carrying device. Explain three patient conditions that might cause you to alter these positions.

CHAPTER 40

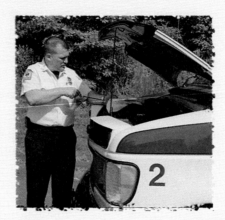

Ambulance Operations

INTRODUCTION

The ambulance is the vehicle that brings care to the patient in times of emergency and transports the patient to a medical receiving facility for follow-up care. It is a crucial part of the EMS system.

An ambulance should be a place of comfort and support to patients suffering from life-threatening problems. It should not pose additional hazards to them. But statistics tell a different story. According to national data, about 10 percent of all ambulances are involved in a collision each year.

To keep from adding to these statistics, the EMT-Basic must learn to drive an ambulance skillfully and safely. The process takes time. But the regulations and guidelines can be learned before getting behind the wheel. This chapter describes how to operate an ambulance safely. It also details other procedures to help ensure the most efficient operation of a properly equipped ambulance.

OBJECTIVES

Numbered objectives are from the United States Department of Transportation 1994 EMT-Basic National Standard Curriculum. Asterisked objectives, if any, pertain to material that is supplemental to the DOT curriculum.

COGNITIVE

7-1.1 Discuss the medical and non-medical equipment needed to respond to a call. (pp. 816–817)

7-1.2 List the phases of an ambulance call. (p. 815)

7-1.3 Describe the general provisions of state laws relating to the operation of the ambulance and privileges in any or all of the following categories: (pp. 812, 815)
- Speed
- Warning lights
- Sirens
- Right-of-way
- Parking
- Turning

7-1.4 List contributing factors to unsafe driving conditions. (pp. 813–814)

7-1.5 Describe the considerations that should be given to: (p. 814)
- Request for escorts
- Following an escort vehicle
- Intersections

7-1.6 Discuss "Due Regard for Safety of All Others" while operating an emergency vehicle. (p. 812)

7-1.7 State what information is essential in order to respond to a call. (pp. 817, 818)

7-1.8 Discuss various situations that may affect response to a call. (pp. 813–814)

7-1.9 Differentiate between the various methods of moving a patient to the unit based upon injury or illness. (p. 818)

7-1.10 Apply the components of the essential patient information in a written report. (p. 822)

7-1.11 Summarize the importance of preparing the unit for the next response. (p. 822)

7-1.12 Identify what is essential for completion of a call. (pp. 822–824)

7-1.13 Distinguish among the terms cleaning, disinfection, high-level disinfection, and sterilization. (p. 824)

7-1.14 Describe how to clean or disinfect items following patient care. (p. 824)

AFFECTIVE

7-1.15 Explain the rationale for appropriate report of patient information. (p. 822)

7-1.16 Explain the rationale for having the unit prepared to respond. (p. 822)

CASE STUDY

THE DISPATCH

Medic One—respond to the rest area at Interstate 80 and the Black Canyon Exit. You have a 33-year-old female patient with labor pains. Time out is 1511 hours.

EN ROUTE

You move quickly to your vehicle. Your partner is driving. You fasten your seat belt. The garage door opens. The engine starts. Your vehicle moves slowly, and then picks up speed. Additional patient information from dispatch crackles over the radio. It's difficult to hear. You inhale deeply and tell yourself, "Relax." You are prepared. You begin to picture in your mind what you need to do and how you should perform throughout the ambulance call.

This chapter will provide you with information on how to prepare yourself, your equipment, medical supplies, and vehicle for an ambulance run. Later, we will return to the case study and apply the steps learned.

DRIVING THE AMBULANCE

As an EMT-B, you have the responsibility for getting an ambulance safely to the scene of an emergency and transporting patients safely in it to medical care. To drive an ambulance well, you need a combination of knowledge, skills, and attitude.

LAWS, REGULATIONS, AND ORDINANCES

As an ambulance operator, you should be familiar with the laws and regulations that apply on both the state and local levels and *consistently obey them.* You have certain privileges under the law as the operator of an emergency vehicle, as do the operators of police vehicles and fire apparatus. At no time is it justified to operate an ambulance in a manner that jeopardizes anyone else. Remember that your first duty to your patient is to arrive at the scene—safely! After that, you must get your patient to definitive care carefully and safely.

While statutes in each state vary slightly, most states give you the privilege, with proper precautions, to do the following while driving the ambulance to an emergency:

- Exceed the speed limit posted for the area as long as you are not endangering lives or property
- Drive the wrong way down a one-way street or drive down the opposite side of the road
- Turn in any direction at any intersection
- Park anywhere as long as you do not endanger lives or property
- Leave the ambulance standing in the middle of a street or intersection
- Cautiously proceed through a red light or red flashing signal
- Pass other vehicles in no-passing zones

In executing the above, you must first signal, ensure that the way is clear, and avoid endangering life and property by driving with due regard for the safety of others.

By law, you must meet several qualifications before you can exercise these privileges:

- You must have a valid driver's license. Some states mandate that you attend an approved driving course.
- You must be responding to an emergency of a serious nature.
- You must use warning devices—red lights, horns, and sirens—so that other vehicles on the road will be aware of you and will have a chance to yield. You must use these devices in the manner prescribed by law.
- *You must exercise due regard for the safety of others.* This means that you may cautiously move through a red light, but you must slow down while entering the intersection so that all traffic can stop to allow you to pass. It means that you may park your ambulance anywhere to care for a patient, but you must not park it just over the crest of a hill on a busy highway unless you post flares and get a police officer or a volunteer to divert traffic out of your line. *The law states that if you do not exercise due regard for the safety of others, you are liable for the consequences.*
- Many EMS systems provide additional guidance. For instance, some specify that your top speed cannot be more than 10 miles per hour over the speed of *traffic,* which may or may not be the posted speed. This allows the emergency vehicle to overtake other moving traffic but promotes safer driving. In some areas, ambulances entering an intersection against the light must come to a complete stop before proceeding.

Be sure that you know the general vehicle code, the regulations for emergency vehicles, and your agency code. Also, know the qualifications in your state for operating an ambulance and be sure that you can qualify. Several states require special licenses and/or special training for ambulance operators.

DRIVING EXCELLENCE

An excellent ambulance operator understands the capabilities and limitations of his vehicle, evaluates weather and road conditions quickly and accurately, appraises and responds to traffic conditions quickly and appropriately, and minimizes risk and discomfort to other members of the crew and to the patient. Notice that fast, dramatic driving is not part of the definition.

BASICS OF GOOD DRIVING

Always wear seat belts when you drive the ambulance. Make sure other team members wear theirs as well.

Hold the steering wheel with both hands at all times. One hand should be in the nine o'clock and the other in the three o'clock position. In turning, one hand pulls while the other slides, paralleling the pulling hand's position. Neither hand should pass the twelve or six o'clock positions to prevent them from becoming tangled. When you reach these limits, the opposite hand begins to grip the wheel and the first hand slides.

You also need to practice enough with your ambulance that you are familiar with how it accelerates and decelerates, the kind of space it requires for its fenders and bumpers, how it brakes, and how it corners.

When driving an ambulance, you must recognize and respond to changes in weather and in road conditions. Adjust your speed to allow for decreased visibility at night and in fog and road handling during rain, snow, and ice storms.

During transport, select the route best suited for safe travel—this is not necessarily the shortest route. Avoid schools, railroad crossings, detours, construction sites, bridges, tunnels, and similar trouble areas whenever you can, even if it means driving a few extra miles. If you are unfamiliar with the roads in your city or area, get a good, detailed local map and study it. Patrolling will help you get a feel for topography. Keep informed about roads undergoing repair or new building sites, and avoid them when you can. Select an alternative route during rush-hour traffic. If you are responding to a traffic collision that can back up traffic on a busy highway, select an alternative route to avoid being caught in the traffic jam.

Maintain a safe following distance. Use headlights to improve your vehicle's visibility. Exercise caution when using red lights and siren.

MAINTAINING CONTROL

For vehicle control, remember the rule about speed: Go the posted limit unless the situation is critical. Speed can complicate patient care by providing a rougher ride, decrease ambulance stability, and risk the safety of everyone in the ambulance.

A number of factors other than speed affect your ability to control the ambulance, and you need to be alert to them to stay in constant control as you drive.

Braking Sudden braking may result in loss of control. The brakes will cause wheels to lock, and you may skid dangerously. Pump your brakes slowly and smoothly. (Newer ambulances may have an antilock braking system in which the brakes should be applied firmly and steadily, not pumped.) Never brake on a curve. Brake when going into the curve and gradually accelerate when going out. When decelerating, rest your foot lightly on the brake. Your stopping distance is the time it takes you to react plus your braking time.

Railroads You may encounter a railroad crossing and have to wait for a long train to crawl along the tracks. Keep calm and monitor the patient. If there is simply no way that you can get around the train, such as an underpass or overpass within a reasonable distance, wait it out instead of trying inappropriate stunts. Plan an alternative route when you can.

School Buses Be especially alert when approaching a stopped school bus with its red lights flashing. You must always be prepared for the possibility that a child will dart out across the road heading to or from the bus. Laws regarding ambulances and school buses vary from state to state. In some, an ambulance must

come to a full stop and remain stopped until signaled ahead by the bus driver. Follow your state law.

Bridges and Tunnels There is little room for passing on bridges or in tunnels. If you are in heavily congested traffic near a bridge or tunnel, consider an alternative route. If there is none, try to get control of the situation before you enter the bridge or tunnel. Remember that you probably will not be able to pass, so go with the flow of traffic at a safe speed until you emerge. Also be sure the height of the bridge or tunnel will accommodate the height of the ambulance.

Day of the Week You can expect less traffic on weekends than on workdays in most areas. Traffic around shopping centers is heaviest on Saturdays, to and from resort areas on Fridays and Sundays, and on commuter routes or in urban and industrialized areas on Monday through Friday. Keep in mind what kind of traffic you are likely to encounter.

Time of Day Rush-hour traffic is more congested in most urban centers than rural areas, so plan accordingly. Watch for school zones and industrial plant shift changes.

Road Surface Always be on the lookout for potholes and bumps. Your goal is to give your patient the smoothest ride possible. The two inner lanes on a four-lane highway are generally the smoothest.

Backing Up Many ambulance collisions occur when the ambulance is backing up. Use all resources (e.g., mirrors, EMT-B in the rear of the ambulance) and back up slowly and carefully.

Higher Speeds At higher speeds, be alert to the following:

- Be especially careful on curves that lead into population pockets (a town or school), curves that lead to intersections, and curves that crest hills. Practice negotiating curves in the ambulance during the early mornings when there is little traffic. Get a good idea of what speed you need to get around the curve safely.
- Brake to the proper speed before you enter a curve. Enter the curve at the outside (or the "high" part), and start turning as early as possible. Go only as fast as feels comfortable while in the curve. Do not accelerate or brake in the curve—the scrubbing action of the tires will slow the ambulance down sufficiently. It is dangerous to brake after you have entered the curve, so make sure that you decelerate to a safe speed before entering.
- Accelerate carefully and gradually as you leave the curve. Too quick an acceleration can cause you to lose control.
- Keep your exit from the curve slow and steady.

- When going down a long hill, use a lower gear instead of riding your brake to maintain control.
- Always use a smooth braking motion. Your stopping distance increases dramatically as your speed increases; allow for it.

Escorts Using a police or other emergency vehicle escort en route to the collision or the hospital should be a last resort. It is dangerous, not only to the escort, but also to the EMT-B driver, to the patient in the ambulance, and to others on the road. All hazards associated with ambulance driving are doubled when an escort is involved, because you are the second vehicle through an intersection and motorists may expect only one.

Use an escort *only* if you are unfamiliar with how to get to the hospital or if you do not think that you can find the victim's location. Allow for a safe distance between the escort vehicle and your ambulance.

Intersection Collisions The most common collisions in which ambulances are involved are those at intersections. There are three main causes of intersection collisions:

- A motorist approaches the intersection just as the light is changing; he does not want to sit through the red light, so he sails through the intersection. Always slow down at each intersection to make sure that it is clear. If you are crossing against the light, come to a complete stop and proceed only when all traffic is clear or appropriately stopped.
- There are two emergency vehicles when motorists expect only one. Maintain a safe distance between your vehicle and the emergency vehicle in front of you, but follow closely enough so that the motorist can see both of you in the same glance. Do not use the same siren mode on both vehicles. Whenever you are using the emergency privileges that allow you to suspend traffic regulations, always use your flashers and siren for the fullest possible warning to the public. In some states, use of your siren when you are driving in the emergency mode is mandated by law.
- Vehicles waiting at an intersection may block your view of pedestrians in the crosswalk. Again, slow down and anticipate people in the crosswalk. Come to a complete stop if you are unsure if pedestrians are entering the intersection.

WARNING DEVICES

Ambulances are equipped with a variety of warning devices. Your agency will have specific protocols for their use. Following are some general guidelines and suggestions.

COLORS AND MARKINGS

Ambulance colors and markings are an aid to traffic safety and reduce the need for excessive dependence on lights and sirens. An early DOT/EMS study, "Ambulance Design Criteria" by the National Academy of Sciences, recommended a nationwide system of specific colors and markings. Later, the General Services Administration and DOT developed and published federal specifications for ambulances (1974:KKK-1822).

The standard color is white; the markings are an orange stripe running around the body, blue lettering, and the "Star of Life" symbol (Figure 40-1). It is recommended that any added lettering be kept below the orange stripe so as not to distract from the basic markings. For maximum effectiveness, these standard colors and markings should not be duplicated on vehicles that are not ambulances.

WARNING LIGHTS AND EMERGENCY LIGHTS

Activate emergency lights on the ambulance at all times when responding to an emergency call. Lights should be used even when you are not using the siren. You should also turn on your headlights during the daytime—in some situations, the warning lights on top of the vehicle are not noticeable because they blend in with traffic lights, signs, Christmas decorations, building colors, and tail lights of vehicles traveling in the opposite direction.

Placement of the ambulance emergency lights on the vehicle is very important. They should be high enough to cast a beam *above* the traffic. Lower lights are needed to be visible in the rear-view mirror of the car ahead of you.

When an ambulance has strobe lights, use them with emergency lights that flash or revolve with a longer duration. White lights can be seen from a longer distance than red or blue, especially at sunrise or sunset. They can also be seen more effectively when wet streets are reflecting.

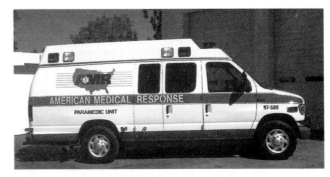

Figure 40-1 Standard colors and markings make ambulances instantly recognizable.

Headlights are a part of the emergency lighting system and should be on whenever you are traveling in an emergency. Specially wired headlights that flash alternately are also effective in gaining attention. (These are not legal in some states—check local protocol.) A spotlight can be used to get the attention of a driver who has not noticed you, but do not panic him. Flash the light across the driver's rear-view mirror so that it gets his attention but is gone before he looks in the mirror. The glare could blind him or oncoming traffic, so be careful.

Use only minimal lighting during heavy fog or when you are parked. Use your emergency lights only when needed, such as when the patient's condition requires rapid transport.

USING YOUR SIREN

Even if you are operating your flashing lights and sirens, do not assume that drivers are aware of you unless they look up to check their interior rear-view mirror, look to the left to check the exterior rear-view mirror, pull over, or stop.

The insulation in newer automobiles can reduce the interior decibel level of an approaching siren by 35 to 40 percent when parked. In motion, the noise of the motor, air-conditioner/heater, and/or radio in the automobile may make the siren completely inaudible. (This also applies to you in the ambulance!) Other sources of interference may be conversation, pelting rain, dense shrubbery or trees, buildings, and thunder. If the driver is wearing headphones, talking on a phone, inattentive, or hearing-disabled, your problem is even more severe. Some drivers may not even recognize a two-tone klaxon as a siren.

Never pull directly behind a car and blast your siren. The driver may panic and slam on the brakes or swerve into another lane. Also, be prepared for the irrational maneuvers of inexperienced, intoxicated, or disoriented drivers.

Since the siren signals "emergency," it can create emotional stress (as well as physical stress from the noise level) for your patient. This is another reason for using your siren sparingly. Always let your patient know before you activate the siren.

Be aware of the siren's effect on you. Even if you can normally drive your own car or the ambulance flawlessly, the siren can have a bizarre effect on your ability to drive the ambulance safely. Studies have shown that ambulance operators tend to increase their speed about 15 miles per hour when the siren is going—an increase that sometimes takes them out of the limits of safe speeds. Some drivers are easily hypnotized by the siren and are unable to negotiate curves, turns, and obstacles; this hypnotic trance makes it seem as though the siren itself were controlling the vehicle. The siren can also prevent you from hearing sirens or horns of other emergency vehicles responding to the same or other incidents.

Follow your state laws and local protocols regarding siren use.

USING YOUR AIR HORN

Avoid overuse of the air horn, but consider it when you need to clear traffic quickly. You can use the air horn with or without the siren, depending on your state law and local protocol. Do not sound your horn when you are close to other vehicles—it may frighten a driver and cause him to slam on the brakes or swerve. (The air horn may, however, be used safely much closer to other cars than may your siren.) Do not assume that other drivers can hear or will heed your horn.

PHASES OF AN AMBULANCE CALL

The major phases of an ambulance call are these:

1. Daily pre-run vehicle and equipment preparation
2. Dispatch
3. En route to the scene
4. At the scene
5. En route to the receiving facility
6. At the receiving facility
7. En route to the station
8. Post run

DAILY PRE-RUN PREPARATION

The key to response readiness is a properly maintained and equipped ambulance. Having a vehicle ready to respond at all times and in all conditions and equipped with all necessary supplies will ensure that you can reach, care for, and transport your patients.

AMBULANCE MAINTENANCE

Basic ambulance maintenance should include oil and filter changes, transmission and differential checks, wheel bearing check, brake check, and tie rod end inspection.

A comprehensive and regularly scheduled preventive vehicle maintenance schedule is essential. Benefits of a professional vehicle maintenance and inspection schedule include:

• Decreased vehicle down time
• Improved response times to the scene
• Safer emergency and non-emergency responses
• Improved transport times to the medical facility
• Safer patient transports to the medical facility

You should know and practice your service's policies and procedures for reporting and correcting vehicle problems. Do not be afraid to take personal responsibility for ensuring that your vehicle is fit for duty. Remember, proper care for your ambulance is part of proper care for your patients.

DAILY INSPECTION OF VEHICLE

Inspect the vehicle systems daily (Figures 40-2a to d). Most ambulance systems have a checklist of the items to be checked, which will typically include the items listed in Table 40-1.

Your service should have a clear protocol for reporting problems with vehicles, taking them out of service if they are deemed unsafe, and performing regular service and maintenance. Legally, you may be within your rights to refuse to use a vehicle that you have reason to believe is unsafe; and incidentally, you may be legally liable for damage caused by a malfunctioning ambulance if you are aware of the problem.

AMBULANCE EQUIPMENT

Your ambulance must contain supplies and equipment for handling medical emergencies, injuries, extrications, and childbirth. Supplies and equipment should be checked each day and restocked, cleaned, or maintained after each run. Table 40-2 lists supplies

ELEMENTS OF THE DAILY VEHICLE INSPECTION

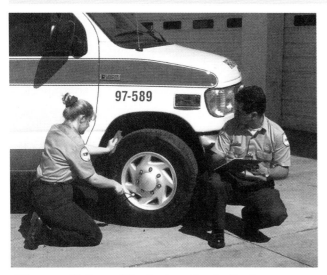

Figure 40-2a Check tires for inflation, wear, or danger spots.

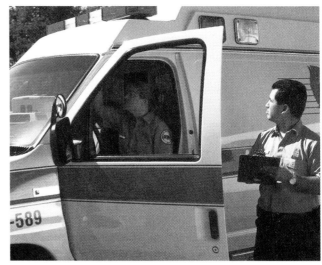

Figure 40-2b Make sure all lights are functional.

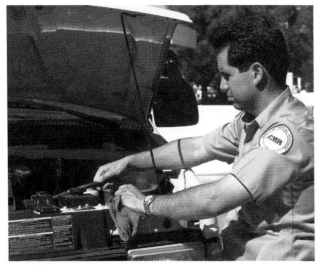

Figure 40-2c Check all belts and hoses.

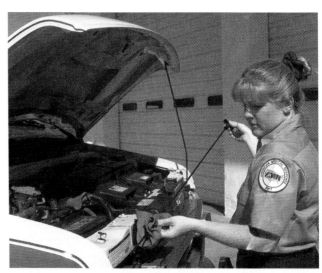

Figure 40-2d Check all fluid levels and keep them up.

TABLE 40-1
Daily Ambulance Inspection

Items Typically Included in a Daily Ambulance Inspection Checklist
Fuel
Oil
Fluid circulation system
Batteries
Brakes
Tires and wheels
Shoreline power connectors
Headlights
Brake lights
Turn signals
Emergency lights
Wipers
Horn
Siren
Windows
Door closing and latching devices
Power systems
Air-conditioning, heating, and ventilation systems
Radiator hoses and fan belts
Seat belts
Dash lights
Radio
Supplies
Interior and exterior cleanliness

TABLE 40-2
Basic Ambulance Supplies

Medical Supplies
Basic supplies
Patient transfer equipment
Airways
Suction equipment
Artificial (positive pressure) ventilation devices
Oxygen inhalation equipment
Automated external defibrillator (AED)
Cardiac compression equipment
Basic wound care supplies
Splinting supplies
Childbirth supplies
Medications
Non-medical Supplies
Personal safety equipment
Pre-planned routes, comprehensive street maps

and equipment as identified in the EMT-B revised curriculum.

PERSONNEL

A properly equipped and maintained ambulance is important to emergency prehospital care. Properly trained personnel to operate the ambulance and make optimum use of its equipment are even more important. Staffing requirements for ambulances vary among states and localities. In some states, one EMT-B in the patient compartment is considered the minimum standard; however, two are preferred. Follow your state laws and local protocols about staffing.

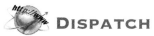 ### DISPATCH

A message from dispatch will start you on your run. The communications component of the EMS system has been discussed in greater detail in Chapter 11,

"Communication." The dispatcher will usually have performed the first assessment of the situation when receiving a call. The dispatcher should provide you with the following information:

• The location of the call
• The nature of the call
• The name, location, and callback number of the caller
• The location of the patient
• The number of patients (if more than one) and the severity of the problem
• Any other special problems or circumstances that may be pertinent

Write this information down so you can refer to it. Use it to prepare yourself physically and mentally for the call. Do not hesitate to ask the dispatcher to repeat or restate information if anything is unclear.

EN ROUTE TO THE SCENE

Your ambulance is checked and ready to respond. The vehicle's medical and non-medical equipment and supplies are clean and operational. You receive a call. Follow these guidelines on your way to the scene:

• Before departure, quickly check the vehicle making sure outside compartment doors are closed and secure, external shoreline cords are disconnected, and any jump kits are retrieved and properly stowed.

- Fasten your seat belt.
- Write down information from the dispatcher on a notepad.
- Confirm the following dispatch information:
  - Location of the call
  - Nature of the call
  - Location of the patient
  - Number of patients and the severity of the problem
  - Any other special conditions or problems
  - If any other units are en route
- Listen for status reports from other units on the scene.
- Think about what equipment you will want to take into the scene.
- Remain relaxed, yet focused. (Studies indicate that fewer than half of all ambulance runs are requested as emergencies. Only half of those are true emergencies with less than 5 percent being life threatening.)
- Drive responsibly, maintaining a 3- to 4-second following distance between your ambulance and the vehicle directly ahead of you.
- Determine what the responsibilities of team members will be before arriving on the scene, and make sure those responsibilities are clear.
- Call for advanced life support if necessary.

AT THE SCENE

Follow these guidelines while at the scene:

- Notify dispatch of arrival on scene.
- Park the ambulance in the safest and most convenient place to load the patient and later depart from the scene, taking into consideration the traffic, the roadway, and any known hazards. Follow local ordinances regarding the use of warning signals and devices at the scene (Figure 40-3).
- Park in front of or behind a collision, but never alongside it. On a narrow, no-parking road, take up the entire road so that no one will try to squeeze past you. Park in a driveway or on the shoulder of the road whenever possible. Stay a minimum of 100 feet from wreckage or a burning vehicle and 2,000 feet from a hazardous materials spill, ideally uphill and upwind (Figure 40-4). Come to a complete stop. Set the parking brake prior to placing the transmission in the "park" position.
- Take the necessary body substance isolation. Determine if you will need eye protection, gloves, mask, and gown before making patient contact.
- Determine if it is safe to approach the patient. Identify and control hazards. If the scene is unsafe, make it safe or do not enter until the scene is secure for you, incoming units, bystanders, and your patient. Review the procedures discussed in Chapter 8, "Scene Size-up."

- If a mechanical failure occurs or you need backup equipment or personnel to help, call the dispatcher immediately.
- Your dispatcher has told you what to expect, but be prepared to shift your perspective quickly. You may encounter an entirely different situation or incident. Remain calm and poised. Unruffled management of the unexpected emergency is part of your job.
- Carefully observe the complete incident or situation as you approach. Look for children, curiosity seekers, or patients who may have wandered away from the scene. Decide if the patient may require immediate movement because of hazardous conditions.
- Determine the patient's mechanism of injury. Follow guidelines from Chapter 8, "Scene Size-up," Chapter 9, "Patient Assessment," and Chapter 28, "Mechanisms of Injury: Kinetics of Trauma."
- Determine the total number of patients. Initiate multiple-casualty-incident response if necessary, following procedures described in Chapter 43, "Multiple-Casualty Incidents." Do this before making patient contact. You are less likely to call for help once you begin intense patient care and treatment. If necessary, begin patient triage.
- Determine your priority of care. Your approach to medical and trauma patients during your initial assessment should be organized. Keep the goal of prompt transport foremost in your mind.
- For motor vehicle crashes, carefully gain access to the patient or patients and extricate them safely. Proper procedures to follow will be discussed in Chapter 41, "Gaining Access and Extrication."
- Take the time needed to properly splint and immobilize injured extremities *before* you move the patient, unless he is unstable and determined to be a high priority for immediate transport. Proper spinal immobilization is critical to appropriate patient care. Review procedures discussed in Chapter 32, "Musculoskeletal Injuries," and Chapter 34, "Injuries to the Spine."
- Carefully remove the patient from any wreckage and move him to the ambulance, choosing methods of moving the patient based on his illness or injury. Follow the patient lifting and moving principles and procedures you learned in Chapter 6, "Preparing to Lift and Move Patients," "Chapter 34, Injuries to the Spine," and Chapter 39, "Moving Patients."
- Transfer the patient to the waiting ambulance. Keep him warm, and watch for any changes in his condition. Make sure the patient is securely strapped on the wheeled stretcher with spinal immobilization performed as necessary. Lock the stretcher securely in place within the ambulance.

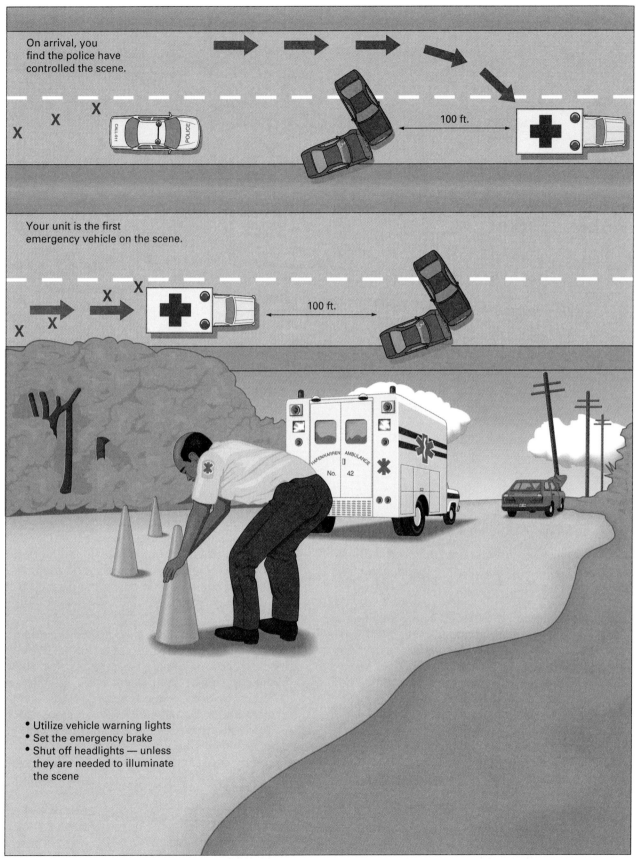

Figure 40-3   Safety at the scene.

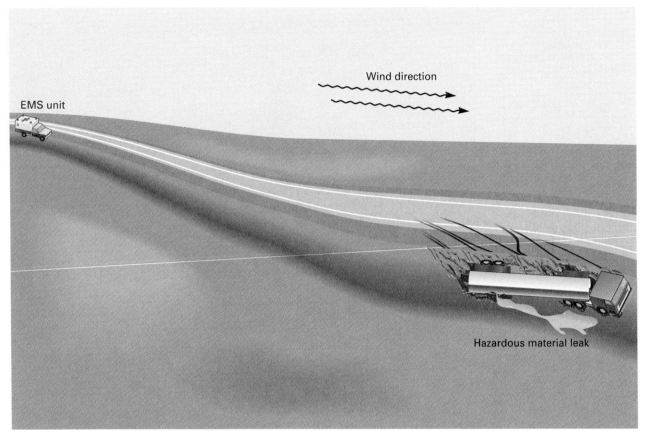

Figure 40-4   Park the EMS unit uphill and upwind from any leaking hazardous materials.

EN ROUTE TO THE RECEIVING FACILITY

Once you are ready to transport your patient to the appropriate medical facility, follow these guidelines (Figures 40-5a to h):

- Make sure your patient is settled before moving the ambulance. Calmly reassure the patient. If you have not already done so, tell him where he is being taken.
- Before departure, the vehicle driver should quickly check the unit, making sure the outside compartment doors are closed and secure.
- Begin your ongoing assessment. This includes a reassessment of the patient's mental status, airway, breathing, and the recording of vital signs. Conduct an ongoing assessment at least every 15 minutes for a stable patient, every 5 minutes for an unstable patient.
- Notify dispatch that you are en route to the hospital. Follow local protocols regarding transmission of additional patient information.
- Check any patient interventions. Make sure oxygen is delivered at the correct flow rate. Check dressings and splints. Continue to reassure the patient.

- If a patient's relative or friend accompanies him, follow local guidelines as to where this person should sit. Allow the companion in the patient compartment only if local protocols permit it and if the relative or friend is in emotional control. If the patient is a child, it is often helpful to have a parent with you.
- Focus on the patient. Smile and reassure him as often as you can. Take advantage of brief stops to monitor blood pressure. Treat each patient like an individual, not a "case." Gentleness, listening, answering questions honestly, and providing as much explanation as the patient wants will make a world of emotional difference—for him and for you.
- The driver should drive prudently, use only the necessary speed, and obey all regulations to keep the patient as comfortable as possible during the trip.
- If you are the EMT-B with the patient, you should keep the driver informed of the patient's condition. Instruct him to slow down or take a different route if the patient is uncomfortable from the speed and bouncing. (If you want to gain a deeper appreciation for how your patient may feel strapped to a stretcher in the back of an ambulance, secure your-

EN ROUTE TO THE RECEIVING FACILITY

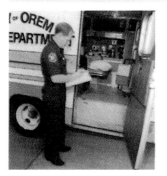

Figure 40-5a Complete, concise records are essential.

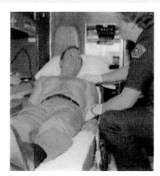

Figure 40-5b Give calming reassurance. Make sure that the patient is stabilized and settled.

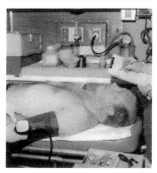

Figure 40-5c Collect patient information with a standard report form while your partner checks vital signs.

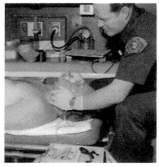

Figure 40-5d Continue your ongoing assessment; reassess vital signs.

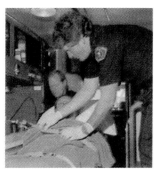

Figure 40-5e Make sure that stretcher and patient are secure. Check straps and adjust any that may be too tight or too loose.

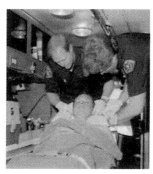

Figure 40-5f Review patient priorities. Check your medical interventions.

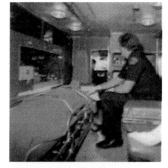

Figure 40-5g The driver should drive prudently. Advise the driver of any changing conditions in the patient.

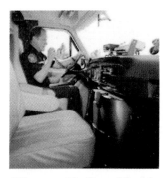

Figure 40-5h Notify dispatch and the hospital of the number of patients you are transporting.

self on the gurney and have your partner drive over bumpy roads. This is a great learning experience.)

- During your ongoing assessment, if the patient's condition worsens and it becomes urgent to reach the hospital immediately, tell your driver so he can proceed as quickly as possible.

- Notify the receiving medical facility as soon as your patient's condition permits you to call in a report. Sometimes this may not be possible. In those situations where the patient's condition demands your full attention, request that your partner notify the hospital. Refer to Chapter 11, "Communication," to review the information that should be radioed to the receiving facility.

- Continue to reassess your patient's condition and notify the receiving facility if that condition deteriorates.

AT THE RECEIVING FACILITY

Once you arrive at the receiving facility you should follow these guidelines:

- Notify dispatch of your arrival at the medical facility.
- The patient is usually presented to the emergency department nurses at the hospital. As you make the transfer of care, continue to concentrate your care on the patient. If the emergency department is crowded, continue to care for your patient until you can transfer your patient care responsibility to emergency department personnel. Never leave the patient unattended!

- When you are able, transfer all records and information about the patient to appropriate emergency department personnel.

- To ensure proper continuity of care, a complete oral report should be given to emergency department personnel at the patient's bedside. You should summarize the information given over the radio:
  - Introduce the patient by name (if known).
  - Repeat the patient's chief complaint.
  - Provide additional vital signs taken en route.
  - Report any history not given previously.
  - Report any additional treatment you provided.

- If requested, assist emergency department personnel in lifting and moving the patient to a hospital gurney or bed.

- Make sure that any valuables or personal effects of the patient are also transferred, and indicate this on your report.

- Once you have released your patient to the care of emergency department personnel, exchange any linens, spine boards, and other equipment you may have to leave at the hospital.

- The written prehospital care report should be completed before you leave the hospital. A copy should be left at the emergency department. Follow local

protocol if your system also requires you to leave a copy of your written report with the patient.

- Before you leave, ask hospital personnel if you are needed further. You may need to transfer the patient to another medical facility or return the patient home if his condition is not serious enough to warrant hospital admission.

EN ROUTE TO THE STATION

In order that your ambulance be available for service as quickly as possible, begin preparation for return to service as soon as possible. Follow these guidelines for returning to the station:

- At the hospital or your station, clean and inspect your ambulance, patient care equipment, reusable supplies, and patient care compartment before notifying dispatch of your availability. During particularly busy shifts, this can be difficult. Always follow your agency's biohazard disposal procedures. Dispose of any contaminated linen. Disinfect any reusable patient care equipment. These steps are essential for you and your patients' safety and health.

- Wash your hands.
- Radio the dispatcher that you are returning to the station (Figure 40-6).
- Buckle your seat belt, then proceed to the station in a safe, cautious manner.
- If a team member is in the patient compartment, he or she can continue to clean as needed from a buckled seat position.
- Refuel according to local protocol.

POST RUN

Follow these guidelines after the run (Figures 40-7a to d):

- Fill out and file any reports as required by local protocol. *Do not* postpone this activity.

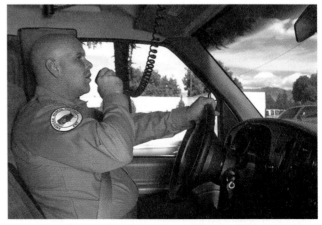

Figure 40-6   Advise dispatch when you are returning to the station.

POST RUN

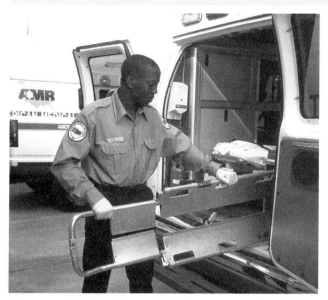

Figure 40-7a   Put all equipment in its proper place.

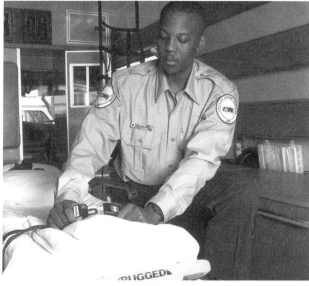

Figure 40-7b   Make up the wheeled stretcher and lock it in place.

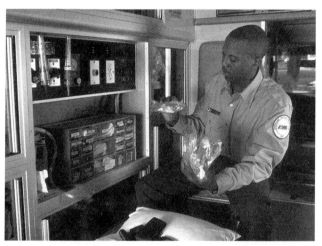

Figure 40-7c   Complete an inventory of equipment and supplies. Replace necessary equipment so that the ambulance is fully stocked.

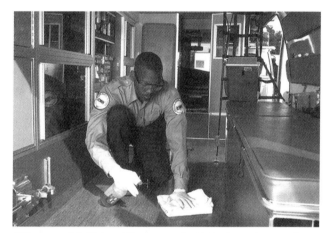

Figure 40-7d   Clean and disinfect the patient compartment.

- After each run, check fuel; if the fuel tank approaches half empty, fill it.
- Complete an inventory of equipment and supplies. Replace what you used during the run, and complete the cleaning and disinfection of nondisposable equipment used.
- Wash the exterior of the ambulance if you were driving in rain or snow or over muddy roads.

- Change soiled uniforms.
- Notify dispatch you are in service, available for calls.

INFECTION CONTROL PROCEDURES

To prevent the spread of infection, follow the procedures outlined next as you ready your unit and yourself for return to service.

Dispose of Sharps   Make sure that needles, blades, and all other disposable sharp items have been placed in clearly labeled, puncture-resistant containers for disposal. (This should have been done immediately after use throughout the call.)

Wash Hands   Use ordinary soap and water to wash your hands at the end of the run and after all cleaning procedures have been completed. (You should also have washed your hands immediately after each contact with a potentially contaminated patient or item.) Use waterless antiseptic hand cleaner if ordinary washing facilities are not available.

Clean, Disinfect, or Sterilize Contaminated Equipment   Use proper procedures to clean (wipe up), disinfect (kill some microbes on), or sterilize (kill all microbes on) contaminated reusable patient care equipment or any items that have or will come in contact with patients. (Review cleaning, disinfecting, and sterilization in Chapter 2, "The Well-being of the EMT-Basic.")

1. *First, clean up visible spills of blood, vomitus, or other body fluids.* Put on protective gloves (use gloves that are heavy enough to resist puncture from sharp edges or while scrubbing). Wear appropriate face and eye protection if you anticipate splashing. If there is a great amount of blood in the area, wear impervious shoe coverings. Use disposable towels or other materials that can be placed in a plastic bag of contaminated laundry after use. After removal of visible material, decontaminate surfaces with a germicide or a 1:100 or 1:10 solution of household bleach and water (see guidelines below). Use clean towels with germicide to wipe the area. Let the area air dry. After the area has been decontaminated, place shoe coverings, gloves, and other contaminated items in a sealed plastic bag for disposal.
2. *Then disinfect reusable patient care equipment.*

For disinfecting surfaces and equipment, choose an appropriate level of disinfection or sterilization as outlined below. Some judgment about the level of disinfection or sterilization required must be exercised.

- *Use low-level disinfection for routine housekeeping on environmental surfaces such as floors, ambulance seats, and countertops when there is no visible blood and contamination by body fluids or a patient with tuberculosis is not suspected.* Use a 1:100 solution of household bleach and water or an EPA-registered "hospital disinfectant" chemical germicide with no claim on the label for tuberculocidal activity, or use. These disinfectants will destroy some viruses, most bacteria, some fungi but not mycobacterium tuberculosis or bacterial spores.

- *Use intermediate-level disinfection for surfaces that come into contact with intact skin, such as stethoscopes, blood pressure cuffs, or splints.* Use a 1:10 solution of household bleach and water or an EPA-registered "hospital disinfectant" chemical germicide with a claim on the label that it is tuberculocidal. These disinfectants will destroy mycobacterium tuberculosis, most viruses, vegetative bacteria, and most fungi, but not bacterial spores.

- *Use high-level disinfection for reusable instruments that come into contact with mucous membranes, such as laryngoscopes, blades, and handles.* Use either hot water pasteurization (80° to 100° Celsius for 30 minutes) or immerse in an EPA-registered chemical sterilant for 10 to 45 minutes. This method will destroy mycobacterium tuberculosis, most viruses, vegetative bacteria, and most fungi, but not bacterial spores.

- *Sterilize equipment that will be used invasively.* Immerse in an EPA-registered chemical sterilant for 6 to 10 hours (only if a heat sterilization process is not available) or expose to steam (autoclave), gas, or dry heat sterilization. This method will destroy all forms of microbial life. It is used primarily in hospitals rather than in prehospital settings. When possible, disposable items are preferred to avoid the need to disinfect or sterilize and to prevent transmission of disease to other patients.

Launder Soiled Clothing and Linens   The risk of disease transmission from soiled clothing or linen is minimal. However, follow these recommendations:

- Handle soiled laundry as little as possible.
- Bag soiled items at the location where they were used. Place items soiled with blood in separate bags and prevent leaking.
- Wash in normal laundry cycles with regular detergent according to the recommendations of the washing machine manufacturer.
- Wear gloves when bagging and placing contaminated clothing into washing machines.
- Launder uniforms according to the label instructions.

Dispose of Infectious Wastes   Place all infectious wastes in clearly labeled and sealed biohazard bags for disposal according to your local protocols.

AIR MEDICAL TRANSPORT

Many medical personnel involved in helicopter rescue consider a helicopter to be not just transport but an extension of the emergency department. Statistics show that many of those transported by helicopter would have died without the accompanying aeromedical support. Airplanes may also be used where transport distances are long.

WHEN TO REQUEST AIR MEDICAL TRANSPORT

Follow local protocols or seek on-line medical consultation when you think air medical transport may be needed. Air transport should be considered according to the following guidelines:

- *Operational guidelines:*
  - The patient needs to be transported to a trauma center or other specialty care facility that is distant from his present location.
  - A high-priority patient is entrapped and a prolonged extrication is expected.
  - Air transport will clearly save time over ground transport.
  - The patient is in a remote area that cannot be reached by ground vehicles.
  - Ground ambulance transport is blocked.
  - The air transport crew possesses medical skills not available with the ground ambulance.
- *Medical guidelines*—The patient is a high priority for air transport where the patient has a time-critical illness or injury, such as the following:
  - Shock
  - Head injury with altered mental status
  - Chest or abdominal trauma with signs of respiratory distress or shock
  - Serious mechanism of injury with alteration of vital signs
  - Penetrating injury to the body cavity
  - Other time-critical illnesses such as severe carbon monoxide poisoning, digit or limb amputation, or heart attack

INFORMATION NEEDED WHEN REQUESTING AIR MEDICAL TRANSPORT

When calling for a helicopter transport, you should be prepared to provide the following information:

- Your name
- Department name
- Call-back number
- Nature of the incident
- Excact location of the incident (landmarks and crossroads are helpful)
- Radio frequency you use, so that you can communicate with the helicopter or plane
- Exact location of the landing zone.

SETTING UP A LANDING ZONE

In setting up a landing zone for a helicopter, keep these guidelines in mind:

- Make sure that the landing area is clear of obstructions. This area should ideally be a flat square with 60-foot sides by day for a small helicopter, but larger—about 100-foot sides—by night. If the helicopter is medium-sized or large, it will need about double that area. Pick up loose debris that might blow up into the rotor system. Choose a landing site at least 50 yards from collision vehicles, if possible, so that noise and rotor wash will not be a problem for rescuers. Contact your local service for landing zone requirements and safety specifications.
- If the landing site is a divided highway, stop the traffic going in both directions, even though the aircraft will land on only one side of the highway.
- Consider the wind direction. Helicopters take off and land into the wind by preference, rather than making vertical descents and ascents. Warn the crew by radio of power lines, poles, antennas, trees, or other obstructions.
- Mark each corner of the landing area with a highly visible device: a flag or surveyor's tapes by day and a flashing or rotating light at night. Use flares either by day or night but only if there is no danger of fire.
- Put a fifth warning device on the upwind side to designate the wind direction.
- If conditions are dusty or dry enough to create a fire hazard, have the area wetted down, if possible.
- Keep the patient and crew clear of the air downwash area. Spectators should be at least 200 feet away. EMT-B personnel should be at least 100 feet away during landing.
- Assign one person to guide the pilot in. He should wear eye and ear protection and should stand near the wind direction marker with his back to the wind, facing the touchdown area, arms raised overhead to indicate the landing direction (Figure 40-8).
- Give primary care to the patient and follow the instructions of the pilot or crew members *exactly* when those instructions relate to the craft's operation. Never try to open a door, for instance, without instructions.
- Be extremely cautious about the rotor-blades. Remember that the tips can dip as low as 4 feet above the ground. Always crouch when approaching or leaving the helicopter (Figure 40-9a), and approach or leave only on the pilot's directions.
- Never approach a helicopter until the pilot indicates it is safe. Never approach from behind the pilot. The pilot cannot see behind the craft, the tail rotor is spinning very quickly, and the pilot sometimes needs to move the tail boom without warning. If you have to go from one side to another, always cross in front of the craft, never behind it or underneath it.
- Secure all loose items so that nothing will blow into the rotor blades when you are approaching or leaving a helicopter.
- No one should smoke within 50 feet of the aircraft. If the helicopter has to land on an incline, always

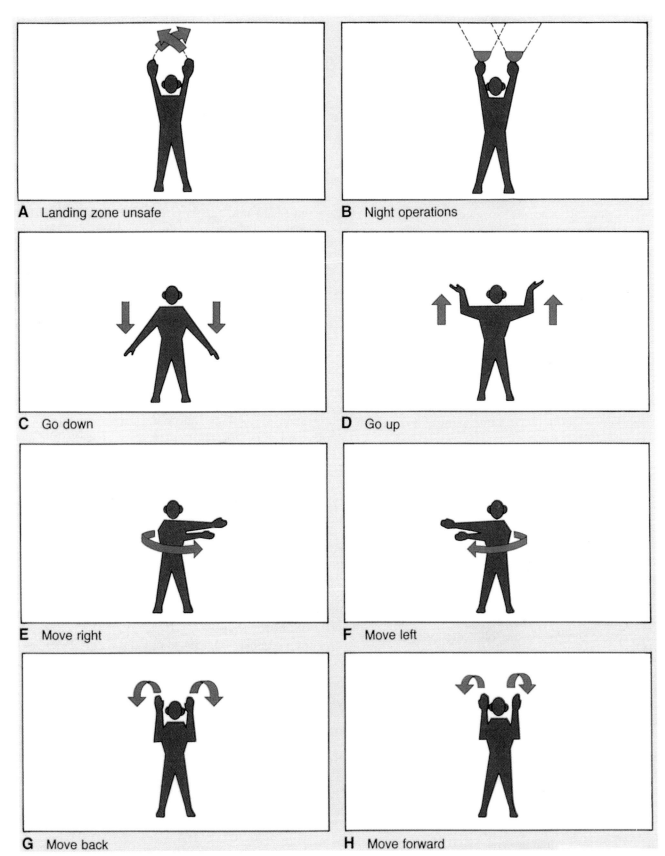

Figure 40-8 Guiding the helicopter pilot in.

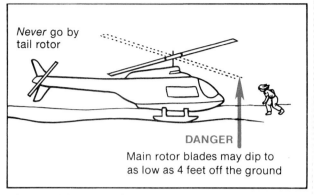

Figure 40-9a Always crouch when approaching or leaving a helicopter.

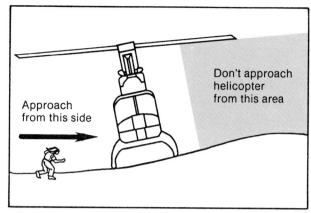

Figure 40-9b Approach a helicopter from downhill.

approach from the downhill side, never from the uphill side (Figure 40-9b).

• Never point spotlights up at a helicopter that is on its final approach at night.

ENRICHMENT

The enrichment section contains information that is valuable as background for the EMT-B but that goes substantially beyond the U.S. Department of Transportation (DOT) EMT-Basic curriculum.

CHANGING CONDITIONS

DRIVING AT NIGHT

While only about one-third of all collisions occur at night, more than half of the fatalities from collisions stem from nighttime driving. In fact, based on miles driven, there are two and a half times more fatal collisions at night than during the day. This is because less light is available and vision is restricted. Night vision varies considerably among people. Older people generally cannot see well in the dark, and eyestrain can substantially reduce night vision. Bright light, such as lightning or high-beam headlights, can cause temporary blindness at night.

Headlights on low beams illuminate the roadside for about 150 feet. On high beams, visibility will be 350 to 400 feet. At 55 miles per hour, it takes 4.5 seconds to cover 350 feet. For night driving, control speed so that your stopping range is within headlight range.

To improve your visibility and the ability of others to see you, do the following:

• Make sure that your ambulance has quartz-halogen headlights, which provide much more light to the road.

• Have your headlights on whenever you are traveling in an emergency.

• Keep your headlights clean and properly aimed. Check them each day before your shift begins. If the weather is bad, especially if there is sleet or snow, stop as necessary during your shift to clean debris off your headlights.

• Replace burned-out bulbs immediately.

• Dim your high beams within 500 feet of an approaching vehicle or within 300 feet of a vehicle in front of you.

• Never stare into the high beams of another car; guide your ambulance by watching the right edge of the road.

• Do not flick your high beams up and down to remind another driver to dim his brights—it can blind him temporarily.

• Never use high beams when going into a curve.

• Keep your windshield clean, inside and out. Keep a bottle of windshield or glass cleaner in the ambulance for mirrors and interior windshields.

• Keep your instrument panels dim.

• Keep your eyes moving; avoid focusing on any one object.

• If the washing solution under your hood does not leave the glass clean after ten wiper cycles, replace the blades and/or use a stronger concentration of washing fluid.

• Be sure that you are rested before you begin a night driving shift. Between 11 P.M. and 3 A.M., be particularly alert for intoxicated or drowsy drivers. If you notice erratic speeds, weaving across lines, or delayed starts at intersections, use extreme care in passing.

DRIVING IN BAD WEATHER

Bad weather affects your ability to control your ambulance. Stopping on wet pavement takes approximately twice the distance as stopping on dry pavement. On ice or sleet, it takes you five times the distance to stop. Leave adequate space between you and the vehicle in front of you in any kind of weather. Nevertheless, 66 percent of ambulance collisions occur in clear or cloudy weather, and 70 percent occur in daylight. Furthermore, 63 percent of ambulance collisions occur on dry roads. Follow these precautions for specific weather situations:

Rainy or Wet Weather   About six times more people are killed on wet roads than on snowy and icy roads combined. Roads are slipperiest as a rain storm begins. When the road is wet, your vehicle can hydroplane—that is, the front tires literally lift so that the vehicle is riding on a film of water rather than on the pavement itself. Hydroplaning can begin at speeds as low as 35 miles per hour if the tires are worn. Do the following when driving on wet roads:

- Keep your mirrors cleared of water.
- Avoid sudden braking and sudden moves of the steering wheel.
- If you are about to go through a large standing puddle, slow down and turn on your wipers before you hit the water. As you leave the water, tap the brake lightly a few times to dry it out. If the ambulance pulls to one side, pump the brake slowly and smoothly to dry the brake out.
- If you begin to hydroplane, hold the wheel steady, take your foot from the accelerator, and gently pump the brake. If you turn the wheel from side to side to try and get down through the water, or if you jam on the brake, you will probably skid.

Winter Driving   Sleet, freezing rain, packed snow, and ice decrease visibility and increase skidding. Powder snow and gusty winds can create a total white-out with zero visibility for several hundred yards. To ensure safety, do the following:

- Make sure that your engine is tuned, your heater and defroster are in good working order, and your battery is charged.
- Carry emergency weather equipment—chains, a shovel, sand, booster cables, and a towing device.
- Equip the ambulance with studded snow tires if you can. Chains are the best insurance against skidding. Follow local and state protocols and laws.
- Stay aware of the temperature. Wet ice and freezing rain, the most hazardous road conditions, occur between 28° and 40°F. Bridges and overpasses freeze sooner than road surfaces.
- Avoid sudden movements of the steering wheel and sudden braking.

Fog, Mist, Dust Storms, Smog   When visibility is poor, do the following:

- Slow down but avoid decelerating suddenly.
- Watch the road ahead and behind carefully for other cars that are traveling slowly.

- Turn on your lights, regardless of the time of day, and use your wipers. Never use the high beams on your headlights. The reflection of the beams from the fog will actually reduce your ability to see. Even if the lights do not improve your ability to see ahead, they will make it possible for other motorists to see you better.
- If you are traveling 15 miles per hour or more below the speed limit, use four-way flashers. (These may not be legal in some states.) Use the four-way flashers if you pull off the road and stop.
- Use the defroster to keep as much fog as possible off the inside of the windshield.
- If you need to slow down, tap your brake pedal several times so that the flash of your brake lights will warn motorists behind you.
- Fog can occur suddenly, and patches of greater density may appear. Vehicles in front may brake suddenly or come to a complete stop when encountering a thicker patch of fog. Be alert for vehicles in front of you.

CARBON MONOXIDE IN AMBULANCES

Another emergency situation that you may encounter while driving an ambulance is the buildup of carbon monoxide gas. Carbon monoxide (CO) is colorless, odorless, tasteless, and deadly. If an ambulance is not properly cared for, a CO level that is harmful to injured or ill patients and even to emergency personnel may build up. Any amount of CO over 10 parts per million above the ambient CO level in the air may be dangerous. Excessive amounts of CO may come from:

- The vehicle's own exhaust gases
- Supplemental gasoline or liquid-petroleum-gas-powered equipment
- The exhaust gases of vehicles parked next to or traveling by the ambulance
- Greater outside air pressure, which forces the CO into the ambulance

Be aware of the symptoms of carbon monoxide poisoning. Low levels of carbon monoxide may cause yawning, dizziness, dimmed vision, headache, irregular heart rhythm, nausea, or vomiting. Extended exposure or high concentrations can lead to seizures, coma, and death. Review the information on carbon monoxide poisoning in Chapter 21, "Poisoning Emergencies."

If any of the indications of the presence of carbon monoxide occur, remove the patient from the ambulance and administer oxygen by nonrebreather mask. Resuscitate the patient if necessary.

Prevent CO poisoning by:

- Having frequent engine tune-ups
- Having an adequate exhaust system that discharges beyond the side of the vehicle

- Keeping rear windows shut
- Making sure that doors shut tightly with proper gaskets and adjustments
- Covering any opening to the outside
- Not using ventilation exhaust fans or static roof vents
- Keeping the heater or air-conditioner on. They create continuous positive interior pressure.

- Not using supplemental gasoline or liquid-petroleum-gas-powered equipment inside the ambulance

A bright light or water spray under pressure will help you identify possible spots where CO can enter. CO testers for the inside of ambulances are available. There are also color-change CO monitors that will stick to the sun visor or dash and audible CO alarms.

CASE STUDY FOLLOW-UP

En Route to the Scene

You've been dispatched to a 33-year-old female patient with labor pains at a highway rest area. You remember that during the patient compartment check you made sure the OB kit was stocked. As your partner drives, you look at your notepad and reconfirm the location of the call. You request a further update from dispatch on the nature of the call. "The mother believes she will have the baby before you arrive!" First Responders at the location give you a report on the radio: "It's a girl!"

At the Scene

You notify dispatch when you reach the rest area. While looking through your vehicle's front window, you begin the scene size-up. Your partner sets the parking brake and then puts the transmission in park. The vehicle is parked so you won't have to back into traffic when leaving. The scene is safe. You put on your body substance isolation gear, turn on the patient compartment heat, and grab the OB kit. You take a deep breath and try to relax.

The First Responders tell you the patient's name is Karen Austin and direct you to the sleeper cab of a semi-tractor and trailer. You in fact have two patients, mother and child. You begin your initial assessment of the mother and baby. After providing initial OB care and treatment, you prepare them for transport. Both are covered with warm blankets and loaded into your warmed ambulance. The truck driver tells you he's Tom Austin, the father, and wants to ride along. You say okay, but politely advise him that your agency requires that he ride in the front seat of the ambulance. You ask a First Responder for assistance en route to the receiving facility. She gladly agrees and jumps in the back.

En Route to the Receiving Facility

In the patient compartment, you complete your focused history and physical exam. Prior to leaving the scene, your partner makes sure all vehicle compartments are secure. He asks for assistance from a police officer in stopping traffic. He then notifies dispatch he is en route to the hospital with two patients. You calmly inform her where she will be transported. She is settled, and baby is resting comfortably.

You are still 30 minutes away from the nearest medical facility. You begin your detailed exam of both mother and baby. After your detailed exam, you begin an ongoing assessment. You reassess the mother's and child's mental status, airway, breathing, and circulation, and all of your medical interventions. You then tell your partner and the father that the mother and baby are doing fine. Your partner decides to continue driving at the posted speed limit. You radio a report on the condition of your two patients to the receiving facility.

At the Receiving Facility

As you arrive at the facility, your partner notifies dispatch. You are greeted at the door by emergency department staff. Mother and baby are immediately wheeled into a patient room. You continue to make sure they are kept warm. Next, you provide your oral report to both the emergency department physician and the nurse.

Meanwhile, your partner has already started to clean and prepare the vehicle for your next run. After transferring the care of your patients to the hospital staff, you ask your partner if he wants help in resupplying the ambulance. He tells you to go ahead and write the prehospital care report while he gets clean linen and disinfects the cot.

You finish your report and leave a copy with the patient's records. Your partner advises you the unit has been cleaned and resupplied. You ask emergency department personnel if they need any further information. They say thanks but everything seems all right. "Good job," they tell you.

En Route to the Station

Your partner has already disposed of contaminated linen and supplies. The vehicle and reusable supplies have been disinfected according to your agency's protocol. Both of you remembered to wash your hands. You advise dispatch you are available for another call and are returning to the station. You and your partner buckle your seat belts and decide to refuel.

POST RUN

Once at the station, you recheck your supplies, and finish cleaning the patient compartment floor. Also, you decide to wash the vehicle's exterior. Your station phone rings. It's Tom Austin calling from the hospital. The baby's name is Sandra. You contact dispatch and let them know.

CHAPTER REVIEW

REVIEW QUESTIONS

1. List some of the privileges that may be granted to an ambulance operator. List the qualifications necessary for using these privileges.
2. Explain when an ambulance operator should use a police escort.
3. List the major causes of intersection collisions.
4. Explain the problems use of a siren can pose for ambulance safety.
5. List the phases of an ambulance run.
6. List information an ambulance crew should receive from dispatch before beginning a run.
7. Describe the procedures you should follow in turning a patient over to a receiving facility.
8. Explain when cleaning and restocking of an ambulance after a run should begin, and why.
9. List the infection control procedures that should be followed.
10. Explain how you should mark a landing area for air ambulance use.

CHAPTER 41

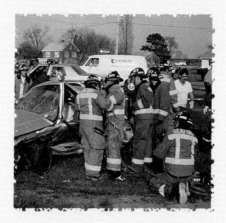

Gaining Access and Extrication

INTRODUCTION

By far the most common rescue situations encountered by the EMT-Basic are motor vehicle collisions. Patient rescue begins with the scene size-up. It includes stabilization of the scene as well as stabilization of the vehicle, gaining access, and safely extricating, packaging, and moving the patient.

Access and extrication are also issues at scenes other than vehicle collisions. Most of the time you will find your patients in safe, easily accessible locations where gaining access requires no more than a knock on a door. However, there will be occasions when advanced rescue techniques must be used to get to and help a patient—for example on a remote mountainside, from a raging river, or from entrapment under machinery or a collapsed building.

Obviously you cannot receive advanced rescue training from this or any other EMT-Basic text. You can, however, become familiar with the situations in which patients are found and the roles you can play in rescue.

The primary role of the EMT-B in a rescue situation is gaining access to the patient as quickly as can be safely accomplished in order to perform patient assessment and care, even as the rescue operation proceeds. Your two major priorities in a rescue situation are (1) to keep yourself and your partner safe, and (2) to prevent further harm to the patient.

OBJECTIVES

Numbered objectives are from the United States Department of Transportation 1994 EMT-Basic National Standard Curriculum. Asterisked objectives, if any, pertain to material that is supplemental to the DOT curriculum.

COGNITIVE

7-2.1   Describe the purpose of extrication. (p. 838)
7-2.2   Discuss the role of the EMT-Basic in extrication. (pp. 838–840)

7-2.3   Identify what equipment for personal safety is required for the EMT-Basic. (p. 833)
7-2.4   Define the fundamental components of extrication. (p. 838)
7-2.5   State the steps that should be taken to protect the patient during extrication. (pp. 839–840)
7-2.6   Evaluate various methods of gaining access to the patient. (pp. 837–838)
7-2.7   Distinguish between simple and complex access. (p. 837)

CASE STUDY

THE DISPATCH

EMS Unit 204—respond to Solzman Road just north of Pin Oak Court—vehicle collision with reported multiple injuries and entrapment. Time out is 2337 hours.

ON ARRIVAL

You find a small red vehicle sitting nose to nose with a large dump truck. The front of the automobile has collapsed and is underneath the front axle of the truck. The front bumper of the truck is even with the windshield of the automobile. You can see two motionless young people in the front seat of the car with a considerable amount of blood coming from multiple facial lacerations. The dash is crushed down onto the patients, pinning them in the vehicle.

How would you proceed?

During this chapter, you will learn about your role as an EMT-B in patient rescue situations. Later, we will return to the case study and put in context some of the information you learned.

PLANNING AHEAD

DISPATCH

As soon as you receive the call from dispatch, you must evaluate whether there are obstacles to patient access and extrication—in other words, whether this is a situation that requires special rescue procedures. Begin with these questions:

• Is the patient ill or injured?
• What is the mechanism of injury?
• What is the location of the incident?
• What time of day is it?
• What is the weather?
• Is there a report of entrapment?
• Is there a report of a leak or a spill?

Most illnesses occur at home and offer little challenge to access and extrication other than an occasional locked door or protective pet dog. However, an incident involving trauma may offer considerable challenge. A trauma patient may be found anywhere under any circumstances. Based upon the dispatch information, the EMT-B can begin to plan for access and extrication problems.

LOCATION

One way to begin to plan is to consider the location of the incident. For example, on a call to a fall in a parking lot at the local mall you may encounter heavy traffic. A cardiac emergency may be easy to handle at a residence, but on the sixteenth green of the local golf course or in the stands at the high school football game, it can be difficult. Access to a home may be easier than access to an industrial site.

Know your territory. Look around your community and begin to identify locations and occupations that may present access difficulties for EMS personnel. For example:

- Utility employees work above and below ground.
- Construction workers work everywhere from ditches to rooftops and around heavy equipment.
- Painters work off ladders and scaffolding, which may be placed on soft, unstable ground.
- Antennas and water towers need periodic maintenance.
- Industrial sites offer all these potential risks and problems and more.

Excluding motor vehicle collisions, most injuries are the result of gravity. People either fall or something falls on them. Consider all the things that can fall on people; for example, a car on top of the weekend mechanic, a tree after a sudden storm, construction material at a new building site, or a few tons of dirt from a cave-in of a ditch or excavation.

People can crawl, climb, and walk to many locations that your ambulance and wheeled stretchers cannot traverse. Be prepared. Have strategies for gaining access in mind, and know the types of specialized rescue teams available through your system.

MOTOR VEHICLE COLLISIONS

Motor vehicle collisions present the most frequent rescue problems. Consider factors such as location and time of day to begin to mentally weigh the odds of patient entrapment and difficult access.

The numbers of accidents are greater during high traffic times, but with more traffic come slower speeds and less chance of entrapment and serious injuries. As traffic thins, speeds increase and so do the number of entrapments, serious injuries, and fatalities. A collision on a freeway holds a greater chance of entrapment than a collision in a parking lot.

The majority of examples discussed in this chapter concern vehicle collisions, because they are the rescue situation you will most commonly encounter as an EMT-B.

SIZING UP THE SCENE

Expect the unexpected. Do not rely solely on the information received from dispatch. It can be sketchy and misleading. Know your territory, and stay alert for potential hazards. For example, when responding in industrial areas or to motor vehicle collisions involving common carriers and other commercial vehicles, stay alert for potential hazardous materials spills and releases. They present special challenges. Be sure your ambulance is equipped with binoculars, so you can assess the scene from a safe distance and position.

Scene size-up is a continual process. Even after you reach your patient, stay alert for changes in your surroundings. Wrecked vehicles can catch fire, the patient in a bar fight may suddenly seek revenge, or the overturned container may begin to leak. Every scene is dynamic and must be approached and continually reviewed until it is stabilized.

PERSONAL PROTECTIVE EQUIPMENT

The scene of a typical motor vehicle collision or other rescue situation is inherently hazardous. Materials such as shattered glass, sharp metal, flammable liquids, battery acid, and blood are commonplace. *Proper protective clothing and equipment must be used at every incident at which such hazards are present.*

The safety of any rescuer must never be jeopardized. Rescuers always must wear the level of protection needed for their particular role in the rescue process. The minimum level of protection for the EMT-B includes eye and head protection, disposable gloves, and any additional protection necessary to prevent direct contact with any blood or body fluid.

Your everyday work uniforms do not provide much protection from the glass and sharp objects usually present at collisions and other rescue scenes. Protective coveralls, for example, may protect you from a patient's body fluids, but they may not protect you from hidden or flying debris. If you need to enter a wrecked vehicle to provide patient care, wear the appropriate protective clothing.

Full turnout gear, including coat, bunker pants, and steel-toed boots are required for personnel involved in the patient extrication process. Head protection, such as a standard fire helmet, will protect your head from impact. The ear flaps and a wide brim will help protect you from shattering glass and falling debris. In addition to goggles or safety glasses, the helmet's face shield offers protection for the face and eyes. Heavy leather gloves worn over disposable gloves will help protect your hands from both sharp objects and body fluids.

Know your local protocols, which may dictate additional precautions.

SCENE SAFETY

As stated earlier, *the most important point to remember in any emergency is that your safety is always the highest priority.* Focus on risk analysis, not risk taking. Never commit yourself to a situation that is not completely secure. Although it may be difficult to remember at times, the biggest difference between you and the average person is your training. Do not compound the emergency or risk other rescuers' lives by becoming part of the problem.

If you are the first to arrive at the scene of an emergency, you may be responsible for scene size-up and scene stabilization until police, fire, and other rescue personnel arrive. The list of hazards that you may encounter at motor vehicle collisions and other emergencies is much too lengthy to address in this chapter. However, common hazards include electrical lines and traffic.

ELECTRICAL LINES

Hazards commonly found at collision scenes are downed electrical lines and damaged poles holding electrical lines and equipment. *Always assume a downed power line is electrically alive.* If you see that electrical lines are down near or in contact with the vehicle, the area must be secured to avoid accidental contact.

Often, the electrical distribution equipment supplying the power to the lines will have automatic resets. This is a method the power companies use to restore power when something such as a fallen tree branch causes a temporary short. When the power is automatically restored to the downed line, it can cause the line to whip and arc. Therefore, if a line is down and broken 75 feet from the pole, the area to be secured should be greater than 75 feet in all directions from the pole. If the power lines are in contact with the vehicle, *stay away*. Request special assistance from your local electric service company.

If patients are still in the vehicle, shout or communicate with them over your unit's PA system. Advise them that the electric company is en route. Tell them to stay inside the vehicle, which is safer than attempting to get out. Vehicle tires provide insulation between the vehicle and the ground. If patients were to climb out of the automobile, the electricity could pass from the vehicle and through them to the ground even before a foot touches the ground.

If the situation is immediately threatening to life, or the electric company is unable to respond, rescue personnel specially trained in handling electrical emergencies may move the downed line using special equipment and techniques designed for that purpose.

TRAFFIC

Traffic must be controlled for scene safety. Directing traffic is primarily the responsibility of the police in most parts of the country. If this job falls to rescue personnel in your area, or if traffic must be controlled prior to police arrival, special prior training in traffic direction and control is necessary.

In general, the safest method for traffic control at a serious vehicle collision is to stop all traffic and reroute it to different roads. This is not only for the safety of patients and bystanders but also for the safety of rescuers at the scene. If the regular flow of traffic must be channeled around the scene, it should be routed at least 50 feet from the wrecked cars (Figures 41-1a-d).

Even specially trained personnel must take extreme care when directing traffic away from an accident scene.

Additional rescue personnel and warning devices such as flares, chemical lights, or reflective cones are needed. All those who are channeling traffic should wear adequate reflective clothing or tape so that they can be clearly seen. Visual signals must be clear, so that approaching drivers can quickly understand exactly what they are being asked to do. Flares or cones should begin far enough from the scene so that a car can safely stop before it hits the scene, *even if the driver did not notice the flares or cones from a distance.*

LOCATING ALL PATIENTS

Most incidents involve a single patient who is easily accessible. Always locate that patient before attempting to gain access. By doing so you will be able to prevent further injury. For example, you can make sure the patient is protected with a blanket before a rescue team breaks a car windshield for emergency extrication. You may also be able to check if an injured or ill patient is behind a bedroom door before the rescue team forces it open.

Some incidents involve more than one patient, and they are not always easy to identify or find. In explosions, building collapses, trench or confined-space rescues, and hazardous materials incidents it is often difficult to locate patients. That is also true in high-impact, roll-over, and off-road vehicle collisions. Look for patients both at the site of the emergency and in the immediate vicinity. Unrestrained automobile occupants, for instance, can be thrown great distances and hidden by uneven terrain, darkness, vegetation, and debris.

Look for clues to "missing" patients. Get information from witnesses and patients about others who may be hurt at the scene. An empty child's car seat or a small sweater and coat in the back seat may be an indication that a child was involved in the incident. If in doubt, have the police contact relatives in an attempt to learn who might have been in the vehicle. Also ask bystanders if a patient walked away from the scene or if a passerby took a patient away. Before leaving the scene, a thorough search of the area for all victims must be conducted by emergency personnel.

It can be frustrating to wait in a safe area while specialized rescue teams locate, extricate, and deliver patients to you. Realize that in difficult and complex rescue situations, a team effort is required to successfully perform a rescue. Follow directions from the scene commander, and provide emergency medical care to patients as necessary and as possible.

VEHICLE SAFETY

If a fire engine company is not yet on the scene, remove the fire extinguisher from your vehicle and place it near the collision in case of fire.

POSITIONING FLARES TO CONTROL TRAFFIC

Posted speed (mph)	Stopping distance for that speed*		Posted speed (in feet)		Distance of the farthest warning device
20 mph	50 feet	+	20 feet	=	70 feet
30 mph	75 feet	+	30 feet	=	105 feet
40 mph	125 feet	+	40 feet	=	165 feet
50 mph	175 feet	+	50 feet	=	225 feet
60 mph	275 feet	+	60 feet	=	335 feet
70 mph	375 feet	+	70 feet	=	445 feet

Figure 41-1a Flares are positioned according to a formula that includes the stopping distance for the posted speed plus a margin of safety.

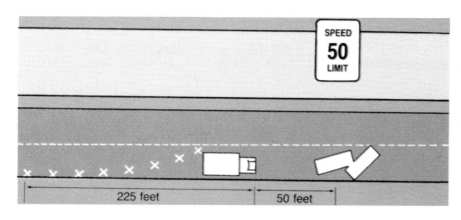

Figure 41-1b Flares positioned on a straight road. Approaching vehicles are moved into the correct lane before they reach the edge of the danger zone.

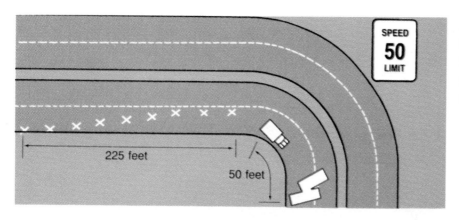

Figure 41-1c Flares positioned ahead of a curved section of road. The start of the curve is considered to be the edge of the danger zone.

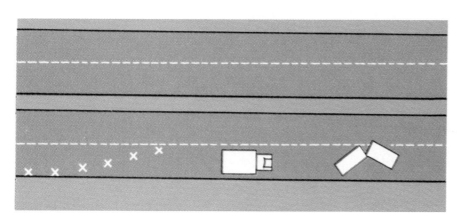

Figure 41-1d Flares positioned on a hill. The flares slow approaching vehicles and make them turn into the correct lane before they reach the top of the hill.

After all hazards are addressed and the scene is secure, the vehicles involved must be properly stabilized. A vehicle is considered stable when it is in a secured position and can no longer move, rock, or bounce. The involved vehicle must be stabilized by specially trained rescue personnel for the safety of everyone at the scene (Figures 41-2a to c). Remember, even a vehicle sitting on its wheels on a level surface may be unstable. Even the slightest movement can further injure a patient.

If necessary, there are steps you can take to stabilize a vehicle without using special equipment. For example, if the vehicle is upright, resting on all four wheels, and safe to approach, you can shut off the engine. Then set the parking brake, and shift the automatic transmission to "park" or the manual transmission to any gear. Also place firm objects such as a spare tire, pieces of wood, or logs in front of and behind a wheel to minimize vehicle movement. These steps usually will prevent a vehicle from rolling until rescue crews can properly and completely stabilize it.

Although rescue personnel may determine it to be necessary to disconnect the vehicle's battery, the majority of electric current and associated hazards can be eliminated by simply turning the ignition off. Before disconnecting power, attempts should be made to lower the power windows, unlock power door locks, and move the power seat to a position that provides the greatest patient access.

If it is necessary to disconnect the car battery, the engine compartment must be accessed. Cut or use a wrench to remove the negative battery cable first. Remove the positive cable last. *Note: If the positive cable is removed first, a spark may occur that could ignite acid fumes from the battery or gasoline spilled from the accident.*

If you determine that the vehicle is in an unstable and unsafe position and you cannot stabilize it with

STABILIZING A VEHICLE WITH CRIBBING

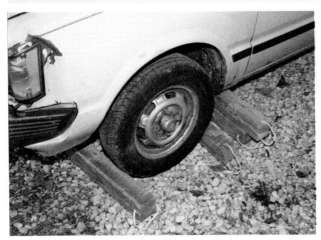

Figure 41-2a Cribbing used to keep a vehicle from moving.

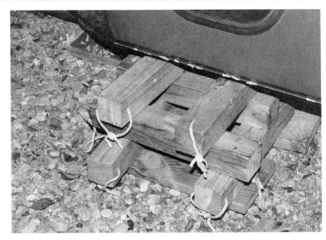

Figure 41-2b Proper use and positioning of cribbing.

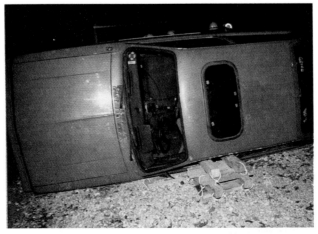

Figure 41-2c Cribbing used to stabilize a vehicle on its side.

available equipment, do not enter it and do not put any weight in or on it. Wait for additional rescue personnel to properly stabilize the vehicle. (See the Enrichment section for more information on vehicle stabilization.)

GAINING ACCESS

There are two basic ways a rescuer can gain access to a patient. **Simple access** is access in which tools are not required. **Complex access** requires the use of tools and specialized equipment.

Fortunately, you will find that most incidents do not present access problems. However, when confronted with one, you must quickly evaluate the situation and decide if a simple or complex access procedure is necessary. If complex access is required, it is best to call for rescuers who have had specialized training. (Specialized training programs available for complex access include trench, high angle, and basic vehicle rescue.)

RESIDENTIAL ACCESS

To gain access to a residence when the door is locked, first walk around the house to check for open windows or doors. Attempt to locate the patient by shouting through doors and windows and looking in windows. If you are able to converse with the patient, ask if a neighbor has a key. If not, ask neighbors if they have a key or if they know someone who does.

You can evaluate the need for a rapid, forced entry based upon dispatch information, what you observe at the scene, and your conversation with the patient. If you need to forcefully enter the scene (break into the house or apartment), have the police and fire department dispatched. If possible, wait for their arrival.

The easiest and least costly method of forceful entry usually is breaking a window. Breaking a pane of glass in or next to a door may permit you to reach in and unlock the door. Kicking the door in is not recommended, since you may be injured and it can cause costly structural damage. It is also more difficult to secure the residence afterward.

After police and fire personnel are on the scene, proceed with a forceful entry as follows:

1. Check all windows and doors for one that is unlocked or open. At the same time, look and shout through each window to try to locate the patient and check for hazards.
2. If a window is open but blocked by a screen, cut through the screen.
3. If you must break a window, choose a room in which there are no patients and a window through which you can see what is on the other side. Locate the smallest and least expensive window that will still allow you access.
4. If the patient is awake and responsive, inform him of what you are going to do.
5. Wear eye protection, heavy work gloves, and coat.
6. Stand alongside the window to be broken (Figure 41-3).
7. Using an object like a flashlight or a tire iron, grasp one end firmly and strike the top corner of the pane nearest you. Do not reach above your head.
8. Clear the broken pieces of glass out of the frame before reaching in to unlock the window or door.

People are becoming more and more security conscious. In many urban areas and areas of high crime, for example, people often cover windows and doors with security bars. As a result, it is difficult to force entry into many homes and apartments. Specialized rescue techniques and tools are constantly being developed and refined. It is best to call on rescue companies within the fire department or other emergency services to gain access in these situations.

 MOTOR VEHICLE ACCESS

By far, the most common access problems encountered by the EMT-B involve motor vehicle collisions. Throughout the process of gaining access, your main function is patient care. Once the scene is secure and you have decided that it is safe to approach the vehicle, walk around it once to identify mechanisms of injury, and approach facing the patient. (If you approach from the side, the patient may attempt to turn his head toward you, possibly aggravating a spinal injury.) If the patient is responsive, it is important to

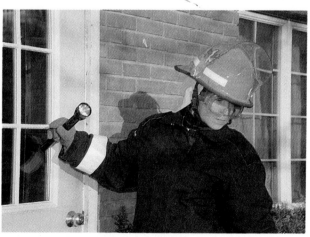

Figure 41-3   The easiest and least costly method of gaining access to a patient inside a house usually is breaking a window.

look directly into his eyes while you tell him not to move his head or neck. Tell the patient about everything you and other rescuers are going to do before you do it. Until you gain access to the patient and are able to stabilize the cervical spine, remind him repeatedly not to move. Tell the patient that focusing on any object directly in front of him will help lessen the chance of neck movement.

The door is always the access of choice because it is the largest uncomplicated opening into the passenger compartment of a car. Always start by testing the door handle to see if will open. If the doors are locked, reach in any open window to unlock one of them. If all windows are intact and rolled up, say to one of the patients: "Without moving your head or neck, try to unlock a door." Be sure to state the instruction not to move the head or neck *first*. If you wait until the end of your request, he may move and injure himself further in his eagerness to help.

If none of these methods of gaining access work, the quickest means of gaining access is by breaking a window. All windows in a modern automobile—except the windshield—are made of tempered safety glass that will break into rounded pieces rather than sharp shards. (The windshield is made of a different kind of safety glass with a layer of plastic between layers of glass.) When breaking windows or using rescue tools near patients or rescuers, cover them with a heavy blanket or tarp whenever possible.

To break a window in an automobile, tell the patient what you are going to do. Then:

1. Wear personal protective equipment. Heavy gloves and eye protection are necessary.
2. Locate the window farthest from the patient and, if time allows, cover it with contact paper or strips of broad tape.
3. Place a sharp tool such as a screw driver against a lower corner of the window and strike the tool with a hammer. Hold the tool with your hand resting against the car so your hand will not go through the window when it breaks.
4. Carefully remove the broken glass, starting at the top and continuing until all has been removed. Broken correctly, although completely shattered, most tempered safety glass will remain in place even if it was not taped.
5. Attempt to unlock the door. If unsuccessful, cover the door edge with a blanket or tarp before crawling into the vehicle to gain access to your patient.

Rescue personnel often carry a spring-loaded punch (Figure 41-4). Available at most hardware stores, this tool can easily be carried in a pocket or equipment holster. It is used in much the same way as described above except that when placed against the lower corner of a tempered safety-glass window, you

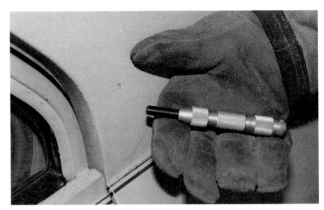

Figure 41-4 A spring-loaded punch.

simply push until the spring causes the tip to punch and break the glass (Figures 41-5a and b). Again, care must be taken to avoid pushing your hand through the window.

A makeshift tool that can be used in an emergency is the car's whip antenna. Snap off the antenna and hold it at one end along the metal of the door frame just below the window, allowing the opposite tip to touch the corner of the glass. Pull the tip away from the glass, causing the antenna to bow. When released, the tip of the antenna will strike the glass with enough force to shatter the window.

Once access is gained, the patient's condition can be evaluated. At that time make the decision to perform rapid or normal extrication (as explained in Chapter 34, "Injuries to the Spine").

EXTRICATION

The purpose of extrication is to remove the patient as rapidly and safely as possible from wreckage—most commonly the wreckage of a vehicle collision—in which he is entrapped.

THE ROLE OF THE EMT-B

The fundamental components of extrication include scene size-up, stabilization, gaining access, disentanglement, and patient removal. The role of the EMT-B in vehicle stabilization and patient extrication is that of patient care provider. Once specialized rescue personnel assure you that the vehicle is stable and the scene is safe to enter, you may approach the patient to initiate assessment and administer emergency care.

Note: Patient care always precedes removal from the vehicle unless delay would endanger the life of the patient, EMS personnel, or other rescuers.

While always bearing in mind that your responsibility is seeing to the welfare of the patient, work with other rescuers. Cooperate in every way possible with personnel who are working to disentangle the

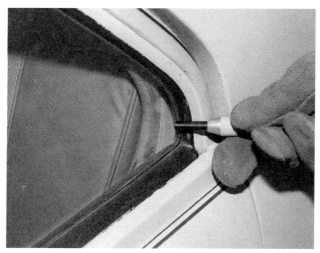

Figure 41-5a   Position the punch in the corner of the side window. Choose the side window farthest from the patient.

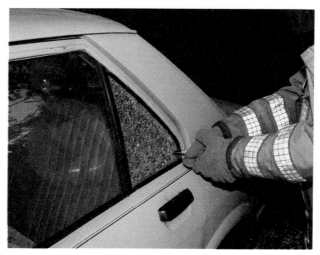

Figure 41-5b   After the tempered glass shatters upon impact of the spring-loaded punch, open the door or crawl through the window.

patient. Help them make certain that the patient is removed from the vehicle in a way that minimizes risk of further injury.

In some EMS systems, EMS providers are both emergency medical care providers and rescuers. In those systems, a chain of command should be established to assure patient care priorities.

CARING FOR THE PATIENT

As in any emergency, your first priority is always your own safety. (You are no good to the patient if you become another casualty.) Be sure the scene is safe, the vehicle is stable, and you are wearing the appropriate personal protective equipment before you try to reach the patient.

After gaining safe access to the patient, provide the same care you would provide to any trauma patient. Stabilize the cervical spine, complete the initial assessment, and provide critical interventions. Be sure you have, or have called for, sufficient personnel to help you provide proper care and to help you protect the patient from hazards.

Once you have access to the patient, establish a rapport. Remain with the patient throughout the rescue. Along with assessment, stabilization, and resuscitation efforts, you are responsible for assisting the patient through the extrication process and preparing him mentally and physically for disentanglement from the wreckage. Often, this requires two EMT-Bs—one to maintain cervical stabilization and communicate with the patient, and another to assess the patient's condition and treat potentially serious injuries.

Before a forcible rescue is initiated, its effect on the patient must be analyzed. The usual approach to rescue is to remove the vehicle from around the pa-

tient. However, when the condition of the patient or the scene dictates speed, the parts of the vehicle that will allow for rapid extrication while protecting the patient's cervical spine should be removed first.

Use heavy blankets, a tarp, or a salvage cover to protect yourself, the patient, and other EMT-Bs from the glass and flying debris that commonly result from disentanglement operations (Figure 41-6). During some extrication procedures, it may be necessary to place a solid object such as a spine board between the tool activity area and the patient.

Continually monitor the patient's condition and position in relation to the extrication tools and procedures. If there is a potential problem, relay this information to the person in charge of the extrication team. If the patient's condition begins to deteriorate or otherwise becomes unstable, advise the rescue crew. They will change the approach to the incident and get the patient out as quickly as possible.

The patient entrapped by a vehicle collision is often in a highly agitated state. He will not be emotionally capable of handling the noise and confusion often associated with extrications and rescues. Even with a diminished level of responsiveness, the patient will be very frightened and may even attempt to move or crawl out of the vehicle.

To avoid this, it is very important that you prepare the patient for the rescue operation. Make him aware of the amount of time that the disentanglement might take and why it is necessary. Explain the activities, movements, and associated noises that are or will be encountered during the extrication process. Give the patient the opportunity to have some control over the process. For example, when the rescue crew asks you if you are ready for them to do a particular function, such as remove the door, check with

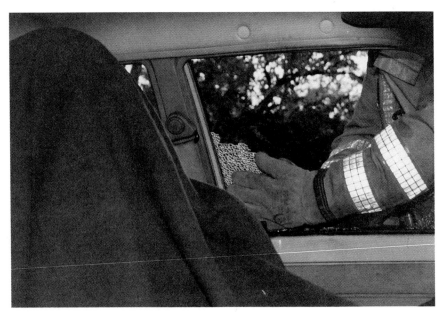

Figure 41-6   Protect the patient from broken glass, sharp metal, and other hazards at the scene.

the patient. Asking if he is ready to have the door or dash removed provides him with a feeling of control. If properly prepared, the patient will readily agree with each step of the extrication.

Stabilize and, if possible, immobilize the spine securely before you remove the patient from the vehicle by normal or rapid extrication procedures. The only exception to this rule is when there is an immediate threat to your patient's life or your own, such as fire, that requires an urgent move without spinal protection.

ENRICHMENT

The enrichment section contains information that is valuable as background for the EMT-B but that goes substantially beyond the U.S. Department of Transportation (DOT) EMT-Basic Curriculum.

STABILIZING A VEHICLE

Vehicle stabilization is carried out by specialized personnel using equipment such as wood cribbing and wedges, step chocks, airbags, hydraulic rams, come-alongs, jacks, chains, and winches (Table 41-1).

UPRIGHT VEHICLE

The first step to properly stabilize an upright vehicle is to immobilize the suspension. This is most easily accomplished by positioning step chocks under the vehicle parallel to each wheel. The chocks can be pushed in until they touch the undercarriage. Then rescuers would either slightly lift the vehicle to set the chocks or let some air out of the tires. If step chocks

are unavailable, a box crib with wedges can function in much the same manner. Either procedure will prevent the vehicle from rocking. Valve stems would be cut and tires would be sliced only when absolutely necessary to release the air.

VEHICLE ON ITS SIDE

Never attempt to enter an upturned vehicle before it is stabilized. A vehicle on its side is likely to continue to roll onto its roof, thereby aggravating a patient's existing injuries and increasing the risk of injury to rescuers both in and around the vehicle.

The first step in stabilizing this vehicle, when the equipment is available, is to attach a pulling device, cable, or chain from the undercarriage of the car to another vehicle or strong immovable object. Rescuers would then crib the length of the vehicle's side where it has contact with the ground. Every void between the ground and the vehicle should be filled with box cribbing and wedges to minimize movement. The 12-inch to 18-inch space between the top of the door frame along the roof line and the ground should also be filled.

If additional support is needed on the undercarriage of the vehicle to prevent rollover back onto its wheels, 3-foot to 6-foot pieces of 4 × 4 cribbing can be wedged from the ground to the undercarriage.

VEHICLE ON ITS ROOF

A vehicle that has landed on its roof usually is in one of two conditions. It will either be held up by its roof posts or, if one or more posts collapse, it may be resting on the hood, trunk lid, or both.

TABLE 41-1

Common Equipment Used for Vehicle Stabilization

Type	Description and Use
Airbag	A rubber bag, found in various shapes and sizes, which, when inflated with air, has great lifting ability
Come-along	A ratcheting cable device used to pull in a straight direction
Cribbing	4 × 4 or 2 × 4 blocks of hardwood cut to approximately 18-inch long sections
Hydraulic cutter	A hydraulic power tool used to cut metal
Hydraulic ram	A hydraulic power tool used to push or pull in a straight direction
Hydraulic spreader	A hydraulic power tool used to open, spread, and separate items such as vehicle doors
Jack	A manual device used much as a ram would be used
Step chock	A set of several 2 × 6 blocks of hardwood cut to varying lengths and secured together to form "steps"
Wedge	A 4 × 4 piece of cribbing tapered to an edge at one end
Winch	A powered cable reel usually electrically or hydraulically driven and mounted to a truck, which is used to pull

Since the roof posts are not designed to support the weight of the vehicle, the vehicle must be stabilized before you can get to the patient. Whether the posts have collapsed or not, the weight of the vehicle must be taken off the posts. This can be accomplished by building a box crib under the hood and trunk and using wedges to remove any remaining space.

Airbags under either the front or the rear of the vehicle can also be used to stabilize the vehicle (Figure 41-7). Low-pressure bags may be used by themselves because of their greater lift height. If high-pressure air bags are used, a box crib should be built to within a couple of inches of the surface of the vehicle. Rescuers would then slide the airbag into that space. When the airbag is inflated and one end of the vehicle begins to lift, the other end will settle onto the box crib and the weight of the vehicle will be totally removed from the roof posts.

Remember, even if the vehicle seems very stable initially, opening or removing doors during patient extrication will reduce the strength of the post. Without proper stabilization, that could lead to collapse.

EXTRICATING A PATIENT

DISENTANGLEMENT

Patient disentanglement is carried out by specialized personnel. The primary goal is to remove the vehicle from around the patient, thus ensuring that the patient's injuries are not aggravated. Key factors in meeting that goal are that all personnel are familiar with extrication procedures and the incident command system (see Chapter 43, "Multiple Casualty Incidents") and that all personnel can communicate with other members of the rescue team.

The most common tool used in vehicle extrication and patient disentanglement is the power hydraulic tool. This tool, along with various attachments, can be used to spread, push, cut, and pull. The power hydraulic rescue tool creates tremendous forces from several thousand pounds of force to well in excess of twenty thousand pounds. In order to prevent injury to rescuers and patients, it should be continually monitored for safety during use.

Methods of removing wreckage from the patient vary. Some common methods are described below.

Door Removal   Normally, the first disentanglement procedure required at a vehicle collision scene is

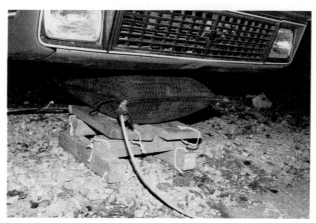

Figure 41-7   Airbags plus cribbing can be used to lift an overturned car off a patient as well as to stabilize the vehicle.

opening or removing a door. *Always* check all doors and confirm that none are able to be opened normally prior to forcing entry.

A rescuer can force a door with manual pry tools, hydraulic spreaders, and air chisels. Protect yourself and the patient from flying debris by covering yourselves with a blanket during the procedure. If possible place a solid object such as a spine board between the tool activity area and the patient. Keep the patient advised of reasons for the noise and any movement that may be encountered.

The front doors are most easily opened by prying at the latch site on the B post. (The A posts are the front posts supporting the car roof. The B posts are the middle posts, and C posts at the rear.) All glass should be broken and removed on the side of the vehicle to be opened.

Often, when using hydraulic spreaders, there is not enough of a gap to fit the tip of the tool in near the latch. The rescuer must begin by widening the gap with a thinner hand pry tool (halligan or hux bar). Another method of widening the gap is by placing the tips of the partially opened hydraulic spreader vertically in the window opening of the door and forcibly enlarging this opening, which will cause the gap near the latch to widen. If the patient position allows clear access to the inside of the door, a third method is to place the partially opened tool over the door with one arm of the tool on each side of the door 6 to 12 inches from the latch. As the arms of the spreader begin to close, pinching the door, the gap near the latch will widen.

Once an opening has been created, the hydraulic spreader will be placed in the gap directly above or below the latch and begin to spread the arms. As long as the metal does not begin to rip, the rescuer should continue to spread the arms. If the metal begins to rip, the rescuer will stop, close the tool as needed, and get another grip nearer the latch.

Once open, the door may need to be removed completely to facilitate patient removal. This can be achieved by placing the tips of the spreader near each hinge and spreading the arms until the hinge fails. When any item is completely separated from the vehicle, such as when you remove the door, the object may suddenly be propelled several feet. This movement can be controlled but not prevented. Care must be taken to secure the object so it will not strike anyone when it becomes detached.

Windshield Removal and Roof Rolling Often it is necessary to displace the roof and windshield of a vehicle to facilitate patient removal (Figures 41-8a and b). Since this procedure involves maneuvers close to the patient, it is very important that you and the patient are well protected from the tools and flying debris.

Before the rescuers displace the roof, the windshield must first be separated from the vehicle. Depending on the type of mounting found, either the mounting or the windshield is cut. Rubber mounts can often be cut with a razor knife and the windshield removed intact. If the windshield is to be cut, it is commonly done with an ax or a special glass cutting saw along the edges. You and the patient should be covered with a heavy blanket or tarp, while the windshield is being cut. Care will be taken not to penetrate the passenger compartment with the cutting tool any farther than necessary. During the cutting process, one of the rescuers must monitor and control the cutting process from a vantage point on the inside of the vehicle.

REMOVING A VEHICLE ROOF

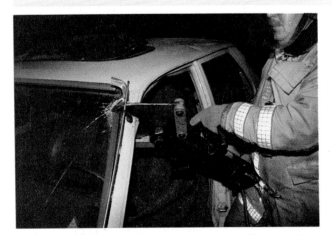

Figure 41-8a *Removal of the roof begins by cutting through the "A" post and then through the "B" post.*

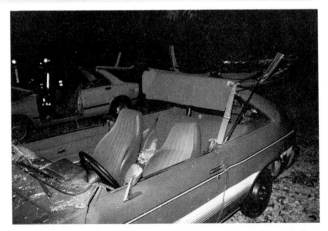

Figure 41-8b *When cutting is complete, fold the roof back like a convertible for greatest access to the patient.*

Next, the A posts and B posts must be cut. Normally either a hack saw, air cutting tool, or hydraulic cutting tool is used. Care must be taken to cut the A posts as close to the dash and the B posts as close to the door as possible. This will increase patient accessibility and minimize potential injury from the remaining post stubs. The roof is then creased just in front of the C posts using a long pry bar, pike pole, or other similar item. The roof can be grasped near the A post on each side and folded up and back toward the trunk.

After the roof is displaced, the stubs of the posts must be covered with duct tape or pieces of old 2½-inch fire hose to protect the patient and rescuers from any exposed sharp metal.

Rolling the Dash Commonly in high speed frontal impact collisions, the front of the vehicle will be pushed in and the passenger compartment area reduced. As a result, the patient can be pinned between the dash, steering wheel, and seat. In this case, a "dash roll" may provide the safest and easiest disentanglement (Figure 41-9).

Although it is not a necessity, it is easier to roll the dash if the doors and roof have already been removed. Rescuers will begin the dash roll by making deep cuts in the base of the A post, just above the rocker panel, with a hydraulic cutter. If the windshield and roof are still intact, rescuers will make a cut at the top of the A post. The hydraulic ram should be placed from the base of the B post to midway on the A post near the dash. As the ram is expanded, the dash will rise and roll forward allowing greater patient access.

Be sure to carefully examine the patient's position before and during this procedure to make certain that no body parts are pinned in the section being moved.

SPECIAL DISENTANGLEMENT PROCEDURES

No two vehicle extrications are exactly alike. Some can be quite complex. Very often, improvisation and common sense must prevail.

One complication occurs when a patient's foot is caught under the brake pedal. In this situation, a pulling device or portable hydraulic tool can be used to force the pedal upward and free the extremity. This procedure involves using tools in very close proximity to the patient, who may have an injury to the trapped part which is causing considerable pain. Therefore, disentanglement must be accomplished with utmost care so as not to disturb the injury. Often

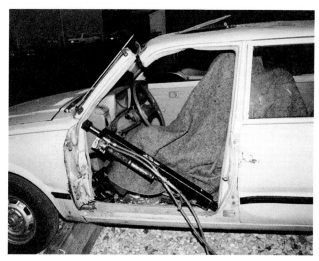

Figure 41-9 The hydraulic rescue tool can be used to roll the dash away from the patient.

the rescuer can simply grab the brake pedal with a hand and pull firmly upward away from the floor, lifting it enough to free the foot.

A patient also may be trapped in a way that requires the seat to be moved or removed, such as a patient in the back seat of a two-door vehicle or a patient with a leg trapped under the seat. Disentanglement may be accomplished by using the seat adjustment lever to gently move the seat. If greater movement is needed, it can be done slowly by using hand tools to remove the nuts securing the seat or quickly by forcing the seat using portable rams or spreaders or a come-along. If the seat is forced, the patient will receive a considerable jolt. If injuries dictate that such movement may be harmful, other options must be considered.

Extricating a patient who is trapped in a vehicle on its side involves some different techniques. Access to the patient is best gained by removing the rear window. Since the passenger compartment is very small to work in, the best way to extricate the patient is to cut the roof of the vehicle on three sides and fold it down. This requires cutting the sheet metal and roof support braces near the patient, usually with a pneumatic chisel. This tool is very loud. Prepare the patient for the noise. It is not only disturbing, but it also makes communication between the interior and exterior of the vehicle difficult.

Once the patient has been disentangled, you will remove him from the wreckage using normal or rapid extrication procedures as discussed in Chapter 34, "Injuries to the Spine."

CASE STUDY FOLLOW-UP

SCENE SIZE-UP

You have been dispatched to a motor vehicle collision between a large dump truck and a small passenger vehicle. You see from your unit that this is a complex rescue situation. You have multiple patients with potentially life-threatening injuries. They are entrapped in the wreckage of what was, minutes before, a bright red sports car.

There are no other emergency personnel immediately responding, so you call for rescue crews and an additional ambulance for each additional patient. Before exiting the unit, you size up the scene, identifying real and potential hazards. You make a mental note of all necessary precautions—including personal protective clothing and equipment—to protect yourself, bystanders, and the patients from further injury.

You position your vehicle 100 feet from the wreckage—the minimum safe distance since there are no electrical lines down or other visible hazards—to provide easy access to your equipment while being out of the way of rescue operations. You review what you and your partner need to do:

- If the patient access is prevented or hampered, attempt to assess the patients' condition based upon the findings of whatever portion of the initial assessment you can perform.
- If you can, establish and maintain an airway, stabilize the cervical spine, and control any serious bleeding from outside the vehicle.
- Provide direction to other responding units as to what the situation is and what you need from them.

Once the rescue crews arrive and the scene is secure, the incident commander and rescue crews assess the situation and direct you in your assignment. This incident will require many very complex rescue operations, so a team approach using an Incident Command System with one commander is vital for success.

You work hard to make sure your attention isn't given only to the patients in the sports car. The driver of the truck may also be injured and many potential hazards must not be overlooked.

DEBRIEFING

It is several days later and you and your partner are at the station, among a group of rescuers who were at the scene. It was a difficult experience for everyone. You were there when the teenager in the passenger side of the sports car died, well before extrication was completed and in spite of all your attempts to keep him alive. You know that the driver of the car, also a teenager, died in the ambulance after prolonged extrication and emergency medical procedures. Neither of the teenagers was wearing a seat belt. Both of them had been drinking. You are grateful to learn that the truck driver will recover.

A health care professional leads the group. He explains that you're all there to talk. You think, "maybe it'll help" and volunteer to start the debriefing session.

The same question is on the mind of everyone in the room. Is there anything we could have done better or faster? Is there any way we could have saved those kids' lives? By the time the session comes to an end, you feel reasonably reassured that you did everything you could. And you and the rescue crew have worked out some refinements in procedure that might make the next rescue just a little faster . . . a little safer . . . a little more effective.

CHAPTER REVIEW

TERMS AND CONCEPTS

You may wish to review the following terms and concepts included in this chapter.

complex access—a way to gain access to a patient that requires the use of tools and specialized equipment.

simple access—a way to gain access to a patient that does not require specialized tools.

REVIEW QUESTIONS

1. Name your first priority in this and any other type of emergency situation.
2. Describe the role of the EMT-B in vehicle stabilization and patient extrication.
3. Identify the first step you should take upon arriving at the site of a motor vehicle collision.
4. Explain how you can locate all the patients involved in an emergency such as a motor vehicle collision.
5. Explain why it is important to approach a motor vehicle collision from the front.
6. Identify which process comes first—patient care or patient extrication—and describe the exceptions.
7. Describe how you can protect the patient from further physical injury during extrication.
8. Describe the minimum level of personal protective equipment required at a motor vehicle collision site.
9. Describe the steps that may be taken after you identify downed electrical lines at the scene.
10. Describe a "stable" vehicle. Then name some simple steps that you can take to stabilize a vehicle in danger of rolling until rescue crews can properly and completely stabilize it.

CHAPTER 42

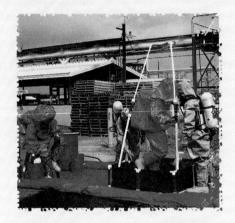

Hazardous Materials Emergencies

INTRODUCTION

More than 50 billion tons of hazardous materials are manufactured in the United States annually. More than 4 billion tons are shipped within this country every year, most commonly including explosives, compressed and poisonous gases, flammable liquids and solids, oxidizers (substances that give off oxygen and stimulate combustion of organic matter), corrosives, and radioactive materials. Hazardous materials spills and other accidents are common problems, the exact extent of which is unknown.

The EMT-Basic is not required to deal with hazardous materials. That takes specialized training. It is more important for you to recognize that a hazardous materials emergency exists.

OBJECTIVES

Numbered objectives are from the United States Department of Transportation 1994 EMT-Basic National Standard Curriculum. Asterisked objectives, if any, pertain to material that is supplemental to the DOT curriculum.

COGNITIVE

7-3.1 Explain the EMT-Basic's role during a call involving hazardous materials. (p. 855)

7-3.2 Describe what the EMT-Basic should do if there is reason to believe that there is a hazard at the scene. (p. 855)

7-3.3 Describe the actions that an EMT-Basic should take to ensure bystander safety. (p. 855)

7-3.4 State the role the EMT-Basic should perform until appropriately trained personnel arrive at the scene of a hazardous materials situation. (p. 855)

7-3.5 Break down the steps to approaching a hazardous situation. (pp. 855–860)

7-3.6 Discuss the various environmental hazards that affect EMS. (pp. 847–850)

7-3.11 Describe basic concepts of incident management. (pp. 855–859)

7-3.12 Explain the methods for preventing contamination of self, equipment, and facilities. (pp. 859–860)

Additional objectives from DOT Lesson 7-3 are addressed in Chapter 43, "Multiple-Casualty Incidents."

CASE STUDY

THE DISPATCH

EMS Unit 101—proceed to the intersection of Route 46 West and Baldwin Road—you have a collision involving a truck and passenger vehicle. No patient information is available. Time out is 1452 hours.

ON ARRIVAL

As soon as you near the collision site, you spot police rerouting traffic. They have cordoned off the scene. Up ahead on the west side of 46 you can just see a passenger vehicle in front of a large tanker truck on the shoulder of the highway.

How would you proceed?

During this chapter, you will learn special considerations related to hazardous materials emergencies. Later, we will return to the case and apply the procedures learned.

IDENTIFYING HAZARDOUS MATERIALS

WHAT IS A HAZARDOUS MATERIAL?

A **hazardous material** is defined as one that in any quantity poses a threat or unreasonable risk to life, health, or property if not properly controlled during manufacture, processing, packaging, handling, storage, transportation, use, and disposal (Table 42-1). Hazardous materials include chemicals, wastes, and other dangerous products. The principal dangers hazardous materials present are toxicity, flammability, and reactivity.

Hazardous materials can asphyxiate, irritate, increase the risk of cancer, act as nerve or liver poisons, or cause loss of coordination or altered mental status. They can cause skin irritation, burns, respiratory distress, nausea and vomiting, tingling or numbness of the extremities, and blurred or double vision. Whether internal or external, the amount of damage depends on the dose, concentration, and amount of time the patient is exposed.

Accidental exposure to hazardous materials can be limited to a few victims, but an accident also can

TABLE 42-1

Hazardous Materials

Classification	Examples	Route of Exposure	Signs & Symptoms	BLS Treatment
1. Explosive	TNT Ammunition Fireworks Black powder	Skin and eyes Inhalation Ingestion Absorption	CARDIOVASCULAR Circulatory collapse and dysrhythmia RESPIRATORY Tachypnea and dyspnea GASTROINTESTINAL Nausea, vomiting, and diarrhea CNS Headache, dizziness, stupor, and coma EYES Chemical conjunctivitis SKIN Dermatitis and skin eruptions	Airway: Consider intubation Oxygen at 15 lpm by nonrebreather mask Monitor for shock Flush skin Flush eyes 8 oz. of water if ingested
2. Poison & Flammable Gas	Chlorine Ammonia Nitrogen Carbon dioxide Acetylene Propane Butane Hydrogen	Skin and eyes Inhalation	CARDIOVASCULAR Circulatory collapse and dysrhythmia RESPIRATORY Tachypnea and dyspnea, respiratory failure, pulmonary edema GASTROINTESTINAL Nausea, vomiting, and diarrhea, irritated mucous membranes CNS Headache, dizziness, seizures, stupor, and coma EYES Chemical conjunctivitis SKIN Dermatitis and skin eruptions	Airway: Consider intubation Oxygen at 15 lpm by nonrebreather mask Monitor for shock Flush skin Flush eyes Treat pulmonary edema Anticipate seizures Treat burns and frostbite
3. Flammable & Combustible	Gasoline Acetone Diesel Brake fluid Oil	Skin and eyes Inhalation Ingestion Absorption	CARDIOVASCULAR Dysrhythmia and tachycardia RESPIRATORY Tachypnea and dyspnea, upper respiratory, and rapid pulmonary edema GASTROINTESTINAL Nausea, vomiting, and diarrhea, irritated mucous membranes CNS Headache, dizziness, seizures, stupor, and coma	Airway: Consider intubation Oxygen at 15 lpm by nonrebreather mask Monitor for shock Flush skin Flush eyes Treat pulmonary edema Anticipate seizures

TABLE 42-1 (CONTINUED)

Hazardous Materials

Classification	Examples	Route of Exposure	Signs & Symptoms	BLS Treatment
			EYES Chemical conjunctivitis and cyanosis **SKIN** Dermatitis, irritation, and cyanosis	8 oz. of water if ingested Treat burns Avoid vomit contact
4. Dangerous Flammable Solid, Spontaneously Combustible	Phosphorus Magnesium Titanium Lithium Calcium resinate	Skin and eyes Inhalation Ingestion Absorption	**CARDIOVASCULAR** Dysrhythmia or shock **RESPIRATORY** Tachypnea and dyspnea, upper respiratory, and rapid pulmonary edema **GASTROINTESTINAL** Nausea, vomiting, abdominal pain, garlic odor **CNS** Headache, dizziness, fatigue, and seizures **EYES** Conjunctivitis and injury **SKIN** Chemical burns and jaundice	Airway: Consider intubation Oxygen at 15 lpm by nonrebreather mask Monitor for shock Flush skin Flush eyes Treat pulmonary edema Anticipate seizures 8 oz. of water if ingested Treat burns Avoid vomit contact
5. Oxidizer & Organic Peroxide	Lithium Peroxide Calcium Chlorite Pool chlorine	Skin and eyes Inhalation Ingestion	**CARDIOVASCULAR** Hypovolemic shock, rapid weak pulse **RESPIRATORY** Acute pulmonary edema, asphyxia, chemical pneumonia, and upper airway obstruction **GASTROINTESTINAL** Acute toxicity, nausea, vomiting, and diarrhea **CNS** Hypoxia, stupor, lethargy, and coma **EYES** Conjunctivitis and blindness **SKIN** Chemical burns, full and partial thickness	Airway: Consider intubation Oxygen at 15 lpm by nonrebreather mask Monitor for shock Flush skin Flush eyes Treat pulmonary edema Anticipate seizures 8 oz. of water if ingested Treat burns Avoid vomit contact
6. Irritant & Poison	Cyanide Arsenic Phosgene Insecticides Pesticides	Skin and eyes Inhalation Ingestion Absorption	**CARDIOVASCULAR** Cardiovascular collapse and dysrhythmia **RESPIRATORY** Acute pulmonary edema, asphyxia, chemical pneumonia, and upper airway obstruction	Airway: Consider intubation Oxygen at 15 lpm by nonrebreather mask Monitor for shock

TABLE 42-1 (CONTINUED)

Hazardous Materials

Classification	Examples	Route of Exposure	Signs & Symptoms	BLS Treatment
			GASTROINTESTINAL Nausea, vomiting, diarrhea, and abdominal pain CNS Coma, depression, and seizures EYES Conjunctivitis and burns SKIN Chemical burns, flushing	Flush skin Flush eyes Treat pulmonary edema Anticipate seizures 8 oz. of water if ingested Treat burns Avoid vomit contact
7. Radioactive	Plutonium Cobalt Uranium 235	Skin and eyes Inhalation Ingestion Absorption	CARDIOVASCULAR Tachycardia RESPIRATORY Dyspnea and cough with irritation and edema to the nose, mouth, and throat GASTROINTESTINAL Nausea, vomiting, and diarrhea CNS Altered mental status, coma, headache, lethargy, tremors, and seizures EYES Conjunctivitis, lacrimation SKIN Chemical burns, irritation	Airway: Consider intubation Oxygen at 15 lpm by nonrebreather mask Monitor for shock Flush skin Flush eyes Treat pulmonary edema Anticipate seizures 8 oz. of water if ingested Avoid vomit contact
8. Corrosive	Hydrochloric acid Sulfuric acid Caustic	Skin and eyes Inhalation Ingestion Absorption	CARDIOVASCULAR Tachycardia and shock RESPIRATORY Dyspnea and cough, burns, and edema to the nose, mouth, and throat GASTROINTESTINAL Nausea, vomiting, and diarrhea, abdominal pain, mouth burns, stomach, and esophagus CNS Altered mental status, coma, headache, lethargy, tremors, and seizures EYES Conjunctivitis and lacrimation SKIN Dermatitis and skin eruptions	Airway: Consider intubation Oxygen at 15 lpm by nonrebreather mask Monitor for shock Flush skin Flush eyes Treat pulmonary edema Anticipate seizures 8 oz. of water if ingested Treat burns Avoid vomit contact Do not induce vomiting

cause widespread destruction and loss of life. Therefore, the primary concern in any hazardous materials emergency is one of safety for the rescuer, the patient, and the public.

PLACARDS AND SHIPPING PAPERS

U.S. Department of Transportation regulations require packages, storage containers, and vehicles containing hazardous materials to be marked with specific hazard labels (Figures 42-1 and 42-2). A vehicle driver also must have shipping papers, which identify the exact substance, quantity, origin, and destination.

A placard is usually a four-sided, diamond-shaped sign. Many are red or orange. A few are white or green. Whatever the color, the placard contains a four-digit identification number and a legend that indicates whether the material is flammable, radioactive, explosive, or poisonous.

The National Fire Protection Association (NFPA) has adopted an internationally recognized diamond-shaped symbol, which is divided into four smaller diamonds (Figure 42-3a). This system—the NFPA 704 system—identifies potential danger with the use of background colors and numbers ranging from 0 to 4. The blue diamond is a gauge of health hazard; the red, fire hazard; and the yellow, reactivity hazard. The white diamond is used for symbols that indicate additional information, such as radioactivity, oxidation, need for protective equipment, and so on. For example, a symbol that has a 1 in the blue diamond and a 4 in the red diamond would present a relatively low health hazard but is extremely flammable. For another example of NFPA 704 labeling, see Figure 42–3b.

Shipping papers are another important means of identifying hazardous materials They will have the name of the substance, the classification (such as flammable or explosive), and a four-digit identification number. With very few exceptions, shipping papers are required to be in the cab of a motor vehicle, in the possession of a train crew member in the engine or caboose, in a holder on the bridge of a vessel, or in the aircraft pilot's possession. Material-safety-data sheets may be found with shipping papers. (Figure 42-4.)

USING YOUR SENSES

Another (but the least reliable) way to determine the presence of hazardous materials at the scene of an accident is to use your senses. Quickly scan the scene looking for signs of potential hazardous materials such as signs restricting entry, storage tanks, or containers with placards (Figures 42-5a and b). A number of visual clues can indicate the probable presence of a hazardous material:

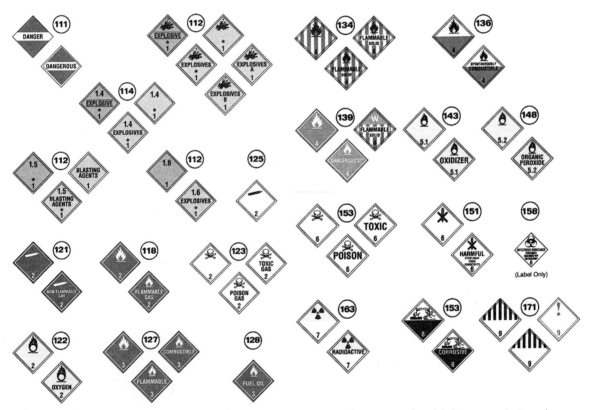

Figure 42-1 DOT requires packages, storage containers, and vehicles containing hazardous materials to be marked with specific hazard labels.

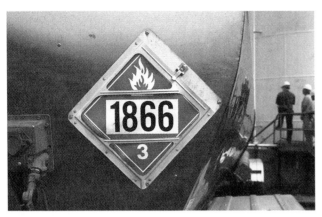

Figure 42-2 Any tank, vehicle, train, or ship that carries hazardous materials must have a placard that identifies the substance.

- Smoking or self-igniting materials
- Extraordinary fire conditions
- Boiling or spattering of materials that have not been heated
- Wavy or unusually colored vapors over a container of liquid material
- Characteristically colored vapor clouds
- Frost near a container leak (indicative of liquid coolants)

- Unusual condition of containers (peeling or discoloration of finishes, unexpected deterioration, deformity, or the unexpected operation of pressure-relief valves)

Remember: you may not be able to see or smell the hazardous material. Some are odorless and colorless, while others have anesthetic properties and will deaden your senses. Never rely on your senses alone—sight, smell, taste, or touch—to detect a hazardous material. Always assume that the area surrounding a spill or leak is dangerous.

RESOURCES

Several resources can assist you in proper identification of hazardous materials emergencies. They include printed materials, the Chemical Manufacturer's Association, and state and local agencies including specialized "hazmat" teams. Poison control centers also provide resources.

One concise print reference is a guidebook published by the U.S. Department of Transportation, Transport Canada, and the Secretariat of Communications and Transportation of Mexico called the *North American Emergency Response Guide* (RSPA P5800). Compact enough to be carried with your usual equipment and supplies, the book lists more than a thousand hazardous materials, each with an identification number cross referenced to complete

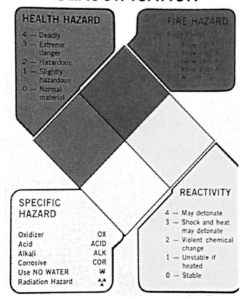

Figure 42-3a NFPA 704 hazardous materials classification.

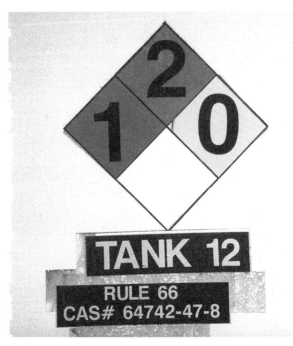

Figure 42-3b NFPA 704 labeling on a tank.

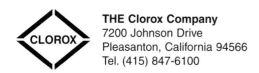

THE Clorox Company
7200 Johnson Drive
Pleasanton, California 94566
Tel. (415) 847-6100

Material Safety Data Sheets

Health	2+
Flammability	0
Reactivity	1
Personal Protection	B

I – CHEMICAL IDENTIFICATION

| Name | regular Clorox Bleach | | CAS No. | N/A |
| Description | clear, light yellow liquid with chlorine odor | | RTECs No. | N/A |

Other Designations	**Manufacturer**	**Emergency Procedure**
EPA Reg. No. 5813-1 Sodium hypochlorite solution Liquid chlorine bleach Clorox Liquid Bleach	The Clorox Company 1221 Broadway Oakland, CA 94612	• Notify your supervisor • Call your local poison control center OR • Rocky Mountain Poison Center (303)573-1014

II – HEALTH HAZARD DATA

• Causes severe but temporary eye injury. May irritate skin. May cause nausea and vomiting if ingested. Exposure to vapor or mist may irritate nose, throat and lungs. The following medical conditions may be aggravated by exposure to high concentrations of vapor or mist: heart conditions or chronic respiratory problems such as asthma, chronic bronchitis or obstructive lung disease. Under normal consumer use conditions the likelihood of any adverse health effects are low. FIRST AID: EYE CONTACT: Immediately flush eyes with plenty of water. If irritation persists, see a doctor. SKIN CONTACT: Remove contaminated clothing. Wash area with water. INGESTION: Drink a glassful of water and call a physician. INHALATION: If breathing problems develop remove to fresh air.

III – HAZARDOUS INGREDIENTS

Ingredients	Concentration	Worker Exposure Limit
Sodium hypochlorite CAS# 7681-52-9	5.25%	not established

None of the ingredients in this product are on the IARC, NTP or OSHA carcinogen list. Occasional clinical reports suggest a low potential for sensitization upon exaggerated exposure to sodium hypochlorite if skin damage (e.g., irritation) occurs during exposure. Routine clinical tests conducted on intact skin with Clorox Liquid Bleach found no sensitization in the test subjects.

IV – SPECIAL PROTECTION INFORMATION

Hygienic Practices: Wear safety glasses. With repeated or prolonged use, wear gloves.

Engineering Controls: Use general ventilation to minimize exposure to vapor or mist.

Work Practices: Avoid eye and skin contact and inhalation of vapor or mist.

V – SPECIAL PRECAUTIONS

Keep out of reach of children. Do not get in eyes or on skin. Wash thoroughly with soap and water after handling. Do not mix with other household chemicals such as toilet bowl cleaners, rust removers, vinegar, acid or ammonia containing products. Store in a cool, dry place. Do not reuse empty container; rinse container and put in trash container.

VI – SPILL OR LEAK PROCEDURES

Small quantities of less than 5 gallons may be flushed down drain. For larger quantities wipe up with an absorbent material or mop and dispose of in accordance with local, state and federal regulations. Dilute with water to minimize oxidizing effect on spilled surface.

VII – REACTIVITY DATA

Stable under normal use and storage conditions. Strong oxidizing agent. Reacts with other household chemicals such as toilet bowl cleaners, rust removers, vinegar, acids or ammonia containing products to produce hazardous gases, such as chlorine and other chlorinated species. Prolonged contact with metal may cause pitting or discoloration.

VIII – FIRE AND EXPLOSION DATA

Not flammable or explosive. In a fire, cool containers to prevent rupture and release of sodium chlorate.

IX – PHYSICAL DATA

Boiling point...................................212°F/100°C (decomposes)
Specific Gravity (H$_2$O = 1).............1.085
Solubility in Water..........................complete
pH..11.4

Figure 42-4   A material-safety-data sheet provides information about the substance being transported and may be found with the shipping papers.

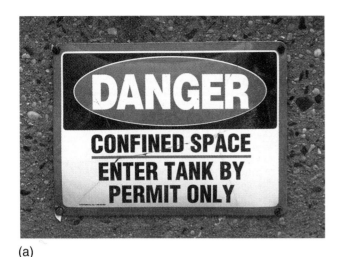

(a)

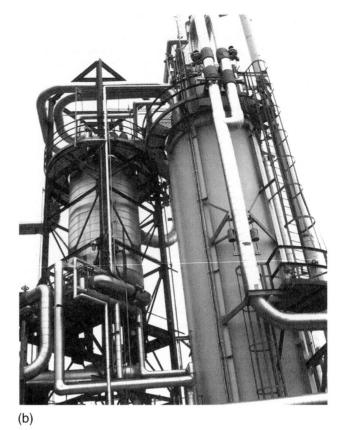

(b)

Figure 42-5   Look for clues to potential hazardous materials, such as (a) signs and (b) storage tanks.

emergency instructions. Other print materials are also available.

CHEMTREC (Chemical Transportation Emergency Center) is a public service division of the Chemical Manufacturer's Association and another important resource. Officials at CHEMTREC can answer any question and advise you on how to handle any emergency involving hazardous materials. They will even locate the shipper of the hazardous materials for appropriate follow-up. You can reach CHEMTREC around the clock, seven days a week, by dialing their toll-free number: 1-800-424-9300.

Chemtrel, Inc. is another emergency response communications service that can be reached at 1-800-255-3924 in the United States and Canada. For calls outside the U.S. or Canada or for collect calls, the number is 813-979-0626. Also, your regional poison control center will be a source of information for hazardous materials incidents.

When contacting an organization, be prepared to provide the following information:

- Your name, call-back number, fax number
- Nature and location of product
- Identification number or name of product
- Name of carrier, shipper, manufacturer, consignee, and point of origin
- Type of container and size (rail, truck, housed open)
- Quantity of material

- Local conditions
- Number of injuries and/or exposures
- Emergency services that are present or are responding

Accidents involving hazardous materials often occur at inconvenient locations, making communication difficult. It is critical that you make every effort to keep a phone line open.

TRAINING REQUIRED BY LAW

Due to the increasing frequency of hazardous materials emergencies, two federal agencies—The Occupational Safety and Health Administration (OSHA) and the Environmental Protection Agency (EPA)—have developed regulations that are meant to enhance the safety of rescuers and bring about a more effective response. The regulations can be found in the OSHA publication "29 CFR 1910.120—Hazardous Waste Operations and Emergency Response Standards (1989)."

The regulations identify four levels of training:

- *First Responder Awareness.* This level is for those who are likely to witness or discover a hazardous materials emergency. They are trained to recognize a problem but are not expected to take any action other than call for proper resources.
- *First Responder Operations.* This level of training is for those who initially respond to hazardous materi-

als emergencies in order to protect people, property, and the environment. They keep at a safe distance and help to stop the emergency from spreading.

- *Hazardous Materials Technician.* This level is for rescuers who actually plug, patch, or stop the release of a hazardous material.
- *Hazardous Materials Specialist.* Rescuers with this training have advanced knowledge and skills. They provide command and support activities at the site of a hazardous materials emergency.

Employers are responsible for determining and documenting the appropriate level of training for each employee. Because training addressed by OSHA usually has a fire-service focus, the National Fire Protection Association has published Standard #473, which also deals with competencies for EMS personnel at hazardous materials emergencies. Refer to the OSHA and NFPA standards for more information on training requirements.

GUIDELINES FOR HAZARDOUS MATERIALS RESCUES

Note: Never attempt a hazardous materials rescue unless you have had the necessary specialized training (to the hazardous materials technician level or better) and have had the proper training in the use of self-contained breathing apparatus (SCBA). If you have had no training, radio immediately for help. While you are waiting for help to arrive, protect yourself and bystanders by keeping uphill, upwind, and away from the danger.

GENERAL RULES

One rule of a hazardous materials rescue is to avoid contact with any unidentified material, regardless of the level of protection offered by your clothing and equipment. In achieving that goal, there are three general priorities in an order that never changes:

1. Protect the safety of all rescuers and victims.
2. Provide patient care.
3. Decontaminate clothing, equipment, and the vehicle.

Another rule of hazardous materials rescue is to *avoid risking your life or your health if the only threat is to the environment.* In other words, if victims are not involved, do not enter the scene. Let specially trained environmental workers clean up the hazard.

Simply cordon off the area and evacuate bystanders. Even if there are victims involved, this is one situation in which you should not automatically begin rescue work. Generally accepted guidelines call

for you to weigh the emergency according to your best judgment, determining whether or not the risk to rescuers is justified by the lives that can be saved. Consider the difficulty of the rescue, the flammability of materials, the possibility of explosion, any time or distance constraints, available escape routes, and the probability of victim survival if they receive medical care. If you decide to begin rescue operations, act quickly—time is critical. But do not work so quickly that you endanger yourself or others or make patient injuries worse.

As a first course of action, secure the scene and limit the exposure of rescuers and bystanders. Then make sure there is enough additional equipment, trained personnel, and whatever else you might need to handle the emergency effectively. Finally, make sure that every rescuer who enters the scene has adequate protective equipment: a positive-pressure self-contained breathing apparatus (SCBA) and a full suit of protective clothing, including a coat and pants, at least two layers of gloves, boots, helmet, eye protection (preferably full-face protection), and lifelines (Figures 42-6a through e). Use wide duct tape to seal off the protective suits at the wrists, ankles, neck, and other gaps or openings. Keep in mind that you will need specialized suits if you are working in high temperatures or areas where you could be splashed with corrosive chemicals.

INCIDENT MANAGEMENT

PRE-INCIDENT PLANNING

The most essential part of hazardous materials rescue is effective pre-incident planning. Before a hazardous materials emergency ever develops, all agencies that would probably be involved in a rescue need to know how various forces will be mobilized to handle the emergency.

Generally, you should prepare for the worst possible scenario. That way, the community will be capable of handling any emergency that arises. Your plan should be specifically tailored to the individual circumstances in the community. However, the following should be included:

- One command officer, who is responsible for all rescue decisions, should be appointed. All rescuers should be aware of who the command officer is. Should the command officer hand over the decision-making power to someone else, all rescuers should be notified of the change in command.
- There should be a clear chain of command from each rescuer to the command officer.
- There should be an established system of communications used throughout the emergency. The system should be one all rescuers are informed about, know how to use, and have access to.

HAZARDOUS MATERIALS PROTECTIVE EQUIPMENT

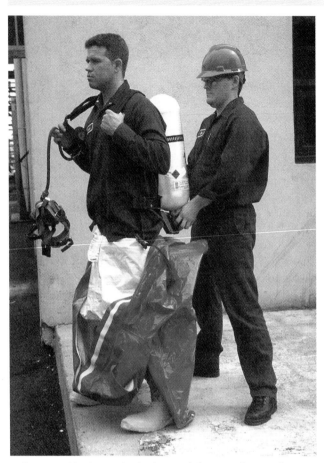

Figure 42-6a   Assisting with an air tank.

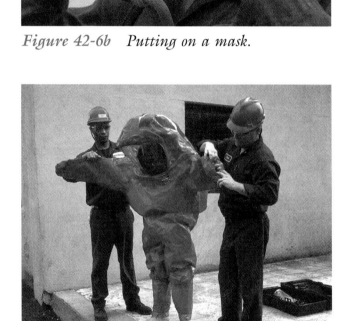

Figure 42-6b   Putting on a mask.

Figure 42-6c   Assisting with a hood.

• Receiving facilities should be predesignated. Choose facilities that are capable of handling large numbers of patients, have surgical capacity and, if possible, have established decontamination procedures.

IMPLEMENTING THE PLAN

The first priority in implementing a plan is to immediately establish a command post from which orders are given and to which information is directed. Then—to help identify the best plan of action under the circumstances—as quickly as possible get the following information:

• Nature of the problem
• Identification of the hazardous materials
• The kind and condition of containers
• Existing weather conditions
• Whether or not there is presence of fire
• Time that has elapsed since the emergency occurred
• What already has been done by people at the scene
• The number of victims
• The danger of victimizing more people

Smoke from hazardous materials fires presents an environmental hazard. It carries toxins and particles of hazardous materials through the air, widening the area of contamination. This "second-hand smoke"

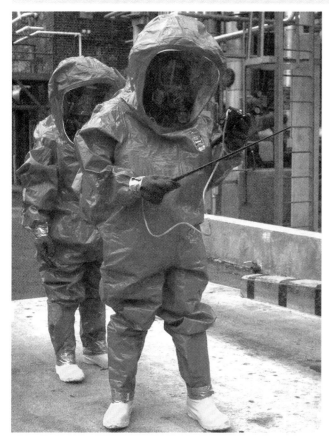

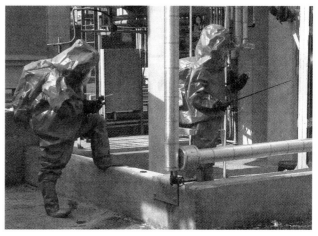

Figure 42-6e   Using sensors to detect hazardous materials.

Figure 42-6d   Hazmat team, fully suited.

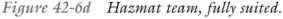

not only threatens the immediate safety of victims and rescuers, it also threatens long-term health, in some cases causing cancer and chronic effects involving the brain, liver, lungs, and kidneys.

Unless you are a trained firefighter, do not attempt to extinguish the fires yourself. Hazardous materials fires often require special techniques. (For example, many cannot be extinguished with water; in fact, water would make them worse.)

ESTABLISHING SAFETY ZONES

As an early priority at the scene of any hazardous materials emergency, **safety zones** are established in which rescue operations and a specific sequence of decontamination procedures (Figure 42-7) take place. Some EMS areas use the circular model for depicting safety zones (Figure 42-8). Remember: you may not be able to see or smell the hazardous material. Always assume that the area surrounding a spill or leak is dangerous and always wear protective gear.

Hot Zone   The **hot zone** (or contamination zone) is where contamination is actually present. It generally is the area that is immediately adjacent to the accident site and where contamination can still occur.

To help limit the spread of contamination, one point at which all rescue personnel enter and exit the hot zone is established. An emergency exit is designated to be used in case the scene deteriorates rapidly (in case of an explosion, for example). Never smoke, eat, or drink in the hot zone, because you would risk inhaling or ingesting the hazardous material.

The hot zone should be restricted. *Only as many trained rescuers as absolutely necessary should enter it.* In areas with a specialized "hazmat" team, only members of that team should enter the hot zone. *Bystanders should never be allowed in the hot zone.* If necessary, cordon off the whole area and appoint people to keep bystanders away.

The only work done in the hot zone is actual rescue, initial decontamination, and treatment for life-threatening conditions by trained personnel who are wearing appropriate protective equipment.

Warm Zone   The **warm zone** (or control zone) is immediately adjacent to the hot zone. While the hazardous materials may not actually be in the warm zone, there is still danger of contamination from the victims and rescue personnel who have exited the hot zone. For that reason, *all personnel in the warm zone must wear appropriate protective gear.*

NINE-STEP DECON PROCEDURE*

ENTER HERE

CLEAN SIDE — **DIRECTION OF TRAVEL** →

CONTAMINATED SIDE

Step	Instructions	#	Title
1	Lay out plastic to contain the contamination. It should be about 12–15 feet wide. Length can vary depending on space available. Personnel enter decon area and drop tools and monitors on the plastic. Move to Step 2.	1	TOOL DROP AREA
2	Position decon pools. Use one to wash gross contaminates off with brushes, soap, and water. Place a portable shower in the second pool to rinse off as much contamination as possible. Dilution is conducted inside the pool and diked area. All rescuers are still wearing suits and SCBA. Move to Step 3.	2	DECON WASH POOL DECON RINSE POOL WITH SHOWER
3	Open the chemical suit and remove the SCBA. Place them on the contaminated side. If the rescuer is returning to the incident, replace the SCBA cylinder, question the rescuer to establish that health conditions are OK, and close the suit. The rescuer should re-enter using the contaminated side. Move to Step 4.	3	SCBA REMOVAL OR REPLACEMENT
4	Remove protective clothing and place on the contaminated side. Move to Step 5 or transport personnel to a fixed decon facility during inclement weather.	4	PROTECTIVE CLOTHING REMOVAL
5	Remove all personal clothing and isolate items on the contaminated side. Bag all personal items. Move to Step 6.	5	PERSONAL CLOTHING REMOVAL
6	Shower and care for personal hygiene using soap and sponges. Dry off and bag cleaning items for disposal, including clothing, sponges, towels, etc. Move to Step 7.	6	PERSONAL HYGIENE & SHOWER
7	Personnel put on clean clothes or paper garments. Move to Step 8.	7	APPLY CLEAN CLOTHES
8	Personnel receive EMS medical evaluation and treatment as necessary. Move to Step 9.	8	EMS MEDICAL EVALUATION
9	Identify personnel and complete exposure records. Transport personnel to hospital, if needed, or to a fixed decon facility for Steps 5 through 9.	9	DOCUMENTATION & EXPOSURE REPORT WRITING

During inclement weather, Steps 5–9 may be moved to a fixed decon facility.

*Written by Kenneth Bouvier, NREMT-I, Hazardous Materials Specialist, New Orleans, Louisiana.

Figure 42-7 Nine-step decontamination procedure.

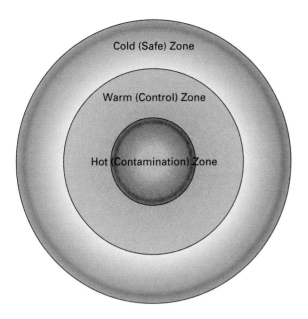

Hot (Contamination) Zone

Contamination is actually present.
Personnel must wear appropriate protective gear.
Number of rescuers limited to those absolutely necessary.
Bystanders never allowed.

Warm (Control) Zone

Area surrounding the contamination zone.
Vital to preventing spread of contamination.
Personnel must wear appropriate protective gear.
Life-saving emergency care is performed.

Cold (Safe) Zone

Normal triage, stabilization, and treatment are performed.
Rescuers must shed contaminated gear before entering
the cold zone.

Figure 42-8   Establishing safety control zones at the site of a hazardous materials emergency.

The warm zone is vital in preventing the spread of contamination. All supplies used in the warm zone must remain there until fully decontaminated. All water used in this area must also be contained here. Rescue work done in the warm zone consists of life-saving emergency care, such as airway management and immobilization.

Cold Zone   The **cold zone** (or safe zone) is immediately adjacent to the warm zone. Before entering the cold zone from the warm zone, rescuers should shed all contaminated protective gear and patients should be as fully decontaminated as possible. Because contamination can still enter the cold zone, you should continue to exercise caution and take measures to protect your equipment and vehicle.

By the time patients enter the cold zone, life-threatening problems should have been initially man-

aged. Continue emergency care. Triage patients to determine the order of care, perform necessary treatment, and stabilize patients prior to transport (see Chapter 43, "Multiple-Casualty Incidents").

EMERGENCY PROCEDURES

Anyone entering the zoned areas must be wearing the proper protective equipment. The type of protective equipment needed is dictated by the type of hazardous material being dealt with and the rescue scene itself.

Initial (gross) decontamination will be performed in the hot zone. The patient will be removed from the actual accident site while any necessary management of immediate life threats is performed. Initial decontamination usually involves the use of soap and copious amounts of water. The patient's clothing, tools, and equipment will be left in the hot zone.

In the warm zone, an initial assessment will be performed. Protective equipment must be worn in the warm zone. Once the immediate life threats are managed, complete decontamination will be performed. Following thorough decontamination in the warm zone, a rapid assessment will be performed. Treat the patient's major injuries, immobilize the spine as appropriate, splint where needed, and move the patient to the cold zone.

All of the protective equipment is removed before entering the cold zone. In the cold zone, take a set of vital signs and SAMPLE history and prepare the patient for transport.

Take precautions to protect your equipment and vehicle during transport, since there may still be some contamination on the patient. Prior to transport, cover the benches, floor, and other exposed areas of your vehicle with thick plastic sheeting. Secure the sheeting with duct tape. Patients should be fully decontaminated before being placed into a helicopter. A contaminated patient in such a closed, tight space could affect the breathing or vision of the air transportation team, resulting in a crash. Contamination of an aircraft can take it out of service for several days.

All clothing and equipment used in the hot or warm zones must be left at the scene so it can be properly contained. Any contaminated equipment or clothing must be sealed in plastic bags or in metal containers with tightly fitting lids. All corpses at the scene need to be decontaminated fully before being transported to a morgue. This must be performed by appropriately trained rescuers.

If you are accidentally exposed to hazardous materials during the rescue, decontaminate yourself thoroughly (Figure 42-9). Contamination occurs most easily in areas of your body where skin is thin or usually moist such as under the arms and in the groin.

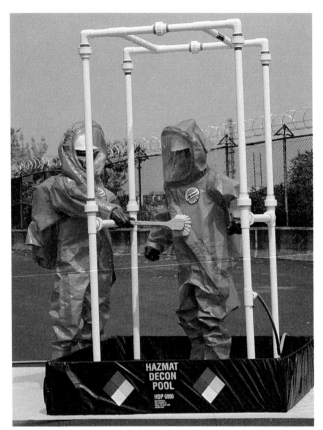

Figure 42-9   Rescuer in decontamination process.

Wash with mild detergent or green soap and plenty of running water. Irrigate exposed skin for at least 20 minutes. Seek medical attention, document the emergency, and report it to your employer.

All rescuers should have a thorough medical examination and medical surveillance to treat any exposure-related injuries or illnesses. Some do not manifest for hours or even days after exposure. Following a hazardous materials emergency, watch yourself for signs of exposure. Seek medical help immediately if you develop headache, nausea and/or vomiting, abdominal cramps and/or diarrhea, difficulty breathing, dizziness, lack of coordination, blurred vision, excessive salivation, or irritation of the skin, eyes, nose, throat, or respiratory tract.

Following rescue, decontaminate your equipment and vehicle by washing them thoroughly inside and out. Caution: if you fail to clean them thoroughly, the result will be chronic chemical exposure. Remember that the clothing under your protective gear also needs decontamination. However, do not take clothing home to launder, since it may contaminate your family and the general sewer system.

ENRICHMENT

The enrichment section contains information that is valuable as background for the EMT-B but that goes substantially beyond the U.S. Department of Transportation (DOT) EMT-Basic curriculum.

RADIATION EMERGENCIES

EXPOSURE AND CONTAMINATION

In a radiation accident, the patient may suffer from exposure, contamination, or both. Exposure occurs when the patient is in the presence of radioactive material without any of the radioactive material actually touching his clothing or body. The rays he receives may be harmful to him, but the patient himself does not become radioactive and does not pose a major threat to rescue personnel. (Remember, however, that the source of the radioactivity may pose a threat to rescuers who come close enough to it.)

Contamination occurs when the patient has come into direct contact with the source of radioactivity or with radioactive gases, liquids, or particles. The radioactive material is present on the patient's clothes or skin, which poses a hazard for the rescuer as well as the patient. The contaminated patient is considered a risk to emergency personnel.

GUIDELINES FOR RADIATION EMERGENCIES

Remember two major principles about radiation-related accidents. One is: *Protect yourself and others from contamination as your first priority.* The second is: *No EMT-B should ever attempt to decontaminate a radiation patient.* If you suspect a patient is contaminated by radiation, you have two choices:

- Wait for a *Radiation Safety Officer (RSO),* an expert specifically trained under federal government provisions to handle such situations. The RSO in your area is probably employed by the county or state health department and will respond to the scene when possible.
- If an RSO cannot come to the site, you can transport the patient to the hospital for decontamination by experts there. To transport, place the patient in a body bag up to the neck, cover the hair completely with a cap or towel, and use disposable wipes to clean the face. Put the disposable wipes in a plastic bag, seal it, and take it to the hospital with you.

Time is the critical factor in managing radiation emergencies. Trained personnel should remove the patient from the source of radiation as quickly as possible before you begin emergency care. Increase distance between you and the source of radiation. Depending on the type of radiation, provide shielding between the patient and the source of radiation. Alpha rays can be stopped by clothing, beta rays by aluminum or like materials. Gamma rays require lead shielding.

PROCEDURES FOR RADIATION EMERGENCIES

Remember to limit your stay in a contaminated area to as little time as possible. Keep as far away from the source as you can and involve as few rescuers as possible. (Exposure to radiation is cumulative and is determined by an inverse square relationship. That is, if you are twice as close, you will receive four times the exposure. If you move twice as far away, you cut your exposure by four times.)

Remember the priorities for hazardous materials emergencies listed earlier in this chapter: *1. Protect the safety of all rescuers and victims; 2. provide patient care; 3. decontaminate clothing, equipment, and the vehicle.* Keeping these priorities in mind, follow the guidelines for scene safety, patient care, and personal decontamination that are outlined below.

Scene Safety First establish scene safety. Follow these guidelines:

1. As you approach the accident scene in your vehicle, visually survey the area for the radiation symbol on the sides of vehicles, machinery, or containers involved (Figure 42-10). Determine the location of a possible source of radiation. Be alert for the presence of other hazardous materials as well. If you determine that radiation is a possibility, park your vehicle upwind of the accident to reduce the chance of radiation particles being blown to your location. Do not park near any

liquid spills or near any transport vehicle that may be leaking. Do not park near any container that might have been cracked or damaged in the accident.

2. As soon as you suspect radiation and before you enter the suspected area of contamination, put on a positive-pressure self-contained breathing apparatus plus protective clothing. Leave no skin or hair exposed. Wear several layers if you can, with an outer layer of tightly woven protective clothing. Seal all openings with duct tape. Wear two pairs of protective gloves under a pair of heavy work gloves. Wear a pair of shoes covered by two pairs of paper shoe covers under a pair of heavy rubber boots.

Personal Protection Protecting yourself from exposure to radiation includes consideration of the following factors:

- *Time*—The less time spent near the radiation source, the less radiation exposure.
- *Distance*—The farther you are from the radiation source, the lower the radiation dose.
- *Shielding*—The denser the material between you and the radiation source, the greater the protection. SCBA and protective clothing or simply examination gloves may be all that is required to adequately shield yourself from the radiation. In some cases, lead shields are required. Increasing the time and distance factors can reduce the amount of shielding needed.
- *Quantity*—Decreasing the amount of radioactive material in the area will decrease exposure. Remove the patient from the radioactive material or remove the radioactive material from the patient.

Patient Care Emergency care for a patient with radiation exposure must center on the patient's life threats and injuries and not on the radiation itself. Remove the patient from the source of radiation as quickly as possible. Conduct an initial assessment and a focused history and physical exam and manage injuries or medical conditions as you normally would. Consult with medical direction when radioactive contamination is a concern.

Personal Decontamination After providing the necessary patient care, transport, and transfer of the patient to the hospital, turn your attention to your own personal decontamination. Report and document your exposure to the radiation source and follow the recommendations of the hospital or local protocol for personal decontamination.

Vehicle/Equipment Decontamination Any equipment that you used to care for the patient—including blankets, towels, bandages, cots, stretchers, or equip-

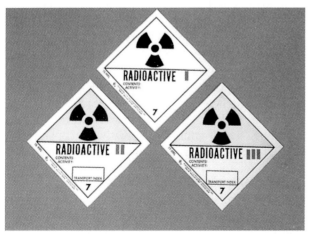

Figure 42-10 Radiation hazard labels.

ment used in transportation—must be checked for radiation contamination before it can be used again. Authorities at the hospital or medical center can arrange for an equipment check.

The vehicle used to transport the patient needs to be washed inside and out before it is placed back in service. Any radioactive dust must be removed from the vehicle. Pay special attention to the tires and other contact points. You may need to use a commercial decontamination solution on your equipment (never use one on the skin). Follow local protocol.

If equipment or tools cannot be completely decontaminated, they will need to be disposed of. Signs of incomplete decontamination include debris adhering to the equipment, discoloration, corrosion, and stains.

PROBLEMS CAUSED BY RADIATION

Radiation is a general term that describes energy transmission. There are three general kinds of problems caused by radiation: radiation sickness, radiation injury, and radiation poisoning.

Radiation sickness is caused by exposure to large amounts of radiation. It starts the day after exposure to the radiation and, depending on the dose, can last anywhere from a few days to 7 or 8 weeks. Common signs and symptoms include nausea and vomiting, diarrhea, hemorrhage, weight loss, appetite loss, malaise, fever, and sores in the throat and mouth. Radiation sickness also affects the immune system, lowering resistance to disease and infection.

Radiation injury is a local injury that is generally caused by exposure to large amounts of less penetrating particles, such as alpha particles. General signs and symptoms include hair loss, skin burns (Figure 42-11), and generalized skin lesions.

Radiation poisoning occurs when the patient has been exposed to dangerous amounts of internal radiation. The result is a host of serious diseases, including cancer and anemia.

While a victim of a radiation accident is not "contagious" or infectious and generally will not endanger a rescuer, you are at risk of becoming contaminated if the patient still has radiation particles on his skin or clothing. Always put on full protective gear as soon as you recognize a radiation accident.

PROTECTION FROM RADIATION

As you approach the scene of an accident, protect yourself and other rescuers if you know ahead of time that radiation sources are present. Immediately contact the Radiation Safety Officer with your federal, state, or county government.

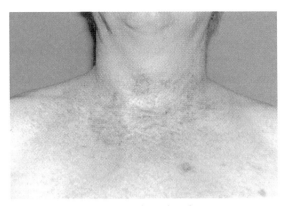

Figure 42-11   Radiation burn.

The following factors determine the amount of radiation damage that you may sustain during a rescue if an unshielded radiation source is present in the vicinity:

- The amount and type of personal shielding you use
- The strength of the radiation source
- Your distance from the radiation source
- The type of radiation
- How long you are exposed
- How much of your body is exposed

You can reduce your risk. The best approach is to divide the rescue work among many rescuers, with teams composed of as few rescuers as possible. The Federal Nuclear Regulatory Commission recommends that an individual in an emergency situation be exposed to no more than a one-time whole-body dose of 25 roentgens. This means that if the Geiger counter at the patient's location indicates 50 roentgens per hour, then a new team of rescuers should move in and relieve the first team after 30 minutes.

Another approach to reducing risk is to shield the radiation source itself (not you or the patient). For example, the best protection against gamma rays (one type of radiation that is extremely dangerous) is lead, preferably 1 to 2 inches thick. If lead is not available, any material that has thick mass (such as bricks, concrete, or several feet of dirt) will do.

Know your community's plan for hazardous materials emergencies. Know how to reach your Radiation Safety Officer. Always wear your protective gear, including a self-contained breathing apparatus as soon as you suspect the involvement of radiation. Never smoke in an area where radiation has contaminated the air, and do not eat food that comes from a contamination site. (Smoking and eating are the two most common ways of become internally contaminated.)

CASE STUDY FOLLOW-UP

SCENE SIZE-UP

You have been dispatched to an MVA involving a tanker truck and passenger vehicle. In addition to the injuries to the patients caused by the impact, you realize that the tanker may pose a possible hazardous materials emergency. As your partner decides on a safe place to park—uphill, upwind, and away from the potential danger—you pull out your Emergency Response Guidebook.

From your present safe position, you note the size and shape of the tank and, with binoculars, search for some form of identification. You finally recognize one—a "Flammable Liquid" placard. Using your Guidebook, you find that danger can come from fire or explosion and you realize that everyone at the scene needs to make sure they don't accidentally start one with an open flame, heat, or sparks. Continuing to size up the scene, you look for signs of damage to the container. You spot a small leak and vapors.

You report to Incident Command. Just as you exit your vehicle, the fire department arrives and begins to set up an entry and decontamination area.

INITIAL ASSESSMENT

You observe the patients as they begin to walk toward the EMS unit. Your general impression is of a male and female in their 40s, neither of whom looks very steady. They were exposed to the vapors, so they are probably dizzy.

Over the loud speaker, Incident Command instructs the patients to stop where they are. Their clothes are contaminated, and they must strip. They don't need much convincing. They can smell the vapors. The patients are soon in the decontamination area being washed down, with rescuers holding manual in-line stabilization.

Once the patients have been decontaminated and are in clean clothes, you and your partner complete the initial assessment while a First Responder continues to hold manual in-line stabilization. Both patients are talking coherently and so you conclude that they are alert and have open airways. Their breathing rates are slightly rapid but adequate. Pulses for both are present, strong, regular, and slightly rapid. Skin color, temperature, and condition are normal. There is no bleeding. You provide both patients oxygen by non-rebreather mask at 15 lpm. You conclude that neither patient is a high priority for immediate transport and you can continue with the focused history and physical exam at the scene.

FOCUSED HISTORY AND PHYSICAL EXAM

You and your partner perform rapid trauma assessments on both patients. Neither appears to have been injured, but since the mechanism of injury was significant (the collision with the truck), you apply cervical spine immobilization collars and immobilize each patient to a long spine board. You take vital signs—all are within normal ranges for both patients—and gather a SAMPLE history. The only symptom either patient reports is dizziness. Neither reports any allergies. The female is taking no medications; the male is taking a medication for high blood pressure. Neither has any pertinent past medical history except for the blood pressure problem. Their last meal was lunch at a fast food restaurant just before the collision. Events leading to the present problem are obvious to all.

Another ambulance arrives at the scene. Both ambulance crews cover the stretchers and other items in the ambulance with thick plastic. Each patient is loaded onto a plastic-covered wheeled stretcher and transferred to one of the ambulances for transport.

DETAILED PHYSICAL EXAM

En route to the hospital, you perform a detailed physical exam on the male patient whom you are transporting. You discover no additional injuries.

ONGOING ASSESSMENT

Since your patient is stable, an ongoing assessment is needed only every 15 minutes. Since transport time is relatively short, you have time to perform only one ongoing assessment en route. You repeat the initial assessment, the rapid trauma assessment, and vital signs measurements. You check that the patient is still securely immobilized and that oxygen is flowing adequately. You arrive at the hospital without any change in the patient's condition. You and your partner transfer the patient to the care of the emergency department personnel, complete your oral and written reports, and then proceed to decontaminate yourselves and the ambulance.

CHAPTER REVIEW

TERMS AND CONCEPTS

You may wish to review the following terms and concepts included in this chapter.

cold zone—the area adjacent to the warm zone in a hazardous materials emergency. Normal triage, treatment, and stabilization are performed here. Also called safe zone.

hazardous material—material that in any quantity poses a threat or unreasonable risk to life, health, or property if not properly controlled during manufacture, processing, packaging, handling, storage, transportation, use, and disposal.

hot zone—the area where contamination is actually present. It generally is the area that is immediately adjacent to the accident site and where contamination can still occur. Also called contamination zone.

safety zones—areas surrounding an accident involving hazardous materials, designated for specific rescue operations. See hot zone, warm zone, and cold zone.

warm zone—the area that is established surrounding or immediately adjacent to the hot zone in a hazardous materials emergency, the purpose of which is to prevent the spread of contamination. Life-saving emergency care is performed here. Also called control zone.

REVIEW QUESTIONS

1. List clues that tell you a hazardous material may be present at an accident scene.
2. Name the first thing an EMT-B should do after recognizing that hazardous materials might be involved in an accident.
3. Explain what qualifies the EMT-B to attempt a hazardous materials rescue.
4. List specific actions you can take to protect bystanders.
5. If you have had no specialized training, explain what you should do while waiting for expert help to arrive.
6. List the resources available to the EMT-B at the site of a hazardous materials emergency.
7. Explain what you can do to protect yourself, others, and your vehicle from contamination.
8. List the "safety zones" and describe what work should be done in each.
9. List the information that is necessary for trained personnel to decide on a course of action at a hazardous materials emergency.
10. Name the required elements of an incident management plan.

CHAPTER 43

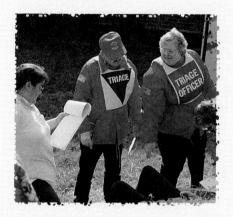

Multiple-Casualty Incidents

INTRODUCTION

This chapter will provide an overview of how to organize and provide emergency medical care when there is an event that involves a number of patients: a multiple-casualty incident, or MCI. MCIs may range from a vehicle collision with several injured passengers to a major disaster such as a hurricane, flood, earthquake, bombing, building collapse, or airliner crash. For a more advanced understanding of MCIs and disaster response, you must regularly practice your community's MCI or disaster response plan.

In this chapter you will learn the fundamentals of MCI response, but these fundamentals must be adapted to your own region. You will learn about the incident management system, EMS sectors, triage, components of a disaster response plan, and—most importantly—how to "get the right patient, to the right hospital, in the right amount of time."

O B J E C T I V E S

Numbered objectives are from the United States Department of Transportation 1994 EMT-Basic National Standard Curriculum. Asterisked objectives, if any, pertain to material that is supplemental to the DOT curriculum.

COGNITIVE

7-3.7 Describe the criteria for a multiple-casualty situation. (p. 866)

7-3.8 Evaluate the role of the EMT-Basic in the multiple-casualty situation. (pp. 866–874)

7-3.9 Summarize the components of basic triage. (pp. 869–874)

7-3.10 Define the role of the EMT-Basic in a disaster operation. (p. 874)

7-3.11 Describe basic concepts of incident management. (pp. 867–868)

7-3.13 Review the local mass casualty incident plan. (pp. 865, 867–868, 869)

* Outline the ways to get help in a multiple-casualty incident. (p. 868)

* Describe various approaches for reducing rescue personnel stress during an MCI or disaster. (pp. 873–874)

PSYCHOMOTOR

7-3.16 Given a scenario of a mass casualty incident, perform triage.

Additional objectives from DOT Lesson 7-3 are addressed in Chapter 42, "Hazardous Materials Emergencies."

C A S E   S T U D Y

THE DISPATCH

EMS Unit 105—respond to the Firebird Raceway—we have reports that two race cars have crashed through a fence into a bleacher full of people. Initial reports indicate as many as ten dead and forty critical injuries. Time out is 1612 hours.

ON ARRIVAL

While en route to the scene, you request dispatch to activate the multiple-casualty incident plan. Dispatch advises you they are contacting appropriate emergency response agencies from the call-up list and that area hospitals have been notified.

On arrival, you see two demolished vehicles in the midst of a collapsed bleacher. Bystanders are helping the injured. People scream for your help. You estimate there are at least fifty injuries. Since you are the senior EMT-B, according to your MCI plan you are the incident manager for EMS operations.

How would you begin your assessment and emergency care in this multiple-casualty incident?

During this chapter you will learn about the roles and responsibilities of an EMT-B during a multiple-casualty incident. Later we will return to the case study and apply the principles you have learned.

MULTIPLE-CASUALTY INCIDENTS

A **multiple-casualty incident (MCI)**—sometimes called a *mass casualty incident* or a *multiple-casualty situation (MCS)*—is any event that places excessive demands on personnel and equipment. Typically, an MCI involves three or more patients. A multiple-patient incident with three patients may be routine in a large metropolitan area, but three critically injured patients can quickly overwhelm a small community or rural area with limited resources and personnel.

Motor vehicle crashes, gang-related violence, or apartment fires are among the situations in which you may encounter multiple patients. But MCIs do not always involve victims of trauma. As an EMT-B your

MCI plan should prepare you to manage the multiple-patient incident involving food poisoning, toxic gas inhalation, and in some parts of the nation, refugee influx.

In any multiple-casualty incident, the key to effective emergency care is to call for plenty of help early (Figure 43-1). Make sure that you call for enough, or more than enough, rescuers with advanced life-saving skills as soon as you encounter the incident. *Remember: It's better to call too many rescuers than too few.*

Getting help, however, is only one aspect of managing the multiple-casualty incident. Effective management of multiple-casualty incidents consists of getting enough help, positioning vehicles properly, giving appropriate emergency medical care, transporting patients efficiently, and providing follow-up care at receiving facilities.

ESTABLISHING INCIDENT MANAGEMENT

Essentially, the senior EMT who arrives at the scene of an MCI or disaster assumes responsibility as the **EMS incident manager,** and that responsibility continues until a predesignated officer, if any, arrives. The EMS incident manager is responsible for seeing that the multiple-casualty incident is responded to in a controlled and orderly way and that all responsibilities are carried out. In many jurisdictions, this is done in accordance with an **incident management system.** An incident management system is a written plan to help control, direct, and coordinate emergency personnel and equipment from the scene of an MCI to the transportation of the patient to definitive care.

An incident management system may describe two methods of determining who is in charge of an MCI. *A unified command system* works best when the MCI involves more than one emergency response agency. Under the unified method, decisions regard-

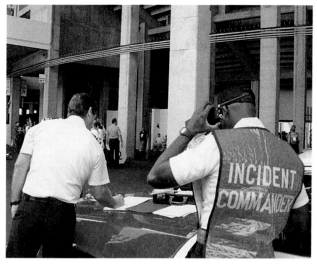

Figure 43-2 The incident manager or commander directs the response and coordinates resources at a multiple-casualty incident (MCI).

ing management of the MCI are made in collaboration by representatives of EMS, the fire service, and law enforcement. In contrast, a *single command system* applies when one agency is given the authority to manage all emergency response resources.

It must be absolutely clear from the beginning who is in charge. That person—the **incident manager,** or *incident commander* (Figure 43-2)—should be stationed in a command center located in a safe area near or at the area where patients will be loaded for transport. The incident manager may, in your jurisdiction, be the EMS incident manager or someone from one of the other emergency response services.

After an incident manager is determined, he should begin to establish the following EMS sectors (Figure 43-3), which will be discussed in detail later in the chapter:

- Mobile command sector
- Supply sector
- Extrication sector
- Triage sector
- Treatment sector
- Staging sector
- Transportation sector

These sectors are established to provide an orderly means of decision making and execution of plans at the scene. The EMT incident manager assigns an officer or team leader to each sector. Each sector officer wears a highly visible reflective vest. Incoming response units will be directed to an EMS sector officer and assigned specific responsibilities. The EMT incident manager must also:

- Rapidly perform a scene size-up for possible hazards to patients or to the surrounding public; mo-

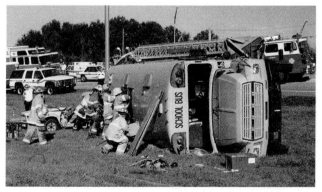

Figure 43-1 Plenty of resources have been called to the scene of this school bus wreck.

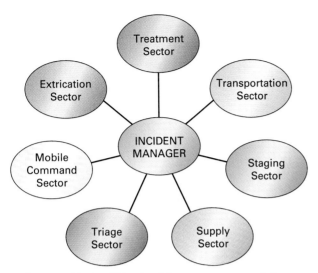

Figure 43-3 The incident manager delegates duties to the various sector officers.

bilize fire and other personnel to reduce those hazards as patient triage and treatment begins.

• Locate and reassure the patients; if the incident involves only a few patients, quickly assess patients, perform triage (sorting patients into treatment priorities, explained later in the chapter), and radio for help as life-saving treatment is begun.

• Radio the communications center (dispatch) for help giving the following information:
  – Name of agency calling
  – Type of incident (e.g., downed aircraft, explosion, bus crash)
  – Location of incident
  – Approximate number of patients
  – Additional EMS personnel needed
  – Additional equipment and supplies needed (transportation, extrication, etc.)
  – Additional emergency agency or expert response required (e.g., fire service, police, utility company)

Those at headquarters who receive the report of the incident should immediately confirm it on all frequencies (ambulance, police, and fire), including exact location and routing instructions. Transmissions should be brief, precise, and in clear, normal language; no codes should be used during transmission.

Communications or dispatch personnel should contact all nearby hospitals to confirm the incident and report the estimated number of patients. Hospital personnel should begin activating their multiple-casualty incident plans.

The community should have a list of ambulances and EMS squads that are predesignated to respond in multiple-casualty incidents. Communications headquarters should contact the ambulances and EMS squads on the call-up list, informing them of the exact location, routing instructions, and estimated number of patients. Predesignated units should be instructed to respond with double crews and multiple-casualty equipment.

Communications should designate which ambulances should stay on standby to cover normal EMS calls during the incident; not all available ambulances should be dispatched to the scene of the incident.

EMT-Bs responding to the scene of an MCI should first report to the mobile command sector for instructions. If you are one of the first EMT-Bs on the scene, you will probably be asked to perform triage. However, if triage has already been completed you may be called upon to provide treatment or assist with moving equipment. Prior to an actual MCI, it is critical that you know and practice the responsibilities for each and every sector. Many agencies include an MCI or Disaster Response Packet in every response vehicle. Typically, these Response Packets outline general duties and responsibilities of responding EMT-Bs for each MCI sector.

POSITIONING ARRIVING VEHICLES

Working closely with fire and police command, the EMS incident manager helps position arriving rescue vehicles. This helps in the smooth transport of patients and prevents accidents and injury.

Arriving personnel are then directed to appropriate sectors. As an EMT-Basic, you will report to the sector officer for specific assignments. Once your task is completed, you will report back to the sector officer for additional duties or reassignment to another sector.

The first ambulance that arrives should be positioned a safe distance from the event itself but near the incident manager. This vehicle can then be used as the **mobile command sector,** which is considered the headquarters or command post for incident management. A flag or other device should be set up to identify the command post. During the early phases of an MCI, one of the functions of a mobile command sector is determining the scope and size of the incident. Some MCIs, such as those that occur on our interstate highways, may stretch for miles. Establish direct radio contact with area hospitals from the ambulance.

Establish a **supply sector,** which is responsible for distributing the medical materials and equipment necessary to render care, and, if needed, an **extrication sector,** which is responsible for freeing patients from wreckage (Figure 43-4) and managing them at the accident site. As fire and rescue personnel arrive, they should be briefed by the extrication sector officer and personnel disbursed where needed. As additional equipment arrives, it should be moved to the

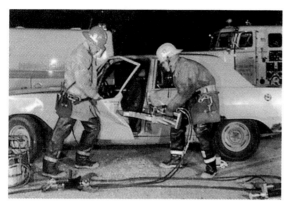

Figure 43-4   Modern extrication equipment is essential for a fast, efficient rescue.

supply sector, where rescue equipment is combined and arranged in orderly piles.

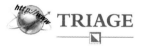 **TRIAGE**

As an EMT-B arriving on scene, you will receive instructions from the incident manager. During the early phases of an MCI, you may be directed to assist in triage. **Triage** is a system used for sorting patients to determine the order in which they will receive medical care or transportation to definitive care. It is performed in the **triage sector.**

The most knowledgeable EMT arriving in the first ambulance should become the triage officer and take charge of the triage sector. Typically, this is a pre-designated individual who has special training in triage. The triage officer assigns care of the patients, updates or changes treatment priority of patients, and coordinates patient transport with the staging and treatment officers.

INITIAL ASSESSMENT

If assigned to the triage sector, you will be expected to perform an initial assessment and begin initial triage. The goals of triage are to assess the patient's condition, determine the urgency of the patient's condition, assign a priority to the patient's treatment, and determine transport to an appropriate hospital.

You will quickly perform an initial assessment, checking for airway, breathing, circulation, and severe bleeding. Perform this initial assessment as follows:

1. If the airway is not open, open it with a manual maneuver. If the patient responds and is talking, move on to the next patient.

2. If the patient is unresponsive, check for breathing and pulse. If there is no breathing or no pulse, do not provide care for that person. Move on to the next patient.

3. If you feel a pulse, check for severe bleeding; if there is severe bleeding, quickly apply a pressure dressing to the wound and move on to the next patient.

As long as there are others still waiting to be triaged, the only initial treatment that should be done is airway management and control of severe bleeding. If there is immediate and obvious danger to the patients, immediately begin moving people, regardless of their injuries. Those who can walk should help evacuate others.

As more EMT-Bs arrive, one is designated as the secondary triage officer, responsible for tagging the patients in order of priority. If the primary triage officer completes the initial triage assessment before other EMT-Bs arrive, he should tag patients for priority treatment.

PRIORITY LEVELS

A triage system typically sets up three priority levels as illustrated in Figure 43-5. The highest priority (those patients whose survival requires care or transport without delay) is also called Level 1 or Priority 1. The second priority (those who will survive even if care is somewhat delayed) is also called Level 2 or Priority 2. The lowest priority (those who do not require or will not benefit from prompt care) is also called Level 3 or Priority 3.

In the three-priority system, the lowest priority includes both those with minor injuries and those who are dead—for obvious reasons. Some multiple-casualty incident plans reserve the third priority level for those with minor injuries and identify a fourth priority level—sometimes known as Priority ∅—for the dead or fatally injured, cardiac arrest patients, decapitation, obvious signs of rigor mortis, severed trunk, and incineration. Become familiar with your local MCI plan so you are fully aware of the classification system you should use.

Although cardiac arrest patients would certainly benefit from swift care, they are usually assigned the lowest triage priority because, in a multiple-casualty incident, the care of a patient in cardiac arrest would take too much time and too many rescuers—time and personnel that can be more effectively used to save a number of other lives. Once the highest priority patients are stabilized or there are enough EMS personnel on the scene, some systems will change cardiac arrest patients to Priority 1 status. The individual EMT-B will not decide what priority to give to cardiac arrest patients (or any other types of patients) but will follow directions from the triage officer.

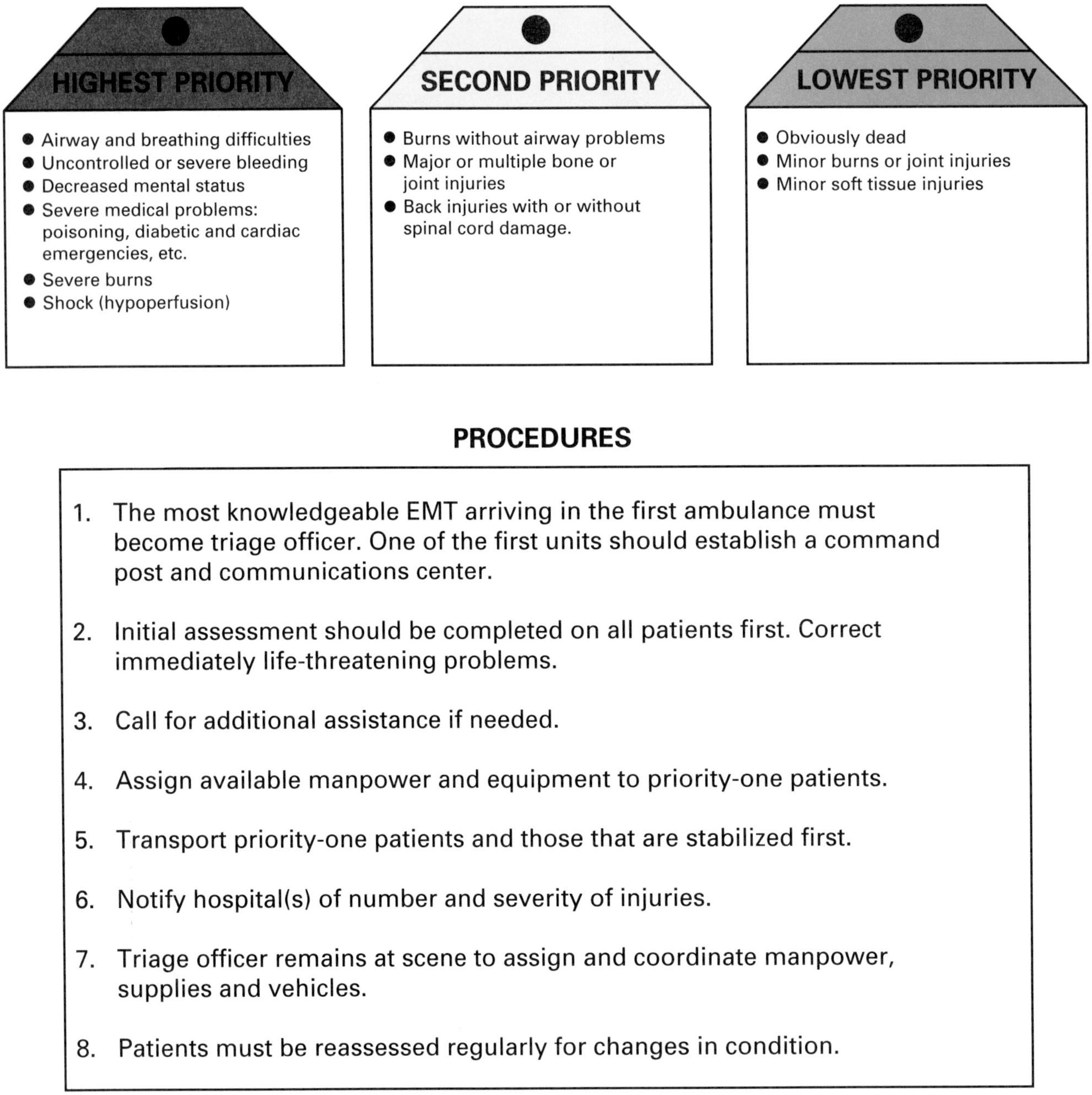

HIGHEST PRIORITY

- Airway and breathing difficulties
- Uncontrolled or severe bleeding
- Decreased mental status
- Severe medical problems: poisoning, diabetic and cardiac emergencies, etc.
- Severe burns
- Shock (hypoperfusion)

SECOND PRIORITY

- Burns without airway problems
- Major or multiple bone or joint injuries
- Back injuries with or without spinal cord damage.

LOWEST PRIORITY

- Obviously dead
- Minor burns or joint injuries
- Minor soft tissue injuries

PROCEDURES

1. The most knowledgeable EMT arriving in the first ambulance must become triage officer. One of the first units should establish a command post and communications center.

2. Initial assessment should be completed on all patients first. Correct immediately life-threatening problems.

3. Call for additional assistance if needed.

4. Assign available manpower and equipment to priority-one patients.

5. Transport priority-one patients and those that are stabilized first.

6. Notify hospital(s) of number and severity of injuries.

7. Triage officer remains at scene to assign and coordinate manpower, supplies and vehicles.

8. Patients must be reassessed regularly for changes in condition.

Figure 43-5 Triage summary.

PATIENT TAGGING

Patient tagging or identification (Figure 43-6) is critical to the successful initial triage of every patient. Tagging the sick or injured helps arriving EMT-Bs quickly and efficiently identify treatment priorities. Also, arriving EMT-Bs know untagged patients will still need initial triage. The tagging system should be easy to understand, standardized, and easily affixed to the patient. One typical patient identification system uses colors to signify priority of care. For example:

- High Priority = Red
- Second Priority = Yellow
- Low Priority = Green
- Priority $\varnothing$ or Fourth Level, if used = Gray or Black

During an MCI, emergency personnel may respond from many miles and across many jurisdictions. If patients are to receive definitive care and transportation, then EMS personnel must have a universally understood triage identification tag system. (See Figure 43-7 for an example of the METTAG patient identification system.)

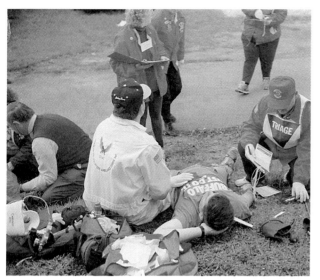

Figure 43-6   Triage tagging is essential in multiple-casualty situations.

TREATMENT

A **treatment sector** (Figure 43-8) should be designated close to the area where ambulances arrive. It should be on high ground, and, if possible, covered and lighted. It should be safe from falling debris, a safe distance from the incident, and clearly marked. Use a tall flag if you have one. Depending on the size and scope of the MCI, it may be necessary to have more than one treatment sector.

Patients should be moved from the triage sector to the patient treatment sector in order of their priority. Immobilize all patients before moving them, and place them in rows according to their triage category.

Each treatment sector should have a treatment officer responsible for the ongoing assessment of patients in his area. Remember that triage is ongoing. Many patients' categories will change as their conditions improve or deteriorate.

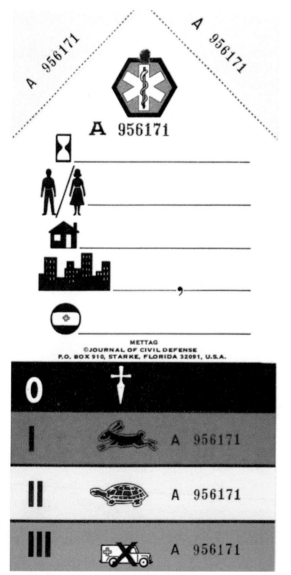

Figure 43-7   The METTAG.

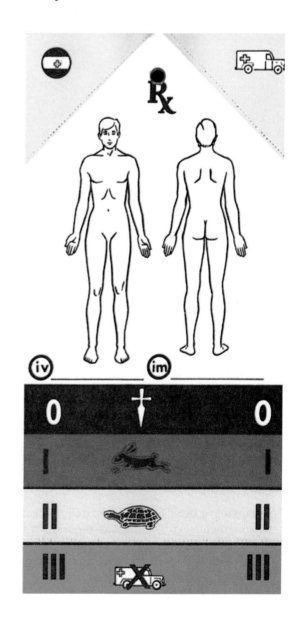

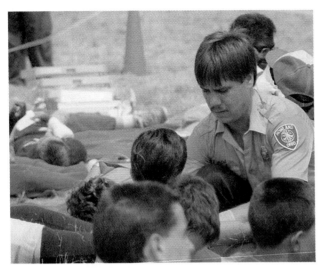

Figure 43-8 Treatment sector at a multiple-casualty incident (MCI).

Treat only salvageable patients. If color-coded triage tags, cards, or ribbons are used, the same colors should be used on color-coded flags that are erected at the triage sectors. Position patients in rows as they await treatment.

Since the dead are the last to be transported, you should set up a morgue in a separate, out-of-sight area. (Some localities establish a Morgue Sector and officer. The Morgue Sector Officer would coordinate the removal of bodies to the morgue with the Coroner's office or its representative.) Again, you should become familiar with your local plan.

If you are working in the treatment sector, a key concept to remember is to *take shortcuts with non-life-threatening injuries.* For example, immobilize patients to a long board instead of trying to splint each individual extremity injury. Give a patient who is able a 4 × 4 dressing and ask him to apply direct pressure to a bleeding wound—his own or someone else's. Once the highest-priority patients have been stabilized, move to the second-priority treatment sector and begin care.

The triage, treatment, and transportation sector officers should remain in constant communication with each other regarding transport availability and needs. Again become familiar with and follow local protocol.

STAGING AND TRANSPORTATION

Once patients have been properly assessed and cared for in the treatment sector, the triage process continues. Working closely together, the treatment, staging, and transportation officers make decisions regarding patient transport priorities.

To begin the process of transporting priority patients to the appropriate medical facility, a staging sector (Figure 43-9) is set up. A **staging sector** officer monitors, inventories, and directs available ambulances to the treatment sector at the request of the transportation sector officer.

The **transportation sector** officer ensures that ambulances are accessible and that transportation does not occur without the direction of the EMS incident manager. The transportation officer also coordinates patient transportation with the triage officer and communicates with the hospitals involved.

To effectively transport patients of a multiple-casualty incident:

- As the highest priority patients are stabilized (airway opened, life-threatening bleeding controlled), begin transport. Before and during transport, one or two triage officers (depending on the number of patients) should move along the rows constantly, monitoring patients for a change in status.
- High-priority patients should be transported first, immediately after treatment; these serious patients should be evenly distributed among available hospitals.
- Before leaving the incident, EMT-Bs should receive specific instructions from the transportation officer or staging officer on how to leave the area (preferred route) and to which hospital to take the patients.
- If the routing in the area is complex, the staging officer should provide EMT-Bs with marked maps to the appropriate hospital.
- As each ambulance leaves, the transportation officer should radio the hospital that the ambulance is en route, briefly describing the injuries involved and giving an estimated time of arrival. Individual EMT-Bs should not try to communicate with the hospital unless an emergency develops during transport. Individual ambulance communication will jam lines and cause confusion.

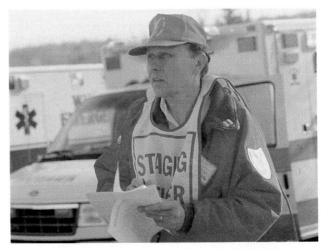

Figure 43-9 Staging sector at a multiple-casualty incident (MCI). (Craig Jackson/In the Dark Photography)

- When the only patients left at the site are ambulatory, load them onto a bus that has been brought to the site for this purpose. Five to ten personnel carrying essential equipment (oxygen masks, suction equipment, emergency kits, and portable radio) should board the bus, and a fully equipped ambulance with its crew should lead the bus slowly and safely to an outlying hospital that has little or no patient load. If a patient on the bus suddenly deteriorates during the trip to the hospital, EMT-Bs on board can handle the situation and, if necessary, call for intercept by another ambulance.

COMMUNICATIONS

Effective communications between emergency responders is one of the most difficult aspects of a multiple-casualty incident. As an EMT-B, you can expect a variety of MCI communication difficulties. Upon your arrival at the scene of an MCI, oral communications between emergency responders may initially appear chaotic. Tasks are not always clear, and duties may not have been assigned.

Once an incident command system and mobile command center are established, the state of confusion will diminish. Throughout an MCI, you may also find radio communications of any kind difficult. Communication "dead spots," frequency unavailability, and channel "gridlock" are a few of the more common radio communications problems you will encounter. These kinds of communication difficulties are mentioned to prepare you for the "real world" of patient care during an MCI. Don't let communication difficulties distract you from your patient care.

FOLLOW-THROUGH

When all patients have been moved from the incident scene, emergency personnel should go to hospitals to assist hospital personnel. However, the incident manager and an assistant should remain at the scene to supervise clean-up and complete restoration.

Once you arrive at the hospital, instructions for care and treatment will come from the facility's incident manager. Depending on the size and nature of the MCI, some facilities may need your help, while other hospitals may have enough personnel to manage the MCI without your assistance. If your services are not needed, you should prepare your vehicle and equipment for other EMS calls. Remember to update your dispatch center regarding your status and availability for response to additional calls.

REDUCING STRESS

Psychological stress is acute at the scene of a multiple-casualty incident. Rescuers, too, react to disaster, often the same way patients do. Common are fears regarding personal safety, crying, anger, guilt, numbness, preoccupation with death, frustration, fatigue, and burnout. Approximately two-thirds of all rescuers suffer long-term reactions. Most rescuer reactions peak within about one week and then diminish. Approximately half of rescuers have recurrent dreams and repeated recollections of the disaster for weeks or months afterward. In some cases, the rescuer may not react at all, then react weeks or months later.

Any rescuer who breaks down or becomes hysterical during the incident operation should be removed immediately to a hospital; a rescuer who is injured or becomes ill during rescue operations should be treated immediately and transported so that other rescuers can continue their work.

To reduce stress on yourself and other rescue personnel who report to you:

- Try not to get overwhelmed by the immensity of the incident. Carefully evaluate injuries and determine which patients should be cared for first. Then set about administering the aid, caring for patients one by one. This will help you maintain some calm and feel that you are making progress.
- As each rescue worker reports to the staffing area for assignment, he should be instructed to rest at regular intervals, maybe as often as once every 1 to 2 hours. *Follow local protocol.* During rest periods, the rescuer should return to the staffing area (preferably an area that is away from the hub of the disaster), sit or lie down, have something to eat or drink, and relax as much as possible.
- If rest periods are effectively rotated, there will always be enough rescue workers to carry on disaster assistance, and the entire team will be rested and relieved periodically.
- Make sure that each rescue worker is fully aware of his exact assignment. Have a well-designed plan that enables you to fully utilize your personnel, and fully explain to each worker what his responsibility is.
- Several workers in the staffing area should circulate among the rescue workers and watch for signs of physical exhaustion or stress. If one of the workers appears to be having problems, he should immediately be required to return to the staffing area and rest for a longer period than usual. After resting, if possible, a less stressful task should be assigned, possibly in another area of the disaster site.
- Make sure that rescue workers are assigned to tasks appropriate for their skills and experience. If there is a question about whether a certain worker can manage a task, don't take the chance.
- Provide plenty of nourishing food and beverages; encourage rescue workers to eat and drink whenever necessary to keep up their strength.
- Encourage rescue workers to talk among themselves; talking helps relieve stress. Discourage light-

hearted conversation and joking, however—some patients as well as workers may be offended by it, increasing the stress level at the scene.

- Make sure that rescuers have the opportunity to talk with trained counselors after the incident. If your team has access to critical incident stress debriefing, make sure that all rescuers who worked on the disaster take advantage of this process.

DISASTER MANAGEMENT

In general, a **disaster** is a sudden catastrophic event that overwhelms natural order and causes great loss of property and/or life.

In a disaster, there is a great disparity between casualties and resources. It exceeds the capabilities of available management resources and may disrupt the community, the medical establishment, or both. It may be designated a "disaster" because of the overwhelming number of patients involved, or because just a few patients are so severely injured.

Disasters may be natural—such as those caused by hurricanes, earthquakes, floods, and tornadoes— or man-made, such as airline crashes, fires, toxic gas leaks, and nuclear accidents.

ENRICHMENT

The enrichment section contains information that is valuable as background for the EMT-B but that goes substantially beyond the U.S. Department of Transportation (DOT) EMT-Basic curriculum.

REQUIREMENTS OF EFFECTIVE DISASTER ASSISTANCE

You think, "It can't happen to me!" Yet, time and time again disasters do happen. Effective disaster assistance begins with emergency responders promoting the need for individual and community disaster preparedness. In general, effective disaster assistance requires:

- Preparation of the entire community; community members at large trained in basic life-supporting first aid and simple rescue procedures
- Careful preplanning
- The ability to quickly implement a plan
- The application of triage skills
- The ability to organize quickly and utilize fully all emergency personnel
- The ability to adapt the plan to meet special conditions, such as inclement weather or isolated locations
- A contingency plan that provides for shelter and transportation of people in an entire area, such as an entire community or county

- The ability to do the greatest good for the greatest number
- A plan that avoids simply relocating the disaster from the scene to the local hospital

WARNING AND EVACUATION

In some cases, such as a hurricane or tornado, you may learn that a disaster is approaching and may have time to evacuate local residents. If you can conduct an orderly evacuation, you can prevent further injury, preserve life, and possibly protect property.

Relocation should, as much as possible, keep people in their natural social groupings. Make every effort to provide home-based relocation instead of relocating people to hospitals and clinics if they are not injured.

Alerts for the evacuation must be repeated often and with clarity. You must convince people that a disaster is really about to occur and that there is a substantial threat to their safety. At a minimum, the evacuation and warning message must contain the following information:

- The nature of the disaster and its estimated time of impact on the area; if possible, a description of the expected severity
- Safe routes to take out of the area
- Appropriate destinations for those who evacuate, indicating where food and shelter will be available

Use whatever means you have available to spread the message frequently and with urgency—by radio, television, roving police cars with loudspeakers, public address systems in buildings, and short-wave radios. Make sure that each message contains all pertinent details concerning the nature and impact of the disaster, how people should evacuate, which routes are safest, and where people should meet for assistance after evacuation.

DISASTER COMMUNICATIONS SYSTEMS

Critical to any successful rescue effort is an efficient communications system that includes a back-up system in case the primary system fails. The specific system that you choose will depend on your area and requirements, but the following general guidelines apply to any disaster communications system:

- Establish details of the system ahead of time. The communications network should be a part of your disaster drill. Decide what radio frequency and kind of system you want, who will be responsible for operating it, and what equipment will be used.
- Appoint only one person at the scene of the disaster who will communicate to those outside the disaster area. It is usually best to use the disaster control chief. That person should be aware at all times

of what is going on and can be a source of reliable information to the outside.

- The person who is designated to communicate should stay in touch with local hospitals and rescue units who may be called on to respond to the disaster. Make sure ahead of time that the person will have access to appropriate equipment to keep in touch with the outside.
- Area-wide communications are vital. They give people warning of an impending disaster as well as help people receive information regarding the status of family members, friends, and the community as a whole.
- Since it may be impossible to restore immediate telephone service to an area, establish a central location where people can register concerning their whereabouts, safety, health status, and so on.
- Make sure that information regarding road conditions, alternative routes, and closed roads is constantly monitored and communicated, especially in the case of a weather-related disaster.
- Constantly monitor and link all hospitals, trauma centers, and clinics in the area so that you can determine which can receive more patients and when those patients can be transported to the specific facility. The status of hospitals will change constantly throughout and after the disaster; therefore, keep communications open.
- Do not allow emergency vehicle operators or EMT-Bs who are en route to the hospital to communicate via radio to the hospital unless an emergency occurs en route. The person designated to take care of communications will contact the appropriate hospital as the ambulance leaves the disaster scene.
- If the disaster area is large, individual rescue workers should be equipped with portable radios so they can communicate with their commands.
- Include a recorder or some other device that will allow you to record crucial communications.

THE PSYCHOLOGICAL IMPACT OF DISASTERS

Faced with the grim physical injuries that can accompany a disaster, it is difficult to remember that the psychological injuries can be severe—even among those not physically injured. The overwhelming reaction to disaster is a reaction to the loss of either life or property.

Almost all people experience fear; many also feel shaky, perspire profusely, become confused, and suffer irritability, anxiety, restlessness, fatigue, sleep disturbances, nightmares, difficulty concentrating, moodiness, suspiciousness, depression, nausea, vomiting, and diarrhea. Survivors of a disaster often experience fear, anxiety, anger, guilt, shock, depression, denial,

feelings of isolation, and vulnerability. All these reactions are normal. As soon as people begin working to remedy the disaster situation, their physical responses usually become less exaggerated, and they are able to work with less tension and fear.

HELPING DISASTER PATIENTS

At high risk for severe emotional reactions are children, the elderly, those in poor physical or emotional health, the handicapped, and those who have an unresolved past loss or crisis.

The reactions of children depend on their age, individual disposition, family support, and community support:

- *Preschoolers* tend to cry, lose control of bowel and/or bladder, become confused, and suck their thumbs.
- *Elementary-age children* suffer extreme fears about their safety and show confusion, depression, headache, inability to concentrate, withdrawal, poor performance, and the tendency to fight with their peers.
- *Preadolescents and adolescents* may show the same reaction as elementary-age children, coupled with extreme aggression and stress that is severe enough to disrupt their lives.

While each disaster presents individual problems, the following are general guidelines that apply to any disaster:

- The families of patients need and deserve accurate information—something that is too often overlooked in the rush to begin emergency medical care. As soon as possible, assign several rescue workers to gather information and disseminate it to local radio and television stations so that psychological stress to other family members may be lessened.
- Reunite families as soon as possible. Emotional stress will be lessened once the patient is with family members, and family members may be able to provide you with critical medical history that may increase your ability to care for the patient.
- If the disaster involved a large number of people, group the patients with their families and neighbors. This will help reduce feelings of fear and alienation.
- Encourage patients to do necessary chores. Work can be therapeutic and should be used to help the patients get over their own problems.
- Provide a structure for the emotionally injured, and let them know your expectations. Tell the patient exactly what is happening—that he is suffering a temporary setback, will probably recover rapidly, and that meanwhile, you expect certain minimal

tasks to be performed. For instance, direct the emotionally traumatized with basic commands such as "Let's walk to the treatment sector."

- Help patients confront the reality of the disaster. Help them work through their feelings. Encourage them to talk about the disaster and its long-term effects. Arrange for a group discussion where patients can exchange ideas as soon as physical needs are taken care of. If you sense that any patients are not facing reality or that expectations are much worse than reality, help them adjust their views.
- Don't give false assurances. The patient needs help in facing problems and deciding how he will react to them, but will need to face facts sooner or later. If the patient finds that you have lied, he may resist any further outside help, and the recovery period will probably be extensive.
- A patient may refuse offers of help because of cultural upbringing, threats to self-image, or an inaccurate concept of the seriousness of the situation. Explain that by accepting help no one is in any way admitting weakness. Make sure it is understood that the help (and, therefore, the patient's dependency) is only temporary and that as soon as things are under control the patient may be needed to help someone else.
- Identify high-risk patients: the elderly, children, the bereaved, those with prior psychiatric illness, those with multiple stresses, those with low or no support systems, those from low socioeconomic backgrounds, and those with severe injuries. Target these people for immediate crisis intervention care.
- Identify people who are in a unique position to help people in need, and recruit them for psychological emergency care.
- Arrange for all those involved in the disaster—including rescuers—to get good follow-up care and support.

CASE STUDY FOLLOW-UP

SCENE SIZE-UP

You have been dispatched to the Firebird Raceway, where two race cars have crashed into a bleacher. As you arrive at the raceway, you perform a quick scene size-up. Raceway officials have extinguished the fires caused by the race cars. However, many people have been seriously burned. You decide the scene is safe to enter. You see bystanders are trying to give aid to the injured on the unstable bleachers. Using your vehicle's PA system, you direct the bystanders off the bleachers. You tell them rescue personnel will be here in moments.

Your local plan has predesignated you the incident manager during an MCI or disaster. You estimate at least fifty patients and begin to establish a mobile command sector within a safe range of the crash. Next you and your partner, Judy Eibers, put on sector officer identification vests and set up the EMS command center flag.

You confirm with dispatch the nature of the event, the precise location, and your best estimate of the total number of patients. You also request at least twenty ambulances. Because many of the patients appear entangled in the metal bleachers you request at least ten rescue units with medium to heavy extrication equipment. This may be more equipment and vehicles than you need, but you know it is better to have too many resources than not enough.

In preparation for arriving vehicles, equipment, and personnel you establish an extrication sector, a treatment sector, a transportation sector, a staging sector, a supply sector, and a triage sector.

Using your vehicle as the mobile command sector, you contact incoming units and begin assigning an officer to each sector.

INITIAL ASSESSMENT AND TRIAGE

While you are busy communicating with incoming emergency personnel, Judy has started initial triage. Using a bullhorn, she directs those patients who are able to walk (priority 3) to a safe area away from the bleachers. She counts at least ten people who are able to walk away. She knows that, for now, these patients have adequate airways and circulation. Additional EMT-Bs arrive and assist in rapidly assessing and classifying the remaining patients. Fortunately, you have enough personnel to manage the priority 1 patients, many of whom have severe burns and airway problems.

SUPPLY AND EXTRICATION SECTORS

While the initial triage phase continues, you work closely with the supply and extrication officers who have been assigned to determine the amount of medical materials and extrication equipment necessary to render care. The supply and extrication officers then direct personnel and equipment to where the need is greatest during the initial triage phase.

TRIAGE AND TREATMENT SECTORS

The initial triage is complete. You next work closely with Vinnie Lorenzo, the triage officer, to separate the triaged patients into treatment groups based on the priority tags attached to each patient. Unfortunately, there have been ten deaths. You know that some MCI systems classify these as priority 0 or 4. In your system, the dead are considered priority 3, as are the patients who were able to walk away from the bleachers.

Vinnie directs a total of thirty patients to the treatment sector. There, Harriet Lerner, the treatment officer, reassesses the patients to determine if there have been any changes in patient condition. She determines that several priority 2 patients have inadequate breathing. She directs these patients to the priority 1 treatment sector. Priority 1 patients are cared for and transported first. In the priority 1 treatment sector there are five patients with inadequate airways and severe burns. Harriet Lerner consults with the supply sector officer to request more blood pressure cuffs, bandages, and oxygen. The remaining twenty-five patients are classified as priority 2 patients and are moved to the priority 2 treatment sector. Some of these patients are suffering from burns without airway problems. Many have multiple bone and back injuries, with or without spinal cord damage.

STAGING AND TRANSPORTATION

The staging officer, Harold Walters, has been working closely with Harriet Lerner of the treatment sector to determine the number and priority of patients in need of transport. Walters has kept a record of the number of available ambulances and EMS personnel. Meanwhile, the transportation officer, John Bukowski, has consulted with the receiving hospitals to determine the number of available beds and to make sure the hospitals have called in additional medical personnel.

Bukowski contacts Walters and requests three ambulances respond to the priority 1 treatment sector. All five patients with severe burns and inadequate breathing are then transported to the appropriate hospitals. Because of heavy radio communications,

EMT-Bs transporting priority 1 patients do not contact the hospital. Bukowski provides patient information and estimated times of arrival. Once the priority 1 patients are released to hospital personnel, the ambulances return with more medical supplies to the staging area.

Bukowski next requests thirteen more ambulances from Walters, the staging officer. Walters directs the ambulances to the priority 2 treatment sectors in a staggered sequence so as to not overload the treatment areas. Priority 2 patients are transported to the appropriate area hospitals.

Again, transporting EMT-Bs do not contact the receiving hospitals. Maintaining only essential communications, John Bukowski has informed the receiving hospitals of only the number of patients and each patient's chief complaint.

Finally, Bukowski requests five ambulances from Harold Walters in staging to transport the remaining ten priority 3 patients. Walters directs the ambulances to the priority 3 treatment sector. As incident manager, you keep a skeleton crew of EMT-Bs to assist in clean-up and scene restoration. You direct remaining EMS personnel to the receiving hospitals to assist in further patient care.

Thoroughly exhausted from managing the MCI at Firebird, you make sure to take time to have something nourishing to eat and to rest for a bit. An MCI is an incredibly stressful experience. Both you, as incident manager, and the EMT-Bs providing direct patient care will inevitably be plagued by doubts and second-guessing in the time following the MCI: "Did I make the right triage decision?" "Should I have started CPR?" "How should I have dealt with the mother begging me to care for her dying child?" You know that the best way to minimize these doubts, and the stress they cause, is to routinely practice your MCI plan. Then, when the unexpected happens, as it did at Firebird raceway, you know how to get the right patient, to the right hospital, in the right amount of time.

CHAPTER REVIEW

TERMS AND CONCEPTS

You may wish to review the following terms and concepts included in this chapter.

disaster—a sudden catastrophic event that overwhelms natural order and causes great loss of property and/or life.

EMS incident manager—in most incident management systems, the senior EMT who is first to arrive at a multiple-casualty scene or a predesignated officer, if any. The EMS incident manager is responsible for seeing that the multiple-casualty incident is responded to in a controlled and orderly way and that all responsibilities are carried out.

extrication sector—responsible for freeing patients from wreckage and managing them at the accident site.

incident management system—a written plan to help control, direct, and coordinate emergency personnel at the scene of an MCI.

incident manager—the person in charge of the incident management system at an MCI. The incident manager may be the EMS incident manager or may be from one of the other emergency response agencies. Also called the *incident commander.*

mobile command sector—coordinates the MCI response activities of all sectors and is the headquarters for the incident manager; the EMS command post.

multiple-casualty incident (MCI)—an event that places excessive demands on EMS personnel and equipment.

staging sector—monitors, inventories, and directs available ambulances to the treatment sector at the request of the transportation officer.

supply sector—responsible for inventory and distribution of the medical materials and equipment necessary to render care.

transportation sector—coordinates patient transportation with the triage and staging sectors and its officer communicates with the hospitals involved.

treatment sector—responsible for collecting and treating patients in a centralized treatment area.

triage—the process of sorting patients to determine the order in which they will receive care or transportation to definitive care.

triage sector—responsible for prioritizing patients for emergency medical care and transport.

REVIEW QUESTIONS

1. Name the criteria for determining that an emergency is a multiple-casualty incident.
2. Describe the criteria for choosing an incident manager and list the responsibilities of an incident manager.
3. Define the role of the EMT-Basic in a multiple-casualty incident or a disaster operation.
4. Name the seven sectors of an incident management system and describe their responsibilities.
5. Explain how to perform the initial assessment of a patient during initial triage.
6. Identify the appropriate triage level (in a system with three levels of triage) for each of the fol-

lowing: (a) a patient with inadequate breathing; (b) a patient who is in cardiac arrest with insufficient EMS personnel to provide care; (c) a patient found with a painful, swollen, and deformed forearm; (d) a patient with a laceration to his back.

7. Explain the reasons for using a patient identification or tagging system and give the criteria for a successful patient identification system.
8. List guidelines for effective transport of patients in a multiple-casualty incident.
9. List at least five ways for reducing stress on EMT-Bs during a multiple-casualty incident or disaster operation.

CHAPTER 44

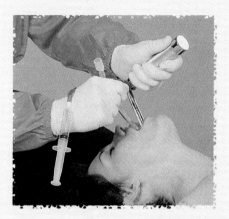

Advanced Airway Management

INTRODUCTION

There are some situations in which manual maneuvers and basic airway adjuncts are not adequate to maintain or possibly even to establish an airway. In those situations, the use of advanced airway adjuncts is necessary.

In the past, performance of advanced airway procedures was reserved for ALS personnel. However, it is the EMT-Basic who is usually first on the scene, and the time required for ALS back-up to arrive and initiate advanced airway care can sometimes spell the difference between life and death for the patient.

For this reason, advanced airway skills are now included as an elective in the EMT-Basic curriculum—to be required of EMT-Bs at the discretion of the medical director. If required in your jurisdiction, you will find learning and maintaining these skills to be challenging but, because they unquestionably offer the opportunity to save lives, well worth the effort.

OBJECTIVES

Numbered objectives are from the United States Department of Transportation 1994 EMT-Basic National Standard Curriculum. Asterisked objectives, if any, pertain to material that is supplemental to the DOT curriculum.

COGNITIVE

8-1.1 Identify and describe the airway anatomy in the infant, child, and the adult. (pp. 881–884)

8-1.2 Differentiate between the anatomy in the infant, child, and the adult. (pp. 883–884)

8-1.3 Explain the pathophysiology of airway compromise. (pp. 881, 883–884)

8-1.4 Describe the proper use of airway adjuncts. (p. 884)

8-1.5 Review the use of oxygen therapy in airway management. (pp. 884, 890, 902, 904)

8-1.6 Describe the indications, contraindications, and technique for insertion of nasal gastric tubes. (pp. 900–902)

8-1.7 Describe how to perform the Sellick maneuver (cricoid pressure). (pp. 889–890)

8-1.8 Describe the indications for advanced airway management. (pp. 885–886)

8-1.9 List the equipment required for orotracheal intubation. (pp. 886–889)

8-1.10 Describe the proper use of the curved blade for orotracheal intubation. (p. 887)

8-1.11 Describe the proper use of the straight blade for orotracheal intubation. (p. 886)

8-1.12 State the reasons for and proper use of the stylet in orotracheal intubation. (pp. 888–889)

8-1.13 Describe the methods of choosing the appropriate size endotracheal tube in an adult patient. (pp. 887–888)

8-1.14 State the formula for sizing an infant or child endotracheal tube. (p. 897)

8-1.15 List complications associated with advanced airway management. (pp. 895–896)

8-1.16 Define the various alternative methods for sizing the infant and child endotracheal tube. (pp. 896–898)

8-1.17 Describe the skill of orotracheal intubation in the adult patient. (pp. 890–895)

8-1.18 Describe the skill of orotracheal intubation in the infant and child patient. (pp. 898–900)

8-1.19 Describe the skill of confirming endotracheal tube placement in the adult, infant, and child patient. (pp. 893–895, 899)

8-1.20 State the consequence of and the need to recognize unintentional esophageal intubation. (pp. 893, 895–896)

8-1.21 Describe the skill of securing the endotracheal tube in the adult, infant, and child patient. (pp. 889, 899)

AFFECTIVE

8-1.22 Recognize and respect the feelings of the patient and family during advanced airway procedures. (p. 884)

8-1.23 Explain the value of performing advanced airway procedures. (pp. 879, 885)

8-1.24 Defend the need for the EMT-Basic to perform advanced airway procedures. (p. 879)

8-1.25 Explain the rationale for the use of a stylet. (p. 888)

8-1.26 Explain the rationale for having a suction unit immediately available during intubation attempts. (p. 889)

8-1.27 Explain the rationale for confirming breath sounds. (pp. 894, 899)

8-1.28 Explain the rationale for securing the endotracheal tube. (pp. 889, 899)

PSYCHOMOTOR

8-1.29 Demonstrate how to perform the Sellick maneuver (cricoid pressure).

8-1.30 Demonstrate the skill of orotracheal intubation in the adult patient.

8-1.31 Demonstrate the skill of orotracheal intubation in the infant and child patient.

8-1.32 Demonstrate the skill of confirming endotracheal tube placement in the adult patient.

8-1.33 Demonstrate the skill of confirming endotracheal tube placement in the infant and child patient.

8-1.34 Demonstrate the skill of securing the endotracheal tube in the adult patient.

8-1.35 Demonstrate the skill of securing the endotracheal tube in the infant and child patient.

CASE STUDY

THE DISPATCH

EMS Unit 206—respond to 3458 LaClede Avenue. You will be responding with the fire department for a three-alarm house fire with possible entrapment. Report to the fire officer in charge. Time out is 1114 hours.

ON ARRIVAL

As you pull up at the fire, you position the ambulance so that it doesn't interfere with the fire apparatus and will allow for rapid exit from the scene. Foul-smelling smoke permeates the air as you step out of the ambulance. You and your partner gather your equipment and are directed by the battalion chief to a stag-ing area safely away from the fire. As you watch the battle against the blaze, you suddenly notice two firefighters struggle out of the thick smoke surrounding the house with a limp body in their arms. You immediately jump to your feet. The firefighters carry the victim a safe distance from the house, and the battalion chief waves you over. As you approach the patient, you note that he is unresponsive and has burns to his face, neck, and upper chest.

How would you proceed to assess and care for this patient?

During this chapter, you will learn about advanced airway management. Later, we will return to this case and apply the procedures learned.

AIRWAY AND RESPIRATORY ANATOMY AND PHYSIOLOGY

The basic anatomy and physiology of the airway and respiratory system have already been discussed in Chapter 4, "The Human Body," Chapter 7, "Airway Management, Ventilation, and Oxygen Therapy," and Chapter 14, "Respiratory Emergencies." However, advanced airway management requires a more detailed understanding of upper airway anatomy, because many anatomical landmarks there must be visualized and identified when performing certain maneuvers. Also, to use various pieces of equipment correctly, it is necessary to understand their relationship to the parts of the upper airway.

AIRWAY ANATOMY

The respiratory system is made up of the upper and lower airway. The upper airway extends from the opening of the nose and mouth down to the larynx. It includes the nasopharynx, oropharynx, and hypopharynx, which is also called the laryngopharynx. The lower airway continues from the inferior (lower) portion of the larynx and consists of the trachea (the "windpipe") and bronchi. The bronchi branch out, tree-like, into the lungs and terminate at the alveoli.

NOSE, MOUTH, AND PHARYNX

The nose is the superior (upper) part of the airway and has several functions: (1) It warms and humidifies the air; (2) it serves as a passageway; and (3) its nasal hairs serve as an initial filter of foreign bodies.

The air entering the nose passes through the nasopharynx, the area of the throat just behind the nose.

The mouth also serves as a conduit for air flow. Air enters the mouth and passes into the oropharynx, the area of the throat just behind the mouth. The reflexes of the oropharynx protect the airway in the responsive patient; however, in the unresponsive patient, the tongue may relax and become an obstruction.

The openings of the esophagus and larynx are at the level of the hypopharynx (or laryngopharynx). The esophagus is an oval, hollow, tube-like structure that lies posterior to (behind) the larynx and trachea. The openings to the esophagus (which leads to the stomach) and the larynx (which is part of the airway to the lungs) are very close together, and this—as you will learn during this chapter—is the reason for a number of the complications involved in establishing an airway and ventilating a patient.

LARYNX

The larynx, which contains the vocal cords and is the major organ of speech, lies inferior to the pharynx and superior to the trachea. It connects and allows air to travel from the pharynx into the trachea. The larynx also contains the thyroid cartilage, the cricoid cartilage, and the epiglottis.

The **thyroid cartilage** is the bulky, shield-like structure commonly known as the Adam's apple that is found at the anterior (front) portion of the neck. The **cricoid cartilage** is a firm circle of cartilage that is located below the thyroid cartilage. The cricoid is attached to the first ring of the trachea. Immediately posterior to the cricoid is the esophagus. When performing advanced airway techniques, it is sometimes useful to occlude, or close off, the esophagus. This can be accomplished by applying pressure directly to the cricoid ring to push it back against the esophagus.

The **epiglottis** is a leaf-shaped cartilaginous structure (consisting of cartilage, a gristle-like tissue) that covers the opening of the larynx during swallowing. When a person swallows, the muscles of the larynx contract and move the epiglottis downward and the larynx upward, closing the opening and preventing food from entering the trachea. A depression that is located between the base of the tongue and the epiglottis is known as the **vallecula.** The **glossoepiglottic ligament,** which helps support and suspend the epiglottis, is found in the center of the vallecula (Figure 44-1). The vallecula and glossoepiglottic ligament are important anatomical structures that are sometimes manipulated to indirectly lift the epiglottis, making it possible to visualize the vocal cords and glottic opening during advanced airway management.

The vocal cords are located in the larynx. The **true vocal cords,** which are normally pale and pearly white, regulate the flow of air into the trachea and produce sounds by vibrating. The space between the true vocal cords is the **glottis** or **glottic opening** (Figure 44-2). It is the glottic area that is covered by the epiglottis during swallowing. The **false vocal**

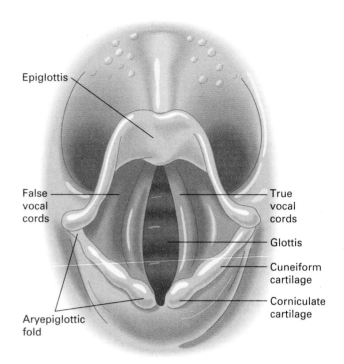

Figure 44-2   *The glottis.*

cords lie above the true vocal cords. The true and false vocal cords can close the glottic opening, preventing air or foreign bodies from entering the trachea. This serves a protective function but can also cause an obstruction by blocking airflow in some conditions.

The larynx also contains three sets of paired cartilages (Figure 44-2). The **arytenoids** are irregular, pyramid-shaped structures located on the top of the posterior aspect of the cricoid ring. The **corniculates** are cone-shaped and are attached to the top of the arytenoids. The **cuneiforms** are more elongated and are attached to the posterior arytenoids. These structures are extremely important in advanced airway maneuvers where visualization of the glottic opening is required.

As noted above, the openings of the larynx and of the esophagus are in close proximity, making incorrect placement of an endotracheal tube a common error. It is also a *serious* error. Inadvertent placement of an endotracheal tube in the esophagus instead of the trachea means that the stomach rather than the lungs will receive the air during ventilation.

Fortunately, the cartilaginous structures described above provide landmarks to differentiate the opening of the larynx from that of the esophagus. One key difference between the two openings is that the esophagus does not have cartilage surrounding its opening as does the larynx. Therefore, before inserting a tube into the larynx, it is imperative to identify the cartilaginous structures and vocal cords to ensure

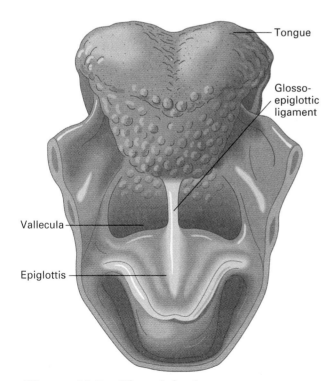

Figure 44-1   *The epiglottis.*

that you are directing the tube into the larynx and trachea, not the esophagus.

TRACHEA AND BRONCHI

The **trachea** extends from the lower portion of the larynx to the bronchi. The trachea has 16 to 20 incomplete C-shaped cartilage rings on its anterior surface that support the airway and prevent it from collapsing. The trachea is shaped like the letter "D" with the straight edge on the posterior side. The C-shaped cartilage rings are joined together by fibrous and elastic tissue. Posteriorly, the **trachealis muscle,** a muscular wall that closes the C-shaped rings, abuts the esophagus, which lies directly posterior.

At about the level of the fifth thoracic vertebra, the trachea splits into the right and left **mainstem bronchi.** This point, where the right and left mainstem bronchi split from the trachea and enter the right and left lungs, is known as the **carina.** The right mainstem bronchus branches from the trachea at a much lesser angle and appears to be almost in a line with the trachea, whereas the left mainstem bronchus branches at a greater angle. Because of this difference, aspiration of food, liquids, or foreign bodies is far more common on the right side than on the left. More important, the lesser angle makes it easier to misdirect an endotracheal tube into the right mainstem bronchus than in the left if it is advanced too far.

The bronchi continue to subdivide into smaller passages known as the **bronchioles.** The bronchioles terminate at the alveoli, the sacs where gas exchange occurs in the lungs.

LUNGS

The right and left lungs are found in the thoracic (chest) cavity. They are separated by the space called the mediastinum which contains the heart and other structures and tissues. The right lung has three lobes and the left lung has two lobes. The lungs contain the alveoli and supporting tissue. Both lungs are covered by the pleura. The pleura consists of two layers, the inner visceral pleura and the outer parietal pleura. Between the layers of the pleura is a small amount of pleural fluid which acts as a lubricant that reduces friction when the lungs move during respiration. The diaphragm is located at the base of the thoracic cavity and separates the chest from the abdominal cavity. The diaphragm is the major muscle of respiration.

The mechanics and physiology of respiration were discussed in Chapter 4, "The Human Body," and Chapter 7, "Airway Management, Ventilation, and Oxygen Therapy."

AIRWAY ANATOMY IN INFANTS AND CHILDREN

There are considerable differences between the airways of adults and those of infants and children. These differences are important to remember when performing advanced airway maneuvers.

HEAD

The head of an infant is much larger in proportion to its body than that of an adult. Because the head is larger, especially the occiput (back of the head), when an infant is placed in a supine position its head tilts forward, flexing the neck and constricting the airway structures. Placing padding under the head in children less than 9 years of age may cause an airflow obstruction. For infants and young children, in fact, it may be necessary to place a small folded towel under the shoulders to keep the airway aligned and assure airflow.

MOUTH, NOSE, AND PHARYNX

In general, all of the structures in these areas are smaller and more pliable in infants and children and thus more easily obstructed by secretions, foreign objects, and swelling. The infant is basically a nose breather during much of his first year because of the more superior location of the epiglottis and anterior location of the larynx, so obstruction of the nasal passages is especially critical.

The most common cause of airway obstruction in the infant or young child is the tongue falling back and blocking the pharynx. This is an even greater problem in infants and children than in adults because the child's tongue is larger in proportion to the mouth and pharynx and the jaw is less prominent. When the muscles of the pharynx relax, the tongue is pulled back like a valve during inspiration, causing an obstruction. The larger tongue also interferes with visualization of anatomical structures during endotracheal intubation.

LARYNX

The airway of the infant and child is narrowest at the level of the cricoid cartilage. Also, that cartilage is less developed and less rigid than in adults. This is especially important to keep in mind during endotracheal intubation. The tube may pass easily through the vocal cords but be too large to fit through the cricoid ring. Therefore, it is necessary to have tubes available that are at least one half-size larger and smaller than the one you estimate is correctly sized when performing this procedure. Pressure on the cricoid and overextension or overflexion of the neck can cause an obstruction.

TRACHEA AND BRONCHI

The major airways are narrower and shorter in infants and children. The trachea is also softer and more flexible. This means that the airway can be more easily occluded by swelling and other obstructions or kinked by flexion or extension of the neck. Small movements of the head or neck may also cause an endotracheal tube to advance into the right mainstem bronchus or out of the glottis in infants and children.

CHEST WALL AND DIAPHRAGM

The chest wall in infants and children is softer and more flexible than in adults. Infants and children also have a tendency to rely more heavily on the diaphragm for breathing.

BASIC AIRWAY MANAGEMENT

One of the situations in which advanced airway management techniques are of great use is when prolonged ventilation of a patient becomes necessary. Some advanced airways reduce problems of poor mask seal and of hand fatigue from holding a mask seal for a prolonged period or performing one- or two-handed bag-valve ventilation. Before using advanced airway management, however, you must first be able to determine whether a patient is breathing adequately or inadequately.

Methods of assessing for adequate or inadequate breathing were discussed in Chapter 7, "Airway Management, Ventilation, and Oxygen Therapy," and Chapter 14, "Respiratory Emergencies."

The first step in airway management is to establish a patent airway by using a manual maneuver. The head-tilt, chin-lift maneuver is used in the patient with no suspected spinal injury. The jaw-thrust is used in a trauma patient or any patient with suspected spinal injury. If any blood, secretions, vomitus, or other substances are in the airway, you must suction them immediately to prevent aspiration. Two basic mechanical airway adjuncts, the oropharyngeal and the nasopharyngeal airways, can be inserted to help maintain the airway. You can review these basic methods of establishing and maintaining an airway in Chapter 7, "Airway Management, Ventilation, and Oxygen Therapy."

It is important to note that basic airway techniques must be employed prior to advanced airway management. There are some conditions where immediate use of an advanced airway technique is necessary, as in upper airway burns and in anaphylaxis, where swelling of the larynx requires immediate insertion of a tube through the larynx and into the trachea. In most situations, however, if the basic steps of airway management and ventilation are omitted and advanced procedures performed instead, the patient can become dangerously hypoxic and suffer irreversible consequences.

For the most part, advanced airway management techniques are used for the following reasons: when it is necessary to protect the patient from aspiration of secretions, blood, or vomitus; when prolonged ventilation by the EMT-B is necessary; or when basic airway management techniques are not adequate. Remember, though, that in these situations, the airway is initially controlled with basic techniques while the patient is being hyperventilated and oxygenated and the necessary equipment is being prepared.

Although advanced airway management is often performed under highly stressful circumstances when the patient's life is threatened by the compromised or potentially compromised airway, bear in mind that airway management procedures can be extremely frightening to the patient (if responsive) or to the patient's family. If possible, offer reassurance by explaining what you are doing and why.

OROPHARYNGEAL SUCTIONING

Before any advanced airway techniques are used, it is necessary to remove any secretions, blood, vomitus, or other substances from the oropharynx with suction. If you hear a gurgling sound during ventilation, it is an indication that some liquid is in the airway and should be suctioned immediately. Some suction units cannot adequately remove heavy vomitus or solid objects, such as teeth, from the airway. You may have to sweep the mouth with your finger, a tongue blade, or the end of the rigid suction catheter to remove the vomitus or object.

A variety of suction units exist. It is vital that a portable suction unit, either electrical or hand operated, be available during airway management, especially when advanced airway procedures are to be performed. Hard, or rigid, suction catheters are used when suctioning the mouth and oropharynx. Soft, or French, suction catheters are useful for suctioning the nose and nasopharynx. Soft suction catheters are also used in clearing secretions from the trachea once an endotracheal tube is in place (a technique that will be discussed later in this chapter). Also note that as the lower structures are visualized, further suctioning may be required. To review oropharyngeal suctioning, refer to Chapter 7, "Airway Management, Ventilation, and Oxygen Therapy."

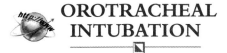

OROTRACHEAL INTUBATION

Orotracheal intubation (from *oro,* meaning "mouth," and *tracheal,* referring to the trachea) is the insertion of a tube through the mouth and along the oropharynx and larynx directly into the trachea. Because the distal end of the tube is designed to be placed in the trachea, it is referred to as an **endotracheal tube** (from *endo* meaning "into," and *tracheal* referring to the trachea). The process of inserting the tube is known as **intubation.** The terms *orotracheal intubation* and *endotracheal intubation* are often used almost interchangeably.

Orotracheal intubation requires the EMT-B to visualize anatomical landmarks with the use of a device called a **laryngoscope.** The laryngoscope, equipped with a light to aid in visualization, is inserted into the mouth and down into the pharynx. It is used to lift, either directly or indirectly, the epiglottis and to expose the vocal cords and glottic opening. The endotracheal tube is then passed through the vocal cords and directly into the trachea.

Visualization of the endotracheal tube as it enters and passes through the vocal cords is extremely important to reduce the risk of improper placement in the esophagus. The EMT-B must be completely familiar with techniques of properly placing the endotracheal tube and must also be able to differentiate immediately between a tracheal intubation and an esophageal intubation. If a tube is inadvertently placed in the esophagus, the patient's lungs will receive no ventilation or oxygen and the patient will die.

ADVANTAGES

Endotracheal intubation is the most effective means of controlling the patient's airway. The following advantages make endotracheal intubation the preferred method for controlling the airway in the apneic patient (patient who is not breathing):

- It provides complete control of the airway. The endotracheal tube is placed into the trachea, establishing a direct route of ventilation and oxygenation. The tongue no longer threatens airway occlusion, so it is not necessary to maintain a head-tilt, chin-lift or jaw-thrust, providing some relief for the EMT-B.
- The endotracheal tube is designed to isolate the trachea, eliminating the risk of aspiration of material into the lower airways and lungs. Secretions, blood, vomitus, and other substances are blocked by the endotracheal tube in the upper portion of the trachea and pharynx and kept from traveling farther. The substances can then be removed by suction.

- The endotracheal tube permits better ventilation and oxygen delivery. The bag-valve device is connected directly to the endotracheal tube, thus allowing more effective ventilation because air goes directly into the trachea and lungs. Because no mask seal is required, only one EMT-B is needed to perform two-handed bagging. Also, hazards associated with air entering the esophagus and subsequently the stomach are eliminated since the tube directs ventilation into the trachea and lungs.
- A suction catheter can be passed through the endotracheal tube to allow for deeper suctioning of the trachea and bronchi. This removes secretions that the patient may not have been able to eliminate otherwise and effectively clears the airway.
- The endotracheal tube with positive pressure ventilation can overcome both mechanical and physiologic problems that compromise normal ventilation.

INDICATIONS

Not every patient requires endotracheal intubation. It should be used only under certain conditions. Indications for its use include the following:

- *The EMT-B is unable to ventilate the apneic patient effectively with standard methods such as mouth-to-mask or bag-valve mask.* Establishing a good mask seal may be very difficult in some patients, especially those with trauma to the mouth or jaws. Sealing the mask may also be difficult in patients who have no teeth or dentures. Finally, a good seal will be difficult to maintain during a long transport.
- *The patient cannot protect his own airway.* This includes patients who are unresponsive or in cardiac arrest. Whenever you determine that a patient is unable to protect his own airway, he should be intubated with an endotracheal tube. The patient who cannot protect his own airway is the patient who:
  - *Is unresponsive to any type of stimulus*—In a completely unresponsive patient, the muscles that control the tongue and epiglottis relax and easily occlude the airway. The patient cannot clear blood, vomitus, secretions, and other substances from his airway, and the risk of aspiration is high.
  - *Has no gag reflex or loses the cough reflex*—The gag and cough reflexes are very important in protecting the airway against foreign body occlusion and aspiration. The loss of these reflexes leaves the airway extremely vulnerable to blockage or foreign body aspiration.

As a general rule, if you are able to insert an oropharyngeal airway in the patient without incident, you can assume that he has lost his gag reflex and cannot protect his airway; he is, therefore, a good candidate for endotracheal intubation. Since the patient is unable to protect his own airway, have a suction device ready in case of vomiting. Be sure to provide adequate ventilation and oxygenation before any attempt at endotracheal intubation.

BODY SUBSTANCE ISOLATION

When performing endotracheal intubation, the EMT-B must get extremely close to the patient's open mouth and visualize deep into the airway. Contact with the patient's secretions, vomitus, and/or blood is likely during intubation. Put on gloves, eye protection, and a mask before attempting the procedure to avoid contact with body fluids.

EQUIPMENT

Several pieces of equipment are required for endotracheal intubation. Be sure to check that the equipment is in proper working order before any attempt at intubation. The equipment needed for intubation includes the following:

- Laryngoscope (handle and blades)
- Endotracheal tube
- Stylet
- Water-soluble lubricant
- 10 cc syringe
- Endotracheal tube securing device
- Suction unit
- Towels or padding
- Stethoscope

LARYNGOSCOPE

The **laryngoscope** is inserted in the mouth and then into the hypopharynx where it is used to lift the epiglottis and provide visualization of the vocal cords and glottic opening. This procedure is known as **laryngoscopy.** Laryngoscopes may be reusable or disposable.

The laryngoscope has two components: the handle and the blade. The laryngoscope handle is a cylindrical device that contains batteries as a source of power. During intubation, the EMT-B holds the laryngoscope handle in his left hand and uses it to control the laryngoscope blade. The laryngoscope blade is the component that directly or indirectly lifts the epiglottis for visualization during intubation. A locking bar and fitting at the top of the handle serve as the connecting point with the blade. A bulb is located in the distal third of the blade and serves as a light source to permit visualization of the glottic opening and the vocal cords. Fiber-optic laryngoscope handles have the light source in the handle and a fiber-optic strand in the blade to provide a bright light.

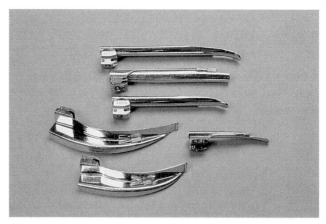

Figure 44-3 Straight and curved laryngoscope blades.

There are two types of laryngoscope blades available: the **straight blade** (Miller, Wisconsin, or Flagg) or the **curved blade** (McIntosh) (Figure 44-3). The name of the blade describes its shape. Both types of blades can lift the epiglottis, but each type does this differently. The choice of blade type is basically a matter of personal preference.

Straight Blade   The straight blade is straight at the distal end and has a more rounded edge. The blade is narrower than the curved blade and has a hollow central channel. The straight blade comes in a variety of sizes ranging from 0, the smallest, to 4, the largest. A size 0 blade would be used on an infant, whereas a size 4 would be used to intubate a large adult.

The end or distal edge of the straight blade is fitted under the epiglottis and directly lifts it to expose the vocal cords and glottic opening (Figure 44-4a). During insertion, the rounded part of the blade is used to push the tongue over to the left side as the blade is brought into the midline of the mouth and oropharynx. The top of the straight blade is then used to gently lift the tip of the epiglottis. The hollow channel is used as a sight as the endotracheal tube is placed between the vocal cords and into the glottic opening. The channel is *not* used to advance the tube. Attempts to force the endotracheal tube through the straight blade channel will likely result in damage to the tube. If the tube is damaged, it is necessary to remove it and repeat the intubation process. During this time, the patient's airway is not protected.

The straight blade is the preferred blade for performing intubation in infants and children. Because of the anatomical differences, the straight blade provides greater displacement of the tongue and allows for better visualization of the vocal cords and glottic opening and causes less tissue damage in this age group. The straight blade is also preferred in larger patients with short, thick necks.

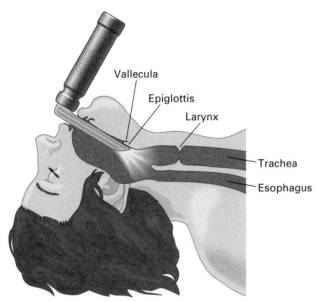

Figure 44-4a   The straight blade is placed under the epiglottis. It directly lifts the epiglottis upward to expose the vocal cords and glottic opening.

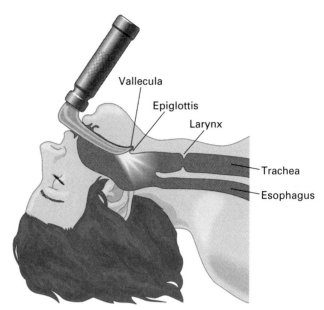

Figure 44-4b   The curved blade is placed into the vallecula and indirectly lifts the epiglottis.

Curved Blade   The curved blade is curved at the distal end and has a beaded or blunt edge. The blade has a broad surface and tall flange that is used to move and hold the tongue out of the way during intubation (Figure 44-4b). The curved blade also comes in a variety of sizes ranging from 0 for the infant to 4 for the large adult.

The beaded end of the curved blade is inserted into the vallecula, the space located between the epiglottis and base of the tongue. When the edge of the blade is placed in the vallecula it presses on the glossoepiglottic ligament, causing the epiglottis to be indirectly lifted upward and exposing the vocal cords and glottic opening.

Assembly   The indentation on the laryngoscope blade is designed to lock onto the bar of the laryngoscope handle. The blade is lifted upward so it is at a right angle to the handle. The electrical connection is then made and the bulb at the end of the blade is lit. Check to be sure that it is on. The light should be tight, bright, and white. If it is not, check that the blade is securely locked. Also, the bulb must be tightly screwed into the socket of the blade. If the bulb is loose, tighten it. If the light is not bright and white, it may be necessary to change the batteries in the handle. It is best to always have an extra bulb and batteries available in case of failure.

In fiber-optic laryngoscope handles and blades, the fiber-optic light source is located in the handle. The blade contains a fiber-optic strand, rather than a bulb, to provide illumination at the end of the blade.

This provides a brighter light source for visualizing the glottic structures.

ENDOTRACHEAL TUBES

The endotracheal tube is a flexible translucent tube made of polyvinyl chloride that is open at both ends. Endotracheal tubes come in a variety of sizes (Figure 44-5). The size noted on the outside of the tube is the tube's internal diameter (i.d.). The external diameter is estimated by adding 2 to 3 mm to the internal

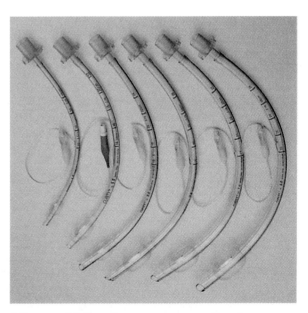

Figure 44-5   An assortment of endotracheal tubes of different sizes.

diameter size. In general, an adult male will require an 8.0 to 8.5 mm i.d. tube and the female adult will take a 7.0 to 8.0 mm i.d. tube. Tube sizes for infants and children range from 2.5 to 6.0 mm i.d.

If you are uncertain what size to use, it is prudent to select a smaller-sized tube. In an emergency, a 7.5 mm i.d. tube will usually fit either an adult male or an adult female. When intubating, it is helpful to have available tubes one size smaller and one size larger than the estimated size.

The endotracheal tube has several components (Figure 44-6). At the proximal end, a 15 mm connector allows attachment of a bag-valve and other ventilation devices. The distal end has a cuff that serves to seal off the trachea. An inflation line extends up the main tube to a pilot balloon that verifies that the cuff is inflated. A one-way inflation valve allows use of a syringe to inflate the cuff. The cuff will hold approximately 10 cc of air. The cuff should be inflated to prevent any leakage of air from around the cuff and the endotracheal tube and between the tube and the tracheal wall. Typically, tubes for infants and children (those less than 6.0 mm i.d.) have no cuff at the distal end and are referred to as uncuffed. Uncuffed tubes are usually used in children younger than 8 years of age, because the narrowest portion of the airway is the cricoid ring and not the vocal cords as in an adult.

At the distal end of the endotracheal tube is a **Murphy eye.** This is a small hole on the side opposite the beveled side. The eye lessens the chance of complete tube obstruction. If the distal end of the tube becomes obstructed by the tracheal wall, blood clots, or secretions, the Murphy eye will still allow air to escape and ventilation to take place.

The length of the tube from the distal end is indicated in centimeter (cm) markings along the tube. The length of the tube for the adult is 33 cm. Following placement of the tube in the adult patient, the 22 cm marker is typically at the level of the teeth. This is only a general rule and does not apply to all patients because of variations in their sizes. Other standard measurements are: 15 cm from the teeth to

the vocal cords; 20 cm from the teeth to the sternal notch; and 25 cm from the teeth to the carina.

The measurements are helpful, but you must rely on good clinical assessment skills to determine that the tube is properly placed. When properly placed, the distal tip of the endotracheal tube is in the trachea and midway between the carina and the vocal cords. The tip of the tube must not extend past the carina. If the tube is inserted beyond the carina, it will most likely enter the right mainstem bronchus (because it is straighter and at a lesser angle from the trachea than the left mainstem bronchus) and only ventilate the right lung. This is referred to as a **right mainstem intubation,** a common complication of endotracheal intubation.

Once you verify that the tube is correctly placed, it is extremely important to note the centimeter level marking on the tube at the teeth. If at any time the level marking has changed, it is an indication that the tube has been inserted deeper or has been pulled back. *You must then immediately reassess tube placement.* The tube can move and become dislodged and end up either in the right mainstem bronchus if pushed farther down or, worse, in the esophagus if pulled upward. Close and continuous reassessment of tube placement is necessary.

STYLET

The malleable **stylet** is a piece of pliable metal wire, typically coated with plastic, that is inserted into the endotracheal tube to alter its shape and provide stiffness (Figure 44-7). The stylet should be lubricated with a water-soluble jelly prior to insertion in the tube to facilitate easy removal. The stylet should not be inserted beyond the Murphy eye and should never extend or project out of the distal end of the endotracheal tube. This could lead to severe trauma to the airway and trachea. The end of the stylet must be recessed at least one-half inch from the distal end of the tube. To ensure proper stylet position, recess the stylet at least one-quarter inch from the cuff or proximal end of the Murphy eye. Once the stylet is in place, it can be used to form the tube into a "hockey stick" shape. This aids in proper insertion of the en-

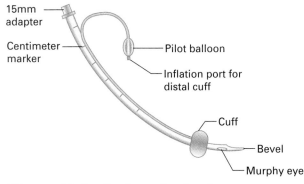

Figure 44-6   Endotracheal tube components.

15mm adapter

Centimeter marker

Pilot balloon

Inflation port for distal cuff

Cuff

Bevel

Murphy eye

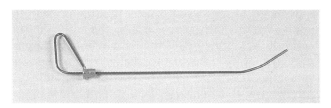

Figure 44-7   The stylet is inserted into the tube to provide stiffness and shape the tube. It should not extend past the end of the tube.

dotracheal tube. After the tube is passed through the vocal cords, the stylet is carefully removed. While removing the stylet, hold the tube securely to avoid accidentally dislodging it.

OTHER INTUBATION EQUIPMENT

Water-soluble lubricant is applied to the end of the endotracheal tube to facilitate insertion into the trachea. Also, lubricant is applied to the stylet to allow for easy removal. Tube displacement may result from pulling out a stylet that is not lubricated. Do not use petroleum-based lubricants. These may cause damage to the endotracheal tube and can irritate and inflame the tracheal lining.

A 10 cc syringe is used to inflate the cuff at the distal end of the endotracheal tube. Prior to insertion, check the cuff to ensure it is working properly by injecting 10 cc of air into the inflation port. It is then necessary to deflate the cuff completely by pulling back on the plunger of the syringe while pushing against the one-way inflation valve before inserting the tube. During intubation, leave the syringe attached to the inflation port. Once the tube is in place, use the syringe to inflate the cuff, and then immediately remove the syringe. The cuff can deflate if the syringe is left attached. Assess cuff inflation by checking the volume of air in the pilot balloon. Being able to seal the trachea through cuff inflation is a primary advantage of the endotracheal tube. Monitor constantly to ensure that inflation is maintained. Keep the syringe close by, since readjustment of the cuff may be needed.

Once the endotracheal tube is properly positioned, you must secure it. Movement of the patient or attachment or removal of the ventilation device can cause the tube to become dislodged and end up in the esophagus or mainstem bronchus. The cuff on the endotracheal tube seals the trachea; it does not secure the tube in place. There are, however, a variety of devices available to do this job. You can employ an elaborate commercial device or simply use tape. Follow your local protocol or medical direction's advice for securing the tube.

The endotracheal tube is flexible enough so that if the patient should bite down or clench his teeth, the tube will be crimped and occluded. An oral airway or bite block should be inserted to avoid this problem, especially if the patient begins breathing on his own or becomes more responsive after being intubated.

A suction unit must be available during endotracheal intubation to clear any fluid, vomitus, blood, secretions, or debris from the oral cavity. A large-bore catheter is needed for suctioning the oropharynx. Once the patient is intubated, a flexible French catheter is used for endotracheal suction (as will be described later).

Towels may be placed under the patient's shoulders or back of the head to raise these areas as needed to align the airway axis for easier visualization during intubation. In patients with suspected spinal injury, you must maintain stabilization of the head in a neutral, in-line position during intubation.

SELLICK'S MANEUVER (CRICOID PRESSURE)

A major complication in both basic and advanced airway management is regurgitation and aspiration of vomitus. Also, during positive pressure ventilation, some air may be forced into the esophagus and stomach causing gastric distention. This increases the risk of regurgitation and may impede effective ventilation.

Sellick's maneuver, also known as **cricoid pressure,** is a technique used during intubation in which slight pressure, directed posteriorly, is applied to the cricoid cartilage. The esophagus lies directly behind the cricoid cartilage; thus, backward pressure on the cricoid cartilage closes off the esophagus. This reduces the amount of air traveling down the esophagus and into the stomach and decreases the chance of vomitus coming up the esophagus and into the airway. This technique should be used in unresponsive patients who do not have a gag or cough reflex to help prevent regurgitation and aspiration during endotracheal intubation.

Another advantage of cricoid pressure is that it pushes the glottic structures into the visual field during intubation. A further advantage is that the endotracheal tube can be felt passing beneath the thumb and index finger, which is another way of confirming correct placement of the tube.

The cricoid cartilage is circumferentially cartilaginous, meaning that it is composed of a complete ring of cartilage. The cricoid cartilage is located inferior to the thyroid cartilage (Adam's apple) and the cricothyroid membrane. To find the cricoid cartilage, palpate the thyroid cartilage with the tip of your finger until you find a depression at the inferior edge. This depression is the cricothyroid membrane. Immediately below the cricothyroid membrane is a prominent bulky ring: the cricoid cartilage.

A third rescuer should locate and apply cricoid pressure while two rescuers are performing the main tasks of spinal stabilization (if necessary) and ventilation. To perform Sellick's maneuver, place the index finger and thumb of one hand on the anterior aspect just lateral to the midline of the cricoid cartilage. Then apply firm backward pressure (Figure 44-8). Maintain the pressure until the endotracheal tube is placed in the trachea and the cuff is inflated and tube placement verified.

Application of backward pressure to upper airway structures other than the cricoid cartilage can cause

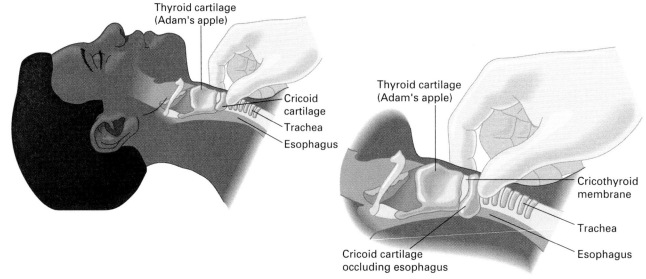

Figure 44-8   To carry out Sellick's maneuver, locate the cricoid cartilage inferior to the thyroid cartilage (Adam's apple). Apply firm posterior pressure with the thumb and index finger.

damage. Be sure that you are completely familiar with the correct anatomy and landmarks associated with the maneuver. It may be difficult to locate the cricoid cartilage in infants, children, and small adults. Tracheal collapse and occlusion may occur in infants if excessive pressure is applied during the maneuver.

A single rescuer should be dedicated to applying cricoid pressure. In some situations, the patient may need immediate advanced airway intervention, and time may not be available to apply cricoid pressure. Remember, use cricoid pressure only if enough personnel are available and the patient's condition permits it.

ENDOTRACHEAL TUBE INSERTION IN AN ADULT

When properly placed, the endotracheal tube is the ultimate airway. However, if it is misplaced, the tube can contribute to rapid deterioration and death. You must become completely competent in orotracheal intubation during your training program. As a certified EMT-B, you must continuously review and practice the technique. This is one of the most critical and complicated skills that you will learn to perform.

The steps for orotracheal intubation are as follows (Figures 44-9a to g):

1. The person performing the intubation should take the necessary body substance isolation precautions, including gloves, eye protection, and a mask.
2. Prior to any intubation attempt, the patient must be adequately ventilated with a bag-valve-mask device and supplemental oxygen.

3. Begin hyperventilating the patient at a rate of 24 breaths per minute for at least 1 to 2 minutes before the intubation attempt.
4. Gather the necessary equipment for inserting and securing the tube, assemble it, and test it.
   a. Test the cuff on the endotracheal tube by injecting 10 cc of air into the inflation port with a syringe and feeling the cuff to ensure that it is inflated fully and does not automatically deflate. Then deflate the cuff by withdrawing all of the air with the syringe. Leave the syringe attached to the inflation port. The endotracheal tube should be kept in its packaging if possible while checking the cuff to avoid any unnecessary contamination.
   b. Assemble the laryngoscope blade and handle. Lift the blade to illuminate the bulb and check the brightness. Also check the bulb to ensure that it is tight and will not become dislodged during the intubation.
   c. If a stylet is to be used, lubricate it with a water-soluble lubricant and insert it into the tube. Check the distal end of the stylet to ensure that it is not projecting out of the endotracheal tube and is recessed adequately.
   d. Lubricate the distal end of the endotracheal tube with a water-soluble lubricant.
   e. Have a suction unit equipped with a large-bore catheter available. Check to make sure that the suction unit works adequately.
   f. Prepare the device that will be used to secure the tube in place.
5. Position yourself at the patient's head. The endotracheal tube and suction unit should be on your right and the laryngoscope on your left.

6. The patient's head must be positioned properly to permit maximum visualization of the vocal cords and glottic opening. The position of the head will depend on whether or not a spinal injury is suspected.

   – *No Spinal Injury Suspected:* Tilt the head backward and lift the chin forward into a "sniffing position." Do not hang the head over the end of a table or bed. If visualization is unsuccessful, it may be necessary to reposition the head. You can place folded towels of approximately one inch thickness under the shoulders or under the back of head to adjust flexion or extension as necessary. The desired position aligns the mouth, pharynx, and trachea and permits better visualization during intubation.

   – *Suspected Spinal Injury:* If a spinal injury is suspected, maintain in-line spinal stabilization throughout the intubation procedure. One EMT-B should hold the head and neck stable from below while the EMT-B who is to intubate secures the head and neck with his thighs (Figure 44-9d). The limited ability to align the head and neck will make visualization more difficult.

7. Stop ventilation and remove the oropharyngeal airway if one has been used. Ventilation must not be interrupted for more than 30 seconds while intubating. The 30-second period begins when positive pressure ventilation is stopped and ends when ventilation is resumed following placement of the tube. If you cannot intubate within 30 seconds, stop the procedure and immediately resume hyperventilating the patient. After a few minutes of hyperventilation, try again to intubate.

8. If enough personnel are available, one EMT-B should apply Sellick's maneuver (cricoid pressure) to reduce the possibility of regurgitation during the intubation procedure. Backward pressure on the cricoid and thyroid cartilage moves the glottic opening slightly posterior and may make visualization of the vocal cords easier.

9. Hold the laryngoscope in your left hand and insert the blade into the right corner of the mouth. You may need to use a crossed-finger (scissors-type) technique to separate the teeth, using the thumb and index finger of the right hand. Move the blade to the midline, sweeping the tongue to the left to allow for more room and better visualization. Advance the blade to the base of the tongue and place it in the proper position, depending on the type of blade used:

   – *Curved blade:* The tip of the curved blade is inserted into the vallecula (the indentation between the base of the tongue and the epiglottis)

   – *Straight blade:* The tip of the straight blade is placed under the epiglottis.

The handle and blade are lifted up and forward, away from the patient's teeth and gums and in the direction of the laryngoscope handle. Do not angle the handle backward in a prying motion or use the teeth as a fulcrum; such actions could cause trauma to the airway and teeth. Do not use a digging motion with the blade and handle in trying to expose the glottic opening. The movement should be smooth and controlled. Exposure should be achieved in three easy movements of the blade: (1) insert the blade in the right corner of the mouth, sweeping the tongue to the left; (2) advance the blade to the base of the tongue; (3) gently lift up and forward to expose the glottic opening.

When using the straight blade, you may see the epiglottis tip when lifting up and forward. Remember, the straight blade is used to get under the epiglottis and lift it up. Drop the blade down slightly and gently advance the blade farther into the hypopharynx to slip the tip of the blade under the epiglottis. Again lift up and forward to expose the glottic opening. The straight blade can easily be advanced past the glottic structures and into the esophagus. In this case, pull back on the blade and again attempt to visualize the structures.

10. Identify the glottic opening by: (1) cartilaginous structures surrounding it, (2) the fact that it is round—not oval like the esophageal opening, (3) the fact that it contains the vocal cords. Once the vocal cords and glottic opening are identified, do not lose sight of them.

11. Insert the endotracheal tube through the right side of the mouth. Guide the endotracheal tube through the vocal cords. *You must actually visualize the tube passing through the vocal cords.* Continue to insert the tube until the proximal end of the cuff is advanced about one-half to one inch beyond the vocal cords. This should place the tip of the endotracheal tube about halfway between the carina and the vocal cords. This position will allow for some movement of the patient's head and neck without displacement of the tube out of the trachea or into a mainstem bronchus. Typically, the tube marker will be at about 22 cm at the level of the teeth.

If you are using a straight blade, do not attempt to advance the tube through the hollowed out area of the blade. This space is for visualization only and will likely cause a tear in the cuff.

12. Remove the laryngoscope blade and fold the blade down so that it is parallel with the handle. This will shut off the light. Hold the tube firmly at all times until it is properly secured in place.

13. If a stylet was used, remove it gently by pulling back. Hold the tube securely with one hand

OROTRACHEAL INTUBATION

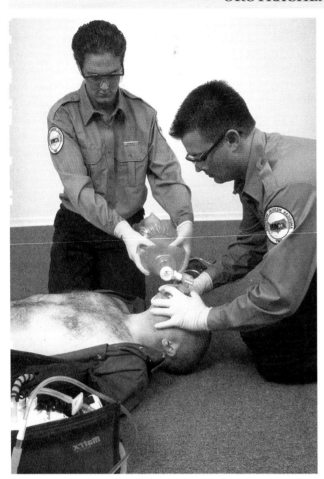

Figure 44-9a Assure adequate ventilation and oxygenation. Prior to any intubation attempt, hyperventilate the patient at a rate of 24 breaths per minute.

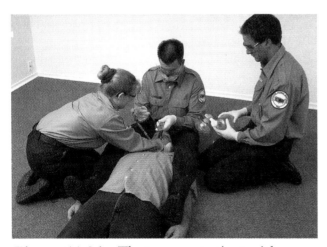

Figure 44-9d The trauma patient with suspected spinal injury must be intubated with in-line spinal stabilization maintained. The EMT-B intubating secures the patient's head with his thighs while the second EMT-B holds the head from a position below the patient's neck.

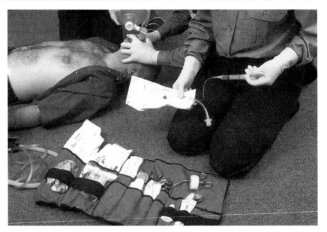

Figure 44-9b Assemble and test the equipment.

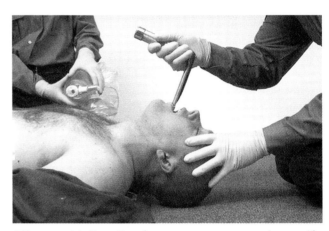

Figure 44-9c In the non-trauma patient, tilt the head and lift the chin into a "sniffing position." Insert the blade on the right and sweep the tongue to the left until the blade is midline.

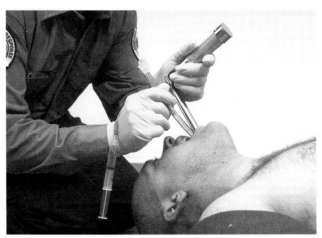

Figure 44-9e Visualize the vocal cords and glottic opening and insert the endotracheal tube through the vocal cords.

OROTRACHEAL INTUBATION continued

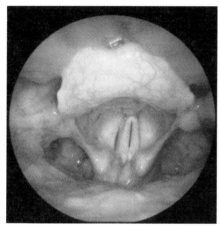

Figure 44-9f   To visualize the glottic opening (shown here), lift the laryngoscope in the direction of the handle.
(Phototake NYC)

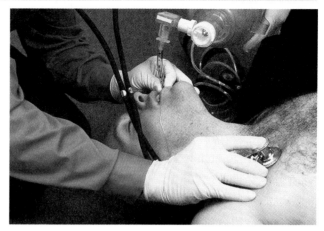

Figure 44-9g   Confirm tube placement.

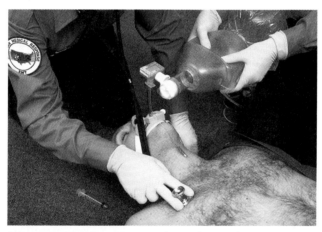

Figure 44-9h   Secure the tube and reassess for tube placement.

while removing the stylet with the other. Pulling the stylet out without holding the tube securely in place may cause accidental **extubation,** removal of the endotracheal tube.

14. With the syringe attached to the inflation port, inflate the cuff by injecting 5 to 10 cc of air. Remove the syringe when you have completed inflation so that the cuff does not deflate.
15. Hold the endotracheal tube in position at all times until it is properly secured. Once the tube is in place, you should not let go of it until after the securing device is applied.
16. Have your partner attach the bag-valve device to the endotracheal tube and begin to deliver positive pressure ventilation.
17. Confirm correct tube placement. *This is one of the most important parts of the intubation process.* You must verify that the tube has been properly

placed in the trachea. As the first ventilation is delivered, you must simultaneously confirm tube placement as follows:
- *Auscultate over the epigastrium.* Gurgling sounds heard while auscultating over the stomach during ventilation are an indication that the tube is improperly placed in the esophagus. Do not deliver any more ventilations, deflate the cuff, and immediately remove the tube. Begin hyperventilating the patient with the bag-valve-mask device at a rate of 24 ventilations per minute. It is common for the patient to vomit after esophageal placement of an endotracheal tube, so have a suction unit ready. Hyperventilate for approximately 2 to 5 minutes and reattempt the intubation. If you are unsuccessful on the second attempt, resume ventilation and contact

medical direction or follow your local protocol to determine if additional intubation attempts should be made.

– *Watch for chest rise and fall during ventilation.*

– *Auscultate breath sounds.* If there are no sounds over the epigastrium and the chest rises with ventilation, auscultate the breath sounds in both lungs. Listen to each apex (top) at about the second intercostal space, midclavicular. Compare the breath sounds heard over the left apex to the sounds over the right apex. Then auscultate at the fourth intercostal space midaxillary and over the bases at about the fourth intercostal space on the anterior side, again comparing the right and left sounds. Breath sounds should be equal on both sides.

If breath sounds are heard on the right, but the breath sounds are diminished or absent on the left, the tube has likely been advanced into the right mainstem bronchus. The problem with a bronchial intubation is that only one lung is being ventilated, which could lead to hypoxia. If a right mainstem intubation is indicated, you should:

a. Deflate the cuff and gently withdraw the tube slightly (1 to 2 cm) while continuing to ventilate the patient and to auscultate for breath sounds on the left side.

b. Be careful not to pull the tube completely out of the trachea. You should pull back on the

tube only enough to restore breath sounds on the left.

c. Once breath sounds become evident on the left, begin to compare the left and right breath sounds. When both sides are equal, reinflate the cuff, secure the tube, and resume positive pressure ventilation.

Other methods that can be used to assess for proper endotracheal tube placement are:

– *Use an end-tidal carbon dioxide detector* (Figure 44-10a) *to measure the concentration of exhaled carbon dioxide.* A lack of carbon dioxide indicates that the tube is improperly placed in the esophagus. There are several different types and models of detectors available, from simple colorimetric devices to more elaborate electronic devices with digital read-out. The end-tidal carbon dioxide detector is used as an adjunct in assessment of endotracheal tube placement, in addition to the methods described above. In some cardiac arrest patients, the extremely low blood flow to the lungs does not produce amounts of carbon dioxide adequate enough to be detected.

– *Use a bulb- or syringe-type esophageal intubation detection device* (Figure 44-10b and c). The function of these devices depends on a key difference between the structure of the trachea and the structure of the esophagus. The trachea is surrounded by rigid cartilage

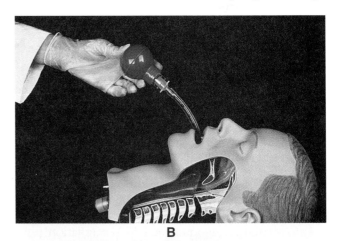

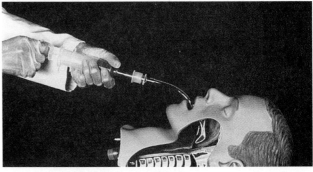

Figure 44-10 **A.** *End-tidal CO$_2$ detector.* (Nellcor Puritan Bennett, Inc.) **B.** *Bulb-type esophageal detection device.* **C.** *Syringe-type esophageal detection device.*

and does not collapse when negative pressure is applied, whereas the esophagus is fibroelastic tissue and collapses easily when negative pressure is applied. The syringe and bulb devices connect to the end of the 15 mm adaptor of the endotracheal tube once the patient has been intubated and the cuff inflated. With the syringe device, the plunger is pulled back. If air enters the syringe, you can assume that the endotracheal tube has been properly placed in the trachea. If resistance is met, you should suspect that the esophagus has been intubated and is collapsing as negative pressure is applied by the syringe. Remove the tube immediately. Similarly, with the bulb device, the bulb is squeezed and allowed to refill. If the refill is swift, you assume that the tube is properly placed in the trachea. If the bulb refills slowly or doesn't refill at all, you presume that the tube is in the esophagus. Immediately remove the tube and ventilate the patient with a bag-valve-mask device.

- *Note a sudden drop in pulse oximeter reading, which may indicate a misplaced endotracheal tube.* (A pulse oximeter is a device attached to a patient's finger or earlobe that "reads" the oxygen saturation of the blood.) Immediately use conventional methods to assess for proper tube placement.
- *Realize that a patient who begins to deteriorate rapidly, becomes combative, or begins to exhibit cyanosis could be suffering from misplaced endotracheal tube placement.* Again, you should immediately use conventional methods to check tube placement.

18. If no sounds are heard over the epigastrium, the chest rises and falls with each ventilation, and breath sounds are equal bilaterally, the tube should be secured in place with tape or a commercial securing device that has been approved by medical direction. Once the tube has been secured, you should do the following:
   a. Ventilate the patient at the appropriate rate based on his age.
   b. Note the centimeter marking on the endotracheal tube at the level of the teeth. This should be included in your written documentation.
   c. Insert an oral airway or other appropriate device to serve as a bite block.

19. Reassess breath sounds as often as possible. It is necessary to reassess breath sounds following any movement of the patient, including movement of the patient onto a stretcher or out to the ambulance. If breath sounds are heard only on the right after a move, assume a right mainstem intubation and reposition the tube as described

earlier to correct the placement. If no breath sounds are heard but sounds are heard over the epigastrium, suspect an esophageal intubation and immediately stop ventilation, remove the tube, and resume ventilation with the bag-valve-mask device. *If you are uncertain that the tube is properly placed after reassessment, remove it. Remember, an esophageal intubation is lethal; therefore, there is no room for error in judgment. Err to benefit the patient.*

Note: If you were the EMT-B who performed the intubation, it is necessary for you to confirm tube placement. Others, such as first responders or EMT-Bs, can help you to check tube placement, but do not rely on them to confirm your placement; they may lack the necessary training. Likewise, if an inexperienced EMT-B has intubated the patient, you must confirm that the endotracheal tube is properly placed. This is a critical skill that requires repetition and experience to produce true competence.

COMPLICATIONS

Many complications, some severe, can occur from endotracheal intubation. The complications are typically associated with either the laryngoscopy (the lifting of the epiglottis to expose the vocal cords and glottic opening with the laryngoscope) or actual tube placement. Some complications can be lethal if not recognized immediately and corrective action taken; other complications are minor. Some of the more common complications of endotracheal intubation include the following:

- *Hypertension (elevated blood pressure), tachycardia (increased heart rate), and dysrhythmias (irregular heart rhythms)* may result from stimulation of the airway during intubation. These conditions can occur during intubation of an adult patient who is not in cardiac arrest.
- *Bradycardia (decreased heart rate) and hypotension (decreased blood pressure) may be seen in infants and children and some adults,* particularly those who are hypoxic, because of stimulation of the airway during intubation, an opposite response from that in adults. Also, heart rates in infants and children may drop as they become hypoxic. Closely monitor the heart rate during intubation.
- *Trauma to the lips, tongue, gums, teeth, and airway* are frequent complications. The blade, the end of the endotracheal tube, and an improperly positioned stylet projecting from the end of the tube can all perforate soft tissue.
- *Inadequate oxygenation and severe hypoxia can result from prolonged attempts at intubation, those lasting longer than 30 seconds.* The apneic patient has no other source of ventilation and oxygenation

except what you are providing. Cessation of positive pressure ventilation during intubation quickly leads to hypoxia. Three minutes without any ventilation can lead to irreversible brain damage in a patient. Therefore, it is important (a) to hyperventilate the patient before the intubation attempt, (b) not to exceed 30 seconds during an intubation attempt from the time you stop ventilating to the point when you resume ventilation, and (c) to hyperventilate after either proper tube placement or a failed attempt.

- *A right mainstem intubation may result in hypoxia,* because only one lung is being ventilated. Closely assess breath sounds and pull back on the tube until bilateral breath sounds are heard equally.
- *Absence of ventilation or oxygenation will result from misplacement of an endotracheal tube in the esophagus.* This is a lethal complication if it is not immediately recognized and corrected. If an esophageal intubation is suspected, immediately deflate the endotracheal tube cuff, remove the tube, and hyperventilate the patient with the bag-valve-mask device and high-flow oxygen.
- *Vomiting may result from stimulation of the gag reflex during intubation.* Be sure to have a suction device readily available when intubating. If the patient begins to vomit and no spinal injury is suspected, turn him on his side to facilitate removal of the vomitus and suction to clear the airway. Prevention of aspiration should be a high priority.
- *The cuff may leak,* requiring reinflation. If the cuff does not stay inflated, extubation and insertion of a new endotracheal tube will be required.
- *Stimulation of the epiglottis or vocal cords during intubation may cause laryngospasm.* The vocal cords will close completely and not allow air to pass through. The vocal cords will eventually relax and allow air to pass through again. Ventilation with a bag-valve-mask device may be necessary if the cords do not relax immediately.
- *The patient may be accidentally extubated during movement or ventilation.* To avoid accidental extubation, secure the tube adequately and limit any unnecessary pulling or pushing on it. If a bag-valve device is connected to the tube and is being used to ventilate the patient, do not drop it while it is still connected to the tube, as for example when clearing during defibrillation. Dropping the bag-valve device while it is connected to the tube puts the weight of the device directly on the tube, greatly increasing the risk of tube displacement. If you have to clear the patient or interrupt ventilations, remove the bag-valve device from the 15 mm adapter at the end of the tube. Reconnect it when you are ready to resume ventilation. After every interruption, check tube placement by assessing chest rise, breath sounds, and gastric sounds during ventilation.

- *The patient may become responsive enough to extubate himself* following resuscitation or intervention. If the patient makes attempts to remove the tube, reassure the patient and restrain his hands.

OROTRACHEAL INTUBATION IN INFANTS AND CHILDREN

The procedure for orotracheal intubation in infants and children is much the same as in adults. However, there are special considerations with infants and children about when and how to intubate.

INDICATIONS IN INFANTS AND CHILDREN

The airway in an infant or child can usually be managed effectively with the proper manual position and an airway adjunct. Most often, a bag-valve-mask device is all that is needed to ventilate the patient adequately. However, there are some situations where ventilation cannot be properly achieved without endotracheal intubation. Endotracheal intubation for the infant and child should be considered in the following circumstances:

- *Prolonged positive pressure ventilation is required.*
- *Artificial ventilation cannot be delivered adequately when using other airway maneuvers and adjuncts.*
- *The patient is completely apneic.* The patient in respiratory arrest or cardiac arrest should be intubated.
- *The patient is unresponsive, with no gag or cough reflex.* If the unresponsive patient accepts an oropharyngeal airway without gagging, consider endotracheal intubation. The infant or child has the same risk of aspiration as the adult in this circumstance. Endotracheal intubation minimizes the risk of aspiration by sealing off the trachea at the level of the cricoid cartilage. Cricoid pressure can be used to reduce the chances of aspiration during the intubation procedure.

ANATOMICAL CONSIDERATIONS

Additional skill is needed when performing intubation in infants and children because of their anatomical differences from adults. Special considerations related to anatomical differences include the following:

- In general, infants' and children's noses, mouths, and jaws are smaller and their tongues disproportionately larger. This makes visualization of the glottic opening and the vocal cords more difficult.
- Sizing of endotracheal tubes for infants and children is based on the internal diameter of the cricoid cartilage and not the glottic opening. Most

often, endotracheal tubes used in infants and in children less than 8 years of age do not have cuffs; the tubes are sealed by the narrow cricoid cartilage. Therefore, ensuring a proper fit of an endotracheal tube is vital.

- The vocal cords and glottic opening are typically more anterior and cephalad (toward the head), making visualization more difficult. It is difficult to create a single, clear visual plane from the mouth through the pharynx to the glottic opening during intubation.
- Bradycardia may result from stimulation of the airway during your intubation attempt. The onset of bradycardia may limit your intubation attempt to even less than 30 seconds. Infants and children are extremely sensitive to hypoxia, which normally results in bradycardia.

EQUIPMENT FOR INFANTS AND CHILDREN

The same basic equipment is used for intubating adults, infants, and children. However, due to the anatomical differences, the equipment has some variations and must be carefully sized prior to the intubation procedure.

LARYNGOSCOPE HANDLES AND BLADES

The same laryngoscope handle used in adult intubation is also used interchangeably with the infant and child laryngoscope blades. A smaller diameter laryngoscope handle is available, if necessary, for infant intubation. The locking mechanism and assembly are the same as in adult equipment.

A straight laryngoscope blade is preferred in infants because it provides greater displacement of the tongue and better visualization of the glottic opening, which is more anterior and cephalad. It also causes less damage to the soft tissues. The straight blade is fitted under the epiglottis and directly lifts it up and forward to expose the vocal cords and glottic opening. The straight blade comes in sizes from 0 to 4. A size 0 blade is usually used in premature infants, whereas a full-term infant would require a 0 or 1. A size 2 blade is usually used to intubate children from 2 to 8 years old. A size 3 straight blade is typically used in adolescent patients.

The curved blade is preferred in older children because its broader base and flange provide better displacement of the tongue in this age group. Curved blades also come in a size range of 0 to 4. A size 2 curved blade is typically used in 8-to-12-year-olds. A size 3 curved blade is used for 12 year olds and adolescents. The curved blade is inserted into the vallecula and indirectly lifts the epiglottis with an upward and forward movement of the handle.

ENDOTRACHEAL TUBES

When intubating an infant or child, an assortment of tube sizes must be available. Tubes at least one-half size above and below the selected size must be immediately available. The tube should be of uniform diameter and not tapered. It should have centimeter distance markings along its length for use as reference points. Some tubes have a vocal cord marker at the distal end to ensure that the tip of the tube is midway between the carina and the level of the vocal cords.

Endotracheal tubes used in infants and children under age 8 are typically uncuffed, with no inflation cuff at the distal end of the tube (Figure 44-11). The cricoid ring is the narrowest portion of the upper airway in infants and children and serves as a functional cuff to seal off the trachea. Therefore, sizing the tube is extremely critical. Cuffed tubes should be used for children older than 8 years. When a cuffed tube is inserted into the trachea, the proximal end of the cuff is inserted approximately one-half inch beyond the level of the vocal cords, since no vocal cord marker may be available on the tube.

The best, most accurate method of selecting the appropriate size endotracheal tube for infants and children is to refer to a sizing chart. You should carry a copy of the chart or keep one in the airway kit containing the infant and child intubation equipment. A commercially available resuscitation tape can be used to determine the appropriate size endotracheal tube. The tape, which is stretched out alongside the infant or child, has reference areas corresponding to the height of the infant or child.

A formula can also be used to estimate the correct size of endotracheal tube for children older than 1 year of age. The formula is: Tube size = (16 + the patient's age in years)/4. For example, the formula for a 4-year-old child would be: (16 + 4 years)/4 = 5.0 mm i.d. endotracheal tube. A half size above and below this range (4.5 and 5.5) should also be available.

Other methods for estimating the size of the endotracheal tube can be used. One method calls for

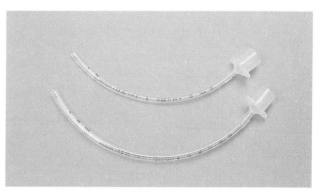

Figure 44-11 Uncuffed endotracheal tubes.

choosing an endotracheal tube with the same outside diameter as the child's little finger. Another method says to select a tube with an outside diameter that is the same as the internal diameter of the child's nares, or nostrils. These methods at best are estimations; therefore, as stated earlier, it is vital to have tubes one-half size larger and one-half size smaller than the one you select available during intubation.

Newborn infants typically require a 3.0 to a 3.5 mm endotracheal tube. A 1-year-old usually requires a 4.0 to 4.5 mm tube size. An 8-year-old child usually requires a 6.0 mm cuffed or uncuffed endotracheal tube. Refer to Table 44-1 for other endotracheal tube sizes.

Both infant- and child-sized endotracheal tubes have centimeter markers as reference points to monitor the depth of tube insertion. The depth also corresponds with age (Table 44-2).

ENDOTRACHEAL TUBE INSERTION IN AN INFANT OR CHILD

Orotracheal intubation in infants and children is basically the same as in adults except for some variations caused by anatomical differences in the upper airway and by the size of the laryngoscope blades and endotracheal tubes. Refer to the step-by-step procedure for orotracheal intubation in adults described earlier, plus the following special considerations for intubating infants and children:

- The patient must be hyperventilated at a rate appropriate for his age before any intubation attempt. Infants should be hyperventilated at a rate of no less than 30 ventilations per minute and children at a rate of no less than 24 ventilations per minute.
- The heart rate should be continuously monitored

during the intubation attempt. Bradycardia is an early sign of hypoxia. (Interruption of ventilation to intubate can drastically reduce the oxygen level and cause severe hypoxia, especially if the intubation attempt lasts longer than 30 seconds.) Stimulation of the airway in infants and young children can also cause bradycardia. If the heart rate drops below 80 beats per minute in the infant or below 60 beats per minute in the child, the intubation procedure should be stopped and the patient hyperventilated with a bag-valve-mask device with supplemental oxygen connected.

- Align the axes of the mouth, pharynx, and trachea to achieve better visualization of the glottic opening. This can be done by tilting the patient's head back, flexing the neck forward, and lifting the chin to place him in a "sniffing position." This should only be done if there is no suspicion of spinal injury. If spinal injury is suspected, the head and neck must be stabilized manually in an in-line position during the intubation attempt. If you are unable to visualize the cords, raise the patient's shoulders 1 inch by placing a folded towel or sheet under them. The height required will vary with the age of the patient and will need to be adjusted accordingly.
- The laryngoscopy should be very gentle. Never use force. Do not use the handle in a prying or levering motion as if digging in the airway. Doing so could cause extensive damage to the upper airway. Also, do not use the teeth or upper gums as a fulcrum.
- The epiglottis is more flexible and less developed in infants and young children. As a result, it is more likely to cause obstruction of your view and may require extra efforts to control when using the straight blade.
- Application of Sellick's maneuver (cricoid pressure) during intubation will reduce the risk of vomiting

TABLE 44-1

Endotracheal Tube Sizes

ENDOTRACHEAL TUBE SIZES BASED ON AGE	
Age	**Endotracheal Tube Size in MM (I.D.)**
Premature	2.5-3.0 uncuffed
Newborn	3.0-3.5 uncuffed
6 months	3.5-4.0 uncuffed
1 year	4.0-4.5 uncuffed
2 years	4.5 uncuffed
4 years	5.0 uncuffed
6 years	5.5 uncuffed
8 years	6.0 cuffed
10 years	6.5 cuffed
12 years	7.0 cuffed
Adolescent	7.0-8.0 cuffed

TABLE 44-2

Measuring the Endotracheal Tube

DISTANCE FROM TUBE TIP PLACED MID-TRACHEA TO LEVEL OF THE TEETH	
Age	Centimeter Marking at the Level of the Teeth
Premature	8
Newborn	10
6 months	12
1 year	12
2 years	14
4 years	16
6 years	16
8 years	18
10 years	18
12 years	20
Adolescent	22

and aspiration. Also, pressure on the cricoid and thyroid cartilage will move the glottic opening slightly posterior, making visualization easier.

- Insert the tube until the vocal cord or glottic marker on the uncuffed tube, if available, is at the level of the vocal cords. If a cuffed tube is being used, insert the tube until the proximal end of the cuff is approximately one-half inch beyond the vocal cords.
- The endotracheal tube must be held in place until it is properly secured. Any movement could easily dislodge it.
- Confirm endotracheal tube placement using the methods described earlier for adults. If corrective action is necessary, follow the procedures that were described. Be aware, however, that observing symmetrical rise and fall of the chest is the best indicator of proper placement in infants and children. Breath sounds could be misleading because sounds are easily referred and transmitted to the other side of the chest and epigastrium due to the small size of the chest cavity.
- Improvement in heart rate and skin color should occur after intubation. If the tube is not placed properly, the patient's heart rate may continue to deteriorate and the cyanosis worsen.
- If the tube is properly placed, secure it by using tape or a commercial securing device approved by medical direction. Insert an oropharyngeal airway as a bite block.
- Note the centimeter marker at the level of the patient's teeth or gums when the tube is properly positioned. Use it as a reference point. If at any time you note a change in insertion depth, immediately reassess tube placement. Remember that small movements of the head or neck of the child can dislodge the tube.

- Once tube placement is confirmed and the tube secured, the patient's head should be immobilized to limit movement that might dislodge the tube.
- If the tube is properly placed but inadequate lung expansion or tidal volume is noted, assess for one of the following causes:
  - *The tube is too small and there is an air leak around the cricoid cartilage.* Such a leak can be heard when auscultating over the neck. If a leak is detected, the tube should be replaced with a larger one. If using a cuffed tube in a child older than 8, inflate the cuff until the air leak is eliminated. Check the pilot balloon to determine if the cuff is still working properly. A defective cuff may leak and deflate.
  - *The pop-off valve on the bag-valve device is not deactivated (as it should be) and air is escaping with ventilation.* This is a problem particularly in children with poor lung compliance or high airway resistance.
  - *The bag-valve device has a leak or is not functioning properly.* Check all its parts, especially the valves, to be sure they are working properly. Remove the bag-valve device from the tube and occlude the tube connection while squeezing the bag to check for any leaks or malfunctions.
  - *The EMT-B performing ventilation is not delivering an adequate volume with each squeeze of the bag.* Have the ventilator increase the volume delivered by squeezing more air out of the bag. Be careful, however, because a pneumothorax can result from too-aggressive ventilation.
  - *The tube has become blocked with secretions or has kinked.* Perform endotracheal suctioning to remove any secretions. Visualize the tube with the laryngoscope to detect any kinks. If the tube remains occluded, remove it and begin positive

pressure ventilation by bag-valve mask. After hyperventilation for 2 to 5 minutes, attempt intubation again.

- Excessive force and/or volume in ventilating an infant or child can easily cause rupture of a lung (barotrauma) and a subsequent pneumothorax (leakage of air into the chest cavity—an extremely dangerous condition). Carefully inspect the chest with each ventilation and watch for rise. As soon as the chest rises adequately, cease your ventilation.

NASOGASTRIC INTUBATION IN INFANTS AND CHILDREN

Gastric distention (air in the stomach) tends to be a greater problem in infants and children than in adults. Because of their small airway structures, it is easy to ventilate them too quickly or too hard, causing air to enter the esophagus and be forced into the stomach. The child's less-developed diaphragm is easily pushed upward by the air in the stomach, compressing the small chest cavity to the point where effective ventilation is impossible, leading to hypoxia. The risk of regurgitation and aspiration of gastric contents is also increased.

In this instance, the gastric air pressure must be relieved by inserting a **nasogastric (NG) tube,** a specialized catheter that is inserted through the nose and down the esophagus into the stomach. The NG tube may also be used to dilute or lavage ingested poisons in the stomach, to remove blood associated with internal gastrointestinal bleeding, or to introduce medications. However, relief of gastric distention in an infant or child patient will be the most common purpose for nasogastric intubation by the EMT-B.

INDICATIONS

The indications for insertion of an NG tube in infants and children include the following:

- *You are unable to provide effective positive pressure ventilation due to gastric distention.*
- *The patient is unresponsive and at risk of vomiting gastric contents or developing gastric distention.*

CONTRAINDICATIONS

An NG tube should not be inserted in a patient who has suffered major facial, head, or spinal trauma. Consult medical direction about using oral insertion with such trauma patients. Also, do not insert the NG tube if you suspect an airway disease such as epiglottitis or croup. This can cause spasms or exacerbate swelling to the point of occluding the airway.

The NG tube is also contraindicated if the patient has ingested certain caustic substances (alkalis) and some hydrocarbons.

EQUIPMENT

The equipment for nasogastric intubation includes the following:

- A nasogastric tube—NG tubes come in a variety of sizes and are measured in units called French. Newborns and infants typically take an 8.0 French; toddlers or preschool children, a 10 French; school-aged children, a 12 French, and adolescents, a 14 to 16 French (Figure 44-12).
- 20 cc syringe to check tube placement
- Water-soluble lubricant to facilitate insertion of the tube
- An emesis basin, in case the patient vomits
- Tape to secure the tube
- Stethoscope to check for proper placement
- Suction unit and suction catheters in case of vomiting and to evacuate the stomach contents following tube placement

INSERTION

Before beginning insertion, take body substance isolation precautions. Gloves, eye protection, and a mask should be worn because of the potential for splatters of secretions, blood, and vomitus. Then insert the NG tube using the following procedure (Figures 44-13a to d):

1. Prepare and assemble the equipment.
2. Determine which nostril appears more patent. If obstruction or other deformity is present in one nostril, select the other.
3. Measure the tube by placing it at the tip of the nose, around the ear, and extending it until the most proximal of the holes at the distal end is just below the xiphoid process. Mark the tube with a piece of tape at the level of the tip of the nose; the tape will serve as a guide, indicating

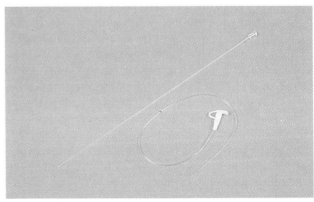

Figure 44-12 Nasogastric tubes.

NASOGASTRIC INTUBATION

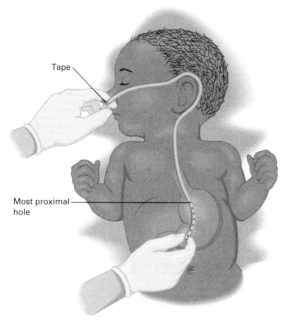

Figure 44-13a *Measure the nasogastric tube by placing the most proximal of the holes slightly below the xiphoid process. The tube is then brought up around the ear and to the tip of the nose. Mark the level at the tip of the nose with a piece of tape.*

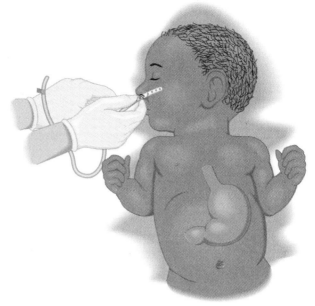

Figure 44-13b *Place the patient supine with the head turned to the side to insert the NG tube.*

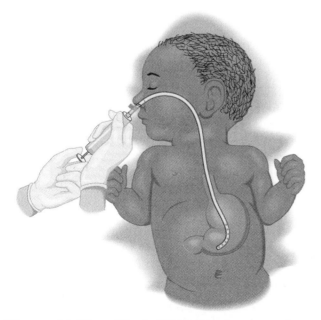

Figure 44-13c *Check NG tube placement by aspirating stomach contents with a syringe.*

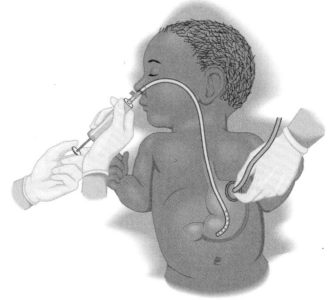

Figure 44-13d *Check NG tube placement by auscultating for air over the epigastrium while injecting 10 to 20 cc of air into the tube.*

when an adequate length of tube has been inserted to enter the stomach.

4. Lubricate 6 to 8 inches of the distal end of the tube with water-soluble lubricant.
5. If trauma is not suspected, place the patient supine with the head turned to the side.
6. Insert the tube gently in one of the nostrils. Advance the tube straight back toward the ear along the floor of the nostril. Continue to advance the tube until the tape marker is at the level of the tip of the nose. If resistance is met when advancing the tube, rotate the tube slightly and continue to advance it. If significant resistance is met, stop, pull back on the tube, and reevaluate its position. Do not force the tube if resistance is found.
7. Check the placement of the nasogastric tube by:
   a. Attaching the 20 cc syringe to the tube, pulling back on the plunger, and aspirating the gastric contents.
   b. Placing your stethoscope over the epigastric region and auscultating while injecting 10 to 20 cc's of air into the tube. A gurgling sound should be heard over the stomach.
8. Secure the tube in place with tape.
9. Attach the tube to low suction and aspirate the gastric contents.
10. Document the tube size, any complications encountered during placement, time of insertion, and assessment of placement.

COMPLICATIONS

There are several possible complications associated with placement of the nasogastric tube:

- Tracheal intubation is possible, with the NG tube entering the larynx and trachea instead of the esophagus. The patient will typically begin severe coughing and choking. Pull back on the tube until it is at the posterior pharynx and reattempt insertion.
- Nasal trauma can occur from insertion of the tube. Be sure the tube is adequately lubricated. Do not insert the tip of the tube in an upward direction in the nose. This commonly causes pain and bleeding.
- Insertion of the NG tube may stimulate the gag reflex and cause the patient to vomit. Be prepared to clear the airway and suction.
- A very rare complication is passage of the tube into the cranium if a basilar skull fracture exists, particularly with mid-facial fractures.
- The tube may become curled in the nose, mouth, or trachea. If insertion becomes difficult, inspect inside the mouth and withdraw the tube to determine its position.
- Perforation of the esophagus may occur.

Medical direction or your local protocol may allow insertion of the NG tube only after endotra-cheal intubation. Once the airway is secured with an endotracheal tube, the risks of misplacing the NG tube in the trachea or of vomiting and aspiration are greatly reduced.

OROTRACHEAL SUCTIONING

Orotracheal suctioning is the process in which a long, soft suction catheter is inserted through the endotracheal tube to clear secretions. The suction catheter is advanced down the endotracheal tube and beyond its tip to the level of the carina. As the catheter is being withdrawn, suction is applied to remove any heavy secretions that could block the airway. In contrast to suctioning of the oropharynx or nasopharynx, where the catheter is never advanced beyond the posterior pharynx, this procedure allows for suctioning at the level of the trachea.

INDICATIONS

There are two major indications for performing orotracheal suctioning:

- *Obvious secretions in the endotracheal tube*—While performing positive pressure ventilation, you may notice secretions in the endotracheal tube. These secretions could reduce the effectiveness of ventilation or obstruct the endotracheal tube.
- *Poor compliance or an increase in resistance when ventilating with the bag-valve device*—These may be signs of obstruction of the endotracheal tube or trachea by heavy, thick secretions that should be cleared by orotracheal suctioning.

Many conditions or illnesses can produce secretions that require suctioning. Patients with respiratory conditions may have problems not only with bronchospasm or inflammation of the lower airways but also with overproduction of mucus. The secretions are usually very thick and heavy and can occlude the trachea and bronchi. The best method for removal, if the patient is unable to remove them himself, is through orotracheal suctioning. Also, trauma may cause bleeding in the trachea, bronchi, or lungs that may require suctioning.

SUCTIONING TECHNIQUE

The procedure for performing orotracheal suctioning is as follows (Figures 44-14a to f):

1. Take the necessary body substance isolation precautions, including gloves and eye protection.
2. Pre-oxygenate the patient using normal positive pressure ventilation with supplemental oxygen. The patient should be hyperventilated at a rate of at least 24 ventilations per minute for 2 min-

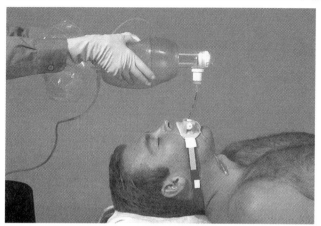

Figure 44-14a   Pre-oxygenate and hyperventilate the patient for 2 minutes prior to orotracheal suctioning.

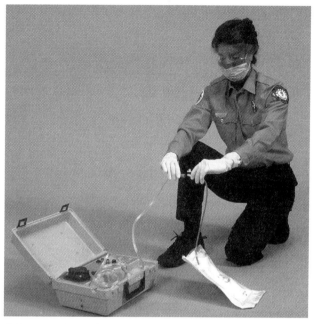

Figure 44-14b   Check the suction equipment. Orotracheal suctioning is a sterile procedure; therefore, do not contaminate the suction catheter.

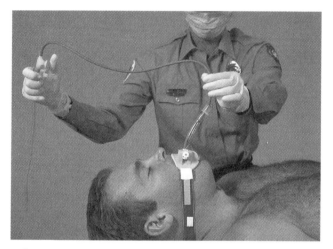

Figure 44-14c   Insert and advance the catheter without suction being applied.

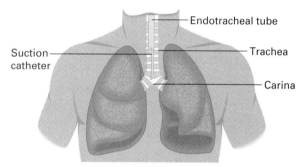

Figure 44-14d   Continue to advance the catheter to the level of the carina.

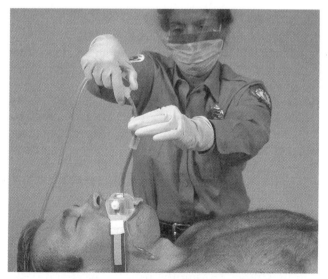

Figure 44-14e   Apply suction by covering the open part on the catheter. Using a twisting motion, withdraw the catheter with suction.

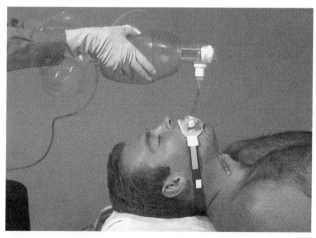

Figure 44-14f   Resume hyperventilation of the patient for 2 minutes following suctioning.

utes before suctioning. This will build up his oxygen reserve and reduce the chances of severe hypoxia.

3. Assemble and check all equipment to be sure it is in working order. Orotracheal suctioning is a sterile procedure; do not contaminate the catheter while assembling or checking it. A sterile glove must be used to handle the catheter. The catheter should remain inside the sterile package until ready for use.

4. Measure the catheter length from the lips to the ear and down to the level of the nipple. This length of catheter should allow placement at about the level of the carina.

5. Set the suction between 80 and 120 mmHg (negative pressure).

6. Insert the catheter down the endotracheal tube with no suction applied.

7. Advance the catheter to the carina or its approximate depth as previously measured.

8. Apply suction. While doing so, withdraw the catheter in a twisting motion. Do not apply suction for longer than 15 seconds.

9. Hyperventilate the patient for 2 minutes. The procedure can be repeated, if necessary, following the same steps.

COMPLICATIONS

As with any advanced invasive maneuver, complications can occur with orotracheal suctioning. Many of those complications result from the interruption of ventilation to perform the procedure. The following are some of the common complications associated with orotracheal suctioning:

- Hypoxia can result from a decrease in lung volume during the application of suction, because you are removing residual air and also interrupting ventilation. (In other words, you are removing whatever air was left in the lungs, and you have stopped providing replacement air.) If hypoxia is severe, it could lead to cardiac arrest. Aggressive hyperventilation for 2 minutes before and after suctioning will reduce the possibility of severe hypoxia. Even more important, do not apply suction for a period greater than 15 seconds.
- Cardiac dysrhythmias can result from suctioning. Tachycardia may occur from stimulation of the airway (or bradycardia in infants and children). Other, more lethal cardiac dysrhythmias may result from a decrease in the supply of oxygen to the heart secondary to hypoxia. Or such dysrhythmias may result from an increase in the oxygen demand due to hypertension and tachycardia. Stimulation of the vagus nerve during suctioning can cause bradycardia and hypotension.
- Coughing may be triggered by the catheter stimu-

lating the mucosa. Coughing can increase pressure within the skull and decrease the blood flow to the brain. This is especially dangerous in a patient with a head injury, stroke, or other condition that had already caused an increase in pressure within the brain.

- The catheter may damage the mucosa, causing swelling, bleeding, and ulcerations that can lead to tracheal infections.
- Bronchospasm can occur if the catheter is inserted beyond the carina and into the bronchi.

ENRICHMENT

The enrichment section contains information that is valuable as background for the EMT-B but that goes substantially beyond the U.S. Department of Transportation (DOT) EMT-Basic curriculum.

ALTERNATIVE INTUBATION TECHNIQUES

You may encounter situations in which you are unable to intubate a patient using the standard techniques described above. There are, however, several ways of inserting an endotracheal tube orally that employ different techniques and equipment. To use these techniques, some of which are described in the following sections, you must be completely familiar with them and the equipment they require. You must also have approval from medical direction before attempting any of the alternative intubation techniques.

DIGITAL INTUBATION

In digital intubation, the EMT-B inserts his fingers into the patient's hypopharynx and uses them to lift the epiglottis. The endotracheal tube is then passed through the glottic opening with the help of the fingers. Digital intubation may be used in a patient who is in cardiac arrest or is unresponsive and has no gag reflex.

Digital intubation is referred to as a "blind" technique, because you do not actually visualize the endotracheal tube passing through the vocal cords. Standard intubation using a laryngoscope is preferred because it permits such visualization. However, you may encounter situations where the patient's position or condition precludes endotracheal intubation with a laryngoscope—for example, when you cannot manipulate the head and neck of an immobilized patient with suspected spinal injury. It is very difficult in such a case to achieve an axis that allows for proper visualization without moving the patient's head and neck. Because digital intubation can be performed without visualizing the vocal cords, it eliminates the need to manipulate the head or neck.

Another situation in which digital intubation might be used is with a patient trapped in a wrecked vehicle. The patient's immediate airway problem may be severe, but the time required for extricating him from the wreck may be long and the position in which he is trapped makes standard intubation with a laryngoscope virtually impossible. Digital intubation may be helpful in such a case.

Finally, digital intubation would allow you to insert an endotracheal tube even if the laryngoscope was not working properly or if its batteries or bulb failed and no spares were available. This should not be performed if the patient has an intact gag reflex or has the ability to bite down.

Equipment   The equipment needed to perform digital intubation includes the following:

- Appropriately sized endotracheal tube
- Malleable stylet
- Water-soluble lubricant
- 10 cc syringe
- Bite block
- Device to secure the endotracheal tube

Procedure   Follow these steps to perform a digital intubation:

1. Take the necessary body substance isolation precautions. Gloves, eye protection, and a mask are recommended.
2. Hyperventilate the patient for approximately 2 minutes before attempting insertion.
3. Check the endotracheal tube as you normally would. Lubricate the tube with a water-soluble lubricant. Lubricate the stylet and insert it to form the tube into a J-shape.
4. If the patient is suspected of having a spinal injury, have an EMT-B or other properly trained rescuer manually stabilize the patient's head and neck. Face the patient and kneel at his left shoulder.
5. Instruct the person ventilating the patient to stop. Quickly place a bite block between the patient's molars to prevent him from biting down on your fingers during the procedure.
6. Insert the middle and index fingers of your left hand into the patient's mouth. Advance your fingers down the mid-line while simultaneously lifting the tongue up and out of the way. Palpate the epiglottis with your middle finger (Figure 44-15a).
7. Press upward and move the epiglottis forward. Insert the endotracheal tube into the mouth with your other hand and advance the tube using your index finger to maintain the tip of the tube against the middle finger. The tip will be directed upward toward the epiglottis. Guide the tip of the tube into the glottic opening with the index and middle fingers (Figure 44-15b).
8. Remove your fingers while holding the tube in place with your other hand. Inflate the cuff with 5 to 10 cc of air. Attach a bag-valve device to the tube. Artificial ventilation must not be interrupted for more than 30 seconds during the insertion.

DIGITAL INTUBATION

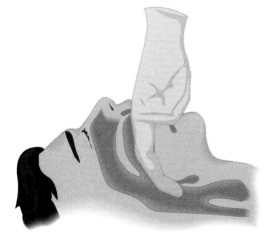

Figure 44-15a   Insert your index and middle finger into the patient's mouth. Elevate the epiglottis with your middle finger.

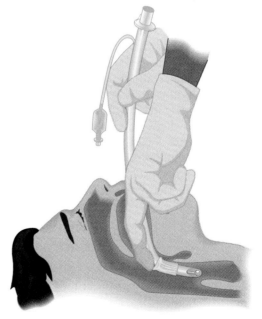

Figure 44-15b   Guide the tube forward and into the glottic opening with your index and middle fingers.

9. As with any endotracheal intubation, assure that the tube is not misplaced in the esophagus or mainstem bronchus. Auscultate over the epigastrium (gurgling should not be heard) and at the apices laterally and at the bases of the lungs (breath sounds should be present and equal). Also watch for equal rise and fall of both sides of the chest with each ventilation. Take the steps described earlier in this chapter to correct any misplacement of the tube. Hyperventilate the patient between attempts to intubate.

10. When correct placement is confirmed, secure the tube as described earlier. Reassess tube position whenever the patient or the ventilating device are moved.

TRANSILLUMINATION (LIGHTED STYLET) INTUBATION

Another method of inserting an endotracheal tube is transillumination, or the "lighted stylet," technique. In this procedure, a special lighted stylet is inserted into the endotracheal tube which is then inserted through the mouth, into the hypopharynx, and on into the larynx and trachea.

Remember that the trachea is anterior to the esophagus, so that the bright light seen through the soft tissues at the front of the neck will indicate that the tube is correctly placed in the trachea. This means that the EMT-B can pass the endotracheal tube through the glottic opening without visualizing the structures directly to ensure correct placement. There is no need to manipulate the head or neck during this procedure. Thus, the transillumination technique can be an effective means of intubating a trauma patient.

The stylet used in this technique is a special device with a high-intensity bulb at the distal end. A small battery housed at the proximal end supplies power for the light and is controlled by an on-off switch. Because tube placement with this method requires seeing the light through the tissues of the neck, the technique is best performed in a darkened room or, if in the sunlight, with the neck shielded or in a shadow. A major problem with this technique is the inability to see the stylet light well in bright ambient light.

Equipment The equipment needed to perform transillumination endotracheal intubation includes the following:

- Appropriately sized endotracheal tube
- Lighted stylet
- Water-soluble lubricant
- 10 cc syringe
- Scissors (to trim the tube)
- Securing device for the endotracheal tube

Procedure Follow these steps to perform a transillumination intubation:

1. Take the necessary body substance isolation precautions including gloves, eye protection, and a mask.
2. Hyperventilate the patient for approximately 2 minutes before attempting to intubate.
3. Assemble and check the equipment. The endotracheal tube should be between 7.5 and 8.5 mm i.d., and will need to be cut to 25 to 27 cm in order to accommodate the stylet. Place the stylet into the tube and bend it just proximal to the cuff.
4. Kneel on one side of the patient, facing his head.
5. Turn on the stylet light.
6. With your index and middle fingers inserted deeply into the patient's mouth and your thumb on the chin, lift the patient's tongue and jaw forward. Insert the tube/stylet combination into the mouth and advance it through the oropharynx and into the hypopharynx. Using a "hooking" motion, lift the epiglottis out of the way (Figure 44-16).
7. When you see a circle of light at the level of the larynx on the anterior neck, hold the stylet stationary (Figure 44-17). Advance the tube off the stylet into the larynx approximately one-half to one inch. The following are indications of misplacement of the stylet and tube:
   - *If the light at the front of the neck is diffuse, dim, or hard to see—or not visible at all—this*

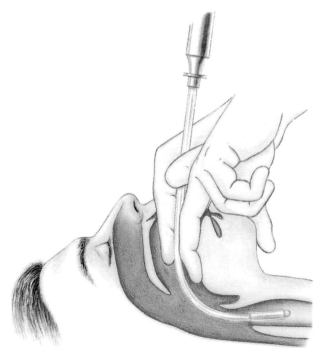

Figure 44-16 Lighted stylet (transillumination) endotracheal tube in position.

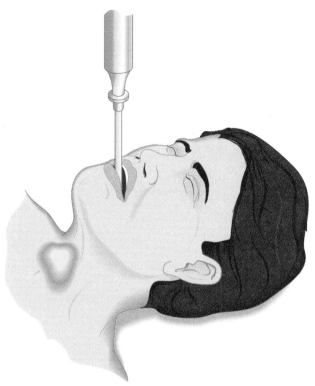

Figure 44-17   The properly positioned stylet should be visible at the front of the patient's neck.

indicates that the tube/stylet combination is incorrectly placed in the esophagus. The tube should be withdrawn immediately and hyperventilation resumed.

- *A bright light appearing lateral to the upper aspect of the thyroid cartilage (Adam's apple)* indicates that the tube/stylet is placed in the right or left pyriform fossa (furrow). Immediately withdraw the tube and resume hyperventilation. Make another attempt after a few minutes.

8. Hold the tube in place with one hand and remove the stylet.
9. Inflate the cuff with 5 to 10 cc of air and attach the bag-valve device to the end of the tube.
10. As with any endotracheal intubation, assure that the tube is not misplaced in the esophagus or mainstem bronchus. Auscultate over the epigastrium and at the apices and bases of the lungs and watch for equal rise and fall of both sides of the chest with each ventilation. Take the steps described earlier in this chapter to correct any misplacement. Hyperventilate the patient between attempts to intubate. Do not interrupt ventilation for more than 30 seconds.
11. When correct placement is confirmed, secure the tube. Reassess tube position whenever the patient or the ventilating device are moved.

ALTERNATIVE ADVANCED AIRWAY ADJUNCTS

Several other devices are available to help control the airway. Some serve a similar purpose to the endotracheal tube but require no visualization during insertion. Even though insertion techniques with these devices are relatively simple, just as with any intubation the ability to assess and differentiate tube placement is the key to using them effectively. Also note that the endotracheal tube is preferred over all of the devices described in the next sections. Medical direction is required prior to use of any of these devices.

PHARYNGEO-TRACHEAL LUMEN (PtL®) AIRWAY

The Pharyngeo-tracheal Lumen (PtL®) airway is a dual-lumen, or two-tube, device designed to be inserted into the airway without direct visualization (Figure 44-18). Actually, the PtL® is a tube within a tube. A long, clear endotracheal-type tube with a cuff at the distal end is situated inside a shorter, wider tube that is designed to fit just proximal to the glottic opening. The shorter tube has a large balloon cuff on the distal third of the device. The balloon is inflated to seal the entire pharynx. The proximal end of the shorter tube is green in color. The longer tube has a cuff at the distal end that can be inserted into either the trachea or the esophagus. That distal cuff is then inflated to seal the trachea or the esophagus. The proximal end of this tube is longer, is clear in color, and it contains a semi-rigid plastic stylet.

When the long, clear tube has been inserted into the trachea, the plastic stylet is removed and ventilation is performed through that tube with a bag-valve or other ventilation device attached to its proximal end. However, if the long tube is placed in the esophagus, the plastic stylet is left in place and ventilation is delivered through the short green tube. Since the long tube and its inflated cuff are sealing off the esophagus, and the balloon cuff on the short tube is sealing off the pharynx, the ventilations delivered through the short tube into the space between the cuffs have nowhere to go but into the trachea.

Inflation lines are provided in order to inflate the two cuffs—the one on the long tube and the one on the short tube—simultaneously or separately. The oropharyngeal cuff on the short tube can be deflated to allow for orotracheal intubation if the long tube has been placed in the esophagus. The short tube also serves as a bite block that keeps the patient from biting down and occluding the tube with his teeth.

This device is only used in an adult patient. Also, only one size is available.

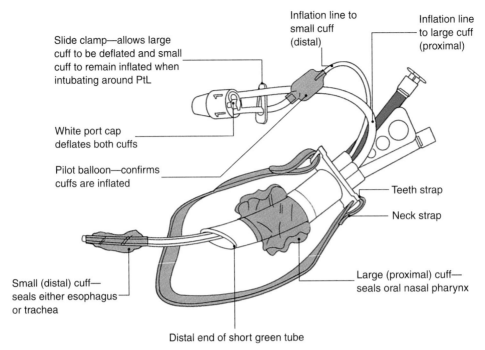

Slide clamp—allows large
cuff to be deflated and small
cuff to remain inflated when
intubating around PtL

Inflation line to
small cuff
(distal)

Inflation line
to large cuff
(proximal)

White port cap
deflates both cuffs

Pilot balloon—confirms
cuffs are inflated

Teeth strap

Neck strap

Small (distal) cuff—
seals either esophagus
or trachea

Large (proximal) cuff—
seals oral nasal pharynx

Distal end of short green tube

Figure 44-18   The pharyngeotracheal-lumen (PtL®) airway.

Advantages   Advantages of the PtL® airway over standard endotracheal intubation include the following:

- The PtL® cannot be improperly placed. It can function when placed in either the trachea or esophagus.
- A mask seal is not required because the large pharyngeal cuff seals the upper airway and does not allow air to escape.
- Insertion is a blind technique that does not require visualization at the level of the glottic opening. Thus, less skill is required for the insertion technique.
- It can be used in a trauma patient with suspected spinal injury because the head or neck does not need to be moved during insertion.
- The pharyngeal cuff helps protect the lower airway from secretions and from blood coming from the nasopharynx or mouth.
- It can be inserted following failed attempts at endotracheal intubation when visualization is hampered by difficult anatomy or position.

Disadvantages   Disadvantages of the PtL® airway include the following:

- The patient must be completely unresponsive and cannot have a gag reflex.
- It cannot be used in a patient younger than 16 years of age or less than 5 feet tall.
- It must be removed when the patient starts becoming responsive or regains a gag reflex.
- If the pharyngeal cuff deflates and the longer tube is in the esophagus, the tube loses its effectiveness.

- The tube requires accurate assessment of tracheal versus esophageal placement for appropriate ventilation.

Indications   Standard endotracheal intubation is the preferred method of airway control. However, you can consider using the PtL® in the following circumstances:

- Endotracheal intubation is not successful after two attempts.
- Endotracheal intubation is indicated but is not allowed or cannot be performed immediately.
- Endotracheal intubation cannot be performed or is unsuccessful because the patient's head is immobilized in a neutral, in-line position because of possible spinal injury.
- The patient's anatomy or profuse bleeding or vomiting are obstructing direct visualization.

Contraindications   The PtL® airway should not be inserted in any of the following situations:

- The patient is younger than 16 years of age.
- The patient is less than 5 feet tall.
- The patient is responsive or has a gag reflex.
- The patient has swallowed a caustic substance.
- Esophageal disease is present.

Equipment   The following equipment is necessary for PtL® insertion:

- Pharyngeal-tracheal lumen (PtL®) airway
- Water-soluble lubricant
- Suction unit

Insertion   Before inserting the PtL® airway, you must ensure that the patient is being adequately ventilated with a bag-valve mask or other acceptable ventilation device.

Gather and prepare the equipment that will be used in insertion. Make sure that both the pharyngeal and distal tube cuffs are completely deflated. The tubes and inflation ports are marked as follows: The inflation port is designated as #1, the green shorter tube is #2, and the long clear tube is #3. Be sure that the white inflation port cap is closed. If the cuffs require further deflation, remove this white cap and compress the cuffs until they are completely flat. A clamp is located on the inflation port allowing deflation of the pharyngeal cuff while the cuff on the distal end of the longer tube remains inflated. Lubricate the long clear #3 tube with a water-soluble lubricant. An adjustable cloth strap is used to secure the PtL® airway in place.

Follow these steps to insert the PtL® airway:

1. Hyperventilate the patient at a rate greater than 24 ventilations per minute for 2 minutes prior to inserting the device.
2. Place the patient's head into a hyperextended position if no spinal injury is suspected. If a spinal injury is suspected, maintain the head in a neutral, in-line position.
3. Insert your thumb deep into the mouth, grasping the tongue and lower jaw between the thumb and index finger, and lift the tongue and lower jaw forward.
4. Insert the PtL® airway into the mouth with your free hand while maintaining the tongue-jaw lift with the other hand. Insert the airway so that it follows the natural curvature of the oropharynx. Insert the tip into the patient's mouth and advance it carefully beyond the tongue until the teeth strap touches the patient's teeth. You will feel modest resistance when passing the tube at the correct angle in the oropharynx. Do not use force during insertion. If the tube is not advancing, either redirect the tip or withdraw it and attempt insertion a second time, following 2 minutes of hyperventilation. Do not interrupt artificial ventilation for more than 30 seconds when inserting the device.
5. When the flange that holds the strap meets the teeth, the tube is in the proper position. Slide the neck strap over the patient's head and tighten it with the hook-and-tape closures on both sides.
6. Inflate both cuffs simultaneously by blowing into the main inflation valve #1 with a sustained breath. If the cuffs are not inflated properly, the pilot balloon will not be inflated or air will rush from the mouth during ventilation. These may be indications that one of the cuffs is defective and the device needs to be replaced. If the pilot balloon is inflated, puffs of air delivered through inflation port #1 can improve the seal if some air leakage is noticed.
7. Attach the bag-valve device to the shorter green #2 tube and deliver a ventilation. If the chest rises with the ventilation and breath sounds are heard over the chest in the apex and base of each lung, you know that the longer #3 tube has been placed in the esophagus and ventilations through the shorter tube are being directed into the trachea. Continue to ventilate through the shorter green #2 tube with a bag-valve or other ventilation device (Figure 44-19).
8. If the chest fails to rise or no breath sounds are heard upon ventilation through the short green #2 tube, you will assume that the longer #3 tube has been placed in the trachea and is blocking ventilations delivered through the short tube. Detach the bag-valve from the #2 tube, remove the plastic stylet from the #3 tube, attach the bag-valve device to the #3 tube, and deliver ventilations through the #3 tube.

   Auscultate the chest for breath sounds, auscultate the epigastrium for gurgling sounds in the stomach, and watch the chest for rise and fall with each breath. Breath sounds should be equal bilaterally, no gurgling sounds should be heard over the stomach, and the chest should rise and fall with each ventilation. If these conditions apply, you have confirmed that the longer #3 tube has been placed in the trachea and is functioning much like an endotracheal tube.
9. Hyperventilate for 2 minutes after insertion and resume normal ventilation thereafter. Continuously reassess the breath sounds and chest rise and fall to ensure correct tube placement. Also, check the pilot cuff periodically to ensure that the cuffs are adequately inflated.

Removal   If either the patient regains responsiveness or his gag reflex returns, the PtL® airway must be removed. Endotracheal intubation is very difficult to perform around the PtL® airway; therefore, in some cases it may be necessary to remove it to achieve proper visualization and oral placement of an endotracheal tube. Follow these steps when removing the PtL® airway:

1. Take the necessary body substance isolation precautions including gloves, eye protection, and a mask. Splatters of secretions and vomitus should be expected.
2. If the patient is not suspected of having any spinal injury, turn him on his side into the lateral recumbent position. If the patient has a suspected spinal injury and is properly secured to a long backboard, turn the entire board on its side.

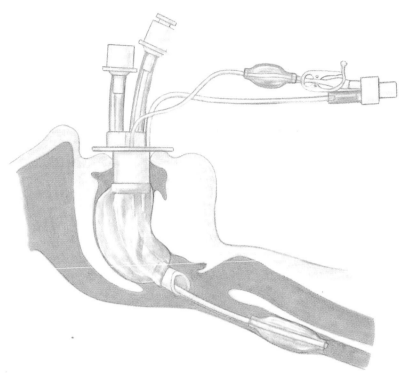

Figure 44-19 The PtL® airway in place. The longer tube is shown placed in the esophagus while ventilations delivered through the shorter tube are directed into the trachea.

3. A gastric tube can be inserted through the tube not being used for ventilation and passed on into the stomach. In this way, you can decompress and evacuate the stomach contents prior to PtL® removal. This should only be done if you are properly trained in the procedure and have received approval from medical direction. You may be asked to remove the PtL® airway in the medical facility where you can suggest that personnel decompress the stomach by insertion of a Levine (gastric) tube down the non-ventilation tube.
4. Remove the white cap from the inflation port #1 to simultaneously deflate both cuffs.
5. Have suction ready. Remove the PtL® gently and discard it. Be alert for vomiting.
6. Reassess the patient's breathing status and resume positive pressure ventilation if necessary.

ESOPHAGEAL TRACHEAL COMBITUBE® (ETC) AIRWAY

The esophageal tracheal Combitube® airway, commonly known simply as the Combitube® or the ETC, is a double-lumen airway that is structurally and functionally very similar to the PtL® airway. Unlike the PtL® lumens, however, the ETC lumens are not placed one inside the other. Instead, the lumens are side by side and separated by a partition wall within a single larger tube (Figure 44-20).

The distal end of the ETC tube has a cuff that is used to seal either the trachea or the esophagus, depending on placement. A proximal pharyngeal cuff is used to seal the pharynx. The #1 tube is slightly longer and is used to deliver ventilations through holes located between the two cuffs. These holes are located just proximal to the glottic opening when the tube is placed in the esophagus. At the proximal end,

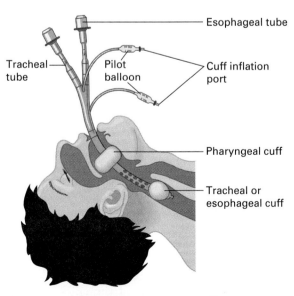

Figure 44-20 The Combitube® airway.

the #2 tube is slightly shorter than the #1 tube and provides ventilation from the end of the tube below the distal cuff, similar to an endotracheal tube. This tube is used when the device has been placed in the trachea. It is more likely that the device will be placed in the esophagus.

Advantages The advantages of the ETC airway over standard endotracheal intubation are similar to those of the PtL® airway. They include the following:

- No visualization is required during insertion, allowing for rapid insertion.
- The device is properly placed whether it is in the esophagus or trachea.
- The inflated pharyngeal cuff prevents ventilations delivered through the tube from escaping through the nose and mouth. This eliminates the need to maintain a mask seal.
- The pharyngeal balloon (cuff) is self-adjusting and self-positioning, an advantage over the PtL®.
- There is no stylet in the distal lumen, allowing for immediate suctioning of the gastric contents. This is another advantage over the PtL® airway.

Disadvantages The complication rate reported with use of the ETC in one limited study group was low. However, complications do exist. Disadvantages to ETC use include the following:

- The ETC requires accurate assessment of tracheal versus esophageal placement.
- Endotracheal intubation is difficult to achieve when the ETC airway is in the esophagus.
- The ETC cannot be used in responsive patients or those with a gag reflex.
- Tracheal suctioning cannot be done with the device in the esophagus.
- The device cannot be used in patients less than 16 years old or less than 5 feet tall.

Indications Standard endotracheal intubation is the preferred method of controlling the airway. However, as with the PtL®, you can consider using the ETC when endotracheal intubation is not successful after two attempts, when endotracheal intubation is not allowed or cannot immediately be performed, although indicated, when in-line immobilization of the patient with possible spine injury prevents successful endotracheal intubation, or when the patient's anatomy, bleeding, or vomiting obstruct the direct visualization required for endotracheal intubation.

Contraindications As with the other airway adjuncts, there are times when the ETC should not be used. Do not use an ETC if the patient is younger than 16 or less than 5 feet tall, the patient is responsive or has a gag reflex, the patient has swallowed a caustic substance, or if esophageal disease is present.

Insertion ETC insertion should be attempted only after the patient has been well ventilated and oxygenated with an appropriate device. Take body substance isolation precautions. Because this is an invasive procedure, gloves, eye protection, and a mask should be used. The procedure for insertion of the ETC is as follows:

1. Hyperventilate the patient at a rate of 24 ventilations per minute for at least 2 minutes before attempting insertion.
2. Assemble and check the equipment. Ensure that the cuffs on the ETC are not leaking. Lubricate the distal end of the tube with a water-soluble lubricant.
3. Place the patient's head and neck in a neutral position. If a spinal injury is suspected, maintain the head in a neutral, in-line position.
4. Perform a tongue-jaw-lift maneuver and insert the device to the level of the black rings. The teeth should be between the two black rings. If the patient has no teeth, use the gum line where the bony structure once held the teeth.
5. Use the large syringe to inflate the pharyngeal cuff with 100 cc of air. The pharyngeal balloon will self-position behind the hard palate in the posterior pharynx. The pharynx will be sealed once the cuff is inflated.
6. Inflate the distal cuff with 10 to 15 cc of air with the smaller syringe.
7. Attach the ventilation device to tube #1, the longer of the two tubes. This is the esophageal tube. It is ventilated first since the tube is most likely in the esophagus (directing ventilations through the holes above the sealed-off esophagus and into the trachea—Figure 44-21). During

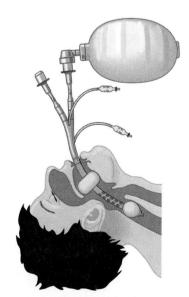

Figure 44-21 Esophageal placement of the Combitube®—ventilating through tube #1.

the ventilation, auscultate over the epigastrium and listen for gurgling sounds. If no sounds are heard, watch for chest rise and auscultate for breath sounds. If equal chest rise and breath sounds are present bilaterally and no gastric sounds are heard over the stomach, continue to ventilate through tube #1.

8. If you hear gurgling sounds in the stomach over the epigastrium, assume that the device has been placed in the trachea and the ventilations exiting through the holes are going into the esophagus. Cease ventilation immediately and reposition the ventilation device on the shorter #2 tube, which will direct the ventilations into the trachea (Figure 44-22). Auscultate over the epigastrium and listen for gurgling. If gurgling is present, remove the tube. If no gurgling is heard, assess the breath sounds. If the breath sounds are equal bilaterally, continue to ventilate through tube #2.

9. Hyperventilate the patient for 2 minutes, then resume normal ventilation. Reassess tube placement after each move involving the patient. Periodically check the pilot balloon located on each tube to ensure the cuffs are adequately inflated.

Removal If the patient regains responsiveness or his gag reflex returns, the ETC airway must be removed. As with the PtL®, removal of the ETC is likely to be followed by vomiting. Remove the tube gently and discard it. Be alert for vomiting. If the patient is not suspected of having any spinal injury, place him in a lateral recumbent position. If the patient has a suspected spinal injury and is properly secured to a long backboard, turn the entire board on its side. Have suctioning equipment ready for use. Reassess the patient's breathing status and resume positive pressure ventilation if necessary.

ESOPHAGEAL OBTURATOR AIRWAY (EOA)

The esophageal obturator airway (EOA) has been used in prehospital care for many years. The device consists of a long esophageal tube that is closed at the distal end and has a series of 16 ventilation holes toward the proximal end. The distal end of the tube also has an inflatable cuff that serves to seal the esophagus. The esophageal tube attaches to a face mask that is sealed over the patient's nose and mouth. An inflation port and line are used to inflate the distal cuff. A pilot balloon on the inflation line is used to verify cuff inflation (Figure 44-23).

As with the PtL® and ETC, insertion of the EOA is a blind technique where no visualization of the glottic opening is required. This eliminates the need for using other devices, such as the laryngoscope, during insertion. When placed properly, the esophageal tube is inserted into the esophagus. The cuff is inflated and the esophagus sealed. The mask is connected to the tube during insertion and a ventilation device is connected to the ventilation port on the mask. During ventilation, the air is forced out of the proximal holes on the tube and into the trachea. Air is prevented from entering the esophagus by the inflated cuff. Also, the risk of aspiration of vomitus is reduced since the esophagus is sealed. A good mask seal must be maintained in order to ventilate the patient effectively.

Complications Many studies have shown that the risk of complications with the EOA is higher than with endotracheal intubation. Also, clinical evaluations have noted that quality of ventilation and oxygenation with the EOA may be inferior to that achieved with the endotracheal tube.

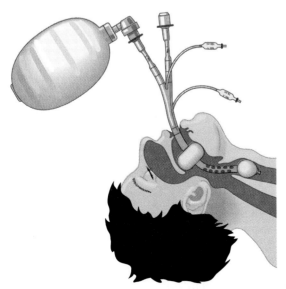

Figure 44-22 *Tracheal placement of the Combitube®—ventilating through tube #2.*

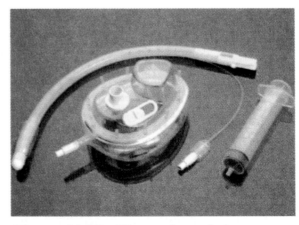

Figure 44-23 *The esophageal obturator airway (EOA).*

The inadvertent placement of the esophageal tube in the trachea during EOA insertion could be a lethal complication. For this reason, the tube must be removed within one-to-two ventilations of recognizing the misplacement. Poor mask seal is the main reason for poorer oxygenation and ventilation. Esophageal lacerations have also been reported with the use of the EOA.

Most of these complications are associated with operator misuse and not with the device itself. Therefore, it is vital that any user of the EOA be thoroughly trained and completely familiar with the insertion technique, assessment for proper placement, and proper ventilation techniques.

Equipment The following equipment must be available when preparing to insert the EOA:

- An EOA complete with mask and esophageal tube
- A 35 cc syringe
- Water-soluble lubricant
- Suction unit
- Stethoscope

Advantages There are several advantages associated with the use of the EOA. They include the following:

- The device permits rapid, blind insertion.
- It prevents air from entering the stomach, thereby eliminating gastric distention.
- It prevents vomitus from traveling up the esophagus, thereby reducing the risk of aspiration. (Remember, however, that blood and secretions from the upper airway can still be aspirated.)
- It allows for insertion of an endotracheal tube with the EOA still in place.
- It can be inserted with the trauma patient's head in a neutral in-line position.

Disadvantages Several disadvantages are associated with EOA use. They include the following:

- A tight mask seal must be maintained the entire time the patient is being ventilated.
- Use of the EOA requires that the patient be completely unresponsive and not have a gag reflex.
- The EOA may lacerate or rupture the esophagus.
- It can be improperly placed in the trachea and may cause asphyxia and trauma to the trachea if placed there.
- It cannot be used for prolonged ventilation.
- It does not prevent the aspiration of blood or secretions coming from the oropharynx or nasopharynx.
- It cannot be inserted in a patient less than 16 years of age, less than 5 feet tall, or greater than 7 feet tall.

Indications Standard endotracheal intubation is the preferred method of controlling the airway. However, as with the PtL® and ETC, you can consider using the EOA, if approved by medical direction, when endotracheal intubation is not successful after two attempts, when endotracheal intubation is not allowed or cannot immediately be performed, although indicated, when in-line stabilization of the patient with possible spine injury prevents successful endotracheal intubation, or when the patient's anatomy, bleeding, or vomiting obstruct the direct visualization required for endotracheal intubation.

Contraindications The EOA should not be inserted in any of the following conditions:

- The patient is alert, responsive, or has a gag reflex.
- The patient has ingested a caustic poison. The weakened and burned esophageal wall may rupture or lacerate.
- The patient is younger than 16 years of age.
- The patient is less than 5 feet tall or more than 7 feet tall.
- The patient has significant bleeding in the oropharynx or nasopharynx.

Insertion The EOA must be completely assembled before insertion. Do not insert the tube without the mask attached because the mask, when seated on the face, provides an indication that the tube is inserted at the proper level. To attach the mask to the tube, position the tube 180 degrees from its correct position. Insert the tube into the ventilation port of the mask and then turn it 180 degrees until it is in the proper position and you hear and feel it lock into place. To remove the tube from the mask, you simply squeeze together the two yellow plastic tips projecting from the ventilation port and pull the tube from the opposite direction of the mask.

Because this is an invasive procedure, you must take the necessary body substance isolation precautions, including gloves, eye protection, and a mask. Then insert the EOA following these steps:

1. Hyperventilate the patient at a rate of 24 ventilations per minute for at least 2 minutes prior to the insertion attempt.
2. Assemble and prepare the equipment. Assemble the mask and esophageal tube ensuring that the tube is securely locked in the mask. Inflate the distal cuff on the tube with 30 cc of air. Check the distal cuff on the tube to ensure that it fills with air and does not leak. Be sure to deflate the cuff completely prior to insertion. Check the mask to be sure it is inflated enough to allow for a seal on the patient's face. If the mask needs to be inflated, take the 35 cc syringe, attach it to the inflation port located on the mask, and add an adequate amount of air. Do not over-inflate the mask; this will make achieving a seal on the patient's face much more difficult. Lubricate the lower two-thirds of the tube with a water-soluble lubricant.

3. Place the patient's head in a neutral or slightly flexed position and have the EMT-B administering the ventilations stop. If a spinal injury is suspected, maintain the head in a neutral, in-line position.

4. Open the patient's mouth and insert your thumb into it, grasping the tongue and mandible and lifting both up and forward to perform a tongue-jaw-lift. Failure to lift the tongue adequately will impede insertion of the EOA. Do not hyperextend the head or neck since doing so may cause the EOA to be inserted into the trachea.

5. Grasp the EOA, with mask attached, in your free hand and insert it in the mouth following the natural curve of the posterior oropharynx and hypopharynx (Figure 44-24a). Doing this should permit the EOA to be passed into the esophagus. Continue inserting the tube until the mask is completely seated on the face (Figure 44-24b). Do not force the tube during insertion. If you meet moderate to severe resistance, the tube is most likely going into the trachea; immediately withdraw it and advance it again. Do not interrupt ventilations for more than 30 seconds during the insertion procedure. You may need to stop, hyperventilate for a few minutes, and then reattempt the insertion.

6. Hold a tight seal with your hands on the mask and have your partner attach the bag-valve device or other ventilation device to the yellow ventilation port on the mask. Then ventilate, watching for the chest to rise and fall while auscultating over the chest for breath sounds. Auscultate over the epigastrium for gurgling sounds from the stomach. If the chest does not rise or fall or breath sounds are not heard, immediately remove the device and begin hyperventilating the patient (Figure 44-24c).

7. Once you confirm placement of the EOA, attach the syringe to the inflation port and inject 30 to 35 cc of air to inflate the distal cuff. Check the pilot balloon to make sure that it is inflated.

8. Reassess breath sounds bilaterally and over the epigastrium, and watch for equal chest rise and fall. You should hear good breath sounds and no sounds over the stomach and observe equal chest expansion. If you are unsure whether the tube is properly placed, deflate the cuff and remove it. Remember, placing an EOA in the trachea can quickly become a lethal mistake.

9. Hyperventilate the patient for 2 minutes following insertion of the EOA, then resume the normal ventilation rate.

INSERTING THE ESOPHAGEAL OBTURATOR AIRWAY

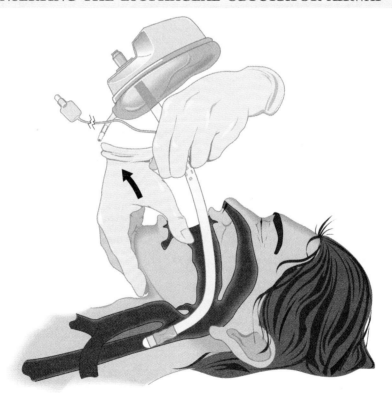

Figure 44-24a Insert the EOA completely assembled. Flex the patient's head forward while grasping the jaw and tongue. Lift up and forward.

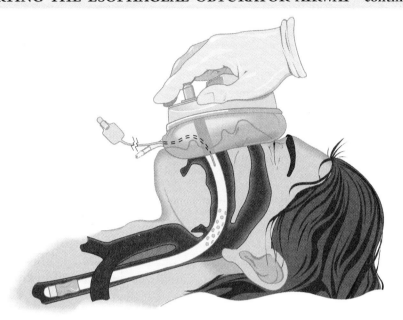

Figure 44-24b *Advance the tube until the face mask fits snugly over the patient's nose and mouth.*

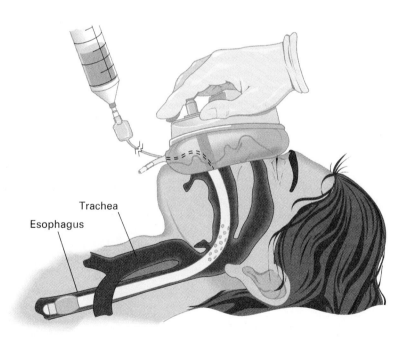

Figure 44-24c *Inflate the distal cuff. Check positioning of the EOA. Watch and auscultate for bilateral expansion of the chest and bilateral breath sounds. If the chest does not rise on both sides and breath sounds are not heard, withdraw the tube, hyperventilate, then reattempt insertion.*

10. Recheck tube placement periodically, especially after any movement of the patient.

Removal Remove the EOA only if the patient is intubated with an endotracheal tube, has regained responsiveness, or the gag reflex returns. It is very likely that the patient will vomit upon removal of the EOA. Be sure the EOA is not removed until you can adequately protect the airway. Ideally, the patient will be intubated with an endotracheal tube and the trachea will be protected by the distal cuff on the tube in the case of vomiting. The procedure for removing the EOA is as follows:

1. Have the suction unit available and next to the patient for immediate access.
2. Turn the patient on his side if there is no suspected spinal injury. If the patient has a suspected spinal injury and is completely and properly immobilized to the backboard, turn the entire board on its side.
3. Detach the mask from the tube.
4. Attach the syringe to the inflation port and withdraw all the air from the cuff.
5. Gently remove the tube. Be alert for vomiting and suction as necessary.
6. Resume ventilation of the patient.

ESOPHAGEAL GASTRIC TUBE AIRWAY (EGTA)

Essentially, the esophageal gastric tube airway (EGTA) is the same as the esophageal obturator airway (EOA). The major difference between the two devices is that the EGTA allows for a gastric tube to be inserted through the esophageal tube and into the stomach. This gastric tube allows for evacuation and decompression of the stomach, which reduces the risk of aspiration of gastric contents and eliminates problems associated with gastric distention. The tube can also be used to remove stomach contents in the case of a poisoning.

The EGTA consists of an inflatable face mask and an esophageal tube that is hollow and has an opening at its distal tip. A gastric tube can be passed through a port in the mask, out the distal end of the esophageal tube, and into the stomach.

The transparent face mask has two ports, one for attachment of the esophageal tube and the other, a standard 15 mm port, for ventilation. The ventilation device cannot be connected to the proximal end of the tube that projects from the mask. Unlike the EOA esophageal tube, the EGTA esophageal tube does not have any holes to facilitate air flow into the trachea. The EGTA esophageal tube merely serves to occlude the esophagus. Ventilation occurs through the mask ventilation port and is forced into the trachea because the esophagus is sealed.

Insertion of the EGTA is the same as with the EOA. The only variation occurs when a gastric tube is to be inserted; in such a case, the gastric tube must first be measured to gauge the proper length. To measure the gastric tube, extend the tubing from the tip of the nose, around the ear, and then to the level of the xiphoid process.

The EGTA has the same advantages, disadvantages, and carries the same complications as the EOA. The indications and contraindications are also the same. The only additional advantage to the use of the EGTA over the EOA is the ability to evacuate and decompress the stomach.

LARYNGEAL MASK AIRWAY (LMA)

The laryngeal mask airway (LMA) (Figure 44-25) was developed by a British anesthesiologist in 1981 and has been widely used by anesthesiologists and prehospital providers in the United Kingdom for several years. For the past few years, the LMA has been used by anesthesiologists and nurse anesthetists in the United States. The LMA is gaining popularity as an adjunct airway device that may be considered for prehospital airway management when difficult endotracheal intubation is encountered or as a primary adjunct to control the airway.

The LMA consists of a tube similar to an endotracheal tube connected to a cuff-like mask at the distal end of the tube. An inflation line is used to inflate the mask, and a pilot balloon monitors the mask inflation. The tube is connected to the mask at a 30-

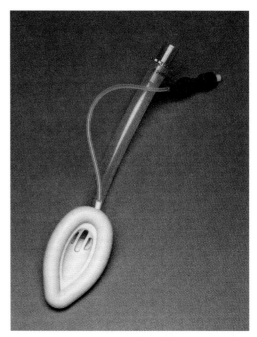

Figure 44-25 The laryngeal mask airway (LMA). (LMA North American, Inc.)

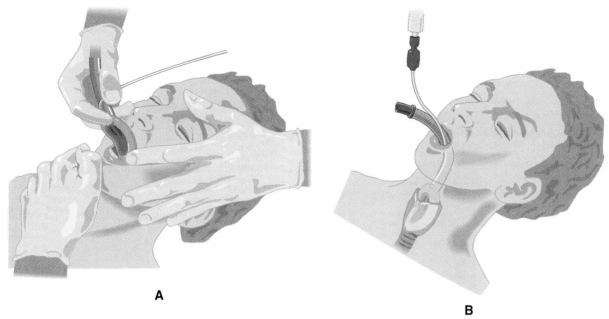

A **B**

Figure 44-26 *A. Inserting the laryngeal mask airway. B. The laryngeal mask airway in place.*

degree angle. Two vertical bars inside the inflatable mask support the epiglottis and prevent it from falling into the opening of the tube. The tube is inserted in the hypopharynx, and the cuff-like mask forms a seal around the laryngeal opening. The LMA comes in a variety of sizes from 1 for neonates to 5 for adults.

Insertion Insert the LMA, following these steps (Figure 44-26):

1. Hyperventilate the patient at a rate of 24 ventilations per minute for 2 minutes prior to insertion of the LMA.
2. Check the LMA mask for leaks. Be sure to completely deflate the mask prior to insertion.
3. Lubricate the posterior portion of the mask with a water-soluble lubricant.
4. If no cervical injury is suspected, place the patient's head in a sniffing position with the head hyperextended and the neck flexed. Hold the occiput of the head with your free hand to ensure the correct position. Another EMT may assist in opening the patient's mouth by lifting the chin forward.
5. Hold the LMA device like a dart as you insert it into the patient's mouth. Make sure the opening of the mask is anterior with the black line on the tube aligned with the middle of the patient's nose.
6. Advance the LMA into the hypopharynx until resistance is met. Do not rotate the tube. Keep

the black line aligned with the middle of the nose. The tube should now be properly placed.

7. Inflate the cuff with the proper volume of air. The tube may rise about 1.5 cm once the mask is inflated. The black line should be midline against the upper lip.
8. Confirm tube placement by assessing for the presence of breath sounds bilaterally and no epigastric sounds.
9. Insert an oropharyngeal airway or a bite block to keep the patient from biting down on the tube.
10. Once you have confirmed proper tube placement, secure the device in place.

Complications The LMA has only a few complications associated with its use. They are:

• Vomiting during the insertion when used in a patient who still has a gag reflex.
• Possible airway obstruction if the mask is improperly aligned in the hypopharynx.
• Ineffective ventilation caused by escape of air around the mouth resulting from mask deflation or improper mask seal.
• Aspiration (Remember that the LMA does not protect the patient from aspiration like an appropriately placed endotracheal tube.)

As previously stated, it is important to remember that an endotracheal tube remains the best device for protecting and controlling the airway.

CASE STUDY FOLLOW-UP

SCENE SIZE-UP

You and your partner have been dispatched to a three-alarm house fire. You arrive on the scene and position the ambulance so it does not interfere with the fire apparatus and also allows you to exit rapidly. You are directed to a staging area by the battalion chief. You and your partner gather the equipment and proceed to the appropriate area safely away from the fire and smoke. You suddenly notice two firefighters emerging from the blazing house carrying someone. When they are a safe distance from the house, the battalion chief waves you over. As you approach, you note that the victim is a man who is unresponsive with obvious burns to his face, neck, and upper chest. It is apparent that his shirt has been burned off his body.

INITIAL ASSESSMENT

As the firefighters gently lay the patient on the ground, you begin your assessment. You note that you have a male patient approximately 40 years of age with reddened, charred burns to the chest, neck, and face. You kneel and ask the patient, "Sir, can you hear me?" When he doesn't respond, you perform a sternal rub which elicits no response.

You perform a head-tilt, chin-lift and open the airway. You look inside the mouth and note a blackened, burned, and swollen oral cavity. The patient's eyebrows and nasal hairs are also singed. On assessing the breathing, you cannot see the chest rise or fall or hear or feel any air movement. You instruct your partner to insert an oropharyngeal airway and immediately begin positive pressure ventilation with a bag-valve mask.

You assess the carotid pulse which is strong and approximately 100 beats per minute. The skin in the unburned area is warm and dry. It is difficult to determine skin color because of the soot on the patient's body.

Your partner indicates that he is beginning to feel a great deal of resistance and is having difficulty in ventilating the patient with the bag-valve mask. You elect to perform endotracheal intubation because of the evidence of an upper airway burn. You have your partner hyperventilate the patient as you prepare the equipment. You perform the laryngoscopy and note swelling to the upper airway. You visualize the glottic opening and insert the endotracheal tube between the vocal cords. You inflate the cuff with 10 cc of air and hold the tube securely as your partner attaches the bag-valve device to the 15 mm adapter on the proximal end of the endotracheal tube.

You instruct your partner to ventilate as you inspect the chest for equal rise and fall and listen for gurgling over the epigastrium. There is no gurgling, so you instruct your partner to continue ventilating as you auscultate over the apices and bases of both lungs. The breath sounds are equal bilaterally. An end-tidal CO_2 detector is attached and is indicating adequate CO_2 levels. You tape the tube securely in place and note that the 22 cm marker is at the level of the teeth. You instruct two firefighters to get the stretcher quickly because you identify this patient as a priority.

FOCUSED HISTORY AND PHYSICAL EXAM

As the firefighters are getting the stretcher, you perform a rapid trauma assessment, paying particular attention to the location and depth of the burns. The hair is singed almost completely off. Partial thickness and full thickness burns are noted to the face, neck, and upper third of the anterior and lateral chest. The breath sounds are equal bilaterally and the chest rises with each ventilation.

No evidence of injury or burns is noted to the abdomen, pelvis, or lower extremities. The pedal pulses are present, and the patient does not respond to a pinch to each foot. Partial thickness and full thickness burns are noted to both upper extremities, covering them almost entirely on both sides. Radial pulses are present, and the patient does not respond to a pinch to either hand. You log-roll the patient and note partial thickness burns to the upper third of the posterior thorax.

You carefully remove the remainder of the shirt and instruct the firefighter to open and lay a burn sheet on a backboard. The patient is log-rolled onto the burn sheet on the backboard.

You quickly reassess endotracheal tube placement by auscultating breath sounds and for epigastric sounds and inspect the rise and fall of the chest. The breath sounds are equal bilaterally and no epigastric sounds are heard. The tube is still at the 22 cm marker.

The burn sheet is wrapped around the patient. The burn is estimated at 44 per cent partial and full thickness. You quickly assess the baseline vital signs as blood pressure 126/62 mmHg, pulse 104, respirations absent and assisted at 20 per minute. The skin remains warm and dry in the unburned area. You are unable to obtain a SAMPLE history because the patient is unresponsive and no one else at the scene can provide any information regarding the patient. You load the patient onto the stretcher, wheel him to the ambulance, and prepare him for transport.

ONGOING ASSESSMENT

Immediately after loading the patient into the ambulance, you reassess endotracheal tube placement. You notice that the tube is now at the 26 cm marker at the level of the teeth. You auscultate the breath sounds and note that the sounds on the left are significantly diminished compared to the right. You remove the tape securing the tube and take the 10 cc syringe and deflate the cuff. You pull back on the tube as you continue to auscultate breath sounds on the left. As soon as you hear good breath sounds you stop pulling and assess breath sounds and note they are now equal bilaterally. You reinflate the cuff with 10 cc of air and resecure the tube with tape.

The breathing is still absent so you continue ventilating at a rate of 20 times per minute. The radial pulse remains at 104 per minute, BP is 120/60 mmHg, and the skin is still warm and dry in the unburned area. You ensure that the bag-valve device is connected to oxygen that is flowing properly. You reassess tube placement every few minutes by watching the chest rise and fall, auscultating the breath sounds, and auscultating for gurgling over the epigastrium. You contact the hospital and provide a report of the patient's condition and your ETA.

Upon arrival at the hospital, you unload the patient from the ambulance. You immediately reassess breath sounds, chest rise and fall, and absence of epigastric sounds. The tube is still at the 22 cm marker, breath sounds are equal bilaterally, no sounds are heard in the stomach, and the chest rises and falls with each ventilation. You transfer care of the patient to the emergency department staff. The physician quickly checks endotracheal tube placement and confirms that the tube is properly placed. You give an oral report to the physician and nurse. You then complete a prehospital care report as your partner cleans and restocks the ambulance.

Before leaving the hospital, you check on the patient's condition. The doctor states, "If you hadn't intubated him, his airway would have swollen completely shut and he would probably be dead. You did a great job controlling the airway. We're going to transfer him by helicopter to the burn center. I don't know if he'll make it, but at least now he has a chance." You clear the hospital and radio that you are back in service.

CHAPTER REVIEW

TERMS AND CONCEPTS

You may wish to review the following terms and concepts included in this chapter.

arytenoids—irregular pyramid-shaped structures located on the top of the posterior aspect of the cricoid ring.

bronchioles—smaller airways that branch from the bronchi and terminate at the alveolar sacs.

carina—the point of division at about the level of the fifth thoracic vertebra where the trachea splits into the right and left mainstem bronchi.

corniculates—cone-shaped cartilage attached to the top of the arytenoids. They are landmarks used when visualizing the glottic opening.

cricoid cartilage—a firm and complete circular ring located below the thyroid cartilage and attached to the first ring of the trachea.

cricoid pressure—pressure applied to the cricoid cartilage, directed posteriorly, to close off the esophagus and help bring the vocal cords and glottic opening into view. Also called Sellick's maneuver.

cuneiforms—elongated cartilage attached to the posterior arytenoids. They are landmarks used when visualizing the glottic opening.

curved blade—a laryngoscope blade that is curved at the distal end. The blade is inserted into the vallecula to indirectly lift the epiglottis and expose the vocal cords and glottic opening.

endotracheal tube—a tube designed to be inserted between the vocal cords, through the larynx, and into the trachea in order to maintain an airway and to facilitate ventilation.

epiglottis—a leaf-shaped cartilaginous structure that covers the opening of the larynx during swallowing.

extubation—the removal of a tube.

false vocal cords—membranous tissue that lies above the true vocal cords.

glossoepiglottic ligament—a ligament that helps support and suspend the epiglottis and is found in the center of the vallecula.

glottic opening—the opening between the vocal cords. Also called the glottis.

glottis—see glottic opening.

intubation—the process of passing a tube, such as an endotracheal tube, into the body.

laryngoscope—a device with a lighted distal end used to lift the epiglottis and provide visualization of the vocal cords and glottic opening.

laryngoscopy—the procedure of using a laryngoscope to lift the epiglottis to visualize the vocal cords and glottic opening.

mainstem bronchi—the main branches of the airway leading from the trachea to the lungs. There are two mainstem bronchi, the *right mainstem bronchus* and the *left mainstem bronchus.*

Murphy eye—a small hole opposite the bevel at the distal end of an endotracheal tube. Its purpose is to lessen the chance of complete tube obstruction.

nasogastric (NG) tube—a specialized catheter that is inserted through the nose and esophagus into the stomach.

orotracheal intubation—the passage of an endotracheal tube through the mouth, along the oropharynx and larynx, and into the trachea.

orotracheal suctioning—the procedure in which a long, soft suction catheter is inserted through the endotracheal tube to clear secretions deep in the airway.

right mainstem intubation—a complication of endotracheal intubation in which the tube is advanced too far down the trachea and into the right mainstem bronchus. This provides for ventilation of only one lung and can lead to severe hypoxia.

Sellick's maneuver—see cricoid pressure.

straight blade—a laryngoscope blade that is straight at the distal end. The blade is fitted under the epiglottis to lift it to expose the vocal cords and glottic opening.

stylet—a piece of pliable metal wire, typically coated with plastic, that is inserted into an endotracheal tube to shape it and provide stiffness.

thyroid cartilage—the bulky shield-like structure, commonly known as the Adam's apple, that forms the anterior surface of the larynx.

trachea—a tubular structure that extends from the lower portion of the larynx to the bronchi; the "windpipe."

trachealis muscle—the muscular wall that closes the C-shaped rings on the posterior side of the trachea and abuts the esophagus.

true vocal cords—strands of fibrous tissue that regulate the flow of air into the trachea and produce sounds by vibrating.

vallecula—a depression located between the base of the tongue and the epiglottis.

REVIEW QUESTIONS

1. List the indications for performing endotracheal intubation in the adult.
2. Describe and contrast the use of straight and curved laryngoscope blades in endotracheal intubation.
3. Explain the following: (a) how to locate the cricoid cartilage, (b) how to perform Sellick's maneuver, and (c) reasons for using Sellick's maneuver.
4. Explain the methods used to assess endotracheal tube placement.
5. Name the laryngoscope blades preferred for intubating infants and for intubating older children.
6. Regarding determining appropriate endotracheal tube size in infants and children: (a) describe techniques that may be used to determine appropriate tube size, and (b) based on the sizing formula, state the size endotracheal tube you would use to intubate a 6-year-old child.
7. Endotracheal tubes for infants and children are usually uncuffed; explain how the trachea is sealed during intubation.
8. Describe the method of measuring the nasogastric tube in the infant and child.
9. List (a) indications and (b) contraindications for insertion of a nasogastric tube in an infant or child.
10. List the complications associated with orotracheal suctioning.

APPENDIX 1
Basic Life Support

INTRODUCTION

Airway, breathing, and circulation are often referred to as the "ABCs" without which life cannot continue. The ability to correct life-threatening compromises to these three essential functions—at least temporarily, until more advanced care can be given—is the primary function of basic life support. Opening the airway, artificial ventilation, cardiopulmonary resuscitation (CPR), and foreign body airway obstruction (FBAO) techniques are the primary basic life-support skills.

BASIC LIFE SUPPORT

When breathing or breathing and pulse (heartbeat) are absent, basic life support procedures must be initiated. These measures consist of artificial ventilation—to support breathing—or the combination of artificial ventilation and chest compressions known as cardiopulmonary resuscitation (CPR)—to support breathing and circulation.

Artificial ventilation and CPR are performed for the purpose of keeping oxygenated blood circulating in order to prevent the death of brain and other body cells. (The cessation of breathing and heartbeat are known as *clinical death*. The death of brain cells resulting in irreversible brain damage is known as *biological death*. Deprived of oxygen, brain cells will begin to die within 4 to 6 minutes after breathing and heartbeat cease.)

Once begun, artificial ventilation and CPR must be continued until one of the following occurs:

- The patient recovers spontaneous breathing and heartbeat (on his own, without support), or . . .
- Advanced life support measures, including defibrillation, are begun, or . . .
- A physician orders that life support measures be discontinued.

ASSESSMENT

According to the American Heart Association, "The assessment phases of basic life support are crucial. No victim should undergo any one of the more intrusive procedures of cardiopulmonary resuscitation (i.e., positioning, opening the airway, artificial ventilation, and external chest compression) until the need for it has been established by the appropriate assessment."

The recommended sequence for basic life support in the adult is:

1. Determine unresponsiveness (assessment).
2. Activate the EMS system.
3. Open the airway.
4. Determine breathlessness (assessment).
5. Perform artificial ventilation.
6. Determine pulselessness (assessment).
7. Deliver chest compressions.

In the infant and child, CPR (Steps 3 through 7) is performed for 1 minute prior to activating the EMS system if the rescuer is working alone. Always remember that you must:

- Open the airway before determining breathlessness.
- Determine breathlessness before providing artificial ventilation.
- Determine pulselessness before delivering chest compressions.

DETERMINE UNRESPONSIVENESS

To determine whether the patient is responsive, tap the patient gently on the shoulder and ask loudly, "Are you OK?" Look for any kind of response—fluttering eyelids, muscle movement, turning from the noise, or other. If there is no response, the patient should be considered unresponsive.

ACTIVATE THE EMS SYSTEM

If the adult patient is unresponsive, *activate the EMS system immediately*. Do not proceed with any other part of the basic life support sequence, including opening the airway, until you have activated the EMS system. However, if the emergency involves an infant (less than 1 year of age) or a child (1 to 8 years of age), artificial ventilation or CPR should be performed for 1 minute prior to activating EMS. These criteria apply if you are a single rescuer working alone; if you have a partner, of course, one can activate EMS while the other performs resuscitation.

There is a reason for the difference—activating EMS immediately for an adult, but after 1 minute of resuscitation for an infant or child: An adult is likely to have suffered cardiac arrest as a result of some failure in heart rhythm that may possibly be corrected by defibrillation or other advanced cardiac care. Therefore it is vital to get advanced cardiac life support to the scene as quickly as possible for the adult. The infant or child, on the other hand, is much more likely to have suffered cardiac arrest as a consequence of an airway obstruction or respiratory arrest rather than from failure of the heart itself. Therefore, first establishing an airway and providing effective ventilation is more likely to be vital for the infant or child.

Note: If you suspect that the patient has sustained neck or spinal injuries, do not move the patient unless absolutely necessary. Provide manual in-line stabilization of the head and neck as taught in Chapter 9, "Patient Assessment."

OPEN THE AIRWAY

If the patient is not breathing, you must first establish an open airway. Place the patient in a supine position. Provide spinal stabilization and roll the patient as a unit if spinal injury is suspected. Open the mouth using the crossed finger technique. Open the airway, relieving any possible obstruction of the airway by the tongue, by using the head-tilt, chin-lift technique (Figure A1-1) or, if spinal injury is suspected, the jaw-thrust technique (Figure A1-2). These techniques, suctioning of fluids and foreign matter from the airway, and the use of airway adjuncts to help maintain an open airway, are discussed in detail in Chapter 7.

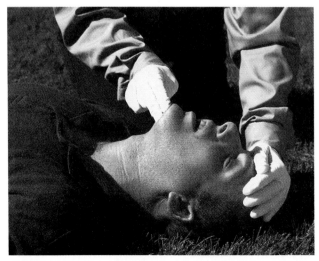

***Figure A1-1** Head-tilt, chin-lift maneuver.*

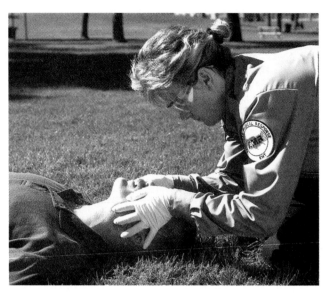

***Figure A1-2** Jaw-thrust maneuver.*

DETERMINE BREATHLESSNESS

Once the airway has been opened, determine that the patient is not breathing (or is not breathing adequately). Place your ear close to the patient's mouth and nose for 3 to 5 seconds, and:

- LOOK for the chest rising and falling.
- LISTEN for air escaping during exhalation.
- FEEL for air flow against your cheek.

It is important to note that the patient may make respiratory efforts while the airway is completely blocked and no air can move in or out of the lungs. Do not mistake this effort to breathe as adequate breathing. (If you merely *look,* you may see the patient's chest moving, but if you *listen* and *feel* for air flow you will realize that the patient is not getting air in and out of the lungs. Assessing for inadequate breathing is covered in Chapter 7, "Airway Management, Ventilation, and Oxygen Therapy.")

If the patient is breathing adequately and has not suffered any trauma that would make you suspect spinal injury, place the patient in the recovery position (Figure A1-3). This is done by rolling the patient onto his side while bringing the knee of the top leg up toward the chest and placing an arm under the head. This position will keep the airway aligned and reduce the chance of airway blockage by the tongue, secretions, blood, or vomitus.

If the patient is still not breathing, or not breathing adequately, initiate artificial ventilation.

PERFORM ARTIFICIAL VENTILATION

The air we breathe contains about 21 percent oxygen; only about 5 percent is used by the body. Because exhaled breath still contains the remaining 16

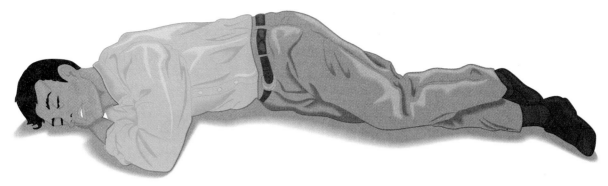

Figure A1-3   *The recovery position.*

percent oxygen, a patient can be oxygenated using only your breath. This can be accomplished by using the techniques of mouth-to-mouth, mouth-to-mask, or mouth-to-stoma ventilation. These techniques are described and illustrated in Chapter 7.

If at all possible, artificial ventilation must be delivered using a barrier device, such as a pocket mask with one-way valve, to protect you and your patient from exchange of body fluids and possible transmission of infectious disease (Figure A1-4).

Administer two slow ventilations over a 1½ to 2-second period for each ventilation. If the chest does not rise with the first ventilation, reposition the patient's head to realign the airway before attempting the second ventilation. If the second ventilation fails, proceed with the foreign body airway obstruction procedures described later in this appendix.

DETERMINE PULSELESSNESS

After you have determined breathlessness and delivered the initial ventilation, also assess the patient's pulse to determine whether the heart is beating. *The*

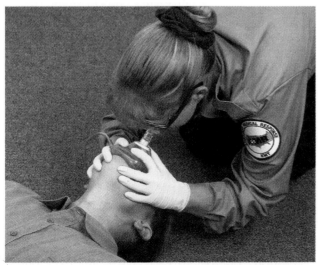

Figure A1-4   *Providing ventilations with a pocket face mask.*

patient must be determined to be pulseless before chest compressions are delivered.

To determine whether the heart is beating, take the adult or child patient's pulse at the carotid artery. (In an infant, assess the brachial pulse, as described later in this appendix.) While maintaining the head tilt with one hand on the patient's forehead, place the first two fingers of your other hand on the patient's larynx. Then slide your fingers down toward the floor, into the groove alongside the larynx, to locate the carotid artery. Exert gentle pressure only, to avoid compressing the carotid artery, and feel for a pulse for as long as 10 seconds (30 to 45 seconds if the patient has been submerged in cool or cold water or is suspected of being hypothermic). Do not use your thumb, which has its own pulse.

If there is no carotid pulse, you can assume that the patient is pulseless—the carotid pulse being one of the last to disappear.

DELIVER CHEST COMPRESSIONS

If the patient has no circulation, as evidenced by a lack of carotid pulse, apply rhythmic compressions over the lower half of the sternum to start the patient's blood circulating again. The compressions, alternated with ventilations, comprise cardiopulmonary resuscitation, or CPR. The technique for CPR varies for the adult, child, and infant and for delivery by one or by two rescuers, as explained on the following pages and summarized in Table A1-1.

Chest compressions work on two principles to help circulate the blood: First, they increase pressure in the chest cavity, causing blood to move through the thorax; and, second, they provide direct compression to the heart itself. Paired with artificial ventilation, chest compressions provide circulation of oxygenated blood until spontaneous breathing and circulation are restored or until advanced cardiac life support procedures can be begun.

The patient must be supine (lying on the back) on a firm, flat surface; the patient's head should not be elevated above the position of the heart.

TABLE A1-1 CPR Summary

	Adult (over 8 years)	Child (1 to 8 years)	Infant (under 1 year)
Hand Position	Two hands on lower half of sternum	Heel of one hand on lower half of sternum	Two or three fingers on lower half of sternum (one finger width below nipple line)
Compressions	Approximately 1½ to 2 inches in depth	Approximately 1 to 1½ inches in depth (equal to ⅓ to ½ the total chest depth)	Approximately ½ to 1 inch in depth (equal to ⅓ to ½ the total chest depth)
Breaths	Slowly, until chest gently rises (about 1½ to 2 seconds per breath)	Slowly, until chest gently rises (about 1 to 1½ seconds per breath)	Slowly, until chest gently rises (about 1 to 1½ seconds per breath
Cycle	15 compressions, 2 breaths (one rescuer) 5 compressions, 1 breath (two rescuers)	5 compressions, 1 breath (one or two rescuers)	5 compressions, 1 breath (one rescuer)
Rate	15 compressions in about 10 seconds or 80-100 per minute	5 compressions in about 3 seconds or 100 per minute	5 compressions in about 3 seconds or at least 100 per minute

Position Your Hands

Proper hand placement on the patient's chest is essential to avoid internal injury from chest compressions (Figures A1-5a to d). To position your hands correctly on the lower half of the sternum:

1. Locate the lower edge of the patient's rib cage on the side of the chest next to where you are kneeling.
2. Using the fingers of your hand that is closest to the patient's feet, locate the notch where the ribs are attached to the lower end of the sternum in the center of the chest. Place your middle finger on the substernal notch and your index finger beside it on the sternum.
3. Place the heel of your hand that is closest to the patient's head on the sternum beside the index finger of the other hand. Have the heel of your hand on the long axis of the sternum. This will distribute the pressure along the sternum, reducing the chance of rib fracture.
4. Place the hand that was closest to the patient's feet on top of the hand whose heel is on the sternum. Keep your hands parallel. (You can grasp the wrist of your first hand, instead, if your hands are weak or arthritic.)
5. Hold your fingers up off the patient's chest by spreading your fingers or interlacing them—also to prevent rib fracture.

DELIVER CHEST COMPRESSIONS

To deliver chest compressions:

1. With your hands properly placed, straighten your arms, lock your elbows, and position your shoulders directly over your hands. In this position, each thrust will be straight down onto the patient's sternum.
2. Press straight down, compressing the patient's sternum approximately 1½ to 2 inches, to force blood from the heart. (You may have to compress the chest more in an obese or very muscular person and less in a very thin or small person.)

HAND PLACEMENT FOR CPR

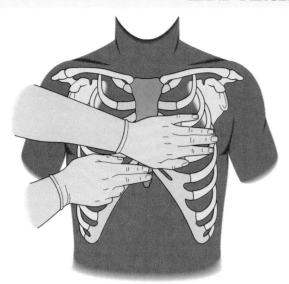

Figure A1-5a *Place the heel of one hand on the lower half of the sternum.*

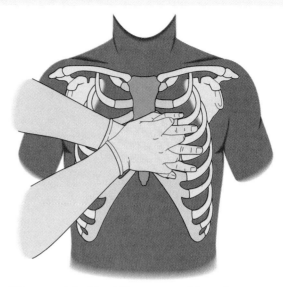

Figure A1-5b *Place second hand on top of first and interlace or spread the fingers.*

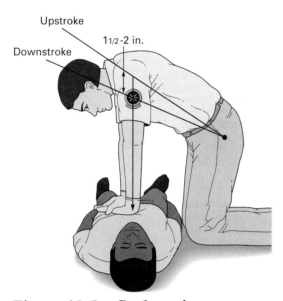

Figure A1-5c *Perform chest compressions.*

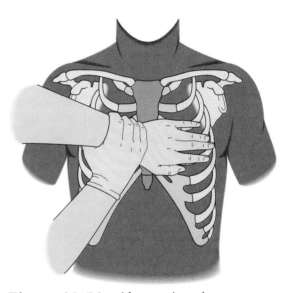

Figure A1-5d *Alternative placement for weak or arthritic hands.*

3. Release the pressure on the sternum completely to allow blood to flow back into the heart. You should allow the chest to return to its normal position between every compression.
4. Keep your hands in contact with the patient's chest at all times during chest compressions; do not lift your hands from the patient's chest or switch their position in any way.
5. Deliver chest compressions at the rate of 80 to 100 per minute.

CPR PERFORMED BY ONE RESCUER

If you do not have a partner, determine unresponsiveness, activate the EMS system, open the airway, determine breathlessness, perform artificial ventilation, and determine pulselessness as described earlier. To perform CPR (Figures A1-6a to d):

1. Position your hands properly on the patient's chest as described previously.
2. Deliver 15 chest compressions at the rate of 80

ONE-RESCUER CPR

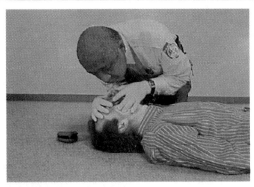

Figure A1-6a   Open the airway, determine breathlessness, and perform artificial ventilation, using a pocket mask if possible.

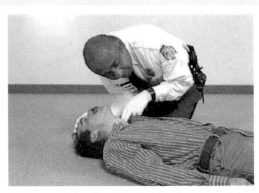

Figure A1-6b   Palpate the carotid to determine pulselessness.

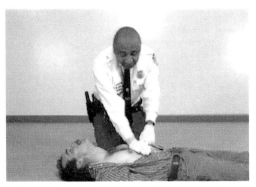

Figure A1-6c   Place hands on the lower half of the sternum.

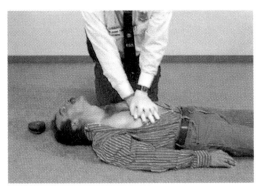

Figure A1-6d   Deliver 15 chest compressions at 80 to 100 per minute to a depth of 1½ to 2 inches. Then deliver 2 ventilations at 1½ to 2 seconds. Continue cycles of 15 compressions and 2 ventilations.

to 100 per minute (approximately 15 compressions over 9 to 11 seconds); count aloud to keep track of the compressions.

3. Remove your hands from the patient's chest, open the patient's airway, and deliver two slow ventilations of approximately 1½ to 2 seconds each.

4. Re-identify the lower half of the sternum. Correctly reposition your hands on the patient's chest, and deliver 15 more compressions at the rate of 80 to 100 per minute.

5. Repeat this cycle, performing four complete cycles of 15 compressions and 2 ventilations.

6. After four complete cycles, reassess the patient for circulation and breathing. If there is still no pulse, resume CPR with another four cycles of 15 chest compressions and 2 ventilations. If there is a pulse but the patient is not breathing, perform artificial ventilation at the rate of 12 breaths per minute but *do not* resume chest compressions. Continue to assess the patient every few minutes to determine whether breathing and pulse are present.

7. Continue CPR until the patient is breathing and has a pulse, until you are relieved by a second rescuer who performs CPR, or until you are relieved by an advanced cardiac life support team, or until you are physically unable to continue.

CPR PERFORMED BY TWO RESCUERS

If you have a partner, one of you should be positioned at the patient's side, the other at the patient's head. (See Figure A1-7, to compare positions for one-rescuer and two-rescuer CPR. Also see Figures A1-8a to h illustrating two-rescuer CPR.)

ONE-RESCUER CPR

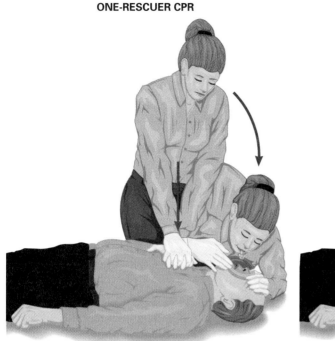

Fifteen chest compressions at a rate of 80-100 per minute.

Two full ventilations. Each breath is full, slow, and 1.5 to 2 seconds in length.

TWO-RESCUER CPR

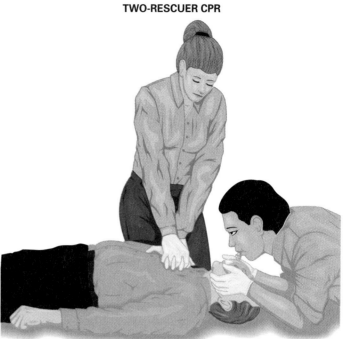

Five chest compressions at a rate of 80-100 per minute. Pause for ventilation.

One ventilation after each 5 compressions. Breaths are full, slow, and 1.5 to 2 seconds in length.

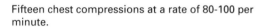

Figure A1-7 Be prepared for any circumstance. Know both one-rescuer and two-rescuer techniques well.

In two-rescuer CPR, the rescuer at the patient's side should deliver 5 chest compressions, as described above, then pause while the rescuer at the patient's head delivers 1 ventilation.

The rescuer at the patient's side who is performing the chest compressions should not remove his hands from the patient's chest. This will prevent losing, or wasting time re-identifying, the correct hand position after the second rescuer delivers the ventilation. The rescuer at the patient's head should maintain an open airway throughout resuscitation.

After 1 minute of CPR and every few minutes thereafter, the rescuer who is delivering ventilations should check for a return of a spontaneous carotid pulse. Since chest compressions will produce a carotid pulse, the pulse check must take place after the pause for ventilation. If there is no pulse, resume CPR with the cycle of chest compressions and ventilation.

When the rescuer delivering chest compressions gets fatigued, the two rescuers can rapidly switch positions on a given command, then resume resuscitation with the cycle of chest compressions and ventilation.

PERFORMING CPR ON INFANTS AND CHILDREN

As explained earlier, because infants and children are more likely to require airway and respiratory support and less likely to require defibrillation, the American Heart Association recommends that you *perform CPR for 1 minute before activating the EMS system—* if you are working alone. As with adults, you should never perform artificial ventilation or deliver chest compressions unless you have determined breathlessness and/or pulselessness. Infant and child CPR is summarized in Figures A1-9a to i.

In Infants under 1 Year of Age

- Determine pulselessness at the brachial pulse, located on the inner side of the upper arm.
- Using your hand that is closest to the infant's feet, place your fingers on the sternum as follows: Place the index finger just below the level of the nipples. Place the middle and ring fingers adjacent to the index finger. Lift the index finger and perform the compressions with the middle and ring fingers that are placed approximately one finger's width below the level of the nipples.

TWO-RESCUER CPR

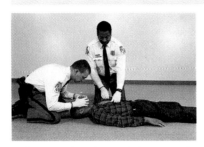

Figure A1-8a *After establishing breathlessness, ventilation rescuer delivers two ventilations, using a pocket mask, while compression rescuer bares chest. If the first ventilation is unsuccessful, reposition the head before reattempting ventilation.*

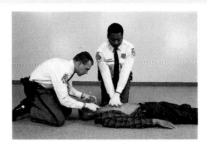

Figure A1-8b *After establishing pulselessness, ventilation rescuer says "No pulse" and other delivers 5 chest compressions at 80 to 100 per minute to a depth of 1½ to 2 inches.*

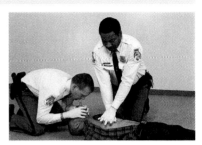

Figure A1-8c *Ventilation rescuer delivers 1 ventilation over 1½ to 2 seconds. Cycle of 5 compressions to 1 ventilation continues.*

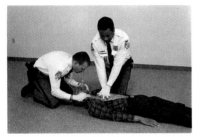

Figure A1-8d *Stop CPR so ventilation rescuer can assess carotid pulse after 1 minute and every few minutes thereafter. Compression rescuer keeps hands in position, ready to resume compressions if there is no pulse.*

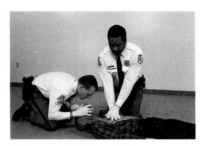

Figure A1-8e *The exhausted compression rescuer asks to switch.*

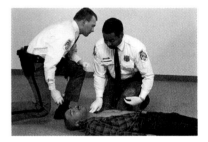

Figure A1-8f *The ventilation rescuer delivers a ventilation as usual, then they switch.*

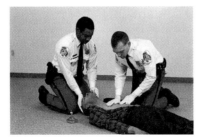

Figure A1-8g *The new ventilation rescuer opens the airway and checks pulse and respiration. The other prepares for compressions.*

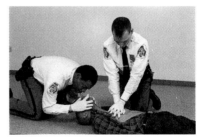

Figure A1-8h *If there is no pulse, the cycle of compressions and ventilations is resumed.*

INFANT AND CHILD CPR

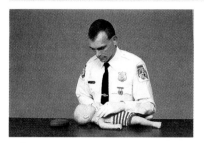

Figure A1-9a Determine unresponsiveness in the infant by shouting or flicking the soles of the feet. Do not shake an infant.

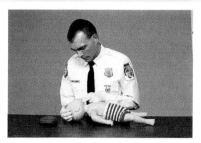

Figure A1-9b Gently open the airway.

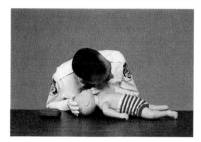

Figure A1-9c Determine breathlessness by the look-listen-feel method.

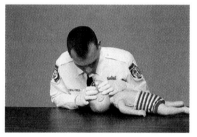

Figure A1-9d Establish a good seal with the pocket mask. Then deliver 2 ventilations at 1 to 1½ seconds per ventilation.

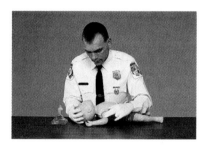

Figure A1-9e Determine pulselessness by palpating the brachial artery in the infant, the carotid artery in the child.

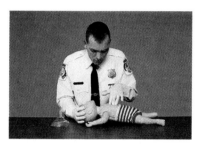

Figure A1-9f Locate the correct hand position for chest compressions.

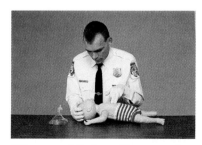

Figure A1-9g Depress the lower sternum one-third to one-half the depth of the chest (approximately ½ to 1 inch in the infant, 1 to 1½ inch in the child). Deliver compressions at a rate of 100 per minute.

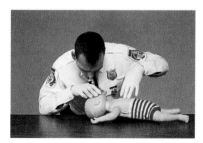

Figure A1-9h Deliver 1 ventilation after every 5 compressions. Activate EMS after 1 minute of CPR.

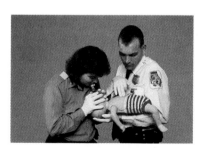

Figure A1-9i Performing infant CPR while carrying the infant.

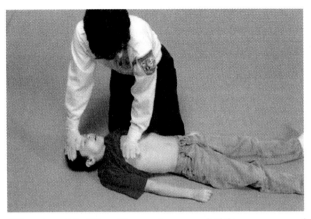

Figure A1-10 For a larger child, compress the sternum one-third to one-half the depth of the chest (approximately 1 to 1½ inches) with the heel of one hand.

- Deliver chest compressions. Depress the sternum about one-third to one-half its total depth, which will be a depth of about ½ to 1 inch.
- Deliver 5 compressions, then 1 ventilation. Continue in cycles of 5 to 1. The compression rate is *at least* 100 times per minute (5 compressions over 3 seconds or less).
- Activate EMS after 1 minute; that is, after 20 cycles of compressions and ventilation.

In Children Aged 1 to 8 Years

- Determine pulselessness at the carotid artery.
- Use the heel of only one hand; *do not* place your second hand on top of your first hand (Figure A1-10).
- Deliver compressions to the lower half of the sternum. Depress the sternum about one-third to one-half its total depth, which will be a depth of about 1 to 1½ inches.
- Deliver 5 compressions, then 1 ventilation. Continue in cycles of 5 to 1. The compression rate is 100 times per minute (5 compressions over 3 seconds).
- Activate EMS after 1 minute; that is, after approximately 20 cycles of compressions and ventilation.

In infants and children under the age of 8, deliver ventilations at the rate of 20 per minute and chest compressions at the rate of 100 per minute. For children over the age of 8, use the same rates as for adults.

OBSTRUCTED AIRWAY EMERGENCIES

An upper airway obstruction is anything that blocks the nasal passages, the oropharynx, or the laryngopharynx; lower airway foreign body obstruction can be caused by breathing in foreign materials or a severe bronchospasm. Airway obstruction is a true emergency. The airway must be cleared so the patient can breathe or so that artificial ventilations can be delivered.

CAUSES OF AIRWAY OBSTRUCTION

The most common source of upper airway obstruction is the tongue; the airway can also be obstructed by foreign bodies, secretions, blood clots, cancerous conditions of the mouth or throat, tonsil enlargement, injury to the face or jaw, acute epiglottitis, aspirated vomitus, and broken dental bridges.

Suspect that the patient choked on food if the patient had been eating or had anything in the mouth prior to collapsing. Elderly people are at particular risk for choking because they have a slower gag reflex and are more frequently misdiagnosed as having coronary disease if they collapse.

SIGNS AND SYMPTOMS OF AIRWAY OBSTRUCTION

Signs and symptoms of airway obstruction include:

- Clutching the neck with the hands
- Audible, noisy breathing, or no breath sounds
- Ability to nod but inability to speak or cough (a person who can't breathe because of a medical problem, such as a heart attack, will usually be able to speak or whisper)
- Labored use of muscles required in breathing
- Flared nostrils
- Strained neck and facial muscles
- Progressive restlessness, anxiety, and confusion
- Cyanosis
- Unresponsiveness

EMERGENCY CARE FOR PARTIAL OBSTRUCTION

A patient who can cough forcefully is getting some air exchange; obstruction is only partial. To treat:

1. Allow the patient time to remove the obstruction himself by encouraging him to cough. Don't interfere with the patient's attempts to expel the foreign object, but monitor him closely.
2. Watch for signs of reduced air passage: a weak, ineffective cough; a high-pitched wheeze during inhalation; increased strain in breathing; clutching the throat; and the beginning of cyanosis. If these signs develop, treat the patient as if he were suffering from a complete airway obstruction (see below).
3. Transport the patient rapidly to a medical facility where the partial obstruction can be removed.

EMERGENCY CARE FOR COMPLETE OBSTRUCTION

To clear the airway of a complete obstruction, use the foreign body airway obstruction (FBAO) maneuvers described in the following sections and in Figures A1-11a and b. Use abdominal thrusts (the Heimlich maneuver) to clear the airway. The maneuver thrusts the diaphragm quickly upward, forcing enough air from the lungs to create an artificial cough that dislodges and expels the foreign object.

Responsive Patient

1. If the patient is standing or sitting, stand behind the patient and wrap your arms around the waist; keep your elbows out, away from the patient's ribs.
2. Make a fist with one hand, and place the thumb side on the midline of the abdomen slightly above the navel and well below the xiphoid process (cartilage extending from the inferior sternum).
3. Grasp your fist with your other hand, thumbs toward the patient.
4. Press your fist into the patient's abdomen with a quick inward and upward thrust.
5. If you need to repeat the thrust, make each thrust separate and distinct. Continue until the object is released or the patient becomes unresponsive.

Be aware of these dangers:

- If you are improperly positioned or perform the thrusts too rapidly and too forcefully, you may lose your balance and fall into the patient.
- If your hands are too high (on the lower edges of the rib cage), you can cause internal injuries.
- The maneuver will often cause vomiting; correct hand placement and force can minimize the risk of vomiting.

Unresponsive Patient

1. If the patient is unresponsive or becomes unresponsive while you are attempting abdominal thrusts, place the patient in a supine position.
2. *If you witness the victim becoming unresponsive or there is reason to suspect that a foreign body is present, perform a finger sweep.* Open the patient's mouth with a tongue-jaw lift (grasp both the tongue and the lower jaw between thumb and fingers and lift the jaw). This maneuver may, itself, partially relieve the obstruction. Insert the index finger of the other hand along the inner cheek and deeply into the throat to the base of the tongue. Use a hooking motion to dislodge the foreign object and move it into the mouth where it can be removed. *Use this maneuver only on an unresponsive adult; a responsive person will*

FOREIGN BODY AIRWAY OBSTRUCTION (FBAO) MANEUVERS

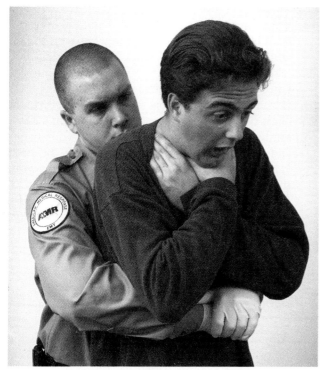

Figure A1-11a *Abdominal thrusts (Heimlich maneuver).*

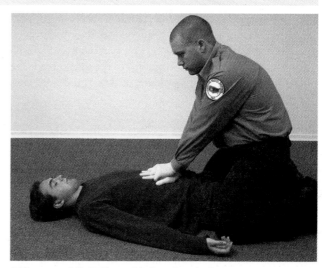

Figure A1-11b *Abdominal thrusts to an unresponsive patient.*

gag, and you may push the object deeper into the throat of a baby or small child.

3. *If the patient is unresponsive when found or no foreign body is immediately suspected, attempt ventilation,* as described earlier in this appendix. If the first ventilation is unsuccessful, reposition the head and attempt a second ventilation. If unsuccessful, perform the Heimlich maneuver, as described in steps 3 to 8.
4. Straddle the patient's thighs or hips.
5. Place the heel of one hand on the midline of the patient's abdomen, slightly above the navel and well below the tip of the xiphoid process to avoid possible laceration of internal organs. Put your second hand directly over the first.
6. Deliver quick upward thrusts. If you are in the correct mid-abdominal position, the thrusts will not veer off to the right or left.
7. If this action does not dislodge the foreign body, perform a tongue-jaw lift and finger sweep to attempt to relieve and dislodge the obstruction, as described in step 2, above. Remove dentures if they are present and loose or are causing difficulties; however, remember that keeping dentures in place can improve mask or mouth seal if artificial ventilations are needed.
8. If the foreign object is still not expelled, try giving ventilations by opening the airway and performing artificial ventilation; if ventilations are unsuccessful, repeat the cycle of abdominal thrusts, finger sweep, and ventilations.

If the patient is responsive and obese or in the late stages of pregnancy, there may be no room between the rib cage and the abdomen to perform abdominal thrusts, or you may be unable to reach around the patient. To treat, perform chest thrusts, as follows (Figures A1-12a to d):

Responsive Patient Who Is Obese or in Late Pregnancy

1. With the patient standing or sitting, stand behind the patient with your arms directly under the armpits; wrap your arms around the chest.
2. Position the thumb side of your fist on the midline of the sternum. If you are near the margins of the rib cage, you are too low.
3. Seize your fist firmly with your other hand and thrust backward sharply.
4. Repeat until the object is expelled or the patient becomes unresponsive.

Unresponsive Patient Who Is Obese or in Late Pregnancy

1. If the patient is unresponsive or becomes unresponsive, place in a supine position and kneel close to the patient's side.

2. Place the heel of your hand directly over the lower half of the sternum, as you would for CPR compressions.
3. Give distinct, separate thrusts downward, as for CPR compressions, until the object is expelled.

OBSTRUCTED AIRWAY IN INFANTS AND CHILDREN

In a child older than 1 year but less than 8 years, for partial obstruction—and assuming there are no cervical or spinal injuries—place the child on the side so that secretions, blood, and vomitus can drain out to the mouth. This position also causes the jaw to fall forward, bringing the tongue and epiglottis away from the airway. For a child older than 1 year with complete airway obstruction, follow the techniques, including the Heimlich maneuver, that were described above for an adult (Figure A1-13).

If an infant 1 year of age or younger is choking but still responsive, transport rapidly and let the infant try to expel the foreign object by coughing. For an infant who cannot expel the foreign object or who is unresponsive, perform the steps that follow.

Responsive Infant Who Is Choking and Cannot Expel the Foreign Object

1. Straddle the infant over one of your arms, with the face down and the head lower than the trunk. Support the infant's head by firmly holding the jaw. Rest your forearm on your thigh for support (Figure A1-14).
2. With the heel of your other hand, deliver five back blows rapidly and forcefully between the infant's shoulder blades. (Back blows are delivered first, since there is some risk of injuring an infant's liver with chest thrusts.)
3. If the foreign body has not been expelled, try chest thrusts. While supporting the infant's head, sandwich the infant's body between your hands and turn the infant on his back, with the head lower than the trunk. Lay the infant on your thigh or over your lap with the head supported. Deliver five quick, firm thrusts in the midsternal region with the same finger placement as for CPR chest compressions.
4. Repeat steps 2 and 3 until the obstruction is expelled or the infant becomes unresponsive.

Unresponsive Infant Who Is Not Breathing

1. Open the airway.
2. Attempt ventilation; if ventilation is unsuccessful, reposition the head and try again.
3. Deliver five rapid, forceful back blows.
4. If the back blows do not dislodge the foreign object, deliver five quick chest thrusts.

FOREIGN BODY AIRWAY OBSTRUCTION (FBAO) MANEUVERS
FOR THE OBESE OR PREGNANT PATIENT

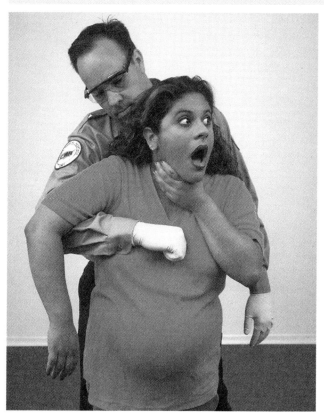

Figure A1-12a *Position thumb side of fist at midline of patient's sternum.*

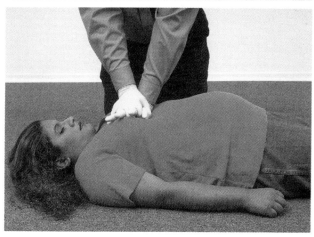

Figure A1-12c *Deliver chest compressions as for CPR to the supine pregnant patient.*

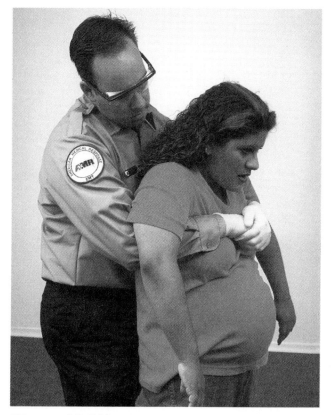

Figure A1-12b *Seize your fist firmly with your other hand and thrust backward sharply.*

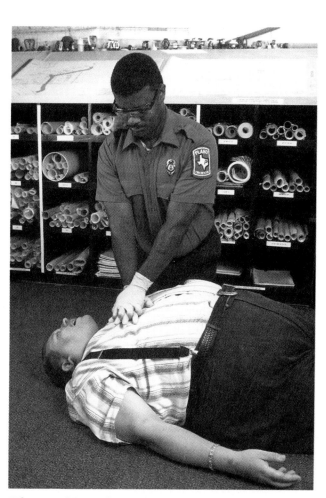

Figure A1-12d *Deliver chest compressions as for CPR to the supine obese patient.*

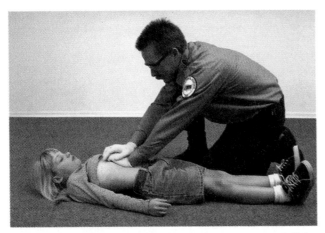

Figure A1-13   Abdominal thrusts on a child.

5. Perform a jaw-thrust maneuver to check for a foreign body; *never perform a blind finger sweep with infants and children;* you must be able to see the foreign object before trying to grasp it with your fingers. For infants and small children, use your little finger to hook and remove the object after you have visually located it.
6. Try ventilation again; repeat steps 2 to 5 as necessary.

After a foreign object is removed from any patient, regardless of age or responsiveness, transport the patient to the hospital. The airway may close again due to swelling, which often follows foreign-body obstruction. The patient should also be routinely evaluated for internal injuries that can be caused by abdominal or chest thrusts.

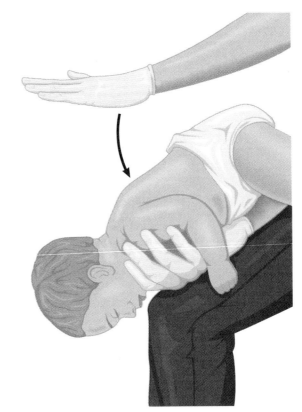

Figure A1-14   Back blows for an infant.

National Registry Skill Sheets

The National Registry of Emergency Medical Technicians is an organization founded in 1970, one of whose goals is to establish nationwide professional standards for EMTs. Many state EMS systems use examinations developed by the National Registry to establish certification of EMTs.

The National Registry has prepared a certification examination correlated to the 1994 Department of Transportation Emergency Medical Technician-Basic: National Standard Curriculum. The examination includes both a written portion and a practical portion that consists of a series of performance-based skill stations.

To assist students in preparing for the skill stations that are part of the EMT-Basic examination, as well as to establish guidelines and parameters for those who will evaluate students' performance at the skill stations, the National Registry has developed a series of skill sheets. Each skill sheet contains a set of directions, the skill criteria, and the critical criteria that result in immediate failure of the station.

In studying for the National Registry examination, these skills sheets should be used in conjunction with the material presented in the textbook and not as the sole means of learning the individual skills. The skill sheets will aid you in organizing the steps necessary to perform each skill and in identifying the criteria that will be used to evaluate your performance. You can use these sheets to evaluate your own performance when practicing these skills and preparing for your practical skills evaluation.

Note: Three skill sheets regarding advanced airway management are included. The use of these skills will vary based on your medical director, training program, and local protocol.

ORGANIZATION OF THE NATIONAL REGISTRY EXAMINATION

The practical examination consists of six stations, five mandatory stations and one random basic skill station consisting of both skill-based and scenario-based testing. The random skill station is conducted so the candidate is totally unaware of the skill to be tested until he or she arrives at the test site.

The candidate will be tested individually in each station and will be expected to direct the actions of any assistant EMTs who may be present in the station. The candidate should pass or fail the examination based solely on his or her actions and decisions.

The following is a list of the stations and their established time limits. The maximum time is determined by the number and difficulty of tasks to be completed.

Station 1:	Patient Assessment/Management—Trauma	10 min
Station 2:	Patient Assessment/Management—Medical	10 min
Station 3:	Cardiac Arrest Management/AED	15 min
Station 4:	Bag-Valve-Mask Apneic Patient	10 min
Station 5:	Spinal Immobilization Station:	
	Spinal Immobilization—Supine Patient	10 min
	Spinal Immobilization—Seated Patient	10 min
Station 6:	Random Basic Skill Verification:	
	Long Bone Injury	5 min
	Joint Injury	5 min
	Traction Splint	10 min
	Bleeding Control/Shock Management	10 min
	Upper Airway Adjuncts and Suction	5 min
	Mouth-to-Mask with Supplemental Oxygen	5 min
	Supplemental Oxygen Administration	5 min

INSTRUCTIONS TO THE CANDIDATE: PATIENT ASSESSMENT/ MANAGEMENT—TRAUMA

This station is designed to test your ability to perform a patient assessment of a victim of multi-system trauma and voice-treat all conditions and injuries discovered. You must conduct your assessment as you would in the field, including communicating with your patient. You may remove the patient's clothing down to shorts or swimsuit if you feel it is necessary. As you conduct your assessment, you should state everything you are assessing. Clinical information not obtainable by visual or physical inspection, for example blood pressure, will be given to you after you demonstrate how you would normally gain that information. You may assume that you have two EMTs working with you and that they are correctly carrying out the verbal treatments you indicate. You have (10) ten minutes to complete this skill station. Do you have any questions?

INSTRUCTIONS TO THE CANDIDATE: PATIENT ASSESSMENT/ MANAGEMENT—MEDICAL

This station is designed to test your ability to perform a patient assessment of a victim with a chief complaint of a medical nature and voice-treat all conditions and injuries discovered. You must conduct your assessment as you would in the field, including communicating with your patient. As you conduct your assessment, you should state everything you are assessing. Clinical information not obtainable by visual or physical inspection, for example, blood pressure, will be given to you after you demonstrate how you would normally gain that information. You may assume that you have two EMTs working with you and that they are correctly carrying out the verbal treatments you indicate. You have (10) ten minutes to complete this skill station. Do you have any questions?

INSTRUCTIONS TO THE CANDIDATE: CARDIAC ARREST MANAGEMENT

This station is designed to test your ability to manage a pre-hospital cardiac arrest by integrating CPR skills, defibrillation, airway adjuncts, and patient/scene management skills. There will be an EMT assistant in this station. The EMT assistant will only do as you instruct him. As you arrive on the scene you will encounter a patient in cardiac arrest. A first responder will be present performing single rescuer CPR. You must immediately establish control of the scene and begin resuscitation of the patient with an automated external defibrillator. At the appropriate time, you must control the airway and ventilate the victim using adjunctive equipment. You may not delegate this action to the EMT assistant. You may use any of the supplies available in this room. You have (15) fifteen minutes to complete this skill station. Do you have any questions?

INSTRUCTIONS TO THE CANDIDATE: AIRWAY, OXYGEN, VENTILATION SKILLS—BAG-VALVE-MASK APNEIC PATIENT WITH PULSE

This station is designed to test your ability to ventilate a patient using a bag-valve mask. As you enter the station you will find an apneic patient with a palpable central pulse. There are no bystanders and artificial ventilation has not been initiated. The only patient intervention required is airway management and ventilatory support using a bag-valve mask. You must initially ventilate the patient for a minimum of 30 seconds. You will be evaluated on the appropriateness of ventilator volumes. I will inform you that a second rescuer has arrived and will instruct you that you must control the airway and the mask seal while the second rescuer provides ventilation. You may use only the equipment available in this room. Do you have any questions?

INSTRUCTIONS TO THE CANDIDATE: SPINAL IMMOBILIZATION—SUPINE PATIENT

This station is designed to test your ability to provide spinal immobilization on a patient using a long spine immobilization device. You arrive on the scene with an EMT assistant. The assistant EMT has completed the scene size-up as well as the initial and focused assessments. As you begin the station there are no airway, breathing, or circulatory problems. You are required to treat the specific, isolated problem of an unstable spine using a long spine immobilization device. When moving the patient to the device, you should use the help of the assistant EMT and the evaluator. The assistant EMT should control the head and cervical spine of the patient while you and the evaluator move the patient to the immobilization device. You are responsible for the direction and subsequent action of the EMT assistant. You may use any equipment available in this room. You have (10) ten minutes to complete this procedure. Do you have any questions?

INSTRUCTIONS TO THE CANDIDATE: SPINAL IMMOBILIZATION SKILLS— SEATED PATIENT

This station is designed to test your ability to provide spinal immobilization on a patient using a half spine immobilization device. You arrive on the scene with an EMT assistant. The assistant EMT has completed the scene size-up, initial and focused assessments. As you begin the station, there are no airway, breathing, or circulatory problems. You are required to treat the specific, isolated problem of an unstable spine using a half spine immobilization device. Continued assessment of airway, breathing, and central circulation is not necessary. You are responsible for the direction and subsequent actions of the EMT assistant.

Transferring the patient to the long spine board should be accomplished verbally. You may use any equipment available in this room. You have (10) ten minutes to complete this procedure. Do you have any questions?

INSTRUCTIONS TO THE CANDIDATE: IMMOBILIZATION SKILLS—LONG BONE

This station is designed to test your ability to properly immobilize a closed, non-angulated long bone injury. You are required to treat only the specific, isolated injury. The scene size-up and initial assessment have been completed and during the focused assessment a closed, non-angulated injury of the _____ (radius, ulna, tibia, fibula) was detected. Ongoing assessment of the patient's airway, breathing, and central circulation is not necessary. You may use any equipment available in this room. You have (5) five minutes to complete this procedure. Do you have any questions?

INSTRUCTIONS TO THE CANDIDATE: IMMOBILIZATION SKILLS—JOINT INJURY

This station is designed to test your ability to properly immobilize a non-complicated shoulder injury. You are required to treat only the specific, isolated injury. The scene size-up and initial assessment have been accomplished on the victim and during the focused assessment a shoulder injury was detected. Ongoing assessment of the patient's airway, breathing, and central circulation is not necessary. You may use any equipment available in this room. You have (5) five minutes to complete this procedure. Do you have any questions?

INSTRUCTIONS TO THE CANDIDATE: IMMOBILIZATION SKILLS—TRACTION SPLINTING

This station is designed to test your ability to properly immobilize a mid-shaft femur injury with a traction splint. You will have an EMT assistant to help you in the application of the device by applying manual traction when directed to do so. You are required to treat only the specific, isolated injury. The scene size-up and initial assessment have been accomplished

on the victim and during the focused assessment a mid-shaft femur deformity was detected. Ongoing assessment of the patient's airway, breathing, and central circulation is not necessary. You may use any equipment available in this room. You have (10) ten minutes to complete this procedure. Do you have any questions?

INSTRUCTIONS TO THE CANDIDATE: BLEEDING CONTROL/SHOCK MANAGEMENT

This station is designed to test your ability to control hemorrhage. This is a scenario-based testing station. As you progress through the scenario, you will be offered various signs and symptoms appropriate for the patient's condition. You will be required to manage the patient based on these signs and symptoms. A scenario will be read aloud to you and you will be given an opportunity to ask clarifying questions about the scenario; however, you will not receive answers to any questions about the actual steps of the procedures to be performed. You may use any of the supplies and equipment available in this room. You have (10) ten minutes to complete this skill station. Do you have any questions?

INSTRUCTIONS TO THE CANDIDATE: AIRWAY, OXYGEN, VENTILATION SKILLS—UPPER AIRWAY ADJUNCTS AND SUCTION

This station is designed to test your ability to properly measure, insert, and remove an oropharyngeal and a nasopharyngeal airway as well as suction a patient's upper airway. This is an isolated skills test comprised of three separate skills. You may use any equipment available in this room. Do you have any questions?

INSTRUCTIONS TO THE CANDIDATE: AIRWAY, OXYGEN, VENTILATION SKILLS—MOUTH-TO-MASK WITH SUPPLEMENTAL OXYGEN

This station is designed to test your ability to ventilate a patient with supplemental oxygen using a mouth-to-mask technique. This is an isolated skills test. You may assume that mouth-to-mouth ventilation is in progress and that the patient has a central pulse. The only patient management required is ventilator support using a mouth-to-mask technique with supplemental oxygen. You must ventilate the patient for at least 30 seconds. You will be evaluated on the appropriateness of ventilatory volumes. You may use any equipment available in this room. Do you have any questions?

INSTRUCTIONS TO THE CANDIDATE: AIRWAY, OXYGEN, VENTILATION SKILLS—SUPPLEMENTAL OXYGEN ADMINISTRATION

This station is designed to test your ability to correctly assemble the equipment needed to administer supplemental oxygen in the pre-hospital setting. This is an isolated skills test. You will be required to assemble an oxygen tank and regulator and administer oxygen to a patient using a nonrebreather mask. At this point you will be instructed to discontinue oxygen administration by the nonrebreather mask because the patient cannot tolerate the mask and start oxygen administration using a nasal cannula. Once you have initiated oxygen administration using a nasal cannula, you will be instructed to discontinue oxygen administration completely. You may use only the equipment available in this room. Do you have any questions?

INSTRUCTIONS TO THE CANDIDATE: ADVANCED AIRWAY SKILLS

This station is designed to test your ability to provide immediate and aggressive ventilatory assistance to an apneic patient who has no other associated injuries. This is a non-trauma situation and cervical precautions are not necessary. You are required to sequentially demonstrate all procedures you would perform, from simple maneuvers and adjuncts to placement of one of the devices present in this station. Since you are testing as an EMT-Basic candidate today, which device will you be using? [Identify the device that is present in the station.] You will have three (3) attempts to successfully place the (EOA, EGTA, Combitube®, PtL®, or ET). You must actually ventilate the mannikin for at least thirty (30) seconds with each adjunct and procedure utilized. The examiner will serve as your trained assistant and will be interacting with you throughout this station. He or she will correctly carry out your orders upon your direction. Do you have any questions?

PATIENT ASSESSMENT/MANAGEMENT
TRAUMA

	Points Possible	Points Awarded
Takes or verbalizes body substance isolation precautions	1	
SCENE SIZE-UP		
Determines the scene is safe	1	
Determines the mechanism of injury	1	
Determines the number of patients	1	
Requests additional help if necessary	1	
Considers stabilization of spine	1	
INITIAL ASSESSMENT		
Verbalizes general impression of patient	1	
Determines responsiveness	1	
Determines chief complaint/apparent life threats	1	
Assesses airway and breathing — Assessment	1	
Initiates appropriate oxygen therapy	1	
Assures adequate ventilation	1	
Injury management	1	
Assesses Circulation — Assesses for and controls major bleeding	1	
Assesses pulse	1	
Assesses skin (color, temperature and condition)	1	
Identifies priority patients/makes transport decision	1	
FOCUSED HISTORY AND PHYSICAL EXAM/RAPID TRAUMA ASSESSMENT		
Selects appropriate assessment (focused or rapid assessment)	1	
Obtains or directs assistant to obtain baseline vital signs	1	
Obtains SAMPLE history	1	
DETAILED PHYSICAL EXAMINATION		
Assesses the head — Inspects and palpates the scalp and ears	1	
Assesses the eyes	1	
Assesses the facial area including oral and nasal area	1	
Assesses the neck — Inspects and palpates the neck	1	
Assesses for JVD	1	
Assesses for tracheal deviation	1	
Assesses the chest — Inspects	1	
Palpates	1	
Auscultates the chest	1	
Assesses the abdomen/pelvis — Assesses the abdomen	1	
Assesses the pelvis	1	
Verbalizes assessment of genitalia/perineum as needed	1	
Assesses the extremities — 1 point for each extremity includes inspection, palpation, and assessment of pulses, sensory and motor activities	4	
Assesses the posterior — Assesses thorax	1	
Assesses lumbar	1	
Manages secondary injuries and wounds appropriately — 1 point for appropriate management of secondary injury/wound	1	
Verbalizes reassessment of the vital signs	1	
	TOTAL:	**40**

CRITICAL CRITERIA
- ____ Did not take or verbalize body substance isolation precautions
- ____ Did not assess for spinal protection
- ____ Did not provide for spinal protection when indicated
- ____ Did not provide high concentration of oxygen
- ____ Did not find or manage problems associated with airway, breathing, hemorrhage or shock (hypoperfusion)
- ____ Did not differentiate patient's needing transportation versus continued on scene assessment
- ____ Does other detailed physical examination before assessing airway, breathing and circulation
- ____ Did not transport patient within ten (10) minute time limit

---

PATIENT ASSESSMENT/MANAGEMENT
MEDICAL

	Points Possible	Points Awarded
Takes or verbalizes body substance isolation precautions	1	
SCENE SIZE-UP		
Determines the scene is safe	1	
Determines the mechanism of injury/nature of illness	1	
Determines the number of patients	1	
Requests additional help if necessary	1	
Considers stabilization of spine	1	
INITIAL ASSESSMENT		
Verbalizes general impression of patient	1	
Determines responsiveness/level of consciousness	1	
Determines chief complaint/apparent life threats	1	
Assesses airway and breathing — Assessment	1	
Initiates appropriate oxygen therapy	1	
Assures adequate ventilation	1	
Assesses Circulation — Assesses/controls major bleeding	1	
Assesses pulse	1	
Assesses skin (color, temperature and condition)	1	
Identifies priority patients/makes transport decision	1	
FOCUSED HISTORY AND PHYSICAL EXAM/RAPID ASSESSMENT		
Signs and Symptoms (Assess history of present illness)	4	

Respiratory	Cardiac	Altered Mental Status	Allergic Reaction	Poisoning/ Overdose	Environmental Emergency	Obstetrics	Behavioral
•Onset?	•Onset?	•Description of the episode	•History of allergies?	•Substance?	•Source?	•Are you pregnant?	•How do you feel?
•Provokes?	•Provokes?	•Onset?	•What were you exposed to?	•When did you ingest/become exposed?	•Environment?	•How long have you been pregnant?	•Determine suicidal tendencies
•Quality?	•Quality?	•Duration?	•How were you exposed?	•How much did you ingest?	•Duration?	•Pain or contractions?	•Is the patient a threat to self or others?
•Radiates?	•Radiates?	•Associated symptoms?	•Effects?	•Over what time period?	•Loss of consciousness?	•Bleeding or discharge?	•Is there a medical problem?
•Severity?	•Severity?	•Evidence of trauma?	•Progression?	•Interventions?	•Effects: General or local?	•Do you feel the need to push?	•Interventions?
•Time?	•Time?	•Interventions?	•Interventions?	•Estimated weight?		•Last menstrual period?	
•Interventions?	•Interventions?	•Seizures?		•Effects?		•Crowning?	
		•Fever?					

	Points Possible	Points Awarded
Allergies	1	
Medications	1	
Past medical history	1	
Last Meal	1	
Events leading to present illness (rule out trauma)	1	
Performs focused physical examination — Assesses affected body part/system or, if indicated, completes rapid assessment	1	
Vitals (Obtains baseline vital signs)	1	
Interventions — Obtains medical direction or verbalizes standing order for medication interventions and verbalizes proper additional intervention/treatment	1	
Transport (Re-evaluates transport decision)	1	
Verbalizes the consideration for completing a detailed physical examination	1	
Ongoing Assessment (verbalized)	1	
Repeats initial assessment	1	
Repeats vital signs	1	
Repeats focused assessment regarding patient complaint or injuries	1	
Checks interventions	1	
	TOTAL:	**34**

CRITICAL CRITERIA
- ____ Did not take or verbalize body substance isolation precautions if necessary
- ____ Did not determine scene safety
- ____ Did not obtain medical direction or verbalize standing orders for medication interventions
- ____ Did not provide high concentration of oxygen
- ____ Did not evaluate and find conditions of airway, breathing, circulation
- ____ Did not find or manage problems associated with airway, breathing, hemorrhage or shock (hypoperfusion)
- ____ Did not differentiate patient's needing transportation versus continued assessment at the scene
- ____ Does detailed or focused history/physical examination before assessing airway, breathing and circulation
- ____ Did not ask questions about the present illness
- ____ Administered a dangerous or inappropriate intervention

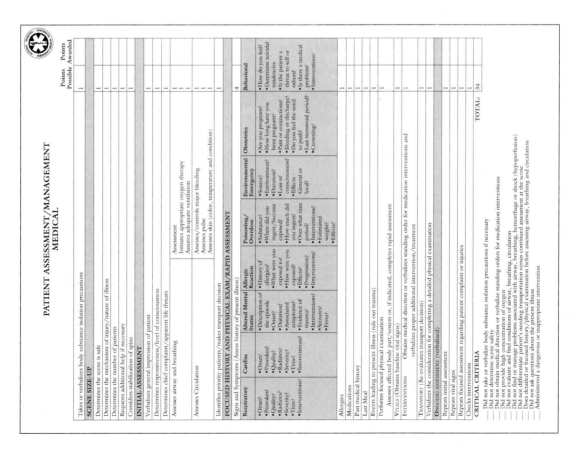

BAG-VALVE-MASK
APNEIC PATIENT

	Points Possible	Points Awarded
Takes or verbalizes body substance isolation precautions	1	
Voices opening the airway	1	
Voices inserting an airway adjunct	1	
Selects appropriate size mask	1	
Creates a proper mask-to-face seal	1	
Ventilates patient at no less than 800 ml volume	1	
(The examiner must witness for at least 30 seconds)		
Connects reservoir and oxygen	1	
Adjust liter flow to 15 liters/minute or greater	1	
The examiner indicates the arrival of second EMT. The second EMT is instructed to ventilate the patient while the candidate controls the mask and the airway.		
Voices re-opening the airway	1	
Creates a proper mask-to-face seal	1	
Instructs assistant to resume ventilation at proper volume per breath	1	
(The examiner must witness for at least 30 seconds)		
	TOTAL: 11	

CRITICAL CRITERIA

___ Did not take or verbalize body substance isolation precautions
___ Did not immediately ventilate the patient
___ Interrupted ventilations for more than 20 seconds
___ Did not provide high concentration of oxygen
___ Did not provide or direct assistant to provide proper volume/breath *(more than 2 ventilations per minute are below 800 ml)*
___ Did not allow adequate exhalation

CARDIAC ARREST MANAGEMENT/AED

	Points Possible	Points Awarded
ASSESSMENT		
Takes or verbalizes body substances isolation precautions	1	
Briefly questions rescuer about events	1	
Directs rescuer to stop CPR	1	
Verifies absence of spontaneous pulse	1	
(skill station examiner states "no pulse")		
Turns on defibrillator power	1	
Attaches automated defibrillator to patient	1	
Ensures all individuals are standing clear of the patient	1	
Initiates analysis of rhythm	1	
Delivers shock (up to three successive shocks)	1	
Verifies absence of spontaneous pulse	1	
(skill station examiner states "no pulse")		
TRANSITION		
Directs resumption of CPR	1	
Gathers additional information on arrest event	1	
Confirms effectiveness of CPR (ventilation and compressions)	1	
INTEGRATION		
Directs insertion of a simple airway adjunct (oropharyngeal/nasopharyngeal)	1	
Directs ventilation of patient	1	
Assures high concentration of oxygen connected to the ventilatory adjunct	1	
Assures CPR continues without unnecessary/prolonged interruption	1	
Re-evaluates patient/CPR in approximately one minute	1	
Repeats defibrillator sequence	1	
TRANSPORTATION		
Verbalizes transportation of patient	1	
	TOTAL: 20	

CRITICAL CRITERIA

___ Did not take or verbalize body substance isolation precautions
___ Did not evaluate the need for immediate use of the AED
___ Did not direct initiation/resumption of ventilation/compressions at appropriate times
___ Did not assure all individuals were clear of patient before delivering each shock
___ Did not operate the AED properly (inability to deliver shock)

SPINAL IMMOBILIZATION
SEATED PATIENT

	Points Possible	Points Awarded
Takes or verbalizes body substance isolation precautions	1	
Directs assistant to place/maintain head in neutral in-line position	1	
Directs assistant to maintain manual immobilization of the head	1	
Reassesses motor, sensory, and distal circulation in extremities	1	
Applies appropriate size extrication collar	1	
Positions the immobilization device behind the patient	1	
Secures the device to the patient's torso	1	
Evaluates torso fixation and adjusts as necessary	1	
Evaluates and pads behind the patient's head as necessary	1	
Secures the patient's head to the device	1	
Verbalizes moving the patient to a long board	1	
Reassesses motor, sensory, and distal circulation in extremities	1	
TOTAL:	**12**	

CRITICAL CRITERIA

_____ Did not immediately direct or take manual immobilization of the head
_____ Releases or orders release of manual immobilization before it was maintained mechanically
_____ Patient manipulated or moved excessively, causing potential spinal compromise
_____ Device moves excessively up, down, left, or right on patient's torso.
_____ Head immobilization allows for excessive movement
_____ Torso fixation inhibits chest rise, resulting in respiratory compromise
_____ Upon completion of immobilization, head is not in the neutral position
_____ Did not reassess motor, sensory, and distal circulation after voicing immobilization to the long board
_____ Immobilized head to the board before securing the torso

---

SPINAL IMMOBILIZATION
SUPINE PATIENT

	Points Possible	Points Awarded
Takes or verbalizes body substance isolation precautions	1	
Directs assistant to place/maintain head in neutral in-line position	1	
Directs assistant to maintain manual immobilization of the head	1	
Assesses motor, sensory, and distal circulation in extremities	1	
Applies appropriate size extrication collar	1	
Positions the immobilization device appropriately	1	
Directs movement of the patient onto device without compromising the integrity of the spine	1	
Applies padding to voids between the torso and the boards as necessary	1	
Immobilizes the patient's torso to the device	1	
Evaluates the pads behind the patient's head as necessary	1	
Immobilizes the patient's head to the device	1	
Secures the patient's legs to the device	1	
Secures the patient's arms to the device	1	
Reassesses motor, sensory, and distal circulation in extremities	1	
TOTAL:	**14**	

CRITICAL CRITERIA

_____ Did not immediately direct or take manual immobilization of the head
_____ Releases or orders release of manual immobilization before it was maintained mechanically
_____ Patient manipulated or moved excessively, causing potential spinal compromise
_____ Patient moves excessively up, down, left, or right on the device.
_____ Head immobilization allows for excessive movement
_____ Upon completion of immobilization, head is not in the neutral in-line position
_____ Did not reassess motor, sensory, and distal circulation after immobilization to the device
_____ Immobilized head to the board before securing torso

IMMOBILIZATION SKILLS
JOINT INJURY

	Points Possible	Points Awarded
Takes or verbalizes body substance isolation precautions	1	
Directs application of manual stabilization of the injury	1	
Assesses motor, sensory, and distal circulation	1	
NOTE: The examiner acknowledges present and normal		
Selects proper splinting material	1	
Immobilizes the site of the injury	1	
Immobilizes bone above injured joint	1	
Immobilizes bone below injured joint	1	
Reassesses motor, sensory, and distal circulation	1	
NOTE: The examiner acknowledges present and normal		
TOTAL:	8	

CRITICAL CRITERIA

___ Did not support the joint so that the joint did not bear distal weight

___ Did not immobilize bone above and below injured joint

___ Did not reassess motor, sensory, and distal circulation before and after splinting

IMMOBILIZATION SKILLS
LONG BONE

	Points Possible	Points Awarded
Takes or verbalizes body substance isolation precautions	1	
Directs application of manual stabilization	1	
Assesses motor, sensory, and distal circulation	1	
NOTE: The examiner acknowledges present and normal		
Measures splint	1	
Applies splint	1	
Immobilizes the joint above the injury site	1	
Immobilizes the joint below the injury site	1	
Secures the entire injured extremity	1	
Immobilizes hand/foot in the position of function	1	
Reassesses motor, sensory, and distal circulation	1	
NOTE: The examiner acknowledges present and normal		
TOTAL:	10	

CRITICAL CRITERIA

___ Grossly moves injured extremity

___ Did not immobilize adjacent joints

___ Did not assess motor, sensory, and distal circulation before and after splinting

BLEEDING CONTROL/SHOCK MANAGEMENT

	Points Possible	Points Awarded
Takes or verbalizes body substance isolation precautions	1	
Applies direct pressure to the wound	1	
Elevates the extremity	1	
NOTE: The examiner must now inform the candidate that the wound continues to bleed.		
Applies an additional dressing to the wound	1	
NOTE: The examiner must now inform the candidate that the wound still continues to bleed. The second dressing does not control the bleeding.		
Locates and applies pressure to appropriate arterial pressure point	1	
NOTE: The examiner must now inform the candidate that the bleeding is controlled.		
Bandages the wound	1	
NOTE: The examiner must now inform the candidate that the patient is showing signs and symptoms indicative of hypoperfusion.		
Properly positions the patient	1	
Applies high concentration oxygen	1	
Initiates steps to prevent heat loss from the patient	1	
Indicates need for immediate transportation	1	
TOTAL:	**10**	

CRITICAL CRITERIA

___ Did not take or verbalize body substance isolation precautions
___ Did not apply high concentration of oxygen
___ Applies tourniquet before attempting other methods of bleeding control
___ Did not control hemorrhage in a timely manner
___ Did not indicate a need for immediate transportation

IMMOBILIZATION SKILLS
TRACTION SPLINTING

	Points Possible	Points Awarded
Takes or verbalizes body substance isolation precautions	1	
Directs application of manual stabilization of the injured leg	1	
Directs the application of manual traction	1	
Assesses motor, sensory, and distal circulation	1	
NOTE: The examiner acknowledges present and normal.		
Prepares/adjusts splint to the proper length	1	
Positions the splint at the injured leg	1	
Applies the proximal securing device (e.g., ischial strap)	1	
Applies the distal securing device (e.g., ankle hitch)	1	
Applies mechanical traction	1	
Positions/secures the support straps	1	
Re-evaluates the proximal/distal securing devices	1	
Reassesses motor, sensory, and distal circulation	1	
NOTE: The examiner acknowledges present and normal.		
NOTE: The examiner must ask candidate how he/she would prepare the patient for transportation.		
Verbalizes securing the torso to the long board to immobilize the hip	1	
Verbalizes securing the splint to the long board to prevent movement of the splint	1	
TOTAL:	**14**	

CRITICAL CRITERIA:

___ Loss of traction at any point after it is assumed
___ Did not reassess motor, sensory, and distal circulation before and after splinting
___ The foot is excessively rotated or extended after splinting
___ Did not secure the ischial strap before taking traction
___ Final immobilization failed to support the femur or prevent rotation of the injured leg
___ Secures leg to splint before applying mechanical traction

NOTE: If the Sager splint or Kendrick Traction Device is used without elevating the patient's leg, application of manual traction is not necessary. The candidate should be awarded 1 point as if manual traction were applied.

NOTE: If the leg is elevated at all, manual traction must be applied before elevating the leg. The ankle hitch may be applied before elevating the leg and used to provide manual traction.

MOUTH-TO-MASK WITH SUPPLEMENTAL OXYGEN

	Points Possible	Points Awarded
Takes or verbalizes body substance isolation precautions	1	
Connects one-way valve to mask	1	
Opens patient's airway or confirms patient's airway is open (manually or with adjunct)	1	
Establishes and maintains a proper mask to face seal	1	
Ventilates the patient at the proper volume and rate (800–1200 ml per breath/10–20 breaths per minute)	1	
Connects mask to high concentration oxygen	1	
Adjusts flow rate to 15 liters/minute or greater	1	
Continues ventilation at proper volume and rate (800–1200 ml per breath/10–20 breaths per minute)	1	
NOTE: The examiner must witness ventilations for at least 30 seconds.		
TOTAL:	8	

CRITICAL CRITERIA

___ Did not take or verbalize body substance isolation precautions
___ Did not adjust liter flow to 15 L/min or greater
___ Did not provide proper volume per breath
   (more than 2 ventilations per minute are below 800 ml)
___ Did not ventilate the patient at 10–20 breaths per minute
___ Did not allow for complete exhalation

AIRWAY, OXYGEN, AND VENTILATION SKILLS
UPPER AIRWAY ADJUNCTS AND SUCTION

OROPHARYNGEAL AIRWAY

	Points Possible	Points Awarded
Takes or verbalizes body substance isolation precautions	1	
Selects appropriate size airway	1	
Measures airway	1	
Inserts airway without pushing the tongue posteriorly	1	
NOTE: The examiner must advise the candidate that the patient is gagging and becoming conscious.		
Removes oropharyngeal airway	1	

SUCTION

	Points Possible	Points Awarded
NOTE: The examiner must advise the candidate to suction the patient's oropharynx/nasopharynx.		
Turns on/prepares suction device	1	
Assures presence of mechanical suction	1	
Inserts suction tip without suction	1	
Applies suction to the oropharynx/nasopharynx	1	

NASOPHARYNGEAL AIRWAY

	Points Possible	Points Awarded
NOTE: The examiner must advise the candidate to insert a nasopharyngeal airway.		
Selects appropriate airway	1	
Measures airway	1	
Verbalizes lubrication of the nasal airway	1	
Fully inserts the airway with the bevel facing toward the septum	1	
TOTAL:	13	

CRITICAL CRITERIA

___ Did not take or verbalize body substance isolation precautions
___ Did not obtain a patent airway with the oropharyngeal airway
___ Did not obtain a patent airway with the nasopharyngeal airway
___ Did not demonstrate an acceptable suction technique
___ Inserts any adjunct in a manner dangerous to the patient

VENTILATORY MANAGEMENT
ENDOTRACHEAL INTUBATION

NOTE: If a candidate elects to initially ventilate with a BVM attached to a reservoir and oxygen, full credit must be awarded for steps denoted by "**" if the first ventilation is delivered within the initial 30 seconds

	Points Possible	Points Awarded
Takes or verbalizes body substance isolation precautions	1	
Opens airway manually	1	
Elevates tongue and inserts simple airway adjunct (oropharyngeal or nasopharyngeal airway)	1	
NOTE: The examiner now informs the candidate no gag reflex is present and the patient accepts the adjunct.		
**Ventilates the patient immediately using a BVM device unattached to oxygen	1	
**Hyperventilates the patient with room air	1	
Note: The examiner now informs the candidate that ventilation is being performed without difficulty.		
Attaches the oxygen reservoir to the BVM	1	
Attaches BVM to high-flow oxygen	1	
Ventilates the patient at the proper volume and rate (800–1200 ml per breath/10–20 breaths per minute)	1	
NOTE: After 30 seconds, the examiner auscultates and reports breath sounds are present and equal bilaterally and medical control has ordered intubation. The examiner must now take over ventilation.		
Directs assistant to hyperventilate patient	1	
Identifies/selects proper equipment for intubation	1	
Checks equipment — Checks for cuff leaks	1	
— Checks laryngoscope operation and bulb tightness	1	
NOTE: The examiner must remove the OPA and move out of the way when the candidate is prepared to intubate.		
Positions the head properly	1	
Inserts the laryngoscope blade while displacing the tongue	1	
Elevates the mandible with the laryngoscope	1	
Introduces the ET tube and advances it to the proper depth	1	
Inflates the cuff to the proper pressure	1	
Disconnects the syringe from the cuff inlet port	1	
Directs ventilation of the patient	1	
Confirms proper placement by auscultation bilaterally and over the epigastrium	1	
NOTE: The examiner must ask, "If you had proper placement, what would you expect to hear?"		
Secures the ET tube *(may be verbalized)*	1	
TOTAL:	21	

CRITICAL CRITERIA

___ Did not take or verbalize body substance isolation precautions
___ Did not initiate ventilations within 30 seconds after applying gloves or interrupts ventilations for greater than 30 seconds at any time
___ Did not voice or provide high oxygen concentrations (15 L/min or greater)
___ Did not ventilate patient at a rate of at least 10/minute
___ Did not provide adequate volume per breath (maximum of 2 errors/minute permissible)
___ Did not hyperventilate the patient prior to intubation
___ Did not successfully intubate within 3 attempts
___ Used the patient's teeth as a fulcrum
___ Did not assure proper tube placement by auscultation bilaterally and over the epigastrium
___ If used, the stylette extended beyond the end of the ET tube
___ Inserts any adjunct in a manner that would be dangerous to the patient
___ Did not disconnect syringe from cuff inlet port

OXYGEN ADMINISTRATION

	Points Possible	Points Awarded
Takes or verbalizes body substance isolation precautions	1	
Assembles regulator to tank	1	
Opens tank	1	
Checks for leaks	1	
Checks tank pressure	1	
Attaches non-rebreather mask	1	
Prefills reservoir	1	
Adjusts liter flow to 12 liters/minute or greater	1	
Applies and adjusts mask to the patient's face	1	
NOTE: The examiner must advise the candidate that the patient is not tolerating the non-rebreather mask. Medical direction has ordered you to apply a nasal cannula to the patient.		
Attaches nasal cannula to oxygen	1	
Adjusts liter flow up to 6 liters/minute or less	1	
Applies nasal cannula to the patient	1	
NOTE: The examiner must advise the candidate to discontinue oxygen therapy.		
Removes the nasal cannula	1	
Shuts off the regulator	1	
Relieves the pressure within the regulator	1	
TOTAL:	15	

CRITICAL CRITERIA

___ Did not take or verbalize body substance isolation precautions
___ Did not assemble the tank and regulator without leaks
___ Did not prefill the reservoir bag
___ Did not adjust the device to the correct liter flow for the non-rebreather mask (12 L/min or greater)
___ Did not adjust the device to the correct liter flow for the nasal cannula (up to 6 L/min)

VENTILATORY MANAGEMENT
ESOPHAGEAL OBTURATOR AIRWAY INSERTION FOLLOWING AN UNSUCCESSFUL ENDOTRACHEAL INTUBATION ATTEMPT

	Points Possible	Points Awarded
Continues body substance isolation precautions	1	
Confirms the patient is being properly ventilated	1	
Directs assistant to hyperventilate the patient	1	
Identifies/selects proper equipment	1	
Assembles airway	1	
Tests cuff	1	
Inflates mask	1	
Lubricates tube (*may be verbalized*)	1	
Removes the oropharyngeal airway	1	
Positions head properly with neck in the neutral or slightly flexed position	1	
Grasps and elevates tongue and mandible	1	
Inserts tube in the same direction as the curvature of the pharynx	1	
Advances tube until the mask is sealed against the face	1	
Ventilates the patient while maintaining a tight mask seal	1	
Confirms placement by observing chest rise and auscultating over the epigastrium and bilaterally over the chest	1	
NOTE: The examiner confirms adequate chest rise, bilateral breath sounds and absent sounds over the epigastrium.		
Inflates the cuff to the proper pressure	1	
Disconnects the syringe	1	
Continues ventilation of the patient	1	
TOTAL:	**18**	

CRITICAL CRITERIA

___ Did not take or verbalize body substance isolation precautions
___ Interrupts ventilation for more than 30 seconds
___ Did not direct hyperventilation of the patient prior to placement of the device
___ Did not assure proper placement of the device
___ Did not successfully ventilate the patient
___ Did not provide high flow oxygen (15 L/min or greater)
___ Inserts any adjunct in a manner that would be dangerous to the patient

---

VENTILATORY MANAGEMENT
DUAL LUMEN AIRWAY DEVICE (PTL OR COMBI-TUBE) INSERTION FOLLOWING AN UNSUCCESSFUL ENDOTRACHEAL INTUBATION ATTEMPT

	Points Possible	Points Awarded
Continues body substance isolation precautions	1	
Confirms the patient is being properly ventilated with high percentage oxygen	1	
Directs assistant to hyperventilate the patient	1	
Checks/prepares airway device	1	
Lubricates distal tip of the device (*may be verbalized*)	1	
Removes the oropharyngeal airway	1	
Positions the head properly	1	
Performs a tongue-jaw lift	1	
Inserts airway device to proper depth	1	
COMBI-TUBE	**PTL**	
Inflates pharyngeal cuff and removes syringe	Secures strap	1	
Inflates distal cuff and removes syringe	Blows into tube #1 to inflate both cuffs	1	
Ventilates through proper first lumen		1	
Confirms placement by observing chest rise and auscultating over the epigastrium and bilaterally over the chest		1	
NOTE: The examiner states: "You do not see rise and fall of the chest and hear sounds only over the epigastrium."			
Ventilates through the alternate lumen		1	
Confirms placement by observing chest rise and auscultating over the epigastrium and bilaterally over the chest		1	
NOTE: The examiner confirms adequate chest rise, bilateral breath sounds, and absent sounds over the epigastrium.			
Secures tube at appropriate step in sequence		1	
	TOTAL:	**16**	

CRITICAL CRITERIA

___ Did not take or verbalize body substance isolation precautions
___ Interrupts ventilation for greater than 30 seconds
___ Did not direct hyperventilation of the patient prior to placement of the device
___ Did not assure proper placement of the device
___ Did not successfully ventilate patient
___ Did not provide high flow oxygen (15 L/min or greater)
___ Inserts any adjunct in a manner that would be dangerous to the patient

Glossary

abandonment—the act of discontinuing emergency care without ensuring that another health care professional with equivalent or better training will take over.

abdominal aorta—a major division of the primary artery that runs through the abdomen.

abdominal cavity—the space located below the diaphragm that extends to the top of the pelvis.

abdominal quadrants—the four parts of the abdomen as divided by imaginary horizontal and vertical lines through the umbilicus.

abortion—*see* spontaneous abortion.

abrasion—an open injury to the outermost layer of the skin (epidermis) caused by a scraping away, rubbing, or shearing away of the tissue.

absorption—passage of a substance through skin or mucous membranes upon contact.

acceleration-deceleration injury—a head injury typical of a car crash in which the head comes to a sudden stop, but the brain continues to move back and forth inside the skull, resulting in bruising to the brain.

acetabulum—the rounded cavity or socket on the lateral surface of the pelvis that receives the head of the femur.

acromion—the lateral triangular projection of the scapula that forms the point of the shoulder.

actions—the therapeutic (helpful) effects of a medication; for example, an action of nitroglycerin is relaxation of the blood vessels.

activated charcoal—a distilled charcoal in powder form that can adsorb many times its weight in contaminants; often administered to patients who have ingested poison to adsorb the poison and help prevent its absorption by the body.

active rewarming—technique of aggressively applying heat to a patient to rewarm his body. *See also* passive rewarming.

acute—severe, with rapid onset.

acute abdomen—an abdominal associated with a medical condition. Acute abdomen can have a number of causes. Also called acute abdominal distress.

acute abdominal distress—*see* acute abdomen.

Adam's apple—*see* thyroid cartilage.

administration—the route and form by which a drug is given.

adolescent—a person 12 to 18 years of age.

advance directive—instructions written in advance, such as a living will or Do Not Resuscitate (DNR) order.

afterbirth—the placenta and other tissues that are expelled shortly after the birth of a child.

agonal respirations—gasping-type respirations that have no pattern and occur very infrequently; a sign of impending cardiac or respiratory arrest.

air embolism—an air bubble that enters the bloodstream and obstructs a blood vessel.

allergen—a substance that enters the body by ingestion, injection, inhalation, or contact and triggers an allergic reaction.

allergic reaction—a misdirected and excessive response by the immune system to a foreign substance or an allergen.

altered mental status—condition in which the patient displays a change in his normal mental state ranging from disorientation to complete unresponsiveness.

alveoli—small air sacs in the lungs that fill with air on inspiration and are the point of gas exchange with the pulmonary capillaries.

Alzheimer's disease—disease characterized by cerebral function loss as seen with diseases that affect the brain.

amniotic sac—a thin, transparent membrane that forms the sac which holds the fetus suspended in amniotic fluid. Also called bag of waters.

amputation—an open injury caused by the ripping or tearing away of a limb, body part, or organ.

anaphylactic shock—a shock (hypoperfusion) state that results from dilated and leaking blood vessels related to severe allergic reaction. The patient also experiences respiratory distress and hives. It is also called anaphylaxis or anaphylactic reaction. *See also* anaphylaxis.

anaphylaxis—a severe allergic reaction that produces respiratory distress and shock (hypoperfusion). *See also* anaphylactic shock.

anatomical planes—imaginary straight-line divisions of the body.

anatomy—the study of the structure of the body and the relationship of its parts to each other.

anterior—toward the front. Opposite of posterior.

anterior chamber—the front chamber of the eye containing the aqueous humor.

anterior fontanelle—the "soft-spot" on the top of an infant's head where the plates of the skull have not yet fused together.

anterior plane—the front, or abdominal side of the body.

antibodies—special proteins produced by the immune system that search out antigens, combine with, and help to destroy them.

antigen—a foreign substance that enters the body and triggers an immune response.

anxiety—a state of painful uneasiness about impending problems characterized by agitation and restlessness.

aorta—major artery that starts at the left ventricle and carries oxygen-rich blood to the body.

apnea—absence of breathing; respiratory arrest.

aqueous humor—the watery fluid that fills the anterior chamber of the eye.

arachnoid—middle layer of protective brain tissue (meninges). *See also* dura mater; meninges; pia mater.

arteriole—smallest branch of an artery, leading to a capillary.

arteriosclerosis—disease process that causes the loss of elasticity in the vascular walls due to thickening and hardening of the vessels.

artery—a blood vessel that carries blood away from the heart.

artificial ventilation—*see* positive pressure ventilation.

arytenoids—irregular pyramid-shaped structures located on the top of the posterior aspect of the cricoid ring.

aspiration—breathing a foreign substance into the lungs.

aspiration pneumonia—inflammation of the lungs caused by the aspiration of vomitus or other foreign matter.

assessment—*see* patient assessment.

asystole—a heart rhythm indicating absence of any electrical activity in the heart, also known as "flatline."

atrium—one of the two upper chambers of the heart.

aura—an unusual sensory sensation that may precede a seizure episode by hours or only a few seconds.

auscultation—the process of listening with a stethoscope for sounds within the body.

auto-injector—a device with a concealed, spring-loaded needle, used for injecting a single dose of medication. An epinephrine auto-injector is often prescribed to patients with a history of anaphylactic reaction.

automated external defibrillator (AED)—a device that can analyze the electrical activity or rhythm of a patient's heart and deliver an electrical shock (defibrillation) if appropriate.

automatic transport ventilator (ATV)—a positive pressure ventilation device that delivers ventilations automatically.

autonomic nervous system—part of the nervous system that influences involuntary muscles and glands.

AVPU—a mnemonic for alert, responds to verbal stimulus, responds to painful stimulus, unresponsive, to characterize levels of responsiveness.

avulsion—an open injury characterized by a loose flap of skin and soft tissue that has been torn loose or pulled completely off.

bag of waters—*see* amniotic sac.

bag-valve-mask device (BVM)—a positive pressure ventilation device that consists of a bag with a nonrebreather valve and a mask. The bag-valve device is connected to the mask or other airway. The bag is squeezed to deliver a ventilation to the patient.

bandage—any material used to secure a dressing in place.

base station—the central dispatch and coordination area of an EMS communications system that ideally is in contact with all other elements of the system.

baseline vital signs—the first set of vital signs measurements to which subsequent measurements can be compared. *See* vital signs.

basilar skull—floor of the skull.

Battle's sign—discoloration of the mastoid, suggesting basilar skull fracture.

behavior—the way a person acts or performs.

behavioral emergency—a situation in which a person exhibits abnormal behavior.

bilateral—on both sides.

bipolar disorder—a psychiatric condition, also known as manic-depressive disorder, characterized by wide swings between periods of depression and periods of elation and manic behavior.

blood pressure—the pressure exerted during circulation of the blood against the arterial walls. *See also* diastolic pressure; systolic pressure.

bloody show—the mucus and blood that are expelled from the vagina as labor begins.

blunt trauma—a force that impacts or is applied to the body but is not sharp enough to penetrate it, such as a blow or a crushing injury.

body mechanics—application of the study of muscles and body movement (kinesiology) to the use of the body and to the prevention and correction of problems related to posture and lifting. Principles of body mechanics focus on the most efficient methods of moving or using the body to gain a mechanical advantage when lifting objects.

body substance isolation (BSI)—a method of preventing infection by disease organisms based on the premise that all blood and body fluids are infectious.

brachial artery—the major artery of the upper arm.

bradycardia—a heart rate that is slower than the normal lower limit.

bradypnea—a breathing rate that is slower than the normal lower limit.

brainstem—the funnel-shaped inferior part of the brain that controls most automatic functions of the body. It is made up of the pons, the midbrain, and the medulla, which is the brain's connection to the spinal cord.

breech birth—a common abnormality of delivery in which the fetal buttocks or lower extremities are low in the uterus and are the first to be delivered.

bronchioles—smaller airways that branch from the bronchi and terminate at the alveolar sacs.

bronchoconstriction—constriction of the smooth muscle of the bronchi and bronchioles causing a narrowing of the air passageway.

bronchodilator—a drug that relaxes the smooth muscle of the bronchi and bronchioles and reverses bronchoconstriction.

bronchospasm—spasm or constriction of the smooth muscle of the bronchi and bronchioles.

burn sheet—commercially prepared sterile, particle-free, disposable sheet used to cover the entire body in severe burns injuries.

burnout—a condition resulting from chronic job stress, characterized by a state of exhaustion and irritability that can markedly decrease effectiveness.

calcaneus—the heel bone.

capillary—tiny blood vessel connecting arterioles to venules; site of gas and nutrient exchange with the body's cells.

capillary refill—the amount of time it takes for capillaries that have been compressed to refill with blood.

cardiac arrest—the cessation of cardiac function with the patient displaying unresponsiveness with no pulse and no breathing.

cardiac conduction system—the specialized contractile and conductive tissue of the heart that generates electrical impulses and causes the heart to beat.

cardiac hypertrophy—an increase in the size of the heart from a thickening of the heart wall, without a parallel increase in the size of the cavity.

cardiac muscle—a kind of involuntary muscle found only in the walls of the heart. Cardiac muscle has automaticity, the ability to generate an impulse on its own, separately from the central nervous system.

cardiopulmonary resuscitation (CPR)—provision of artificial ventilation and external chest compressions in patients with absent pulse (in cardiac arrest) to provide circulation of oxygenated blood to support life.

cardiovascular system—*see* circulatory system.

carina—the point of division at about the level of the fifth thoracic vertebra where the trachea splits into the right and left mainstem bronchi.

carotid artery—the major artery in the neck.

carpals—the eight bones that form the wrist.

cavitation—a cavity formed by a pressure wave resulting from the kinetic energy of a bullet traveling through body tissue; also called pathway expansion.

central nervous system—the brain and the spinal cord. Abbr. CNS.

cerebellum—second largest part of the brain, responsible for controlling equilibrium and muscle coordination.

cerebrospinal fluid (CSF)—a clear fluid that surrounds and cushions the brain and the spinal cord. Leakage of cerebrospinal fluid is evidence of a fractured skull.

cerebrovascular accident—*see* stroke.

cerebrum—largest part of the brain, responsible for most conscious and sensory functions, the emotions, and the personality.

cervical spine—the first seven vertebrae; the neck.

cervix—the neck of the uterus.

chain of survival—term used by the American Heart Association for the series of four interventions—early access, early CPR, early defibrillation, and early ACLS—that provides the best chance for successful resuscitation of a cardiac arrest victim.

chief complaint—the patient's answer to the question "Why did you call the ambulance?"

chronic—long term, progressing gradually.

chronic obstructive pulmonary disease (COPD)—umbrella term used to describe pulmonary diseases such as emphysema or chronic bronchitis.

circulatory system—the body system that transports blood to all parts of the body. Includes the heart, blood vessels, and blood. Also called the cardiovascular system.

circumferential burn—burn that encircles a body area, e.g., arm, leg, or chest.

clavicle—the collarbone, attached to the superior portion of the sternum.

cleaning—the process of washing a soiled object with soap and water. *See also* disinfecting; sterilization.

closed injury—any injury in which the skin remains unbroken.

coccyx—the four fused vertebrae that form the lower end of the spine; the tailbone.

cold zone—the area adjacent to the warm zone in a hazardous materials emergency. Normal triage, treatment, and stabilization are performed here. Also called safe zone. *See also* hot zone; warm zone.

compensated respiratory distress—*see* early respiratory distress.

complex access—a way to gain access to a patient that requires the use of tools and specialized equipment.

concussion—temporary loss of brain function.

conduction—transfer of heat through direct physical touch with nearby objects.

congestive heart failure (CHF)—a cardiac disease in which the heart cannot pump blood sufficiently to meet the needs of the body.

conjunctiva—the thin covering of the inner eyelids and exposed portion of the sclera of the eye.

constricted—narrowed, made small.

contraindications—situations in which a medication should not be used; for example, because nitroglycerin lowers blood pressure, existing low blood pressure in a patient is a contraindication for nitroglycerin.

contusion—a closed injury to the cells and blood vessels contained within the dermis that is characterized by discoloration, swelling, and pain; a bruise.

convection—loss of body heat to the atmosphere when air passes over the body.

convulsion—unresponsiveness accompanied by a generalized jerky muscle movement affecting the entire body.

cornea—the clear front portion of the eye that covers the pupil and the iris.

corniculates—cone-shaped cartilage attached to the top of the arytenoids. They are landmarks used when visualizing the glottic opening during endotracheal intubation.

coronary arteries—blood vessels that supply the heart with blood.

coup-contrecoup injury—a brain injury in which there may be damage at the point of a blow to the head and/or damage on the side opposite the blow as the brain is propelled against the opposite side of the skull.

cranial skull—*see* cranium.

cranium—the bones that form the top, back, and sides of the skull plus the forehead.

crepitus—the sound or feel of broken fragments of bone grinding against each other.

cricoid cartilage—the most inferior portion of the larynx and only full cartilaginous ring of the upper airway. It is felt immediately below the thyroid cartilage.

cricoid pressure—pressure applied to the cricoid cartilage, directed posteriorly, to close off the esophagus and help bring the vocal cords and glottic opening into view. Also called Sellick's maneuver.

critical incident—any situation that causes unusually strong emotions that interfere with the ability to function.

critical incident stress debriefing (CISD)—a session usually held within 24 to 72 hours of a critical incident, where a team of peer counselors and mental health professionals help rescuers work through the emotions that normally follow a critical incident.

crossed-finger technique—a technique in which the thumb and index finger are crossed with the thumb on the lower incisors and the index finger on the upper incisors. The fingers are moved in a snapping or scissors motion to open the mouth.

crowing—a sound similar to that of a cawing crow that indicates that the muscles around the larynx are in spasm and beginning to narrow the opening into the trachea.

crowning—the stage in delivery of a baby when the fetal head presents at the opening of the vagina.

crush injury—a closed or open injury to soft tissues and underlying organs that is the result of a crushing force applied to the body.

cuneiforms—elongated cartilage attached to the posterior arytenoids. They are landmarks used when visualizing the glottic opening.

curved blade—a laryngoscope blade that is curved at the distal end. The blade is inserted into the vallecula to indirectly lift the epiglottis and expose the vocal cords and glottic opening.

Cushing's reflex—a protective reflex by the body to try to maintain perfusion of the brain in a head-injured patient with an increase in intracranial pressure. The systolic blood pressure increases, heart rate decreases, and respiratory pattern changes. This collective change in vital signs indicates a severe head injury.

cyanosis—a bluish color of the skin and mucous membranes that indicates poor oxygenation of tissue.

decerebrate posturing—a posture in which the patient extends the arms and legs and sometimes arches the back; a nonpurposeful response to painful stimulus; a sign of deep unresponsiveness and serious brain injury.

decoder—device that recognizes and responds to only certain codes imposed on radio broadcasts.

decompensated respiratory failure—when the respiratory compensatory mechanisms have begun to fail and respiration becomes inadequate.

decorticate posturing—a posture in which the patient flexes the arms across the chest and extends the legs; a nonpurposeful response to painful stimulus; a sign of deep unresponsiveness and serious brain injury.

defibrillation—electrical shock or current delivered to the heart through the patient's chest wall to help the heart restore a normal rhythm.

defusing—a session held for rescuers most directly involved in a critical incident, prior to a critical incident stress debriefing (CISD), to provide an opportunity to vent emotions and get information before the CISD.

dementia—condition resulting in the malfunctioning of normal cerebral processes.

deoxygenated—containing low amounts of oxygen, as with venous blood.

depression—one of the most common psychiatric conditions, one characterized by deep feelings of sadness, worthlessness, and discouragement, feelings that often do not seem connected to the actual circumstances of the patient's life.

dermis—the layer of skin below the epidermis. *See also* epidermis and subcutaneous layer.

detailed physical exam—a head-to-toe physical assessment for injuries and medical conditions that may follow the focused history and physical exam and is more thorough than the rapid trauma assessment or rapid medical assessment.

diabetes mellitus—a disease in which the normal relationship between glucose and insulin is altered.

diaphragm—the major muscle of respiration that separates the chest cavity from the abdominal cavity.

diastolic pressure—pressure exerted against the arterial walls during relaxation of the left ventricle of the heart.

dilated—expanded, made large.

direct force—a direct blow. Injuries from direct force occur at the point of impact.

disaster—a sudden catastrophic event that overwhelms natural order and causes great loss of property and/or life.

disc—fluid-filled pad of cartilage between two vertebrae.

disinfecting—using a substance such as alcohol or bleach to kill many of the microorganisms that may be present on the surface of an object. *See also* cleaning; sterilization.

dissipation of energy—the way energy is transferred to the human body by the forces acting upon it.

distal—distant, or far from the point of reference. Opposite of proximal.

dorsal—toward the back or spine. Opposite of ventral.

dorsalis pedis artery—artery of the foot, palpable at the top of the foot on the great toe side.

dose—the amount of a medication that is given to a patient at one time; for example a dose of nitroglycerin may be one tablet and a dose of epinephrine may be the contents of one auto-injector.

drag—the factors that slow a projectile.

dressing—a sterile covering for an open wound that aids in the control of bleeding and prevention of further damage and contamination.

drowning—death from suffocation due to submersion.

drug—a chemical substance that is used to treat or prevent a disease or condition.

drug abuse—self-administration of drugs (or of a single drug) in a manner that is not in accord with approved medical or social patterns.

drug toxicity—an adverse or toxic reaction to a drug or drugs.

dura mater—outer layer of protective brain tissue (meninges). *See also* arachnoid; meninges; pia mater.

duty to act—the obligation to care for a patient who requires it.

dyspnea—shortness of breath or perceived difficulty in breathing.

early respiratory distress—increased respiratory effort due to impaired respiratory function.

edema—collection of fluid in the body tissues; swelling.

embolism—blockage of a blood vessel by an air bubble, blood clot, or other foreign matter. *See also* air embolism; pulmonary embolism.

emergency move—a technique for moving a patient that should be performed when there is immediate danger to the patient or to the rescuer.

EMS incident manager—in most incident management systems, the senior EMT who is first to arrive at a multiple-casualty scene or a predesignated officer, if any. The EMS incident manager is responsible for seeing that the multiple-casualty incident is responded to in a controlled and orderly way and that all responsibilities are carried out.

EMS system—Emergency Medical Services system. An organization that provides emergency prehospital or out-of-hospital care and ambulance transport to hospitals.

EMT-Basic—emergency medical technician trained to the basic level. Also EMT-B.

EMT-Intermediate—emergency medical technician trained to the intermediate level. Also EMT-I.

EMT-Paramedic—emergency medical technician trained to the paramedic level. Also EMT-P.

encoder—device that breaks down sound waves into unique digital codes for radio transmission.

endocrine system—a system of ductless glands that produce hormones which regulate body functions.

endotracheal intubation—placement of a tube down the trachea to facilitate air flow into the lungs and aid in breathing. *See also* orotracheal intubation.

endotracheal tube—a tube designed to be inserted between the vocal cords, through the larynx, and into the trachea in order to maintain an airway and to facilitate ventilation.

epidermis—the outermost layer of the skin. *See also* dermis and subcutaneous layer.

epidural—between the dura mater and the skull.

epiglottis—a leaf-shaped cartilaginous structure that covers the opening of the larynx during swallowing.

epilepsy—a medical disorder characterized by recurrent seizures.

epinephrine—a medication that constricts blood vessels to improve blood pressure, reduces leakage from capillaries, and relaxes smooth muscle in the bronchioles; often prescribed in single-dose auto-injector form to patients with a history of anaphylactic reaction.

epistaxis—bleeding from the nose resulting from injury, disease, or environment; a nosebleed.

eschar—the hard, tough, leathery dead soft tissue formed as a result of a full thickness burn.

esophagus—a tubular structure that serves as a passageway for food and liquids to enter the stomach.

evaporation—conversion of a liquid or solid into a gas; evaporation of sweat is a means by which the body is cooled.

evisceration—a protrusion of organs from a wound.

exhalation—the passive process of breathing air out of the lungs. It is also known as expiration.

expiration—*see* exhalation.

expressed consent—permission which must be obtained from every responsive, mentally competent adult before emergency treatment may be provided.

extremities—the limbs of the body. The lower extremities include the hips, thighs, legs, ankles, and feet. The upper extremities include the shoulders, arms, forearms, wrists, and hands.

extrication sector—responsible for freeing patients from wreckage at a multiple-casualty incident under an incident management system.

extubation—the removal of a tube.

face—the area of the skull between the brow and the chin.

false vocal cords—membranous tissue that lies above the true vocal cords.

femoral artery—the major artery of the thigh.

femur—the thigh bone.

fetus—the child in the uterus from the third month of pregnancy to birth; prior to that time it is called an embryo.

fibula—the lateral, smaller long bone of the lower leg.

First Responder—a person typically trained to the first responder level who is likely to be the first person on the scene with emergency care training.

flail segment—two or more adjacent ribs that are fractured in two or more places and thus move independently from the rest of the rib cage.

flow-restricted, oxygen-powered ventilation device (FROPVD)—a device that consists of a ventilation valve and trigger or button and is driven directly by oxygen. It is used to provide positive pressure ventilation.

flushing—abnormally red skin color.

focused history and physical exam—the portion of patient assessment conducted after the initial assessment, for the purpose of identifying additional serious or potentially life-threatening injuries or conditions and as a basis for further emergency care.

focused medical assessment—a physical exam that is focused on the parts of the body indicated by a responsive patient's chief complaint, signs, or symptoms.

focused trauma assessment—a physical exam that is focused on a specific injury site, performed on a responsive patient with no significant mechanism of injury.

form—the size, shape, consistency, or appearance of a medication; for example nitroglycerin may be in pill or spray form; oral glucose is in gel form.

Fowler's position—a position in which the patient is lying on the back with upper body elevated at a 45° to 60° angle.

French catheter—*see* soft catheter.

frostbite—*see* local cold injury.

full thickness burn—burn that involves all of the layers of the skin and can extend beyond the subcutaneous layer into the muscle, bone, or organs below; also called a third degree burn. *See also* partial thickness burn; superficial burn.

gastric distention—inflation of the stomach.

generalized cold emergency—*see* generalized hypothermia.

generalized hypothermia—an overall reduction in body temperature, affecting the entire body; also called hypothermia or generalized cold emergency.

generalized tonic-clonic seizure—a common type of seizure that produces unresponsiveness and a generalized jerky muscle activity. It is also known as a grand mal seizure.

genitalia—the external sex organs.

Glasgow Coma Scale—a method of evaluating a patient's level of responsiveness.

glossoepiglottic ligament—a ligament found in the center of the vallecula that helps support and suspend the epiglottis.

glottic opening—the opening between the vocal cords. Also called the glottis.

glottis—*see* glottic opening.

glucose—a form of sugar that is the body's basic source of energy.

Good Samaritan laws—laws written to provide some protection from liability to emergency care personnel who provide emergency care in good faith according to the standard of care.

grand mal seizure—*see* generalized tonic-clonic seizure.

grunting—a sound heard in infants during exhalation when suffering from a respiratory problem that causes collapsed lungs.

guarded position—a position with knees drawn up and hands clenched over the abdomen, generally assumed by patients with acute abdominal pain.

guarding—protective tensing of the abdominal muscles by a patient suffering abdominal pain; may be voluntary or involuntary (reflexive).

gurgling—a gargling sound that indicates a fluid is in the mouth or pharynx.

gynecological—having to do with the female reproductive system.

hard catheter—*see* rigid catheter.

hazardous material—material that in any quantity poses a threat or unreasonable risk to life, health, or property if not properly controlled during manufacture, processing, packaging, handling, storage, transportation, use, and disposal.

head-tilt, chin-lift maneuver—a manual airway technique used to open the airway. The head is tilted back by one hand. The tips of the fingers of the other hand lift the chin up and forward.

heart—the muscular organ that contracts to force blood into circulation through the body.

hematoma—a closed injury to the soft tissues characterized by swelling and discoloration caused by a collection of blood beneath the epidermis.

hemoglobin—a complex protein molecule found on the surface of the red blood cell that is responsible for carrying a majority of oxygen in the blood.

high-pressure regulator—a one-gauge regulator that is used to power the flow-restricted, oxygen-powered ventilation device. The flow rate cannot be adjusted.

hives—raised, red blotches associated with some allergic reactions.

hot zone—the area where contamination is actually present at a hazardous materials emergency. It generally is the area that is immediately adjacent to the accident site and where contamination can still occur. Also called contamination zone. *See also* cold zone; warm zone.

humane restraints—padded soft leather or cloth straps used to tie a patient down to keep him from hurting himself or others.

humerus—the largest bone in the upper extremity, located in the proximal portion of the upper arm.

hyperglycemia—high blood sugar.

hyperthermia—high body temperature.

hyperventilation—provision of ventilations at an increased rate to provide increased oxygen to the body.

hypoglycemia—low blood sugar.

hypoperfusion—the insufficient delivery of oxygen and other nutrients to some of the body's cells and inadequate elimination of carbon dioxide and other wastes that results from inadequate circulation of blood. Also called shock. *See also* perfusion.

hypothermia—low body temperature. *See also* generalized hypothermia.

hypoxia—the absence of sufficient oxygen in the body cells.

iliac crest—the upper margin of the bones of the pelvis.

immune response—production of antibodies by the immune system to fight off invasion by foreign substances.

immune system—the body's defense mechanism against invasion by foreign substances.

impaled object—an object embedded in an injury to the body.

implied consent—the assumption that—in a true emergency where a patient who is unresponsive or unable to make a rational decision is at significant risk of death, disability, or deterioration of condition—that patient would agree to emergency treatment.

in-line stabilization—bringing the patient's head into a neutral position in which the nose is lined up with the navel, and holding it there manually.

incident management system—a written plan to help control, direct, and coordinate emergency personnel at the scene of a multiple-casualty incident.

incident manager—the person in charge of the incident management system at a multiple-casualty incident. The incident manager may be the EMS incident manager or may be from one of the other emergency response agencies. Also called the incident commander.

index of suspicion—an anticipation that certain types of accidents and mechanisms will produce specific types of injuries.

indications—the common reasons for using a medication to treat a specific condition; for example, chest pain is an indication for nitroglycerin.

indirect force—a force that causes injury some distance away from the point of impact.

infant—a child up to 12 months of age.

inferior—beneath, lower, or toward the feet. Opposite of superior.

inferior plane—everything below the transverse line. Opposite of superior plane.

ingestion—swallowing a substance, allowing it to reach the stomach.

inhalation—the active process of breathing air into the lungs. It is also known as inspiration.

initial assessment—the portion of patient assessment conducted immediately following scene size-up for the purpose of discovering and treating immediately life-threatening conditions. Initial assessment also includes determining whether the patient is injured or ill and making decisions about priorities for further assessment, care, and transport.

injection—forced introduction into the body through the skin, possibly into a muscle or blood vessel, usually via a syringe, bite, or sting.

inspiration—*see* inhalation.

insulin—a hormone secreted by the pancreas that promotes the movement of glucose into the cells.

intercostal muscles—the muscles between the ribs.

intracranial pressure (ICP)—the amount of pressure within the skull.

intubation—the process of passing a tube, such as an endotracheal tube, into the body.

involuntary guarding—an abdominal wall muscle contraction, due to inflammation of the peritoneum, that the patient cannot control.

involuntary muscle—muscle that carries out the automatic muscular functions of the body. Also called smooth muscle.

iris—the colored portion of the eye that surrounds the pupil.

ischium—the posterior and inferior portion of the pelvis.

jaundice—a condition characterized by yellowness of skin, whites of eyes, mucous membranes, and body fluids.

jaw thrust maneuver—a manual technique used to open the airway in the patient with a suspected spinal injury. The fingers are placed at the angles of the jaw and used to lift the jaw up and forward without extending the head or neck.

joint—a place where one bone meets another.

jugular vein distention (JVD)—engorgement of the neck veins; a sign of serious injury to the chest, lungs, or heart.

kinetic energy—the energy contained by an object in motion. Kinetic energy equals mass (weight in pounds), times the velocity (feet per second) squared, divided by two.

kinetics of trauma—the science of analyzing mechanism of injury.

kyphosis—abnormal curvature of the spine with convexity backward. Also called slouch.

labor—the physiological process by which the fetus is expelled from the uterus into the vagina and then to the outside of the body. Also called childbirth.

laceration—an open injury usually caused by forceful impact with a sharp object and characterized by a wound whose edges may be linear (smooth and regular) or stellate (jagged and irregular) in appearance.

laryngectomy—a surgical procedure in which a patient's larynx is removed. A stoma (opening in the neck) is created for the patient to breathe through.

laryngoscope—a device with a lighted distal end used to lift the epiglottis and provide visualization of the vocal cords and glottic opening.

laryngoscopy—the procedure of using a laryngoscope to lift the epiglottis to visualize the vocal cords and glottic opening to aid in correct placement of an endotracheal tube.

larynx—the part of the airway that connects the pharynx with the trachea and contains the vocal cords.

lateral—refers to the left or right of the midline, or away from the midline of the body. *See also* medial.

lateral recumbent—a position in which the patient is lying on the side. Also called recovery position.

left—refers to the patient's left.

left plane—everything to the left of the midline.

lens—the portion of the eye behind the pupil that focuses light on the retina.

ligaments—bands of fibrous tissue that connect bones about a joint and support organs.

limb presentation—when an arm or a leg is the first fetal part to protrude from the vaginal opening.

local cold injury—damage to body tissues in a specific part of the body resulting from exposure to cold. Also called frostbite.

lordosis—abnormal anterior convexity of the spine. Also called swayback.

lumbar spine—the five vertebrae that form the lower back, located between the sacral and the thoracic spine.

lungs—the principal organs of respiration.

mainstem bronchi—the two main branches leading from the trachea to the lungs.

malaise—a general feeling of weakness or discomfort.

malleolus—the knobby surface landmark of the ankle. There is a medial malleolus and a lateral malleolus.

mammalian diving reflex—the body's natural response to submersion in cold water in which breathing is inhibited, the heart rate decreases, and blood vessels constrict in order to maintain cerebral and cardiac blood flow.

mandible—the lower jaw.

manubrium—the superior portion of the sternum where the clavicle is attached.

maxillae—the fused bones of the upper jaw.

mechanism of injury (MOI)—factor involved in producing an injury to a patient, including the strength, direction, and nature of the forces that caused the injury.

meconium staining—a greenish or brownish yellow staining of the amniotic fluid, caused by a fetal bowel movement resulting from distress. The meconium-stained fluid must be suctioned before the newborn takes its first breath or it may be aspirated.

medial—toward the midline or center of the body. *See also* lateral.

medical director—physician who is legally responsible for the clinical and patient care aspects of an EMS system.

medication—a drug or other substance that is used as a remedy for illness.

medulla—*see* brain stem.

meninges—layers of tissue protecting the brain. They include the dura mater, the arachnoid, and the pia mater.

metacarpals—the bones of the hand.

metatarsals—the bones that form the arch of the foot.

metered dose inhaler (MDI)—device consisting of a plastic container and a canister of medication that is used to inhale an aerosolized medication.

midaxillary—refers to the center of the axilla (armpit).

midaxillary line—an imaginary line that divides the body into anterior and posterior planes; the imaginary line from the middle of the armpit to the ankle.

midclavicular—refers to the center of the clavicle (collarbone).

midclavicular line—the imaginary line from the center of either clavicle down the anterior thorax.

midline—an imaginary line drawn vertically through the middle of the patient's body, dividing it into right and left planes.

minimum data set—the minimum information the U.S. Department of Transportation has determined should be included on all prehospital care reports.

minor consent—permission obtained from a parent or legal guardian for emergency treatment of a minor or a mentally incompetent adult.

miscarriage—*see* spontaneous abortion.

mobile command sector—coordinates the MCI response activities of all sectors at a multiple-casualty incident under an incident management system; the headquarters for the incident manager; the EMS command post.

mucous membrane—a thin layer of tissue that lines various structures within the body.

multiple-casualty incident (MCI)—an event that places excessive demands on EMS personnel and equipment.

Murphy eye—a small hole opposite the bevel at the distal end of an endotracheal tube. Its purpose is to lessen the chance of complete tube obstruction.

musculoskeletal system—the system of bones and muscle plus connective tissue that provides support and protection to the body and permits motion.

nasal airway—*see* nasopharyngeal airway.

nasal bones—the bones that form the bed of the nose.

nasal cannula—an oxygen delivery device that consist of two prongs that are inserted into the nose of the patient. The oxygen concentration delivered is from 24 to 44 percent.

nasogastric (NG) tube—a specialized catheter that is inserted through the nose and esophagus into the stomach.

nasopharyngeal airway—a curved, hollow rubber tube that is inserted into the nose, through the nasopharynx, and into the pharynx, providing a passage for air. Also called a nasal airway.

nasopharynx—the portion of the pharynx that extends from the nostrils to the soft palate.

nature of illness (NOI)—the type of medical condition or complaint a patient is suffering from.

near-drowning—survival for at least 24 hours from near suffocation due to submersion.

neglect—the provision of insufficient attention or respect to someone who has a claim to that attention.

negligence—the act of deviating from the accepted standard of care through carelessness, inattention, disregard, inadvertence, or oversight, which results in further injury to the patient.

neonate—an infant in the first 30 days of life.

nervous system—the body system including the brain, spinal cord, and nerves, that controls the voluntary and involuntary activity of the human body.

neurogenic shock—type of shock common in cases of damage to the brain or spinal cord that results in vasodilation and relative hypovolemia. *See also* spinal shock.

neurologic deficit—any deficiency in the nervous system's functioning.

nitroglycerin—medication often prescribed for patients with a history of heart problems for the relief of chest pain.

nonpurposeful response—*see* decerebrate posturing; decorticate posturing.

nonrebreather mask—an oxygen delivery device that consists of a reservoir and one-way valve. It can deliver up to 100 percent oxygen to the patient.

nontraumatic brain injury—a medical injury to the brain which is not caused by external trauma. Stroke is an example of a nontraumatic brain injury.

nonurgent move—a technique for moving a patient that is used when no immediate threat to life exists.

normal anatomical position—a position in which the patient is standing erect, facing forward, with arms down at the sides and palms forward.

obstetric—having to do with pregnancy or childbirth.

occlusive dressing—a dressing that can form an airtight seal over a wound.

olecranon—the part of the ulna that forms the bony prominence of the elbow.

ongoing assessment—the assessment that is conducted following the rapid or focused assessment, or following the detailed physical exam if one is conducted, to detect any changes in the patient's condition, to identify any missed injuries or conditions, and to adjust emergency care as needed. The initial assessment is repeated, baseline vital signs reassessed and recorded, focused assessment conducted for additional complaints, and interventions checked. The ongoing assessment is repeated every 5 minutes for an unstable patient, every 15 minutes for a stable patient.

open injury—any injury in which the skin is broken as a result of trauma.

oral airway—*see* oropharyngeal airway.

oral glucose—a form of sugar often given as a gel, by mouth, to help correct a glucose-insulin imbalance in patients with an altered mental status and a history of diabetes.

oral mucosa—mucous membranes of the mouth.

orbits—the bony structures that surround the eyes; the eye sockets.

oropharyngeal airway—a semicircular hard plastic device that is inserted in the mouth and holds the tongue away from the back of the pharynx. Also called an oral airway.

oropharynx—a portion of the pharynx that extends from the mouth to the oral cavity at the base of the tongue with the mouth as the opening.

orotracheal intubation—the passage of an endotracheal tube through the mouth, along the oropharynx and larynx, and into the trachea. *See also* endotracheal intubation.

orotracheal suctioning—the procedure in which a long, soft suction catheter is inserted through the endotracheal tube to clear secretions deep in the airway.

osteoporosis—loss of bone minerals that results in bones becoming brittle.

overdose—an emergency that involves poisoning by drugs or alcohol.

oxygen—a gaseous element required by the body's tissues and cells to sustain life; often provided as a medication to patients whose injuries or medical conditions may lead to or may be caused or exacerbated by a lack of oxygen.

oxygen humidifier—a container that is filled with sterile water and connected to the oxygen regulator to add moisture to the dry oxygen prior to being delivered to the patient.

oxygenated—containing high amounts of oxygen, as with arterial blood.

oxygenation—the process by which the blood and the cells become saturated with oxygen.

pallor—pale or abnormally white skin color.

palmar—relates to the palm of the hand.

palpation—feeling, as for a pulse.

paradoxical movement—when a section of the chest moves in the opposite direction to the rest of the chest during the phases of respiration; typically seen with a flail segment.

paranoia—a highly exaggerated or unwarranted mistrust or suspiciousness.

paresthesia—a prickling or tingling feeling that indicates some loss of sensation.

parietal pleura—the outermost pleural layer (tissue surrounding the lungs) that adheres to the chest wall.

partial thickness burn—burn that involves the epidermis and portions of the dermis; also called a second degree burn. *See also* full thickness burn; superficial burn.

passive rewarming—the use of the patient's own heat production and conservation mechanisms to rewarm him, for example simply placing the patient in a warm environment and covering him with blankets. *See also* active rewarming.

patella—the kneecap.

patent—open and clear of any obstructions, as a patent airway.

pathogens—microorganisms such as bacteria and viruses that cause disease. Bloodborne pathogens can spread disease by way of the blood. Airborne pathogens can spread disease by way of spraying droplets through the air.

patient assessment—procedures performed to find out what is wrong with a patient, on which decisions about emergency medical care and transport will be based. *See also* the entries for the separate steps of the patient assessment: scene size-up, initial assessment, focused history and physical exam, detailed physical exam, and ongoing assessment.

pelvis—the bones that form the floor of the abdominal cavity: the sacrum and coccyx of the spine, the iliac crests, the pubis, and the ischium.

penetrating trauma—a force that pierces the skin and body tissues, for example a knife or gunshot wound.

perfusion—the delivery of oxygen and other nutrients to the cells and elimination of waste products of all organ systems, which results from the constant adequate circulation of blood through the capillaries. *See also* hypoperfusion.

perineum—the area of skin between a female's vagina and anus.

peripheral nervous system—that portion of the nervous system located outside the brain and spinal cord. Abbr. PNS.

peritoneum—the lining of the abdominal cavity.

personal protective equipment—equipment an emergency rescuer uses or wears to protect against injury and spreading infectious disease.

pertinent negatives—signs or symptoms that might be expected in certain circumstances, based on the chief complaint, but are denied by the patient.

phalanges—bones of the fingers, thumbs, and toes.

pharmacology—the study of drugs.

pharynx—the common passageway for the respiratory and digestive tract; the throat.

phobia—an irrational fear of specific things, places, or situations.

physical abuse—improper or excessive action taken so as to injure or cause harm.

physiology—the study of the function of the living body and its parts.

pia mater—inner layer of protective brain tissue (meninges).

placenta—the fetal organ through which the fetus exchanges nourishment and waste products during pregnancy.

plantar—refers to the sole of the foot.

plasma—the serum, or fluid, component of the blood.

platelet—component of the blood essential to the formation of blood clots.

pleura—two layers of connective tissue that surround the lungs.

pleural space—a small space between the visceral and parietal pleura that is at negative pressure and filled with serous fluid.

pneumonia—infection of the lungs, usually from a bacterium or virus.

pneumothorax—air in the pleural space causing collapse of the lungs.

pocket mask—a plastic mask placed over the patient's nose and mouth through which ventilations can be delivered.

poison—any substance—liquid, solid, or gas—that impairs health or causes death by its chemical action when it enters the body or comes into contact with the skin.

positive pressure ventilation (PPV)—method of aiding a patient whose breathing is inadequate by forcing air into his lungs, for example by mouth-to-mask ventilation or bag-valve-mask-unit ventilation.

posterior—toward the back. Opposite of anterior.

posterior plane—the back or dorsal side of the body.

posterior tibial artery—artery of the calf, palpable behind the medial ankle bone.

postictal state—the recovery period that follows the clonic phase of a generalized seizure. In a postictal state the patient commonly appears weak, exhausted, and disoriented and progressively improves.

power grip—recommended gripping technique. The palm and fingers come in complete contact with the object and all fingers are bent at the same angle.

power lift—recommended technique for lifting. Feet are apart, knees bent, back and abdominal muscles tightened, back as straight as possible, lifting force driven through heels and arches, upper body rising before hips.

prehospital care—emergency medical treatment given to patients before they are transported to a hospital or other facility. Also out-of-hospital care.

prehospital care report (PCR)—documentation of an EMT-B's contact with a patient.

premature infant—an infant weighing less than 5½ pounds, or an infant born before its 38th week of gestation.

preschooler—a child 3 to 6 years of age.

pressure point—the point where an artery lies close to the surface over a bony prominence. By compressing an artery at a pressure point, arterial blood flow can be reduced in an extremity.

profile—refers to the size and shape of a bullet's point of impact; the greater the point of impact the greater the injury.

prolapsed cord—when the umbilical cord, rather than the head of the fetus, is the first part to protrude from the vagina.

prone—lying on the stomach.

proximal—near the point of reference. Opposite of distal.

pubis—inferior bone of the pelvis.

pulmonary artery—vessel carrying oxygen-depleted blood from the heart's right ventricle to the lungs.

pulmonary edema—fluid in the lungs.

pulmonary embolism—occlusion of the pulmonary vessels by a clot.

pulmonary vein—vessel carrying oxygen-rich blood from the lungs to the left atrium of the heart.

pulse—the wave of blood propelled through the arteries as a result of each contraction of the left ventricle.

pulseless electrical activity (PEA)—a condition in which the heart generates relatively normal electrical rhythms but fails to perfuse the body adequately because of a decreased or absent cardiac output from cardiac muscle failure or blood loss.

pupil—the dark center of the eye; the opening that expands or contracts to allow more or less light into the eye.

purified protein derivative (PPD) test—a test for tuberculosis.

quality improvement—a system of internal and external reviews and audits of an EMS system to ensure a high quality of care.

raccoon sign—discoloration of tissue around the eyes suggestive of basilar skull injury.

radial artery—major artery of the forearm.

radiation—transfer of heat from the surface of one object to the surface of another without physical contact between the objects.

radius—the lateral bone of the forearm.

rapid extrication—a technique using manual stabilization rather than application of an immobilization device for the purpose of speeding extrication when the time saved will make the difference between life and death.

rapid medical assessment—a head-to-toe physical exam that is swiftly conducted on an unresponsive medical patient or a medical patient who is suspected to also have injuries.

rapid trauma assessment—a head-to-toe physical exam that is swiftly conducted on a trauma patient who is unresponsive or who has a significant mechanism of injury.

reasonable force—the minimum amount of force required to keep a patient from injuring himself or others.

red blood cell—component of the blood that carries oxygen to the body's cells and carries carbon dioxide away from the body's cells.

referred pain—pain that is felt in a body part removed from its point of origin.

repeaters—devices that receive transmissions from a relatively low-powered source such as a mobile or portable radio and rebroadcast them at another frequency and a higher power.

respiration—the exchange of oxygen and carbon dioxide that takes place during inhalation and exhalation.

respiratory arrest—when breathing stops completely; apnea.

respiratory distress—*see* early respiratory distress.

respiratory failure—inadequate oxygenation of the blood and elimination of carbon dioxide.

respiratory system—the organs involved in the exchange of gases between an organism and the atmosphere.

restraints—*see* humane restraints.

retina—the back of the eye.

retractions—depressions seen in the neck, above the clavicles, between the ribs, or below the rib cage from excessive muscle use during breathing. It is an indication of respiratory distress.

right—refers to the patient's right.

right plane—everything to the right of the midline.

right mainstem intubation—a complication of endotracheal intubation in which the tube is advanced too far down the trachea and into the right mainstem bronchus. This provides for ventilation of only one lung and can lead to severe hypoxia.

rigid catheter—a rigid plastic tube that is part of a suctioning system, commonly referred to as a "tonsil tip" or "tonsil sucker."

route—the means by which a medication is given or taken; for example sublingual (under the tongue), oral (by mouth), inhalation (breathed in), injection (inserted by needles into a muscle or vein).

rule of nines—standardized format to quickly identify the amount of skin or body surface area (BSA) that has been burned.

sacral spine—the five vertebrae that are fused together to form the rigid part of the posterior side of the pelvis. Also sacrum.

safety zones—areas surrounding an accident involving hazardous materials, designated for specific rescue operations. *See* hot zone, warm zone, and cold zone.

SAMPLE history—a type of patient history. SAMPLE is an acronym used to remember categories of information necessary to the patient history: signs and symptoms, allergies, medications, pertinent past history, last oral intake, and events leading to the injury or illness.

scapula—the shoulder blade.

scene safety—an assessment of the scene for safety hazards to ensure the safety and well-being of the EMT-B, his partners, patients, and by-standers.

scene size-up—an overall assessment of the scene to which an EMT-B has been called to gain useful information that includes ensuring scene safety; determining whether a patient is suffering from trauma or a medical problem; and determining the total number of patients and whether additional resources are needed to handle them.

schizophrenia—the name given to a group of mental disorders characterized by debilitating distortions of speech and thought, bizarre delusions, hallucinations, social withdrawal, and lack of emotional expressiveness.

school age—a child 6 to 12 years of age.

sclera—the outer coating of the eye; the exposed portion is "the white of the eye."

scope of practice—the actions and care that are legally allowed to be provided by an EMT-Basic.

seizure—a sudden and temporary alteration in the mental status caused by massive electrical discharge in a group of nerve cells in the brain.

self-contained breathing apparatus (SCBA)—a unit designed to provide uncontaminated air to a person who must enter an area in which toxic fumes are present.

Sellick's maneuver—*see* cricoid pressure.

sensitization—the process by which antibodies are produced after exposure to an antigen.

serous fluid—fluid that acts as a lubricant to reduce the friction between the parietal and visceral pleura.

shock—*see* hypoperfusion.

side effects—the undesired effects of a medication; for example, side effects of epinephrine are increased heart rate and increased anxiety.

signs—any objective evidence of a medical or trauma condition that can be seen, heard, felt, or smelled in a patient. See also symptoms.

silent heart attack—a myocardial infarction (heart attack) that does not cause chest pain.

simple access—any way to gain access to a patient that does not require specialized tools.

skeletal system—the bony framework of the body.

skull—the bony structure at the top of the spinal column that houses and protects the brain. The skull has two parts, the cranium and the face.

sniffing position—a position that aligns the airway, neck flexed and head extended.

snoring—a sound that is heard when the base of the tongue or relaxed tissues in the pharynx partially block the upper airway. Also called a *sonorous* sound.

soft catheter—flexible tubing that is part of a suctioning system, the "French" catheter.

soft tissue—the tissues of the body that are not bone or cartilage, including the skin, muscles, blood vessels, nerves, and tissues of the organs.

spacer—a chamber that is connected to the metered dose inhaler to collect the medication until it is inhaled.

sphygmomanometer—instrument used to measure blood pressure. Also called a blood pressure cuff.

spinal column—the column of vertebrae that encloses the spinal cord.

spinal cord—a column of nervous tissue that exits from the brain and extends down the spinal column. All nerves to the trunk and extremities originate from the spinal cord.

spinal shock—shock caused by injury to the spinal cord, causing vasodilation and relative hypovolemia (neurogenic shock) as well as paralysis and loss of sensation below the level of the injury.

splint—any device used to immobilize a body part.

spontaneous abortion—without apparent cause, the termination of a pregnancy before the fetus reaches the stage of viability, generally before the 20th week of pregnancy. Also called miscarriage.

staging sector—monitors, inventories, and directs available ambulances to the treatment sector at the request of the transportation officer at a multiple-casualty incident under an incident management system.

standard of care—emergency care that would be expected to be given to a patient by any trained EMT-B under similar circumstances.

status epilepticus—a seizure lasting longer than 10 minutes or seizures that occur consecutively without a period of responsiveness

between them. This is a serious medical emergency that may be life threatening.

sterile—free from living microorganisms such as bacteria, viruses, or spores that may cause infection.

sterilization—the process by which an object is subject to certain chemical or physical substances (typically, superheated steam in an autoclave) that kill all microorganisms on the surface of the object. *See also* cleaning; disinfecting.

sternum—the breastbone.

stethoscope—instrument that aids in auscultating (listening) for sounds within the body; used by the EMT-B primarily to auscultate for breath sounds, heart sounds, and in taking the blood pressure.

stoma—a surgical opening into the neck and trachea; *See also* tracheostomy.

straight blade—a laryngoscope blade that is straight at the distal end. The blade is fitted under the epiglottis to lift it to expose the vocal cords and glottic opening.

stridor—a harsh, high-pitched sound heard on inspiration that indicates swelling of the larynx.

stroke—a disruption of blood flow to the brain that occurs when a blood vessel in the brain becomes blocked or ruptures. Also called *cerebrovascular accident (CVA)*.

stylet—a piece of pliable wire that is inserted into an endotracheal tube to shape it and provide stiffness.

subarachnoid hemorrhage—bleeding that occurs between the arachnoid membrane and the surface of the brain.

subarachnoid space—a lattice of fibrous, spongy tissue filled with cerebrospinal fluid that separates the arachnoid membrane and the pia mater.

subcutaneous layer—a layer of fatty tissue just below the dermis. *See also* dermis and epidermis.

subdural—beneath the dura mater.

sucking chest wound—an open wound to the chest that permits air to enter the thoracic cavity.

sudden infant death syndrome (SIDS)—the sudden and unexpected death of an infant or young child in which an autopsy fails to identify the cause of death. SIDS typically occurs while the infant is asleep.

suicide—a willful act designed to end one's own life.

superficial burn—burn that involves only the epidermis; also called a first-degree burn. *See also* full thickness burn; partial thickness burn.

superior—above; toward the head. Opposite to inferior.

superior plane—everything above the transverse line. Opposite to inferior plane.

supine—lying on the back.

supine hypotensive syndrome—inadequate return of venous blood to the heart, reduced cardiac output, and lowered blood pressure resulting from pressure on the inferior vena cava, caused by the weight of the uterus and fetus when the patient in late pregnancy is in a supine position.

supply sector—responsible for inventory and distribution of the medical materials and equipment necessary to render care at a multiple-casualty incident under an incident management system.

symptoms—conditions that must be described by the patient because they cannot be observed by another person. *See also* signs.

syncope—a brief period of unresponsiveness caused by a lack of blood flow to the brain; fainting.

systolic pressure—pressure exerted against the arterial walls during contraction of the left ventricle of the heart.

tachycardia—a heart rate that is faster than the normal upper limit.

tachypnea—a breathing rate that is faster than the normal upper limit.

tarsals—the bones of the ankle, hind foot, and midfoot.

tenderness—pain in response to palpation.

tension pneumothorax—a condition in which the build-up of air and pressure in the thoracic cavity of the injured lung is so severe that it begins to shift to the uninjured side, resulting in compression of the heart, large vessels, and the uninjured lung.

therapy regulator—a device that controls the flow and pressure of oxygen from the tank to allow for a consistent delivery of oxygen by liters per minute.

thoracic spine—the twelve vertebrae directly below the cervical vertebrae that comprise the upper back.

thorax—the chest, or that part of the body between the base of the neck and the diaphragm.

thyroid cartilage—the bulky shield-like structure, commonly known as the Adam's apple, that forms the anterior surface of the larynx.

tibia—the medial, larger bone of the lower leg; the shin bone.

tidal volume—the volume of air breathed in and out in one respiration.

toddler—a child 1 to 3 years of age.

tonsil tip or tonsil sucker—*see* rigid catheter.

toxin—a poison of animal, plant, or bacterial origin.

trachea—a tubular structure that serves as the passageway for air to enter the lungs; the windpipe.

tracheal deviation—a shifting of the trachea to either side of the midline as a result of pressure from air trapped in the chest cavity.

trachealis muscle—the muscular wall that closes the C-shaped rings on the posterior side of the trachea and abuts the esophagus.

tracheostomy—a surgical opening into the trachea in which a tube inserted for the patient to breath through. *See also* stoma.

tracheostomy tube—a hollow tube that is inserted into a tracheostomy to allow the patient to breathe.

trajectory—the path of a projectile during its travel; a trajectory may be flat or curved.

transient ischemic attack (TIA)—temporary disturbance in cerebral blood flow, causing an oxygen deficit to a portion of the brain. The difference between TIA and stroke is that the TIA will subside within 24 hours of onset.

transportation sector—coordinates patient transportation with the triage and staging sectors and communicates with the hospitals involved at a multiple-casualty incident under an incident management system.

transverse line—an imaginary line drawn horizontally through the waist to divide the body into the superior and inferior planes.

trauma—a physical injury or wound caused by external force or violence.

treatment sector—responsible for collecting and treating patients in a centralized treatment area at a multiple-casualty incident under an incident management system.

Trendelenburg position—lying on the back with the lower part of the body elevated up to 12 inches.

triage—the process of sorting patients to determine the order in which they will receive care or transportation to definitive care.

triage sector—responsible for prioritizing patients for emergency medical care and transport at a multiple-casualty incident under an incident management system.

triage tag—a tag containing key information about a patient that is attached to a patient during a multiple-casualty incident.

tripod position—a position in which the patient sits upright, leans slightly forward, and supports the body with the arms in front and elbows locked. This is a common position found in respiratory distress.

true vocal cords—strands of fibrous tissue that regulate the flow of air into the trachea and produce sounds by vibrating.

twisting force—a force that twists a bone or extremity while one end is held stationary.

ulna—the medial bone of the forearm.

umbilical cord—an extension of the placenta through which the fetus receives nourishment while in the uterus.

umbilicus—the navel.

urgent move—a move made because there is an immediate threat to life due to the patient's condition and the patient must be moved quickly for transport.

uterus—an organ of the female reproductive system for containing and nourishing the embryo and fetus from the time the fertilized egg is implanted to the time of birth.

vagina—the passageway through which the fetus is delivered. The lower part of the birth canal.

vallecula—a depression located between the base of the tongue and the epiglottis.

valves—structures within the heart and circulatory system that keep blood flowing in one direction and prevent backflow.

vein—a blood vessel that carries blood toward the heart.

venae cavae—the principal veins that carry deoxygenated blood to the heart. Pl. of vena cava. The superior vena cava carries blood from the upper body; the inferior vena cava carries blood from the lower body.

ventilation—the passage of air into and out of the lungs.

ventral—toward the front, or toward the anterior portion of the body. Opposite of dorsal.

ventricle—one of the two lower chambers of the heart.

ventricular fibrillation (VF or V-Fib)—a continuous, uncoordinated, chaotic rhythm which does not produce pulses.

ventricular tachycardia (V-Tach)—a very rapid ventricular heart rhythm which may or may not produce a pulse and is generally too fast to adequately perfuse the body's organs.

venule—smallest branch of a vein, leading from a capillary.

vertebrae—bones of the spinal column.

visceral pleura—innermost layer of the pleura that covers the lung.

vital signs—the traditional signs of life; assessments related to breathing, pulse, skin, pupils, and blood pressure. *See also* baseline vital signs.

vitreous body—the large chamber of the eye, containing the vitreous humor.

vitreous humor—the clear jelly that fills the large chamber of the eye.

voluntary guarding—a deliberate abdominal wall muscle contraction.

voluntary muscle—any muscle that can be consciously controlled by the individual. Also called skeletal muscle.

voluntary nervous system—part of the nervous system that influences voluntary muscles and movements of the body.

warm zone—the area that is established surrounding or immediately adjacent to the hot zone in a hazardous materials emergency, the purpose of which is to prevent the spread of contamination. Life-saving emergency care is performed here. Also called control zone. *See also* cold zone; hot zone.

water chill—the increase in rate of cooling in the presence of water or wet clothing.

white blood cell—component of the blood that provides part of the body's immune system.

wind chill—the combined cooling effect of wind speed and environmental temperature.

withdrawal—a syndrome that occurs after a period of abstinence from the alcohol or drugs to which a person's body has become accustomed.

xiphoid process—inferior portion of the sternum.

zygomatic bones—the cheek bones.

Index